ExpertDDX

Chest

SECOND EDITION

Carter | Rosado-de-Christenson
Lichtenberger | Martínez-Jiménez

BETANCOURT-CUELLAR • BUENO • CARRILLO-BAYONA
FRANQUET • GARRANA • NIRATTISAIKUL

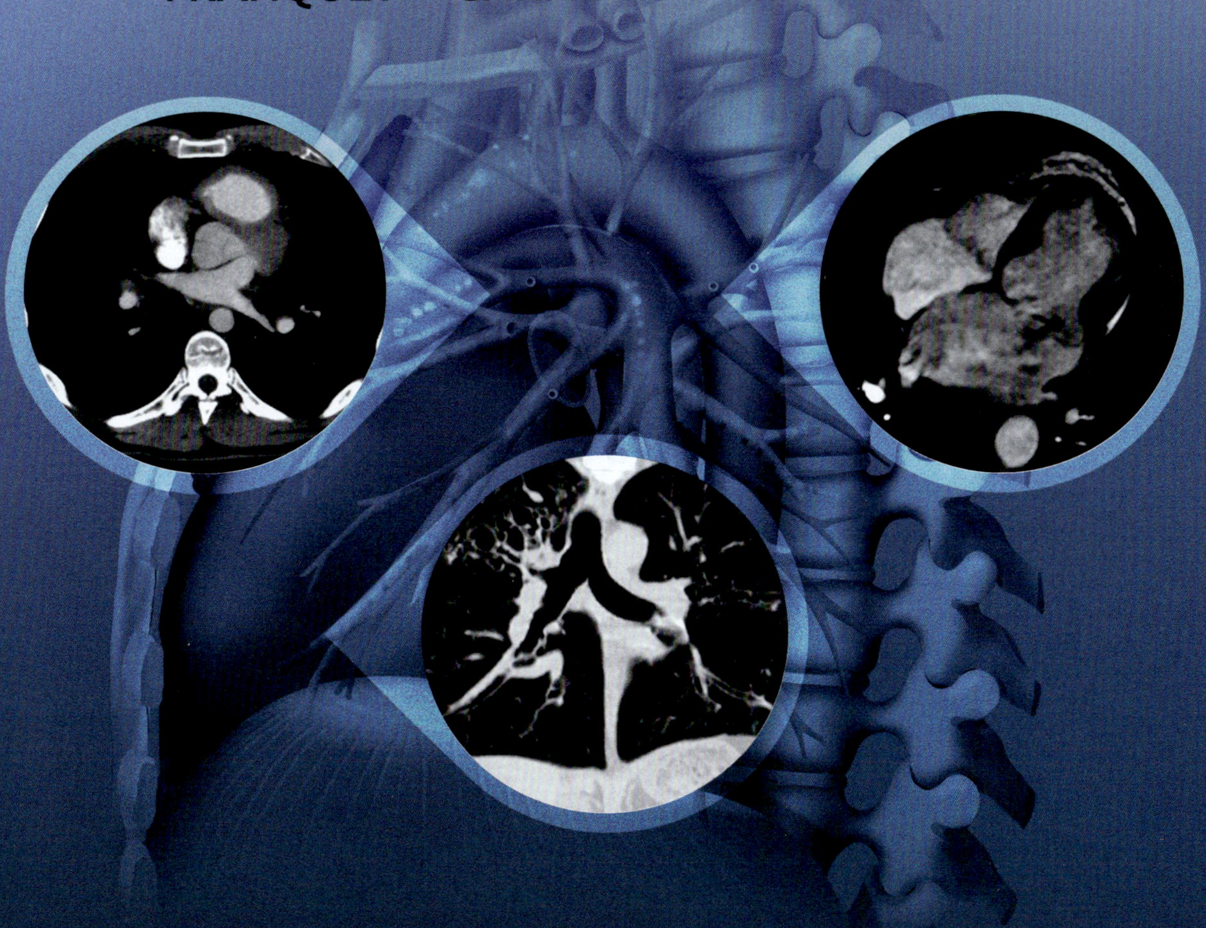

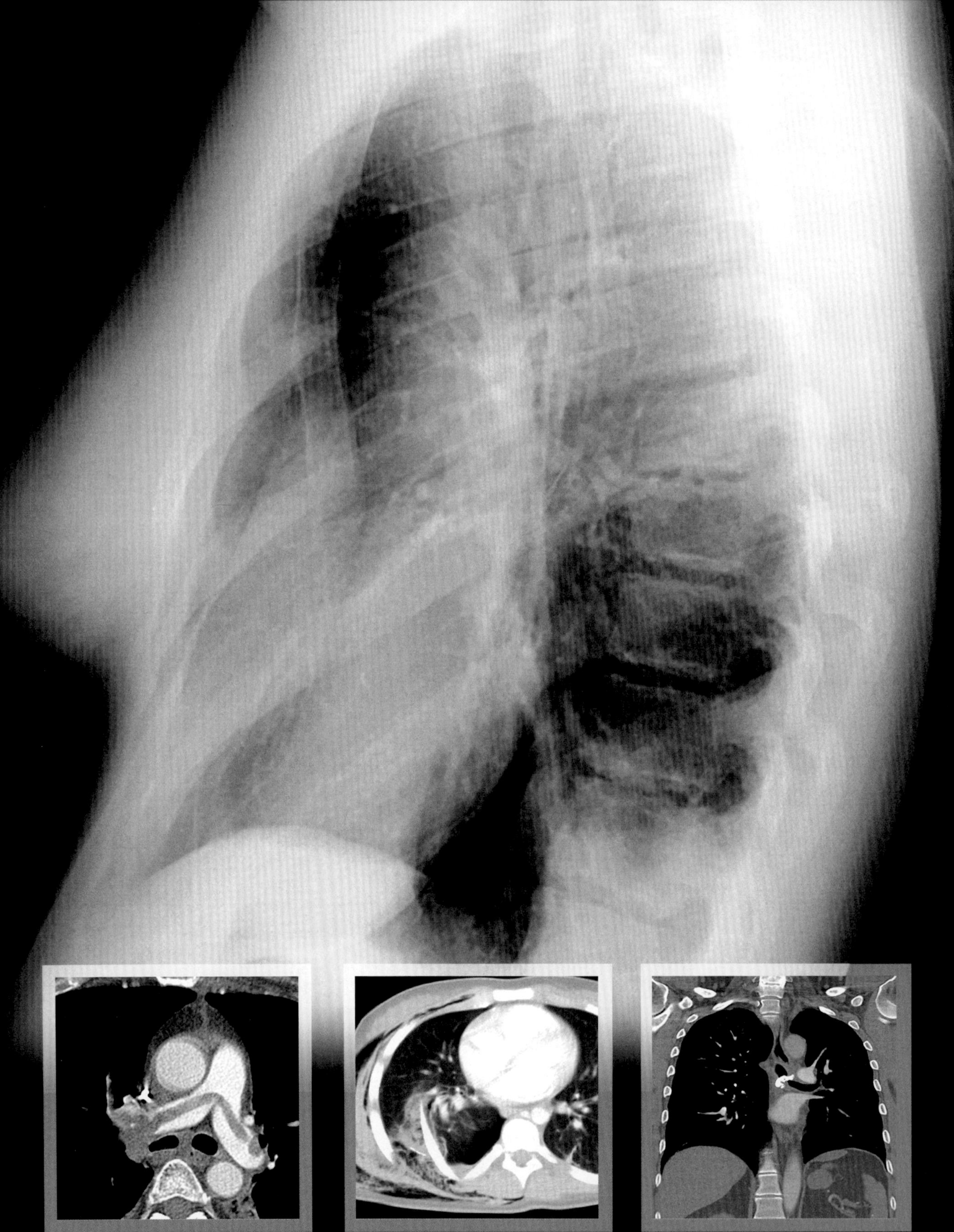

ExpertDDX

Chest

SECOND EDITION

Brett W. Carter, MD
Director of Clinical Operations
Chief Patient Safety and Quality Officer
Diagnostic Imaging
Associate Professor, Thoracic Imaging
The University of Texas MD Anderson Cancer Center
Houston, Texas

Melissa L. Rosado-de-Christenson, MD, FACR
Section Chief, Thoracic Radiology
Department of Radiology
Saint Luke's Hospital of Kansas City
Professor of Radiology
University of Missouri-Kansas City School of Medicine
Kansas City, Missouri

John P. Lichtenberger, III, MD
Associate Professor of Radiology
The George Washington University School of Medicine
Chief of Thoracic Radiology
Department of Radiology
The George Washington University Hospital
Washington, DC

Santiago Martínez-Jiménez, MD
Department of Radiology
Saint Luke's Hospital of Kansas City
Kansas City, Missouri

Elsevier
1600 John F. Kennedy Blvd.
Ste 1800
Philadelphia, PA 19103-2899

EXPERTDDX: CHEST, SECOND EDITION ISBN: 978-0-323-52482-7

Copyright © 2020 by Elsevier. All rights reserved.

No part of this publication may be reproduced or transmitted in any form or by any means, electronic or mechanical, including photocopying, recording, or any information storage and retrieval system, without permission in writing from the publisher. Details on how to seek permission, further information about the Publisher's permissions policies and our arrangements with organizations such as the Copyright Clearance Center and the Copyright Licensing Agency, can be found at our website: www.elsevier.com/permissions.

This book and the individual contributions contained in it are protected under copyright by the Publisher (other than as may be noted herein).

Notices

Practitioners and researchers must always rely on their own experience and knowledge in evaluating and using any information, methods, compounds or experiments described herein. Because of rapid advances in the medical sciences, in particular, independent verification of diagnoses and drug dosages should be made. To the fullest extent of the law, no responsibility is assumed by Elsevier, authors, editors or contributors for any injury and/or damage to persons or property as a matter of products liability, negligence or otherwise, or from any use or operation of any methods, products, instructions, or ideas contained in the material herein.

Previous edition copyrighted 2011.

Library of Congress Control Number: 2019941288

Printed in Canada by Friesens, Altona, Manitoba, Canada

Last digit is the print number: 9 8 7 6 5 4 3 2 1

Working together to grow libraries in developing countries

www.elsevier.com • www.bookaid.org

dedication, honesty, and integrity, and who worked really hard for me to have the privilege of education. Para mis queridos padres, Fernando y Gloria, quienes me enseñaron la perseverancia, la dedicación, la honestidad y la integridad, y quienes trabajaron durísimo para darme el privilegio de la educación. GRACIAS!

SMJ

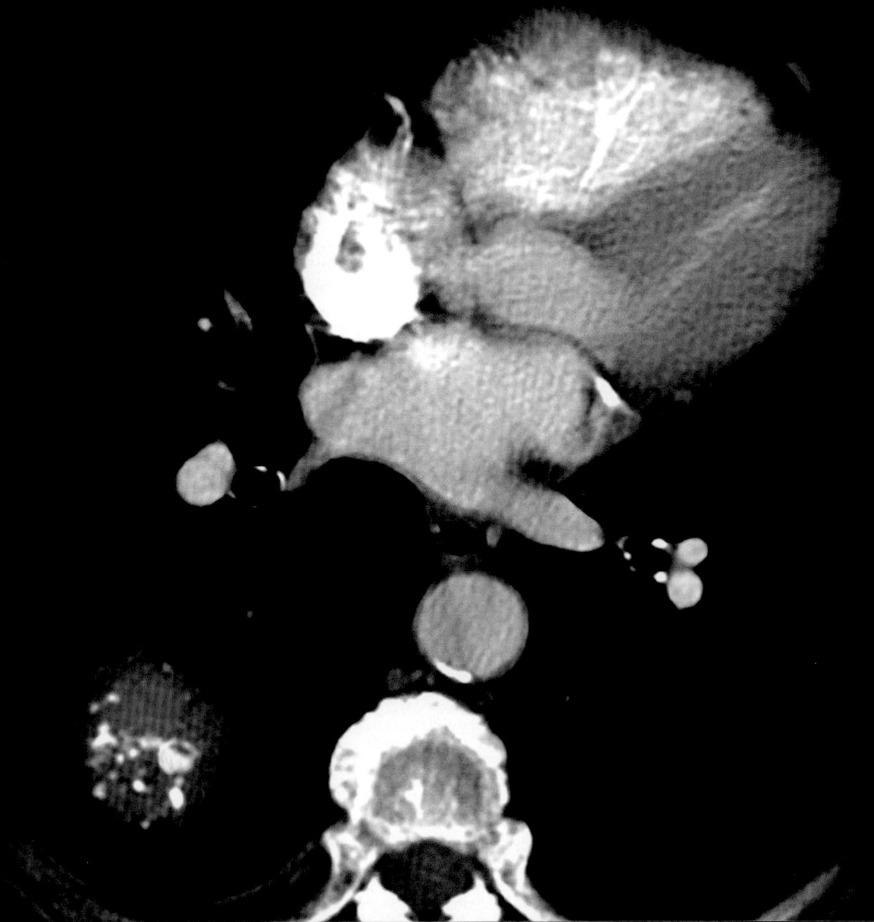

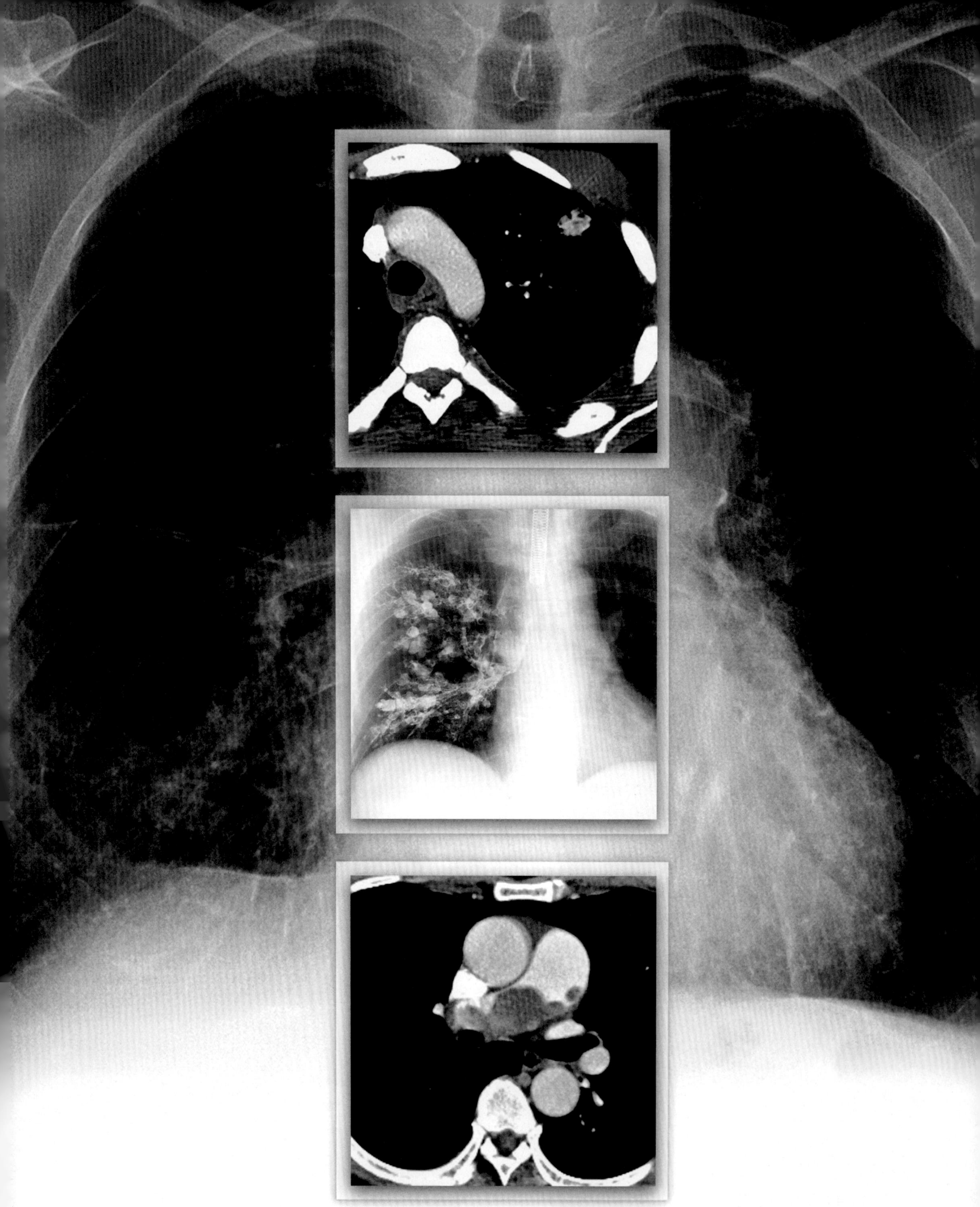

Contributing Authors

Sonia L. Betancourt-Cuellar, MD
Associate Professor
Department of Diagnostic Radiology
The University of Texas MD Anderson Cancer Center
Houston, Texas

Juliana Bueno, MD
Associate Professor of Radiology
Department of Radiology and Medical Imaging
University of Virginia Health System
Charlottesville, Virginia

Jorge Alberto Carrillo-Bayona, MD
Associated Professor of Radiology
Universidad Nacional de Colombia
Hospital Universitario Mayor Mederi
RIMAB
Bogotá, Colombia

Tomás Franquet, MD, PhD
Chief of Thoracic Imaging
Department of Radiology
Hospital de Sant Pau
Universidad Autónoma de Barcelona
Barcelona, Spain

Sherief Garrana, MD
Fellow, Thoracic Imaging and Intervention
Department of Radiology
Massachusetts General Hospital / Harvard Medical School
Boston, Massachusetts

Sitang Nirattisaikul, MD
Instructor
Radiology Department
Songklanagarind Hospital
Prince of Songkla University
Hatyai, Songkhla
Thailand

Additional Contributors

Jud W. Gurney, MD, FACR

Gregory Kicska, MD, PhD

Sudhakar Pipavath, MD

Christopher M. Walker, MD

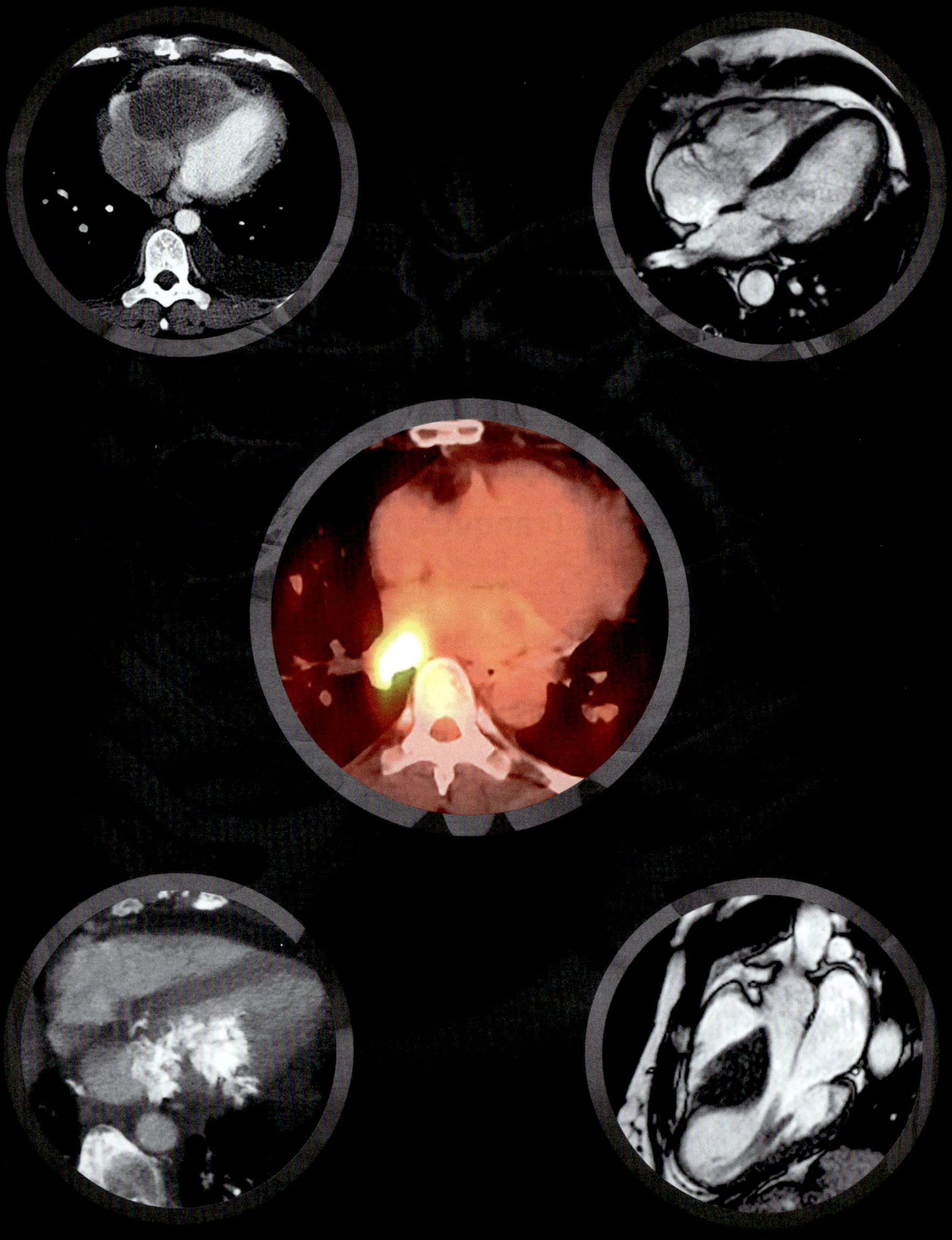

Preface

The differential diagnosis is one of the most fundamental and important concepts in radiology and typically refers to the section of the report that contains conditions potentially responsible for abnormalities identified on imaging examinations &/or patient symptoms. The formulation of a relevant differential diagnosis is one of the most significant contributions that a radiologist can make to the care of a patient and demonstrates, in part, the value added by the specialty to the overall patient experience.

Similar to the first edition of ***Expert Differential Diagnosis*** (***ExpertDDx***): ***Chest*** and other titles in the series, this second edition focuses on observable findings on imaging studies, often in combination with specific clinical symptoms evident at the time of patient presentation, that can be used to construct a focused and appropriate differential diagnosis. Specific entities are presented in order of greatest relevance, mirroring the approach in clinical practice. Our goal is not to present a comprehensive list of all possible conditions for each imaging finding, but to emphasize the most important and practical considerations.

The second edition of ***ExpertDDx: Chest*** has been both revised and expanded. The table of contents has been reorganized into eleven sections: An introductory section that includes chapters devoted to several of the most common presentations encountered in clinical practice, and ten following sections dedicated to individual anatomic regions of the chest, focusing on the lungs and airspaces, interstitium, airways, mediastinum and hila, pulmonary arteries, thoracic aorta, pleura, chest wall and diaphragm, heart, and pericardium. There has been an increase in the number of chapters, now totaling 130, that are organized into subsections titled "General Imaging Patterns" and "Modality-Specific Imaging Findings," the former referring to findings or patterns typically identifiable on multiple modalities, such as radiography, CT, MR, &/or FDG PET/CT, and the latter referring to those on individual imaging modalities, principally CT or MR. For example, in the section on the mediastinum and hila, there are multiple chapters that approach mediastinal masses by location based on complementary imaging modalities, as well as separate, more limited chapters focusing on the composition of mediastinal lesions on CT alone.

I am incredibly grateful to the other three leads, Drs. Melissa Rosado-de-Christenson, John P. Lichtenberger, III, and Santiago Martínez-Jiménez, for the everlasting enthusiasm, energy, wisdom, and guidance imparted during the writing and editing of this book. Finally, I would like to thank the Elsevier team for the opportunity to helm this project.

Brett W. Carter, MD
Director of Clinical Operations
Chief Patient Safety and Quality Officer
Diagnostic Imaging
Associate Professor, Thoracic Imaging
The University of Texas MD Anderson Cancer Center
Houston, Texas

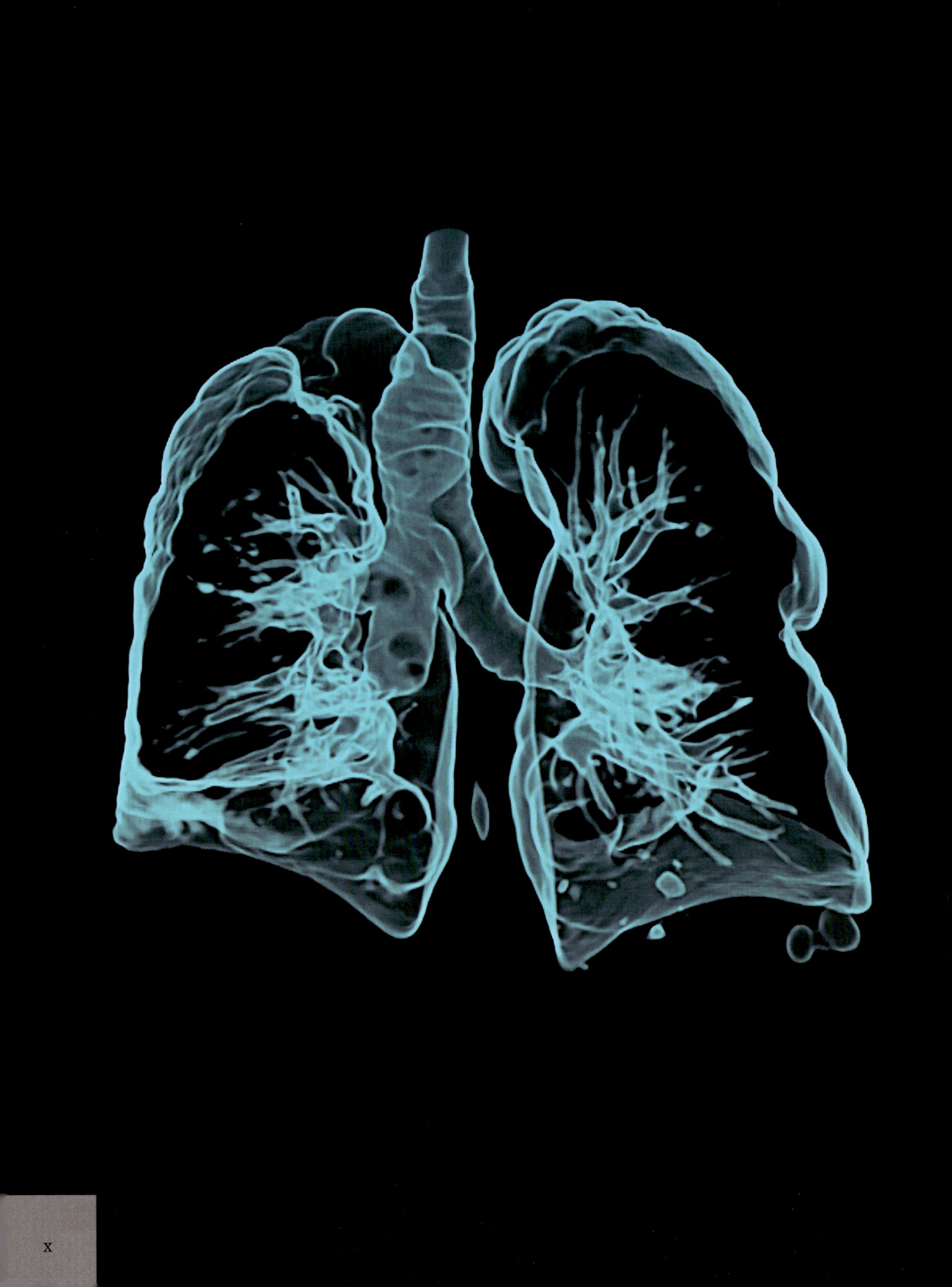

Acknowledgments

LEAD EDITOR
Terry W. Ferrell, MS

TEXT EDITORS
Arthur G. Gelsinger, MA
Rebecca L. Bluth, BA
Nina I. Themann BA
Megg Morin, BA
Kathryn Watkins, BA

IMAGE EDITORS
Jeffrey J. Marmorstone, BS
Lisa A. M. Steadman, BS

ILLUSTRATIONS
Richard Coombs, MS
Lane R. Bennion, MS
Laura C. Wissler, MA

ART DIRECTION AND DESIGN
Tom M. Olson, BA

PRODUCTION COORDINATORS
Emily C. Fassett, BA
John Pecorelli, BS

ELSEVIER

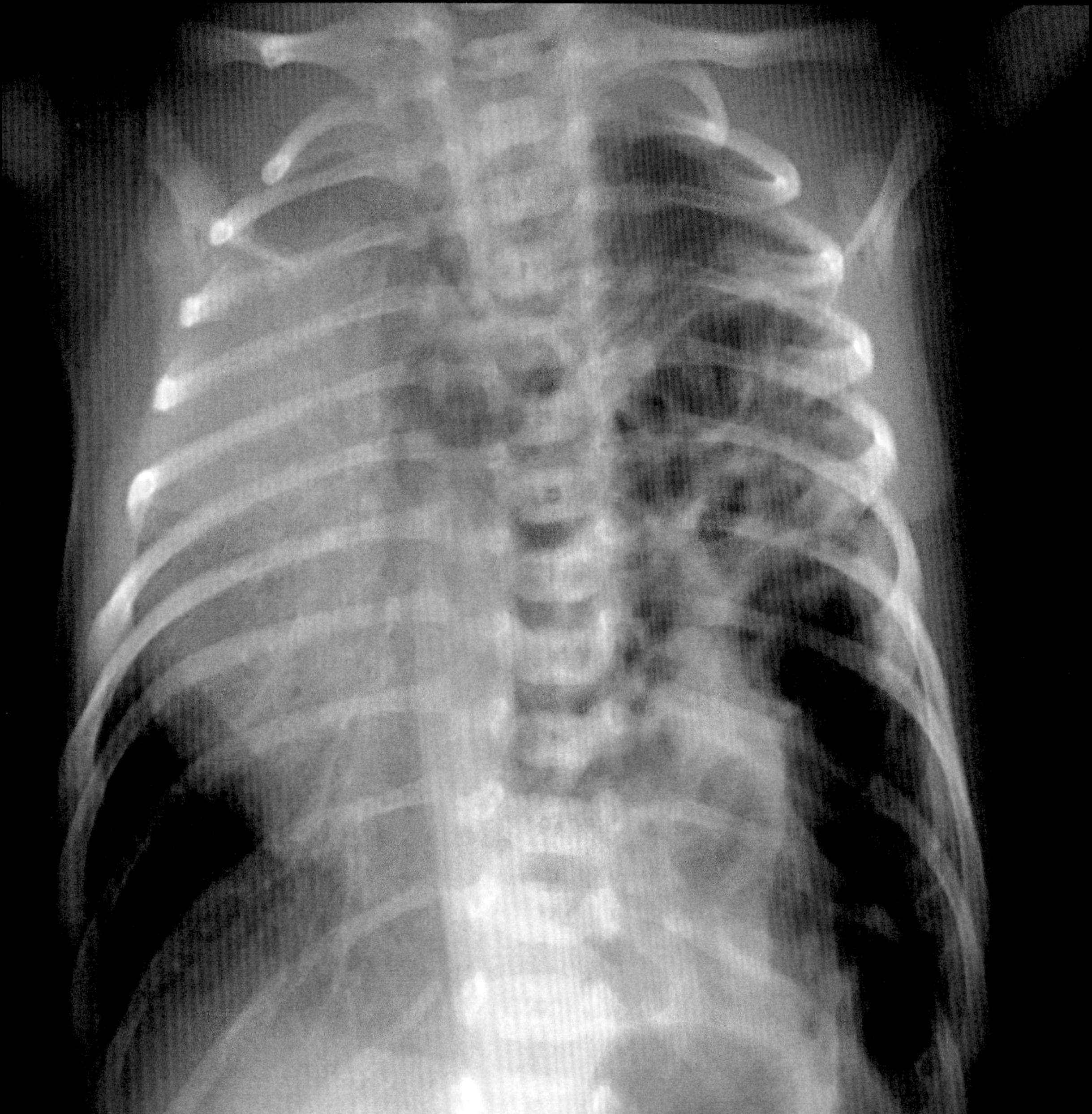

Sections

TABLE OF CONTENTS

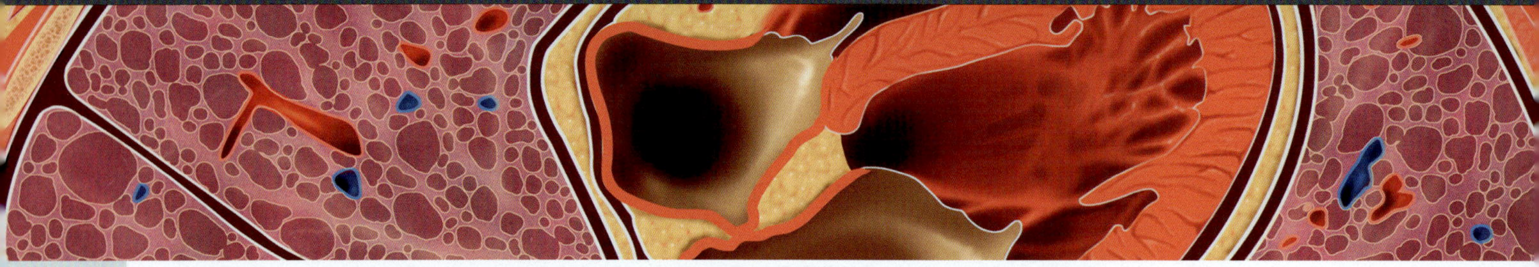

TABLE OF CONTENTS

SECTION 3: INTERSTITIUM

APPROACH TO INTERSTITIUM

GENERAL IMAGING PATTERNS

MODALITY-SPECIFIC IMAGING FINDINGS: COMPUTED TOMOGRAPHY

SECTION 4: AIRWAYS

APPROACH TO AIRWAYS

GENERAL IMAGING PATTERNS

MODALITY-SPECIFIC IMAGING FINDINGS: COMPUTED TOMOGRAPHY

SECTION 5: MEDIASTINUM AND HILA

APPROACH TO MEDIASTINUM AND HILA

GENERAL IMAGING PATTERNS

MODALITY-SPECIFIC IMAGING FINDINGS: RADIOGRAPHY

MODALITY-SPECIFIC IMAGING FINDINGS: COMPUTED TOMOGRAPHY

TABLE OF CONTENTS

TABLE OF CONTENTS

ExpertDDX
Chest

SECOND EDITION

Carter | Rosado-de-Christenson
Lichtenberger | Martínez-Jiménez

BETANCOURT-CUELLAR • BUENO • CARRILLO-BAYONA
FRANQUET • GARRANA • NIRATTISAIKUL

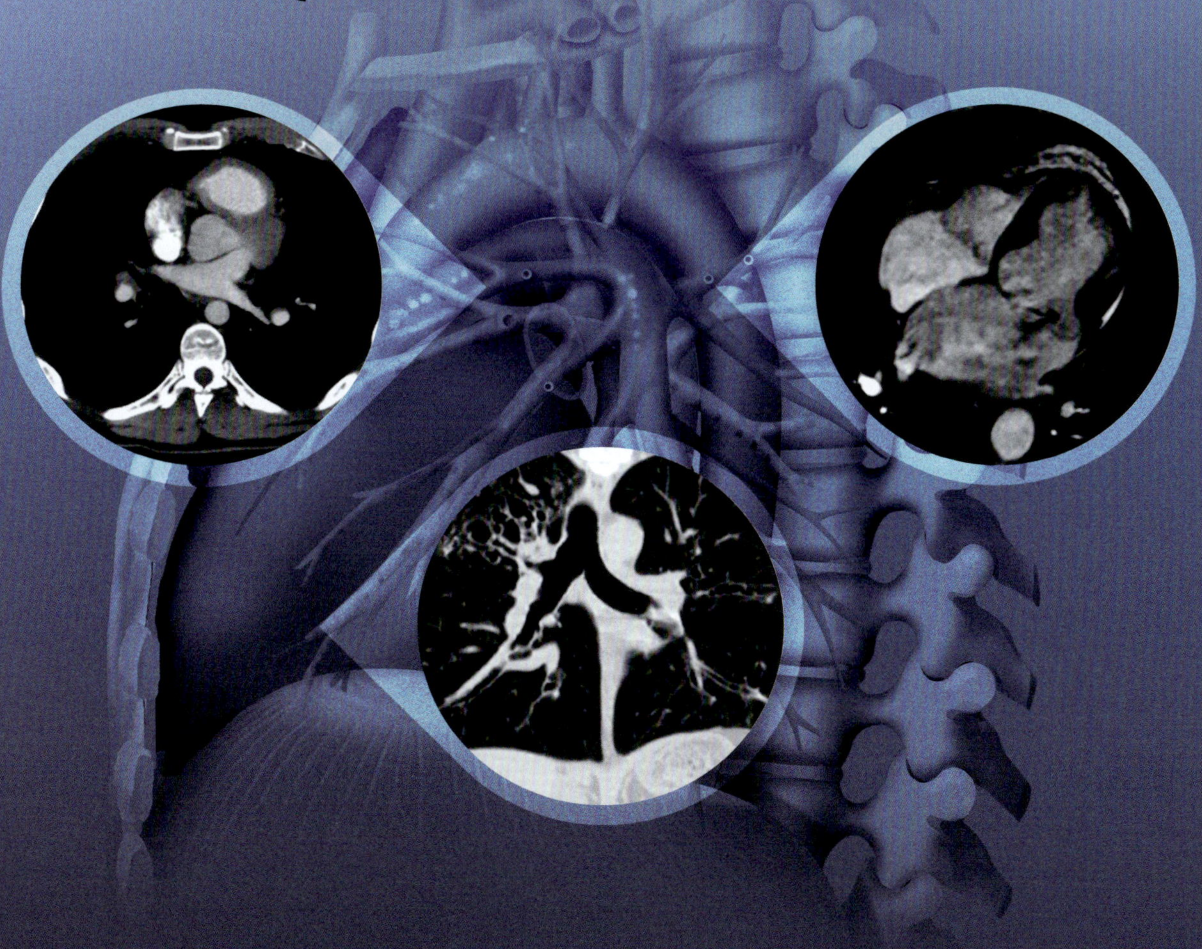

SECTION 1

Introduction

Approach to Clinical Presentation

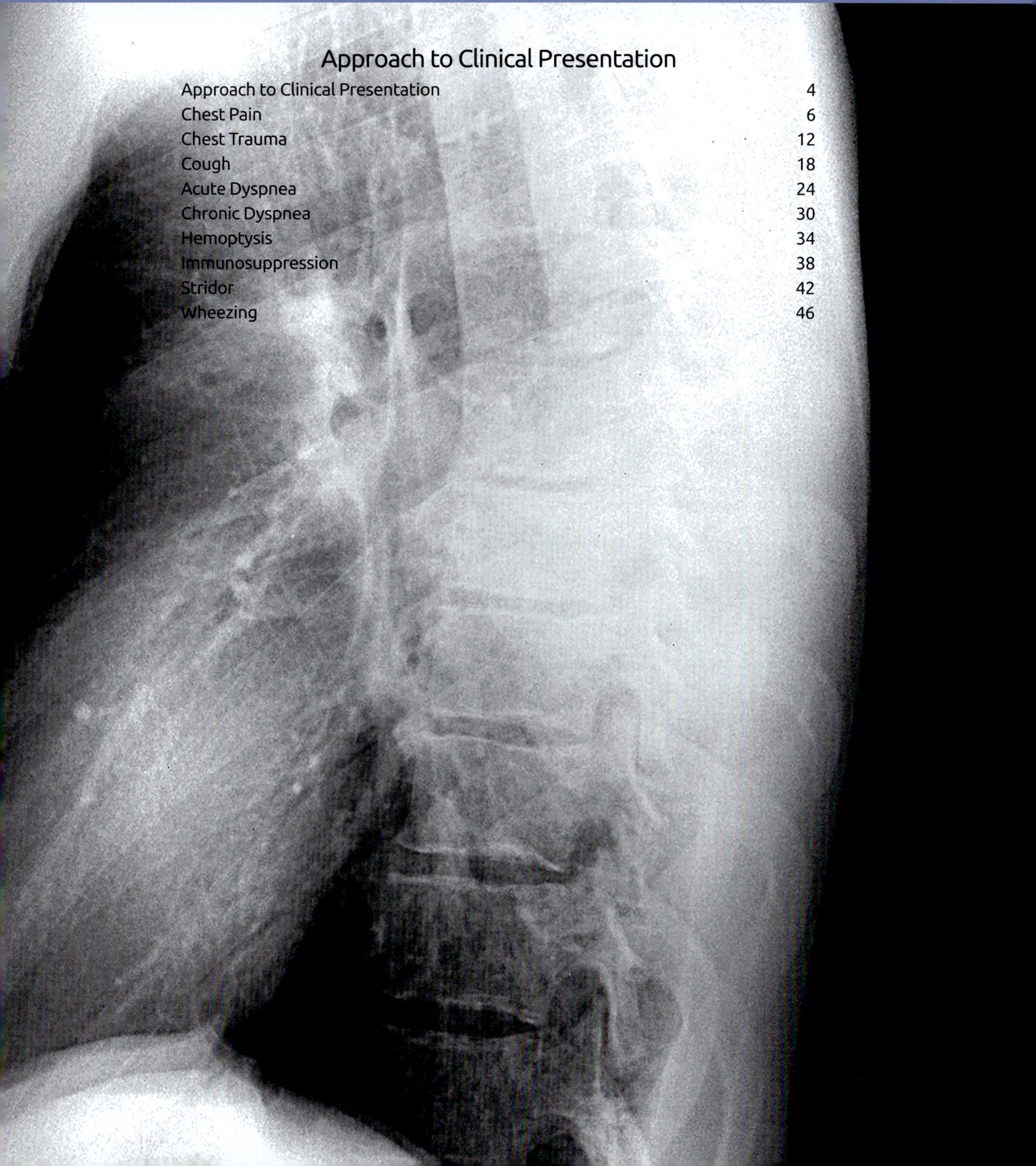

Introduction

Patients with thoracic disease may present with a variety of complaints and are typically initially imaged with radiography. Presenting symptoms may include chest pain, cough, dyspnea, wheezing, and stridor. Patients may also present for assessment of minor or major thoracic trauma. In some instances, thoracic imaging is ordered in asymptomatic patients, including those undergoing routine physical examination or elective extrathoracic surgery. Patients with extrathoracic complaints may also undergo chest imaging as part of their evaluation. While imaging of such asymptomatic patients is generally discouraged, this practice is common and many such imaging studies demonstrate no abnormalities. However, chest imaging of asymptomatic patients may reveal incidental abnormalities that require additional assessment and definitive management.

Clinical Presentation

Chest Pain

Chest pain is a common presenting complaint both in the Emergency Department and in the outpatient setting. Because it may occur as a symptom of both life-threatening and relatively benign conditions, it often poses a diagnostic challenge for the clinician. Chest pain may be due to numerous etiologies. Important life-threatening conditions that manifest with chest pain include myocardial ischemia and infarction, pulmonary thromboembolism, acute aortic syndrome, heart failure, and pneumothorax. In some cases, the clinical history provides helpful clues to the etiology of chest pain. For example, patients with pulmonary thromboembolism may have well-known risk factors or complain of lower extremity symptoms of deep venous thrombosis. Patients with acute aortic syndrome are typically in the seventh decade of life, present with acute chest pain, and exhibit systemic hypertension. Patients with sickle cell anemia may present with chest pain from acute chest syndrome.

Several non-life-threatening conditions may initially manifest with chest pain and include pneumonia, chronic obstructive pulmonary disease, asthma, and pulmonary hypertension. Patients with pulmonary &/or cardiac sarcoidosis may also present with chest pain, often in association with dyspnea and cough. Some patients with thoracic malignancy may initially present with chest pain. While chest pain is typically associated with cardiopulmonary disease, other conditions may also produce this symptom, including esophageal and other gastrointestinal disorders and diseases of the thoracic musculoskeletal system.

Chest radiography allows rapid identification of pulmonary consolidation, pleural effusion, and pneumothorax. In many cases, chest CT follows and is usually tailored to the clinical presentation, with specific techniques including CT pulmonary angiography, CT aortography, and cardiac CT. MR is often reserved for patients in whom iodinated contrast administration is contraindicated and those with suspected cardiac disease.

Cough

Cough is a very common complaint in the outpatient setting and is classified based on its duration as acute (< 3 weeks), subacute (3-8 weeks), or chronic (> 8 weeks). Acute cough is often due to pulmonary infection, but other conditions may also cause it, including pulmonary embolism and exacerbation of chronic lung disease. Subacute and chronic cough may be related to upper airway cough syndrome, which is associated with postnasal drip and characteristically affects women. Additional etiologies include asthma, gastroesophageal reflux disease, and viral, mycoplasma, and chlamydia infections. *Bordetella pertussis* is associated with subacute or chronic persistent cough. Important etiologies of chronic cough include bronchitis (cough and sputum production for at least 3 months in the absence of another explanation) and bronchiectasis. Lung cancer may also manifest with cough, particularly when the neoplasm involves the central airways.

Acute cough is typically evaluated with chest radiography, the preferred imaging modality for diagnosing pneumonia, which may manifest with sublobar, lobar, &/or multifocal consolidations. In cases in which the radiograph is normal or nearly normal, chest CT may demonstrate acinar opacities &/or cellular bronchiolitis, which allows the radiologist to suggest pulmonary infection. Patients with pulmonary infection should be stratified as immunocompetent or immunocompromised, as the latter may be affected by atypical infections &/or neoplastic disorders.

Patients with subacute or chronic cough may have normal or nearly normal chest radiographs. In such cases, chest CT is often performed to exclude morphologic airway abnormalities that include bronchiectasis and bronchial wall thickening characteristic of bronchitis.

Dyspnea

Dyspnea refers to subjective breathing discomfort and may be acute (hours to days) or chronic (> 4-8 weeks). It may be caused by both cardiovascular and respiratory disorders. Cardiovascular disorders that produce dyspnea include heart failure, anemia, and deconditioning. Respiratory causes of dyspnea include chronic obstructive pulmonary disease that may manifest with emphysema and restrictive disease related to pulmonary fibrosis. Neuromuscular disorders such as myasthenia gravis and Guillain-Barré syndrome may also manifest with dyspnea. Evaluation of affected patients usually includes both chest radiography and CT. In patients with suspected chronic fibrosing interstitial lung disease, chest CT and high-resolution CT are invaluable imaging tools for determining the distribution of pulmonary fibrosis, formulating a differential diagnosis, and assessing disease progression.

Wheezing

Patients who present with wheezing are often suspected of having either asthma or chronic obstructive pulmonary disease. However, "all that wheezes is not asthma," and other entities must be considered in the differential diagnosis. These include anaphylaxis, upper airway stenosis, cervical or mediastinal mass (including vascular rings), upper airway neoplasms, tracheomalacia/tracheobronchomalacia, constrictive bronchiolitis, and diffuse idiopathic pulmonary neuroendocrine cell hyperplasia, among many others.

Stridor

Stridor refers to a high-pitched, monophonic sound made during inspiration or expiration. It typically signifies large airway obstruction located in supraglottic, glottic, subglottic, or intrathoracic regions. Stridor often suggests foreign body aspiration but may also be secondary to centrally obstructive inflammatory or neoplastic conditions. While radiography is usually initially performed, CT allows optimal assessment of central airway obstructive lesions.

Acute Aortic Syndrome

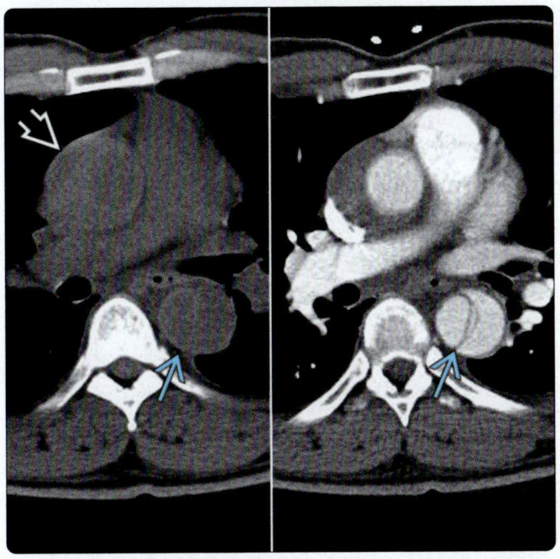

Pulmonary Thromboembolism

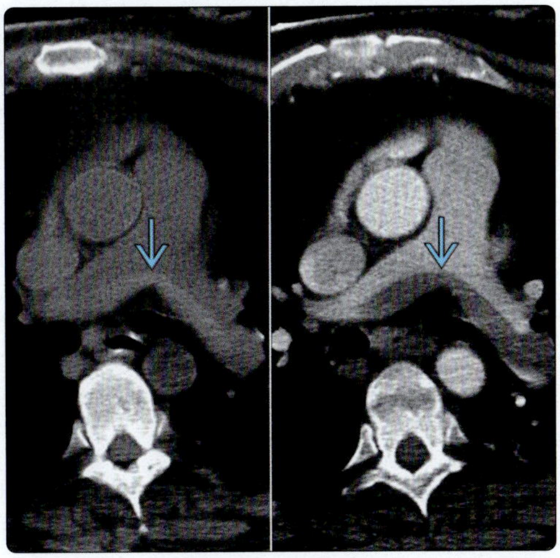

(Left) *Composite image with axial NECT (left) and CECT (right) of a 68-year-old man with chest pain and hypertension shows an ascending aortic intramural hematoma and a descending aortic dissection.* **(Right)** *Composite image with axial NECT (left) and CECT (right) of a patient with suspected acute aortic syndrome shows a saddle pulmonary embolus that exhibits high attenuation on NECT. CT angiography tailored to the clinical history is valuable for evaluating patients with acute chest pain.*

Pneumonia

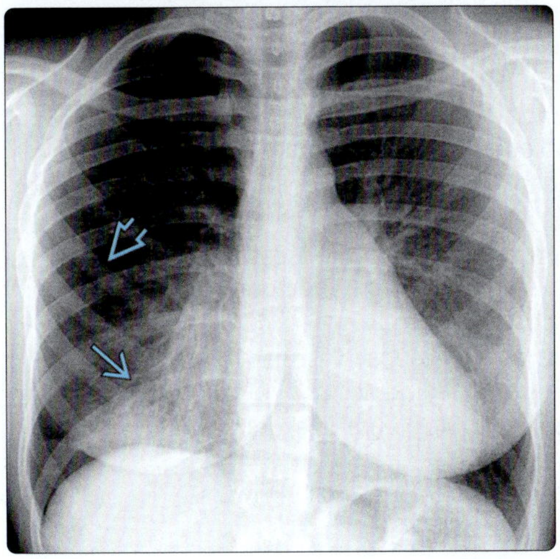

Pneumonia

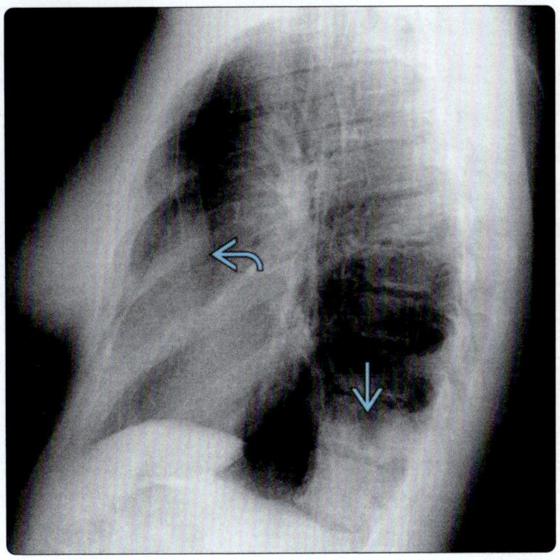

(Left) *PA chest radiograph of a 45-year-old woman who presented with productive cough and fever shows airspace consolidation in the right lung base, consistent with pneumonia. Note oblique orientation of the anterior ribs characteristic of pectus excavatum deformity.* **(Right)** *Lateral chest radiograph of the same patient confirms both pectus excavatum deformity and a right lower lobe pneumonia that produces the spine sign. Chest radiography is the study of choice for the diagnosis of pneumonia.*

Emphysema

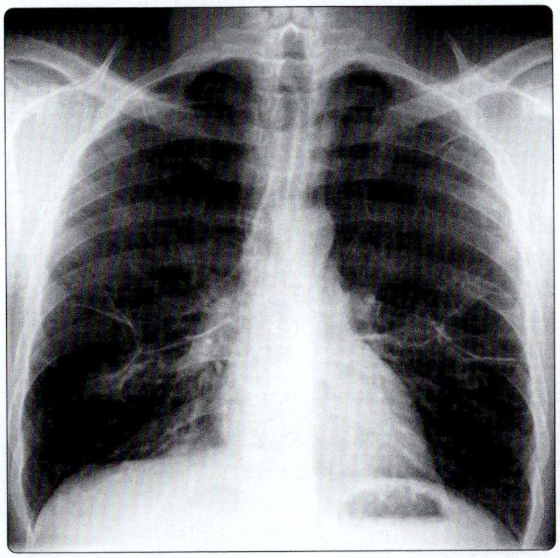

Usual Interstitial Pneumonia

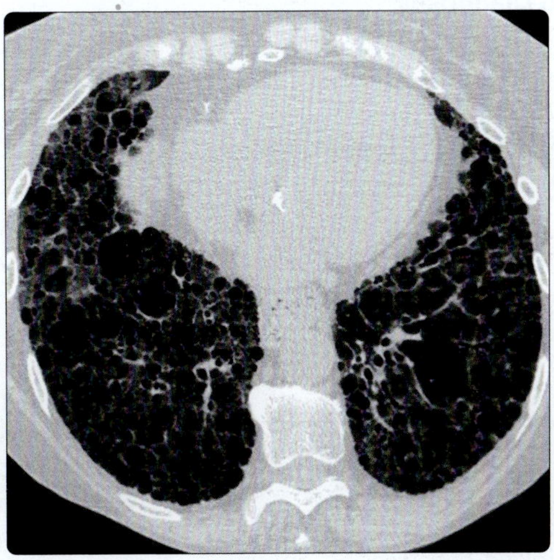

(Left) *PA chest radiograph of a 48-year-old man who presented with dyspnea shows severe bilateral upper and mid lung zone-predominant bullous emphysema.* **(Right)** *Axial HRCT of a 58-year-old woman with scleroderma and dyspnea shows basilar predominant fibrosing interstitial lung disease, consistent with usual interstitial pneumonia (UIP) pattern. Imaging is very useful in the assessment of patients with chronic dyspnea and often allows evaluation and assessment of obstructive and restrictive lung diseases.*

DIFFERENTIAL DIAGNOSIS

Common

- Heart Failure
- Myocardial Ischemia/Infarction
- Pulmonary Thromboembolism
- Pneumothorax
- Chest Wall Trauma
- Thoracic Malignancy
- Pneumonia
- Gastroesophageal Disease

Less Common

- Acute Aortic Syndrome
- Acute Chest Syndrome
- Cardiomyopathy
- Pleuritis

Rare but Important

- Pericardial Disease
- Esophageal Rupture
- Sarcoidosis
- Mediastinal Fat Necrosis

ESSENTIAL INFORMATION

Key Differential Diagnosis Issues

- Chest pain: 2nd most common complaint of patients presenting to emergency departments in USA; ~ 6 million annual visits
- Diagnostic challenge as numerous and diverse conditions manifest with chest pain: Cardiovascular, pulmonary, pleural, gastroesophageal, chest wall
    - Identification and exclusion of life-threatening entities
- Assessment and diagnosis relies on history, physical examination, laboratory findings, and imaging
- Imaging
    - PA and lateral chest radiography; AP chest radiography in traumatized, debilitated, &/or critically ill patients
    - Chest CT or CT angiography for specific indications

Helpful Clues for Common Diagnoses

- **Heart Failure**
    - Etiologies: Coronary atherosclerosis, cardiomyopathy, valvular disease, uncontrolled hypertension
    - Progressive chest pain/discomfort, dyspnea, cough, fatigue, peripheral edema
    - Radiography/CT
        - Subpleural edema, perihilar haze, peribronchial cuffing, Kerley lines
        - Cardiomegaly, wide vascular pedicle
        - Ground-glass and acinar opacities, consolidation
        - Pleural effusion
- **Myocardial Ischemia/Infarction**
    - Angina: Chest pain/pressure, heaviness; may radiate to left arm &/or jaw
    - Male > female; males > 45 years, females > 55 years
    - Risk factors: Cigarette smoking, hypertension, obesity, hypercholesterolemia, hyperlipidemia, diabetes, family history
    - Diagnosis: Cardiac biomarkers, elevated &/or rising troponin; ST segment and Q wave abnormalities
    - Imaging
        - Luminal occlusion or filling defect on catheter angiography or CT coronary angiography
        - New perfusion abnormality on CT/MR indicating loss of viable myocardium
            - ↑ T2 signal, delayed myocardial enhancement
        - New wall motion abnormality
- **Pulmonary Thromboembolism**
    - Dyspnea, pleuritic chest pain, deep venous thrombosis
    - Risk factors: Hypercoagulable state, recent surgery, pregnancy, prolonged immobilization, malignancy, HIV infection, oral contraceptive use, deep vein thrombosis
    - Radiography: Nonspecific abnormalities, Fleischner sign (enlarged pulmonary artery), Hampton hump (peripheral wedge-shaped opacity), Westermark sign (oligemia)
    - CT
        - Endoluminal filling defects on CT or MR pulmonary angiography
        - ± pulmonary infarct, pulmonary hypertension, right heart strain, pleural effusion
- **Pneumothorax**
    - Traumatic: Blunt or penetrating trauma
    - Spontaneous
        - Primary
            - Young adult; male > female; asthenic body habitus, subpleural blebs/bullae, cigarette smoking
        - Secondary: Cystic, cavitary, or infiltrative lung disease
            - Male > female; > 55 years
            - Emphysema, cystic lung disease, primary and metastatic malignancy, necrotizing infection
    - Illicit drug use
    - Iatrogenic: Surgery, biopsy, vascular catheterization/medical device placement, barotrauma
    - Radiography: Visible pleural line, deep sulcus sign on supine imaging
    - CT: Assessment of underlying lung disease
- **Chest Wall Trauma**
    - Blunt or penetrating injury
    - Skeletal fracture: Rib, sternum, thoracic spine
    - Soft tissue injury: Contusion, hematoma
- **Thoracic Malignancy**
    - Lung cancer: Chest pain, cough, dyspnea, hemoptysis
        - Older adult, cigarette smoker
        - Mediastinal, parietal pleura, &/or chest wall involvement
        - Central neoplasm with postobstructive pneumonia
        - Pancoast syndrome: Superior sulcus tumor with osseous destruction, pain/atrophy of upper extremity musculature, Horner syndrome
    - Metastases to lung, mediastinum, pleura, chest wall
    - Imaging
        - Identification of pulmonary &/or thoracic mass
        - ± lymphadenopathy, pleural effusion, chest wall involvement
- **Pneumonia**
    - Chest pain (may be pleuritic), fever, cough
    - Leukocytosis, ↑ procalcitonin in bacterial infection
    - Focal or multifocal consolidation(s)
    - Cellular bronchiolitis, acinar ground-glass opacities
    - ± cavitation, pleural effusion

- **Gastroesophageal Disease**
  - Gastroesophageal reflux disease: May mimic angina pectoris; substernal chest pain radiating to back
    - Mucosal thickening, ulcers, erosions, strictures
  - Esophageal spasm: Mid/distal esophageal smooth muscle contractions
  - Nutcracker esophagus: High amplitude distal esophageal peristalsis (not imaging diagnosis)

Helpful Clues for Less Common Diagnoses

- **Acute Aortic Syndrome**
  - Aortic dissection, incomplete dissection, penetrating ulcer, intramural hematoma
  - Male > female; acute chest pain and hypertension
  - CT aortography
    - Unenhanced chest CT: Identification of intramural hematoma
    - Contrast-enhanced chest CT: Identification of dissection and penetrating ulcer
- **Acute Chest Syndrome**
  - Sickle cell anemia
  - Chest pain, dyspnea, fever, hypoxemia
  - Imaging: Atelectasis, consolidation, &/or pleural effusion
- **Cardiomyopathy**
  - Etiologies: Ischemic, nonischemic, restrictive, hypertrophic, inflammatory, valvular, hypertensive
  - Takotsubo or stress cardiomyopathy
    - History of recent emotional/physical stress
    - Chest pain and dyspnea
    - Electrocardiographic abnormalities
    - Cardiogenic shock, ventricular fibrillation
  - Regional wall motion abnormalities; apical ballooning, narrow mouth and broad base of left ventricle resemble Japanese octopus pot
- **Pleuritis**
  - Pleurisy or pleural inflammation
  - Pleuritic pain
  - Pleural effusion &/or thickening
  - Etiologies: Infection, pneumoconiosis, collagen vascular disease (rheumatoid arthritis), autoimmunity

Helpful Clues for Rare Diagnoses

- **Pericardial Disease**
  - Pericarditis: Serous, purulent, tuberculous, fibrinous, hemorrhagic
    - Pericardial effusion, thickening
  - Pericardial tamponade: Jugular vein distension, hypotension, muffled heart sounds
    - Pericardial effusion, compression of right heart chambers
- **Esophageal Rupture**
  - Laceration, tear
  - Boerhaave syndrome: Esophageal rupture after forceful emesis
  - Mallory-Weiss tear: Partial-thickness tear after emesis
  - Pneumomediastinum, extraluminal contrast
  - Pleural effusion, consolidation
- **Sarcoidosis**
  - Systemic granulomatous disease of unknown etiology
    - Noncaseating epithelial granulomas: Thoracic lymph node and lung involvement; may involve skin, joints, eyes
  - Affected patients may present with chest pain
    - Pulmonary sarcoidosis: Chest pain frequently associated with cough and dyspnea
    - Cardiac sarcoidosis: Chest pain related to cardiac arrhythmia and heart block; may be associated with palpitations and syncope
  - Imaging
    - Bilateral hilar and mediastinal lymphadenopathy
    - Perilymphatic distribution of pulmonary nodules, micronodules, masses, ground-glass opacities
- **Mediastinal Fat Necrosis**
  - Synonym: Epipericardial fat necrosis; not always adjacent to pericardium
  - Acute pleuritic chest pain
  - CT: Ovoid juxtapericardial/mediastinal lesion
    - Fat attenuation lesion surrounded by soft tissue rind
    - Stranding of adjacent mediastinal fat

Heart Failure

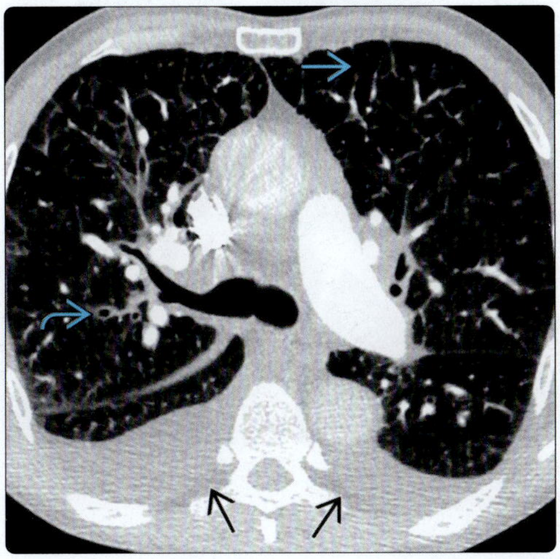

Heart Failure

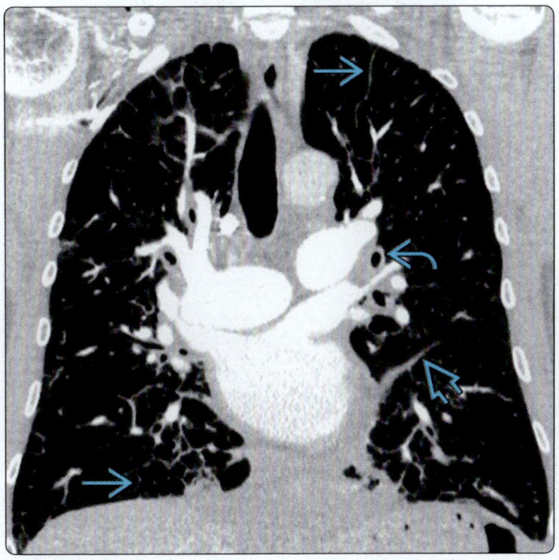

(Left) *Axial CECT of a 69-year-old man with chest pain and dyspnea and suspected pulmonary thromboembolism shows profuse bilateral smooth interlobular septal thickening → on a background of centrilobular emphysema, diffuse bronchial wall thickening ↪, and small bilateral pleural effusions ➔.* **(Right)** *Coronal CECT of the same patient shows smooth interlobular septal thickening →, bronchial wall thickening ↪, and subpleural edema ⇨, consistent with interstitial edema secondary to acute heart failure.*

(Left) *Two-chamber coronary CTA of a patient with chest pain shows left anterior descending coronary artery noncalcified plaque with severe stenosis* ➔ *and a perfusion defect of the anterior wall of the left ventricle* ➔. **(Right)** *Composite image with axial CECT at baseline (left) and 4 months later (right) of a 95-year-old woman with chest pain shows hypoperfusion* ➔ *of the left ventricular septum secondary to myocardial infarction complicated by acquired ventricular septal defect* ➔ *in the same area.*

Myocardial Ischemia/Infarction

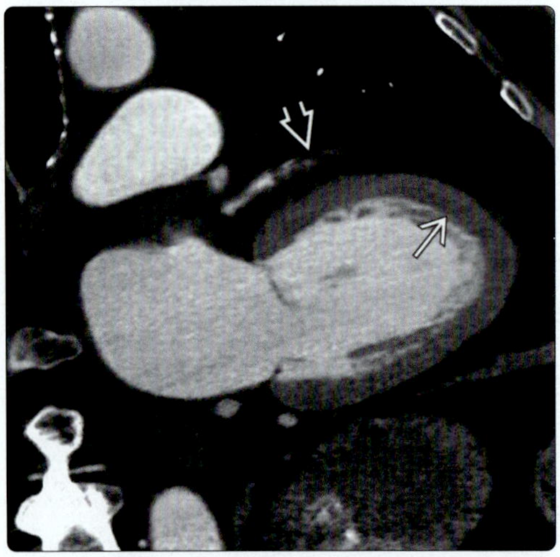

Myocardial Ischemia/Infarction

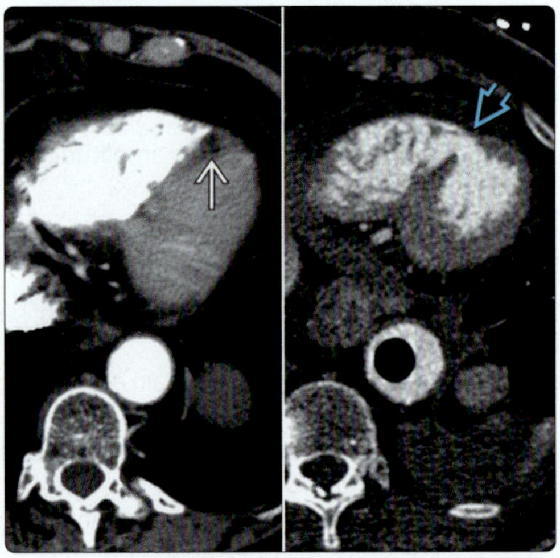

(Left) *AP chest radiograph of a 43-year-old man with acute chest pain and dyspnea shows right perihilar hyperlucency and paucity of vascular markings concerning for the Westermark sign of pulmonary thromboembolism. Note enlargement of the right interlobar pulmonary artery* ➔. **(Right)** *Coronal CECT of the same patient shows a large occlusive right pulmonary artery thromboembolus* ➔ *and a right basilar peripheral subpleural wedge-shaped consolidation* ➔, *consistent with a pulmonary infarct.*

Pulmonary Thromboembolism

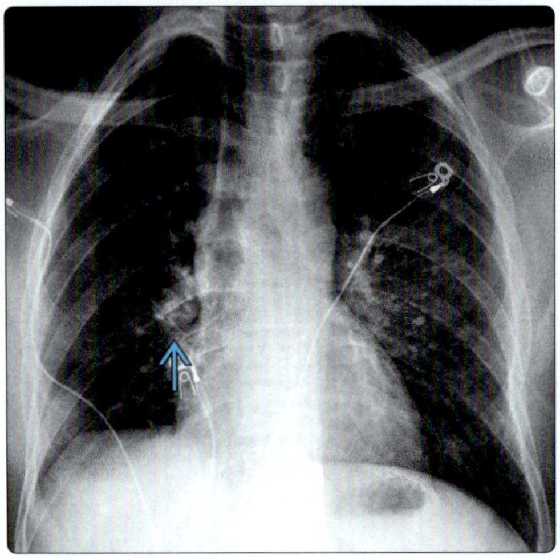

Pulmonary Thromboembolism

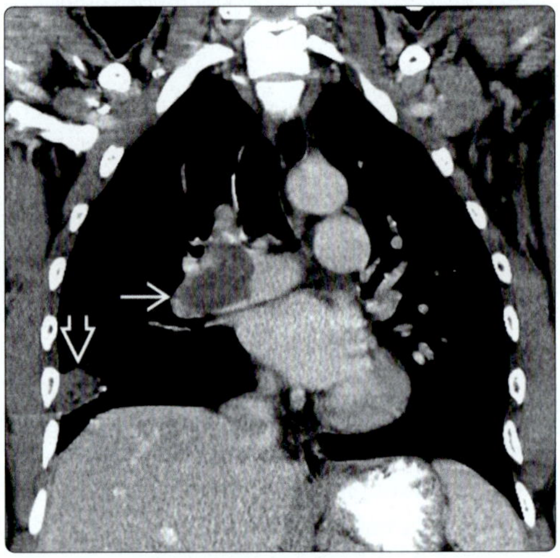

(Left) *PA chest radiograph of a 20-year-old man who presented to the emergency department with acute left-sided chest pain and dyspnea shows a large left pneumothorax with apical, lateral, and basilar components. Note tiny left apical subpleural bulla or bleb* ➔. **(Right)** *Coronal CECT of the same patient after chest tube placement shows a small left apical pneumothorax adjacent to small left apical pulmonary bullae or blebs* ➔. *The findings are typical of primary spontaneous pneumothorax.*

Pneumothorax

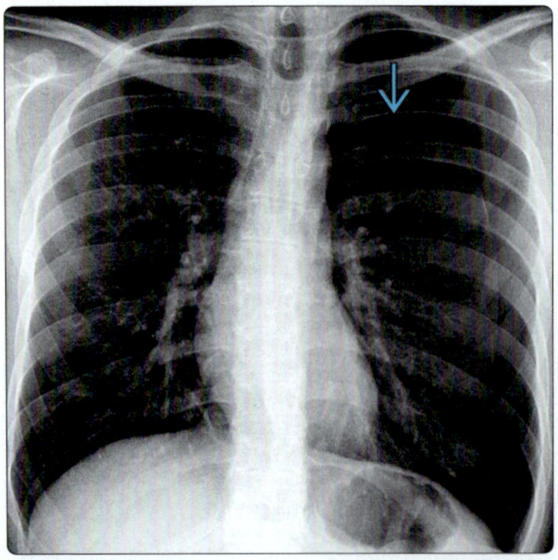

Pneumothorax

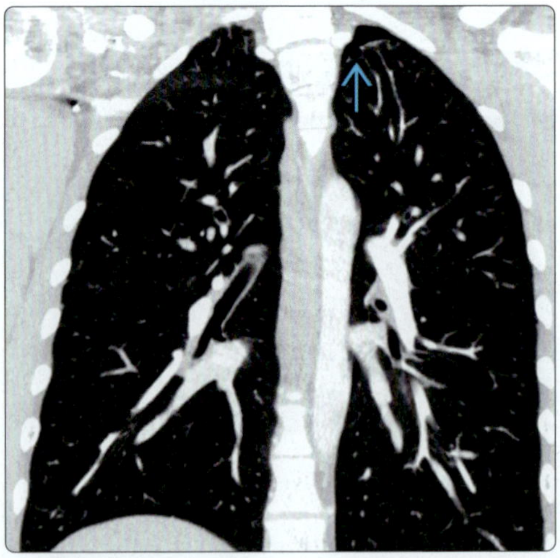

Chest Wall Trauma

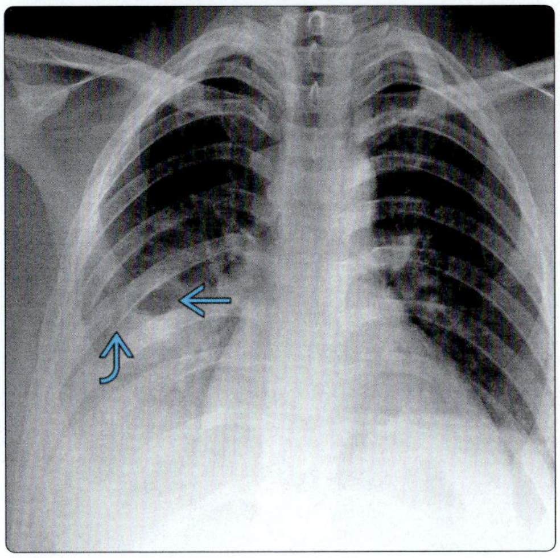

Chest Wall Trauma

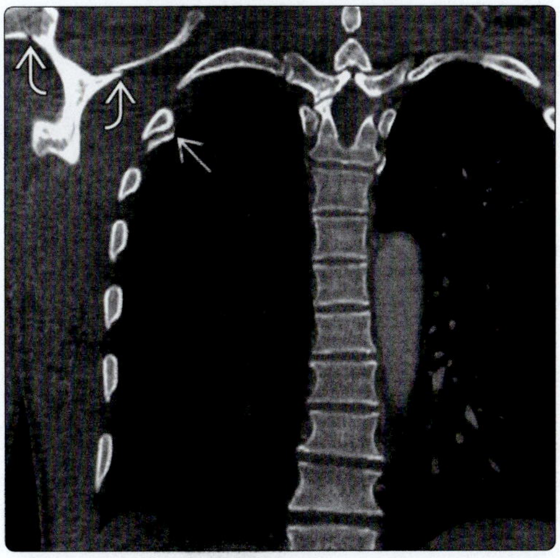

(Left) *AP chest radiograph of a 40-year-old man who presented with right-sided chest pain after a fall shows right basilar and mid lung zone airspace disease and a focal ovoid lucency that represented a pulmonary laceration secondary to multifocal displaced right posterolateral rib fractures.* **(Right)** *Coronal CECT of a 21-year-old man who sustained blunt right chest trauma shows a displaced fracture of the right posterolateral 3rd rib and a comminuted right scapular fracture.*

Thoracic Malignancy

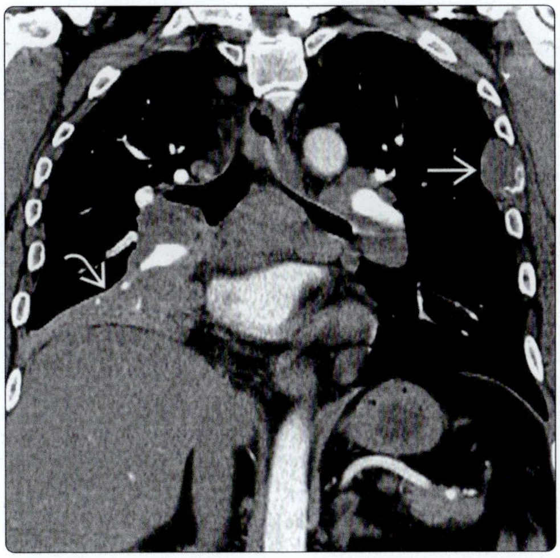

Thoracic Malignancy

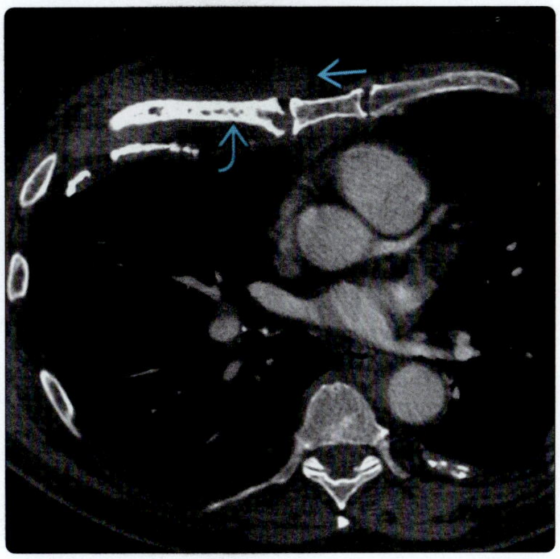

(Left) *Coronal CECT of a 53-year-old man with metastatic squamous cell lung cancer who presented with chest pain shows right lower lobe postobstructive atelectasis, diffuse mediastinal and hilar lymphadenopathy, and a lytic lesion of the left lateral 6th rib.* **(Right)** *Axial CECT of a 72-year-old man with metastatic prostate cancer who presented with right anterior chest wall pain shows a permeative sclerotic lesion of a right anterior rib surrounded by infiltrative soft tissue tumor, consistent with metastatic disease.*

Pneumonia

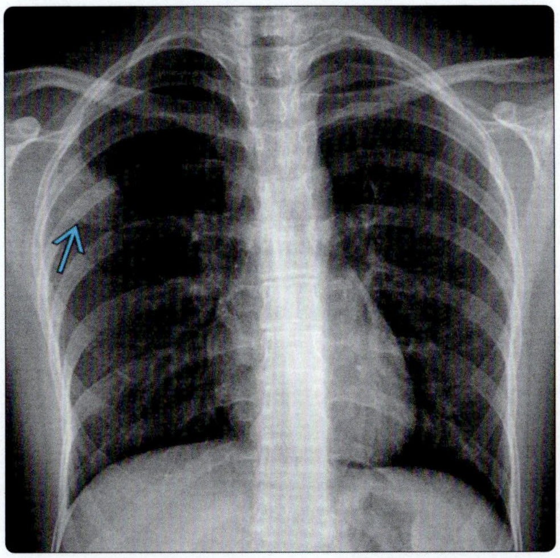

Pneumonia

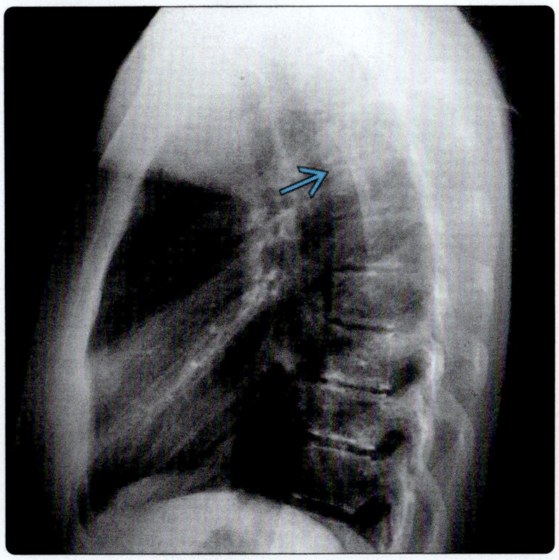

(Left) *PA chest radiograph of a 22-year-old woman who presented to the emergency department with right scapular pain shows a rounded peripheral right upper lobe consolidation.* **(Right)** *Lateral chest radiograph of the same patient shows that the consolidation is located in the posterior segment of the right upper lobe. On further questioning, a history of fever and cough was elicited compatible with the diagnosis of pneumonia. Patients with pneumonia may present with chest pain.*

(Left) *Barium esophagram of a 65-year-old man with intermittent chest pain shows a small hiatus hernia with gastric folds ➡ extending above the diaphragm and a stricture ⇨ at the gastroesophageal junction with associated mucosal ulceration.* **(Right)** *Barium esophagram of a 50-year-old man with AIDS who presented with chest pain and painful swallowing shows innumerable raised plaques and mucosal ulcerations of the distal esophagus secondary to Candida esophagitis.*

Gastroesophageal Disease

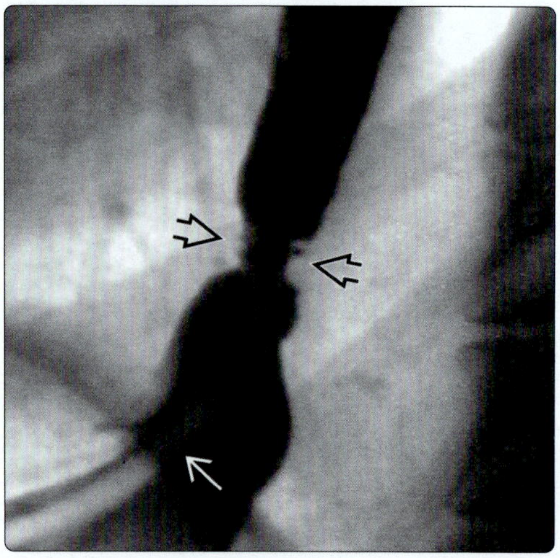

Gastroesophageal Disease

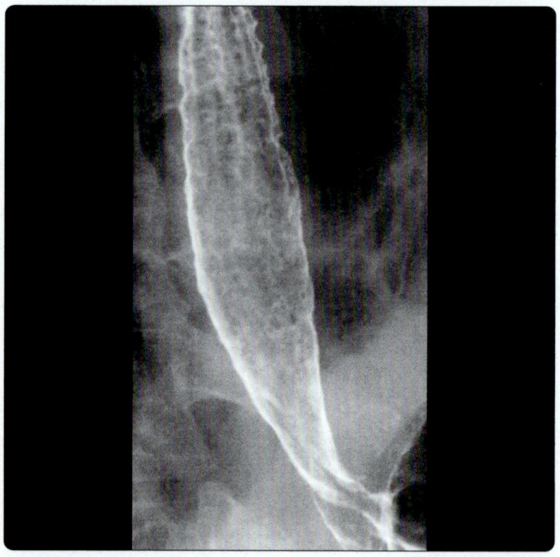

(Left) *Composite image with axial NECT of a 79-year-old hypertensive woman who presented with acute chest pain shows an intramural hematoma of the ascending aorta and a descending aortic aneurysm with surrounding soft tissue stranding concerning for aortic rupture.* **(Right)** *Composite image with axial CECT of the same patient confirms the presence of an ascending aorta type A intramural hematoma and demonstrates rupture of the descending thoracic aorta as a complication of the acute aortic syndrome.*

Acute Aortic Syndrome

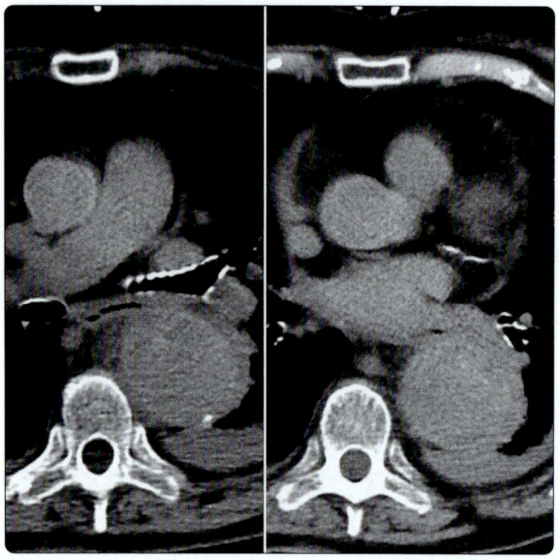

Acute Aortic Syndrome

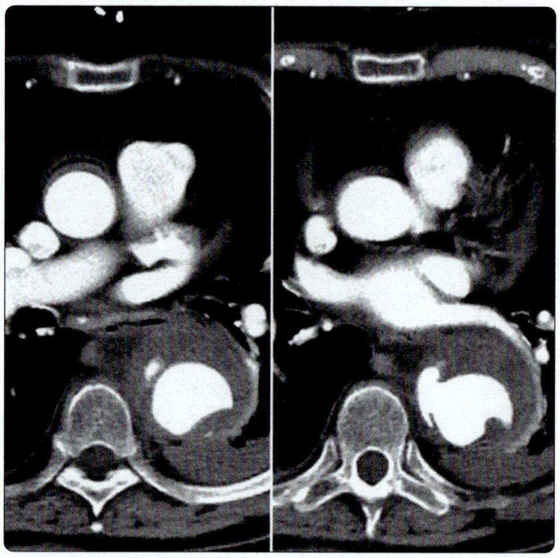

(Left) *PA chest radiograph of a 25-year-old man with sickle cell disease who presented with acute chest pain and fever shows a left lower lobe consolidation and a small left pleural effusion.* **(Right)** *Axial CECT of the same patient performed for exclusion of acute pulmonary thromboembolism shows a left lower lobe consolidation ➡ and small bilateral pleural effusions ⇨. Patients with acute chest syndrome may demonstrate lower lobe-predominant consolidations and pleural effusions, as in this case.*

Acute Chest Syndrome

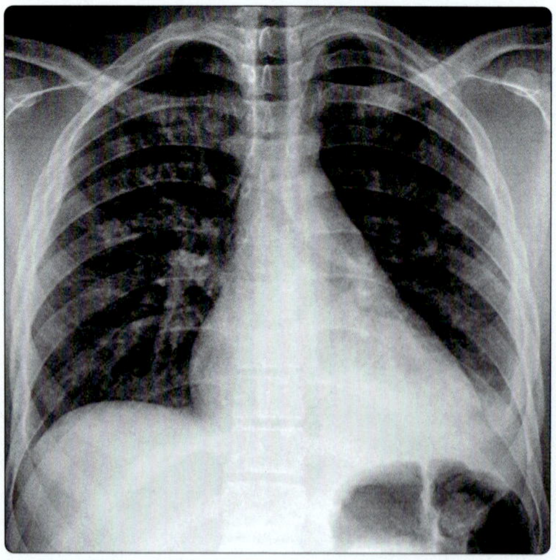

Acute Chest Syndrome

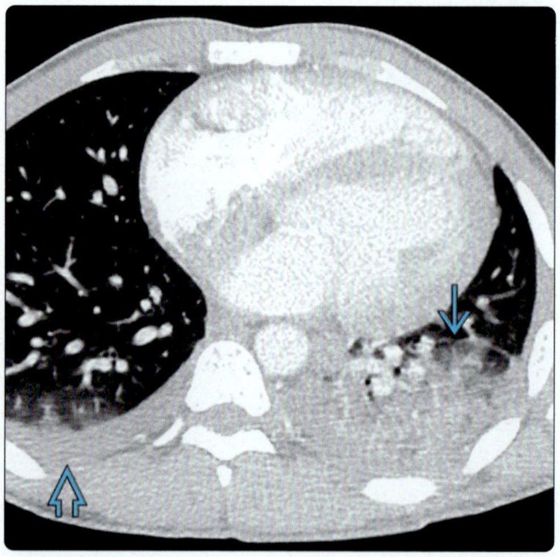

Cardiomyopathy

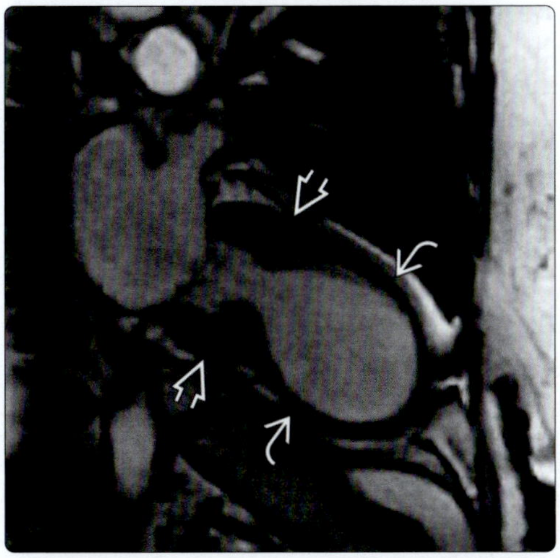

Cardiomyopathy

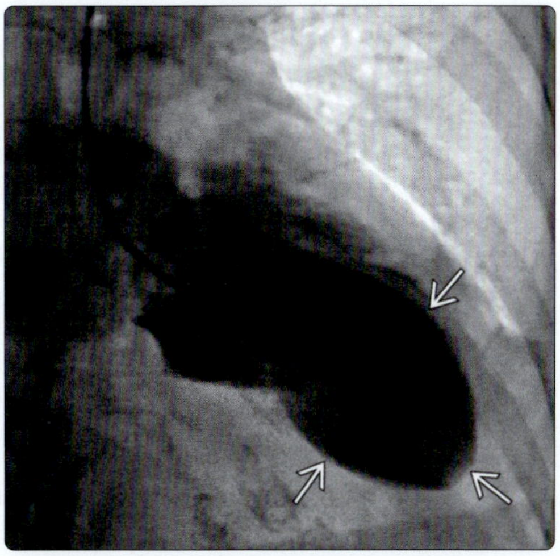

(Left) *Two-chamber SSFP MR of a patient who presented with chest pain and dyspnea secondary to stress cardiomyopathy shows characteristic features of ballooning of the left ventricular apex* ➡ *and normal contraction of the base of the left ventricle* ➡. **(Right)** *Left ventriculogram obtained during diastole shows ballooning of the left ventricular apex* ➡, *typical of stress or takotsubo cardiomyopathy. Affected patients present with acute chest pain that mimics acute coronary syndrome.*

Pleuritis

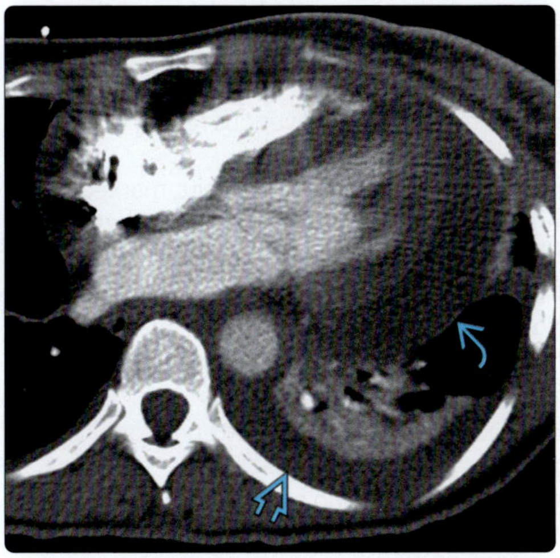

Esophageal Rupture

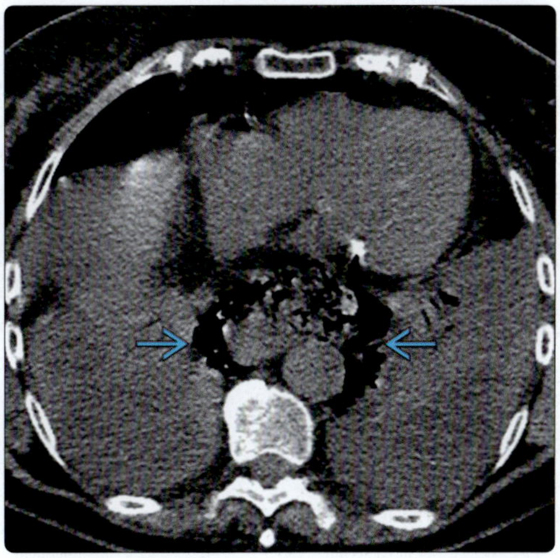

(Left) *Axial CECT of a 42-year-old woman with systemic lupus erythematosus and pleuritic chest pain shows small bilateral pleural effusions* ➡ *and a moderate pericardial effusion* ➡, *consistent with lupus pleuritis and pericarditis.* **(Right)** *Axial NECT of an 89-year-old woman with acute chest pain after forceful vomiting shows large pleural effusions, bibasilar consolidations, and pneumomediastinum* ➡ *centered about a dilated and thickened distal esophagus, consistent with esophageal rupture.*

Sarcoidosis

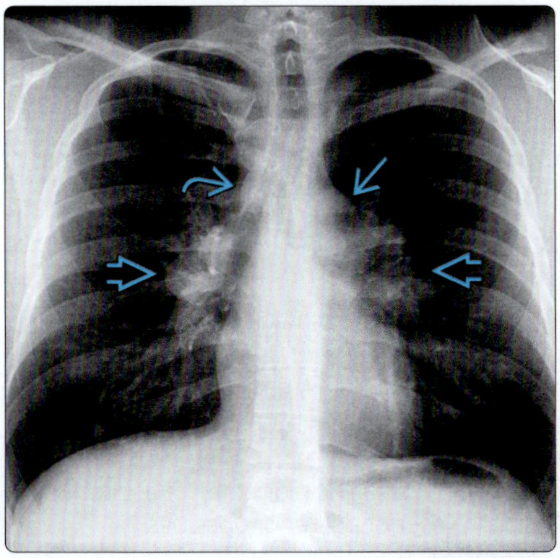

Mediastinal Fat Necrosis

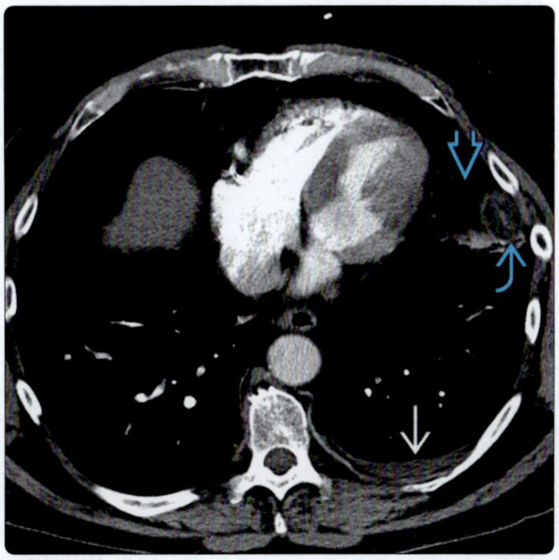

(Left) *PA chest radiograph of a 37-year-old man who presented with chest pain shows bilateral hilar* ➡, *right paratracheal* ➡, *and aortopulmonary window* ➡ *lymphadenopathy, typical of sarcoidosis. Affected patients may present with chest pain.* **(Right)** *Axial CECT of a 40-year-old man with acute chest pain shows an ovoid fat attenuation lesion* ➡ *surrounded by a thin soft tissue rim and stranding of the adjacent mediastinal fat* ➡, *characteristic of mediastinal fat necrosis. Note small left pleural effusion* ➡.

DIFFERENTIAL DIAGNOSIS

Common

- Soft Tissue Injury
- Rib Fracture
- Pneumothorax
- Hemothorax
- Pulmonary Contusion

Less Common

- Aspiration
- Pulmonary Laceration
- Sternal Fracture
- Vertebral Fracture
- Traumatic Aortic Injury

Rare but Important

- Diaphragmatic Rupture
- Pneumomediastinum
- Cardiac/Pericardial Injury
- Tracheobronchial injury
- Sternoclavicular Dislocation
- Esophageal Rupture

ESSENTIAL INFORMATION

Key Differential Diagnosis Issues

- Chest trauma: 10% fatality rate among survivors
- Motor vehicle collisions are most common cause of blunt thoracic trauma
- Mechanisms
  - Blunt trauma: 90% of thoracic injuries
  - Penetrating trauma: Stabbing, gunshot injuries
- Imaging plays critical role in diagnosis and management
  - Supine portable chest radiography is usually initial study
  - CT: Imaging modality of choice
    - IV contrast mandatory for assessment of traumatic vascular injury
    - Injuries demonstrated in up to 20% of patients with normal chest radiographs
- Imaging findings are variable and evolve over time
  - Injuries in multiple thoracic structures may coexist
  - Imaging helps differentiate acute, subacute, and chronic traumatic injuries
  - Knowledge of site and mechanism of injury is critical for accurate imaging interpretation

Helpful Clues for Common Diagnoses

- **Soft Tissue Injury**
  - Contusion
    - Induration of subcutaneous fat due to soft tissue bruising
    - Seat belt sign: Clinical and radiologic
      - Bruising (induration of subcutaneous fat) diagonally in chest, horizontally in abdomen
  - Hematoma
    - Associated with rib fractures and venous/arterial injury
    - Soft tissue mass with intrinsic high attenuation &/or blood products
    - May be life-threatening in anticoagulated patients and require embolization
- **Rib Fracture**
  - Most frequent skeletal injury
    - 1st-3rd rib fractures (sternum and scapula) indicate high-energy trauma
    - Nondisplaced or displaced, may be comminuted; fracture fragments with sharp cortical edges
    - Surrounding hematoma
    - Segmental fractures
      - ≥ 2 fractures of same rib
    - Flail chest
      - May occur with ≥ 3 segmental fractures or > 5 contiguous rib fractures
      - Paradoxical motion of flail segment during respiration
      - May require surgical fixation in patients with respiratory failure
- **Pneumothorax**
  - Variable volume; occult on radiography in up to 50% of cases
  - Visible pleural line, absence of peripheral markings
  - Frequent associated rib fractures
  - Supine radiography: Basilar hyperlucency, deep sulcus sign
  - Tension pneumothorax
    - Clinical diagnosis: Decreased venous return to heart with hemodynamic compromise
    - Imaging: Contralateral mediastinal shift, marked ipsilateral atelectasis, hemidiaphragmatic inversion, splayed ipsilateral intercostal spaces
- **Hemothorax**
  - Variable volume pleural effusion
  - Frequent associated displaced rib fractures
  - Variable attenuation on CT
    - Heterogeneous, may exhibit low attenuation, dependent hyperdense blood clots
    - Hematocrit effect: Layering of blood products of different age and degree of coagulation
    - Active bleeding may demonstrate blush of contrast
- **Pulmonary Contusion**
  - Most common type of lung injury
  - Capillary disruption with alveolar/interstitial hemorrhage
  - Peripheral ground-glass opacities/consolidations
    - Geographic, nonsegmental, do not respect anatomic boundaries, may exhibit air bronchograms
    - May be imperceptible in first 6 hours post trauma
    - Complete resolution after 3-14 days

Helpful Clues for Less Common Diagnoses

- **Aspiration**
  - Dependent distribution; may coexist with pulmonary contusion in trauma patients
  - Ground-glass acinar nodules if small volume aspiration
  - Dependent consolidations and bronchial impaction if large volume aspiration
  - Assessment of airway opacification to favor aspiration over contusion in cases of posterior opacities
- **Pulmonary Laceration**
  - Lung disruption and tearing; may exhibit tubular morphology
  - Surrounding pulmonary contusion may initially obscure underlying laceration

- Solitary or multiple: Spherical or ovoid cavity with intrinsic air, fluid, air-fluid level
- **Sternal Fracture**
  - Anterior chest wall trauma
  - Visualization of cortical discontinuity: Lateral radiography, CT
  - Increased sensitivity on sagittal and coronal CT and coronal MIP reformations
  - Associated retrosternal and presternal hematoma
- **Vertebral Fracture**
  - Most common between T9 and T12
  - May be missed on radiography
  - CT with multiplanar imaging: High sensitivity
  - Cortical disruption, various degrees of compression
- **Traumatic Aortic Injury**
  - High morbidity and mortality, frequently fatal
  - Fixed aortic segments most frequently injured
    - Aortic isthmus > aortic arch > aortic root > distal descending aorta
  - Mediastinal widening on radiography
    - Periaortic mediastinal hemorrhage
  - CT aortography: Imaging study of choice
    - Indirect signs: Obliteration of tissue planes, periaortic hematoma, mediastinal hematoma
    - Direct signs: Active contrast extravasation, traumatic dissection, pseudoaneurysm, intimal tear, endoluminal thrombus, abrupt caliber change

Helpful Clues for Rare Diagnoses

- **Diaphragmatic Rupture**
  - More common in abdominal than in chest trauma; L > R
  - Diagnosis may be delayed
  - Radiography: Intrathoracic abdominal contents
  - CT: Diaphragmatic discontinuity, waist-like constriction of herniated viscus (collar sign), abdominal viscera abut posterior chest wall (dependent viscera sign)
    - Multiplanar imaging increases sensitivity
- **Pneumomediastinum**
  - Associated airway or esophageal injury
  - Macklin effect: Alveolar rupture with air dissection along bronchovascular interstitium into mediastinum
- **Cardiac/Pericardial Injury**
  - More common in penetrating trauma; high morbidity/mortality
  - Difficult diagnosis, requires high index of suspicion
  - Cardiac injury: Low-attenuation myocardium on contrast CT, hemopericardium
  - Pericardial injury: Pneumopericardium, hemopericardium, cardiac herniation
- **Tracheobronchial Injury**
  - Uncommon, high mortality
  - Typically affects distal trachea and proximal mainstem bronchi
    - Tracheal laceration typically perpendicular to cartilage rings; bronchial laceration typically parallel to cartilage rings
    - Bronchial laceration more common
  - Pneumomediastinum, pneumothorax
  - Direct CT finding: Airway lumen cutoff/disruption surrounded by extraluminal gas
  - Indirect CT findings
    - Atelectatic lung located away from hilum in dependent hemithorax (fallen lung sign)
    - Persistent pneumothorax after chest tube placement
    - Persistent pneumomediastinum
    - Herniation/overdistension of endotracheal tube balloon through site of tracheal laceration
- **Sternoclavicular Dislocation**
  - Anterior dislocation is more common; palpable, easier to diagnose
  - Posterior dislocation may be silent on clinical exam, may be missed on imaging
  - Associated injuries of adjacent mediastinal structures
- **Esophageal Rupture**
  - Rare; more common in penetrating trauma and iatrogenic injury
  - Mediastinal hemorrhage, pneumomediastinum
  - Extraluminal contrast on esophagography

Soft Tissue Injury

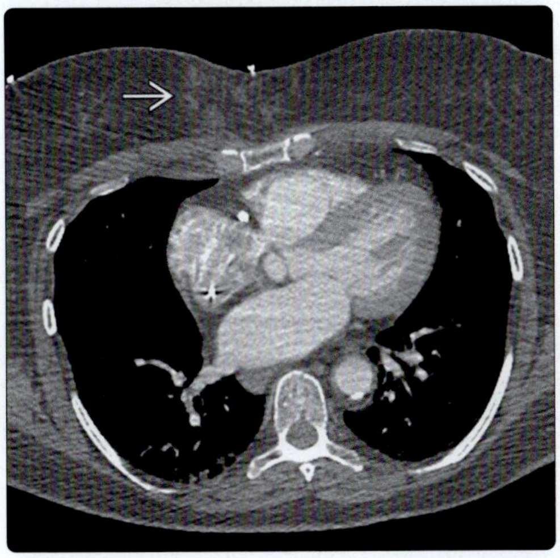

Rib Fracture

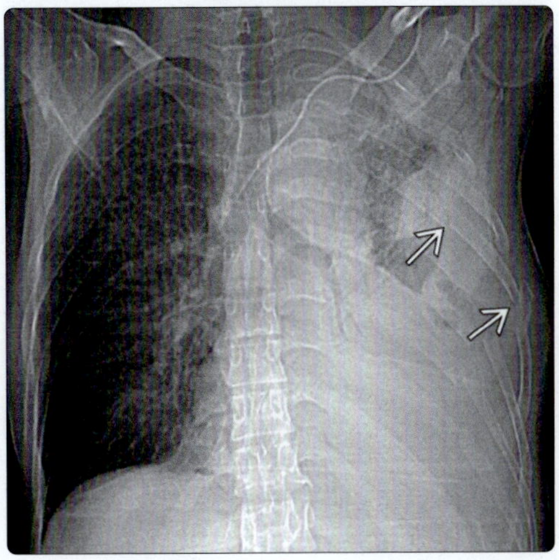

(Left) *Axial CECT of a 30-year-old restrained passenger who sustained blunt chest trauma during a motor vehicle collision shows induration of the right anterior chest wall subcutaneous fat ➡ at the site of a visible bruise secondary to seat belt injury.* **(Right)** *CT scout view of a patient who sustained severe blunt left chest trauma shows displaced comminuted segmental ➡ fractures of the left 2nd-10th ribs and underlying left lung contusions. Such fractures predispose the patient to flail chest physiology.*

(Left) *CECT volume-rendered image of the same patient demonstrates multiple displaced and comminuted left rib fractures. Although this image is not necessary for diagnosis, it may help surgeons visualize the extent of skeletal injury in preparation for intraoperative fixation.* **(Right)** *Axial CECT of a patient who sustained severe left right chest trauma shows an elephant trunk-shaped rib fragment that punctures the right lung with resultant hemopneumothorax, lung laceration, and subcutaneous gas.*

Rib Fracture

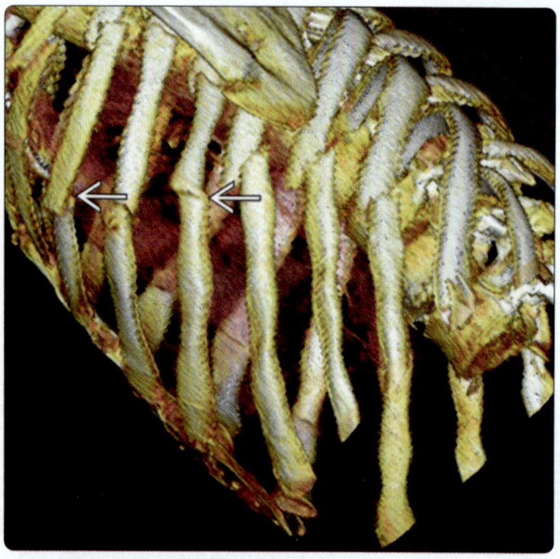

Rib Fracture

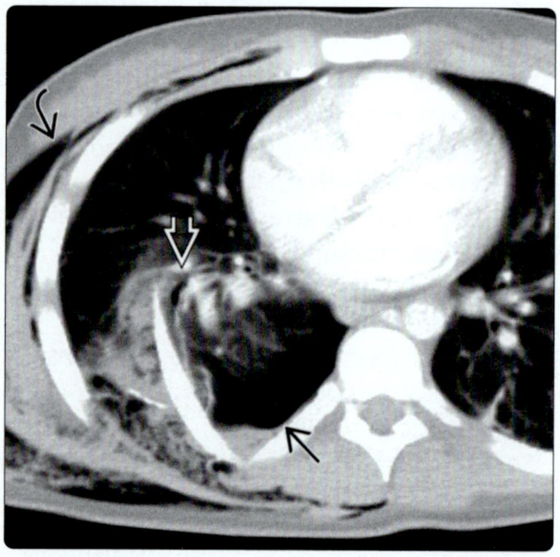

(Left) *AP chest radiograph of a patient who sustained blunt chest trauma shows a right pleural line and absence of peripheral markings consistent with right pneumothorax and a right chest tube in place. Ipsilateral subcutaneous gas should prompt the radiologist to look for pneumothorax.* **(Right)** *AP chest radiograph of a 19-year-old man who sustained blunt chest trauma and presented with a clinical tension pneumothorax shows a large right pneumothorax, complete right lung atelectasis, and shift of the mediastinum to the left.*

Pneumothorax

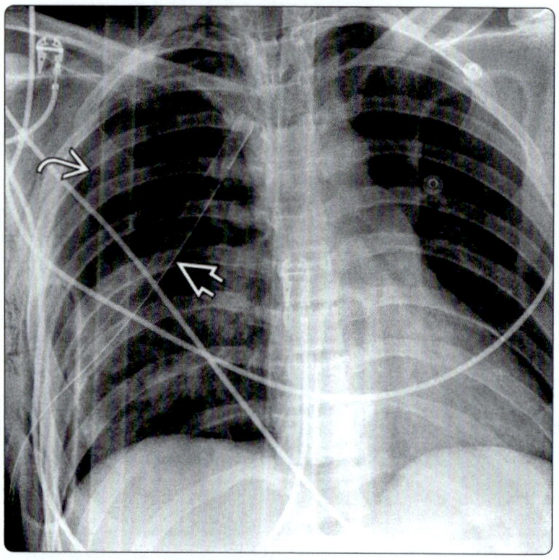

Pneumothorax

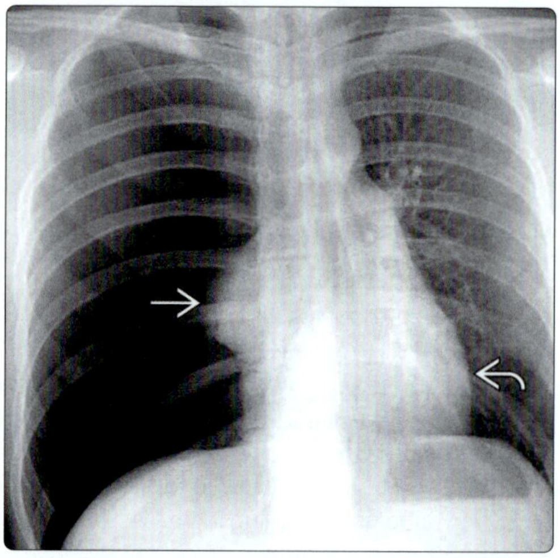

(Left) *Axial NECT of a patient who sustained blunt chest trauma shows heterogeneous, hyperattenuating right pleural fluid consistent with a hemothorax. Blood products in various stages of coagulation may produce a heterogeneous pleural fluid attenuation.* **(Right)** *Axial CECT of a patient with trauma and left rib fractures (not shown) shows a free left hemothorax and a left loculated subpleural hemothorax. The latter likely relates to disruption of intercostal vessels and may continue to grow if there is active bleeding.*

Hemothorax

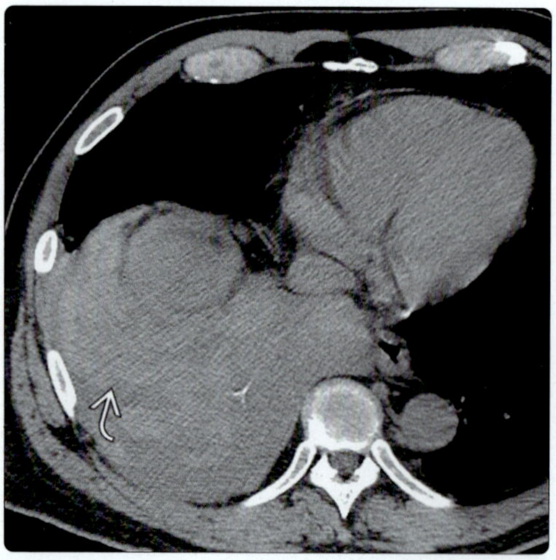

Hemothorax

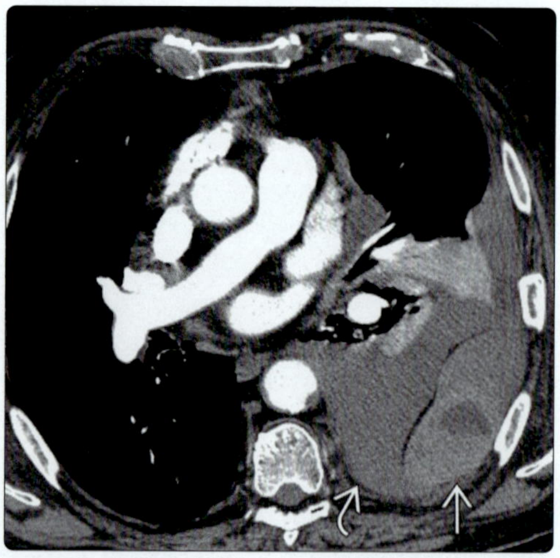

Pulmonary Contusion

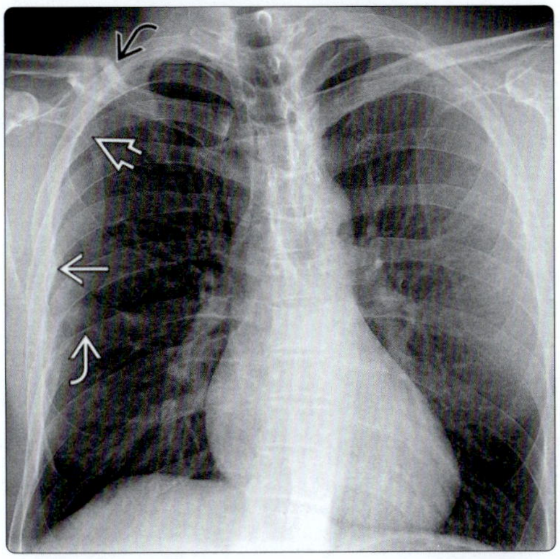

Pulmonary Contusion

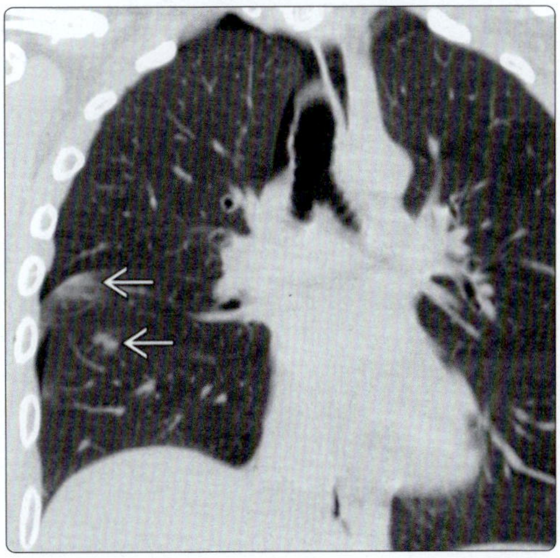

(Left) *AP chest radiograph of a 51-year-old man who sustained blunt chest trauma shows a comminuted right clavicle fracture, right rib fractures, a small right pneumothorax, and an ill-defined right mid lung zone opacity concerning for a pulmonary contusion.* **(Right)** *Coronal NECT of the same patient shows the right pneumothorax and several pulmonary contusions in the middle and right lower lobes, which manifest as multifocal ground-glass opacities.*

Aspiration

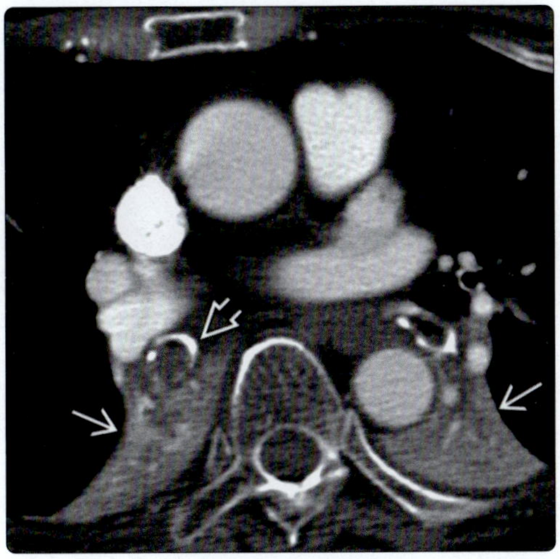

Pulmonary Laceration

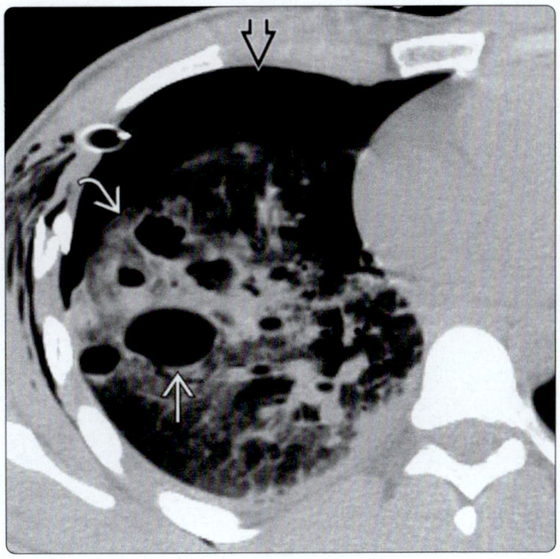

(Left) *Axial CECT of a trauma patient with large volume aspiration shows fluid-filled lower lobe bronchi and bilateral lower lobe consolidations. Aspiration may mimic pulmonary contusion.* **(Right)** *Axial NECT of a patient who sustained multiple displaced comminuted right rib fractures shows multifocal right lung "cystic" lesions that represent pulmonary lacerations and a moderate right pneumothorax. Surrounding ground-glass opacities represent pulmonary contusions.*

Sternal Fracture

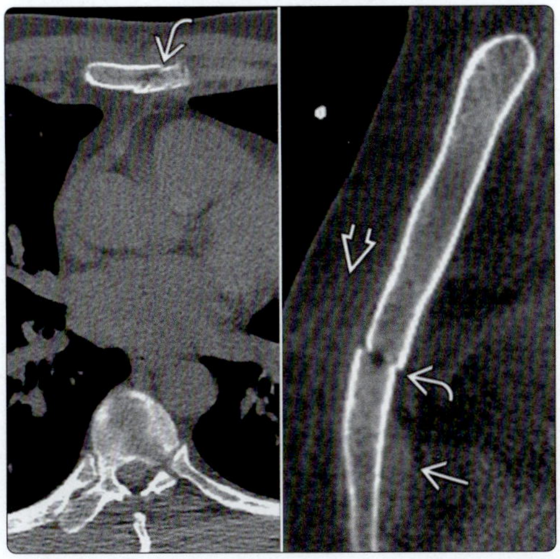

Sternal Fracture

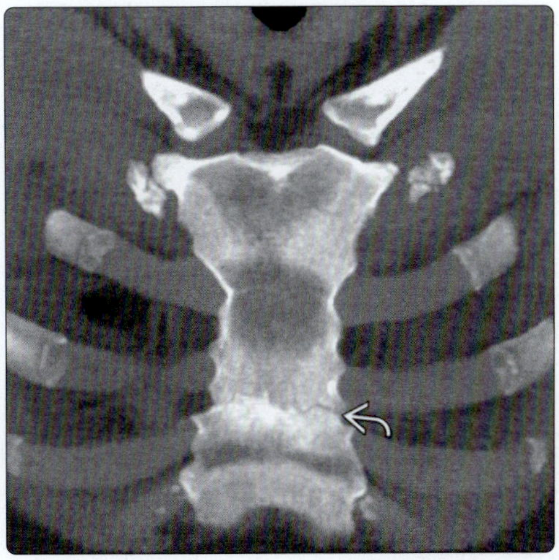

(Left) *Composite image with axial (left) and sagittal (right) NECT of a 35-year-old man who sustained blunt chest trauma shows a comminuted mildly displaced mid sternal body fracture and associated presternal and retrosternal hematomas.* **(Right)** *Coronal NECT (MIP reformatted image) of the same patient shows the mid sternal body fracture manifesting as a jagged horizontal sternal lucency. Coronal MIP reformations may allow detection of subtle sternal fractures.*

(Left) *Coronal CECT of a 53-year-old man who sustained a fall from height shows a comminuted compression fracture of T4 with surrounding mediastinal hematoma.* **(Right)** *Sagittal CECT of the same patient shows the T4 fracture and retropulsion of the fracture fragments as well as a subtle fracture of the T3 superior end plate. Note associated comminuted fracture of the upper sternal body with adjacent presternal and retrosternal hematoma. Trauma victims may have injuries of multiple sites.*

Vertebral Fracture

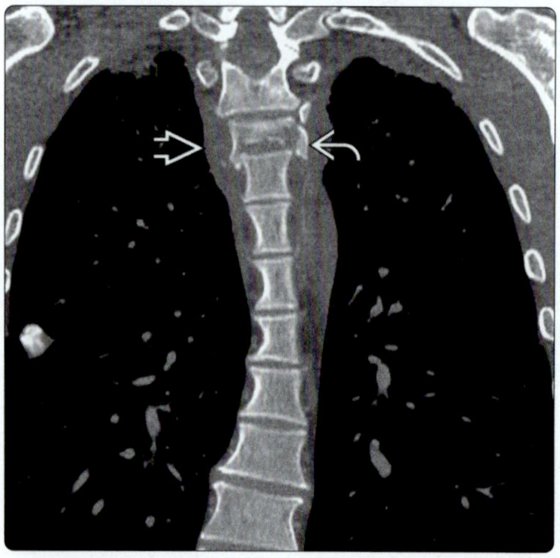

Vertebral Fracture

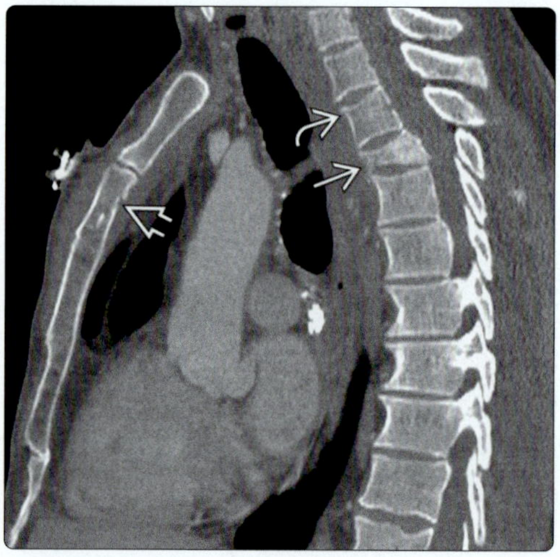

(Left) *AP chest radiograph of a patient who sustained blunt chest trauma during a motor vehicle collision shows a wide featureless superior mediastinum, which is highly concerning for traumatic vascular injury confirmed at CT aortography. Note large right pneumothorax and right rib fractures.* **(Right)** *Composite image with coronal (left) and sagittal (right) CECT of a patient who sustained blunt chest trauma shows traumatic aortic rupture with pseudoaneurysm formation and pneumomediastinum.*

Traumatic Aortic Injury

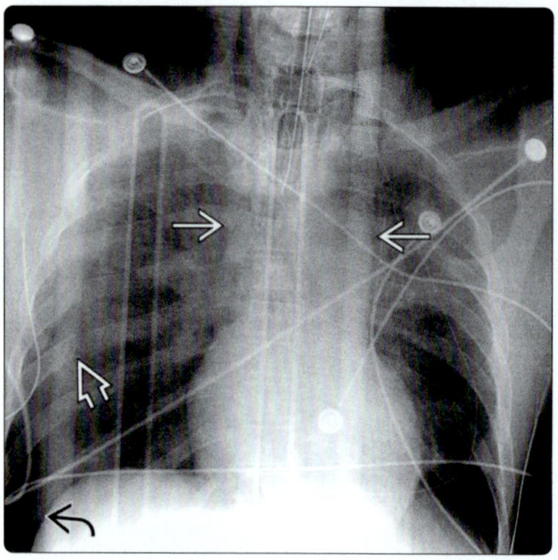

Traumatic Aortic Injury

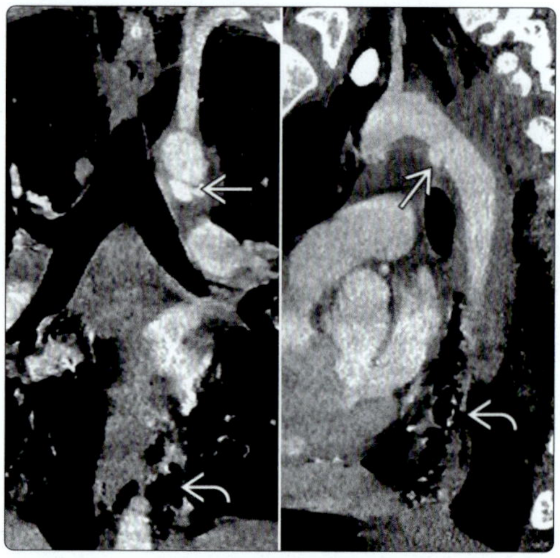

(Left) *Axial CECT of a patient who sustained severe blunt chest trauma and demonstrated a wide superior mediastinum on radiography (not shown) demonstrates diffuse periaortic mediastinal hemorrhage and disruption of the aortic contour consistent with traumatic aortic injury.* **(Right)** *CECT 3D surface-rendered display of the thoracic aorta demonstrates the complex aortic pseudoaneurysm located at the aortic isthmus, the most common site of traumatic aortic injury.*

Traumatic Aortic Injury

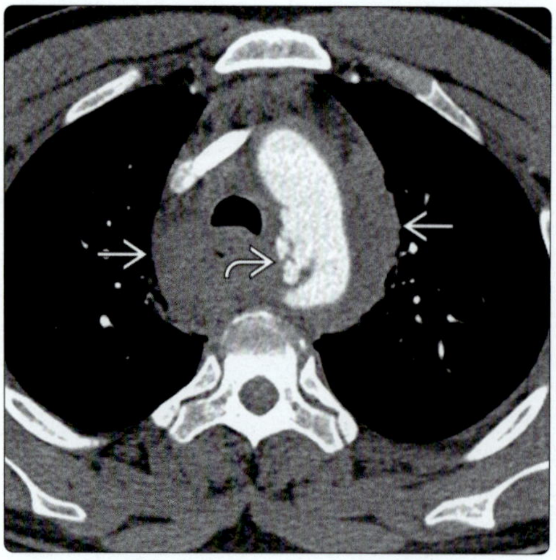

Traumatic Aortic Injury

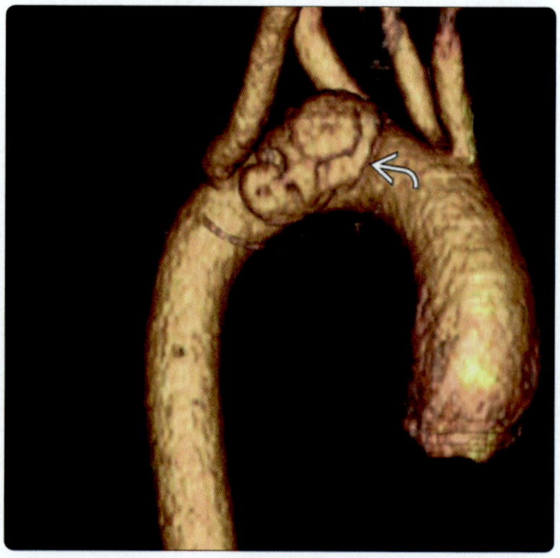

Diaphragmatic Rupture

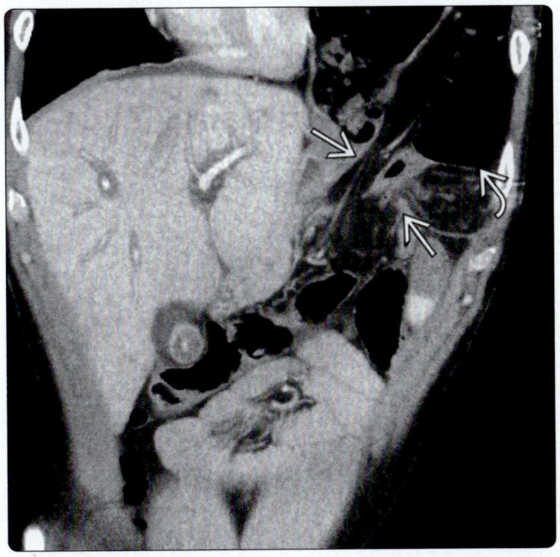

Pneumomediastinum

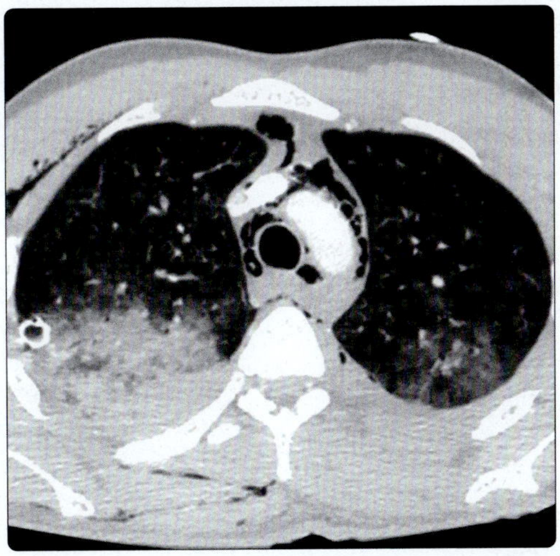

(Left) *Coronal oblique CECT of a 39-year-old man with blunt trauma to the chest and abdomen during a motor vehicle collision shows traumatic diaphragmatic rupture with herniation of mesenteric fat and colon into the thorax. The herniated contents are constricted at the level of the diaphragmatic tear, the so-called collar sign.* **(Right)** *Axial CECT of a 22-year-old man who sustained severe blunt chest trauma shows traumatic pneumomediastinum, for which airway and esophageal injuries should be excluded.*

Cardiac/Pericardial Injury

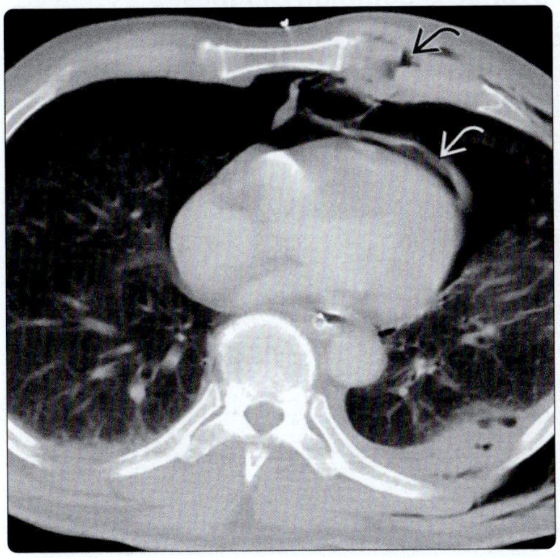

Tracheobronchial injury

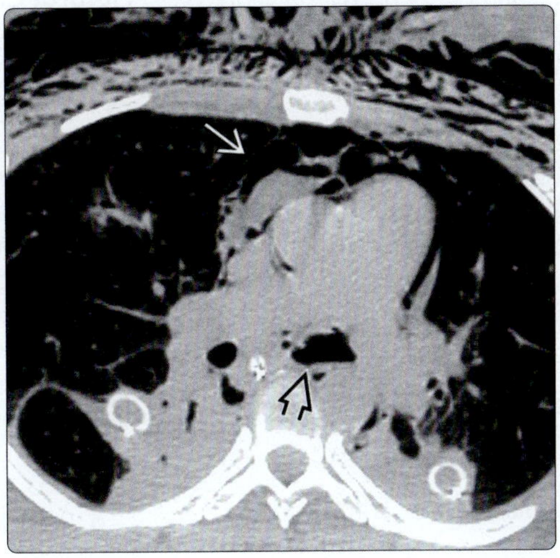

(Left) *Axial CECT of a patient who sustained severe blunt chest trauma shows bilateral hemopneumothoraces, pneumomediastinum, pneumopericardium, and a comminuted left anterior costal cartilage fracture.* **(Right)** *Axial NECT of a patient who sustained severe blunt chest trauma shows extensive pneumomediastinum, subcutaneous gas, and an asymmetric distorted left mainstem bronchus consistent with large airway injury, a rare but life-threatening traumatic thoracic injury.*

Sternoclavicular Dislocation

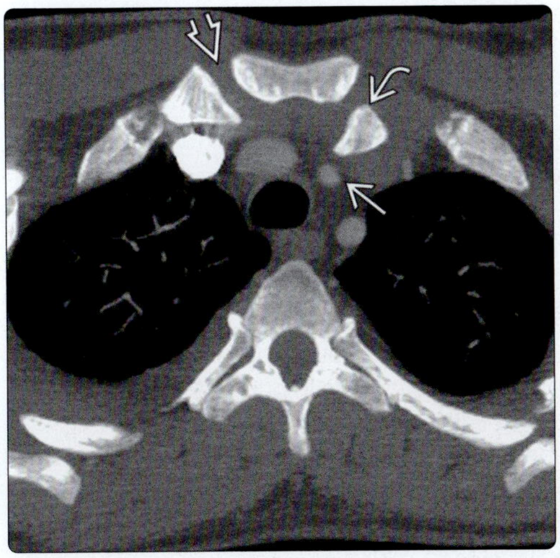

Esophageal Rupture

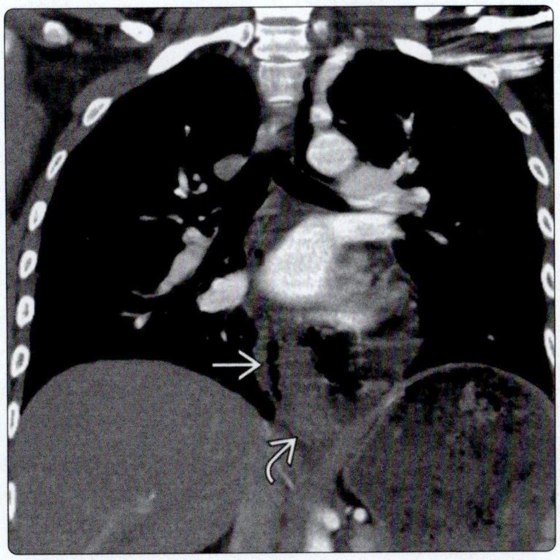

(Left) *Axial CECT (MIP reformation) of a young man who sustained blunt anterior chest wall trauma shows a left posterior sternoclavicular dislocation, which compressed the left common carotid artery. Note the normal right sternoclavicular joint.* **(Right)** *Coronal CECT of a 31-year-old woman involved in a motor vehicle collision shows pneumomediastinum centered about the lower esophagus. Esophageal rupture was confirmed on esophagram (not shown).*

DIFFERENTIAL DIAGNOSIS

Common

- Pneumonia
- Chronic Obstructive Pulmonary Disease
- Heart Failure
- Asthma

Less Common

- Pulmonary Malignancy
- Mycobacterial Infection
- Sarcoidosis
- Bronchiectasis
- Pulmonary Thromboembolism
- Interstitial Lung Disease
- Airway Foreign Body
- Pneumothorax

ESSENTIAL INFORMATION

Key Differential Diagnosis Issues

- Cough is responsible for large number of outpatient visits
- Acute cough: < 3 weeks duration
  - Typically secondary to acute infection
- Subacute cough: 3-8 weeks duration
  - Typically postinfectious etiology
- Chronic cough: > 8 weeks duration
  - Common etiologies: COPD, upper airway cough syndrome (postnasal drip), gastroesophageal reflux disease

Helpful Clues for Common Diagnoses

- **Pneumonia**
  - Causative organisms: Bacteria, viruses, fungi
  - Acute cough, fever, leukocytosis
  - Imaging
    - Consolidation, centrilobular nodules, tree-in-bud opacities
      - Lobar, segmental, subsegmental, multifocal
    - ± pleural effusion
- **Chronic Obstructive Pulmonary Disease (COPD)**
  - Airflow limitation with chronic symptoms due to airway/alveolar abnormalities caused by noxious substance exposure
    - Affects > 5% of population, 4th most common cause of death in USA
    - Cigarette smoking is most common risk factor
  - Chronic cough, dyspnea, sputum production
  - Subtypes
    - Emphysema
      - Centrilobular: Lucencies with imperceptible borders and central "dot" representing lobular artery
      - Paraseptal: Single row of subpleural cysts with intervening interlobular septa
      - Panlobular: Hyperlucent lung with paucity of vascular markings; α-1-antitrypsin deficiency
    - Chronic bronchitis: Bronchial wall thickening
    - Chronic obstructive asthma
- **Heart Failure**
  - Extravascular lung water; typically worsening chronic heart failure
  - Acute air hunger, anxiety, cough productive of pink frothy sputum in severe pulmonary edema
  - Imaging
    - Perihilar opacities, peribronchial thickening, interlobular septal thickening, subpleural edema
    - Alveolar edema: Ground-glass opacities, consolidation
    - Cardiomegaly, wide vascular pedicle, pleural effusion
- **Asthma**
  - Reversible airway obstruction, airway inflammation, airway hyperreactivity
  - Sporadic chronic cough in adults and children, ± wheezing and dyspnea
  - Imaging
    - Hyperinflation
    - Bronchial wall thickening, mosaic attenuation, expiratory air-trapping
    - Complications: Atelectasis, pneumomediastinum, pneumothorax, pneumonia

Helpful Clues for Less Common Diagnoses

- **Pulmonary Malignancy**
  - Chronic cough (up to 75% of patients) ± hemoptysis, chest pain, dyspnea; may clinically mimic pneumonia
    - Cough typically relates to central lung cancers: Squamous cell carcinoma, small cell carcinoma
    - Invasive mucinous adenocarcinomas may produce bronchorrhea
  - Lung cancer
    - Leading cause of death in men and women in USA
    - Associations: Cigarette smoking, carcinogens (e.g., asbestos), interstitial fibrosis
    - Imaging
      - Lung nodule, mass, consolidation, atelectasis
      - Lymphadenopathy
  - Bronchial carcinoid
    - Central airway involvement: Postobstructive atelectasis, pneumonia, bronchiectasis
    - ± calcification, contrast enhancement
  - Metastatic disease
    - Angiocentric basilar predominant nodules, masses
    - Lymphangitic carcinomatosis: Smooth or nodular interlobular septal thickening
    - Mediastinal/hilar lymphadenopathy
- **Mycobacterial Infection**
  - Chronic cough ± hemoptysis, dyspnea, fever
  - *Mycobacterium tuberculosis* (postprimary pattern)
    - Upper lobe apical segments, lower lobe superior segments
    - Nodule(s), mass(es), consolidation(s) ± cavitation
    - Centrilobular nodules, tree-in-bud opacities
    - Cavitation + cellular bronchiolitis should raise suspicion for active tuberculosis
  - Nontuberculous mycobacterial infection
    - Bronchiectatic pattern
      - Female, elderly, white, nonsmoker
      - Imaging: Middle lobe and lingular volume loss, bronchiectasis, cellular bronchiolitis
    - Classic pattern
      - Older, white, male, chronic lung disease

        - Imaging: Upper lobe thin-walled cavity(ies), cellular bronchiolitis
- **Sarcoidosis**
    - Young adults, peak age of 20-29 years; 2nd peak at 50 years
    - Chronic dry cough, dyspnea, chest pain
    - Constitutional symptoms, lymphadenopathy, eye/skin lesions
    - Imaging
        - Lymphadenopathy: Bilateral hilar, right paratracheal, AP window, subcarinal
        - Perilymphatic micronodules, nodules, masses, ground-glass opacities
        - Peribronchovascular mass-like fibrosis, cystic changes
- **Bronchiectasis**
    - Chronic cough, frequent recurrent infection
    - Numerous etiologies
        - Fungal hypersensitivity
        - Mucociliary clearance disorders: Cystic fibrosis, primary ciliary dyskinesia
        - Structural airway abnormalities
        - Systemic disease: Inflammatory bowel disease, autoimmunity
        - Primary and secondary immunodeficiencies
    - Imaging
        - Radiography: Tram-track opacities
        - CT: Abnormal bronchoarterial ratio
            - Cylindrical, varicose, cystic/saccular
            - Bronchial wall thickening, endoluminal content, ± cellular or constrictive bronchiolitis
- **Pulmonary Thromboembolism**
    - Dyspnea, pleuritic chest pain, cough, deep venous thrombosis
        - Cough is not dominant symptom
    - Imaging
        - CT pulmonary angiography
            - Pulmonary artery filling defect: Surrounded by contrast, arterial occlusion, enlarged vessel caliber
            - Pulmonary hypertension: Pulmonary trunk diameter > 29 mm
            - Right heart strain: Right ventricle:left ventricle diameter ≥ 1, flat or leftward bowed interventricular septum, reflux of contrast into inferior vena cava and hepatic veins
        - Ventilation-perfusion scintigraphy
            - ≥ 2 unmatched segmental perfusion defects
- **Interstitial Lung Disease**
    - Progressive dyspnea, chronic nonproductive cough
    - Chronic fibrotic interstitial pneumonias
        - Usual interstitial pneumonia (UIP), nonspecific interstitial pneumonia
        - Imaging
            - Basilar and subpleural fibrosis with honeycombing
            - Honeycombing is distinguishing feature of UIP
- **Airway Foreign Body**
    - Choking event followed by acute cough and dyspnea
    - Imaging
        - Most foreign bodies are radiolucent (organic)
        - Predilection for right tracheobronchial tree
        - Pulmonary hyperlucency on expiratory imaging
        - Postobstructive pneumonia, atelectasis
- **Pneumothorax**
    - Acute dyspnea and pleuritic chest pain ± cough
    - Primary spontaneous: Young, tall, thin male smokers
    - Secondary spontaneous: Underlying emphysema and cystic, cavitary, or diffuse infiltrative lung disease
    - Traumatic or iatrogenic
    - Imaging
        - Visible pleural line, no peripheral lung markings
        - Assessment of lung parenchyma
            - Bullae, blebs, emphysema
            - Interstitial lung disease, cavitary disease

Other Essential Information

- Numerous other etiologies of cough
    - Pneumoconiosis
    - Hypersensitivity pneumonitis
    - Lipoid pneumonia
    - E-cigarette or vaping product use-associated lung injury (EVALI)

Pneumonia

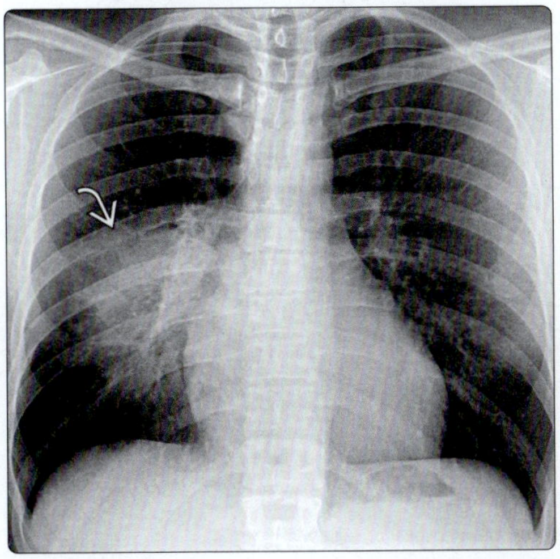

Pneumonia

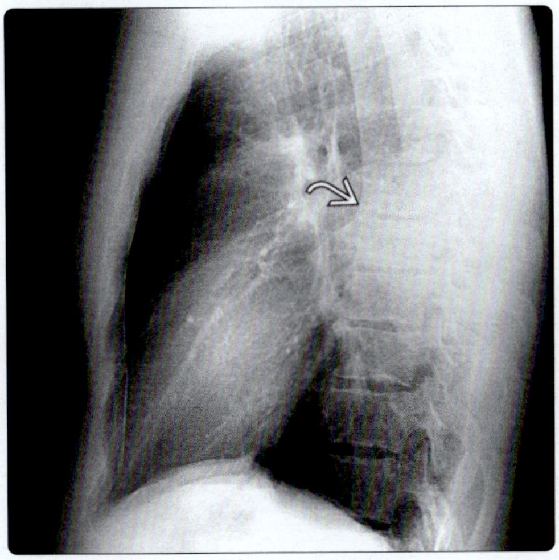

(Left) *PA chest radiograph of a 23-year-old man who presented acutely with cough, fever, and leukocytosis shows a mass-like consolidation* ➔ *in the right lower lobe consistent with pneumonia.* **(Right)** *Lateral chest radiograph of the same patient confirms that the consolidation* ➔ *is in the right lower lobe, specifically in the superior segment. Infections of the upper respiratory tract, airways, and lungs are common etiologies of acute cough. Pneumonia may be lobar, segmental (as in this case), or subsegmental.*

(Left) *Axial CECT of a 35-year-old woman who presented with cough, low-grade fever, and malaise shows middle lobe nodular consolidations* ⇨ *and scattered centrilobular nodules* ➔ *consistent with multifocal pneumonia. Note mosaic attenuation of the lung parenchyma.* **(Right)** *Axial CECT of the same patient shows bilateral lower lobe band-like opacities* ➔*, clustered centrilobular nodules, and tree-in-bud opacities* ⇨*. Mycoplasma pneumoniae was confirmed on sputum polymerase chain reaction (PCR).*

Pneumonia

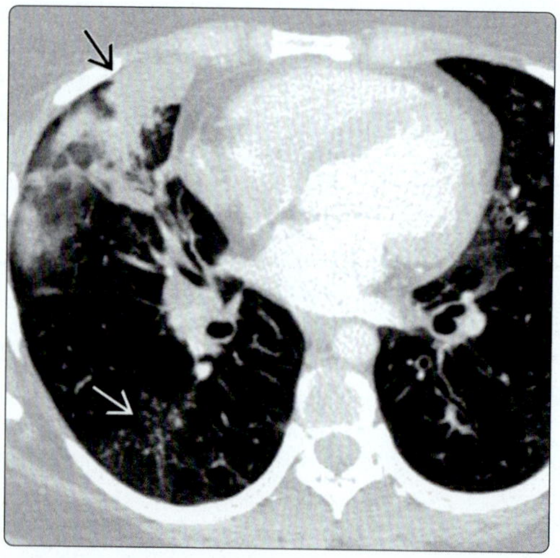

Pneumonia

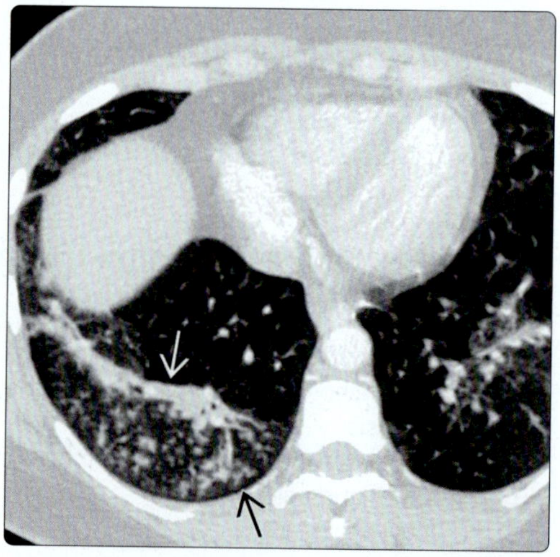

(Left) *Axial NECT of a 72-year-old life-long smoker shows centrilobular emphysema manifesting as centrilobular lucencies with imperceptible borders. Note the central "dot"* ➔*, which corresponds to the central lobular artery.* **(Right)** *Axial NECT of a 74-year-old woman with chronic productive cough and dyspnea shows diffuse bronchial wall thickening* ➔ *consistent with chronic bronchitis. COPD is defined as persistent airflow limitation and may manifest with emphysema, chronic bronchitis, or chronic asthma.*

Chronic Obstructive Pulmonary Disease

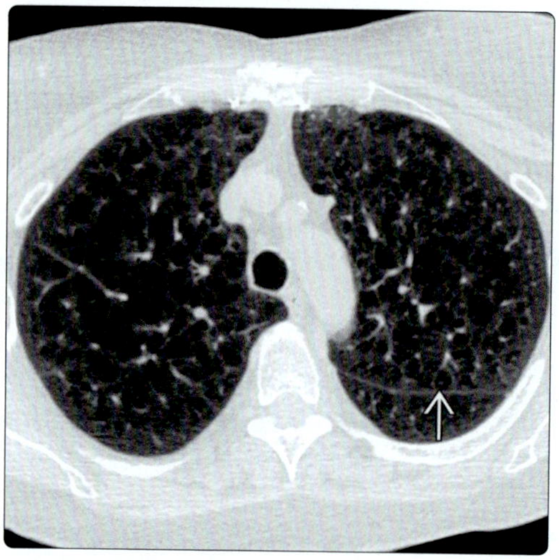

Chronic Obstructive Pulmonary Disease

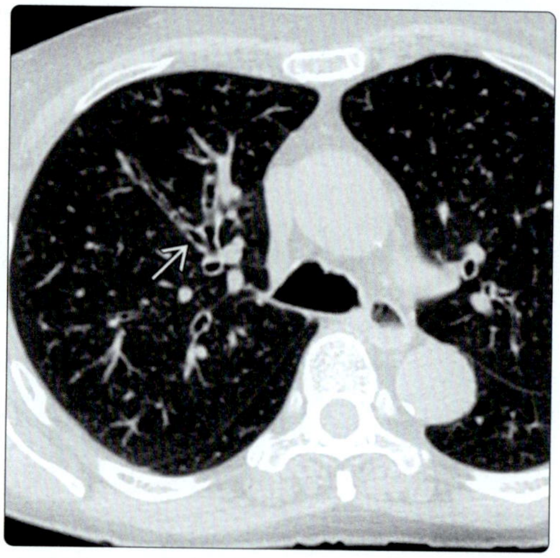

(Left) *AP chest radiograph of a 62-year-old man with acute dyspnea and cough shows asymmetric right lung predominant interlobular septal thickening* ➔ *and peribronchial cuffing* ↪ *consistent with interstitial edema.* **(Right)** *Axial NECT of a 72-year-old man with acute dyspnea and cough productive of a frothy pink sputum shows bilateral perihilar consolidations consistent with the batwing pattern of alveolar pulmonary edema. Cough is common in patients with acute decompensated heart failure.*

Heart Failure

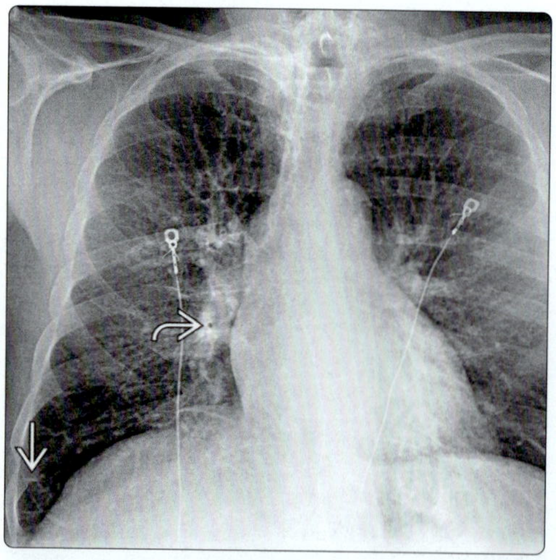

Heart Failure

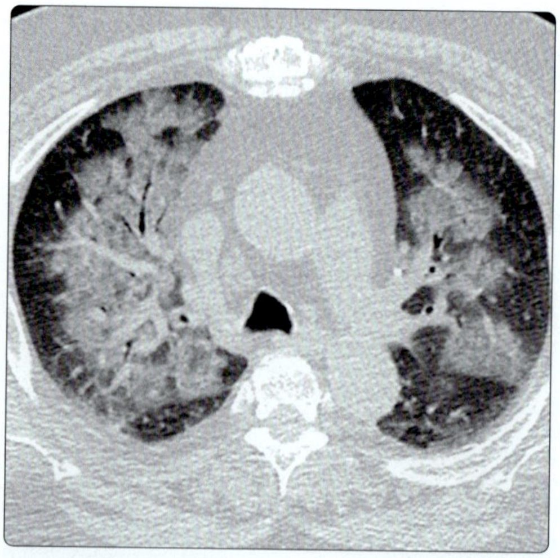

Asthma

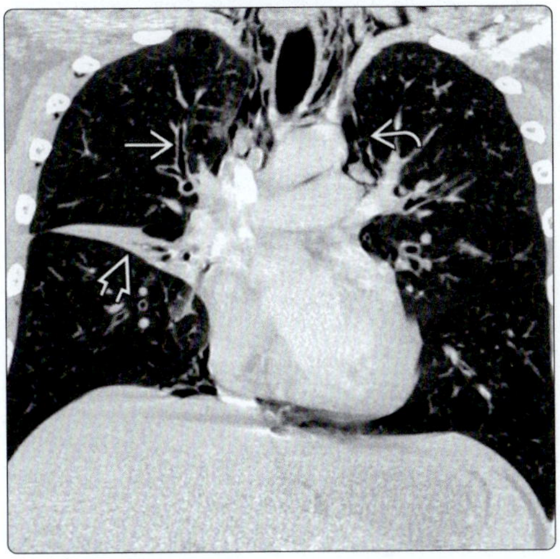

Asthma

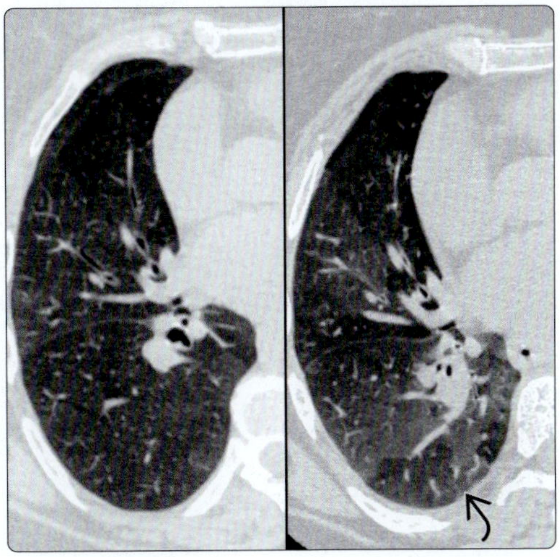

(Left) *Coronal CECT of a 23-year-old asthmatic man who presented with acute wheezing, dyspnea, cough, and chest pain shows bronchial wall thickening →, middle lobe atelectasis →, and pneumomediastinum →. Atelectasis and pneumomediastinum are known complications of asthma.* **(Right)** *Composite image with inspiratory NECT (left) and expiratory HRCT (right) of a 58-year-old woman with asthma shows mosaic lung attenuation and expiratory air-trapping →.*

Pulmonary Malignancy

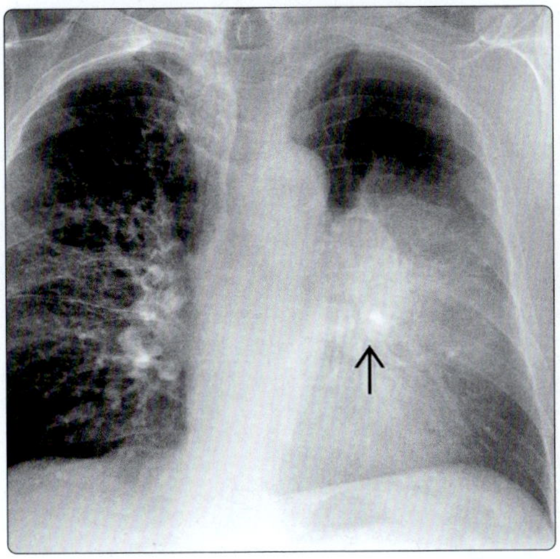

Pulmonary Malignancy

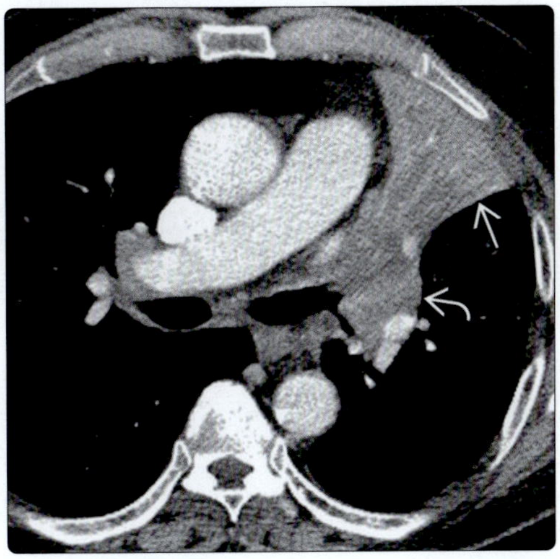

(Left) *PA chest radiograph of a 68-year-old man who presented with chronic cough, dyspnea on exertion, and chest pain shows left upper lobe atelectasis secondary to a centrally obstructing mass →.* **(Right)** *Axial CECT of the same patient confirms complete left upper lobe atelectasis → secondary to a central mass → with an endobronchial component. Biopsy confirmed squamous cell carcinoma. Patients with central lung cancers frequently present with cough.*

Pulmonary Malignancy

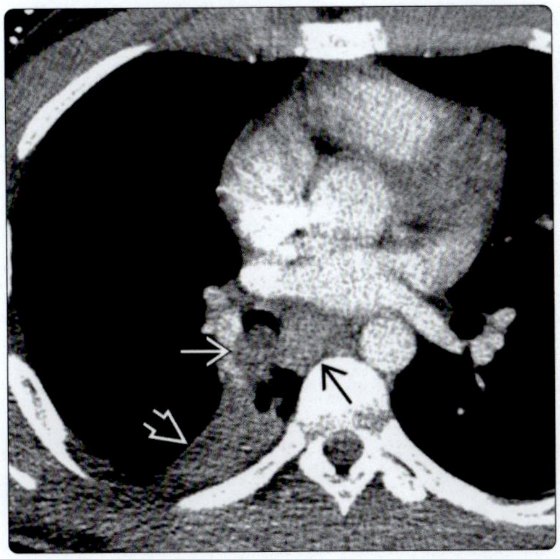

Pulmonary Malignancy

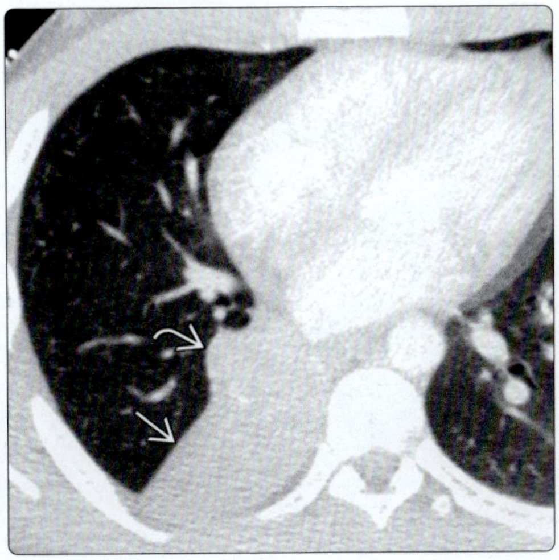

(Left) *Axial CECT of a 20-year-old woman with cough and hemoptysis shows right lower lobe atelectasis → due to a central mass → with an endoluminal component that partially obstructs the right lower lobe bronchus. Note adjacent mediastinal lymphadenopathy →.* **(Right)** *Axial CECT of the same patient shows right lower lobe atelectasis → and a central convexity → that corresponds to the extraluminal portion of the mass. Carcinoid tumor was confirmed at surgery. Patients with central lung malignancies may present with cough.*

(Left) *PA chest radiograph of an 83-year-old woman with chronic cough shows multifocal bilateral small pulmonary nodules and obscuration of the right heart border secondary to middle lobe airspace disease.* **(Right)** *Axial NECT of the same patient shows classic findings of nontuberculous mycobacterial infection, including middle lobe and lingular bronchiectasis, bilateral clustered centrilobular nodules, and tree-in-bud opacities.*

Mycobacterial Infection

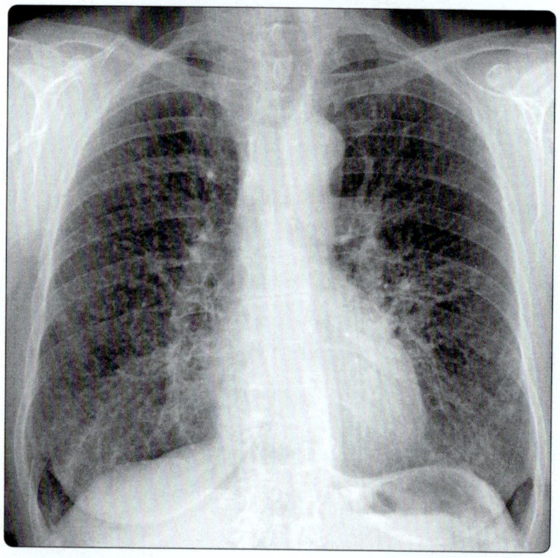

Mycobacterial Infection

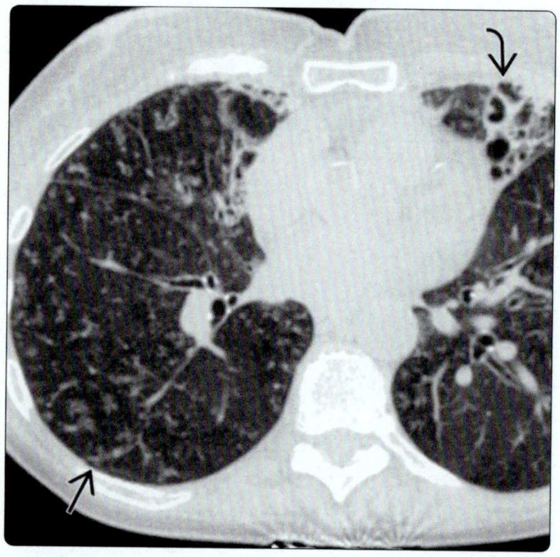

(Left) *PA chest radiograph of a 36-year-old woman who presented with dry cough and mild dyspnea shows bilateral hilar and right paratracheal lymphadenopathy secondary to pulmonary sarcoidosis.* **(Right)** *Coronal CECT of the same patient shows relatively symmetric mediastinal and bilateral hilar lymphadenopathy. Note subtle right upper lobe nodular bronchial wall thickening. Sarcoidosis is a diagnosis of exclusion.*

Sarcoidosis

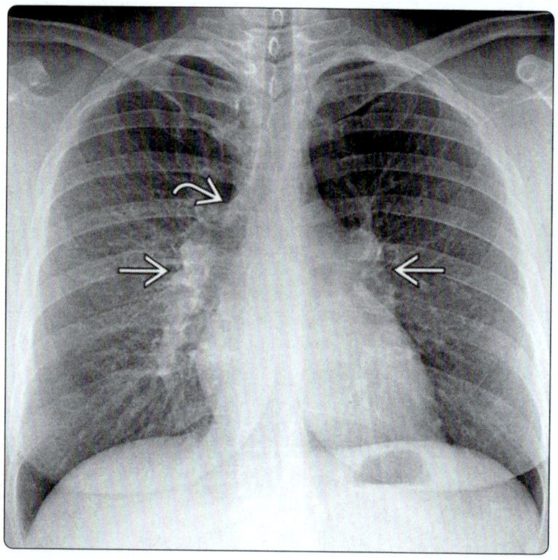

Sarcoidosis

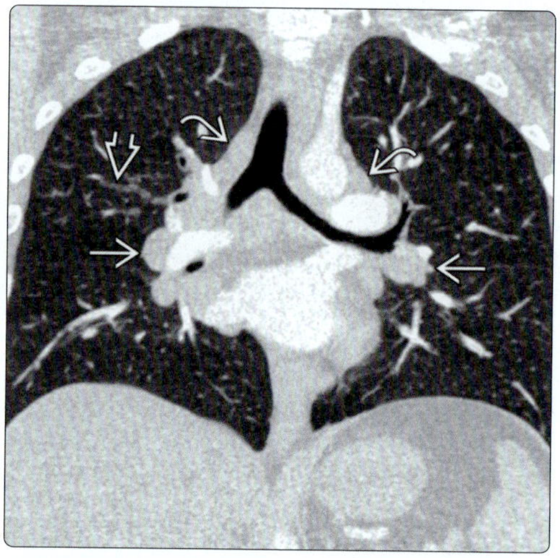

(Left) *Axial CECT of a 72-year-old man with primary ciliary dyskinesia, chronic cough, and recurrent infections shows basilar predominant bronchiectasis, bronchial wall thickening, and scattered tree-in-bud opacities.* **(Right)** *Axial CECT of a 59-year-old woman with deep venous thrombosis who presented with acute dyspnea, chest pain, and cough shows large burden bilateral central pulmonary thromboemboli and trace bilateral pleural fluid. There were also right basilar pulmonary infarcts (not shown).*

Bronchiectasis

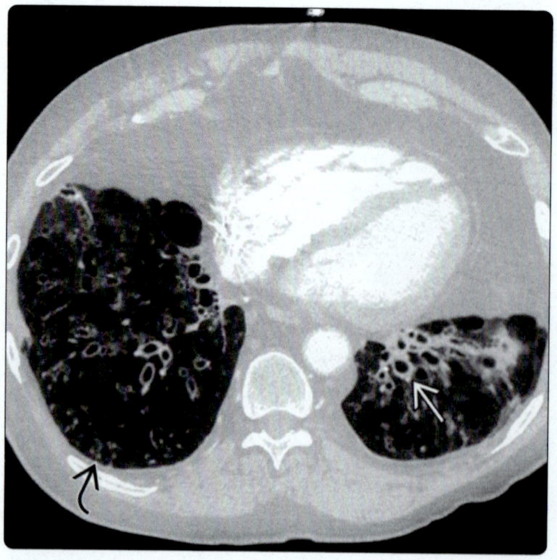

Pulmonary Thromboembolism

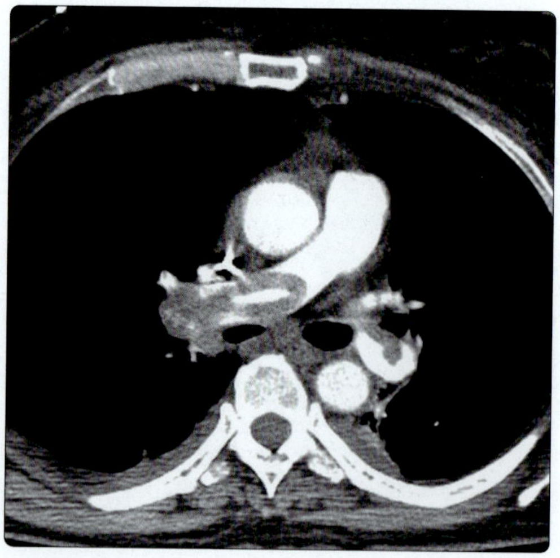

Interstitial Lung Disease

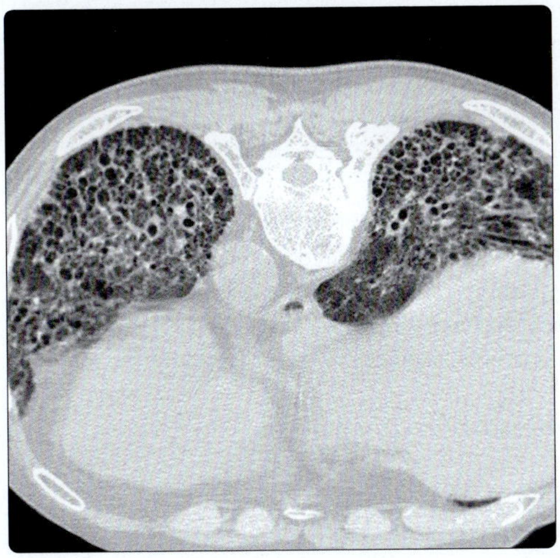

Interstitial Lung Disease

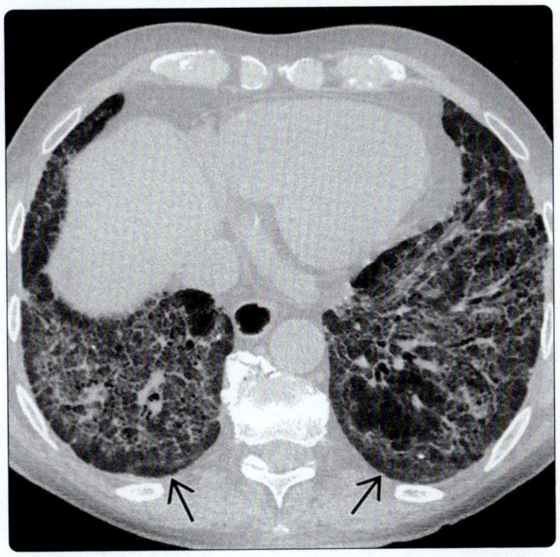

(Left) *Axial prone HRCT of a 71-year-old man with chronic progressive dyspnea and dry cough shows typical CT features of usual interstitial pneumonia, characterized by basilar honeycombing and traction bronchiectasis.* **(Right)** *Axial HRCT of a 73-year-old man with scleroderma, chronic cough, and dyspnea shows basilar predominant fibrosing interstitial lung disease with subpleural sparing ⇨, a well-described feature of nonspecific interstitial pneumonia.*

Airway Foreign Body

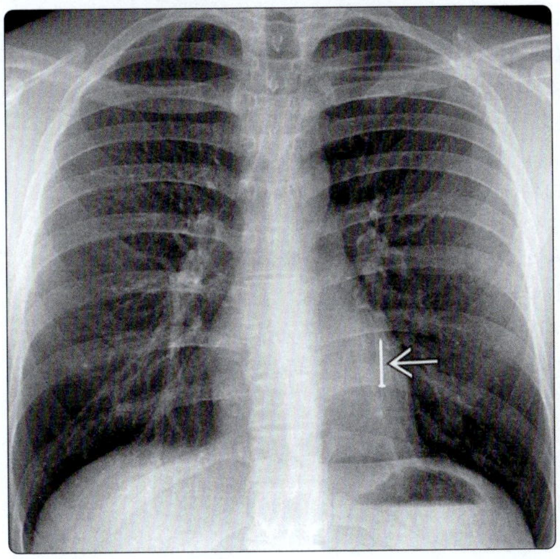

Airway Foreign Body

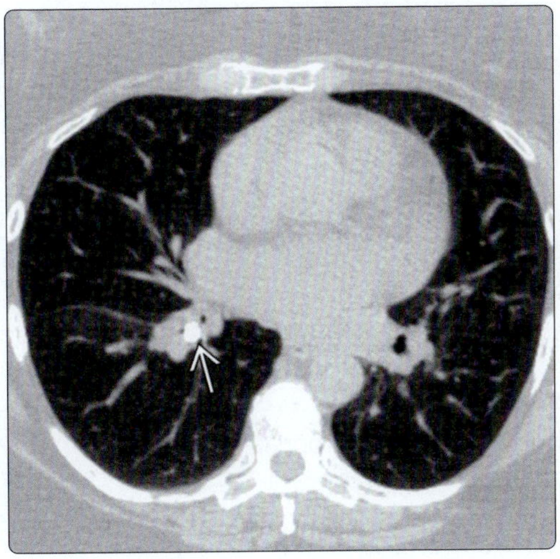

(Left) *PA chest radiograph of an 18-year-old man who experienced choking followed by cough after aspirating a nail shows the aspirated foreign body ➡ lodged in a branch of the left lower lobe bronchus. Metallic foreign bodies are easily identified on radiography.* **(Right)** *Axial NECT of a 62-year-old woman who developed cough after aspirating a pill shows the radiopaque foreign body ➡ in the distal right lower lobe truncus basalis and mild hyperlucency of the peripheral lung. The pill was not radiopaque on radiography.*

Pneumothorax

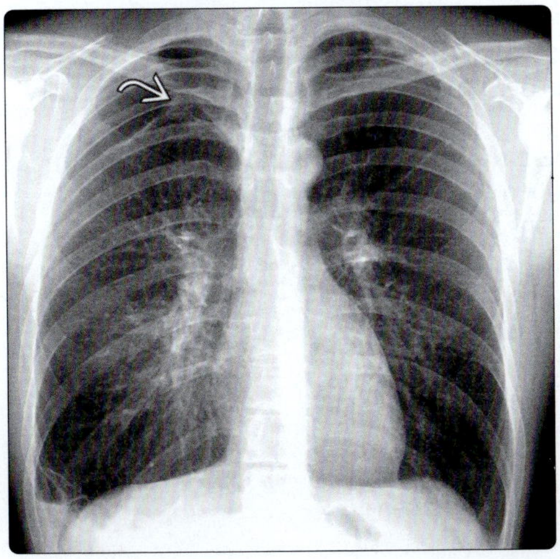

Pneumothorax

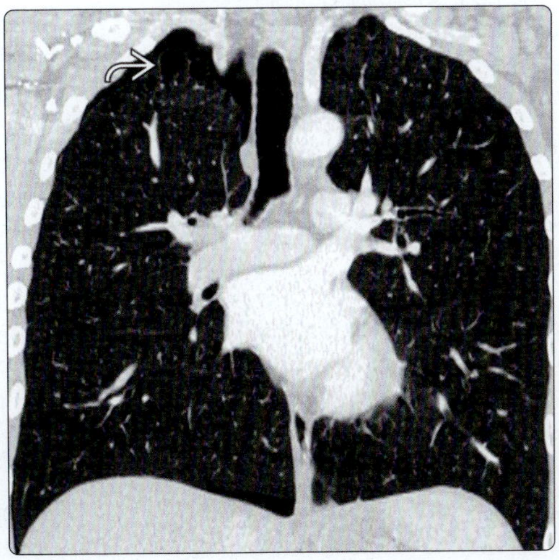

(Left) *PA chest radiograph of a 26-year-old man who presented with acute right chest pain, dyspnea, and cough shows a spontaneous right hydropneumothorax and apical bullae or blebs ↪, characteristic of primary spontaneous pneumothorax.* **(Right)** *Coronal CECT of the same patient shows the right pneumothorax and right > left apical bullae or blebs ↪. Patients with spontaneous pneumothorax often present with acute chest pain and dyspnea. Cough may also be present but is not common.*

DIFFERENTIAL DIAGNOSIS

Common

- Heart Failure
- Pneumonia
- Chronic Obstructive Pulmonary Disease
- Pulmonary Embolism
- Asthma

Less Common

- Airway Foreign Body
- Angioedema
- Infections of Pharynx and Neck
- Airway Trauma
- Spontaneous Pneumothorax
- Pneumomediastinum
- Acute Respiratory Distress Syndrome
- Pleural Effusion
- Diffuse Alveolar Hemorrhage
- Acute Coronary Syndrome
- Cardiomyopathy
- Cardiac Arrhythmia
- Valvular Dysfunction
- Pericardial Tamponade
- Acute Chest Syndrome
- Pulmonary Contusion/Laceration

Rare but Important

- High-Altitude Pulmonary Edema
- Near Drowning

ESSENTIAL INFORMATION

Key Differential Diagnosis Issues

- Dyspnea: Perception of inability to breathe appropriately
- Acute dyspnea may also result from nonthoracic &/or systemic processes
  - Abdominal processes: Ascites, bowel obstruction, ruptured viscus/peritonitis
  - Obesity, anemia, sepsis
  - Neuromuscular disorder: Multiple sclerosis, Guillain-Barré, myasthenia gravis, amyotrophic lateral sclerosis
  - Metabolic acidosis, diabetic ketoacidosis, poisoning (organophosphates, carbon monoxide, salicylates)

Helpful Clues for Common Diagnoses

- **Heart Failure**
  - May result from numerous etiologies among which coronary artery disease is common
  - Interstitial edema
    - Interlobular septal thickening (i.e., Kerley B lines)
    - Peribronchial and perivascular thickening
  - Alveolar edema
    - Patchy peribronchovascular and acinar opacities
  - Ancillary findings
    - Pleural effusions
    - Cardiomegaly
- **Pneumonia**
  - May result from bacterial, viral, or fungal infections
  - Common community acquired pneumonias: *Streptococcus pneumoniae*, *Staphylococcus aureus*, *Mycoplasma pneumoniae*, *Legionella pneumophila*, viruses
  - Lobar pneumonia
    - Classically seen in *Streptococcus pneumoniae* pulmonary infection
    - Focal segmental or subsegmental consolidations
  - Bronchopneumonia
    - More frequent in children and elderly patients
    - Classically seen in *Staphylococcus aureus*
    - Patchy multifocal peribronchovascular consolidations
- **Chronic Obstructive Pulmonary Disease (COPD)**
  - Comprises emphysema and chronic bronchitis, which often coexist
  - Associated with cigarette smoking
  - Emphysema
    - Radiography: Hyperinflation, attenuated lung markings
    - CT: Emphysema, initially centrilobular ± paraseptal, may progress to panlobular; bullae are common
  - Chronic bronchitis
    - Strictly clinical diagnosis
    - Nonspecific findings (e.g., bronchial wall thickening)
- **Pulmonary Embolism**
  - Often related to embolism from lower extremity deep venous thrombosis
  - Radiography
    - Poor sensitivity
    - Westermark sign: Regional oligemia
    - Fleischner sign: Enlarged central pulmonary artery
    - Hampton hump: Peripheral wedge-shaped consolidation; implies pulmonary infarct
    - Ancillary findings
      - Subsegmental atelectasis
      - Pleural effusion
  - CT angiography
    - Pulmonary arterial filling defects ± luminal expansion of affected vessel
    - Large burden disease may exhibit dilated pulmonary trunk from pulmonary hypertension and right ventricular strain (right ventricle:left ventricle ratio > 1); implies worse prognosis
    - Pulmonary infarct: Peripheral wedge-shaped opacity
- **Asthma**
  - Reversible airway inflammation and obstruction from airway hyperreactivity
  - Radiography
    - Hyperinflation
    - Peribronchial cuffing
    - Complications
      - Pneumothorax
      - Pneumomediastinum
      - Pneumonia
  - CT
    - Bronchial wall thickening
    - Mosaic attenuation
    - Expiratory air-trapping
    - Bronchiectasis

Helpful Clues for Less Common Diagnoses

- **Spontaneous Pneumothorax**
  - Primary: Tall young adults
  - Secondary: Preexistent lung disease (e.g., COPD, asthma, cystic lung disease)
  - Radiography: Visible thin pleural line, deep sulcus sign on supine imaging
  - CT: Identification of underlying structural lesions
- **Pneumomediastinum**
  - Common complication of asthma and drug abuse
  - Mediastinal streak-like lucencies
  - Macklin effect: Air dissecting along bronchovascular bundles and interstitium into mediastinum
- **Acute Respiratory Distress Syndrome (ARDS)**
  - Noncardiogenic pulmonary edema resulting from myriad of inflammatory, infectious, or traumatic conditions
  - Radiography and CT: Heterogeneous opacities involving 4 pulmonary quadrants
- **Pleural Effusion**
  - Obliteration of costophrenic sulci, meniscus sign
  - ± loculation, pleural nodules, nodular thickening
  - Large pleural effusion in elderly individual should always prompt exclusion of malignant pleural effusion
- **Diffuse Alveolar Hemorrhage**
  - May be idiopathic but often associated with autoimmunity (e.g., Goodpasture syndrome, systemic lupus erythematosus, granulomatosis with polyangiitis)
  - Hemoptysis is common but may be absent
  - ↓ hemoglobin and hematocrit
  - Radiography: Diffuse and relatively symmetric opacities
  - CT: Peribronchovascular ground-glass/airspace opacities; may exhibit crazy-paving pattern
- **Pericardial Tamponade**
  - Radiography
    - Enlarged cardiac silhouette
    - Fat pad (Oreo cookie) sign: Retrosternal soft tissue stripe outlined by mediastinal fat anteriorly and by subepicardial fat posteriorly
  - CT
    - Fluid-filled pericardial space
    - Pericardial thickening implies inflammatory or infectious process
    - Flattening of right ventricular wall, bowing of interventricular septum, dilated SVC and IVC, retrograde contrast flow into IVC and hepatic veins
- **Acute Chest Syndrome**
  - Respiratory symptoms + new opacities on chest radiography in patient with sickle cell disease
  - Osseous findings: Avascular necrosis of humeral heads, H-shaped vertebrae, osseous sclerosis
  - Extramedullary hematopoiesis: Paravertebral soft tissue nodules or masses
- **Pulmonary Contusion/Laceration**
  - Occur in setting of thoracic trauma
  - Contusion
    - No anatomic disruption of lung parenchyma
    - Ground-glass or acinar opacities; may transgress fissures
    - Often associated with other stigmata of trauma (e.g., rib fractures, pneumothorax, hemothorax)
    - May coexist with laceration
  - Laceration
    - Anatomic disruption of lung parenchyma
    - Nodules with intrinsic or developing cavitation; may be referred to as traumatic pneumatocele
    - Surrounding ground-glass opacities representing contusions

Helpful Clues for Rare Diagnoses

- **High-Altitude Pulmonary Edema**
  - History of significant change in altitude
  - Radiography: Asymmetric heterogenous opacities bilaterally
  - CT: Peribronchovascular and acinar opacities distributed asymmetrically throughout both lungs
- **Near Drowning**
  - History is ultimately required for diagnosis
  - Imaging: Patchy opacities bilaterally

Heart Failure

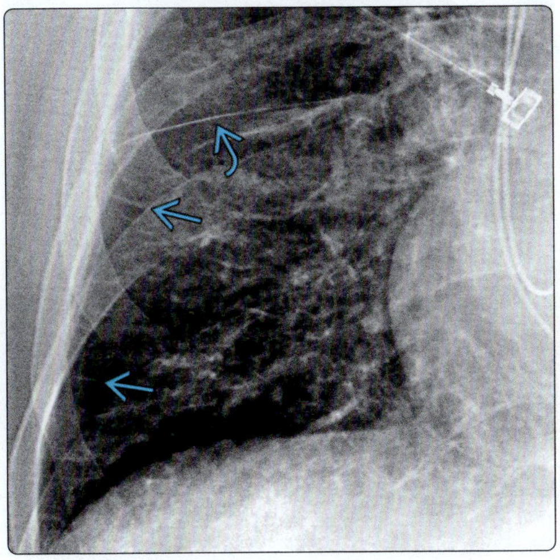

Heart Failure

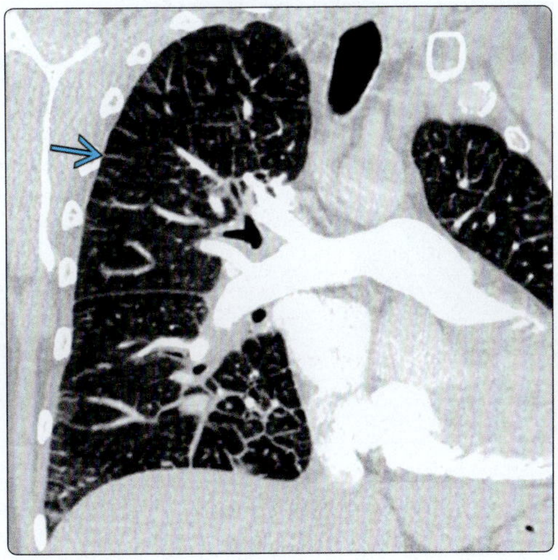

(Left) *PA chest radiograph of a patient with interstitial pulmonary edema shows right perihilar haze and interlobular septal thickening that manifests as Kerley B lines →. Note subpleural edema, which manifests as thickening of the minor fissure ↗.* **(Right)** *Coronal CECT of a patient with interstitial edema shows extensive interlobular septal thickening → bilaterally. This finding is typical of interstitial pulmonary edema, but can also be seen in lymphangitic carcinomatosis and other conditions.*

(Left) *AP chest radiograph of a patient with alveolar pulmonary edema shows extensive, symmetric, peribronchovascular consolidations. When there is sparing of the peripheral subpleural lung, as in this case, this appearance is often referred to as the "bat-wing" pattern of alveolar edema. As edema progresses from interstitial to alveolar, opacities become more confluent and diffuse.* **(Right)** *Axial NECT of the same patient shows dense bilateral peribronchovascular consolidations.*

Heart Failure

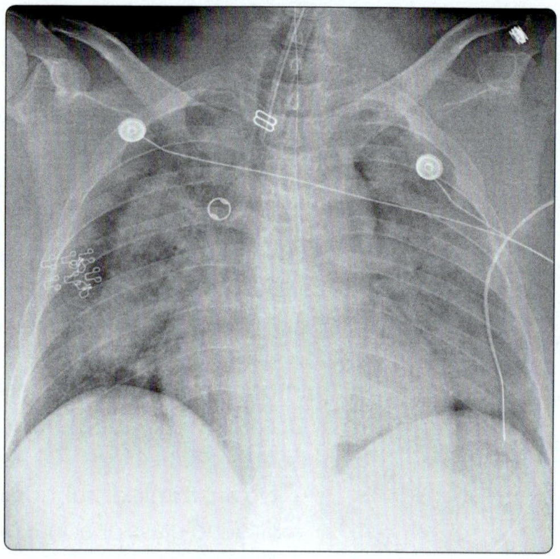

Heart Failure

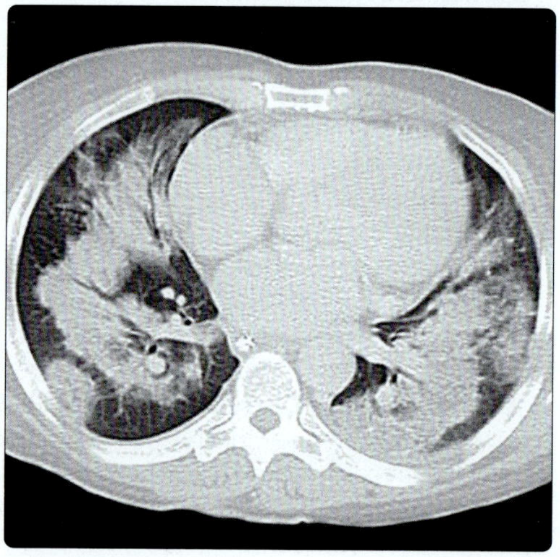

(Left) *AP chest radiograph of a patient with pneumonia secondary to Streptococcus pneumoniae shows a large right upper lobe consolidation.* **(Right)** *Axial NECT of the same patient shows a typical right upper lobe consolidation with intrinsic air-bronchograms ➙. Lobar and segmental consolidations are common radiologic manifestations of community acquired pneumonia, with Streptococcus pneumoniae being one of the most common causative microorganisms.*

Pneumonia

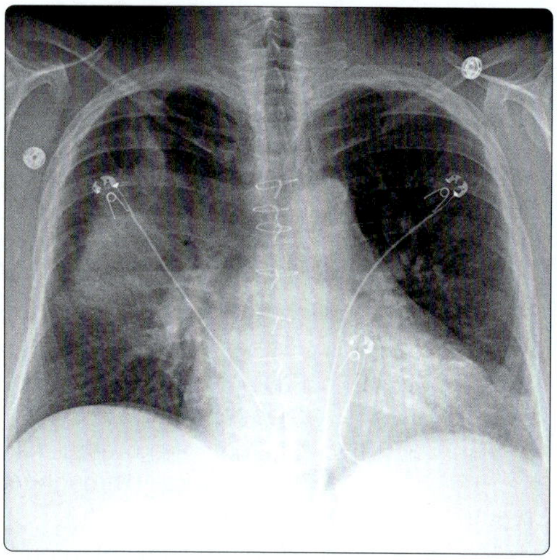

Pneumonia

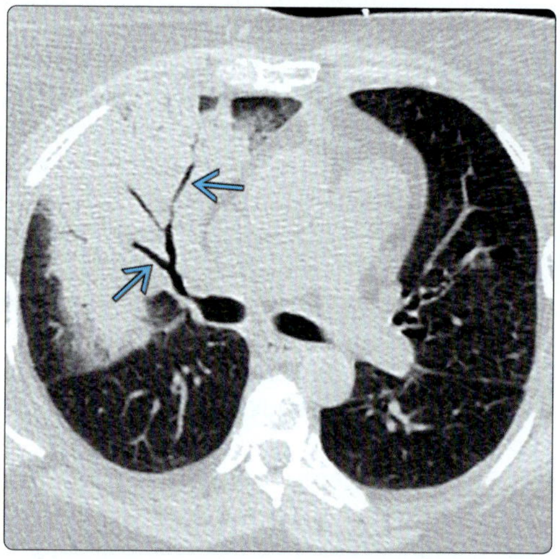

(Left) *PA chest radiograph of a patient with bronchopneumonia secondary to Staphylococcus aureus shows multifocal bilateral patchy peribronchovascular opacities ➙.* **(Right)** *Axial NECT of the same patient shows multifocal peribronchovascular nodular consolidations. This pattern of pulmonary infection, also referred to as bronchopneumonia, is commonly seen in Staphylococcus aureus pneumonia, and is also common in children and elderly patients.*

Pneumonia

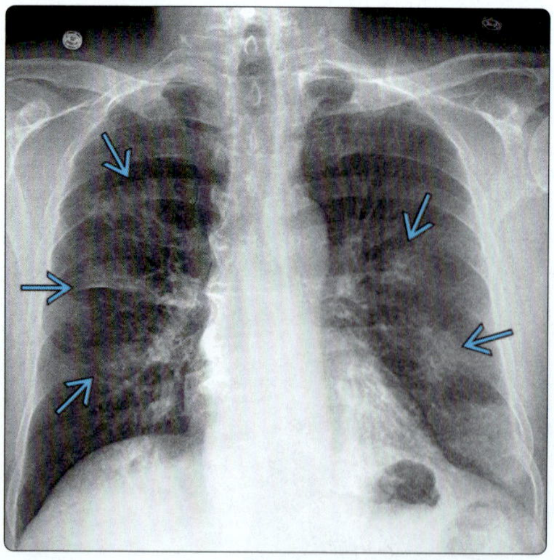

Pneumonia

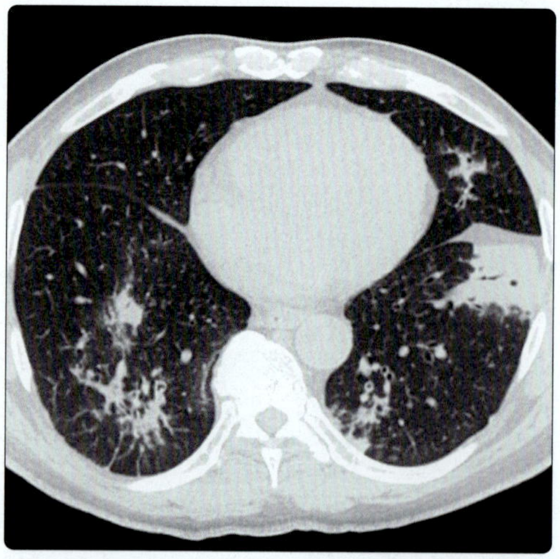

Chronic Obstructive Pulmonary Disease

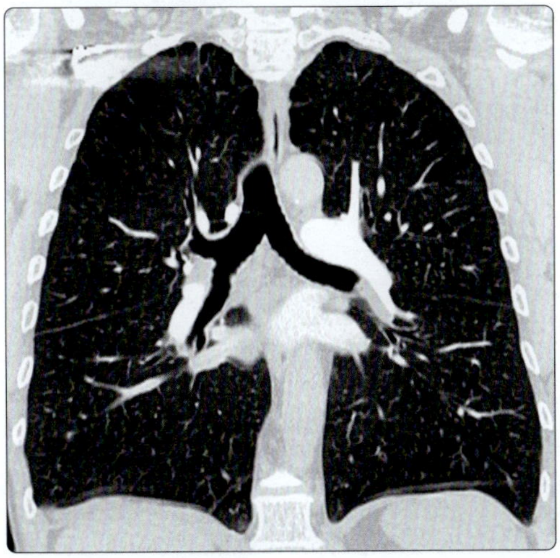

Pulmonary Embolism

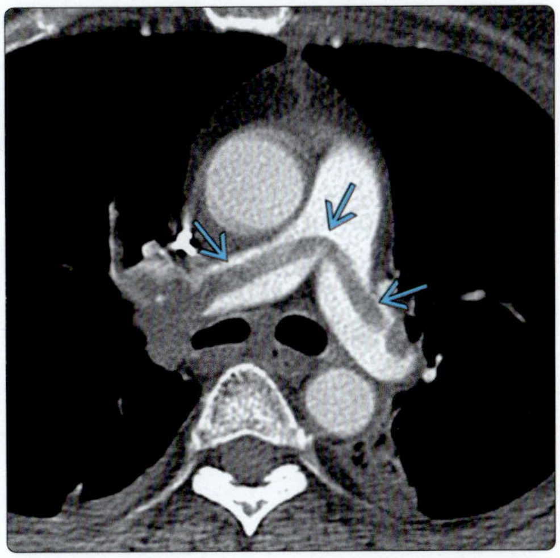

(Left) *Coronal CECT shows upper lobe predominant centrilobular emphysema manifesting as hypoattenuating areas with imperceptible walls representing areas of lung destruction. Emphysema is mostly related to smoking and is part of the spectrum of chronic obstructive pulmonary disease together with chronic bronchitis.* **(Right)** *Axial CECT of a patient with pulmonary embolism shows a large saddle pulmonary thromboembolus ➔ involving the pulmonary trunk and the bilateral pulmonary arteries.*

Pulmonary Embolism

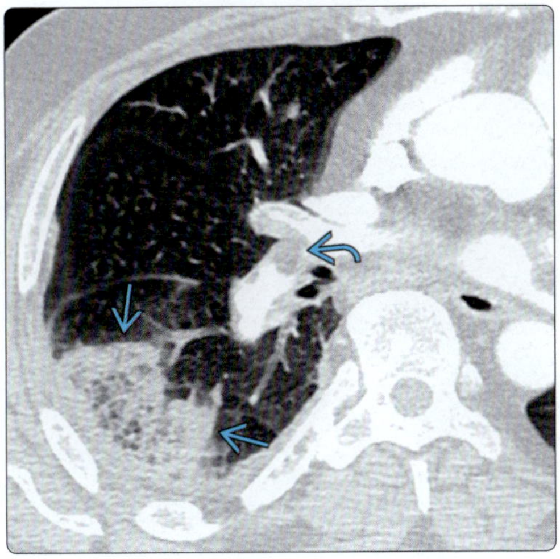

Asthma

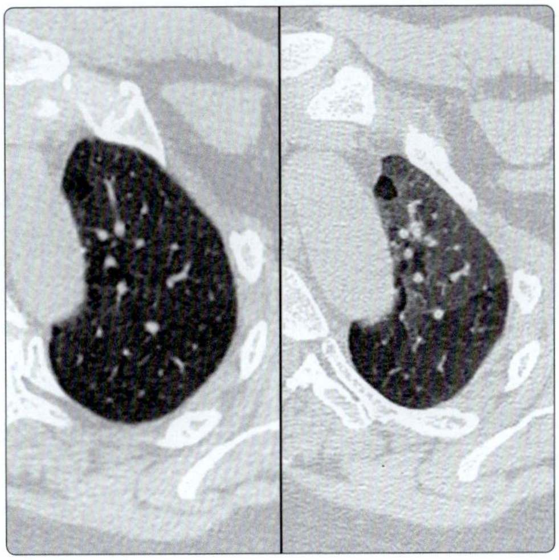

(Left) *Axial CECT of a patient with pulmonary thromboembolism shows a right lower lobe peripheral wedge-shaped consolidation with central lucencies typical of a pulmonary infarct ➔. Note arterial filling defects ➔ representing pulmonary thromboemboli.* **(Right)** *Composite image with axial inspiratory (left) and axial expiratory (right) HRCT of a patient with asthma shows mosaic attenuation (left) and air-trapping (right) on expiratory imaging. Air-trapping occurs in diseases involving the small airways.*

Spontaneous Pneumothorax

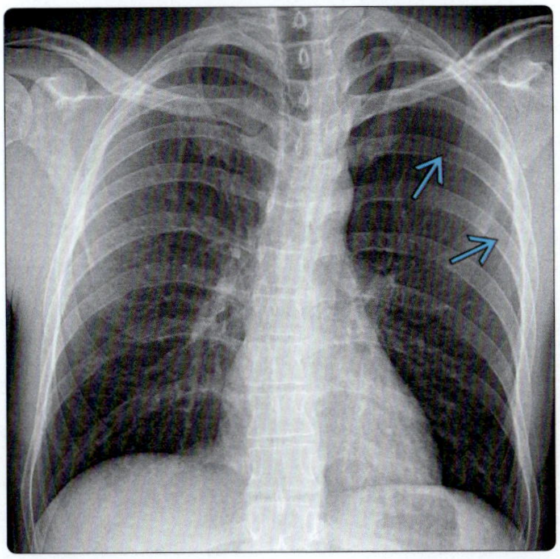

Pneumomediastinum

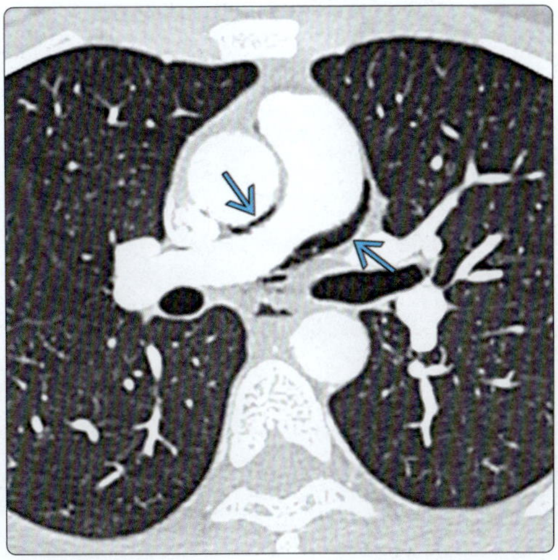

(Left) *PA chest radiograph of a young man who presented with acute chest pain and dyspnea shows a primary spontaneous left pneumothorax manifesting with a visible pleural line ➔ and absence of peripheral lung markings.* **(Right)** *Axial CECT of a patient with a spontaneous pneumomediastinum shows abnormal mediastinal air ➔ adjacent to the aorta and pulmonary trunk. Spontaneous pneumomediastinum typically occurs in patients with asthma and in patients with a history of illicit drug abuse.*

(Left) *AP chest radiograph of a patient with acute respiratory distress syndrome following esophageal surgery shows diffuse bilateral heterogeneous opacities and small bilateral pleural effusions.* **(Right)** *Axial NECT of the same patient shows diffuse bilateral ground-glass opacities and a background of septal thickening, the so-called "crazy-paving" CT pattern. Acute respiratory distress syndrome is a lung reaction to a variety of insults that results in acute respiratory failure requiring aggressive respiratory support.*

Acute Respiratory Distress Syndrome

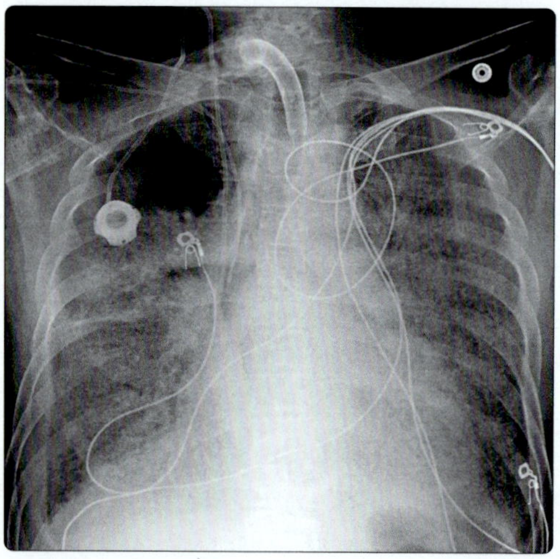

Acute Respiratory Distress Syndrome

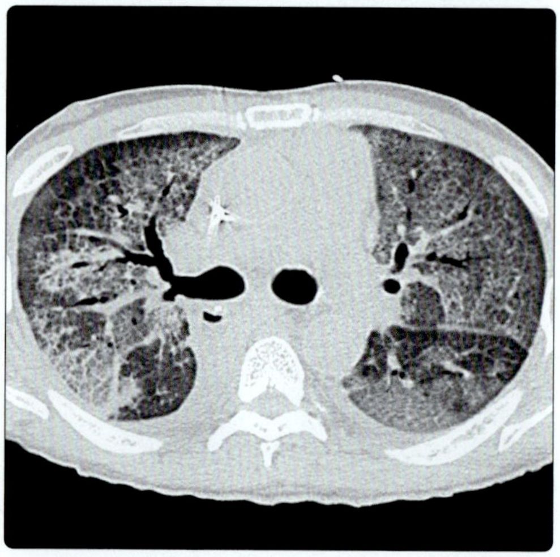

(Left) *AP chest radiograph of a patient with a massive malignant left pleural effusion secondary to metastatic breast cancer shows complete opacification of the left hemithorax and contralateral displacement of the cardiomediastinal silhouette* ➔. **(Right)** *Axial NECT of the same patient shows a massive left pleural effusion with nodular pleural thickening* ➔ *secondary to solid pleural metastases. A large pleural effusion in an elderly individual should always suggest the possibility of malignancy.*

Pleural Effusion

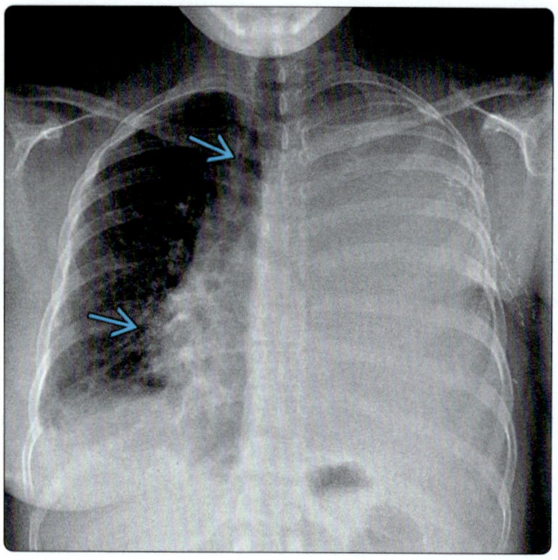

Pleural Effusion

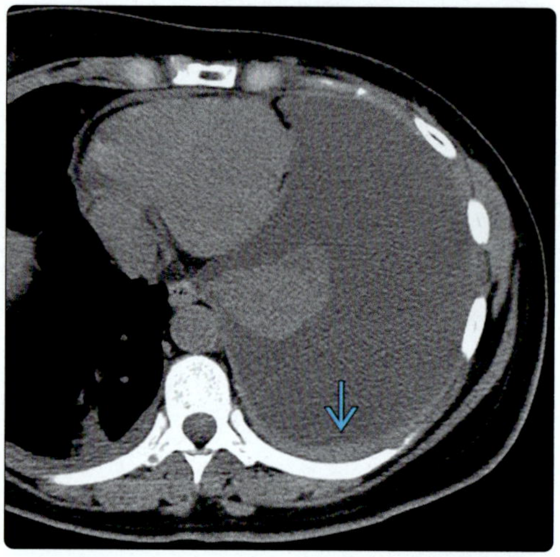

(Left) *Axial CECT of a patient with diffuse alveolar hemorrhage shows extensive bilateral patchy peribronchovascular airspace opacities. Patients with diffuse alveolar hemorrhage may present with hemoptysis and decreased hemoglobin levels.* **(Right)** *Axial NECT of a patient with acute myocardial infarction complicated by a left ventricular pseudoaneurysm (not shown) shows a moderate to large high-attenuation pericardial effusion secondary to hemopericardium* ➔.

Diffuse Alveolar Hemorrhage

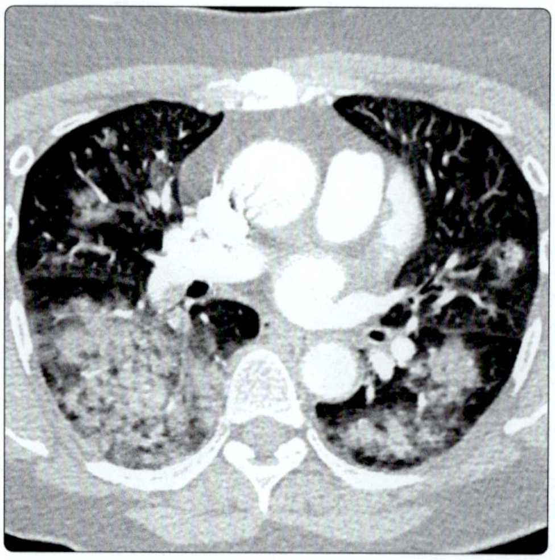

Pericardial Tamponade

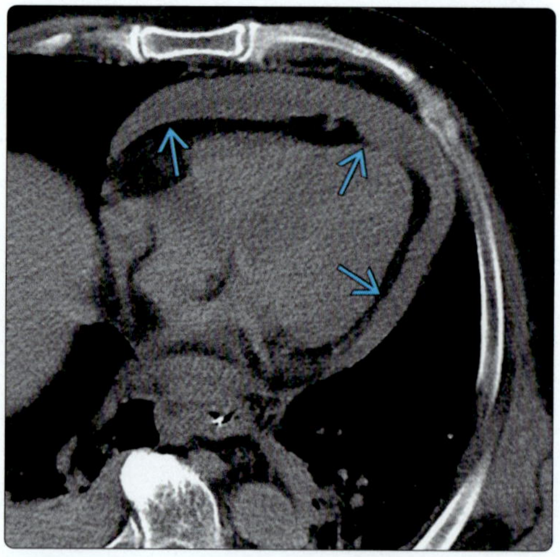

Bronchiectasis

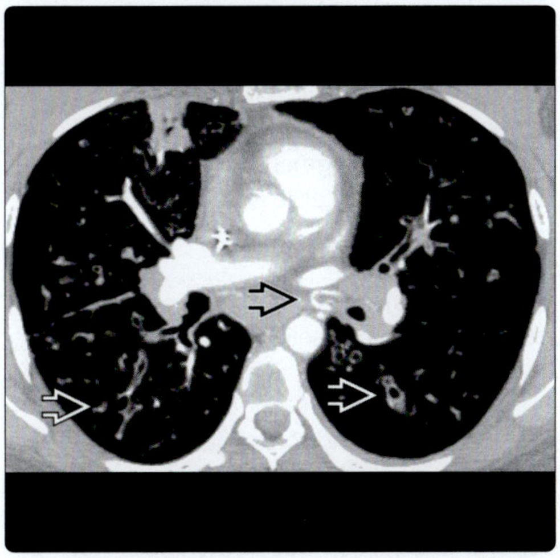

Bronchitis

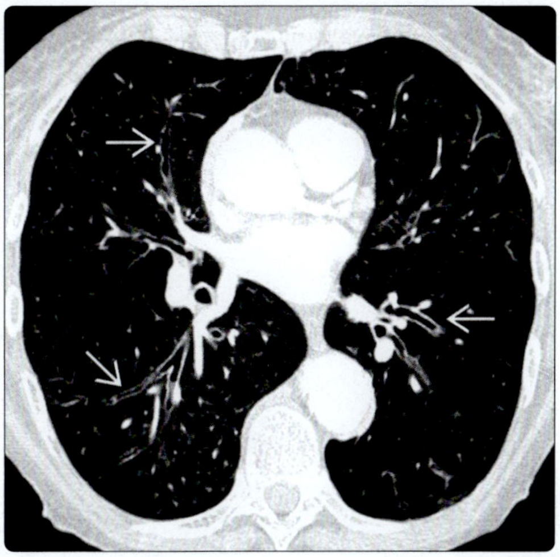

(Left) *Axial CECT shows bronchial wall thickening, bronchiectasis, and mucus plugging of both large and small airways ➔ in a patient with cystic fibrosis. Note the enlarged left bronchial artery ➔.* **(Right)** *Axial CECT shows thickened and irregular bronchial walls with slight bronchial dilatation ➔. This patient was a long-term smoker with chronic cough and hemoptysis. Bronchitis may manifest as bronchial wall thickening or focal ground-glass opacities and consolidation representing active hemorrhage.*

Pulmonary Emboli

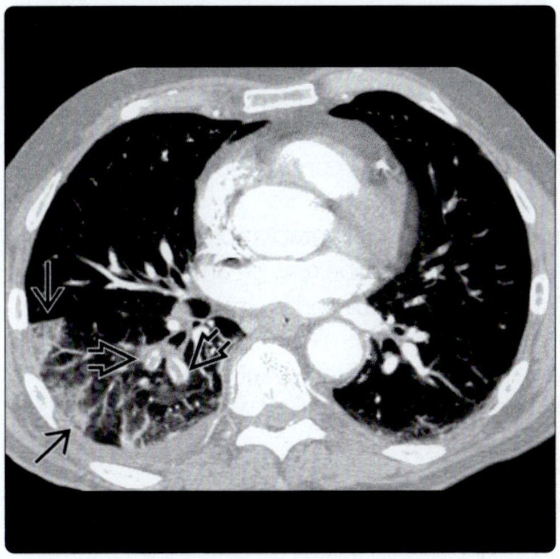

Pulmonary Emboli

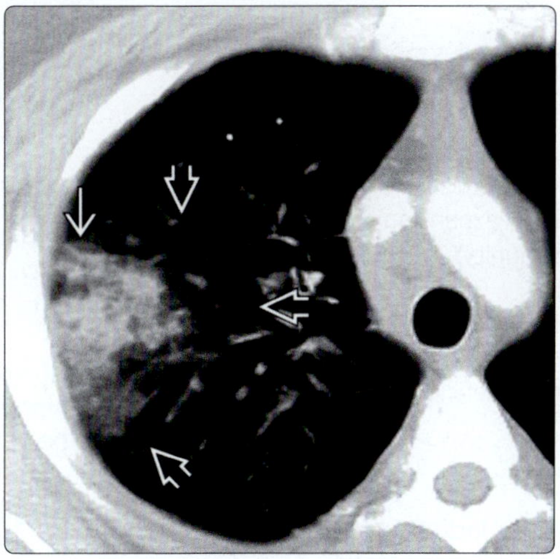

(Left) *Axial CECT of a patient with pulmonary emboli in the right lower lobe pulmonary arteries demonstrates pulmonary infarcts ➔ in regions fed by affected branches ➔.* **(Right)** *Axial CECT of a patient with pulmonary emboli shows wedge-shaped consolidation in the right upper lobe ➔. The central consolidation surrounded by ground-glass opacities ➔ is the classic imaging manifestation of pulmonary infarct.*

Diffuse Alveolar Hemorrhage

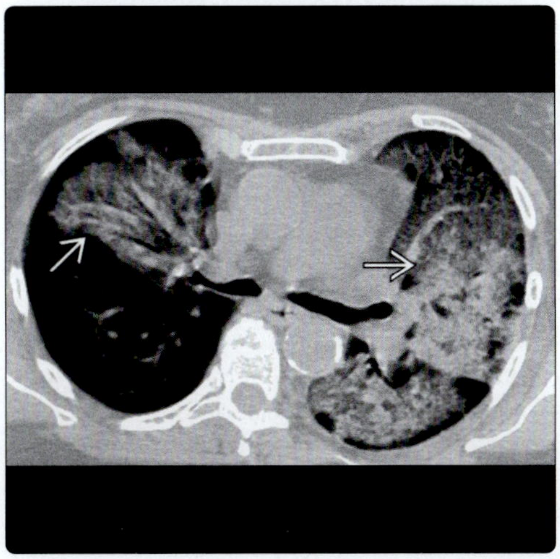

Diffuse Alveolar Hemorrhage

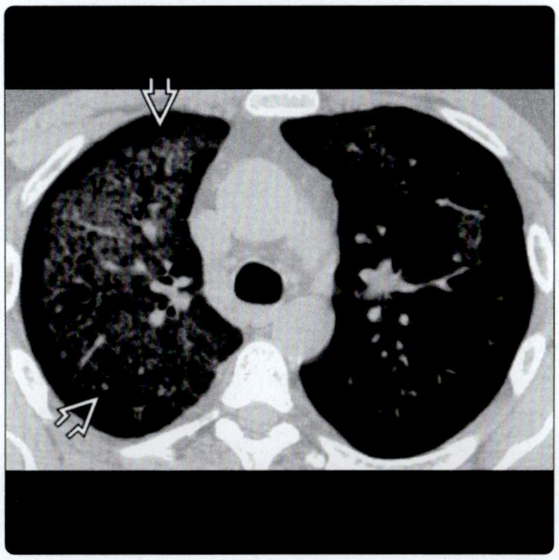

(Left) *Axial NECT of a patient presenting with hemoptysis and a history of vasculitis shows asymmetric consolidation and ground-glass opacities from hemorrhage ➔.* **(Right)** *Axial CECT shows diffuse ground-glass opacities throughout the right lung with peripheral sparing ➔ and lobular involvement of the left lung. Renal biopsy showed Goodpasture syndrome. Diffuse alveolar hemorrhage typically results in lobular ground-glass opacities admixed with consolidation.*

DIFFERENTIAL DIAGNOSIS

Common

- Bacterial Pneumonia
- Viral Pneumonia
- Tuberculosis
- Aspergillosis
- *Pneumocystis jirovecii* Pneumonia

Less Common

- Cryptococcosis
- Mucormycosis

Rare but Important

- Strongyloidiasis
- Candidiasis

ESSENTIAL INFORMATION

Key Differential Diagnosis Issues

- Immune response: Innate or adaptive
- Innate response: Rapid nonspecific host defense mechanism
  - Anatomic barriers (skin and mucous membranes), epithelial barriers, humoral components (complement and acute phase reactants), cells (monocyte-macrophage, granulocytes, and natural cytotoxic cells)
- Adaptive response: Antigenic specificity, immune memory, recognition of one's own, clonal expansion
  - T lymphocytes (cellular immunity), B lymphocytes (humoral immunity)
- Immunosuppression: Inhibition of 1 or more immune system components (innate &/or adaptive)
- Immunosuppression or immunodeficiency: Primary or secondary
  - Primary
    - Rare
    - ~ 300 alterations identified, including defects of cellular and humoral immunity, combined immunodeficiency, and defects in phagocytosis and complement (cytokine defects)
- Secondary
  - HIV infection, malnutrition, metabolic disease (diabetes mellitus), pharmacologic immunosuppression (management of autoimmune disease, neoplasia, or solid organ or stem cell transplantation), genetic alterations, environmental conditions, surgery, and trauma
- Clinical manifestations: Unexpected increased complications of common infections, opportunistic infections
- Specific defects may be associated with certain infections, but immune defects may be multiple, and coinfections may occur
- Differential diagnosis of lung disease in immunosuppressed patient
  - Infection
  - Noninfectious entities
    - Pulmonary edema, drug toxicity, organizing pneumonia pattern, idiopathic pneumonia syndrome, and neoplasms

Helpful Clues for Common Diagnoses

- **Bacterial Pneumonia**
  - Most common infection in HIV-infected patients
  - Frequent in non-HIV/AIDS immunosuppressed patients
  - Imaging: Similar manifestations as those that occur in immunocompetent patients
    - Consolidation (lobar or segmental)
    - Bronchopneumonia (scattered patchy consolidation)
    - Cavitation
- **Viral Pneumonia**
  - Cytomegalovirus (CMV): Most common viral pathogen in hematopoietic stem cell and solid organ transplant recipients
  - Imaging
    - Ground-glass opacities and consolidation
    - Centrilobular nodules
    - Interlobular septal thickening
    - Bronchial &/or bronchiolar wall thickening
    - Cavitary mass-like consolidation in non-HIV/AIDS patients
- **Tuberculosis**
  - HIV-infected patients
    - 50-200x higher risk of developing tuberculosis compared to general population
    - Advanced immunosuppression (CD4 < 200 cells/mm³): Manifestations formerly considered atypical in adults, primary pattern of tuberculosis
      - Lymphadenopathy (several lymph node stations)
      - Consolidation (any lobe may be affected)
      - Miliary or random pulmonary micronodules (hematogenous dissemination)
  - Non-AIDS patients: Organ transplant recipients, hemodialysis, and patients treated with antitumor necrosis factor drugs
    - Nonspecific radiologic manifestations
- **Aspergillosis**
  - Most frequent cause of invasive fungal infection in solid organ or stem cell transplant recipients
  - Angioinvasive aspergillosis
    - Invasion of small blood vessels with hemorrhagic necrosis and pulmonary infarct(s)
    - Single or multiple lung nodules surrounded by ground-glass opacity (halo sign)
    - Peripheral wedge-shaped consolidation (corresponding to pulmonary infarct)
  - Airway invasive aspergillosis
    - Invasion of airway basement membrane
    - Centrilobular nodules and tree-in-bud opacities
    - Bronchial/bronchiolar wall thickening
    - Peribronchovascular consolidation
- ***Pneumocystis jirovecii* Pneumonia**
  - Decreased incidence in AIDS population
    - Introduction of highly active antiretroviral therapy (HAART)
    - Widespread use of pneumocystis pneumonia prophylaxis
  - Most common AIDS-defining illness
  - CD4(+) cell count < 200 cell/mm³
  - HIV-infected patients
    - Subacute clinical course

- Radiography
  - Bilateral perihilar or diffuse symmetric ill-defined or reticular opacities
- HRCT
  - Ground-glass opacities with variable distribution
    - Central distribution with relative peripheral sparing (41%)
    - Mosaic attenuation (29%)
    - Diffuse involvement (24%)
  - Crazy-paving pattern
  - Lung cysts (10-34%)

Helpful Clues for Less Common Diagnoses

- **Cryptococcosis**
  - Infection caused by fungi of genus *Cryptococcus*
    - Most infections caused by *C. neoformans* or *C. gattii*
  - May affect immunocompetent and immunocompromised patients
  - HIV-infected patients
  - Non-AIDS patients
    - Pharmacologic immunosuppression (management of autoimmune disease, neoplasia or solid organ or stem cell transplantation)
  - Similar imaging manifestations in HIV-infected patients compared to patients without HIV infection
    - Solitary or multiple nodules or masses (91%)
      - Soft tissue density
      - Variable contours (well or ill defined)
      - Halo sign
      - Cavitation
    - Ground-glass opacities/consolidation
- **Mucormycosis**
  - Infection caused by fungi of class Zygomycetes (most commonly order Mucorales)
  - Non-AIDS immunocompromised patients
    - Diabetes mellitus, hematologic malignancy, and transplant recipients
  - Lung and airway involvement: Pulmonary vessel thrombosis from fungal angioinvasion and secondary lung necrosis
    - Solitary or multiple nodules or masses
      - Halo sign
      - Reversed halo sign
      - Air crescent sign: Thin rim of air between necrotic and nonnecrotic lung
      - 10 or more nodules are more frequent in mucormycosis than in aspergillosis
    - Ground-glass opacities/consolidation
    - Cavitation

Helpful Clues for Rare Diagnoses

- **Strongyloidiasis**
  - Infection caused by *Strongyloides stercoralis* (microscopic nematode)
  - HIV-infected patients
  - Non-AIDS patients
    - Pharmacologic immunosuppression by glucocorticoid therapy
  - Continuous autoinfection may lead to massive parasitic infestation (hyperinfection syndrome)
  - Imaging: Diffuse random micronodular pattern, multilobar consolidation
- **Candidiasis**
  - Infection caused by *Candida* spp. (*C. albicans*, *C. glabrata*)
  - Mechanisms of infection: Hematogenous spread and aspiration
  - Risk factors
    - Neutropenia (> 10 days), *Candida* colonization, necrotizing pancreatitis, immunosuppressive therapy (corticosteroids), central venous catheters, diabetes mellitus
  - Imaging
    - Multiple nodules (88-95%); halo sign (33%)
    - Consolidation (65%)
    - Ground-glass opacities (35%)
    - Tree-in-bud opacities

Bacterial Pneumonia

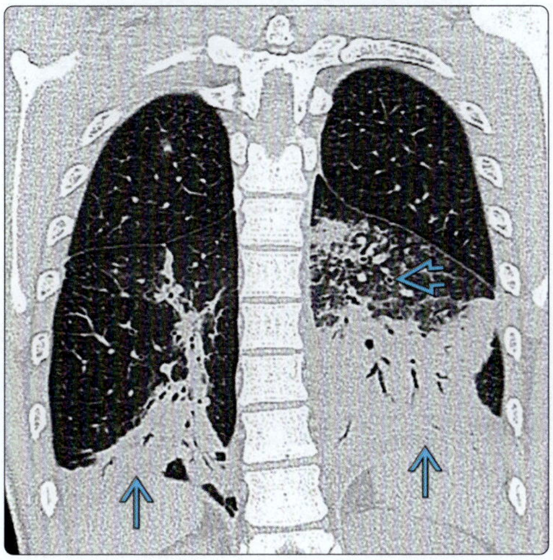

Bacterial Pneumonia

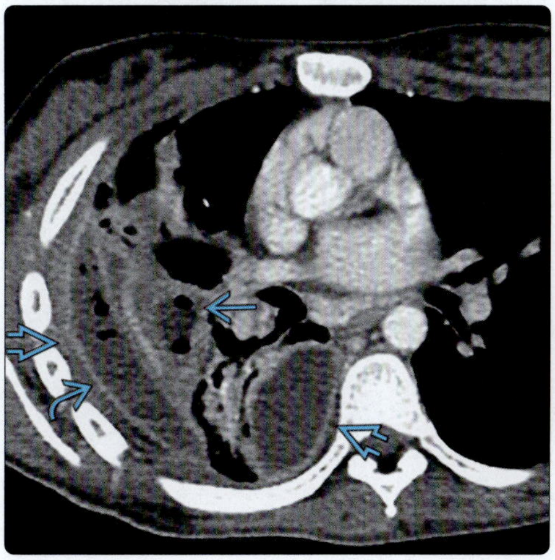

(Left) *Coronal NECT of a patient with AIDS who became infected with pulmonary Pneumococcus pneumoniae shows bilateral lower lobe consolidations ➡, left greater than right, with intrinsic air bronchograms. Note bronchial wall thickening ➡.* **(Right)** *Axial CECT of a patient with systemic lupus erythematosus and staphylococcal pneumonia shows a heterogeneous right lower lobe consolidation with areas of cavitation ➡, a multilocular right pleural effusion ➡, and a thick enhancing parietal pleura ➡.*

(Left) *Axial CECT of a patient with HIV/AIDS and cytomegalovirus pneumonia shows multifocal right lung predominant centrilobular micronodules ➡ and tree-in-bud opacities ⇨.* **(Right)** *Axial CECT of a patient with leukemia and cytomegalovirus pneumonia shows a left upper lobe mass-like consolidation with intrinsic cavitation ➡ and a thick cavity wall. Note trace bilateral pleural effusions. Viral pneumonias may exhibit a wide variety of imaging abnormalities that range from micronodules to cavitary disease.*

Viral Pneumonia

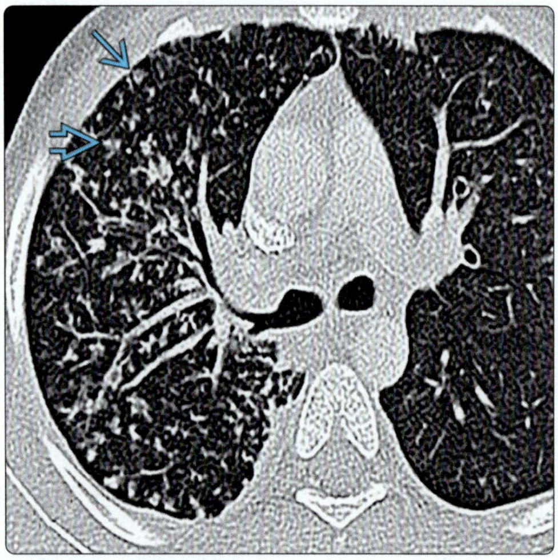

Viral Pneumonia

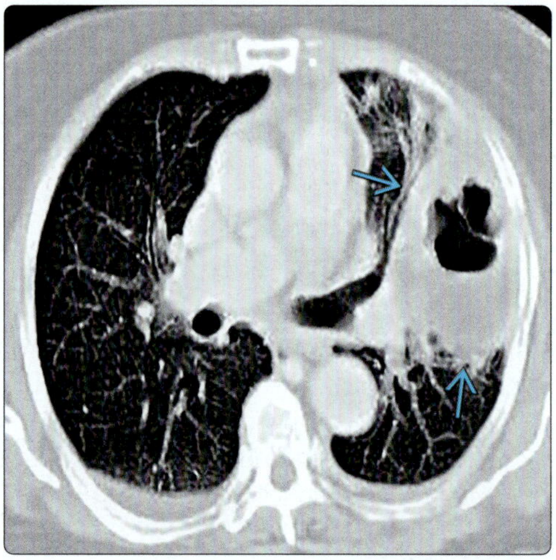

(Left) *PA chest radiograph of a patient with rheumatoid arthritis undergoing corticosteroid treatment shows pulmonary tuberculosis characterized by a heterogeneous right upper lobe consolidation ➡ with volume loss, intrinsic cavitation, and multifocal ill-defined pulmonary nodules ⇨.* **(Right)** *Coronal NECT of the same patient shows the right upper lobe heterogeneous consolidation ➡ and bilateral multifocal and multilobar clustered centrilobular nodules ⇨.*

Tuberculosis

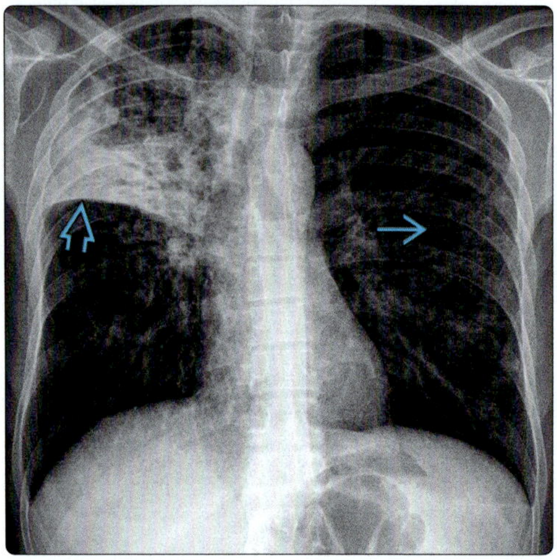

Tuberculosis

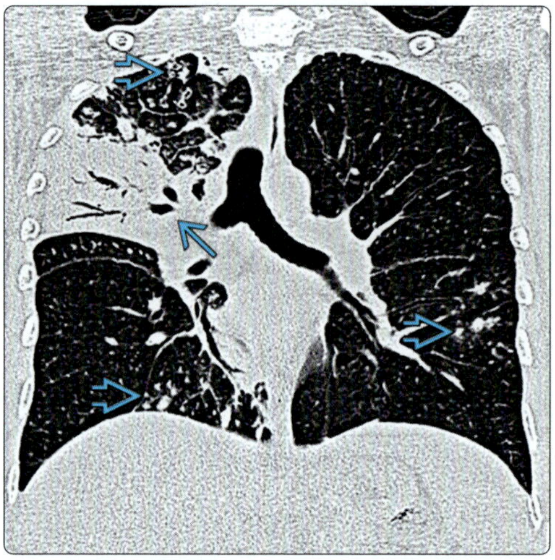

(Left) *Coronal CECT of a patient with leukemia who presented with febrile neutropenia shows typical features of angioinvasive pulmonary aspergillosis, which manifests with multiple bilateral pulmonary nodules surrounded by ground-glass opacity halos ➡, the so-called halo sign.* **(Right)** *Coronal NECT of a nonneutropenic kidney transplant recipient with airway invasive aspergillosis shows multifocal bilateral centrilobular nodules ➡ and tree-in-bud opacities ⇨.*

Aspergillosis

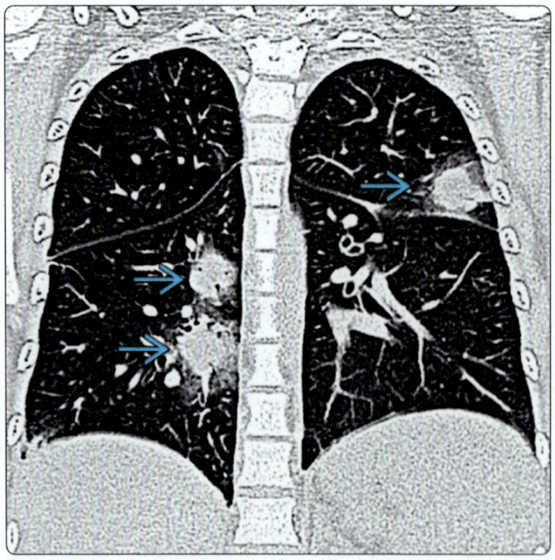

Aspergillosis

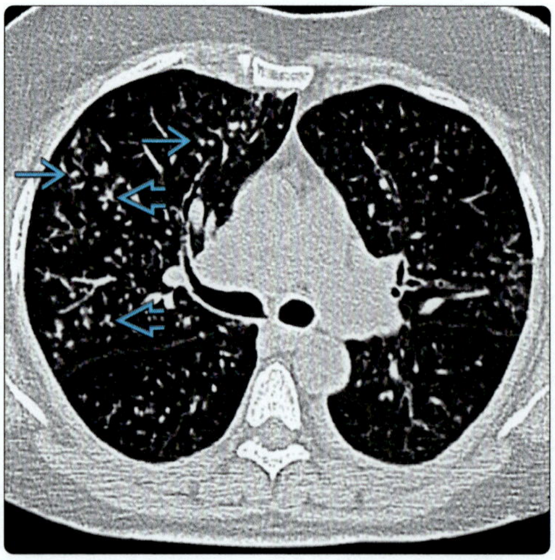

***Pneumocystis jirovecii* Pneumonia**

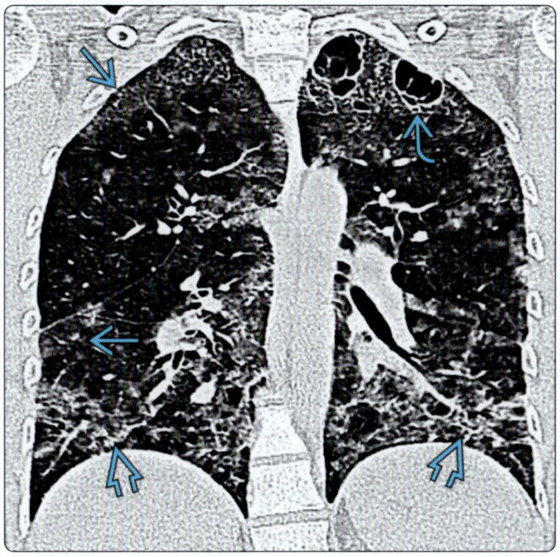

***Pneumocystis jirovecii* Pneumonia**

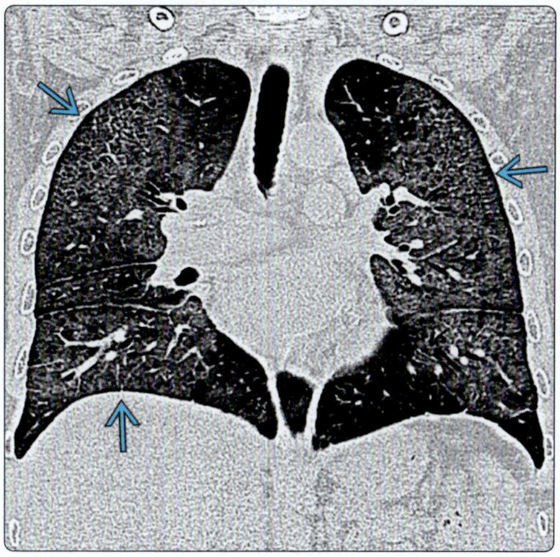

(Left) *Coronal NECT of an HIV-infected patient who developed pneumocystis pneumonia shows bilateral patchy ground-glass opacities →, basilar reticular opacities →, and left upper lobe peripheral pulmonary cysts →.* **(Right)** *Coronal NECT of a kidney transplant recipient who developed Pneumocystis jirovecii pneumonia shows diffuse bilateral ground-glass opacities →. Pneumocystis pneumonia often manifests with pulmonary ground-glass opacities.*

Cryptococcosis

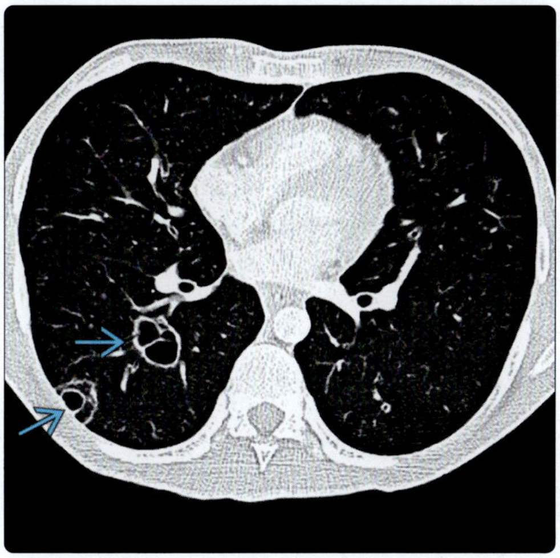

Mucormycosis

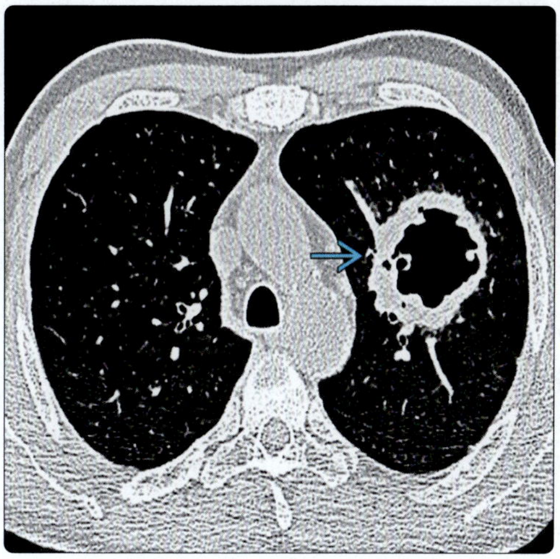

(Left) *Axial CECT of an HIV-infected patient who developed pulmonary cryptococcosis shows right lower lobe cavitary nodules → with relatively thin cavity walls. Cryptococcosis may affect both immunocompetent and immunocompromised subjects.* **(Right)** *Axial NECT of a kidney transplant recipient who developed pulmonary mucormycosis shows a large left upper lobe cavitary mass → with thick and nodular cavity walls. Mucormycosis typically affects solid organ transplant recipients and diabetics.*

Strongyloidiasis

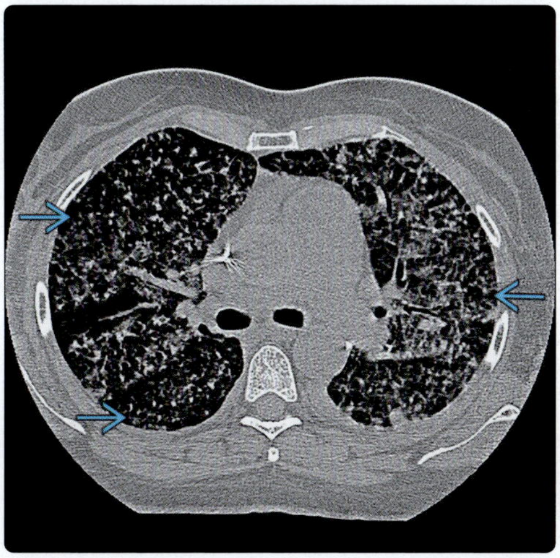

Candidiasis

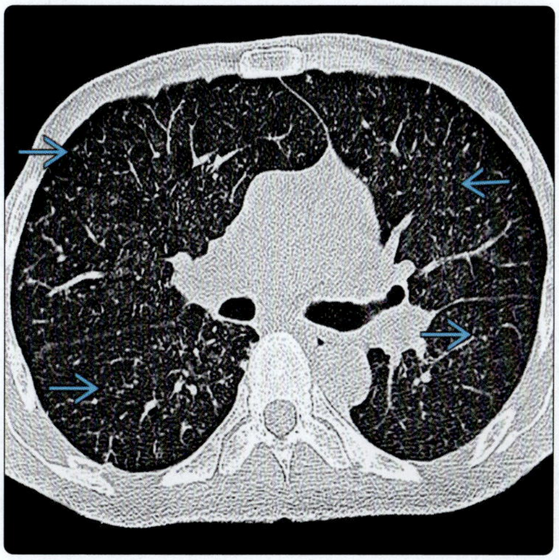

(Left) *Axial NECT of a patient with rheumatoid arthritis on corticosteroid treatment who developed disseminated strongyloidiasis shows diffuse pulmonary micronodules → that exhibit a random distribution. Note trace bilateral pleural effusions and scattered ground-glass opacities.* **(Right)** *Axial NECT of a patient with leukemia who became infected with pulmonary candidiasis shows diffuse bilateral pulmonary micronodules → that exhibit a random distribution.*

DIFFERENTIAL DIAGNOSIS

Common

- Tracheobronchomalacia
- Saber-Sheath Trachea
- Laryngeal/Pharyngeal Tumor
- Thyroid Mass

Less Common

- Trauma
- Tracheal Stenosis
- Foreign Body
- Granulomatosis With Polyangiitis

Rare but Important

- Tracheobronchopathia Osteochondroplastica
- Infection
- Tracheal Neoplasm
- Tracheobronchial Amyloidosis
- Relapsing Polychondritis

ESSENTIAL INFORMATION

Key Differential Diagnosis Issues

- Stridor
  - High-pitched sound secondary to turbulent flow in upper airway
  - Indicates pathology in trachea or larynx
- Primary imaging modalities used in directing differential diagnosis
  - Radiography and CT
- Final diagnosis may require bronchoscopy with biopsy

Helpful Clues for Common Diagnoses

- **Tracheobronchomalacia**
  - Congenital or acquired causes
    - Intubation
    - External mass or vessel causing compression
    - Infection
    - Chronic obstructive pulmonary disease (COPD)
  - Imaging
    - Abnormal tracheal or bronchial cartilage
      - ≥ 50% decrease in cross-sectional area with expiration
      - Trachea may appear normal on inspiratory images
- **Saber-Sheath Trachea**
  - Strong association with COPD
  - Cartilage damage through repeated coughing
  - Imaging
    - Coronal tracheal diameter ≤ 2/3 sagittal diameter
    - Normal tracheal wall thickness
- **Laryngeal/Pharyngeal Tumor**
  - Squamous cell carcinoma is most common etiology
  - Imaging
    - Document extent of disease
      - Influences surgical and therapeutic plan
- **Thyroid Mass**
  - May externally compress trachea
  - Etiology
    - Mediastinal extension of thyroid goiter
    - Ectopic goiter
    - Thyroid carcinoma
  - Imaging
    - Goiter
      - High attenuation on unenhanced CT due to iodine content
      - Direct connection to thyroid is usually evident on CT
      - Cystic regions, calcifications may be present
    - Thyroid malignancy
      - Invasion of adjacent structures
      - Lymphadenopathy
      - Metastatic disease

Helpful Clues for Less Common Diagnoses

- **Trauma**
  - Hematoma compressing airway
  - Secondary tracheal stenosis from remote trauma
- **Tracheal Stenosis**
  - Imaging
    - Focal stricture with circumferential wall thickening
    - ± cartilage damage with resulting tracheomalacia
    - Prolonged endotracheal intubation
      - Subglottic tracheal stenosis at cuff site
      - Reduced incidence with low-pressure balloon cuffs
    - Tracheostomy tube placement
      - Stenosis at stoma site
  - Other etiologies
    - Complete cartilaginous tracheal ring
    - Sarcoidosis
  - Treatment
    - Mechanical dilatation
    - Stenting
- **Foreign Body**
  - History essential for diagnosis
  - Imaging
    - Foreign body rarely radiopaque
    - CT necessary for visualization
- **Granulomatosis With Polyangiitis**
  - Laboratory evidence of glomerulonephritis (microscopic hematuria and proteinuria)
  - Imaging
    - Circumferential subglottic tracheal wall thickening with luminal narrowing
    - ± cavitary lung nodules
    - ± pansinus disease

Helpful Clues for Rare Diagnoses

- **Tracheobronchopathia Osteochondroplastica**
  - Benign disease occurring in older men
  - Often incidental at bronchoscopy
  - Rarely leads to symptoms
  - Imaging
    - Small and irregularly shaped calcified nodules arising from cartilage
    - Spares noncartilaginous posterior tracheal membrane
- **Infection**
  - Tuberculosis
    - Circumferential wall thickening with tracheal narrowing
    - Mediastinal lymphadenopathy

  - Epiglottitis
    - More indolent than pediatric epiglottitis, secondary to larger hypopharynx
  - Rhinoscleroma
    - Chronic granulomatous infection by *Klebsiella rhinoscleromatis*
    - Central America, Africa, and India
    - Nasal cavity involved in 95% with polyps and soft tissue thickening
    - Spares paranasal sinuses
    - 25% have subglottic tracheal involvement with concentric or nodular narrowing
    - Air-filled crypts in tracheal lumen nearly diagnostic
- **Tracheal Neoplasm**
  - 3 different forms
    - Primary malignancy
    - Metastatic disease
    - Primary benign neoplasm
  - 3 growth patterns
    - Sessile
    - Polypoid
    - Circumferential growth
  - Imaging of primary tracheal malignancies
    - Advantages of CT
      - Extent of disease involving trachea
      - Detection of disease that has spread beyond trachea
    - Squamous cell carcinoma
      - Most common primary malignancy of trachea
      - Strong association with smoking
      - 10% multifocal at presentation
    - Adenoid cystic carcinoma
      - Posterolateral tracheal wall
      - ± growth along airways
  - Metastatic disease
    - Hematogenous metastases
      - Melanoma
      - Breast
      - Colon
      - Renal cell
    - Secondary invasion from lung or esophageal carcinomas
    - Imaging of tracheal metastasis
      - ± single or multiple endotracheal lesions
      - External compression
  - Tracheobronchial papillomatosis
    - HPV infection of tracheal and bronchial tree
    - Small well-circumscribed noncalcified tracheal nodules
    - ± cystic lung lesions
- **Tracheobronchial Amyloidosis**
  - Nodular or concentric wall thickening of trachea and mainstem bronchi
    - ± nodular calcification
  - ± atelectasis or lobar collapse
  - Usually no lung nodules
  - Treatment
    - Stenting
    - Corticosteroids
- **Relapsing Polychondritis**
  - Systemic disorder associated with repeated bouts of cartilaginous inflammation
  - Trachea and bronchi affected late in disease course
  - Also affects cartilage of
    - Ears
    - Nose
    - Joints
  - Imaging
    - Tracheobronchial wall thickening with sparing of noncartilaginous posterior wall
    - Severe disease may affect posterior wall
  - Stenosis leads to recurrent pneumonia
  - Treatment
    - Stenting
    - Corticosteroids

Tracheobronchomalacia

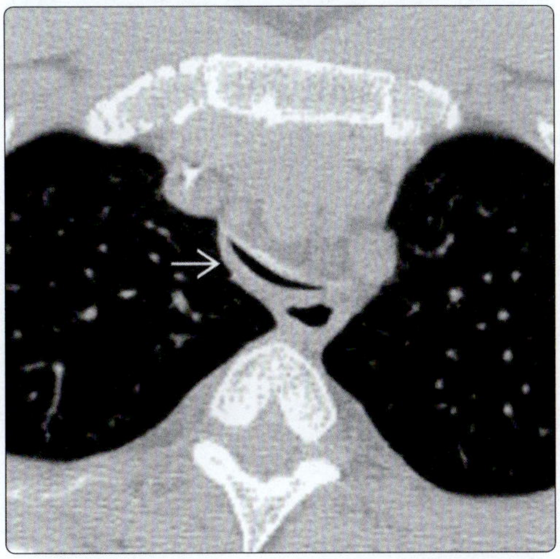

Tracheobronchomalacia

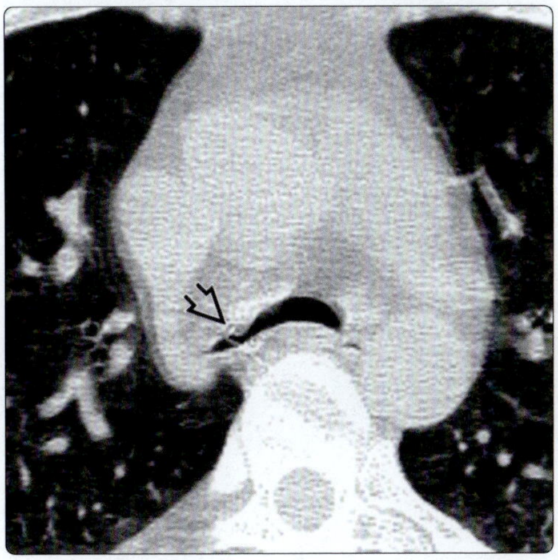

(Left) *Axial NECT shows diffuse intrathoracic tracheal narrowing* ➡ *with more than 50% reduction in cross-sectional area when compared to inspiratory images, which is diagnostic of tracheomalacia.* **(Right)** *Axial HRCT shows collapse of the bronchus intermedius and right upper lobe bronchus* ⇨ *from tracheobronchomalacia. This patient required stenting secondary to persistent respiratory symptoms.*

(Left) *Sagittal CECT shows tracheal compression by an aberrant left subclavian artery ➔ with right aortic arch. In this patient with a cervical arch, the vascular structures are crowded into a narrow thoracic inlet causing compression and resultant tracheomalacia.* **(Right)** *Axial CECT shows saber-sheath intrathoracic trachea ➔ with the sagittal diameter greater than the coronal diameter. There is severe centrilobular emphysema ➔, a common associated finding.*

Tracheobronchomalacia

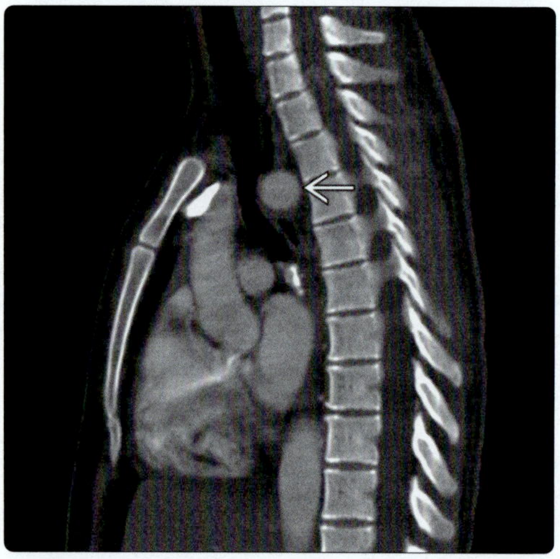

Saber-Sheath Trachea

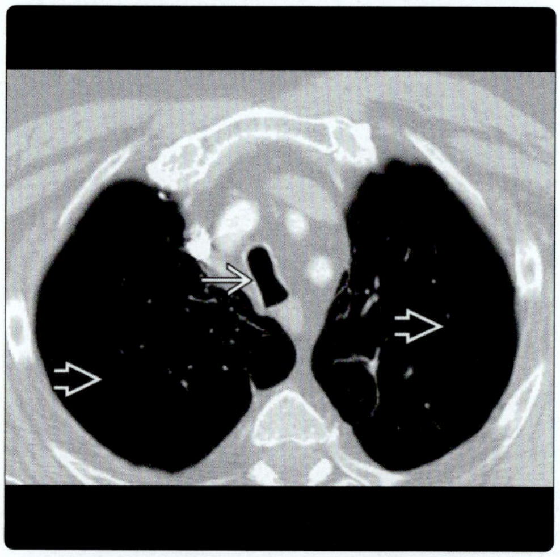

(Left) *Axial NECT shows a mass ➔ located superior to the left true vocal cord. This proved to represent a squamous cell carcinoma. The vocal cord was not involved on lower sections, an important finding to report as this influences surgical therapy.* **(Right)** *Fused axial FDG PET/CT of a different patient demonstrates increased FDG uptake in a left supraglottic mass ➔. This proved to be a primary squamous cell carcinoma on resection.*

Laryngeal/Pharyngeal Tumor

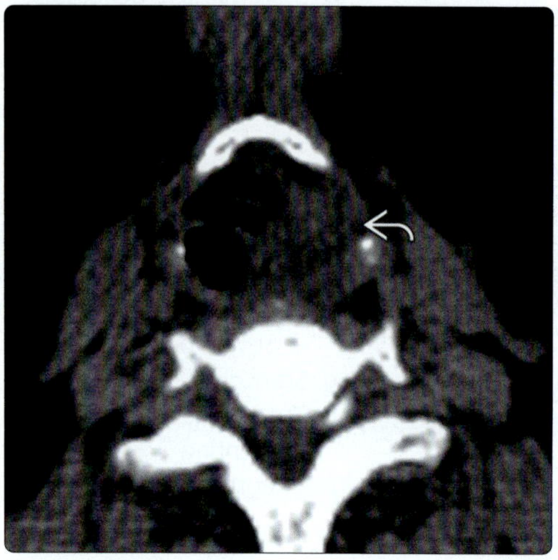

Laryngeal/Pharyngeal Tumor

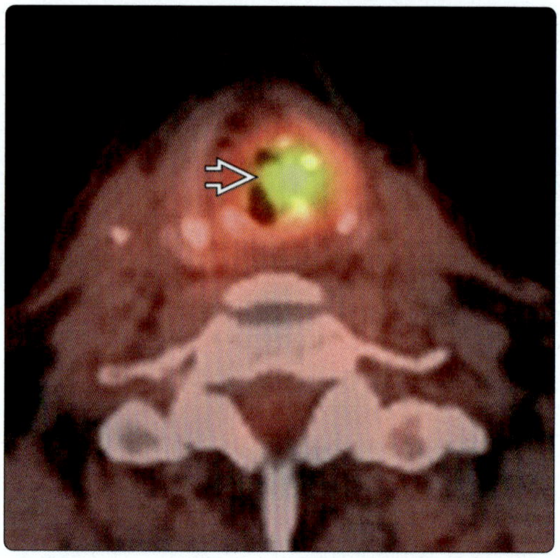

(Left) *Frontal radiograph demonstrates a large right paratracheal mass ➔ with narrowing and leftward displacement of the trachea ➔. This was a large substernal goiter without evidence of malignancy.* **(Right)** *Coronal CECT shows a high-density heterogeneously enhancing mass ➔ in the thoracic inlet deviating the trachea to the right. There is associated tracheal narrowing. This proved to be a thyroid goiter, and connection to the thyroid was revealed on axial images.*

Thyroid Mass

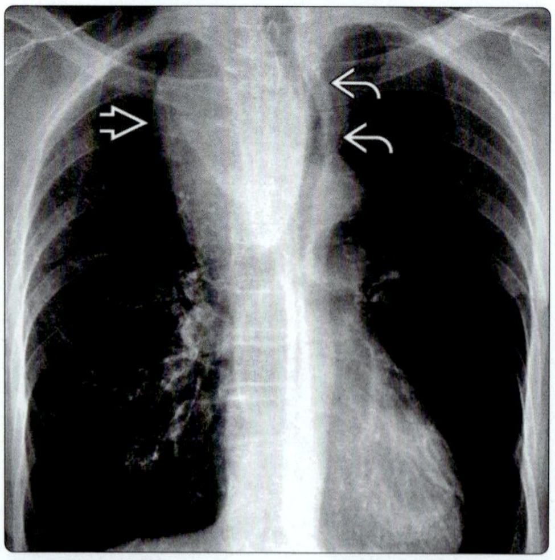

Thyroid Mass

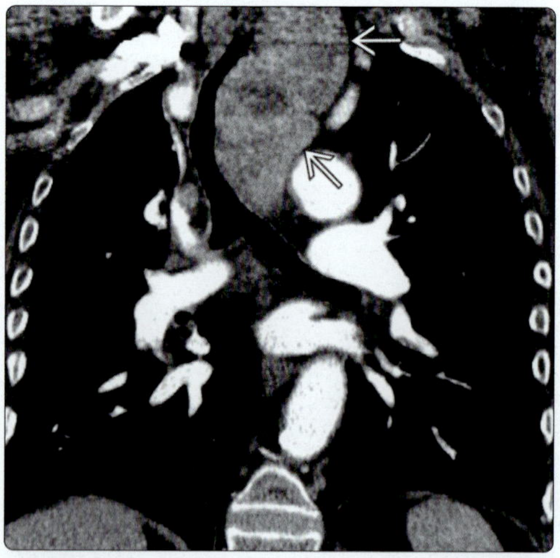

Tracheal Stenosis

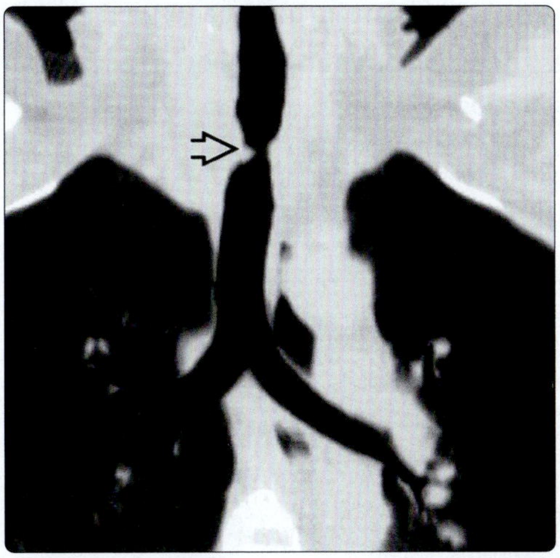

Tracheal Stenosis

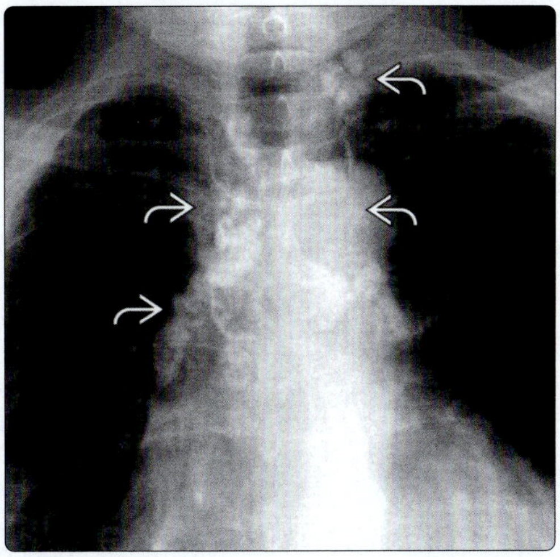

(Left) *Coronal NECT demonstrates short segment tracheal narrowing at the level of the thoracic inlet in this patient with postintubation stenosis.* **(Right)** *Frontal radiograph shows extensive calcified bilateral hilar, paratracheal, and cervical lymph nodes. Note external compression of the trachea caused by lymphadenopathy in this patient with sarcoidosis. This required treatment with stenting.*

Tracheal Stenosis

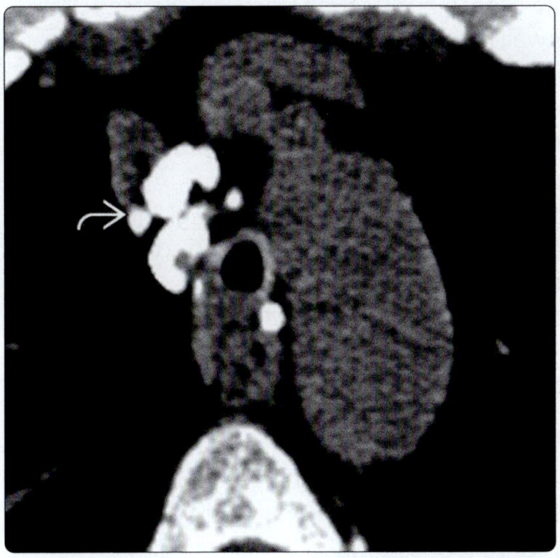

Foreign Body

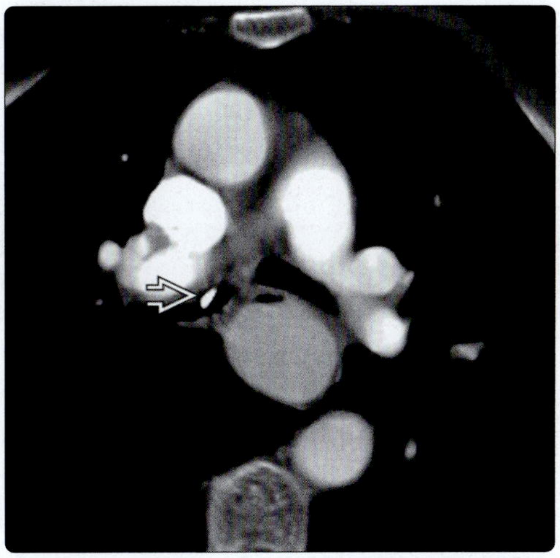

(Left) *Axial NECT shows multiple calcified paratracheal lymph nodes with extrinsic tracheal stenosis secondary to sarcoidosis. Tracheal stenosis from sarcoidosis can be from extrinsic compression, as in this case, or intrinsic compression secondary to luminal granulomas.* **(Right)** *Axial CECT shows an aspirated wire in the bronchus intermedius. Lung windows (not shown) revealed tree-in-bud opacities from postobstructive pneumonia.*

Granulomatosis With Polyangiitis

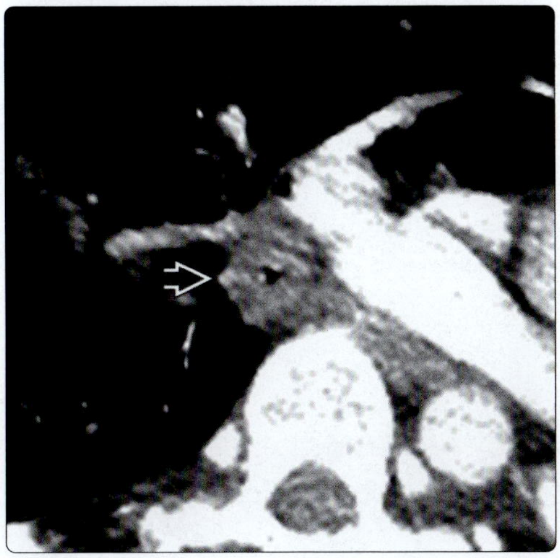

Tracheobronchopathia Osteochondroplastica

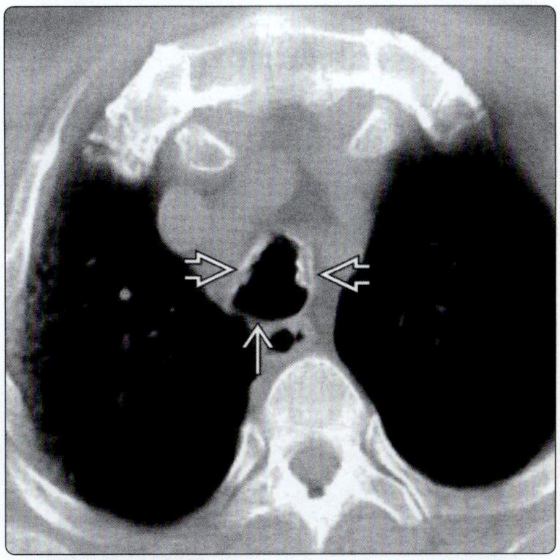

(Left) *Axial CECT shows severe circumferential tracheal narrowing with near complete obliteration of the lumen. This patient had a left pneumonectomy for complications related to granulomatosis with polyangiitis.* **(Right)** *Axial NECT shows calcified nodules along the anterior and lateral wall of the trachea. Nodules arise from cartilage; the posterior tracheal wall is thus spared, as it does not contain cartilage.*

Wheezing

DIFFERENTIAL DIAGNOSIS

Common

- Asthma/Chronic Obstructive Pulmonary Disease
- Pulmonary Edema
- Aspiration

Less Common

- Airway Obstruction
- Tracheobronchomalacia
- Bronchiectasis
- Bronchiolitis

Rare but Important

- Eosinophilic Granulomatosis With Polyangiitis

ESSENTIAL INFORMATION

Key Differential Diagnosis Issues

- High-pitched sound while breathing (inspiratory or expiratory)
- Occurs when air flows through narrowed bronchi

Helpful Clues for Common Diagnoses

- **Asthma/Chronic Obstructive Pulmonary Disease (COPD)**
  - Airway obstruction associated with underlying chronic airway inflammation
  - Bronchial wall thickening/bronchiectasis
  - Emphysema
  - Centrilobular nodules/tree-in-bud pattern
  - Air-trapping
- **Pulmonary Edema**
  - Peribronchovascular edema can cause narrowing of bronchi with wheezing
  - Interlobular septal thickening (i.e., Kerley B lines)
  - Ancillary imaging finding: Cardiomegaly, pleural effusions
- **Aspiration**
  - Recurrent aspiration with aspirated material narrows airway lumen
  - Most common in dependent segments
    - Posterior segments of upper lobes and superior segments of lower lobes (aspiration on decubitus)
    - Lower lobe basal segments (aspiration on upright)

Helpful Clues for Less Common Diagnoses

- **Airway Obstruction**
  - Extrinsic (airway compression)
    - Mediastinal mass, vascular rings
  - Intrinsic (airway narrowing)
    - Focal or diffuse
    - Postintubation stenosis, tracheal neoplasms
    - Tracheobronchopathia osteochondroplastica, relapsing polychondritis, granulomatosis with polyangiitis and amyloidosis
- **Tracheobronchomalacia**
  - Excessive airway collapsibility caused by weakness of airway walls
  - Excessive collapse (> 70%) of expected luminal area during expiratory CT scan
  - Typical morphology: Crescent, lunate, or "frown" sign
- **Bronchiectasis**
  - Irreversible bronchial dilatation usually associated with bronchial wall inflammation
  - Bronchial dilatation
  - Lack of bronchial tapering
  - Visualization of airway within 1 cm of pleura
- **Bronchiolitis**
  - Diverse diseases involving bronchioles (e.g., infectious, aspiration, inflammation, neoplasms, and congenital abnormalities)
  - Centrilobular nodules ± tree-in-bud opacities
  - Bronchial wall thickening
  - Mosaic attenuation/air-trapping

Helpful Clues for Rare Diagnoses

- **Eosinophilic Granulomatosis With Polyangiitis**
  - Granulomatous vasculitis involving small vessels
  - Occurs in context of asthma
  - Patchy ground-glass opacities &/or consolidation (± migratory opacities)

Asthma/Chronic Obstructive Pulmonary Disease

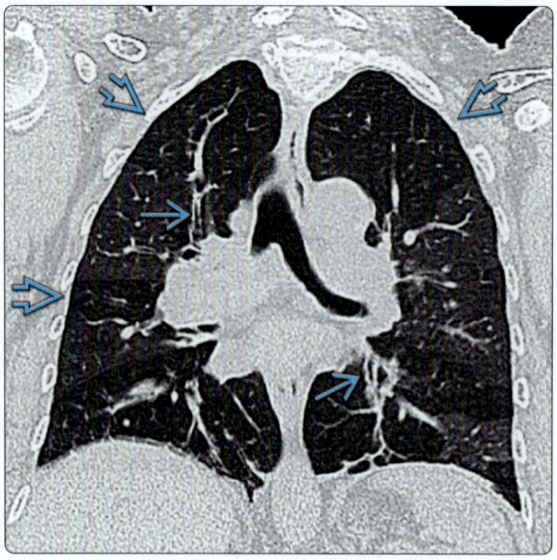

Pulmonary Edema

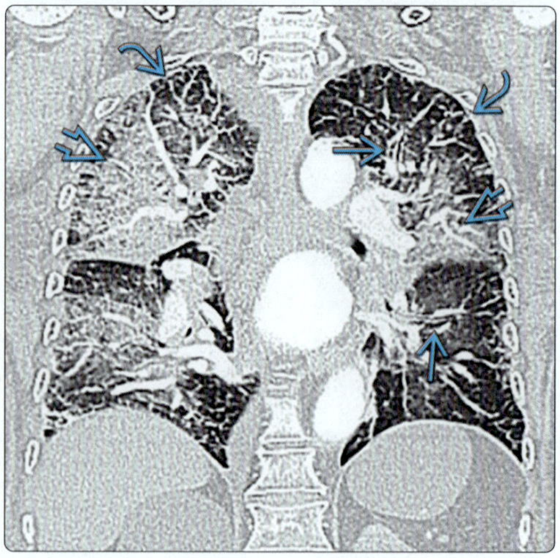

(Left) *Coronal HRCT of a patient with asthma shows diffuse bronchial wall thickening and scattered areas of lucency from mosaic attenuation, which are secondary to air-trapping, characteristic of small airways disease. Asthma is the most classic example of diseases associated with wheezing.* **(Right)** *Coronal CECT of a patient with pulmonary edema (cardiogenic) shows extensive peribronchovascular thickening, interlobular septal thickening, and upper lobe predominant ground-glass opacities.*

Aspiration

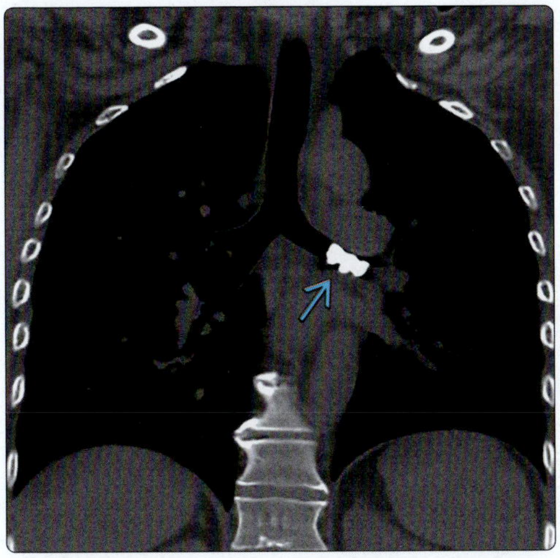

Aspiration

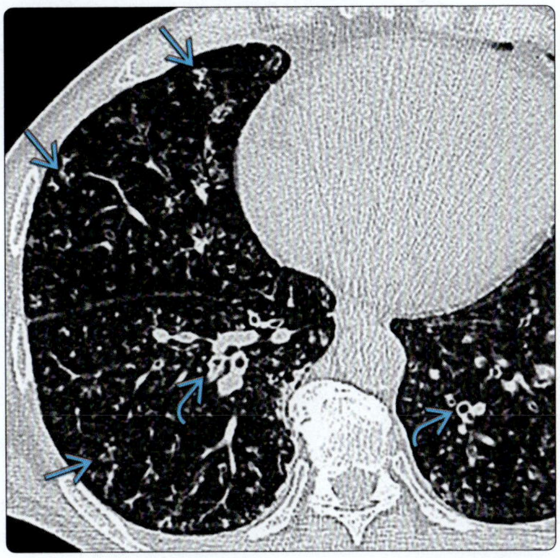

(Left) *Coronal NECT of a patient with an aspirated foreign body (i.e., dental crown) lodged in the left upper lobe bronchus* ➡ *is shown. Foreign bodies are a common source of wheezing.* **(Right)** *Axial HRCT of a patient with diffuse aspiration bronchiolitis shows extensive tree-in-bud opacities* ➡ *and bronchial wall thickening* ➡*. Diffuse aspiration bronchiolitis often results from recurrent small quantities of aspiration, which may not be clinically apparent. A high index of suspicion is often required for the diagnosis.*

Airway Obstruction

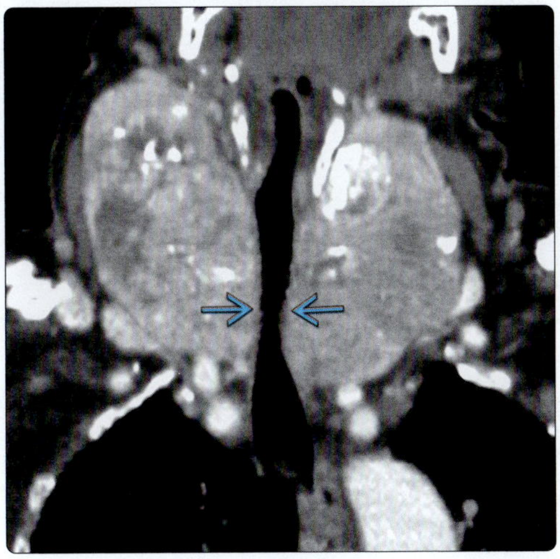

Airway Obstruction

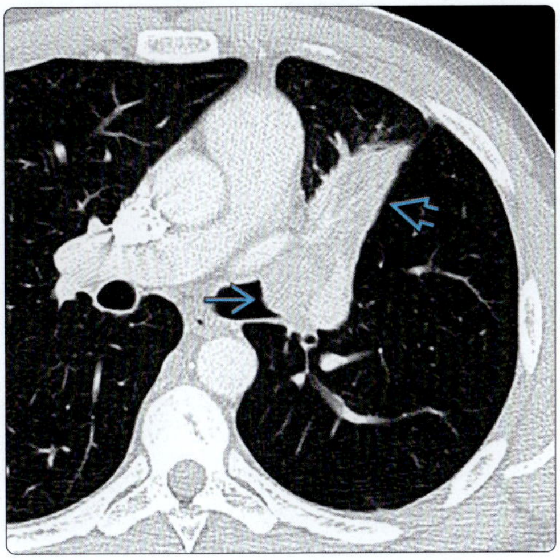

(Left) *Curved planar reformation CECT of a patient with goiter shows extrathoracic smooth segmental tracheal narrowing* ➡*, which is surrounded by heterogeneously enhancing thyroid tissue with intrinsic calcifications.* **(Right)** *Axial CECT of a patient with carcinoid tumor shows an endoluminal mass* ➡ *with left upper lobe atelectasis* ➡*. Carcinoid tumors typically exhibit an endoluminal component often referred to as the "tip of the iceberg" sign.*

Bronchiectasis

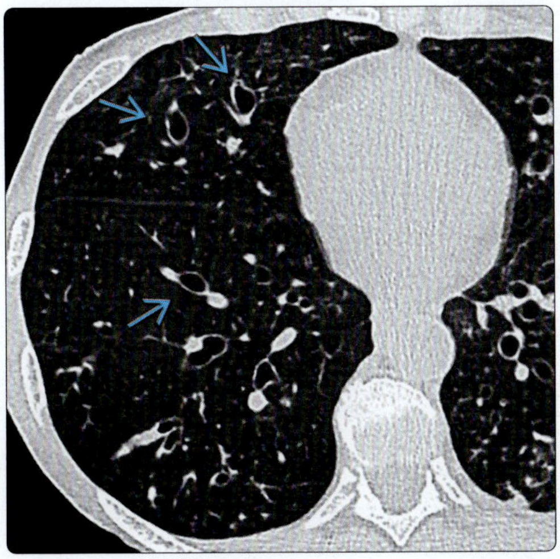

Eosinophilic Granulomatosis With Polyangiitis

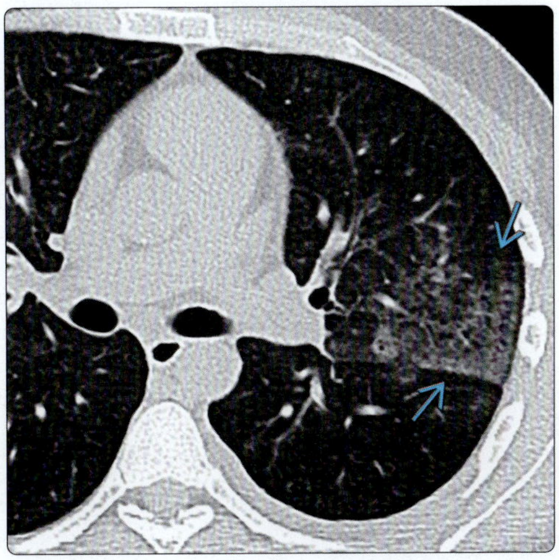

(Left) *Axial HRCT of a patient with bronchiectasis shows diffuse bronchial dilatation with loss of the normal bronchoarterial ratio* ➡*.* **(Right)** *Axial NECT of a patient with eosinophilic granulomatosis with polyangiitis shows left upper lobe ground-glass opacities* ➡*. This entity occurs almost always in the context of asthma and often demonstrates migratory opacities, which are evident on serial imaging. Interlobular septal thickening is also a common feature.*

SECTION 2

Lungs and Airspaces

Approach to Lungs and Airspaces

General Imaging Patterns

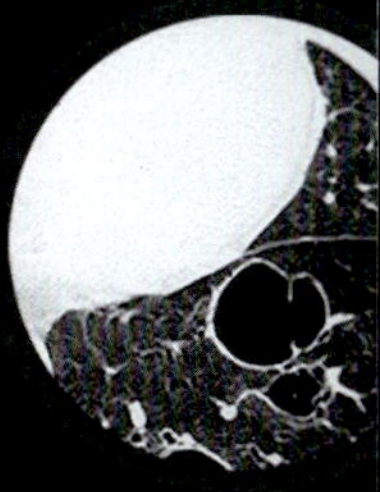

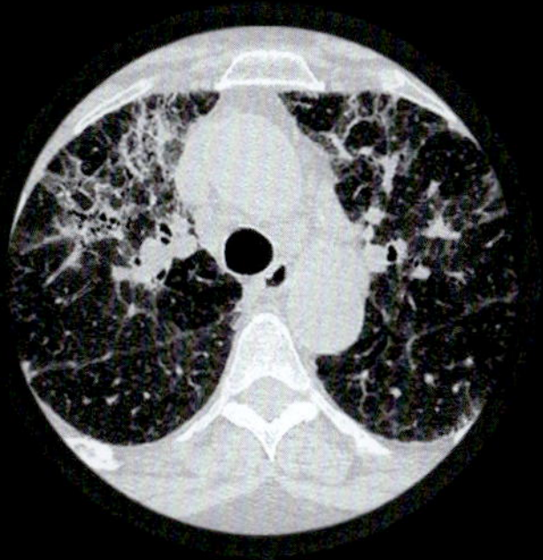

Modality-Specific Imaging Findings: Radiography

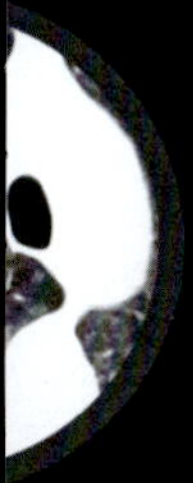

Modality-Specific Imaging Findings: Computed Tomography

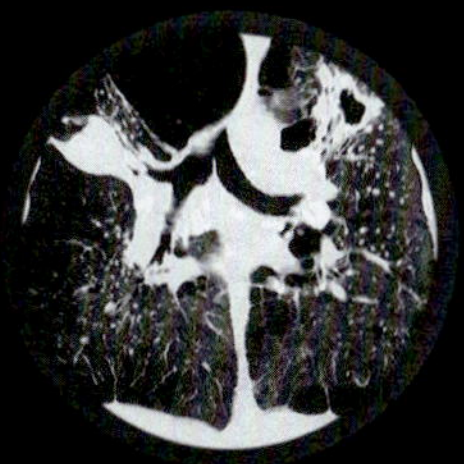

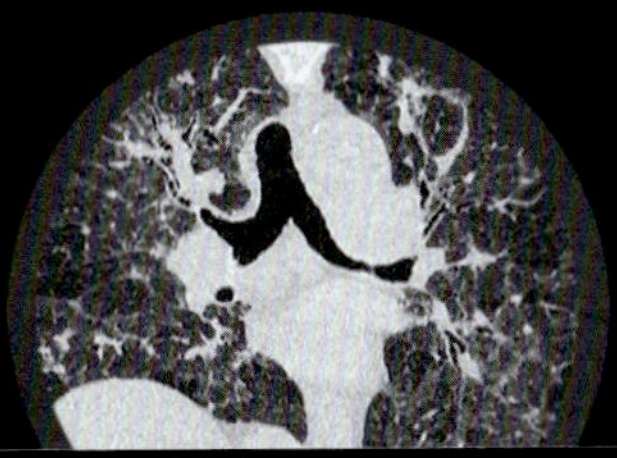

Anatomic Considerations

The lungs are paired structures located on either side of the mediastinum. The lungs are lined by visceral pleura, are freely mobile within the pleural space, and are anchored medially at the hila and pulmonary ligaments. Each lobe is supplied by a lobar bronchus and its accompanying pulmonary artery. Lobes are divided into segments supplied by segmental bronchi and their accompanying pulmonary arteries.

Imaging Normal Lungs

The normal lungs are radiographically lucent. Pulmonary vessels are visible as branching tapered tubular structures that become inconspicuous as they approach the lung periphery. Large airways are visible in the central lung and manifest as thin-walled air-filled tapered tubular branching structures. Airways are not normally visible in the lung periphery. The right lung is larger than the left. Lobar anatomy may be visualized on radiography via identification of interlobar fissures. As chest radiographs are obtained at end inspiration, they provide an imaging assessment of total lung capacity.

CT allows assessment of the pulmonary parenchyma and optimal visualization of the airways and their accompanying vessels. The normal lung exhibits air attenuation and its underlying architecture (airways, vessels, fissures) is easily identified and characterized.

Imaging Abnormal Lungs: Radiography

Emphysema and chronic obstructive pulmonary disease may manifest with large or hyperexpanded lung volume on radiography. Interstitial edema and chronic infiltrative fibrotic lung diseases may manifest with low lung volume. Volume loss may be focal and secondary to subsegmental, segmental, &/or lobar atelectasis. Lobar atelectasis may manifest as decreased ipsilateral lung volume, increased pulmonary opacity, fissural displacement, and hyperexpansion of the unaffected ipsilateral lobe/lobes. Signs of neoplastic lobar collapse include the *Luftsichel sign* and the *reverse S-sign of Golden*. Recognition of these radiographic signs should prompt further assessment for exclusion of a centrally obstructing tumor.

Abnormalities of the lungs and airspaces may be focal or diffuse and may manifest as consolidations, masses, and nodules that may demonstrate calcification &/or cavitation. Consolidations may exhibit air bronchograms in which branching tubular lucent airways course through opaque lung parenchyma. Pulmonary opacities may also demonstrate the *silhouette sign* in which mediastinal &/or diaphragmatic interfaces are obscured by adjacent airspace disease. The pulmonary airspaces are the gas-containing portions of the lung, and their opacification generally signifies alveolar filling with disease products, such as edema fluid, purulent material, hemorrhage, lipoprotein, and inflammatory or neoplastic cells.

Imaging Abnormal Lungs: CT

Chest CT allows accurate localization and characterization of diseases of the lungs and airspaces and determination of the anatomic distribution of these pulmonary diseases. Atelectatic lung generally exhibits high attenuation, particularly in contrast-enhanced CT. Low-attenuation areas within atelectatic lung should raise suspicion for intrinsic pulmonary abnormalities, including pneumonia and pulmonary nodules or masses. CT allows direct visualization and assessment of centrally obstructing lesions in patients with lobar collapse and enables identification of endoluminal content related to mucus plugging as the cause of the central obstruction.

Consolidations may exhibit intrinsic air bronchograms, low attenuation, &/or cavitation. Consolidation may be associated with normal lung volume, volume loss, or lobar expansion. The latter characteristically occurs in cases of bacterial pneumonia secondary to *Klebsiella* and may occur in postobstructive pneumonia distal to endobronchial malignancy. In the past, the term "infiltrate" has been used to signify consolidation, but its use is not currently recommended. CT allows further characterization of consolidations detected on radiography and identification of useful imaging signs. These include the *halo sign* in which a nodule or consolidation is surrounded by ground-glass opacity, which usually correlates with hemorrhage, the *reversed halo sign* in which ground-glass opacity is surrounded by a ring of consolidation characteristic of organizing pneumonia, and perilobular distribution in which airspace disease is distributed about the periphery of secondary pulmonary lobules, also characteristic of organizing pneumonia.

Pulmonary masses are defined by their size > 3 cm and are often of malignant etiology. Pulmonary nodules are rounded opacities ≤ 3 cm that may exhibit variable border characteristics and are generally classified as solid, part-solid or nonsolid (or ground-glass). Solid nodules may exhibit intrinsic calcification, which may help categorize them as benign. Nodule spiculation and polylobular morphology raise suspicion for malignancy. Many solid nodules remain indeterminate. Acinar nodules exhibit poorly defined borders and may demonstrate ground-glass attenuation. Micronodules refer to rounded opacities that measure 3 mm or less and are often described based on their distribution with respect to the secondary pulmonary lobule as centrilobular, perilymphatic, or random.

CT also allows identification of abnormal pulmonary lucencies and the characterization and quantification of emphysema, which can be categorized as centrilobular, paraseptal, or panlobular. Centrilobular emphysema is the most common type and manifests as upper lobe-predominant pulmonary lucencies with imperceptible walls and a central "dot" that represents the lobular artery within the affected secondary pulmonary lobule. Centrilobular emphysema must be distinguished from cystic lung disease in which the pulmonary lucencies are bound by a soft tissue wall, which may be thin and smooth or thick and nodular. Additional pulmonary lucencies include pneumatoceles and pulmonary bullae. In the case of cystic lung disease, the distribution and morphologic characteristics of the cysts help formulate an appropriate differential diagnosis. Basilar subpleural cysts that occur in layers with associated architectural distortion and traction bronchiectasis/bronchiolectasis are characteristic of honeycombing, the imaging hallmark of usual interstitial pneumonia. Clustered basilar bronchiectasis may mimic honeycomb cysts when viewed on axial images.

Summary

Chest imaging is of paramount importance in the detection and characterization of diseases of the lungs and airspaces. Many airspace diseases are readily diagnosed on radiography. Chest CT is reserved for further characterization of confounding pulmonary opacities and helps identify important underlying findings, such as malignancy.

Consolidation | **Consolidation**

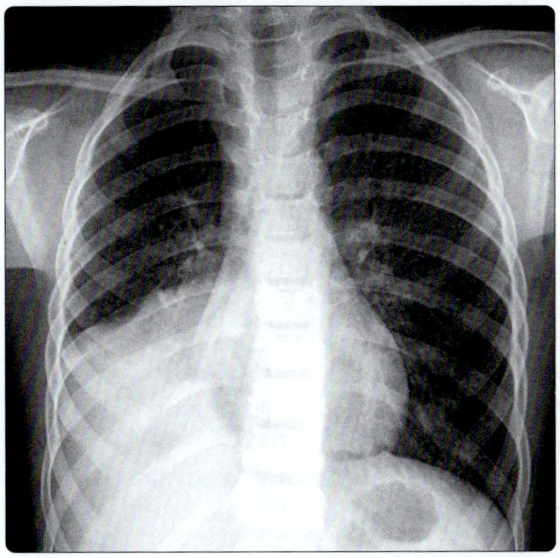

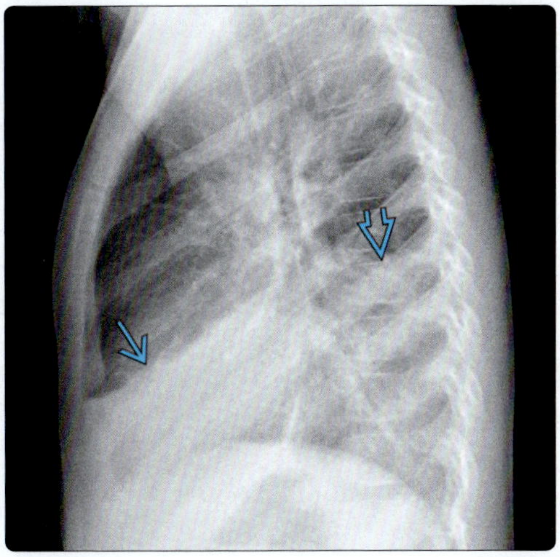

(Left) *PA chest radiograph of a 6-year-old boy with cough and fever shows middle and right lower lobe consolidations that exhibit the silhouette sign with obscuration of the right hemidiaphragm and right cardiac border.* **(Right)** *Lateral chest radiograph of the same patient shows middle → and right lower lobe ⇨ consolidations, consistent with pneumonia. The right hemidiaphragm is completely obscured by adjacent airspace disease. Recognition of the silhouette sign allows identification and localization of airspace abnormalities.*

Halo Sign | **Cavitation and Cellular Bronchiolitis**

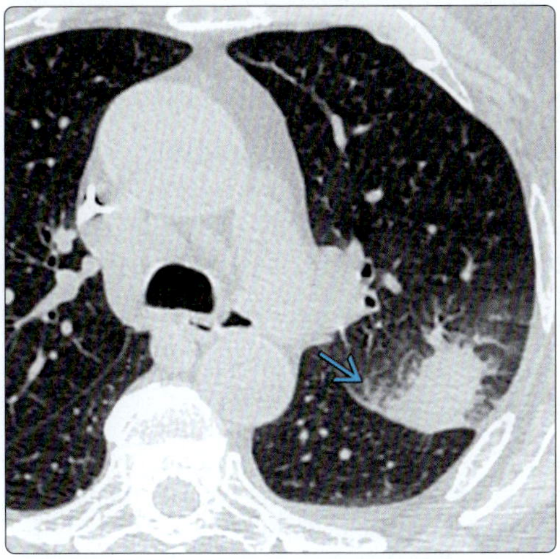

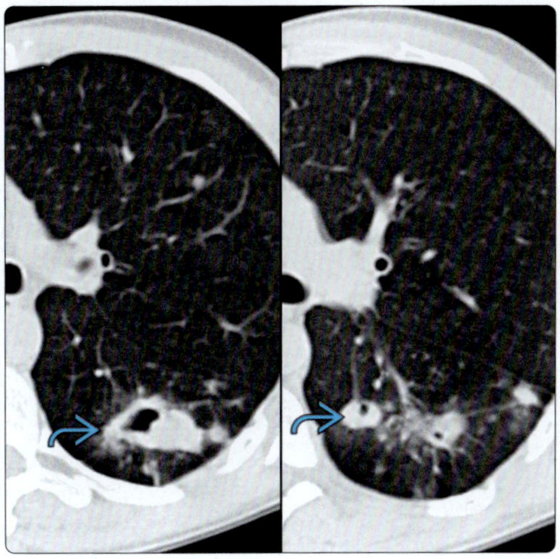

(Left) *Axial NECT of an 80-year-old man with leukemia, febrile leukopenia, and angioinvasive fungal disease shows a left upper lobe consolidation with surrounding ground-glass opacity →, the so-called halo sign. Recognition of the halo sign in this setting helps suggest the diagnosis.* **(Right)** *Axial NECT of a 32-year-old man with HIV shows left lower lobe cavitary nodules ↪ with surrounding cellular bronchiolitis concerning for active tuberculosis but diagnosed as nontuberculous mycobacterial infection.*

Acinar Nodules | **Cysts and Nodules**

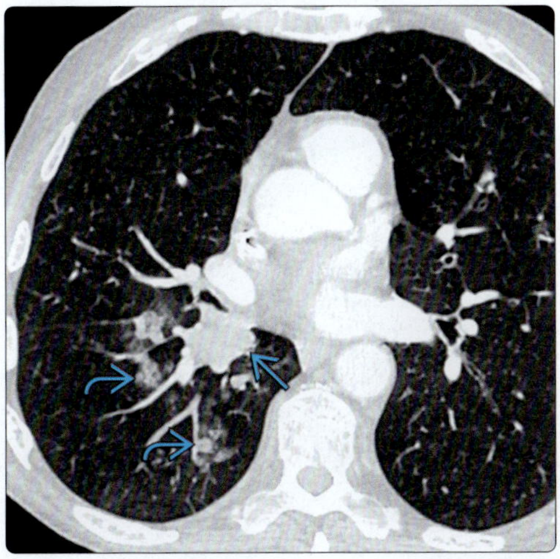

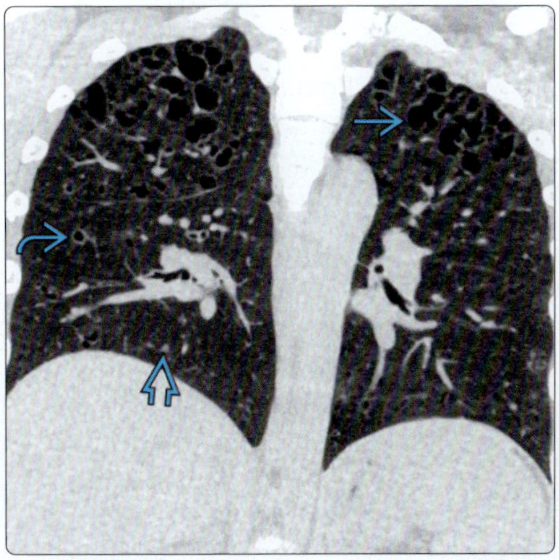

(Left) *Axial CECT of a 56-year-old man with right lower lobe lung cancer → shows a polylobular soft tissue mass that obstructs the right lower lobe bronchi. Note surrounding clustered acinar nodules ↪, consistent with postobstructive pneumonia.* **(Right)** *Coronal NECT of a 22-year-old woman smoker with chest pain and dyspnea shows bilateral upper lung zone-predominant bizarre-shaped → and thick-walled cysts ↪ and small solid nodules ⇨. The CT findings are typical of pulmonary Langerhans cell histiocytosis.*

DIFFERENTIAL DIAGNOSIS

Common

- Pneumonia
- Aspiration
- Edema

Less Common

- Hemorrhage

Rare but Important

- Lung Cancer

ESSENTIAL INFORMATION

Key Differential Diagnosis Issues

- Acinus
  - Synonyms: Acinar shadow, airspace nodule
  - Anatomy
    - Lung structures distal to terminal bronchiole; supplied by 1st-order respiratory bronchioles
      - Respiratory bronchioles
      - Alveolar ducts
      - Alveolar sacs
      - Alveoli
      - Accompanying vessels and connective tissue
      - 2-25 acini in secondary pulmonary lobule
  - Function
    - Largest lung structural unit in which all airways participate in gas exchange
  - Size
    - Diameter of 5-10 mm
  - Imaging
    - Poorly-marginated nodular opacities
      - Consolidation within multiple acini
    - 5-8 mm
    - Poorly visualized on radiography
    - Optimally evaluated on thin-section CT/HRCT
      - Centrilobular location
      - Consolidation &/or ground-glass opacity

Helpful Clues for Common Diagnoses

- **Pneumonia**
  - Acinar nodules may be early manifestation of infection
    - Clustered or multifocal
  - May be identified adjacent to pulmonary consolidation related to pneumonia
  - Bronchopneumonia
    - Multifocal inflammatory exudate
    - Centered on inflamed airways
    - Involvement of some acini and sparing of others
- **Aspiration**
  - Synonyms: Aspiration pneumonia, aspiration bronchiolitis
  - Focal or multifocal consolidation; gravitational distribution
  - Endoluminal content related to aspirated material
  - Centrilobular distribution: Nodules, tree-in-bud opacities, acinar nodules
- **Edema**
  - Pulmonary edema: Extravascular lung water
  - Alveolar edema
    - Central perihilar consolidations
    - Solid or ground-glass attenuation acinar nodules
  - ± Septal thickening, pleural effusion, cardiomegaly

Helpful Clues for Less Common Diagnoses

- **Hemorrhage**
  - Dyspnea, cough, ± hemoptysis
  - Bilateral multifocal consolidations and ground-glass opacities
  - Diffuse, localized, centrilobular
    - May be associated with acinar nodules

Helpful Clues for Rare Diagnoses

- **Lung Cancer**
  - Invasive mucinous adenocarcinoma: Typically manifests with consolidation ± subsolid nodules
  - Tracheobronchial dissemination may manifest with multifocal multilobar consolidations &/or acinar nodules

Pneumonia

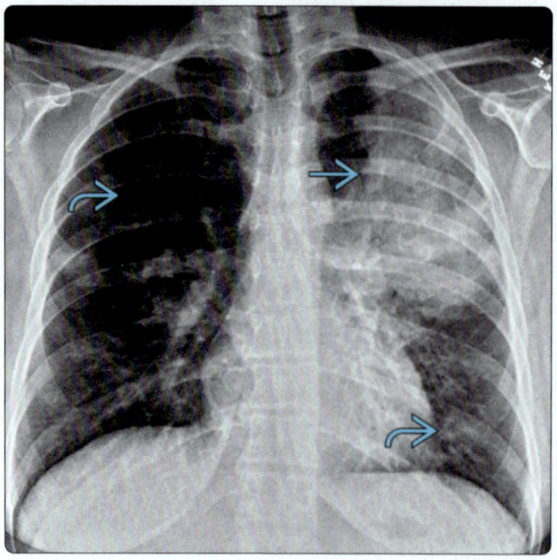

Pneumonia

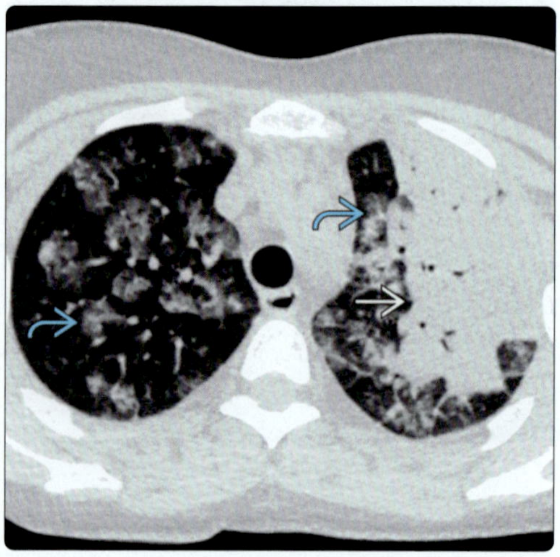

(Left) *PA chest radiograph of a 45-year-old woman with cough, fever, and leukocytosis due to Streptococcus aureus pneumonia shows a left upper lobe consolidation ➔ and multifocal bilateral ill-defined nodules ➔.* **(Right)** *Axial NECT of the same patient shows a dense left upper lobe consolidation ➔ and multifocal acinar nodules ➔ that manifest as centrilobular poorly-marginated ground-glass nodular opacities and consolidations. Acinar nodules may be associated with consolidations related to pulmonary infection.*

Pneumonia

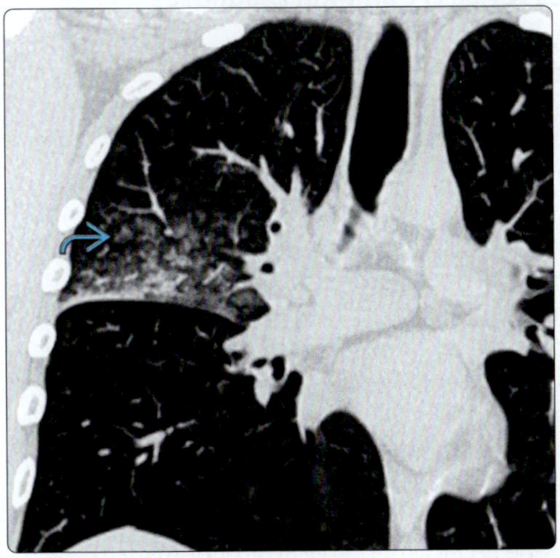

Pneumonia

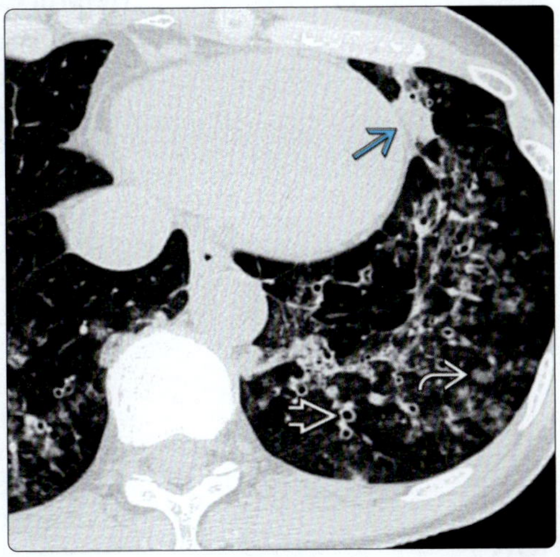

(Left) *Coronal NECT of a 36-year-old man with fever and cough shows right upper lobe bronchopneumonia that manifests with clustered centrilobular acinar nodules ⇨.* **(Right)** *Axial NECT of a 67-year-old woman with fever, cough, and chest pain shows multifocal pulmonary infection manifesting with basilar consolidations ⇨, acinar nodules ⇨, and bronchial wall thickening ⇨. Bronchopneumonia denotes a multifocal exudate centered on inflamed airways with patchy involvement of adjacent acini.*

Aspiration

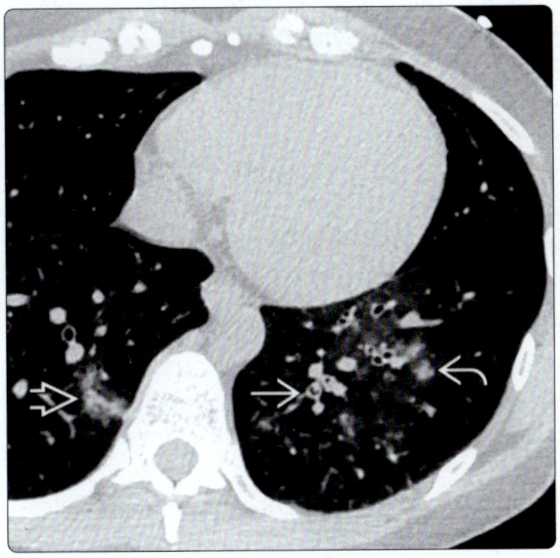

Edema

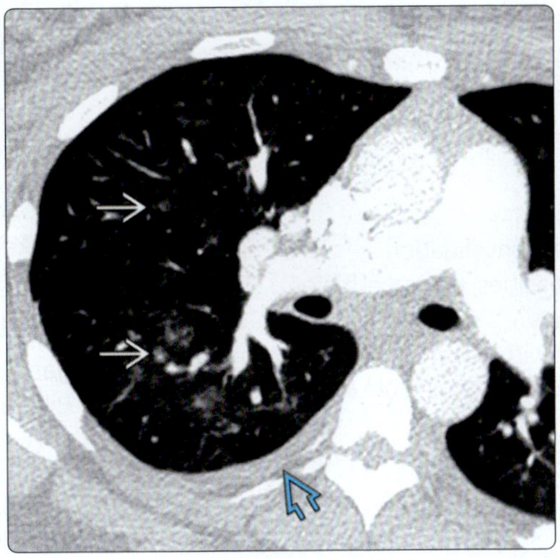

(Left) *Axial NECT of a 46-year-old man with aspiration pneumonia shows multifocal lower lobe consolidations ⇨ and acinar nodules ⇨ on a background of ground-glass opacity. Note right lower lobe bronchial wall thickening and endoluminal content ⇨ related to aspirated material.* **(Right)** *Axial NECT of a 32-year-old woman with post-partum cardiomyopathy and pulmonary edema shows multifocal acinar nodules that manifest as rounded centrilobular ground-glass opacities ⇨. Note small right pleural effusion ⇨.*

Hemorrhage

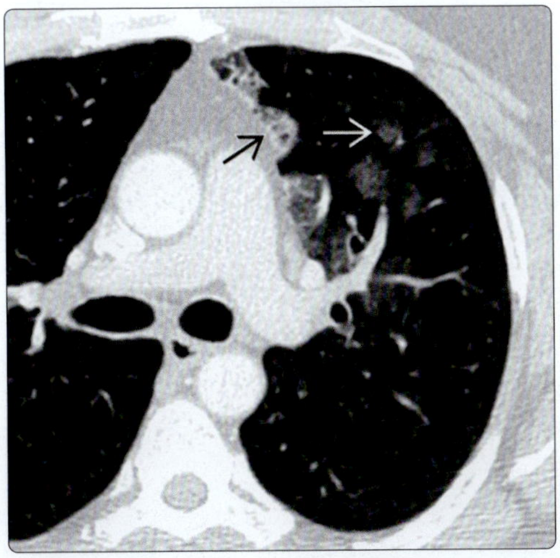

Lung Cancer

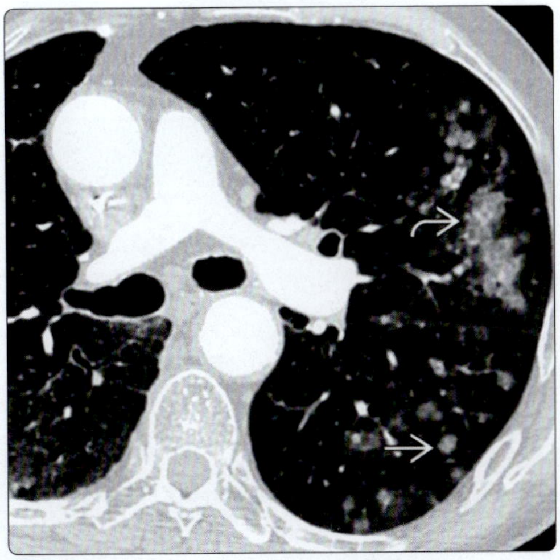

(Left) *Axial CECT of a 50-year-old man with hemoptysis and alveolar hemorrhage shows multifocal peripheral heterogeneous consolidations ⇨ and ground-glass opacity acinar nodules ⇨ that represent intraalveolar blood products.* **(Right)** *Axial CECT of a 70-year-old man with diffuse tracheobronchial dissemination of a right lower lobe invasive acinar and papillary adenocarcinoma (not shown) shows multifocal tumor in the left lung that manifests with scattered ⇨ and coalescent ⇨ acinar nodules.*

DIFFERENTIAL DIAGNOSIS

Common

- Pneumonia
- Non-Obstructive Atelectasis
- Pulmonary Edema

Less Common

- Malignancy
  - Adenocarcinoma
  - Lymphoma
- Pulmonary Hemorrhage
- Acute Respiratory Distress Syndrome

Rare but Important

- Organizing Pneumonia
- Sarcoidosis

ESSENTIAL INFORMATION

Key Differential Diagnosis Issues

- Air bronchograms more frequent in malignant solitary pulmonary nodules or masses than in benign processes
- Persistent consolidation with air bronchogram ± respiratory symptoms should be investigated to exclude malignancy

Helpful Clues for Common Diagnoses

- **Pneumonia**
  - Acute respiratory symptoms
  - Dense lobar or segmental consolidation
    - Associated airspace opacities, pleural effusion
- **Non-Obstructive Atelectasis**
  - Consolidation associated with volume loss (displacement of fissures, elevated ipsilateral hemidiaphragm, vessel and airway crowding)
  - Etiologies: Pleural effusion, pneumothorax, radiation, surfactant deficiency
- **Pulmonary Edema**
  - Alveolar edema: Central consolidations with "batwing" configuration
  - Perihilar haze, peribronchial cuffing, septal lines
  - Cardiomegaly, pleural effusions

Helpful Clues for Less Common Diagnoses

- **Malignancy**
  - **Adenocarcinoma**
    - Subsolid (ground-glass or part-solid) or solid nodule
      - Air bronchograms represent intrinsic distorted/dilated airways
    - Pneumonic-type adenocarcinoma (invasive mucinous)
      - Multilobar bilateral dense consolidation ± peripheral nodules, ground-glass opacities, cavitation, bulging fissures
    - Air bronchogram is much less frequent in squamous cell carcinoma
  - **Lymphoma**
    - Primary: Rarely non-Hodgkin lymphoma, secondary Hodgkin and non-Hodgkin lymphoma relatively common
    - Low-grade B-cell lymphoma, 80% of primary pulmonary lymphoma
    - Nodule(s)/mass(es), consolidation(s)
    - Lymphadenopathy: Secondary lymphoma
- **Acute Respiratory Distress Syndrome**
  - Diffuse bilateral coalescent opacities; may persist for days to weeks
- **Pulmonary Hemorrhage**
  - Postbiopsy hemorrhage ~ 40% of cases, segmental or lobar opacities
  - Leukemia, lymphoma: Bilateral airspace opacities with central and basilar predominance, spare lung bases

Helpful Clues for Rare Diagnoses

- **Organizing Pneumonia**
  - Bilateral or unilateral, patchy airspace consolidation, peribronchial, perilobular, reversed halo sign
- **Sarcoidosis**
  - Alveolar sarcoidosis; mass-like peribronchial opacities
  - Peribronchovascular, subpleural, and septal nodules
  - Bilateral, symmetric hilar and mediastinal lymphadenopathy

Pneumonia

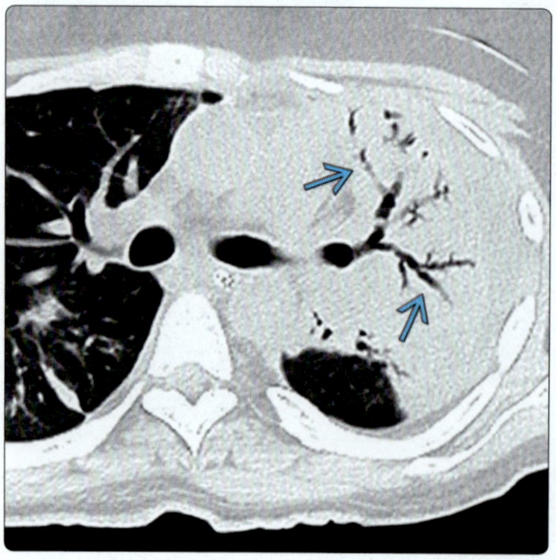

Non-Obstructive Atelectasis

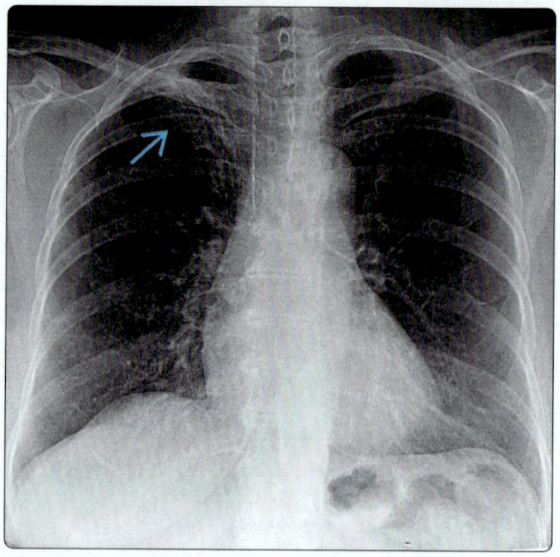

(Left) *Axial NECT of a 45-year-old woman with acute respiratory symptoms shows a dense left upper lobe consolidation with intrinsic air bronchograms ➔, consistent with pneumonia.* **(Right)** *PA chest radiograph of a 62-year-old man with tongue carcinoma shows a right upper lobe opacity ➔ with an intrinsic air bronchogram and volume loss, consistent with non-obstructive cicatricial atelectasis secondary to prior irradiation. Pleural effusion and pneumothorax are also commonly associated with non-obstructive atelectasis.*

Pulmonary Edema

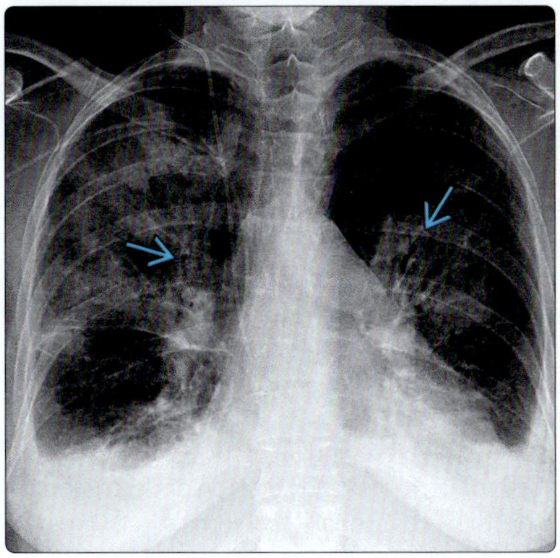

Adenocarcinoma

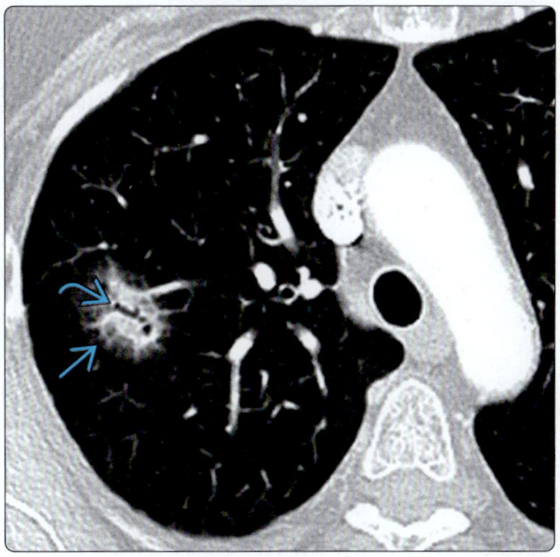

(Left) *PA chest radiograph shows multifocal bilateral predominantly central pulmonary consolidations with intrinsic air bronchograms, consistent with the "batwing" pattern of alveolar pulmonary edema. Note cardiomegaly and small bilateral pleural effusions.* **(Right)** *Axial CECT of a 42-year-old woman shows a part-solid nodule with an intrinsic air bronchogram. Biopsy confirmed adenocarcinoma. The presence of an air bronchogram within a lung nodule may indicate a high likelihood of malignancy, specifically adenocarcinoma.*

Adenocarcinoma

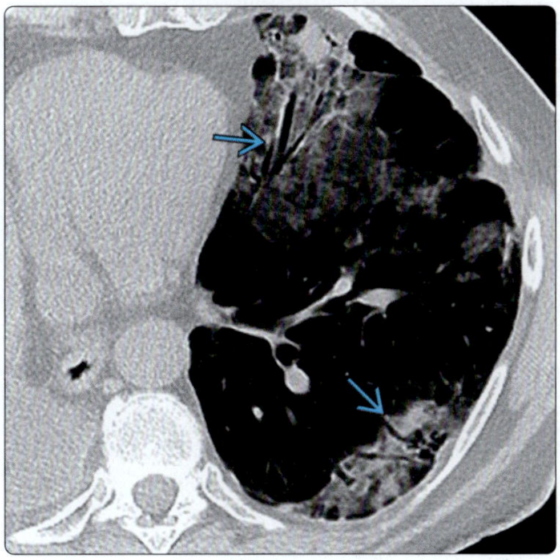

Lymphoma

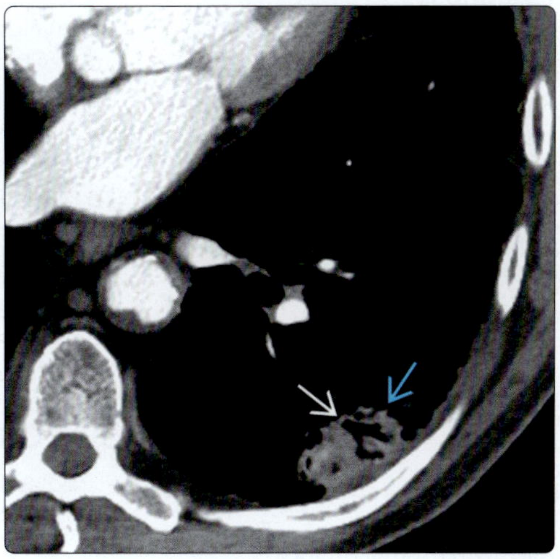

(Left) *Axial NECT of a 63-year-old woman shows multifocal ground-glass opacities and consolidations with intrinsic air bronchograms in the left lung. Biopsy confirmed multifocal pneumonic-type adenocarcinoma, frequently confused with pneumonia.* **(Right)** *Axial CECT of a 60-year-old man shows a left lower lobe nodule with an intrinsic air bronchogram. Biopsy confirmed a low-grade B-cell non-Hodgkin lymphoma, the most common type of primary pulmonary lymphoma.*

Pulmonary Hemorrhage

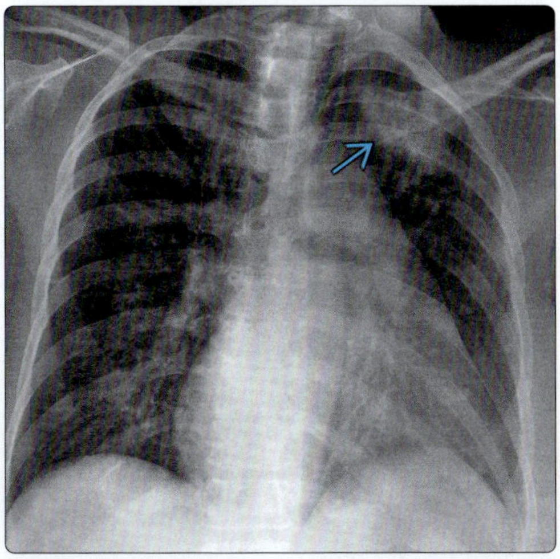

Organizing Pneumonia

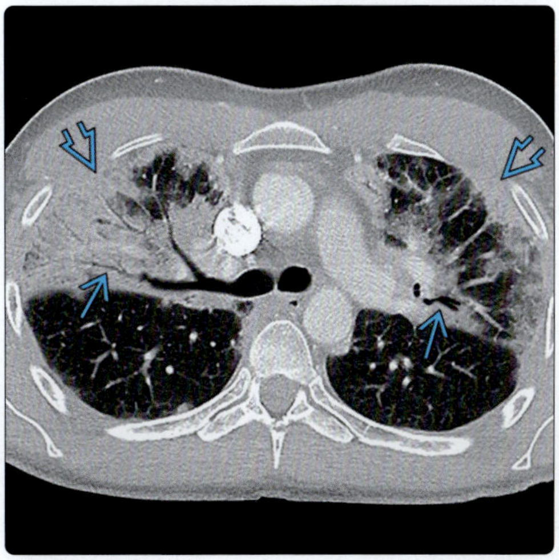

(Left) *AP chest radiograph of 54-year-old woman who underwent biopsy of a left upper lobe nodule shows a dense left upper lobe consolidation with air bronchograms, consistent with pulmonary hemorrhage, which is frequently seen after biopsy.* **(Right)** *Axial CECT of a 46-year-old woman with ovarian cancer undergoing targeted therapy shows bilateral upper lobe subpleural consolidations with intrinsic air bronchograms, consistent with biopsy-proven organizing pneumonia.*

Apical Opacity

DIFFERENTIAL DIAGNOSIS

Common

- Apical Scarring
- Pneumonia

Less Common

- Radiation Fibrosis
- Pancoast Tumor

Rare but Important

- Metastasis
- Hematoma

ESSENTIAL INFORMATION

Key Differential Diagnosis Issues

- Bilateral, symmetric apical opacities are highly suggestive of a benign process
- Unilateral or asymmetric opacity associated with rib destruction &/or neurologic symptoms suggest malignancy

Helpful Clues for Common Diagnoses

- Apical Scarring
  - Associated with advanced age or previous infection
  - Wedge-shaped, triangular, or crescentic fibrous subpleural opacity
  - Prominence of extrapleural fat
  - Sequela of tuberculosis (TB)
    - Peribronchial fibrosis, architectural distortion, traction bronchiectasis, volume loss, residual cavitation, pleural and parenchymal calcification
- Pneumonia
  - Acute onset
  - Patchy opacities + air bronchograms, bilateral or unilateral
    - May be obscured by upper ribs
    - Pleural effusion
  - Atypical infection can be mistaken for malignancy
    - Mass-like opacity, cavitation, and chest wall involvement
      - □ Nocardiosis, actinomycosis: Immunocompromised patients, chronic bronchitis, emphysema, alcoholism, poor oral hygiene
  - TB: Cavitation, consolidation, tree-in-bud opacities

Helpful Clues for Less Common Diagnoses

- Radiation Fibrosis
  - Chronic consolidation associated with air bronchograms
  - Volume loss, bronchiectasis, pleural thickening
    - Unilateral: History of radiated supraclavicular malignancy; breast and lung cancer
    - Bilateral: Head and neck carcinoma, lymphoma
- Pancoast Tumor
  - Non-small cell lung cancer (adenocarcinoma, squamous cell carcinoma)
  - Apical mass, pleural thickening
  - Rib (1st-3rd) &/or vertebral body erosion or destruction
  - Horner syndrome: Ptosis, miosis, anhidrosis

Helpful Clues for Rare Diagnoses

- Metastasis
  - Direct extension from supraclavicular or mediastinal malignancy or hematogenous metastasis
  - Solitary pulmonary nodule/opacity + known malignancy: Probability of metastasis ~ 25%
  - Likelihood of metastasis increases if additional nodules are present
  - Associated pleural thickening &/or bone erosion
- Hematoma
  - Posttraumatic or iatrogenic extrapleural dissection of blood from mediastinal hemorrhage
  - Look for 1st rib or upper thoracic spine fracture or recent central line placement

SELECTED REFERENCES

1. Nachiappan AC et al: Pulmonary tuberculosis: role of radiology in diagnosis and management. Radiographics. 37(1):52-72, 2017
2. Ghaye B et al: Imaging after radiation therapy of thoracic tumors. Diagn Interv Imaging. 97(10):1037-52, 2016

Apical Scarring

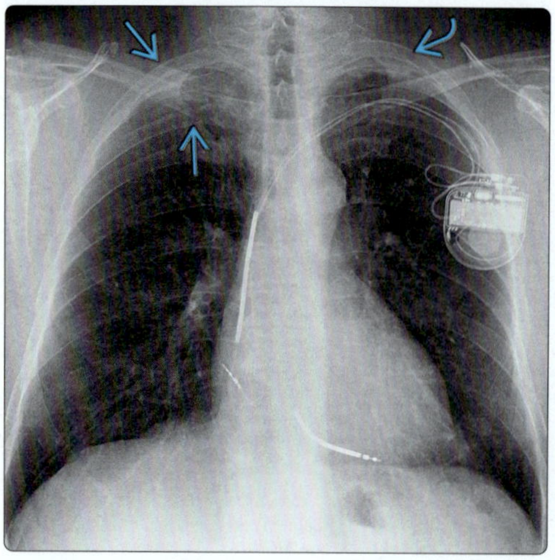

Apical Scarring

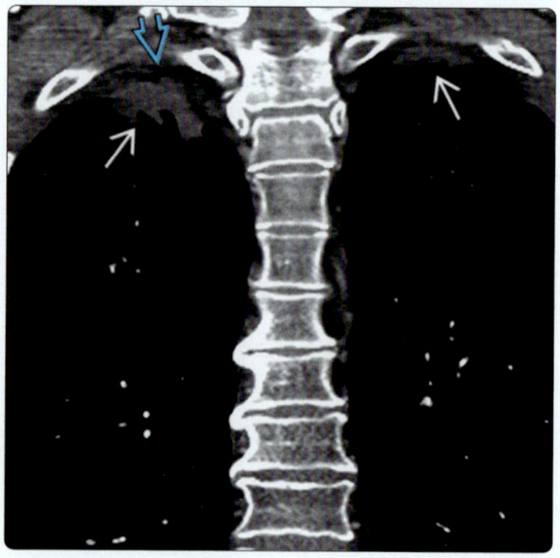

(Left) *PA chest radiograph of a 57-year-old man shows subtle opacity in the right lung apex ⇨ and an irregular opacity in the left lung apex ⇨.* **(Right)** *Coronal NECT of the same patient shows irregular opacities in the lung apices, consistent with fibrosis ➡. Note the presence of prominent extrapleural fat ⇨ that is frequently associated with fibrotic changes in the lung parenchyma. Apical scarring is related to advanced age and previous infection.*

Pneumonia

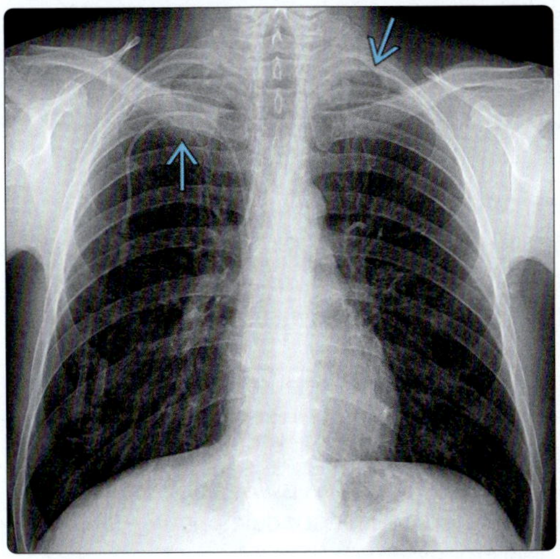

Pneumonia

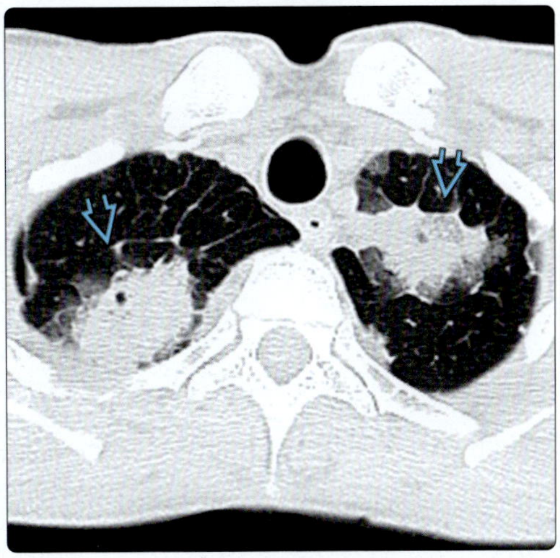

(Left) *PA chest radiograph of a 38-year-old man with a history of leukemia and presenting with acute respiratory symptoms shows subtle opacities in the lung apices ➡ suspicious for multifocal pneumonia.* **(Right)** *Axial NECT of the same patient shows focal dense consolidations in the lung apices surrounded by ground-glass opacities ➡, consistent with multifocal pneumonia. CT is the imaging modality of choice for identifying pneumonia, as apical opacities may be obscured by ribs on radiography.*

Pneumonia

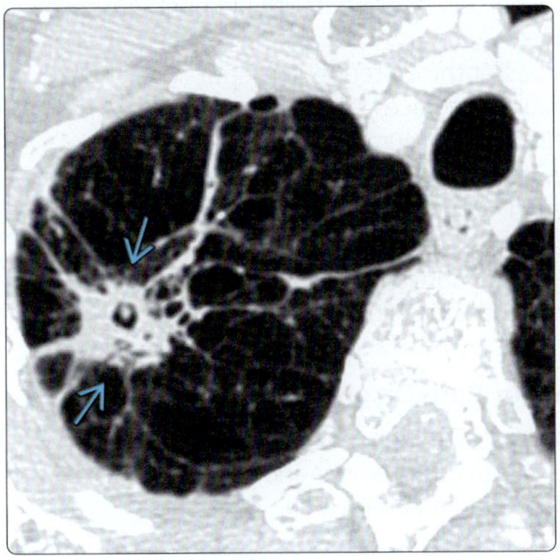

Radiation Fibrosis

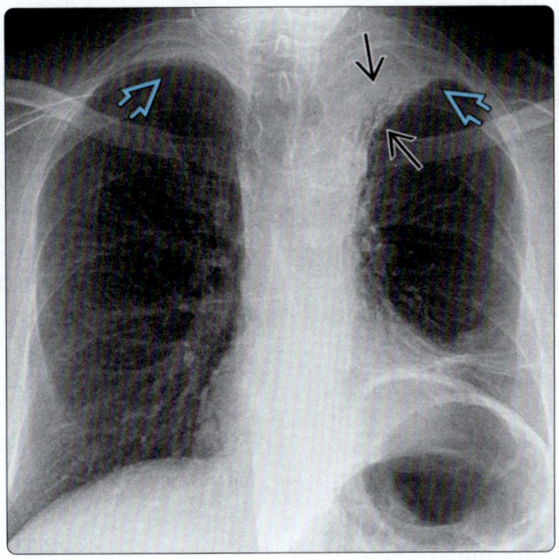

(Left) *Axial CECT of a 58-year-old woman shows a cavitary nodular opacity in the right lung apex ➡. Biopsy demonstrated Nocardia infection, which most commonly affects immunocompromised patients.* **(Right)** *PA chest radiograph of a 63-year-old patient with a history of squamous cell carcinoma of the neck treated with radiation therapy shows dense opacities in the apices ➡ associated with air bronchograms ➡ and volume loss in the left upper lobe, consistent with radiation fibrosis.*

Pancoast Tumor

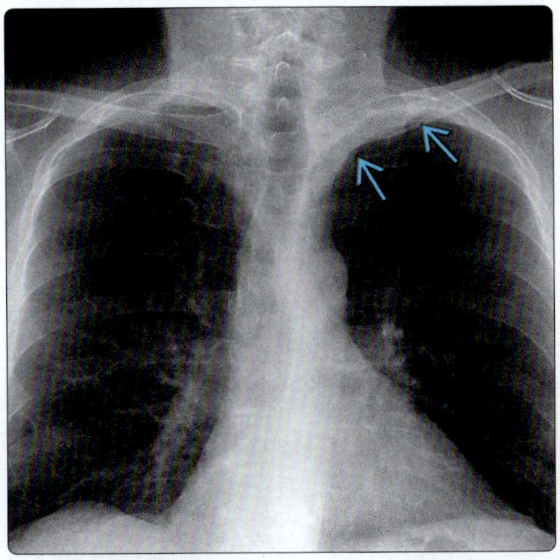

Pancoast Tumor

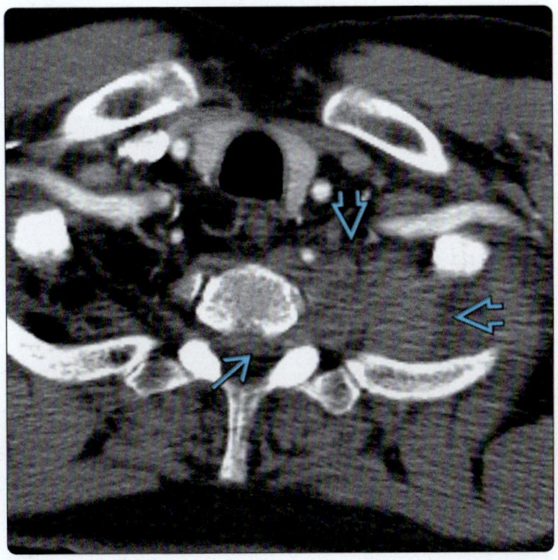

(Left) *PA chest radiograph of a 49-year-old patient with a history of shoulder pain shows a dense and homogeneous opacity in the left lung apex ➡.* **(Right)** *Axial CECT of the same patient shows a soft tissue mass in the left lung apex ➡ extending into the spinal canal ➡. Biopsy demonstrated lung adenocarcinoma. Neurologic symptoms involving the shoulder &/or upper extremity in a patient with an apical opacity strongly suggests malignancy.*

DIFFERENTIAL DIAGNOSIS

Common

- Radiation Fibrosis
- Idiopathic Pulmonary Fibrosis
- Nonspecific Interstitial Pneumonia
- Sarcoidosis

Less Common

- Hypersensitivity Pneumonitis
- Complicated Silicosis
- Asbestosis
- Drug-Induced Lung Disease

Rare but Important

- Acute Respiratory Distress Syndrome
- Tuberculosis

ESSENTIAL INFORMATION

Key Differential Diagnosis Issues

- Architectural distortion: Abnormal displacement of pulmonary structures (bronchi, vessels, fissures, septa) with volume loss; diffuse or localized pulmonary fibrosis

Helpful Clues for Common Diagnoses

- **Radiation Fibrosis**
  - Typically 6-12 months after radiation therapy
  - Consolidation, volume loss, traction bronchiectasis, subpleural reticulation
  - Conforms to radiation pattern: Apical in neck irradiation, apical and along mediastinum in mantle irradiation, subpleural in tangential breast irradiation
- **Idiopathic Pulmonary Fibrosis**
  - Basilar predominant subpleural reticulation, traction bronchiectasis/bronchiolectasis
  - Basilar honeycombing: Subpleural 3- to 10-mm cysts
  - Histology: Usual interstitial pneumonia
- **Nonspecific Interstitial Pneumonia**
  - Basilar ground-glass and reticular opacities, traction bronchiectasis/bronchiolectasis
  - ± subpleural sparing and peribronchovascular fibrosis
  - Absence of honeycombing
- **Sarcoidosis**
  - Upper and mid lung zone predominant volume loss, reticulation, traction bronchiectasis ± honeycombing
  - Peribronchovascular mass-like fibrosis
  - Upper lung zone bullae, cysts

Helpful Clues for Less Common Diagnoses

- **Hypersensitivity Pneumonitis (HP)**
  - Inflammatory response to inhaled organic antigens
  - Cluster 2 HP: Clubbing, hypoxemia, restrictive pulmonary function
  - Peribronchovascular &/or subpleural reticulation ± honeycombing
- **Complicated Silicosis**
  - Progressive massive fibrosis: Mass-like coalescent upper lung zone lesions with silicotic nodules, fibrosis, and paracicatricial emphysema
  - Lymphadenopathy; may exhibit Ca++, ± eggshell Ca++
- **Asbestosis**
  - Pulmonary fibrosis associated with pulmonary asbestos bodies/fibers
  - Posterior basilar thick interlobular septa, intralobular lines, irregular interfaces, parenchymal bands
  - Pleural thickening, pleural plaques
- **Drug-Induced Lung Disease**
  - Patterns of disease: Diffuse alveolar damage, HP, eosinophilic pneumonia, diffuse alveolar hemorrhage
  - Nonspecific interstitial pneumonia: Basilar ground-glass and reticular opacities, traction bronchiectasis/bronchiolectasis, no honeycombing

Helpful Clues for Rare Diagnoses

- **Acute Respiratory Distress Syndrome (ARDS)**
  - Late phase: Reticular opacities and architectural distortion in nondependent lung
- **Tuberculosis**
  - Chronic upper lung zone bronchiectasis and volume loss
  - Cavitation + bronchiolitis should suggest active disease

Radiation Fibrosis

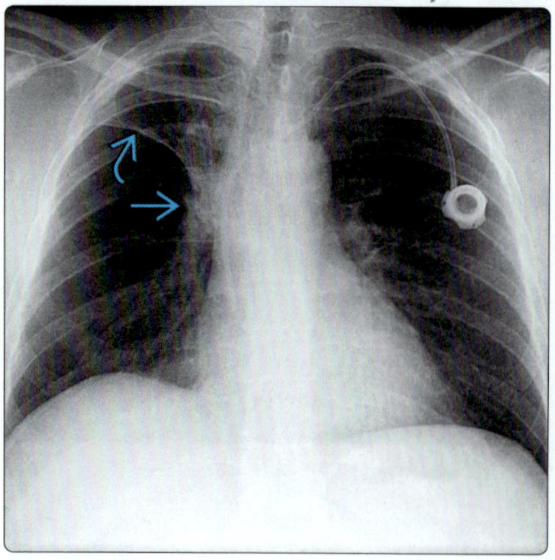

Radiation Fibrosis

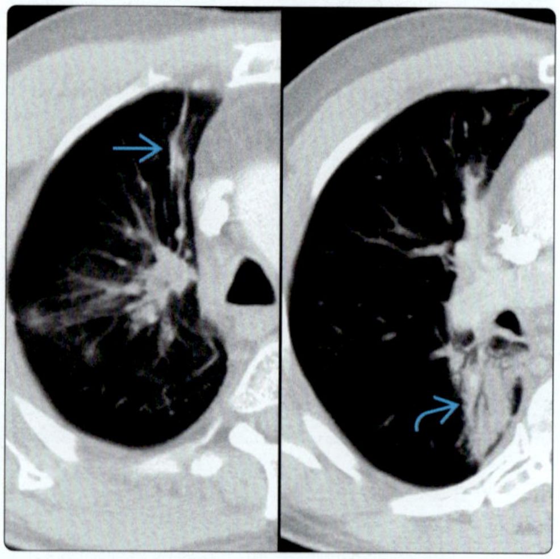

(Left) *PA chest radiograph of a 48-year-old man with right upper lobe lung cancer shows changes related to radiation therapy. Right upper lobe volume loss manifests with elevation of the right hilum* ➡ *and minor fissure* ⮫ *and increased density of the affected lobe.* **(Right)** *Composite image with axial CECT of the same patient shows right lung paramediastinal radiation fibrosis that manifests with linear* ➡ *and mass-like* ⮫ *fibrosis, the latter with intrinsic air bronchograms.*

Idiopathic Pulmonary Fibrosis

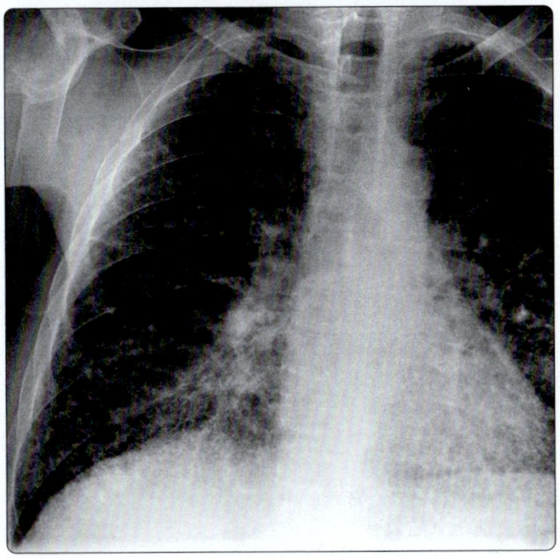

Idiopathic Pulmonary Fibrosis

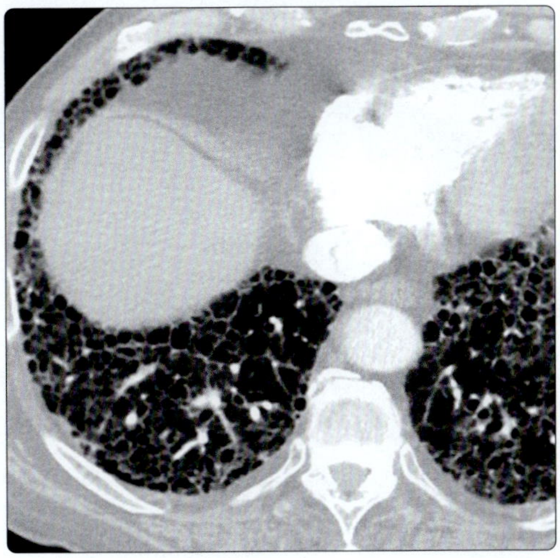

(Left) *Coned-down PA chest radiograph of a 74-year-old man with insidious onset of chronic dyspnea shows profuse, bilateral, peripheral, and basilar predominant reticular opacities.* **(Right)** *Axial CECT of the same patient shows basilar predominant interlobular septal thickening, intralobular lines, and honeycombing. The findings are best characterized as the typical usual interstitial pneumonia CT pattern and are consistent with the clinically suspected diagnosis of idiopathic pulmonary fibrosis.*

Nonspecific Interstitial Pneumonia

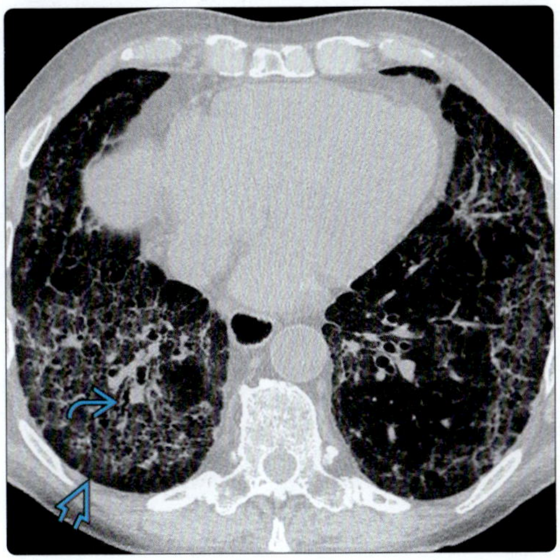

Nonspecific Interstitial Pneumonia

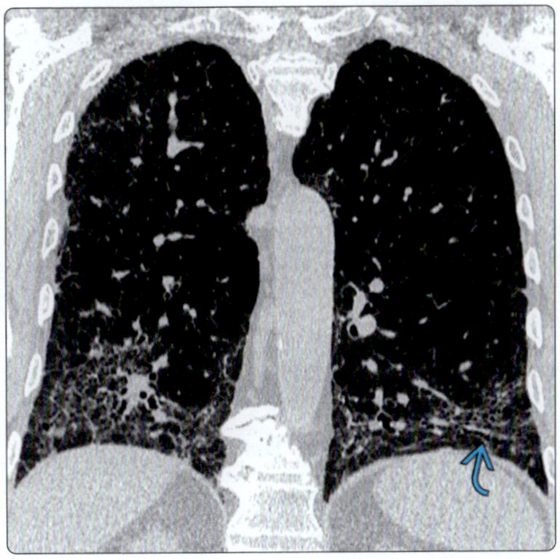

(Left) *Axial NECT of a 76-year-old man with scleroderma shows asymmetric basilar predominant interstitial fibrosis characterized by interlobular septal thickening, intralobular lines, and traction bronchiolectasis. Note sparing of the subpleural lung parenchyma in the absence of honeycombing.* **(Right)** *Coronal NECT of the same patient shows basilar predominant pulmonary involvement characterized by basilar reticulation and traction bronchiolectasis, typical of nonspecific interstitial pneumonia.*

Sarcoidosis

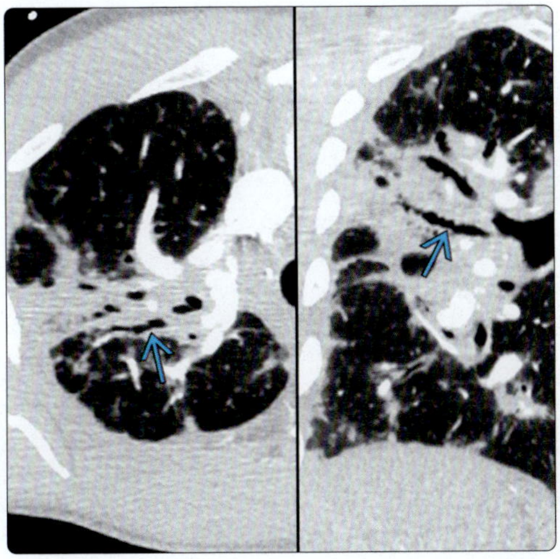

Sarcoidosis

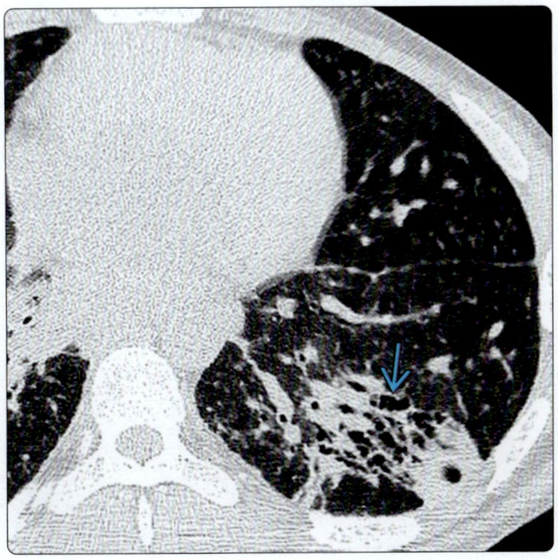

(Left) *Composite image with axial (left) and coronal (right) CECT of a 38-year-old man with sarcoidosis shows upper and mid lung zone peribronchovascular mass-like fibrosis with intrinsic traction bronchiectasis.* **(Right)** *Axial HRCT of a 29-year-old man with end-stage sarcoidosis shows peribronchovascular architectural distortion manifesting as basilar mass-like fibrosis with traction bronchiectasis. Note sparing of most of the visualized subpleural lung and absence of honeycombing.*

(Left) *Axial NECT of a 70-year-old bird fancier with cluster 2 hypersensitivity pneumonitis shows upper lobe predominant peribronchovascular fibrosis and architectural distortion manifesting with reticulation, traction bronchiolectasis →, and mosaic attenuation.* **(Right)** *Coronal NECT of the same patient shows central and upper lung zone predominant peribronchovascular architectural distortion, traction bronchiectasis →, and mosaic attenuation, typical of cluster 2 hypersensitivity pneumonitis.*

Hypersensitivity Pneumonitis

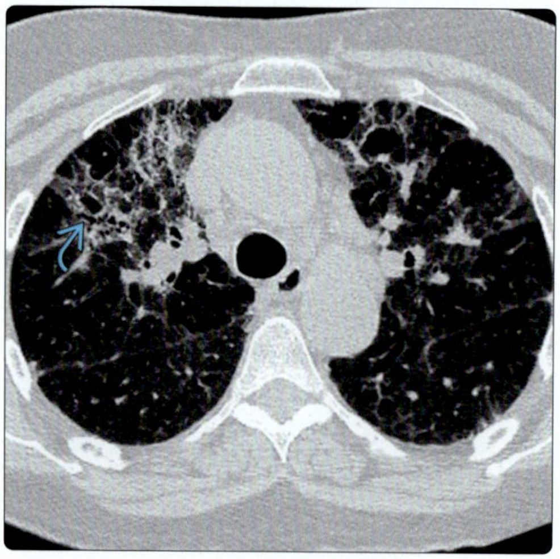

Hypersensitivity Pneumonitis

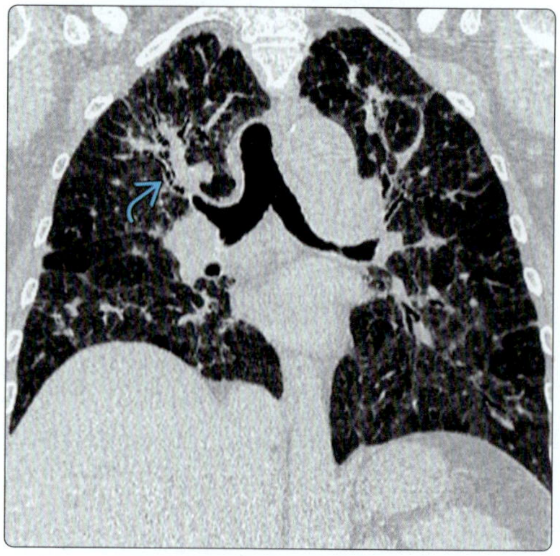

(Left) *Axial NECT of a 70-year-old sandblaster with complicated silicosis shows upper lobe architectural distortion, aggregates of centrilobular micronodules →, calcified subpleural micronodules, and paracicatricial emphysema →.* **(Right)** *Coronal NECT of a 63-year-old man with complicated silicosis shows bilateral progressive massive fibrosis →, left upper lobe cavitation →, mid and upper lung zone micronodules, apical bullous and paracicatricial → emphysema, and basilar panlobular emphysema.*

Complicated Silicosis

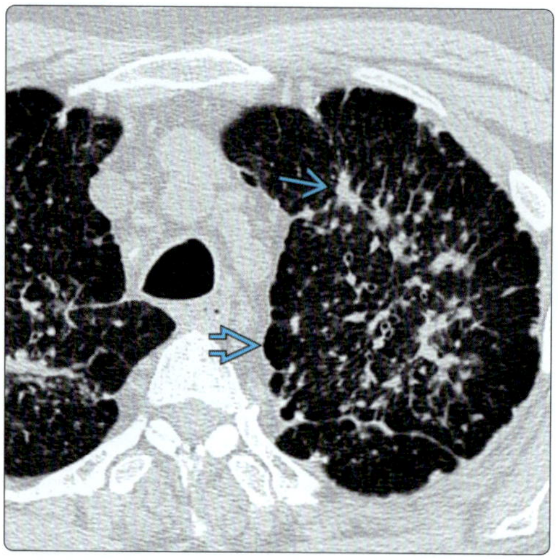

Complicated Silicosis

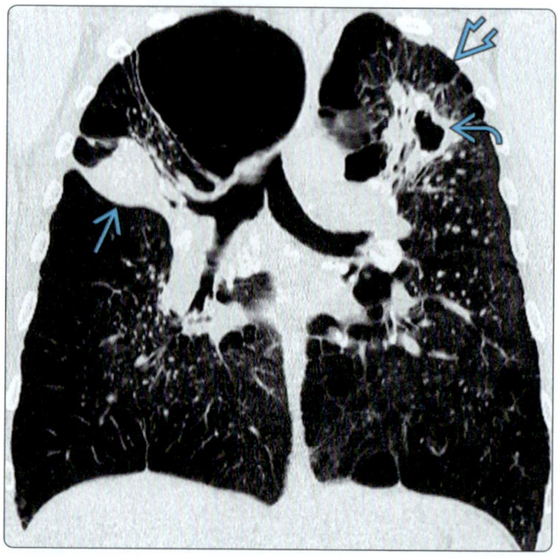

(Left) *Axial prone HRCT of a 79-year-old man with asbestosis shows bilateral basilar pleural plaques →, subpleural architectural distortion with interlobular septal thickening, intralobular lines, early honeycombing, and parenchymal bands.* **(Right)** *Axial NECT of a 60-year-old man with asbestosis shows diffuse bilateral architectural distortion and honeycombing with areas of mass-like fibrosis → and traction bronchiectasis →. Note bilateral calcified pleural plaques → from asbestos-related pleural disease.*

Asbestosis

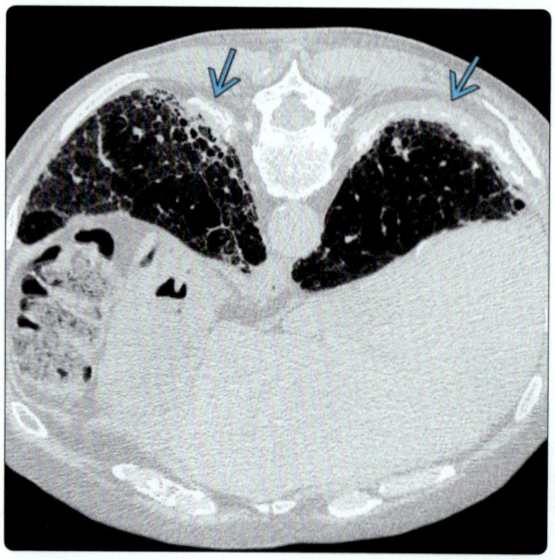

Asbestosis

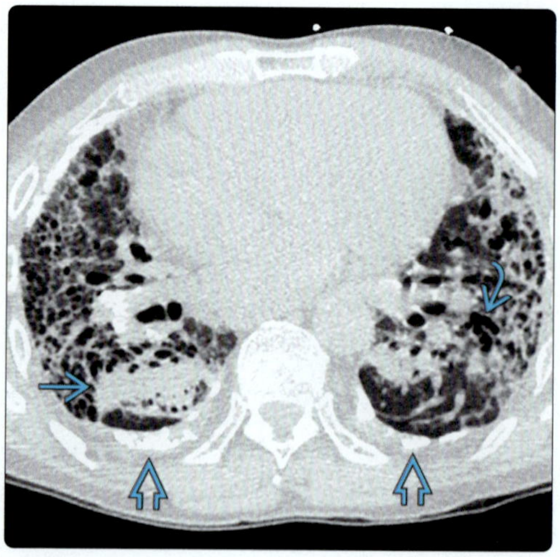

Drug-Induced Lung Disease

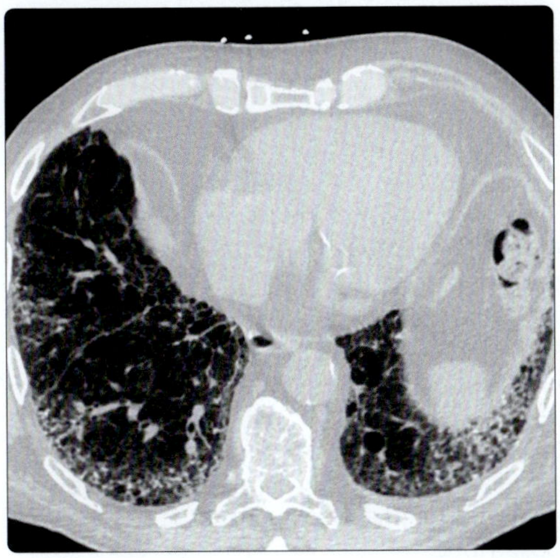

Drug-Induced Lung Disease

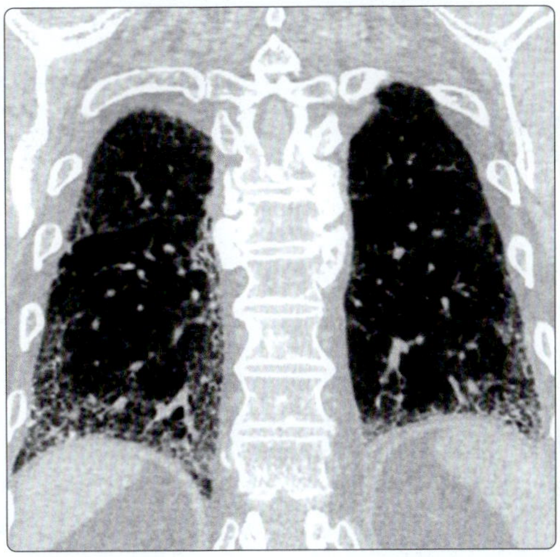

(Left) *Axial NECT of a 74-year-old man with amiodarone toxicity shows architectural distortion that manifests with basilar predominant subpleural reticulation with interlobular septal thickening and intralobular lines but no honeycombing. The findings are consistent with the nonspecific interstitial pneumonia pattern of injury associated with fibrotic drug-induced lung disease.* **(Right)** *Coronal NECT of the same patient demonstrates bilateral basilar predominant reticular opacities in the absence of honeycombing.*

Acute Respiratory Distress Syndrome

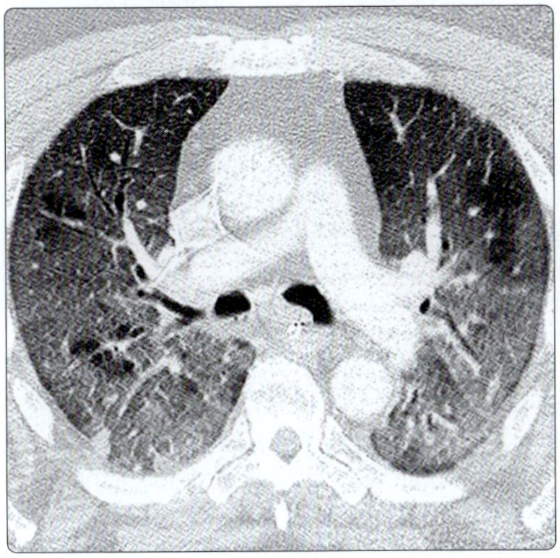

Acute Respiratory Distress Syndrome

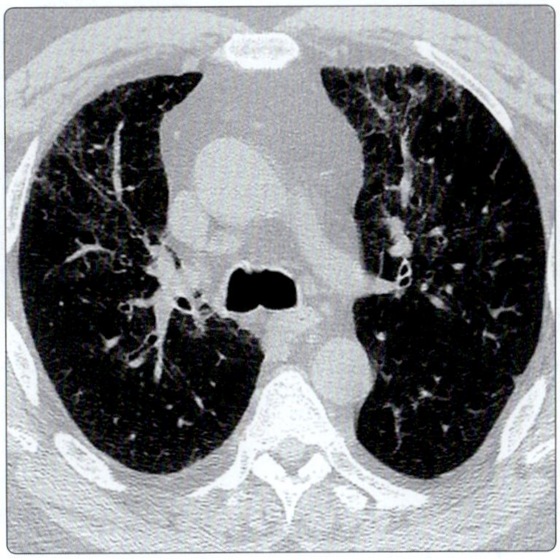

(Left) *Axial NECT of a 59-year-old man with acute respiratory distress syndrome (ARDS) shows bilateral basilar posterior ground-glass opacities on a background of interlobular septal thickening and relative sparing of the anterior lung parenchyma.* **(Right)** *Axial NECT of the same patient after discharge and recovery shows bilateral anterior and subpleural architectural distortion typical of post-ARDS fibrosis. Edema and atelectasis may protect the posterior lung parenchyma from chronic sequela of acute pulmonary injury.*

Tuberculosis

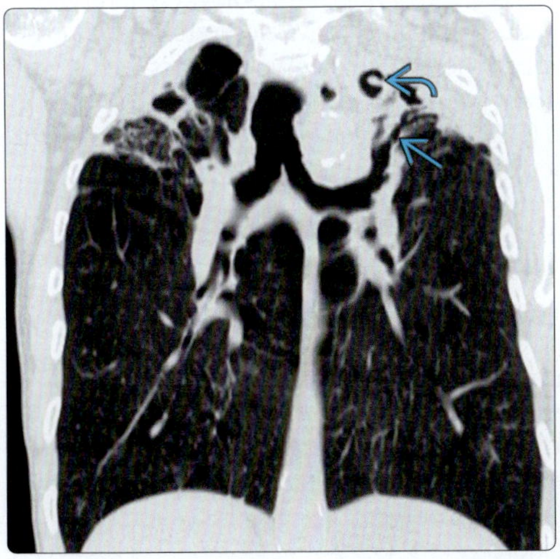

Tuberculosis

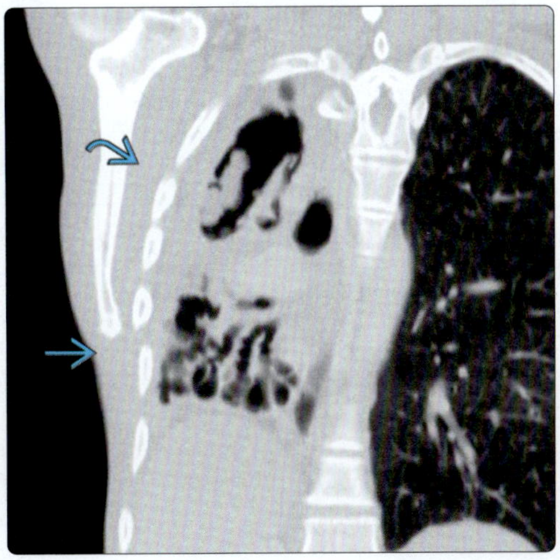

(Left) *Coronal NECT of a 76-year-old man with old tuberculosis shows bilateral upper lobe architectural distortion and volume loss with intrinsic traction bronchiectasis* → *and a left apical cavity with a soft tissue nodule* ↷ *that likely represents a mycetoma.* **(Right)** *Coronal NECT of a 57-year-old man with old right lung tuberculosis shows CT findings of autopneumonectomy characterized by marked right lung volume loss, traction bronchiectasis* →*, cavitation* ↷*, and mycetoma formation.*

DIFFERENTIAL DIAGNOSIS

Common

- Lung Cancer
- Endobronchial Secretions
- Malpositioned Endotracheal Tube
- Pleural Effusion/Pneumothorax/Pleural Thickening

Less Common

- Foreign Body
- Radiation Therapy

Rare but Important

- Endobronchial Neoplasm

ESSENTIAL INFORMATION

Key Differential Diagnosis Issues

- Atelectasis
  - Incomplete expansion of all or part of lung with corresponding diminution in lung volume
    - *Collapse* should be reserved for complete atelectasis
- Mechanism
  - Obstructive (resorptive)
    - Mucus plug, malpositioned endotracheal tube, foreign body, tumor, airway rupture, bronchial stenosis
    - Resorption of air
      - Complete within 24 hours; no air bronchogram
      - Obstructive pneumonitis: Consolidation limits volume loss
  - Compressive/passive
    - Volume loss secondary to space-occupying process
      - Pleural effusion, pneumothorax, pleural mass
  - Adhesive
    - Surfactant deficiency
      - Reduces alveolar surface tension
    - Radiation pneumonitis
      - Limited to irradiated lung
      - 1-6 months after completion of radiation
    - Ischemia distal to thromboembolism
      - Subsegmental, segmental
  - Cicatrization (scar)
    - Volume loss associated with retraction of fibrotic lung (irreversible) and traction bronchiectasis
      - Tuberculosis, idiopathic pulmonary fibrosis, radiation fibrosis
- Radiographic signs of atelectasis
  - Direct signs
    - Displacement of interlobar fissures
      - Most easily recognized sign of atelectasis
    - Crowding of vessels and bronchi
  - Indirect signs
    - Localized increased opacity
    - Hemidiaphragm elevation
    - Mediastinal shift
    - Compensatory overinflation of unaffected lung
    - Hilar displacement
- Patterns
  - Lobar atelectasis
    - Right upper lobe
      - Superior and medial collapse
      - Obscures right superior mediastinal contours
      - Elevation of horizontal fissure
      - Complete collapse: Lobe marginated against mediastinum
      - Juxtaphrenic peak: Triangular opacity extending cephalad from diaphragm
      - S sign of Golden: Centrally obstructing mass, downward concavity of lateral minor fissure, downward convexity of medial minor fissure, reverse S configuration on frontal radiography
    - Left upper lobe
      - Anterior and superior displacement toward anterior chest wall, hyperexpanded left lower lobe superior segment migrates upward and behind upper lobe
      - Luftsichel sign: Left upper lobe collapse, upward and medial migration of hyperexpanded left lower lobe superior segment between aortic arch and collapsed lobe
    - Middle lobe
      - Medial collapse toward heart, downward displacement of minor fissure, superior displacement of major fissure
      - CT: Triangular or trapezoidal opacity with apex directed toward hilum
      - Middle lobe syndrome: Recurrent or chronic atelectasis (neoplasm, inflammation, infection)
    - Lower lobes
      - Similar on right and left because of symmetric anatomy
      - Left lower lobe: Obscured left hemidiaphragm, retrocardiac opacity
      - CT: Triangular or rounded opacity in costovertebral angle
  - Linear (plate-like) atelectasis
    - Subsegmental atelectasis with linear shape, almost always abuts pleura
      - Oriented in any plane
      - Variable thickness: Few millimeters to centimeters
  - Rounded atelectasis
    - Pleural thickening or fluid tethers adjacent lung with invagination or pleural groove along atelectatic lung
    - Chronic peripheral subpleural volume loss
      - Adjacent pleural abnormality: Thickening (88%), fluid (60%), calcification (40%)
      - Asbestos-related pleural disease
      - May mimic lung cancer
  - Complete atelectasis
    - Opaque hemithorax, ipsilateral mediastinal shift
    - Hilar mass + lobar atelectasis: Highly suggestive of primary lung cancer
  - Cicatricial atelectasis
    - Volume loss associated with retraction of fibrotic lung parenchyma
      - Increased elastic recoil: Traction bronchiectasis and bronchiolectasis
    - Associations
      - Granulomatous infection
      - Noninfectious granulomatous disease
      - Radiation fibrosis

Helpful Clues for Common Diagnoses

- **Lung Cancer**
  - Squamous cell carcinoma: Most important neoplastic cause of large airway obstruction
  - Centrally-obstructing endobronchial mass
    - Lobar or segmental atelectasis ± consolidation
      - CECT: Typically delineates low-attenuation central neoplasm against enhancing atelectatic lung
    - Squamous cell carcinoma: Most important neoplastic cause of large airway obstruction
      - 2/3 of squamous cell carcinomas manifest as endobronchial mass
  - Identification of lobar collapse in outpatient population should prompt exclusion of centrally obstructing lung cancer
- **Endobronchial Secretions**
  - Common etiology of atelectasis in hospitalized patients
    - Sudden onset of lobar or total lung collapse; typically identified on radiography
    - Usually relieved with respiratory therapy &/or bronchoscopy
- **Malpositioned Endotracheal Tube**
  - Common cause of volume loss and atelectasis in critically ill patients
  - Diagnosis confirmed on portable radiography
- **Pleural Effusion/Pneumothorax/Pleural Thickening**
  - Massive pleural effusion should raise concern for malignancy
    - Opaque hemithorax; variable mediastinal shift
    - CECT: Pleural thickening, nodules, or masses in malignant effusion; assessment of atelectatic lung
  - Large pneumothorax may produce passive atelectasis of adjacent lung
  - Rounded atelectasis
    - Peripheral subpleural mass-like lesion
      - Comet tail sign: Curvilinear orientation of bronchovascular structures toward mass
    - High specificity: 92%

Helpful Clues for Less Common Diagnoses

- **Foreign Body**
  - Most common cause of endobronchial abnormality in childhood
    - Food, tooth fragment
      - Radiopaque foreign body in only 5-15% of cases
    - Early diagnosis in childhood; may be delayed in adults
  - Imaging: Chronic volume loss, recurrent pneumonia, bronchiectasis
    - Chronic inflammatory reaction about foreign body; endobronchial lesion with lobar or segmental collapse
    - Must be differentiated from lung cancer
- **Radiation Therapy**
  - History of treated thoracic malignancy
  - Consolidation ± volume loss, well-defined curvilinear margins that conform to therapy port, band-like opacity
    - 12 months after therapy completion: Evolution to cicatricial atelectasis
    - Architectural distortion with traction bronchiectasis

Helpful Clues for Rare Diagnoses

- **Endobronchial Neoplasms**
  - Malignant
    - Carcinoid: Completely or partially endobronchial, may exhibit enhancement ± Ca++
    - Mucoepidermoid carcinoma
    - Metastasis
      - 2% of autopsies of patients with solid tumors
      - Most commonly associated with renal and colorectal carcinomas
      - Sessile or polypoid endobronchial lesion, narrowing or irregularity of airway lumen, lobar/segmental/subsegmental atelectasis, and postobstructive pneumonia
  - Benign: Hamartoma, lipoma, neurofibroma, fibroepithelial polyp

Lung Cancer

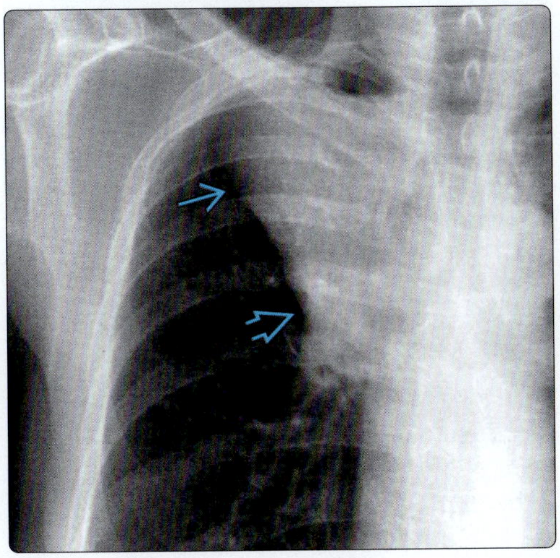

Lung Cancer

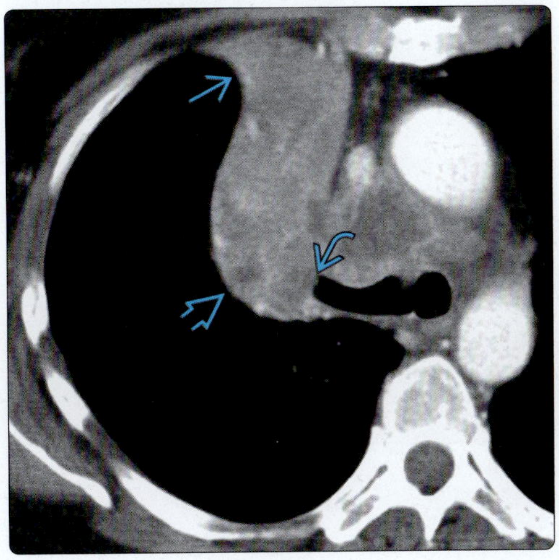

(Left) *Coned-down PA chest radiograph of a 50-year-old man shows right upper lobe collapse due to a centrally obstructing squamous cell carcinoma that produces the radiographic S sign of Golden with superior migration of the minor fissure and a central convexity corresponding to the mass.* **(Right)** *Axial CECT of the same patient shows a heterogeneously enhancing right hilar mass that obstructs the right upper lobe bronchus. The minor fissure is concave adjacent to the atelectatic lung and convex adjacent to the mass.*

(Left) *PA chest radiograph of a 73-year-old man with small cell lung cancer shows left upper lobe atelectasis due to central mass that produces convex interface at the hilum. The hyperinflated left lower lobe superior segment forms a crescent-shaped radiolucency that outlines the aortic arch and manifests with the Luftsichel sign.* **(Right)** *Coronal CECT of the same patient shows the atelectatic left upper lobe, the central tumor mass, and the hyperinflated left lower lobe located between the aortic arch and the collapsed lung.*

Lung Cancer

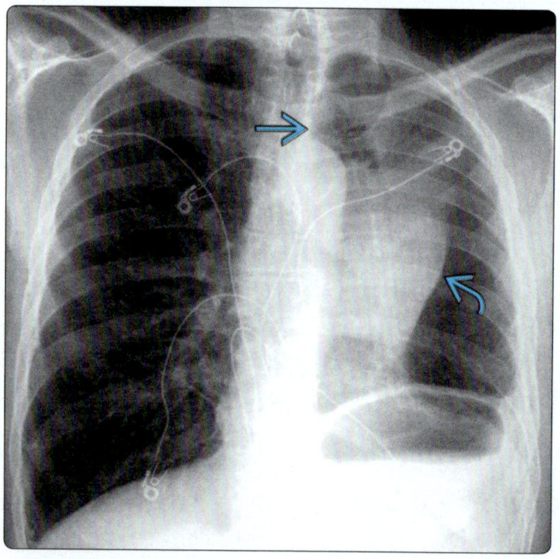

Lung Cancer

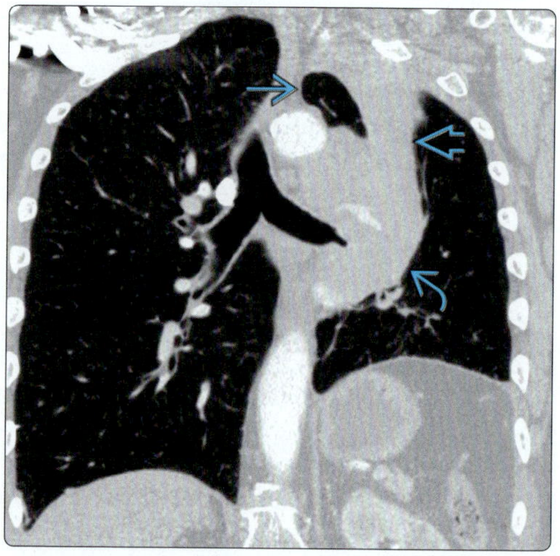

(Left) *PA chest radiograph of a patient with obstructing bronchial secretions shows middle and right lower lobe atelectasis with intrinsic bronchiectasis, obscuration of the right heart border and medial right hemidiaphragm, and inferior displacement of the minor and major fissures.* **(Right)** *AP chest radiograph of a 35-year-old woman found unresponsive and intubated in the field shows a malpositioned endotracheal tube with tip in the right lower lobe bronchus and resultant left lung and right upper lobe atelectasis.*

Endobronchial Secretions

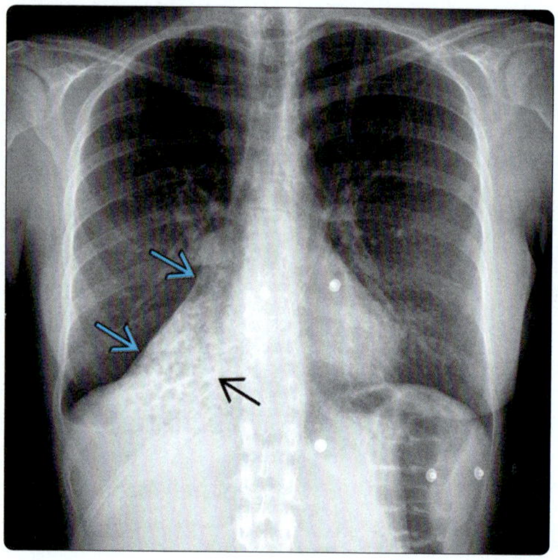

Malpositioned Endotracheal Tube

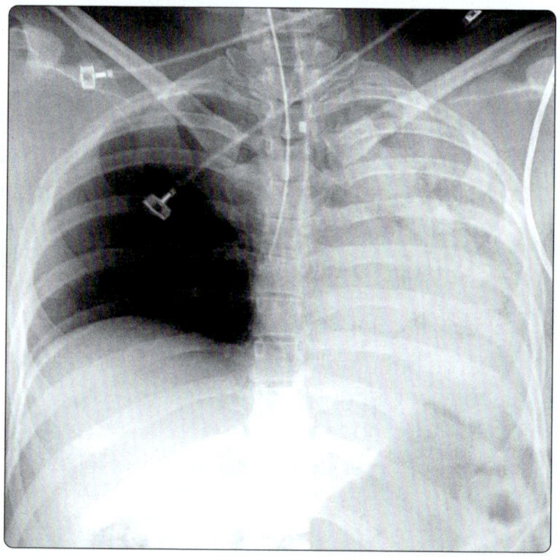

(Left) *AP chest radiograph shows an opaque right hemithorax secondary to complete right lung atelectasis adjacent to a massive malignant right pleural effusion. Note contralateral mediastinal shift due to mass effect.* **(Right)** *Coned-down AP chest radiograph of a patient with acute pain and dyspnea shows a large left tension pneumothorax, marked left lung atelectasis, and mass effect on the mediastinum. Although suggested on imaging, tension physiology is a clinical diagnosis.*

Pleural Effusion/Pneumothorax/Pleural Thickening

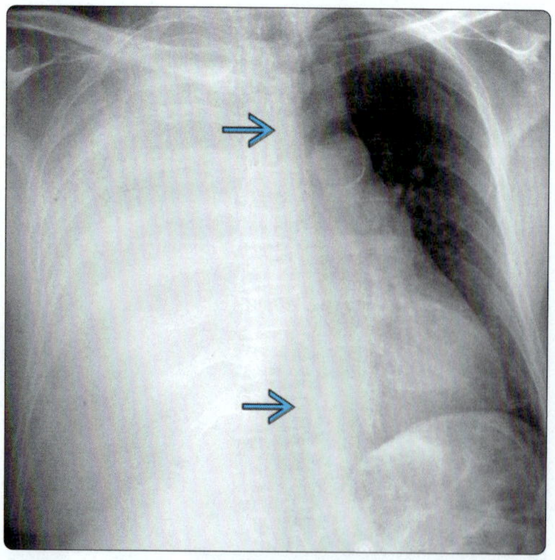

Pleural Effusion/Pneumothorax/Pleural Thickening

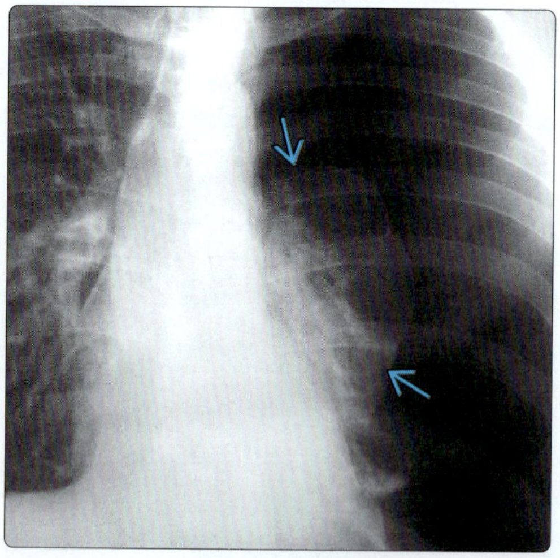

Pleural Effusion/Pneumothorax/Pleural Thickening

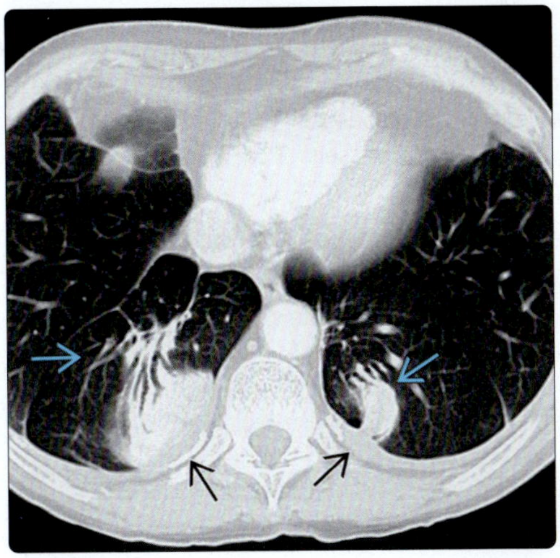

Foreign Body

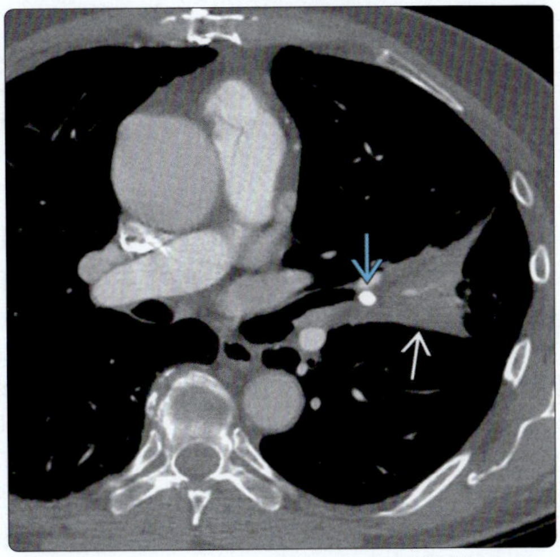

(Left) *Axial CECT of a patient with asbestos-related pleural disease shows bilateral lower lobe rounded atelectasis that exhibits the comet tail sign, characterized by the curvilinear morphology of the bronchovascular bundles. Note adjacent calcified pleural plaques.* **(Right)** *Axial CECT (bone window) of an 80-year-old man who aspirated a dental filling and presented with a new left upper lobe opacity shows the metallic foreign body in the lumen of the superior lingular segmental bronchus and surrounding atelectasis.*

Foreign Body

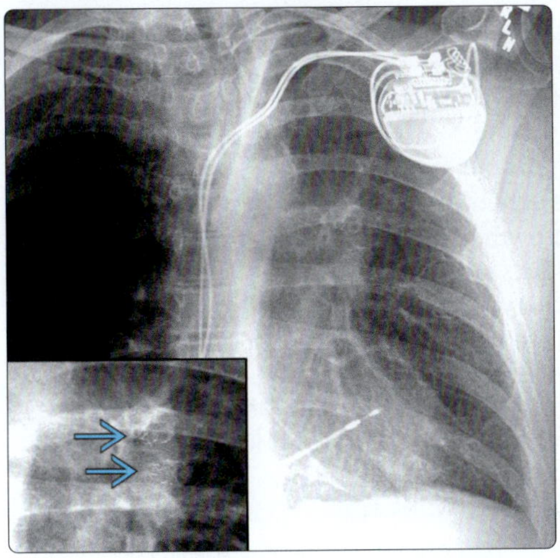

Radiation Therapy

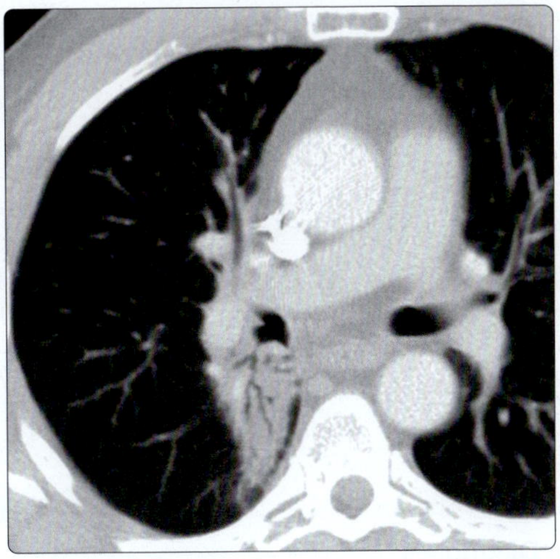

(Left) *Coned-down PA chest radiograph of a 61-year-old woman who underwent volume reduction therapy with bronchial valves (inset shows the bronchial valves) shows resultant left upper lobe atelectasis. The bronchial valves act as an obstructing foreign body to achieve volume reduction.* **(Right)** *Axial CECT of a 58-year-old man status post radiation therapy for primary lung cancer shows cicatricial atelectasis affecting the superior segment of the right lower lobe and the medial segment of the middle lobe.*

Endobronchial Neoplasm

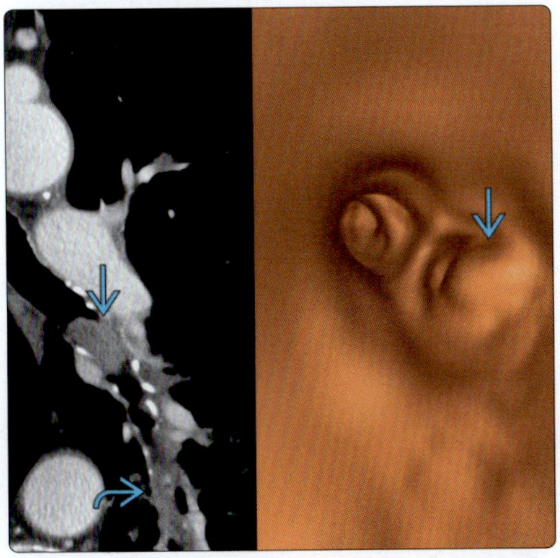

Endobronchial Neoplasm

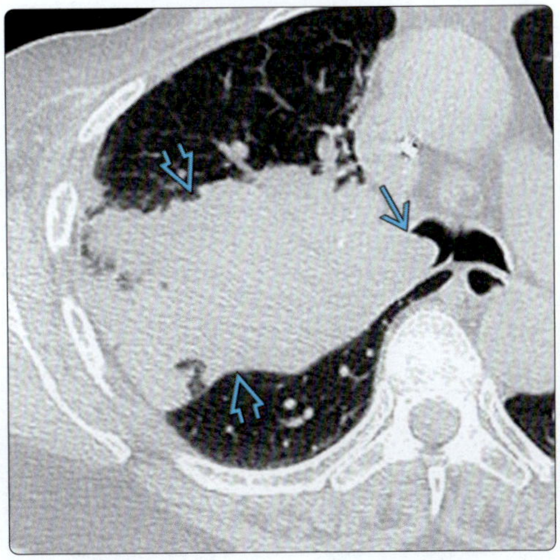

(Left) *Composite image with coronal CECT (left) and virtual bronchoscopy (right) shows a centrally obstructing left lower lobe carcinoid tumor and resultant peripheral lower lobe atelectasis. Carcinoid tumor may be entirely endobronchial, as in this case.* **(Right)** *Axial NECT of a 63-year-old woman with renal cell carcinoma shows right upper lobe consolidation and volume loss secondary to a centrally endobronchial metastasis that obstructs the right mainstem bronchus.*

DIFFERENTIAL DIAGNOSIS

Common

- Bullous Emphysema

Less Common

- Giant Bullous Emphysema

Rare but Important

- Sarcoidosis
- Proteus Syndrome

ESSENTIAL INFORMATION

Key Differential Diagnosis Issues

- Terminology
  - Bulla: Permanent air-containing space in lung parenchyma
    - Etiology: Destruction, dilatation, and confluence of airspaces distal to terminal bronchioles
    - At least 1 cm in diameter, thin- or poorly-defined wall
  - Genetic factors that increase susceptibility to smoking-related bullous emphysema
    - Alpha-1 antitrypsin deficiency
    - Marfan and Ehlers-Danlos syndromes
    - Neurofibromatosis 1
    - Birt-Hogg-Dubé syndrome
    - HIV infection
  - Must be distinguished from other air-filled spaces
    - Bleb, cyst, pneumatocele, cavity
- Imaging
  - Radiography: Hyperlucent lung, bullae may be perceptible
  - CT: Detailed characterization
    - Number, size, location of bullae
    - Assessment of adjacent lung
    - Suggestion of alternate diagnosis

Helpful Clues for Common Diagnoses

- **Bullous Emphysema**
  - Cigarette smoking (90%)
  - 80% of patients with bullae have associated emphysema
  - Alpha-1 antitrypsin deficiency
  - Imaging
    - Hyperinflated lung; ↑ retrosternal clear space, diaphragmatic flattening
    - Thin-walled air-filled spaces
      - No intrinsic blood vessels
      - Upper lobe predominance

Helpful Clues for Less Common Diagnoses

- **Giant Bullous Emphysema (Vanishing Lung Syndrome)**
  - Rare, usually affects young male smokers
    - Progressive dyspnea
  - Bullae involve > 30% of affected hemithorax
    - Bullae fill on inspiration, cause atelectasis of adjacent lung
    - Apical giant bullae may mimic pneumothorax

Helpful Clues for Rare Diagnoses

- **Sarcoidosis**
  - Similar to giant bullous emphysema (vanishing lung syndrome)
    - Non-caseating and non-necrotizing granulomas found adjacent to bullae
  - Differentiation from localized cystic airspaces seen in stage IV disease
- **Proteus Syndrome**
  - Very rare genetic disease
    - Overgrowth of bone, connective tissue, and adipose tissue
    - Pulmonary involvement
      - Unilateral or bilateral severe bullous disease and vein varicosities
      - Excessive growth of bullae: Mediastinal shift, compression of contralateral lung

SELECTED REFERENCES

1. Kligerman S et al: Clinical-radiologic-pathologic correlation of smoking-related diffuse parenchymal lung disease. Radiol Clin North Am. 54(6):1047-63, 2016

Bullous Emphysema

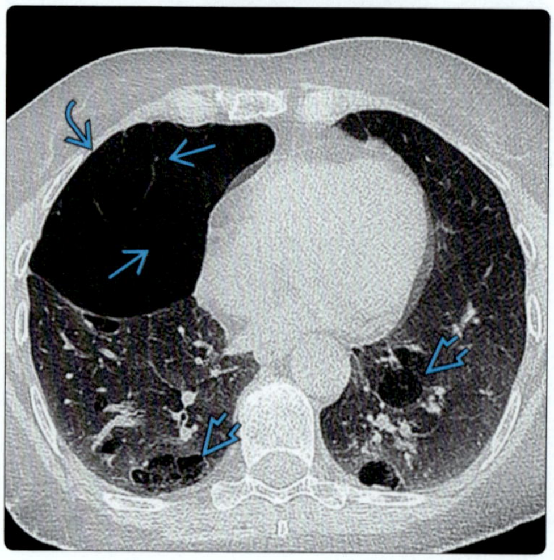

Bullous Emphysema

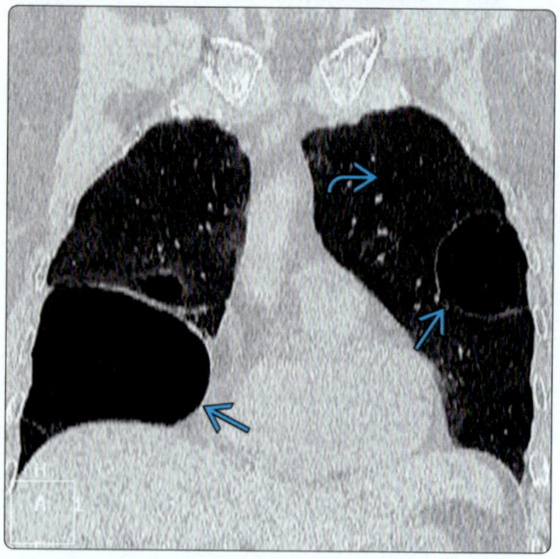

(Left) *Axial HRCT of a patient with dyspnea shows a large middle lobe bulla that exhibits thin internal septations. Note the well-defined lucent lesions in the lower lobes that involve the entirety of the secondary lobule with an imperceptible wall, characteristic of centrilobular emphysema.* **(Right)** *Coronal NECT (minIP reformatted image) of the same patient shows bilateral pulmonary bullae with thin internal septa. Diffuse centrilobular emphysema is also demonstrated in the upper lobes.*

Bullous Emphysema

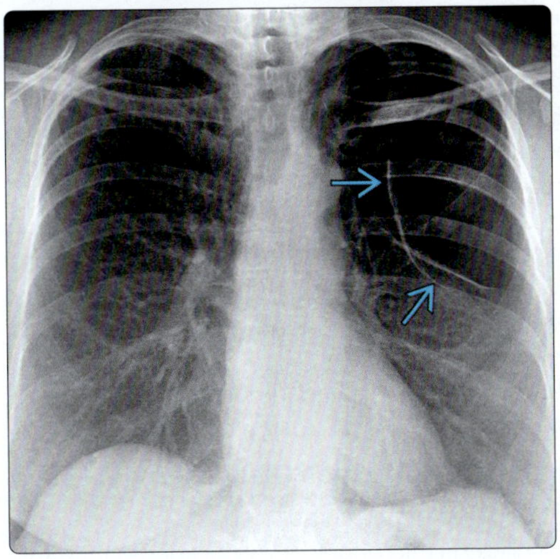

Bullous Emphysema

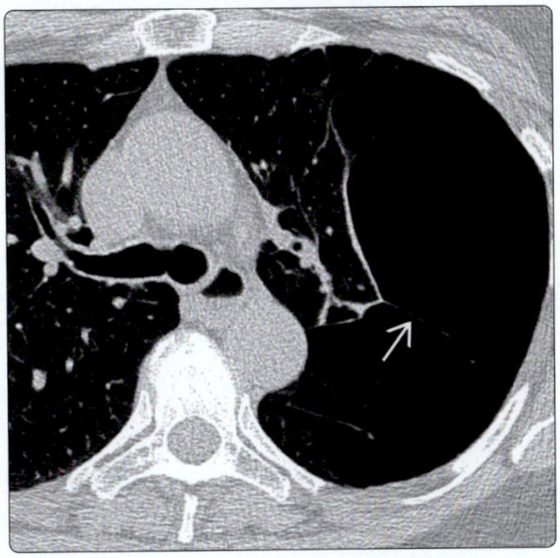

(Left) *PA chest radiograph of a 75-year-old woman never smoker who developed exertional dyspnea shows large left upper lobe thin-walled pulmonary bullae* → *that manifest as pulmonary hyperlucency. The remaining lung appears normal.* **(Right)** *Axial HRCT of the same patient shows the large left upper lobe bullae. Note thin soft tissue septa* ➡ *that represent the bullae walls. The patient underwent surgical bullectomy with symptomatic relief.*

Giant Bullous Emphysema

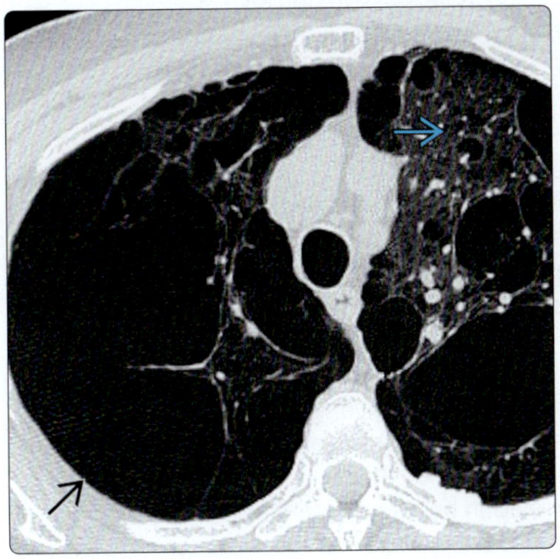

Giant Bullous Emphysema

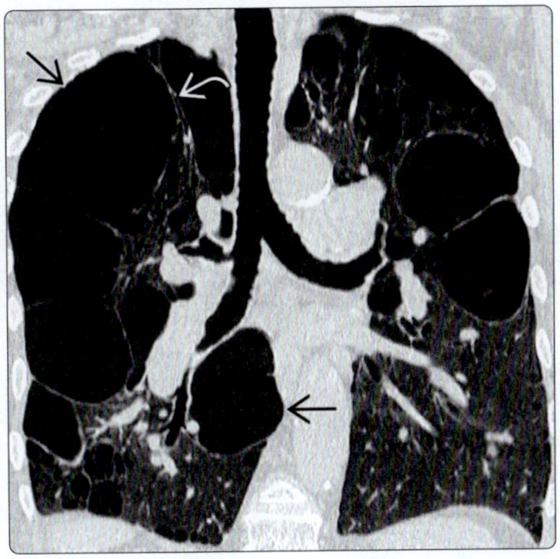

(Left) *Axial HRCT of a 58-year-old man with dyspnea shows bilateral upper lobe predominant thin-walled giant bullae* → *of varying sizes and centrilobular emphysema* →. **(Right)** *Coronal HRCT of the same patient shows asymmetric right greater than left pulmonary involvement by giant bullous disease* → *that produces mass effect* ➡ *on the adjacent lung. Progressive bullous disease may result in the so-called vanishing lung syndrome characterized by decreased lung density on radiography.*

Proteus Syndrome

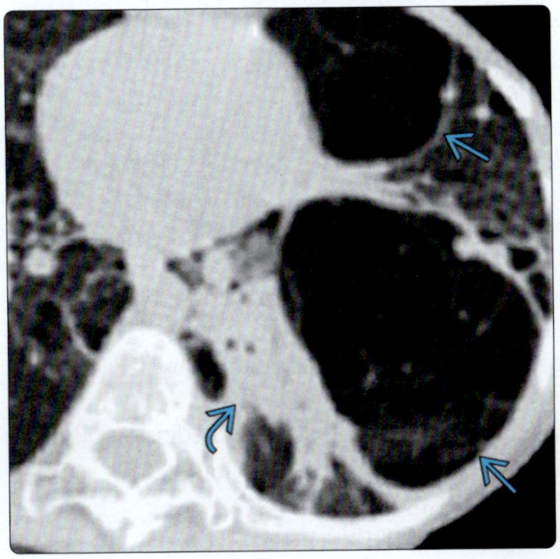

Proteus Syndrome

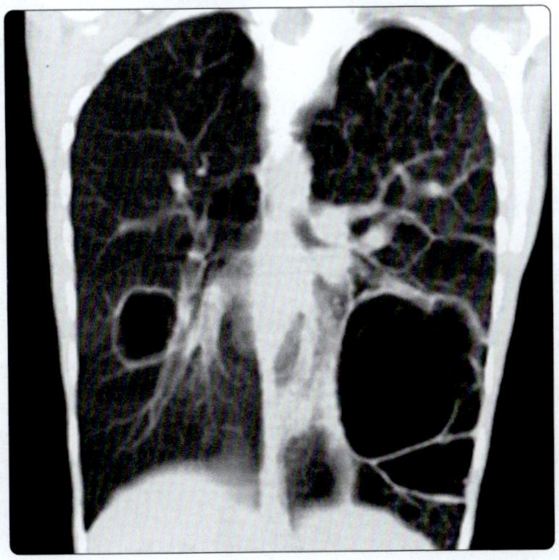

(Left) *Axial NECT of an 11-year-old girl with a history of recurrent pneumonia, enlarged left middle finger, and hypertrophied left leg secondary to Proteus syndrome shows lower lobe predominant thick-walled pulmonary cysts* → *and adjacent compressive atelectasis* ↗. *(Courtesy K. Irion, MD.)* **(Right)** *Coronal NECT of the same patient shows left greater than right thick-walled pulmonary cysts and atelectasis in the adjacent left lower lobe. (Courtesy K. Irion, MD.)*

DIFFERENTIAL DIAGNOSIS

Common

- Healed Infection
  - Tuberculosis
  - Histoplasmosis
  - Varicella

Less Common

- Silicosis
- Coal Workers' Pneumoconiosis
- Sarcoidosis
- Metastatic Calcinosis
- Amyloidosis
- Calcified/Ossified Metastases
- Primary Lung Neoplasm

Rare but Important

- Alveolar Microlithiasis
- Diffuse Pulmonary Ossification

ESSENTIAL INFORMATION

Key Differential Diagnosis Issues

- Calcification: Deposition of calcium salts in tissues
  - Dystrophic calcification with calcium deposits in previously injured lung tissue
    - Sequela of tuberculosis, fungal, or viral infection
    - Silicosis and coal worker's pneumoconiosis
    - Amyloidosis
    - Sarcoidosis
    - Hemosiderosis
  - Metastatic calcification in setting of hypercalcemia
    - Chronic renal insufficiency
    - Hyperparathyroidism (primary and secondary)
    - Multiple myeloma
  - Idiopathic calcification
    - Pulmonary alveolar microlithiasis
- Ossification: Alveolar or interstitial mature bone formation
  - Congestive heart failure
    - Mitral stenosis
    - Chronic left ventricular failure
    - Idiopathic hypertrophic subaortic stenosis
  - Idiopathic pulmonary ossification in patients with pulmonary fibrosis
- Metastatic lung nodules
  - Ossification and calcification may coexist
  - Calcification: Thyroid cancer, synovial sarcoma, gastrointestinal and breast mucinous adenocarcinomas, treated metastases, and lymphoma
  - Ossification: Osteosarcoma and chondrosarcoma

Helpful Clues for Common Diagnoses

- Healed Infection
  - Tuberculosis
    - Calcified granulomas + architectural distortion, fibroparenchymal lesions, bronchiectasis, emphysema, and fibroatelectatic bands
    - Calcified granulomas + calcified hilar or mediastinal lymph nodes: Ranke complex
    - Diffuse nodular calcifications
  - Histoplasmosis
    - Nodules with central, target, or diffuse Ca++
    - Calcified histoplasmoma may be surrounded by smaller calcified and noncalcified nodules
    - Broncholithiasis
    - Calcified hilar and mediastinal nodes: Calcifications may be small and multifocal (mulberry calcifications)
    - Calcified splenic and hepatic granulomas
    - Localized mediastinal fibrosis: Calcified mass, typically subcarinal &/or right paratracheal
  - Varicella (chicken pox)
    - Numerous, well-defined, randomly distributed calcified nodules (2-3 mm)
    - Absence of lymph node, hepatic, or splenic calcifications

Helpful Clues for Less Common Diagnoses

- Silicosis and Coal Workers' Pneumoconiosis
  - Numerous bilateral micronodular calcifications (1-3 mm) with upper and mid lung zone predominance
  - Upper lobe and perihilar calcified irregular conglomerate masses (progressive massive fibrosis)
  - Mediastinal &/or hilar calcified lymph nodes; may exhibit eggshell calcification
- Sarcoidosis
  - Upper and mid lung zone conglomerate masses with punctate or coarse calcification + calcified bilateral mediastinal and hilar lymph nodes
  - May mimic progressive massive fibrosis, but conglomerate masses typically posteriorly located
- Metastatic Calcinosis
  - Patients with chronic renal failure, hyperparathyroidism, multiple myeloma, leukemia, lymphoma
    - Upper lobe primarily involved due to higher ventilation:perfusion ratio producing lower end capillary PCO2 and higher pH
    - No correlation between extent of macroscopic calcifications and clinical symptoms
  - Radiography: Upper lobe confluent dense opacities with progressive calcification
    - Diffuse or localized opacities, may mimic air space disease
      - Stability over time allows differentiation from pulmonary infection
  - HRCT: Centrilobular ground-glass nodules, ill-defined lung nodules (up to 10 mm), may exhibit calcification
  - Calcification of tracheobronchial walls, chest wall vessels, pulmonary arteries, superior vena cava, and dorsal spine dura
  - Technetium Tc 99m methylene diphosphonate (99mTc-MDP)
    - Bilateral, symmetric increased pulmonary radiotracer uptake
      - May be present in the absence of radiographic or CT abnormalities
- Amyloidosis
  - Types: Diffuse septal or nodular
  - Diffuse septal amyloidosis
    - Associated with systemic amyloidosis
    - Patients may present with dyspnea, cough, or hemoptysis

- HRCT: Punctate parenchymal calcifications associated with micronodules, reticular opacities, interlobar septal thickening
- Pulmonary nodules most numerous in lung bases, large lobulated subpleural calcifications
- Pulmonary hypertension

- Nodular amyloidosis
  - Localized lung process associated with hematologic malignancies
    - Asymptomatic patients
  - HRCT: Lower lobe-predominant solitary or multiple calcified lung nodules or masses and diffusely or coarsely calcified lymph nodes
    - Calcified lung nodules of different shapes/sizes (0.5-15.0 cm)
    - Lung nodule calcification often central or irregular
  - Large lobulated subpleural calcifications
- Calcified/Ossified Pulmonary Metastases
  - Sarcoma (osteosarcoma, chondrosarcoma, synovial sarcoma) and carcinoma (mucin-producing carcinoma, adenocarcinoma, thyroid malignancy)
  - Calcified or ossified metastatic nodules may be indistinguishable from granulomas or hamartomas
  - Follow-up imaging to document stability or growth in patients with malignancy
- Primary Lung Neoplasm
  - Ca++ pattern may be useful for determining etiology
  - Lung cancer: Nodule or mass with stippled, amorphus or eccentric calcification in 10% of cases
  - Carcinoid: Well-defined nodule or mass, eccentric calcification in 30%, enhances with contrast
    - Calcification more common in central carcinoids
  - Hamartoma: Popcorn calcification (virtually diagnostic) in 20-30%, fat attenuation in 60%, fat + calcification in 20%

Helpful Clues for Rare Diagnoses

- Alveolar Microlithiasis
  - Autosomal recessive, familial occurrence
  - Male > female, 30-40 years
  - Diffuse intraalveolar accumulation of calcium deposits: Microliths or calcospherites
  - Radiography: Diffuse mid and lower lung zone-predominant reticular and nodular opacities
    - Diffuse sand-like micronodular calcifications: "Sandstorm lung"
  - HRCT
    - Crazy-paving pattern: Diffuse ground-glass opacities + thick interlobular septa
    - Calcifications along interlobular septa, bronchovascular bundles, fissures, and pleura
    - Numerous small calcified lung nodules
    - Dense consolidations, subpleural nodules, and cysts
- Diffuse Pulmonary Ossification
  - Associated with cardiovascular disease: Chronic mitral stenosis, congestive heart failure, chronic pulmonary edema, and pulmonary venous hypertension
    - Nodular ossification
      - Small calculi within alveolar spaces, may coalesce into larger nodules
  - Associated with idiopathic pulmonary fibrosis
    - Dendriform ossification
      - HRCT: Small nodules < 4 mm or branching bronchovascular linear calcifications
      - Calcifications superimposed on pulmonary fibrosis: Subpleural and lower lobe predominance

Other Essential Information

- NECT (specially HRCT) better than radiography for demonstrating calcified or ossified lung nodules
- Microscopic calcification or ossification may exhibit soft tissue attenuation due to volume averaging

SELECTED REFERENCES

1. Egashira R et al: Diffuse pulmonary ossification in fibrosing interstitial lung diseases: prevalence and associations. Radiology. 284(1):255-63, 2017
2. Belém LC et al: Metastatic pulmonary calcification: state-of-the-art review focused on imaging findings. Respir Med. 108(5):668-76, 2014

Tuberculosis

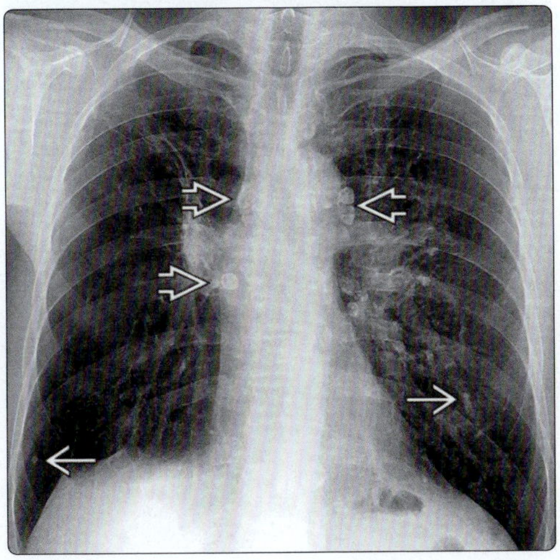

Silicosis

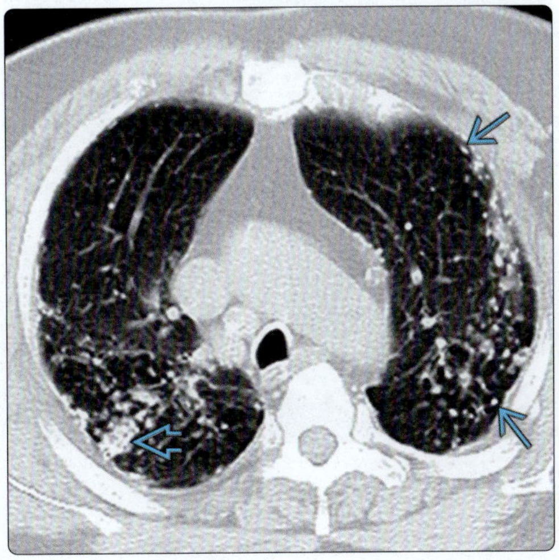

(Left) *PA chest radiograph of a 60-year-old man with treated tuberculosis shows calcified hilar and mediastinal lymph nodes ➡ and small calcified lung nodules ➡. Dystrophic calcifications are frequently seen in patients with healed tuberculosis, fungal or viral infection.* **(Right)** *Axial NECT of a 57-year-old man with exposure to silica dust shows multiple bilateral subpleural calcified small nodules ➡ and a conglomerate of nodules ➡ in the right upper lobe that are common findings in silicosis and coal worker's pneumoconiosis.*

(Left) *Axial CECT of a 65-year-old man with lymphoma and sarcoidosis shows bilateral zone perilymphatic micronodules . Note conglomerate right perihilar mass with coarse calcifications . The findings are typical of sarcoidosis.* **(Right)** *Coronal CECT of a 29-year-old woman with breast cancer and hypercalcemia shows a left upper lobe nodular consolidation with intrinsic calcification secondary to metastatic calcinosis, an entity that typically affects the upper lobes.*

Sarcoidosis

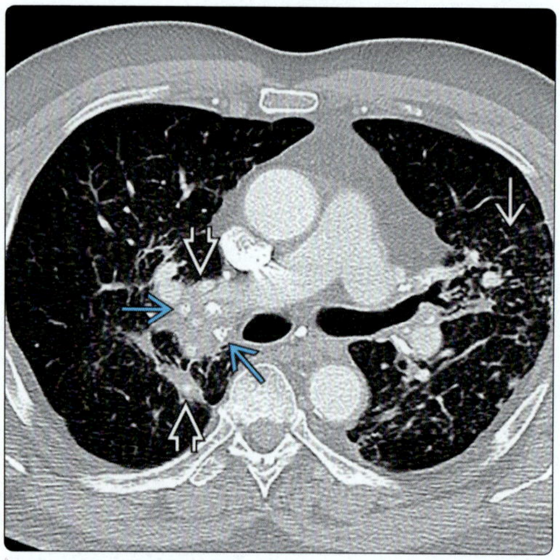

Metastatic Calcinosis

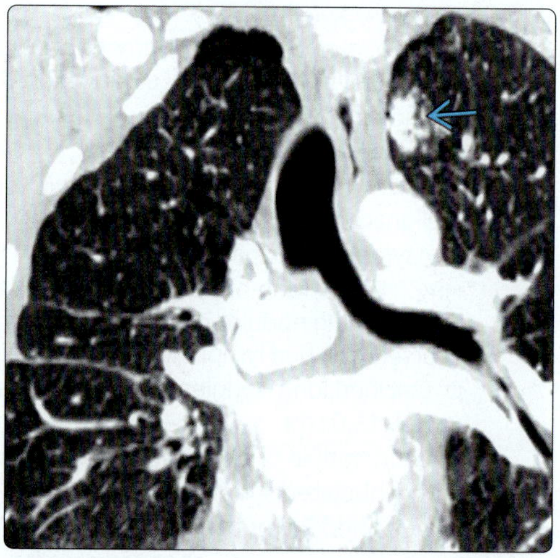

(Left) *Axial CECT (lung window) of a 65-year-old woman with lymphoma demonstrates a left upper lobe heterogeneous opacity with multiple foci of high attenuation related to calcification.* **(Right)** *Axial CECT (soft tissue window) of the same patient shows the dense central component of the lesion, consistent with calcification . Biopsy demonstrated amyloidosis. Small areas of calcification or ossification may be difficult to identify secondary to volume averaging and may manifest as high attenuation.*

Amyloidosis

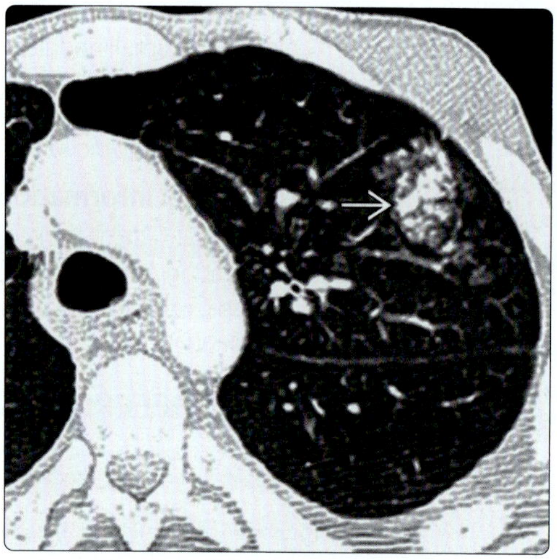

Amyloidosis

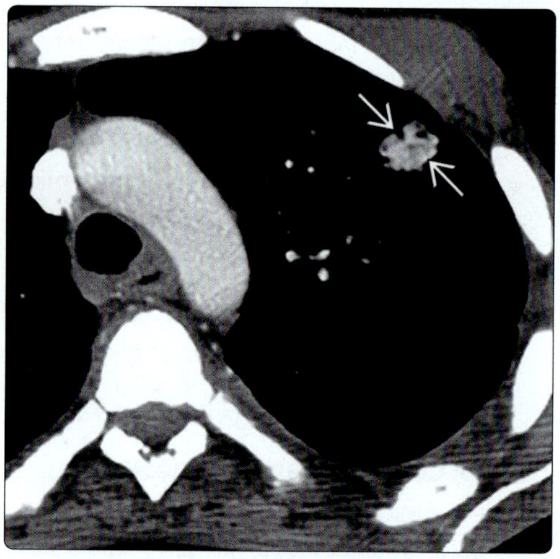

(Left) *Axial CECT of a 32-year-old woman with osteosarcoma demonstrates a small calcified nodule in the right lower lobe.* **(Right)** *Axial CECT of the same patient shows significant increase in the size of the right lower lobe nodule , consistent with a growing metastasis. Note a new noncalcified left posterior pleural metastasis . Calcified nodules in patients with osteosarcoma, chondrosarcoma, synovial sarcoma, and mucin-producing carcinoma require serial imaging to exclude metastatic disease.*

Calcified/Ossified Metastases

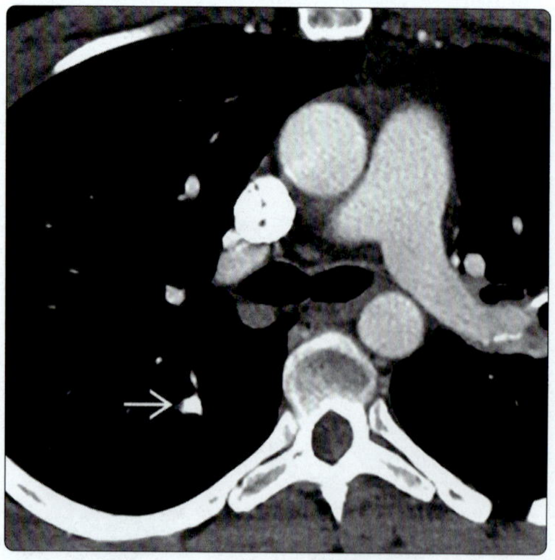

Calcified/Ossified Metastases

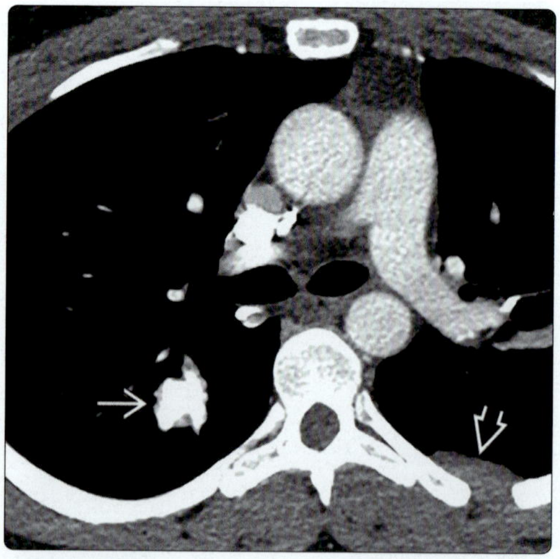

Primary Lung Neoplasm

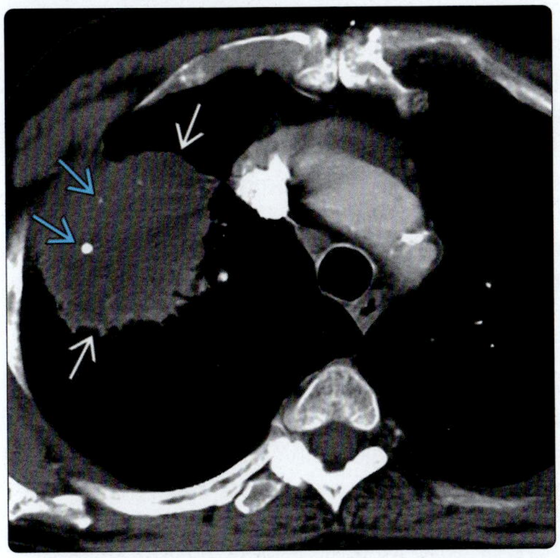

Primary Lung Neoplasm

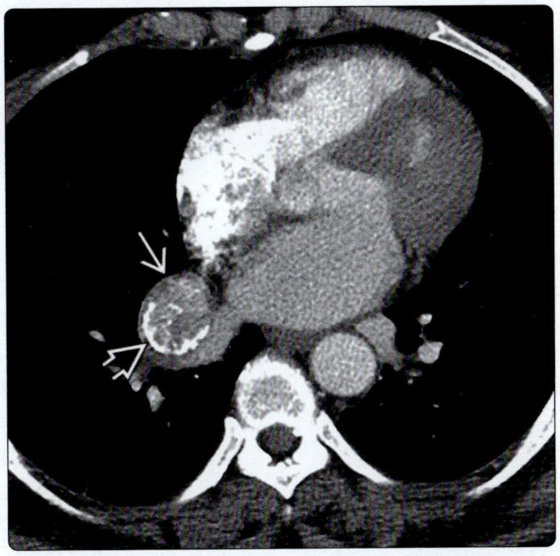

(Left) *Axial CECT of a 69-year-old man with primary lung adenocarcinoma shows a spiculated right upper lobe mass with intrinsic punctate classifications. Punctate, eccentric, and amorphus calcifications are detected in ~ 10% of all lung cancers.* **(Right)** *Axial CECT of a 40-year-old woman shows a well-defined, right perihilar mass with coarse peripheral calcifications. Biopsy demonstrated carcinoid tumor. Eccentric calcifications are present in 30% of cases of centrally located carcinoid tumors.*

Primary Lung Neoplasm

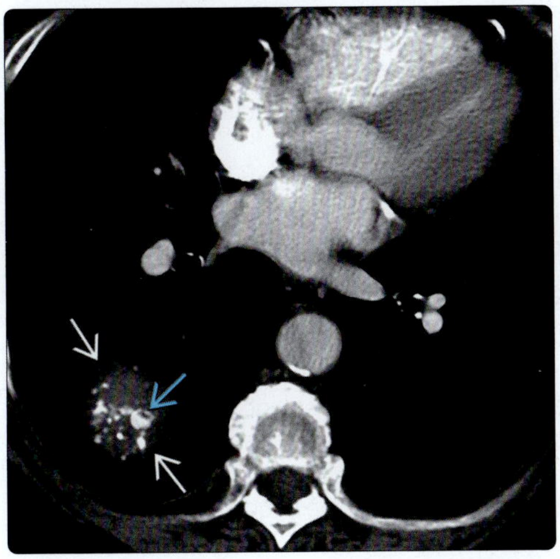

Alveolar Microlithiasis

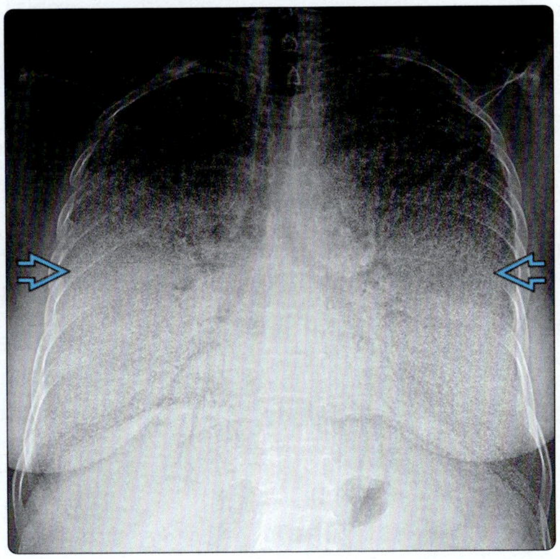

(Left) *Axial CECT of a 62-year-old woman shows a soft tissue mass with intrinsic popcorn calcification, consistent with a hamartoma. The presence of popcorn calcification is virtually diagnostic of hamartoma.* **(Right)** *PA chest radiograph of a 42-year-old woman with progressive cough shows diffuse and confluent bilateral micronodular opacities with a "sandstorm lung" pattern, consistent with alveolar microlithiasis, an autosomal recessive disorder characterized by intraalveolar accumulation of calcium.*

Diffuse Pulmonary Ossification

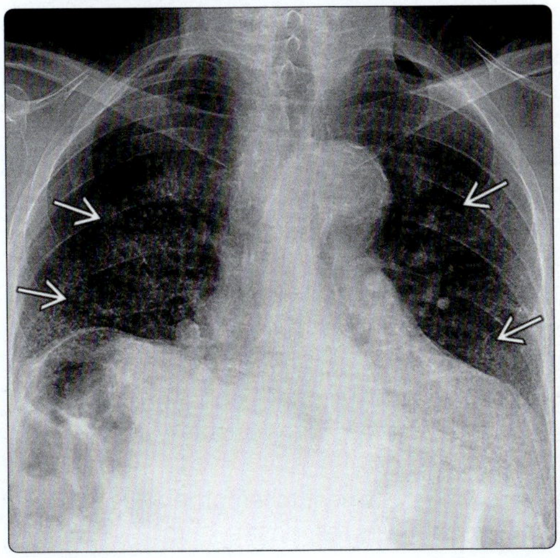

Diffuse Pulmonary Ossification

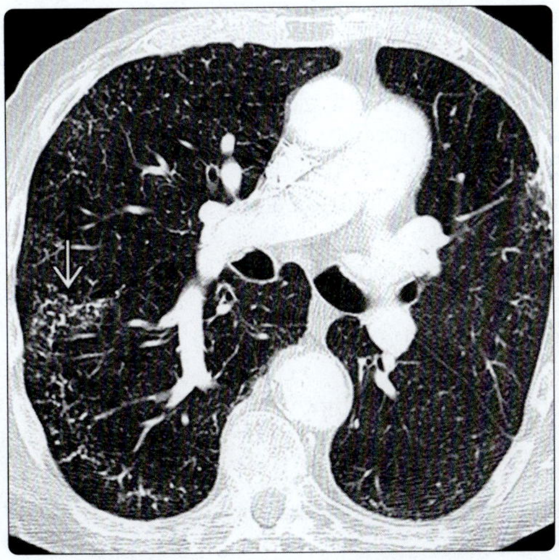

(Left) *PA chest radiograph of a 57-year-old man with a history of mitral stenosis demonstrates bilateral calcified nodules in the lower two-thirds of the lungs.* **(Right)** *Axial CECT of the same patient demonstrates clustered calcified micronodules, consistent with pulmonary ossification secondary to chronic venous congestion associated with chronic mitral valvular dysfunction. Diffuse pulmonary ossification may occur in cardiovascular disease, pulmonary fibrosis, and chronic acid reflux.*

DIFFERENTIAL DIAGNOSIS

Common

- Lung Abscess
- Lung Cancer
- Tuberculosis

Less Common

- Nontuberculous Mycobacterial Infection
- Metastasis
- Fungal Infection
- Pulmonary Infarct
- Septic Embolism
- Granulomatosis With Polyangiitis

Rare but Important

- Rheumatoid Arthritis

ESSENTIAL INFORMATION

Key Differential Diagnosis Issues

- Differential diagnosis includes infection, malignancy, and autoimmune conditions
- Acute/subacute process (≤ 12 weeks) suggests infection or infarct: Lung abscess, septic embolism, pulmonary infarct
- Chronic process (> 12 weeks) suggests mycobacterial infection, malignancy (primary or secondary), autoimmune disease (vasculitis, rheumatoid arthritis)
- Wall thickness
    - Cavitary lesions with wall thickness > 1 mm and < 4 mm are usually benign
    - Lesions with maximal wall thickness of 5-15 mm are equally divided between benign and malignant etiologies
    - 95% of cavitary lesions with maximal wall thickness of > 15 mm are malignant
    - Overlap in wall thickness of malignant and benign lesions (e.g., lung abscess)
- Solitary cavitary lesion suggests lung abscess or primary lung cancer

Helpful Clues for Common Diagnoses

- **Lung Abscess**
    - Complication of pneumonia
        - Associated with aspiration (elderly patient, alcoholism, drug abuse, stroke, esophageal dysmotility, impaired swallowing, history of head and neck cancer)
        - Productive cough, fever, chest pain, night sweats, weight loss, leukocytosis
    - Solitary lesion: Predominantly in upper lobe posterior segments and lower lobe superior segments
    - Thick-walled cavity, irregular inner and outer borders, air-fluid level
    - Association with tree-in-bud opacities or patchy consolidations
    - Pleural effusion in 25% of cases
        - Peripherally located abscess may be associated with pleural thickening &/or empyema
- **Lung Cancer**
    - Cavitation in 2-25% of cases
    - 80% of cavitary neoplasms are squamous cell carcinomas; 20% are adenocarcinomas and large cell carcinomas
    - Upper lobe predominance
    - Worse prognosis than that of non-cavitary tumors
    - Wall thickness > 24 mm
    - Irregular internal wall (49% vs. 26%) and indentation of outer wall (54% vs. 29%) more common in malignancy than in benign cavitary lesions
    - Development of solid component in pre-existing thin-walled lesion requires close imaging follow-up to exclude malignancy
    - Cavitation may develop after radiation treatment secondary to necrosis
- **Tuberculosis**
    - Risk factors: Endemic region, HIV(+) patient
    - Symptoms: Chronic cough, weight loss, fever, night sweats
    - Upper lobe solitary or multiple cavitary lesions on chest radiography in 20-45% of patients
    - Cavities often seen within consolidations; may be multifocal
    - Satellite centrilobular nodules surrounding cavity identified in 50% of cases
    - Cavity walls typically thick and irregular
    - Pleural effusion in 25% of cases
    - Cavities may persist after treatment
        - Intracavitary air-fluid level may be related to tuberculosis or superimposed bacterial infection

Helpful Clues for Less Common Diagnoses

- **Nontuberculous Mycobacterial Infection**
    - Immunocompromised patient or patient with structural lung disease [HIV(+), post transplant, prior tuberculosis, chronic obstructive pulmonary disease, cystic fibrosis] and elderly women
    - Symptoms: Chronic productive cough, hemoptysis, malaise, weight loss
    - Immunocompromised patient: Upper lobe solitary or multiple cavitary lesions: Classic pattern
    - Elderly women: Bronchiectasis, nodules, atelectasis, middle lobe and lingula consolidation and cavitation: Nonclassic or bronchiectatic pattern
        - Cavitary lesions and mediastinal lymphadenopathy are rare in nonclassic or bronchiectatic pattern
- **Metastases**
    - Most commonly associated with squamous cell carcinoma (lung, head and neck); also with renal, pancreas, colon, rectum, cervix, and breast malignancies
        - Weight loss, absence of acute symptoms
    - May affect any region of lung
    - Rounded or irregularly shaped lesions
    - Cheerio sign: Multiple, diffuse, and confluent cavitary nodules; typically associated with gastrointestinal malignancies
    - Cavitation following treatment (chemotherapy, immunotherapy) suggests response
- **Fungal Infection**
    - Invasive aspergillosis
        - Lymphoma, leukemia, myelodysplastic syndrome
        - Fever, cough, dyspnea, hemoptysis, neutropenia

- Solitary or multiple nodules or consolidations surrounded by ground-glass opacity (halo sign) secondary to hemorrhage
- Response to treatment &/or host neutrophil count recovery manifests as cavitation ± air crescent sign
- Aspergilloma
  - Fungus ball that develops in pre-existing cavity
  - May be completely asymptomatic, most common symptom is hemoptysis secondary to vascular invasion
  - Solitary cavitary lesion with air crescent sign; thin or thick cavity walls
  - Documentation of mobility of intracavitary solid component helps confirm diagnosis

- **Pulmonary Infarct**
  - Cavitation in 7% of cases
  - Cavitation secondary to aseptic necrosis more common in upper lobes; infected cavitary infarcts more frequent in lower lobes
  - Well-defined borders, variable wall thickness (1-20 mm)
  - Air-fluid levels in infected infarcts
- **Septic Embolism**
  - Immunosuppressed patient, intravenous drug use, alcoholism, endocarditis, arterial/intravenous catheter
    - Septic patient with cough, dyspnea, chest pain, tachycardia
  - Multiple peripheral nodules or wedge-shaped opacities with broad base against pleura; cavitation develops within days
  - Frequent pleural effusions
  - Hilar and mediastinal lymphadenopathy may be present
  - Pulmonary artery enlargement may occur due to increased pressure
  - Associated infarct in abdominal organ, brain, skin
- **Granulomatosis With Polyangiitis**
  - Formerly Wegener granulomatosis
  - Demographics
    - Caucasian patients
    - Age at presentation of ≈ 40 years
    - Males and females equally affected
  - Lungs and kidneys involved in 90% and 80% of cases, respectively
  - Lung nodules in 40-70% of cases
    - Patients may present with respiratory signs and symptoms, including cough, hemoptysis, dyspnea, nosebleed
    - ↑ serum c-antineutrophil antibodies against protease 3 in cytoplasmic granules (c-ANCA)
  - Nodules are usually multiple and bilateral without zonal predilection; lesion size between 2-4 cm, but may be larger
  - Cavitation in ~ 25% of lesions > 2 cm
  - Thin, thick, smooth, or nodular cavity walls
  - Perilesional hemorrhage may occur; manifests as surrounding ground-glass opacity (halo sign)

Helpful Clues for Rare Diagnoses

- **Rheumatoid Arthritis**
  - Cavitary necrobiotic nodules are rare; usually only few nodules are present
  - Typically seen in conjunction with subcutaneous nodules and high rheumatoid factor
    - Asymptomatic patient, nodules resolve without treatment
  - Multiple peripheral subpleural lesions
  - Variable size: Few mm to 7 cm
  - Cavitation may lead to hemoptysis, spontaneous pneumothorax, bronchopleural fistula

SELECTED REFERENCES

1. Gafoor K et al: Cavitary lung diseases: a clinical-radiologic algorithmic approach. Chest. 153(6):1443-65, 2018
2. Scapa JV et al: Diffuse alveolar hemorrhage and pulmonary vasculitides: histopathologic findings. Semin Respir Crit Care Med. 39(4):425-33, 2018
3. Nachiappan AC et al: Pulmonary tuberculosis: role of radiology in diagnosis and management. Radiographics. 37(1):52-72, 2017
4. Orlowski HLP et al: Imaging spectrum of invasive fungal and fungal-like infections. Radiographics. 37(4):1119-34, 2017
5. Parkar AP et al: Differential diagnosis of cavitary lung lesions. J Belg Soc Radiol. 100(1):100, 2016

Lung Abscess

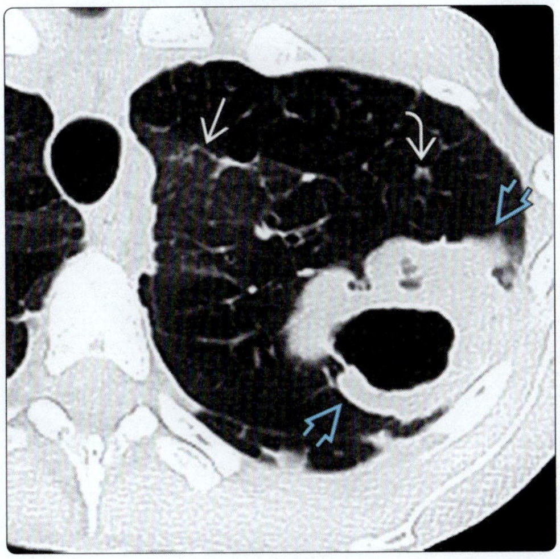

Lung Abscess

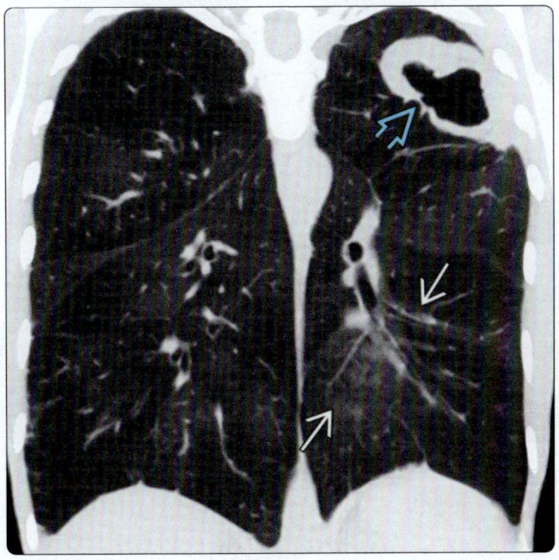

(Left) *Axial CECT of a patient with a history of head and neck cancer shows a left upper lobe cavitary mass with thick irregular nodular walls. Note associated ground-glass opacity and a small irregular nodule adjacent to the cavitary mass, which suggests infection.* **(Right)** *Coronal CECT of the same patient shows the thick-walled left upper lobe cavitary mass and peribronchial ground-glass opacities in the left lower lobe, consistent with infection/aspiration. The differential diagnosis for this lesion includes malignancy.*

(Left) *PA chest radiograph of a patient who presented with hemoptysis shows a large right upper lobe mass with intrinsic cavitation and a nodular opacity in the left upper lobe.* **(Right)** *Axial CECT of the same patient shows a right upper lobe thick-walled cavitary mass and a left upper lobe solid nodule. The findings are consistent with primary lung cancer with metastatic disease. Percutaneous biopsy showed squamous cell carcinoma. Up to 80% of cavitary lung neoplasms are squamous cell carcinomas.*

Lung Cancer

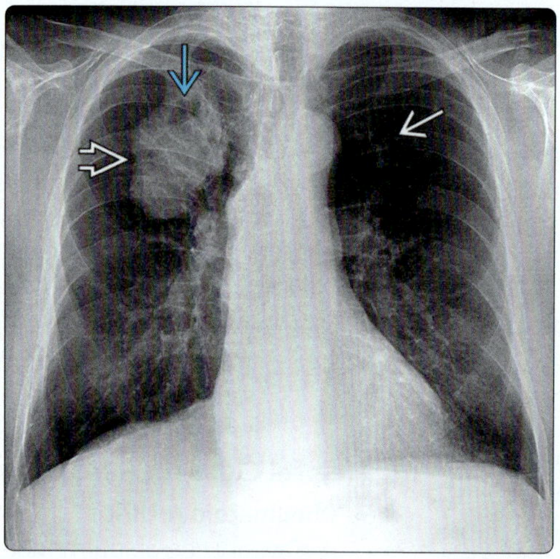

Lung Cancer

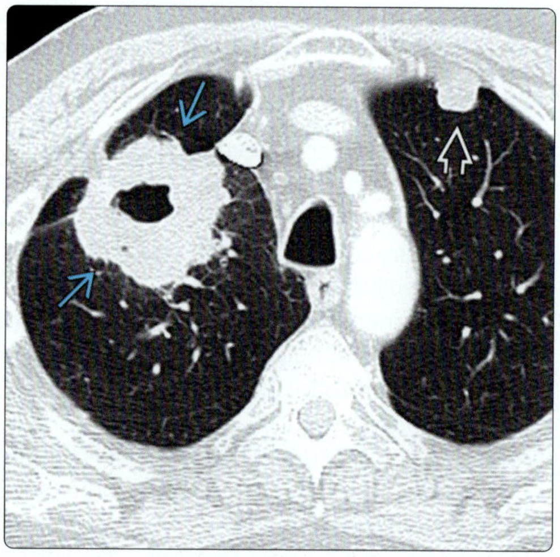

(Left) *Axial CECT of a patient who was previously treated with radiation for primary lung adenocarcinoma shows dense left upper consolidation.* **(Right)** *Axial CECT of the same patient obtained 4 months later for evaluation of severe respiratory symptoms and fever shows a left upper lobe air-fluid level secondary to cavitation, which may be secondary to tumor/parenchymal necrosis &/or superimposed infection. Tissue sampling is necessary for differentiating infection from simple necrosis.*

Lung Cancer

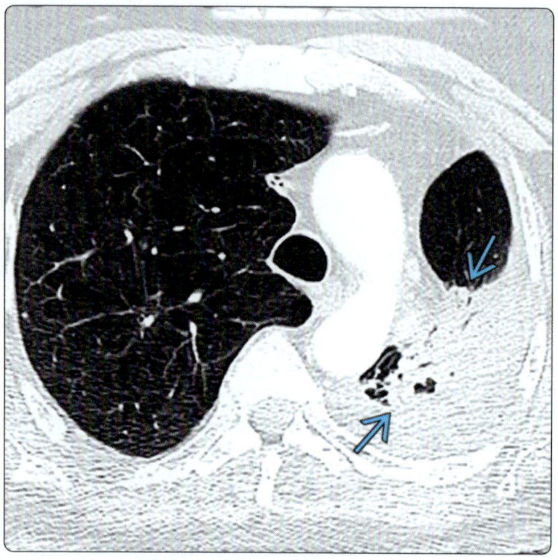

Lung Cancer

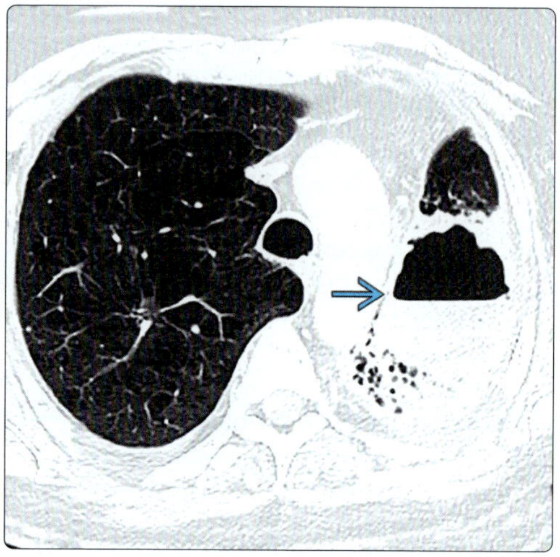

(Left) *PA chest radiograph of a patient with hemoptysis shows a left upper lobe cavitary lesion with adjacent pleural thickening and multiple small nodules in the right lower lung.* **(Right)** *Axial NECT of the same patient shows a left upper lobe cavitary nodule, multifocal tree-in-bud opacities, and patchy nodular consolidations, consistent with the post-primary pattern of tuberculosis. The diagnosis was confirmed by examination of sputum smears.*

Tuberculosis

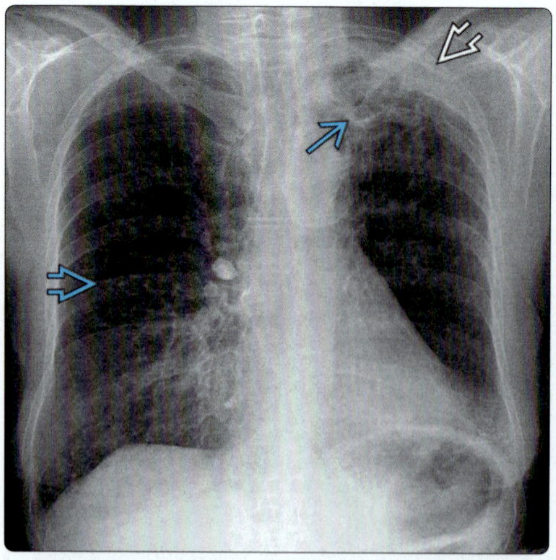

Tuberculosis

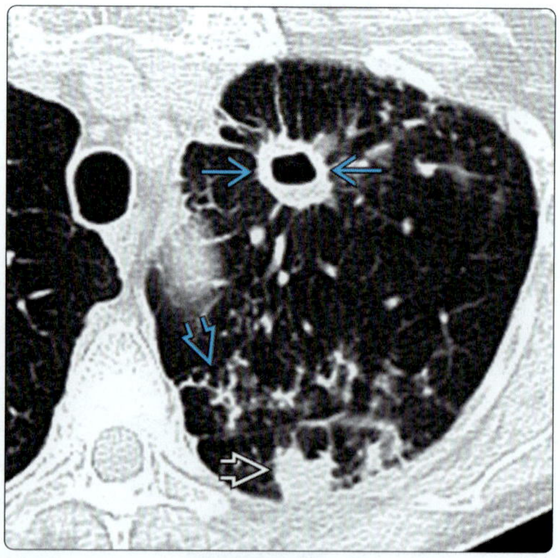

Metastasis

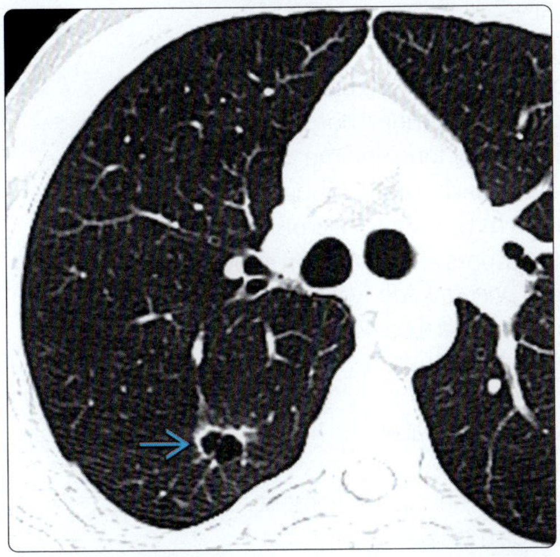

Metastasis

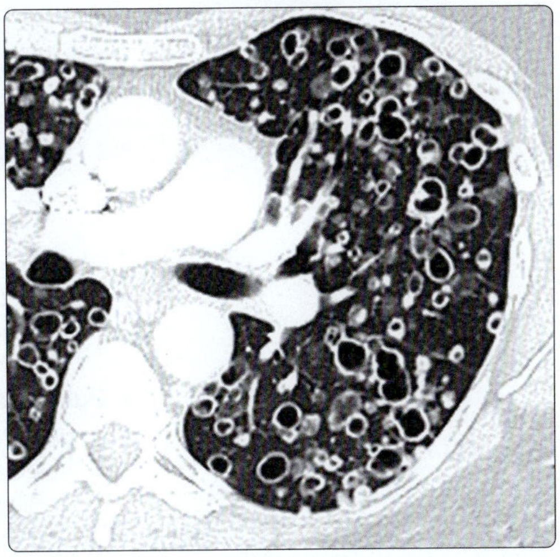

(Left) *Axial NECT of a patient with head and neck cancer shows a right lower lobe cavitary nodule with thin asymmetric walls . Biopsy demonstrated metastatic disease. Cavitary metastases are most commonly associated with squamous cell carcinoma.* **(Right)** *Axial CECT of a patient with colon adenocarcinoma shows multiple, diffuse cavitary lesions of variable sizes that demonstrate the so-called cheerio sign, named for the resemblance to the cereal Cheerios. These findings are associated with metastatic gastrointestinal malignancies.*

Fungal Infection

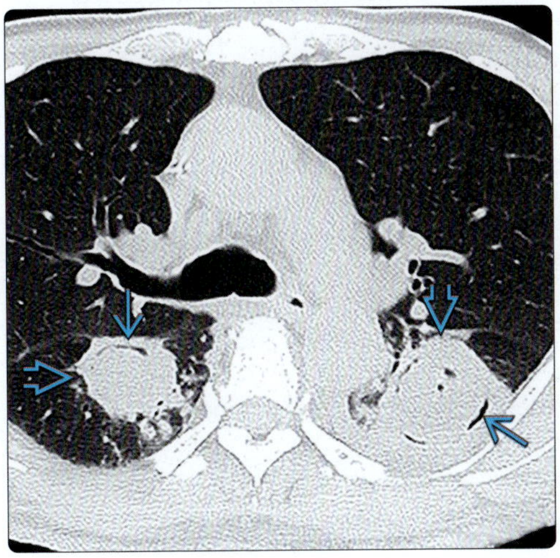

Fungal Infection

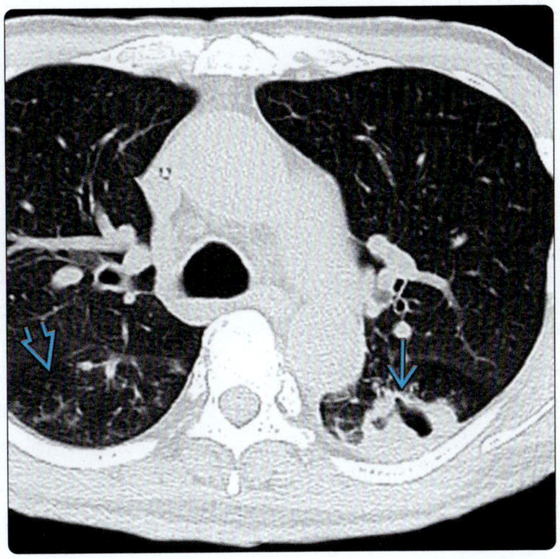

(Left) *Axial CECT of a patient with leukemia and invasive aspergillosis shows lower lobe masses that exhibit the air crescent sign produced by tissue necrosis and intrinsic cavitation.* **(Right)** *Axial NECT of the same patient obtained 3 weeks later shows progression of cavitation within the left lower lobe lesion and near complete resolution of the right lower lobe lesion . The presence of cavitation is associated with return to normal neutrophil function and response to treatment.*

Pulmonary Infarct

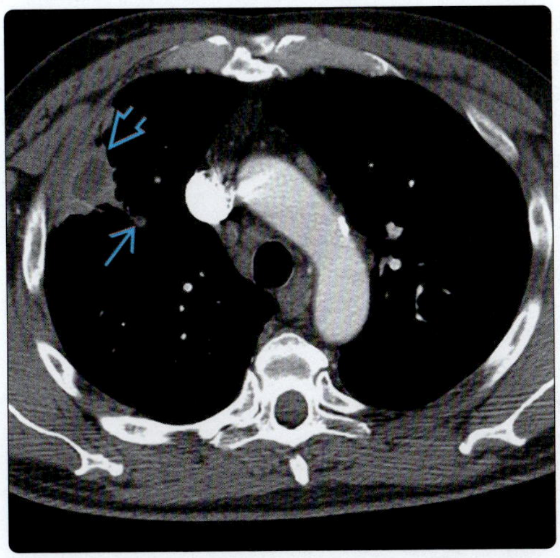

Septic Embolism

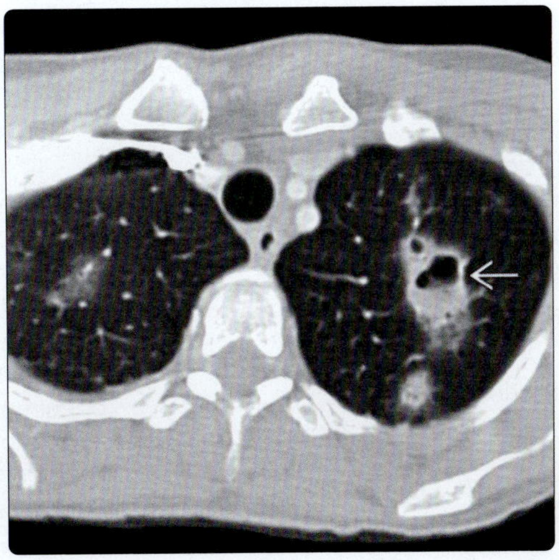

(Left) *Axial CECT of a patient with sarcoidosis who presented with pleuritic pain shows a right upper lobe peripheral wedge-shaped consolidation with central low attenuation from necrosis . Note an occlusive embolus in a right upper lobe pulmonary artery branch . Cavitation in infarcts is usually due to aseptic necrosis and is most frequent in the upper lobes.* **(Right)** *Axial CECT of a patient who presented with fever and positive blood cultures shows multifocal pulmonary nodules, some with cavitation , consistent with septic emboli.*

DIFFERENTIAL DIAGNOSIS

Common

- Pneumonia
- Pulmonary Edema
- Aspiration

Less Common

- Hemorrhage
- Infarction
- Contusion
- Organizing Pneumonia

Rare but Important

- Eosinophilic Pneumonia
- Lung Cancer
- Lymphoma
- Lipoid Pneumonia
- Intralobar Sequestration

ESSENTIAL INFORMATION

Key Differential Diagnosis Issues

- Definition
  - Alveolar filling process that produces increased pulmonary density or attenuation
    - Fluid
    - Blood
    - Purulent material
    - Cells
      - Neoplastic
      - Inflammatory
  - Obscures underlying vessel and airway margins
  - May exhibit intrinsic air bronchograms
  - May demonstrate sign of silhouette: Obscuration of normal anatomic interfaces on radiography
  - May demonstrate CT angiogram sign: Enhanced vascular structures coursing and branching within pulmonary consolidation
- Distribution
  - Lobar
  - Multilobar
  - Diffuse
  - Multifocal
- May exhibit intrinsic cavitation
- Consolidation in patient with signs and symptoms of infection should suggest pneumonia
- Consolidations in adults should be followed to complete imaging resolution to exclude underlying malignancy

Helpful Clues for Common Diagnoses

- **Pneumonia**
  - Common cause of consolidation
  - Affected patients often present with signs and symptoms of infection
  - May exhibit lobar, nonsegmental, or lobular distribution
  - Causative organisms
    - Bacteria: ↑ procalcitonin levels
    - Fungi
    - Mycoplasma
    - Viruses
  - Imaging
    - Homogeneous or heterogeneous pulmonary opacity
      - Focal
      - Multifocal
      - Lobar: Limited by pleura
    - Well- or poorly-defined borders
    - Preservation of lung volume
    - Signs: Air bronchogram, silhouette, CT angiogram
    - Cavitation may occur in necrotizing pneumonia
    - Bulging fissures and cavitation should suggest *Klebsiella pneumoniae*
    - Cavitation associated with bronchiolitis should suggest tuberculosis
- **Pulmonary Edema**
  - Extravascular lung water
  - Alveolar edema
    - Bilateral, symmetric involvement
    - Batwing distribution
      - Perihilar consolidations
      - Spare lung periphery
    - Asymmetric and unilateral distribution may occur
      - Decubitus position
      - Re-expansion edema
      - Right upper lung zone involvement in myocardial infarction with papillary muscle rupture
  - Acute respiratory distress syndrome (ARDS)
    - Diffuse pulmonary involvement
    - Dependent consolidations and airspace disease
    - Mechanical ventilation
- **Aspiration**
  - Clinical: Critically ill, endotracheal and gastric intubation, supine position
  - Consolidation in dependent lung parenchyma
  - Rapid progression
  - May be complicated by pulmonary infection

Helpful Clues for Less Common Diagnoses

- **Hemorrhage**
  - Clinical
    - Hemoptysis is helpful clue but is not always present
    - Specific diseases
      - Idiopathic pulmonary hemorrhage
      - Goodpasture syndrome: Antiglomerular basement membrane disease
      - Vasculitis: Granulomatosis with polyangiitis
      - Systemic lupus erythematosus
  - Imaging
    - Patchy or diffuse consolidations, ground-glass opacities
    - May exhibit central or perihilar distribution
- **Infarction**
  - Pulmonary ischemia and hemorrhage secondary to pulmonary thromboembolism
  - Up to 15% of patients with pulmonary embolism
  - Imaging
    - Hampton hump: Wedge-shaped subpleural consolidation
    - Consolidation with central lucency
    - ± feeding vessel coursing into affected lung
    - Halo sign from surrounding alveolar hemorrhage

- Slow resolution (months); healing with scar formation

- **Contusion**
  - Blunt traumatic lung injury
    - Damage to alveolar capillaries with resultant intraalveolar blood and fluid
    - No disruption of underlying pulmonary architecture
    - Extensive pulmonary contusion may interfere with gas exchange and lead to hypoxia
  - Imaging
    - Nonsegmental consolidation; lung involvement not restricted by anatomic or fissural boundaries
    - Diffuse, multifocal, patchy
    - Affected lung adjacent to point of impact; spares subpleural lung parenchyma
    - Imaging abnormality visible within 6 hours after injury
    - Rapid resolution: 3-10 days
- **Organizing Pneumonia**
  - Chronic non-productive cough, dyspnea, fever, malaise, weight loss; typically responds to steroid therapy
  - Imaging
    - Multifocal ground-glass opacities and consolidations
    - May exhibit migratory behavior
    - Peribronchovascular and perilobular distribution
    - Curvilinear and polygonal morphology
    - Reversed halo sign

Helpful Clues for Rare Diagnoses

- **Eosinophilic Pneumonia**
  - Clinical syndromes
    - Loeffler: Acute presentation; migratory peripheral consolidations
    - Chronic eosinophilic pneumonia
    - Associated conditions: Drug treatment, parasitic disease, fungal disease
    - Peripheral eosinophilia in 2/3 of cases
  - Pathology
    - Alveolar and interstitial accumulation of eosinophils
  - Imaging
    - Peripheral confluent or patchy consolidations
    - Upper lobe predominant, outer 2/3 of lung
- **Lung Cancer**
  - Invasive mucinous adenocarcinoma
    - Lepidic growth pattern
  - Consolidation
    - CT angiogram sign: Pulmonary vessels coursing through and branching within consolidation
    - Bronchus sign: Bronchus coursing into consolidation
    - May exhibit multifocal pulmonary involvement: Consolidation, ground-glass opacities, crazy-paving pattern, acinar nodules
- **Lymphoma**
  - Primary pulmonary lymphoma
    - Typically non-Hodgkin lymphoma
    - Low-grade lymphoma of bronchus-associated lymphoid tissue
    - No evidence of extrapulmonary disease for at least 3 months after diagnosis
  - Focal pulmonary consolidation; may exhibit intrinsic air bronchograms
- **Lipoid Pneumonia**
  - Chronic aspiration or inhalation of oils or fats; most commonly mineral oil
  - Imaging
    - Typically lower lobe predominant consolidations; unilateral or bilateral
    - May manifest as pulmonary nodule or mass
    - May exhibit the crazy-paving pattern
    - Low attenuation within consolidation; ± fat attenuation
- **Intralobar Sequestration**
  - Sequestered lung: No normal communication with tracheobronchial tree + systemic blood supply
  - Clinical: Signs and symptoms of infection, chest pain, may be asymptomatic
  - Imaging
    - Lower lobe consolidation, mass, cystic changes
    - Left > right
    - Identification of systemic blood supply for imaging diagnosis

Pneumonia

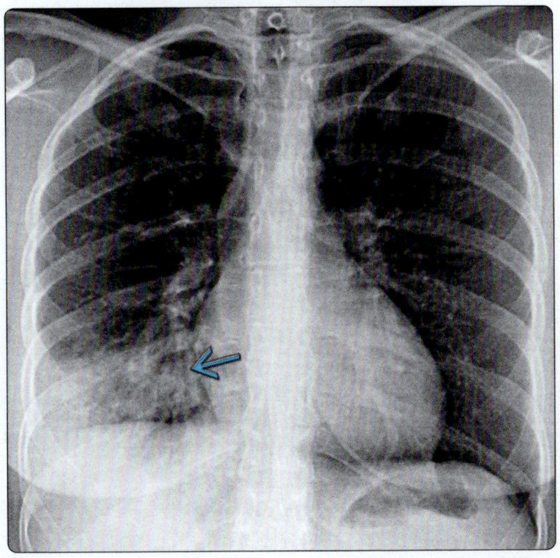

Pneumonia

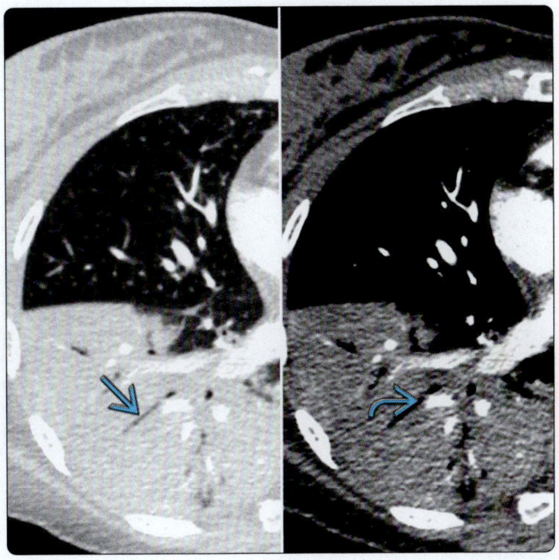

(Left) *PA chest radiograph of a 34-year-old woman with Streptococcus pneumoniae pulmonary infection shows a right lower lobe consolidation that obscures the lateral aspect of the right hemidiaphragm and exhibits the air bronchogram sign →.* **(Right)** *Composite image with axial CECT in lung (left) and soft tissue (right) window of the same patient shows right lower lobe pneumonia that exhibits low attenuation of the consolidated lung as well as the air bronchogram → and the CT angiogram ↪ signs.*

(Left) *PA chest radiograph of a 78-year-old man with cough, low-grade fever, and weight loss shows a large right upper lobe consolidation that produces lobar enlargement and bulging of adjacent interlobar fissures, consistent with Klebsiella pneumonia, diagnosed on sputum culture.* **(Right)** *Coronal CECT of the same patient shows that the right upper lobe consolidation produces lobar expansion and bulging of adjacent interlobar fissures. Lucencies within the consolidation indicate early tissue necrosis.*

Pneumonia

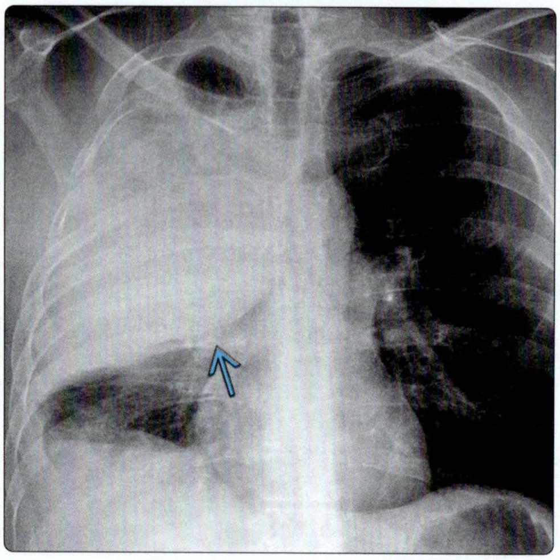

Pneumonia

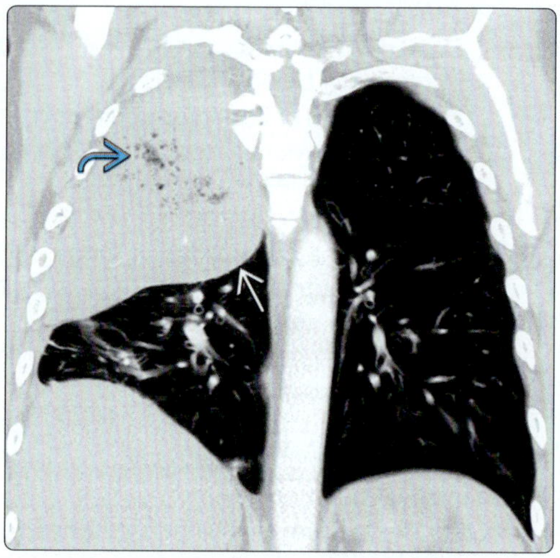

(Left) *Axial CECT of a 47-year-old man with postobstructive right lower lobe pneumonia secondary to a centrally obstructing broncholith in the right lower lobe bronchus shows a heterogeneous right lower lobe consolidation with volume loss and an adjacent moderate pleural effusion.* **(Right)** *Coronal CECT of the same patient (soft tissue window) shows the consolidated right lower lobe distal to the obstructing right lower lobe broncholith. Note the endobronchial mucus plugs and the adjacent right pleural effusion.*

Pneumonia

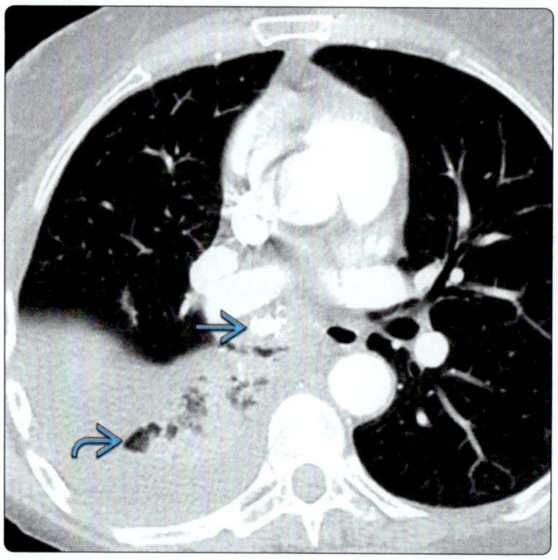

Pneumonia

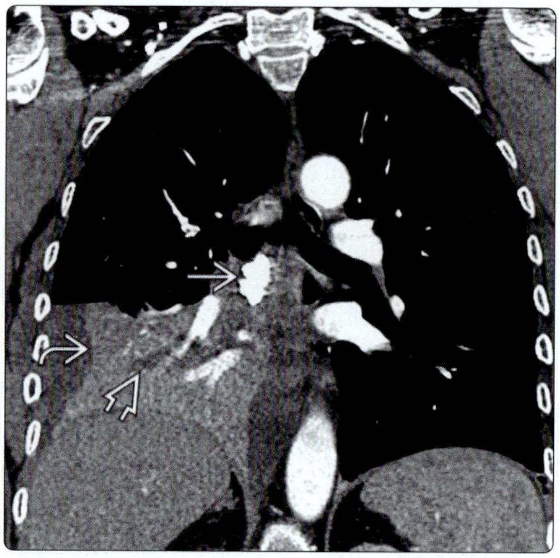

(Left) *AP chest radiograph of a 65-year-old man with chronic heart failure who presented acutely with severe dyspnea secondary to pulmonary edema shows the batwing pattern of alveolar edema, which manifests with bilateral perihilar consolidations that spare the lung periphery.* **(Right)** *Axial CECT of the same patient shows bilateral perihilar consolidations and minimal interlobular septal thickening. Note small bilateral pleural effusions, consistent with the diagnosis of pulmonary edema.*

Pulmonary Edema

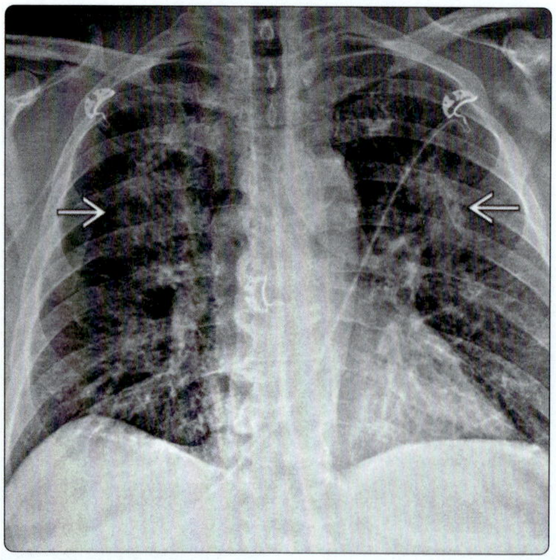

Pulmonary Edema

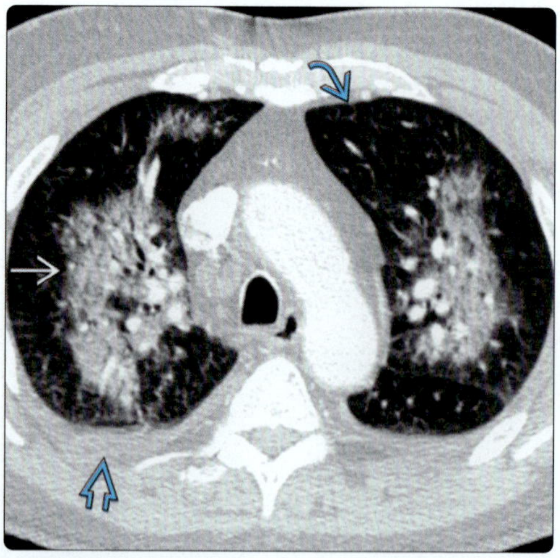

Pulmonary Edema

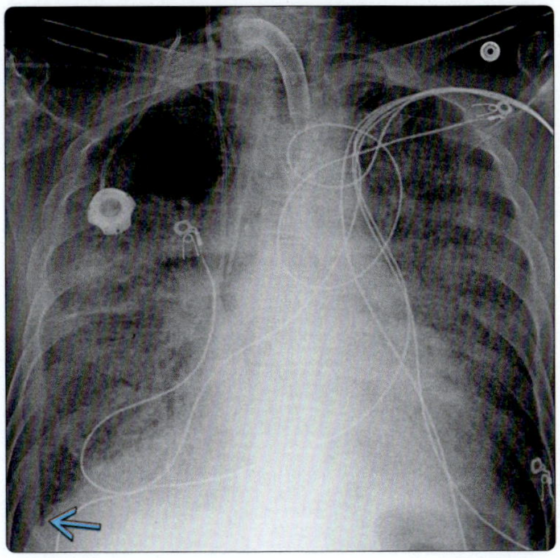

Pulmonary Edema

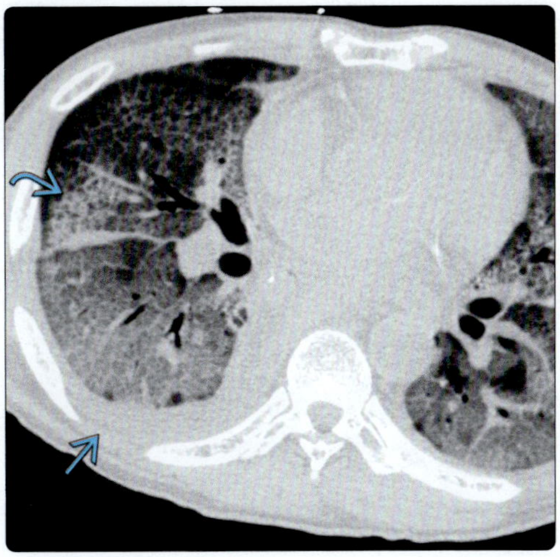

(Left) *AP portable chest radiograph of a 53-year-old man admitted to the intensive care unit for management of acute respiratory distress syndrome (ARDS) secondary to multifocal pulmonary infection shows diffuse bilateral consolidations, a small right pleural effusion, and a tracheostomy required for mechanical ventilation.* **(Right)** *Axial NECT of the same patient shows diffuse bilateral ground-glass opacities that demonstrate the crazy-paving pattern, small consolidations, and a small right pleural effusion.*

Aspiration

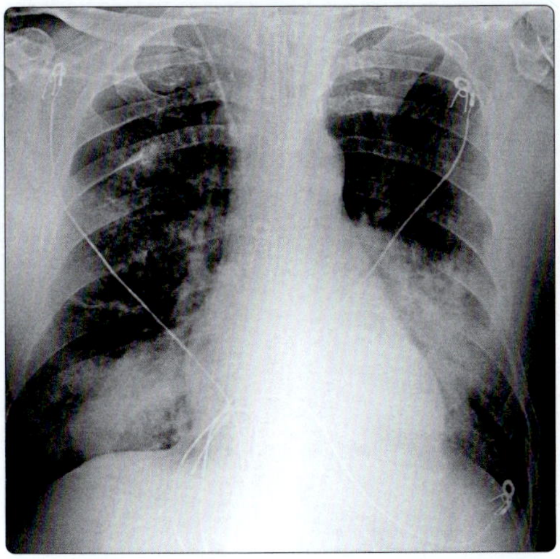

Hemorrhage

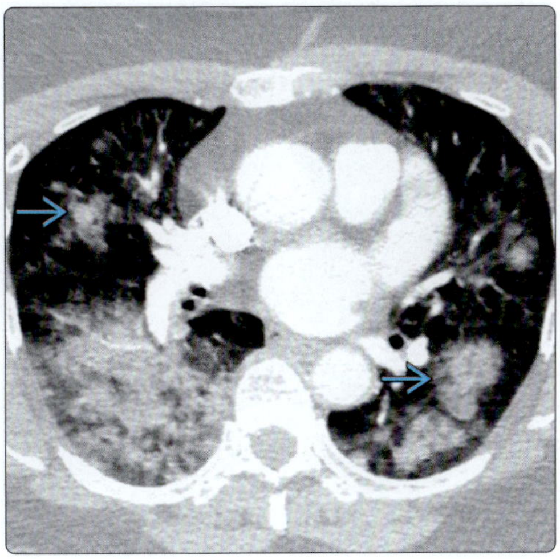

(Left) *AP portable chest radiograph of an 83-year-old patient obtained status post a witnessed episode of aspiration shows bilateral lower lobe dense mass-like consolidations. Consolidations from aspiration preferentially affect the dependent portions of the lungs.* **(Right)** *Axial CECT of a 67-year-old woman who presented with hemoptysis secondary to idiopathic pulmonary hemorrhage shows alveolar hemorrhage that manifests with multifocal nodular consolidations and ground-glass opacities.*

Infarction

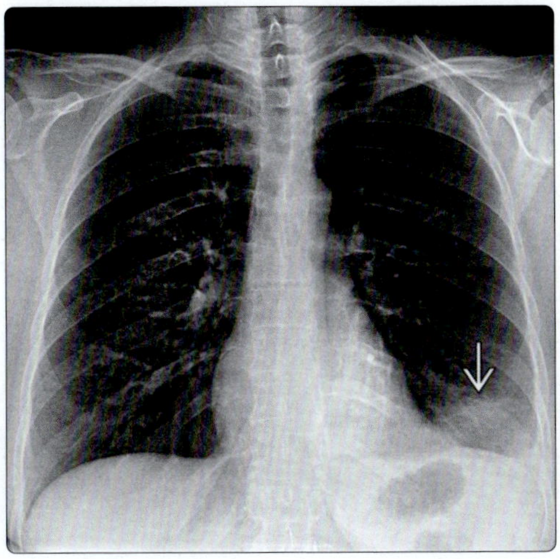

Infarction

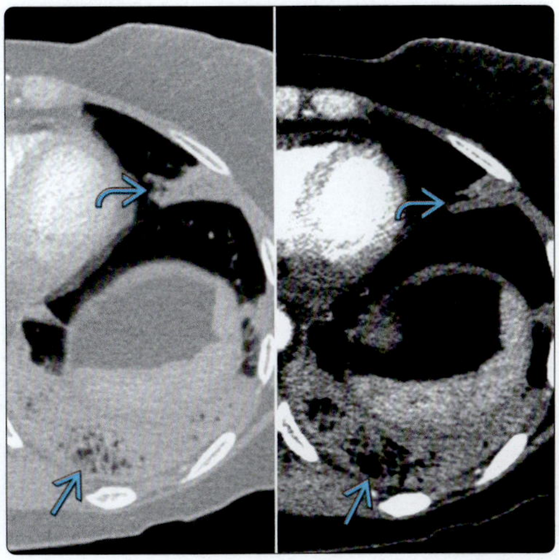

(Left) *PA chest radiograph of a 49-year-old woman who presented to the emergency department with acute onset of chest pain and dyspnea shows a left lower lobe consolidation and a small left pleural effusion.* **(Right)** *Composite image with axial CECT in lung (left) and soft tissue (right) window of the same patient shows that the consolidation corresponds to a left lower lobe pulmonary infarct that exhibits internal lucency. Note the lingular wedge-shaped consolidation, also consistent with pulmonary infarction.*

Infarction

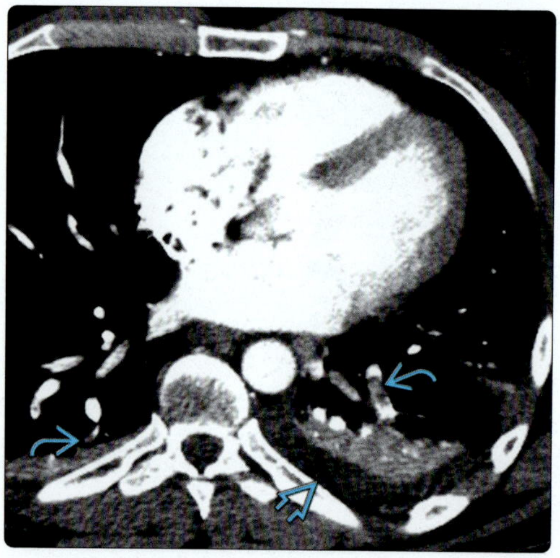

Infarction

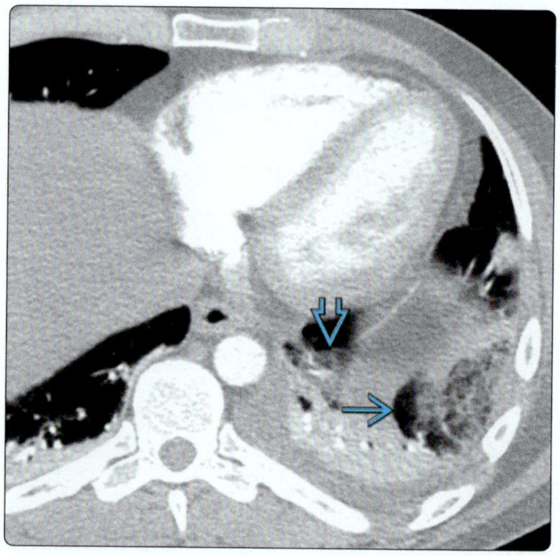

(Left) *Axial CECT of a 37-year-old man who presented with acute chest pain shows bilateral lower lobe pulmonary thromboemboli, bibasilar consolidations that exhibit poor contrast enhancement, and a small left pleural effusion.* **(Right)** *Axial CECT of the same patient shows a dominant left lower lobe consolidation with areas of intrinsic lucency, consistent with the CT findings of pulmonary infarction. Note the small left pleural effusion. Areas of ground-glass opacity likely represent adjacent alveolar hemorrhage.*

Contusion

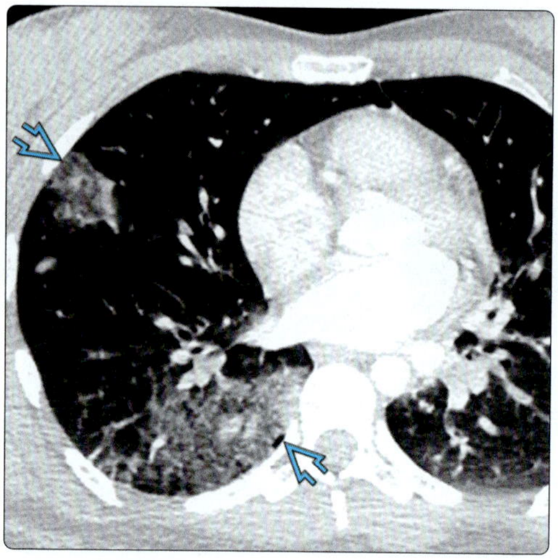

Contusion

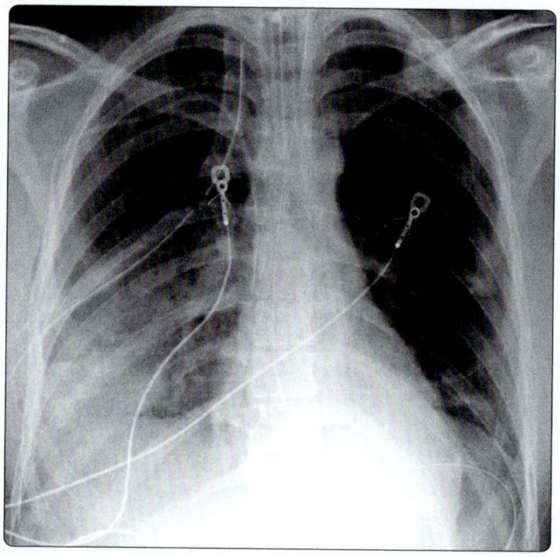

(Left) *Axial CECT of a 38-year-old woman who sustained right chest trauma during a motor vehicle collision shows multifocal right lung consolidations and ground-glass opacities, consistent with pulmonary contusions.* **(Right)** *AP chest radiograph of the same patient obtained hours later shows endotracheal intubation, right chest tube placement, and progression of right basilar consolidation related to contusion, which resulted in hypoxemia that required mechanical ventilatory support.*

Organizing Pneumonia

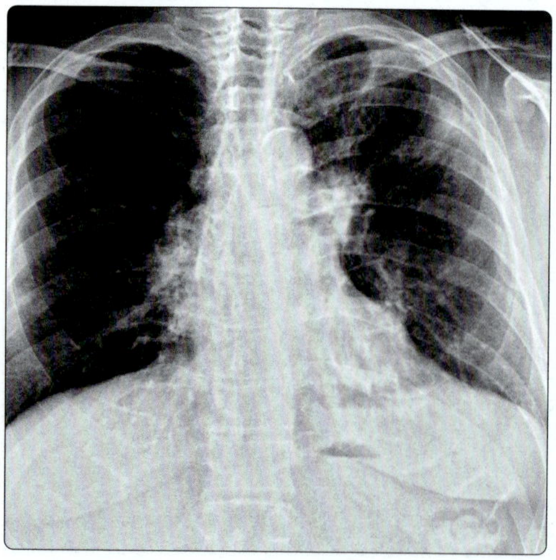

Organizing Pneumonia

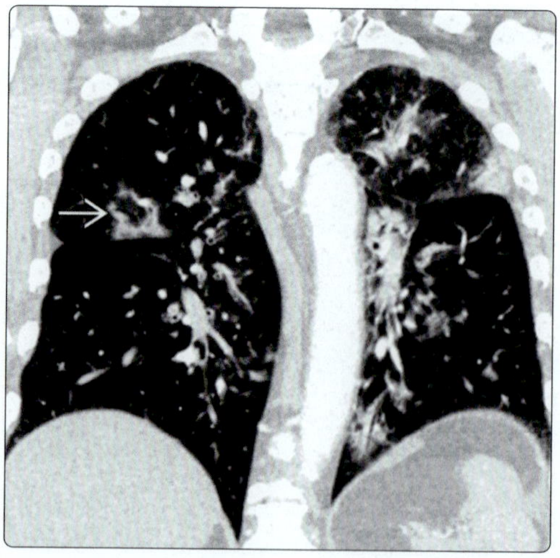

(Left) *PA chest radiograph of a 59-year-old man who presented with cough and fever shows multifocal left lung-predominant patchy consolidations that were initially thought to represent multifocal bacterial pneumonia.* **(Right)** *Coronal CECT of the same patient shows multifocal bilateral, left greater than right, nodular consolidations. Note that the right upper lobe consolidation exhibits the atoll or reversed halo sign suggestive of organizing pneumonia. The patient responded to steroid therapy.*

Eosinophilic Pneumonia

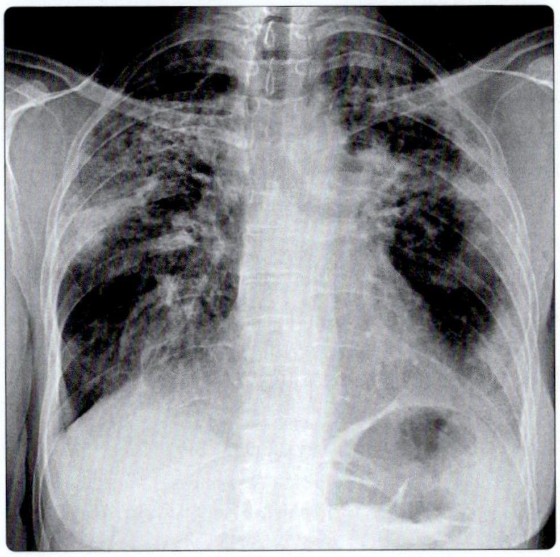

Eosinophilic Pneumonia

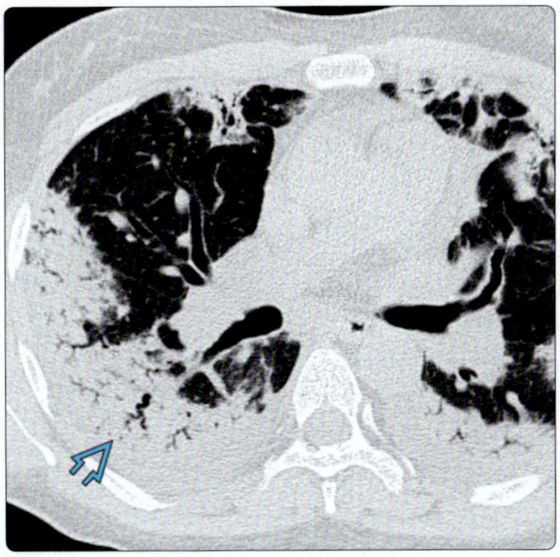

(Left) *PA chest radiograph of a 59-year-old woman who presented with cough and dyspnea shows low lung volume and upper lung zone-predominant peripheral subpleural opacities.* **(Right)** *Axial NECT of the same patient demonstrates peripheral subpleural consolidations with intrinsic air bronchograms. Given the pattern of lung involvement and the presence of peripheral eosinophilia, the diagnosis of eosinophilic pneumonia was suggested. Steroid treatment was successfully instituted.*

Lung Cancer

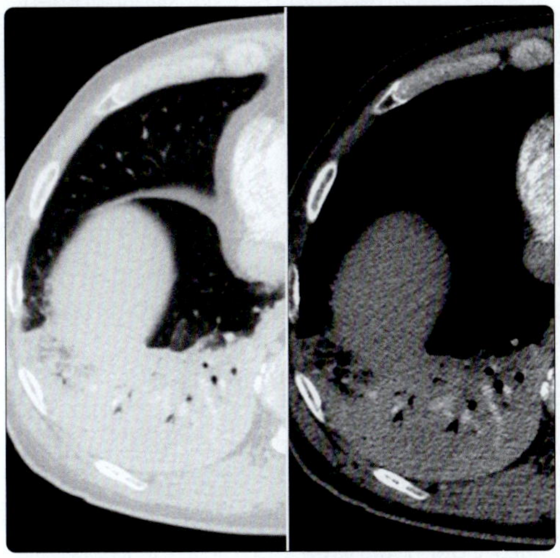

Lymphoma

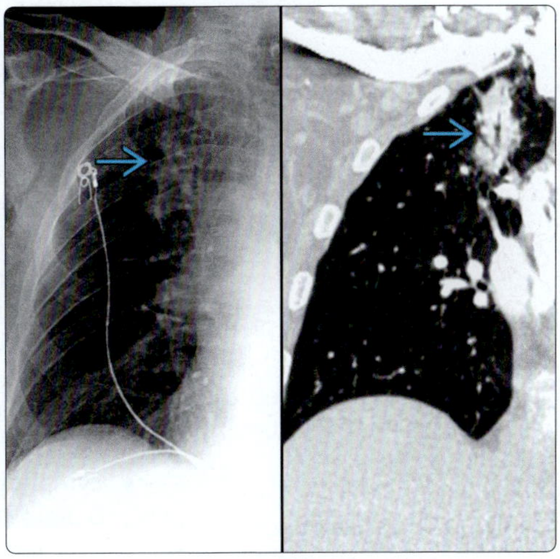

(Left) *Composite image with axial CECT in lung (left) and soft tissue (right) window shows a right lower lobe consolidation that exhibits the air bronchogram and CT angiogram signs. Failure to respond to antimicrobials prompted biopsy, which revealed primary pulmonary invasive adenocarcinoma.* **(Right)** *Composite image with AP chest radiograph (left) and coronal CECT (right) of an 83-year-old man shows a chronic right upper lobe consolidation with air bronchograms, which was a biopsy-proven primary pulmonary lymphoma.*

Lipoid Pneumonia

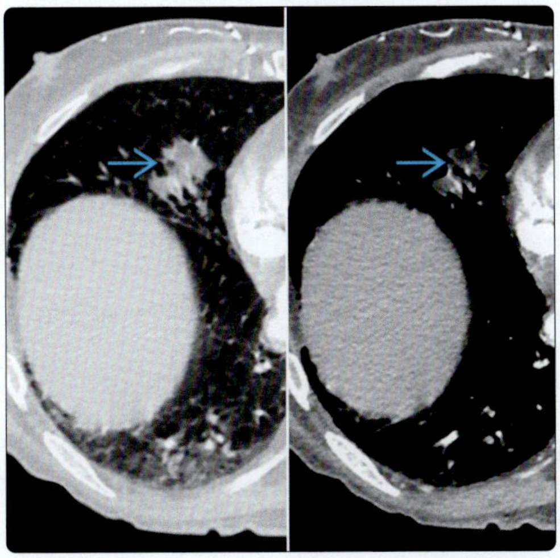

Intralobar Sequestration

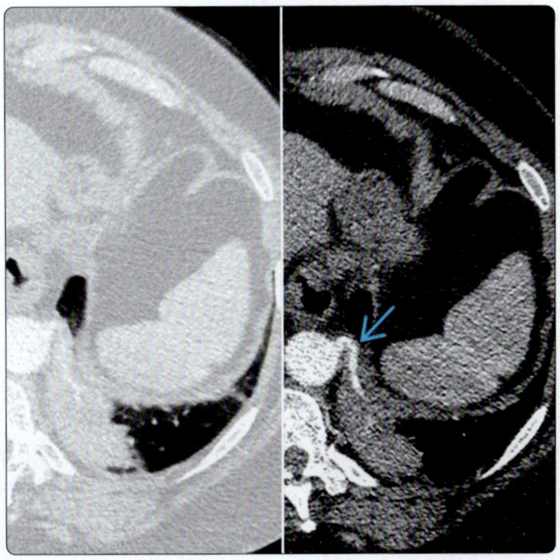

(Left) *Composite image with axial CECT in lung (left) and soft tissue (right) window of a 98-year-old man who used mineral oil for constipation shows an irregular nodular middle lobe consolidation, which demonstrates internal fat attenuation, diagnostic of lipoid pneumonia given the history.* **(Right)** *Composite image with axial CECT in lung (left) and soft tissue (right) window of a 70-year-old man shows a chronic left lower lobe consolidation with systemic blood supply from descending aorta, diagnostic of intralobar sequestration.*

DIFFERENTIAL DIAGNOSIS

Common

- Pneumatocele
- Honeycombing
- Incidental Cyst

Less Common

- Pulmonary Langerhans Cell Histiocytosis
- Lymphangioleiomyomatosis
- Lymphoid Interstitial Pneumonia
- Desquamative Interstitial Pneumonia

Rare but Important

- Birt-Hogg-Dubé Syndrome
- Light-Chain Deposition Disease
- Tracheobronchial Papillomatosis
- Congenital Pulmonary Airway Malformation
- Neurofibromatosis Type 1

ESSENTIAL INFORMATION

Key Differential Diagnosis Issues

- Definition: Cyst on CT
  - Thin-walled (< 2 mm) spherical lucency with perceptible wall
    - Not applicable to bulla, bleb, pneumatocele, or cavity
      - Bulla: Rounded lucency or focal decreased attenuation > 1 cm (usually several centimeters), thin-walled < 1 mm, often with associated emphysema
      - Bleb: Thin-walled cystic space within visceral pleura, typically < 1 cm in size
      - Pneumatocele: Round or spherical, thin-walled, air-filled space; typically caused by infection, trauma, or hydrocarbon fluid aspiration
      - Cavity: Gas-filled space within pulmonary consolidation, mass, or nodule; typically thick walled (> 2 mm) and more irregularly shaped than cyst

Helpful Clues for Common Diagnoses

- **Pneumatocele**
  - Transient, thin-walled, gas-filled space in lung
    - Acute pneumonia
      - Parenchymal necrosis and check-valve airway obstruction
      - *Pneumocystis jirovecii* pneumonia; Staphylococcal pneumonia (children)
      - HIV(+) patients: Ground-glass opacities with coexistent thin-walled cysts should raise possibility of lymphoid interstitial pneumonia or pneumocystis pneumonia
- **Honeycombing**
  - End-stage fibrosis; typical feature of usual interstitial pneumonia
    - Single or multiple layers of subpleural cysts
      - Represent dilated bronchioles
- **Incidental Cyst**
  - Found in 25% of asymptomatic subjects > 75 years
  - Normal spectrum of senescent lung
  - May be associated with bilateral basilar subpleural reticular opacities

Helpful Clues for Less Common Diagnoses

- **Pulmonary Langerhans Cell Histiocytosis**
  - Strong association with cigarette smoking (> 90%)
    - M = F; increasing number of women smokers
  - Pneumothorax: Initial manifestation in 15% of affected patients; recurrent pneumothorax in 60%
  - Radiography: Normal or increased lung volume; upper lung zone predominant reticular opacities, nodules, and cysts; spares lung bases
  - CT
    - Small bronchiolocentric nodules with irregular/stellate borders (1-10 mm)
    - Cysts of variable size, bizarre shapes, and thin or thick nodular walls
    - Upper/mid lung zone predominance, spares lung bases
    - End-stage disease: Fibrosis and cystic spaces
- **Lymphangioleiomyomatosis**
  - Systemic disease that affects almost exclusively women of childbearing age
  - Sporadic disease prevalence: ~ 5 per million
  - Symptoms and signs
    - Dyspnea often exacerbated by exertion, fatigue
    - Pneumothorax: Initial manifestation in 40-50% of affected patients; recurrent in 77%
    - Chylous pleural effusion: 22-39%
    - Extrapulmonary manifestations (76%): Bleeding from renal angiomyolipoma, lymphangioleiomyoma (16%), ascites/chylous ascites (10%)
  - Radiography: Widespread fine reticular opacities from superimposition of thin-walled cysts
  - CT: Diffuse thin-walled cysts of uniform size
- **Lymphoid Interstitial Pneumonia**
  - Rare condition limited to lungs
    - Inflammatory pulmonary reaction of bronchus-associated lymphoid tissue (BALT)
      - Diffuse polyclonal lymphocytic infiltration of alveolar septa
  - Common associations
    - Autoimmune disorders
      - Sjögren syndrome
      - Rheumatoid arthritis
      - Systemic lupus erythematosus
    - Infection: HIV (children), Epstein-Barr virus
  - Complications
    - Monoclonal gammopathy or hypogammaglobulinemia: Low-grade marginal zone lymphoma (BALT type)
    - Pulmonary amyloidosis
  - CT
    - Ground-glass attenuation, ill-defined centrilobular and subpleural nodules, thick bronchovascular bundles
    - Thin-walled cysts (80%): Variable size and variable shape
    - Airspace consolidation, large soft tissue/calcified pulmonary nodules
      - Lymphoma (BALT type)
      - Amyloidosis

- **Desquamative Interstitial Pneumonia**
  - Association with cigarette smoking and passive exposure to cigarette smoke
    - Smokers: 58-91%
      - Accumulation of pigmented macrophages in distal airspaces
    - DIP-like histology
      - Component of connective tissue disease-associated interstitial lung disease (rheumatoid arthritis)
      - Environmental exposure
      - Infection
      - Drug reaction
  - Imaging
    - Patchy ground-glass opacities interspersed with normal lung
      - Lower-lung zone and peripheral predominance
      - Small cystic spaces

Helpful Clues for Rare Diagnoses

- **Birt-Hogg-Dubé Syndrome**
  - Autosomal dominant inherited genodermatosis
  - Cutaneous folliculomas and diverse types of kidney tumors
  - Pulmonary cysts: 80% of cases
- **Pulmonary Light-Chain Deposition Disease**
  - Systemic accumulation of immunoglobulin light chains, most commonly in lymphoproliferative disorders and autoimmune conditions
    - Uncommon
    - Indolent or slowly progressive disease
  - CT
    - Thin-walled pulmonary cysts and nodules
    - Purely cystic lung disease
    - Cysts with mural pulmonary vessels are uncommon
- **Tracheobronchial Papillomatosis**
  - Infectious disease of upper aero-digestive tract
    - Human papillomavirus
    - Most infections occur at birth; contaminated birth canal
    - Clinical symptoms: Chronic cough, hoarseness, wheezing, voice change, chronic dyspnea
  - CT
    - Tracheobronchial and pulmonary lesions
      - Focal or diffuse airway narrowing; nodular vegetant lesions
      - Scattered numerous multilobulated pulmonary nodules of various sizes
      - Nodules may enlarge, become air-filled cysts, and form large cavities
      - Malignant transformation: Squamous cell carcinoma, enlarged airways and nodules/masses, lymphadenopathy
- **Congenital Pulmonary Airway Malformation**
  - Rare developmental abnormality of lower respiratory tract
    - Prenatal diagnosis during routine obstetrical ultrasound
    - Incidence: 1:25,000-1:35,000 births
    - Risk of malignant transformation
      - Adults with pulmonary airway malformation not resected in childhood
  - Imaging
    - Unilocular or multilocular cysts
    - Retained fluid within cysts, air-fluid levels
- **Neurofibromatosis Type 1**
  - Autosomal dominant inherited neurocutaneous disorder
  - Multiple (> 6) café-au-lait spots and cutaneous neurofibromas
  - Diffuse interstitial fibrosis and bullae in 6-12% of patients (> 40 years of age)
  - Asymmetric, upper lung predominant cysts

SELECTED REFERENCES

1. Raoof S et al: Cystic lung diseases: algorithmic approach. Chest. 150(4):945-65, 2016
2. Gupta N et al: Diffuse cystic lung disease. Part II. Am J Respir Crit Care Med. 192(1):17-29, 2015
3. Jawad H et al: Cystic interstitial lung diseases: recognizing the common and uncommon entities. Curr Probl Diagn Radiol. 43(3):115-27, 2014

Pneumatocele

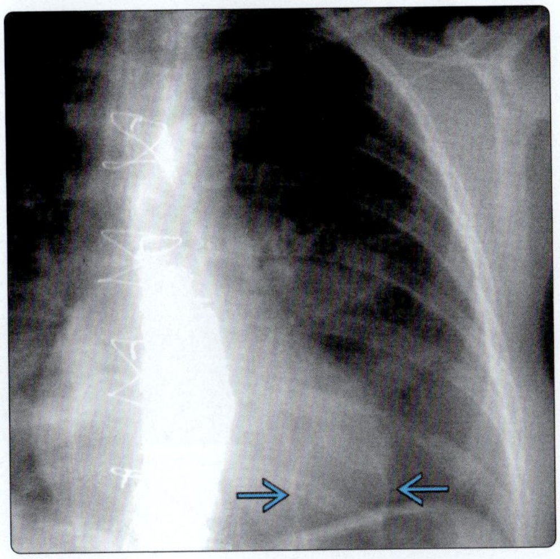

Pneumatocele

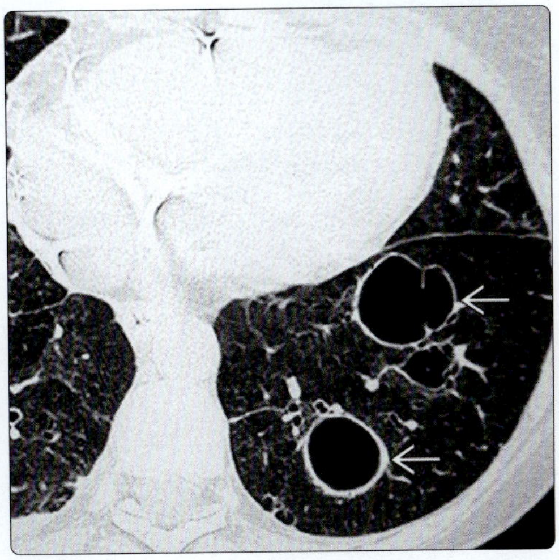

(Left) *Coned-down PA chest radiograph of a man with a history of prior pneumococcal pneumonia shows multiple cystic lesions ➡ in the left lower lobe.* **(Right)** *Axial NECT of the same patient shows multiple left lower lobe pulmonary cysts ➡ with uniform relatively thin walls consistent with postinfectious pneumatoceles. Pneumatoceles are associated with staphylococcal infection, trauma, and hydrocarbon aspiration, and typically resolve spontaneously.*

(Left) *Axial NECT of a patient with human immunodeficiency virus infection and Pneumocystis jirovecii pneumonia shows diffuse bilateral basilar predominant ground-glass opacities and multifocal upper lobe predominant thin-walled pulmonary cysts.* **(Right)** *Axial NECT of a patient with chronic dyspnea and idiopathic pulmonary fibrosis shows bilateral peripheral subpleural multilayered pulmonary honeycomb cysts on a background of reticulation.*

Pneumatocele

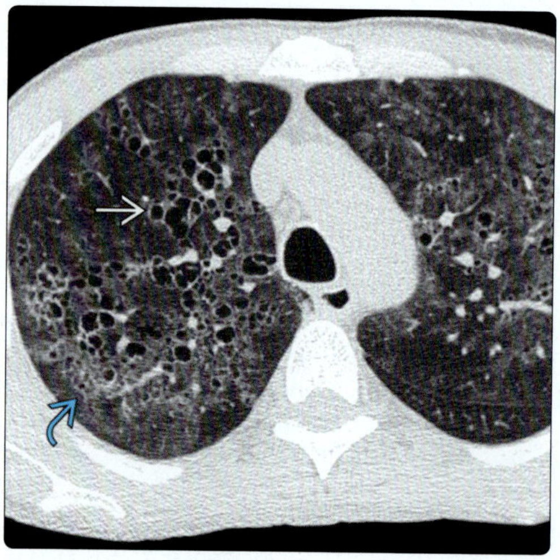

Honeycombing

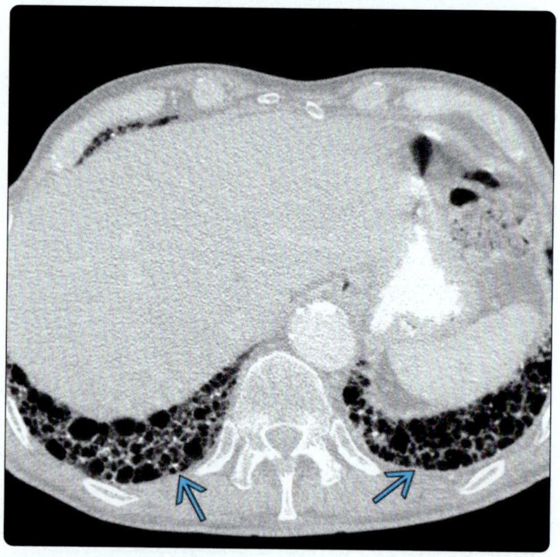

(Left) *Axial NECT of a smoker who presented with cough and dyspnea secondary to pulmonary Langerhans cell histiocytosis shows upper lobe-predominant cysts of variable wall thickness, some with nodular walls and bizarre shapes, and small pulmonary nodules, some with cavitation.* **(Right)** *Axial NECT of a patient with lymphangioleiomyomatosis shows diffuse multifocal thin-walled lung cysts of variable size with intervening normal lung parenchyma.*

Pulmonary Langerhans Cell Histiocytosis

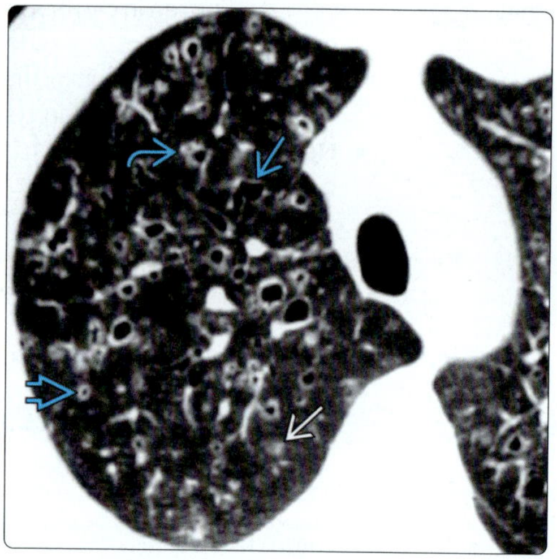

Lymphangioleiomyomatosis

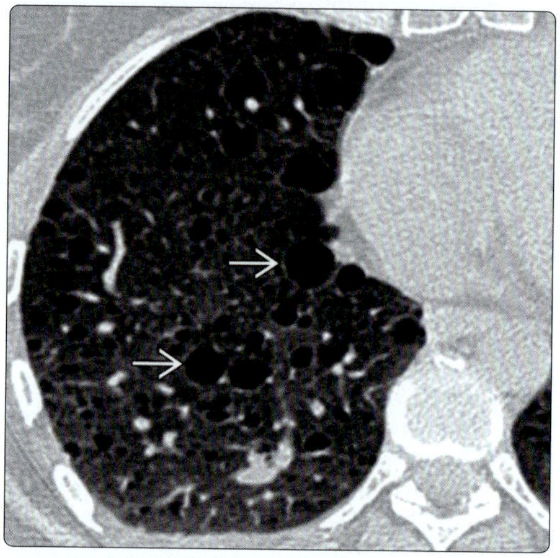

(Left) *Axial NECT of a patient with Sjögren syndrome and lymphoid interstitial pneumonia shows multiple perivascular and subpleural thin-walled cysts on a background of subtle ground-glass opacity and bronchial wall thickening.* **(Right)** *Axial HRCT of a life-long smoker with desquamative interstitial pneumonia shows multiple thin-walled cysts on a background of basilar ground-glass opacity and coexistent basilar paraseptal emphysema. (Courtesy D. Hansell, MD.)*

Lymphoid Interstitial Pneumonia

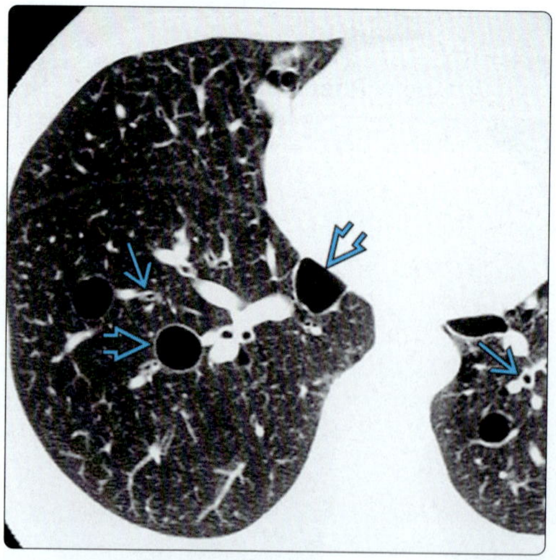

Desquamative Interstitial Pneumonia

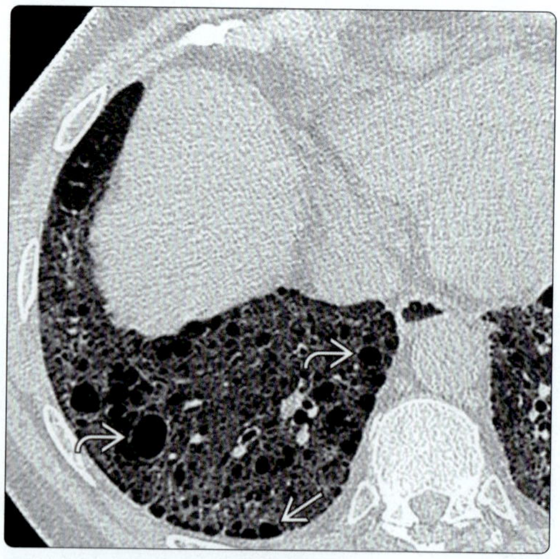

Birt-Hogg-Dubé Syndrome

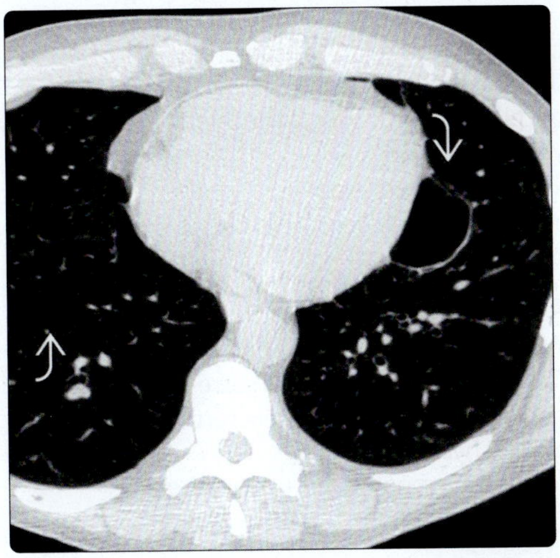

Light-Chain Deposition Disease

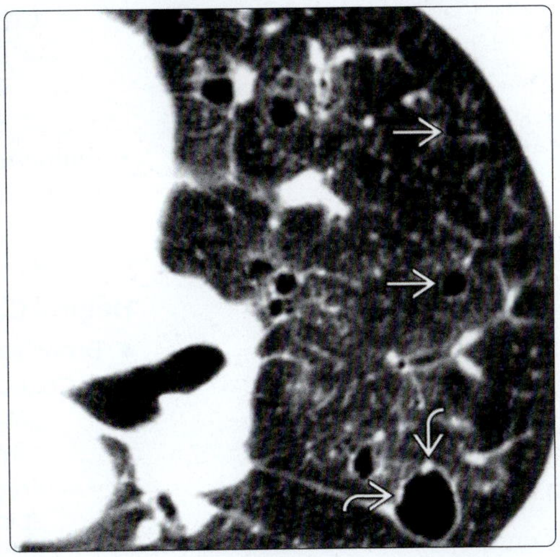

(Left) *Axial NECT of a 71-year-old man with Birt-Hogg-Dubé syndrome shows basilar predominant thin-walled pulmonary cysts with normal intervening lung. Note the characteristic ovoid morphology* ↪ *of some of the cysts.* **(Right)** *Axial NECT of a 62-year-old man with light-chain deposition disease shows multiple thin-walled cysts* ➡ *of varying sizes. Pulmonary vessels* ↪ *coursing in the cyst walls are a characteristic finding of light-chain deposition disease. Note multiple ill-defined centrilobular nodules.*

Tracheobronchial Papillomatosis

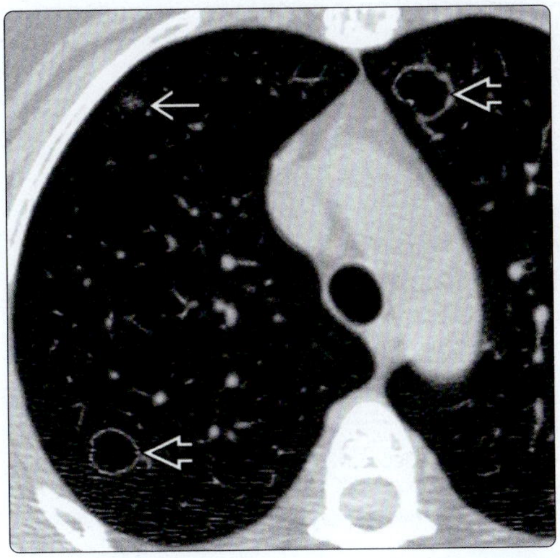

Congenital Pulmonary Airway Malformation

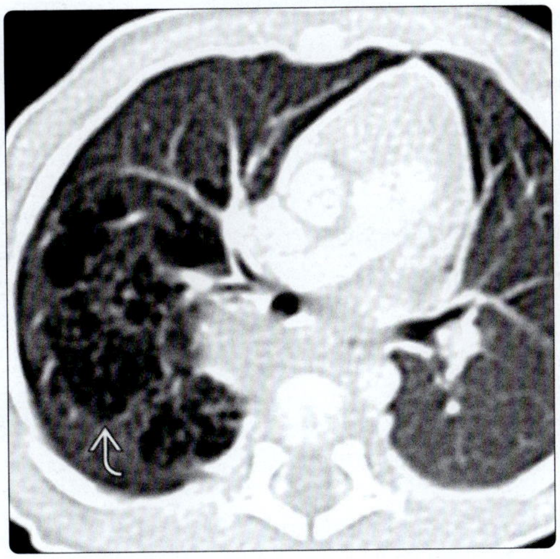

(Left) *Axial NECT of a patient with tracheobronchial papillomatosis shows multifocal bilateral pulmonary cysts, some with nodular walls* ➡*. Note the small part-solid indeterminate right upper lobe nodule* ➡*. Affected patients are at risk of developing squamous cell lung cancer.* **(Right)** *Axial CECT of a 4-week-old infant with type II congenital pulmonary airway malformation shows multiple clustered small pulmonary cysts* ↪ *in the right lung. Unresected lesions in adults have an increased risk of malignant transformation.*

Neurofibromatosis Type 1

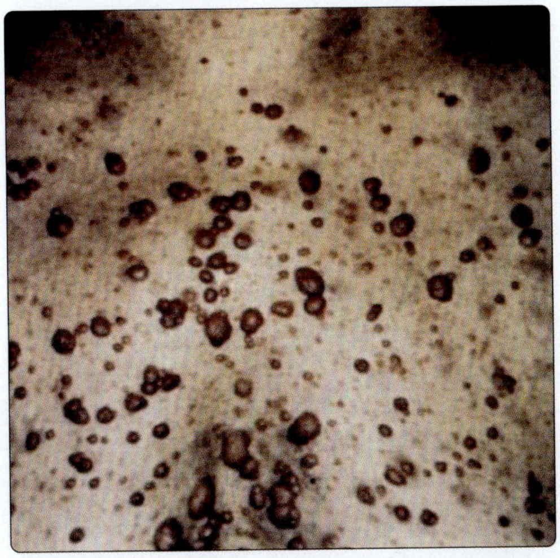

Neurofibromatosis Type 1

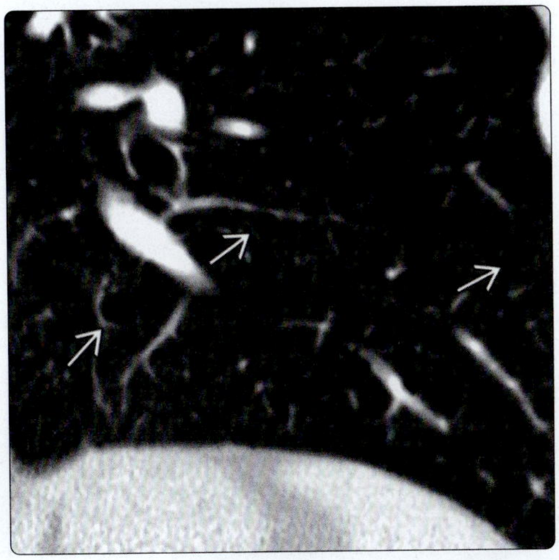

(Left) *Clinical photograph of a 45-year-old woman with neurofibromatosis shows multiple cutaneous neurofibromas of varying sizes widely distributed over the patient's trunk.* **(Right)** *Coned-down coronal NECT of the same patient shows multiple left lower lobe thin-walled cysts* ➡*. Neurofibromatosis is a rare etiology of cystic lung disease that characteristically affects the upper lung zones.*

DIFFERENTIAL DIAGNOSIS

Common

- Emphysema

Less Common

- Pneumatocele
- Constrictive Bronchiolitis
- Pulmonary Hypertension

Rare but Important

- Bronchial Atresia
- Pulmonary Sequestration
- Pulmonary Airway Malformation

ESSENTIAL INFORMATION

Helpful Clues for Common Diagnoses

- **Emphysema**
  - Centrilobular
    - Upper lobe predominant smoking-related disease
    - Centrilobular lucency, imperceptible wall, central "dot" represents lobular artery
  - Paraseptal
    - Single row of subpleural pulmonary cysts
    - May manifest with giant bullous disease
  - Panlobular
    - α-1-antitrypsin deficiency
    - Basilar hyperlucent lung, paucity of vessels

Helpful Clues for Less Common Diagnoses

- **Pneumatocele**
  - Thin-walled, air-filled space (may be multifocal), surrounded by lung parenchyma
  - Associated conditions: Pneumonia (*Pneumocystis*, *Staphylococcus*), trauma, hydrocarbon aspiration
- **Constrictive Bronchiolitis**
  - Concentric luminal narrowing of membranous and respiratory bronchioles: Submucosal and peribronchial fibrosis
    - Chronic airflow obstruction
    - Causes: Infection, inhalation of noxious fumes, graft-vs.-host disease, rheumatoid arthritis
    - CT
      - Expiratory air-trapping: Present in 15% of cases with normal inspiratory CT
      - Bronchial wall thickening, bronchiolar dilatation
- **Pulmonary Hypertension**
  - Mosaic attenuation/perfusion
  - Diminished vascular caliber in areas of decreased lung attenuation

Helpful Clues for Rare Diagnoses

- **Bronchial Atresia**
  - Congenital focal airway obstruction/atresia
    - Enlarged distal bronchi, mucocele formation, surrounding hyperlucent lung
    - Frequent involvement of left upper lobe apicoposterior segment
    - Clinical
      - Incidental finding in asymptomatic patient (50%)
      - Recurrent infection, wheezing, dyspnea
  - CT: Round tubular or branching opacity surrounded by hyperlucent lung
- **Pulmonary Sequestration**
  - No normal communication with tracheobronchial tree + systemic blood supply
  - May manifest as hyperlucent lung, bronchiectatic airways, pulmonary cysts
- **Pulmonary Airway Malformation**
  - Congenital lesion with normal blood supply
  - Cystic lung parenchyma: Clustered cysts of variable size, dominant cyst with internal septations

SELECTED REFERENCES

1. Alsumrain M et al: Pulmonary sequestration in adults: a retrospective review of resected and unresected cases. BMC Pulm Med. 18(1):97, 2018
2. Nemec SF et al: Pulmonary hyperlucency in adults. AJR Am J Roentgenol. 200(2):W101-15, 2013
3. Abbott GF et al: Imaging of small airways disease. J Thorac Imaging. 24(4):285-98, 2009

Emphysema

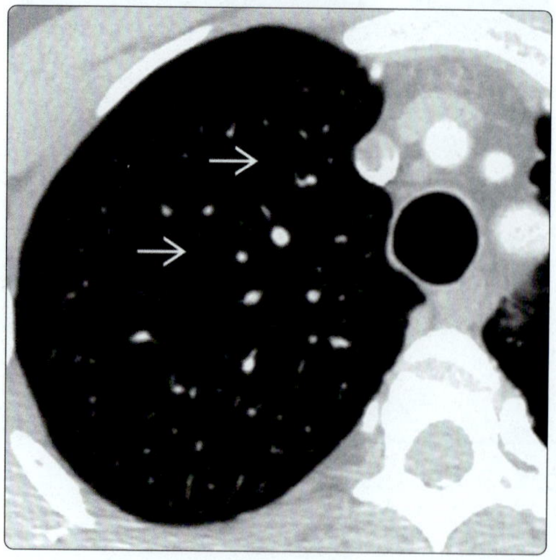

Emphysema

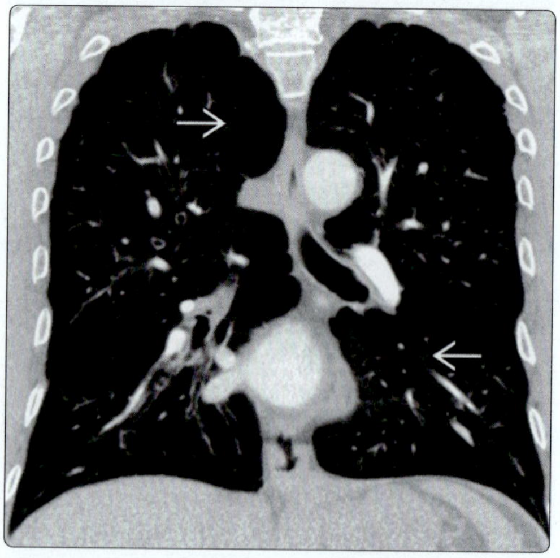

(Left) *Axial CECT of a 52-year-old smoker shows centrilobular emphysema manifesting as multifocal upper lobe centrilobular rounded lucencies with imperceptible borders. Dot-like structures within the lucencies ➡ correlate with normal central lobular arteries.* **(Right)** *Coronal CECT of a 56-year-old male smoker shows extensive bilateral paraseptal emphysema and large bullae manifesting as a single row of subpleural cystic spaces ➡ of various sizes separated by intact interlobular septa.*

Emphysema

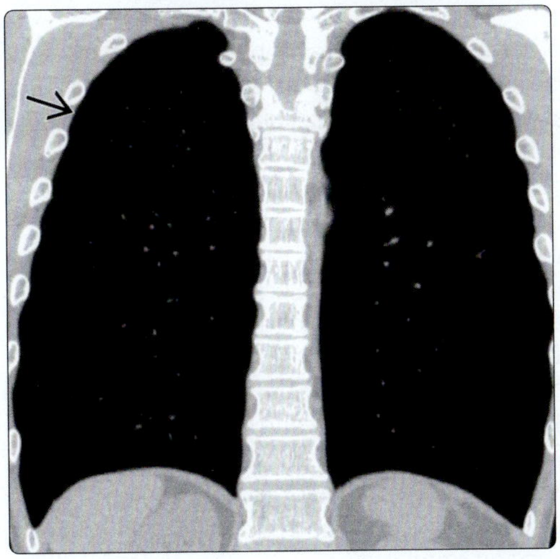

Pneumatocele

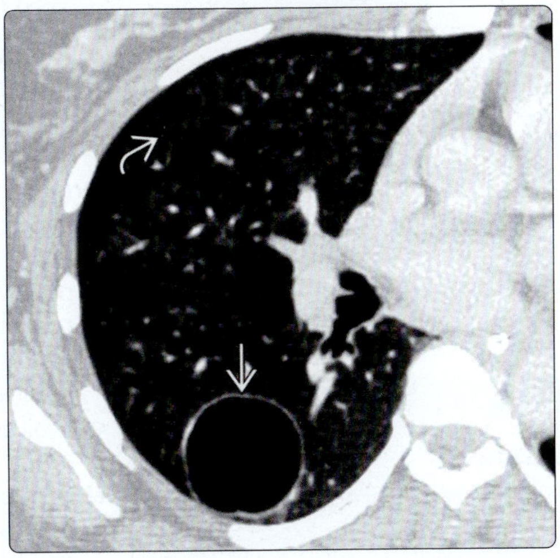

(Left) *Coronal NECT of a 55-year-old man with a-1 antitrypsin deficiency shows bilateral lower lobe predominant pulmonary lucencies and paucity of vascular markings. Note near normal upper lobe lung parenchyma ⇒ with normal distribution of vascular markings.* **(Right)** *Axial NECT of an asymptomatic patient evaluated for resolving pulmonary infection shows a right lower lobe thin-walled pneumatocele ➡. Note patchy middle lobe centrilobular ground-glass acinar opacities ➡.*

Constrictive Bronchiolitis

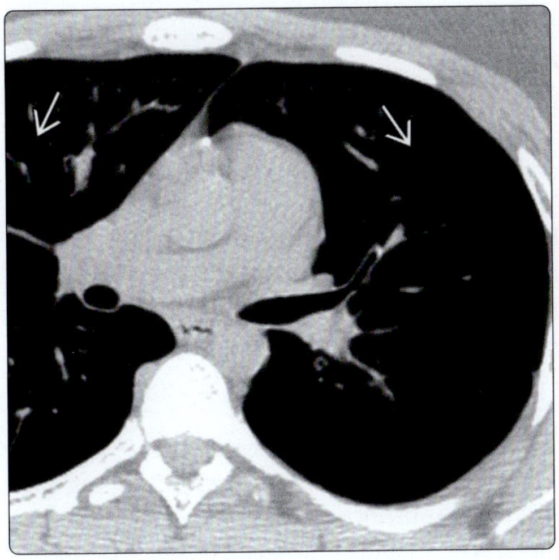

Pulmonary Hypertension

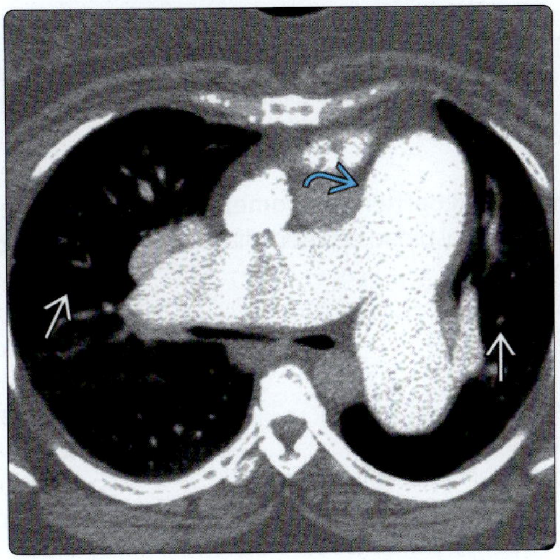

(Left) *Axial NECT of a 21-year-old man with Swyer-James-McLeod syndrome due to childhood adenovirus infection shows constrictive bronchiolitis manifesting with areas of hyperlucent lung ➡ amid areas of normal lung. Air-trapping was demonstrated on expiratory CT (not shown).* **(Right)** *Axial CECT of a 51-year-old woman with severe pulmonary hypertension shows mosaic perfusion characterized by diminished caliber of pulmonary vessels ➡ in areas of low pulmonary attenuation and markedly enlarged pulmonary trunk ⇒.*

Bronchial Atresia

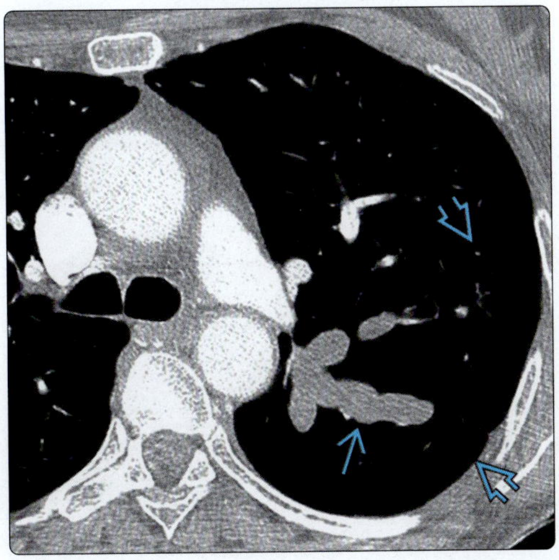

Pulmonary Sequestration

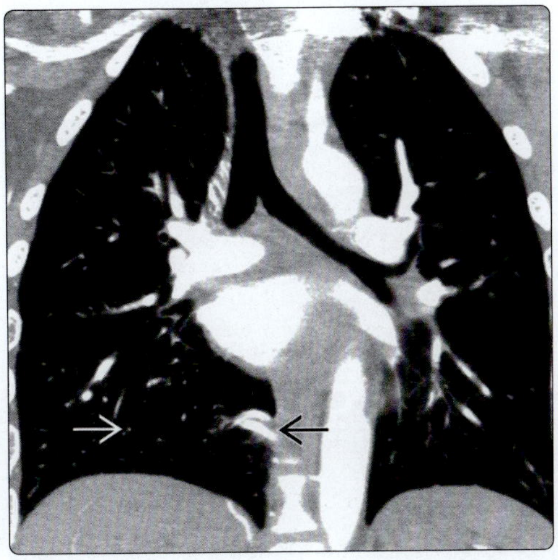

(Left) *Axial CECT of a patient with left upper lobe apicoposterior segment congenital bronchial atresia shows characteristic imaging findings of a branching mucocele ⇒ surrounded by hyperlucent lung parenchyma ⇒. These imaging findings are considered diagnostic of bronchial atresia.* **(Right)** *Coronal CECT of a 34-year-old man with an incidentally found right lower lobe pulmonary sequestration shows right lower lobe posterior basilar hyperlucent lung ➡ supplied by systemic arteries ⇒.*

DIFFERENTIAL DIAGNOSIS

Common

- Recurrent Aspiration

Less Common

- Eosinophilic Lung Disease
- Organizing Pneumonia
- Nontuberculous Mycobacterial Infection

Rare but Important

- Pulmonary Vasculitis
- Pulmonary Hemorrhage

ESSENTIAL INFORMATION

Key Differential Diagnosis Issues

- Migratory opacities: Infectious/inflammatory etiology favored over malignancy
- Clinical history is essential for accurate diagnosis

Helpful Clues for Common Diagnoses

- **Recurrent Aspiration**
  - Cellular bronchiolitis/consolidations in dependent lung
  - ± subsegmental or lobar atelectasis

Helpful Clues for Less Common Diagnoses

- **Eosinophilic Lung Disease**
  - **Simple Pulmonary Eosinophilia (Loeffler Syndrome)**
    - Mild or no symptoms, peripheral blood eosinophilia, resolution within 1 month
    - Migratory mid and upper lung zone peripheral ground-glass opacities &/or consolidations ± centrilobular nodules
  - **Chronic Eosinophilic Pneumonia**
    - Insidious onset, peripheral eosinophilia
    - High percentage of eosinophils on bronchoalveolar lavage
    - Upper lobe-predominant peripheral consolidations
    - Less frequently: Ground-glass opacity, centrilobular nodules, reticulation
  - **Allergic Bronchopulmonary Aspergillosis**
    - Hypersensitivity to *Aspergillus* antigens; cystic fibrosis, asthma
    - Early: Migratory opacities, endobronchial high-attenuation mucoid impaction, upper and central lung
    - Advanced: Bronchiectasis, cellular bronchiolitis, patchy consolidations
- **Organizing Pneumonia**
  - Types: Cryptogenic (idiopathic), secondary
  - Lower lobe-predominant, peribronchovascular/peripheral ground-glass opacities, consolidation, ± centrilobular nodules
  - Perilobular pattern: Poorly-defined polygonal opacities outline interlobular septa, subpleural distribution
  - Atoll and reversed halo signs: Central ground-glass opacity surrounded by rim of consolidation
- **Nontuberculous Mycobacterial Infection**
  - Volume loss, bronchiectasis, and mucus plugs involving middle lobe and lingula
  - Waxing and waning migratory cellular bronchiolitis and nodular consolidations

Helpful Clues for Rare Diagnoses

- **Pulmonary Vasculitis**
  - **Granulomatosis With Polyangiitis**
    - Multifocal lung nodules/masses ± cavitation
    - Less common: Ground-glass opacities ± septal thickening, consolidations, airway wall thickening
  - **Eosinophilic Granulomatosis With Polyangiitis**
    - Bilateral peripheral transient consolidations, lobular distribution
    - Frequent centrilobular nodules within ground-glass opacities
- **Pulmonary Hemorrhage**
  - Idiopathic, vasculitis, Goodpasture syndrome
  - Affected patients may present with hemoptysis, but hemoptysis may be absent
  - Focal or multifocal waxing and waning airspace disease
    - Consolidation, ground-glass opacities ± crazy-paving pattern

Recurrent Aspiration

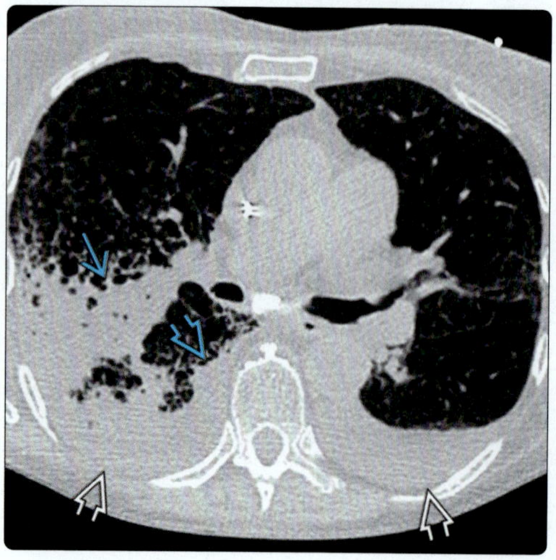

Eosinophilic Lung Disease

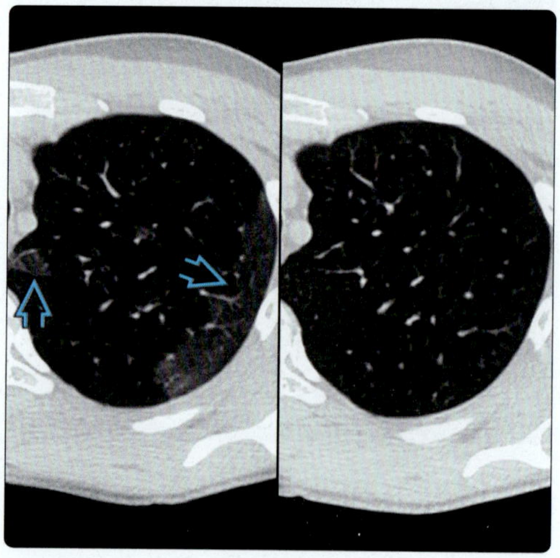

(Left) *Axial NECT shows recurrent aspiration manifesting as multifocal dense consolidations in the dependent right upper ➡ and superior segment of the right lower lobes ➡ and acinar ground-glass opacities. Note centrilobular emphysema and small pleural effusions ➡.* **(Right)** *Composite image with axial NECT obtained at baseline (left) and 2 months later (right) of a patient with simple peripheral eosinophilia shows left upper lobe peripheral ground-glass opacities ➡ that exhibit spontaneous resolution.*

Eosinophilic Lung Disease

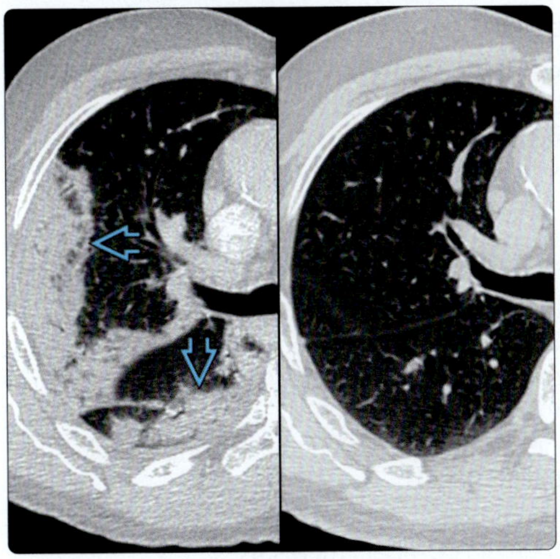

Eosinophilic Lung Disease

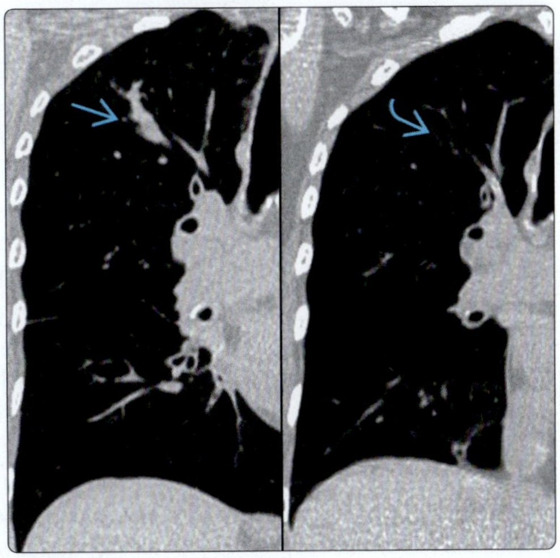

(Left) *Composite image with axial NECT obtained at presentation (left) and after steroid treatment (right) of a patient with chronic eosinophilic pneumonia shows peripheral subpleural consolidations that exhibit complete resolution after treatment.* **(Right)** *Composite image with coronal NECT at presentation (left) and months later (right) of a patient with allergic pulmonary aspergillosis shows upper lobe bronchiectasis with endoluminal plugs that resolved on follow-up.*

Organizing Pneumonia

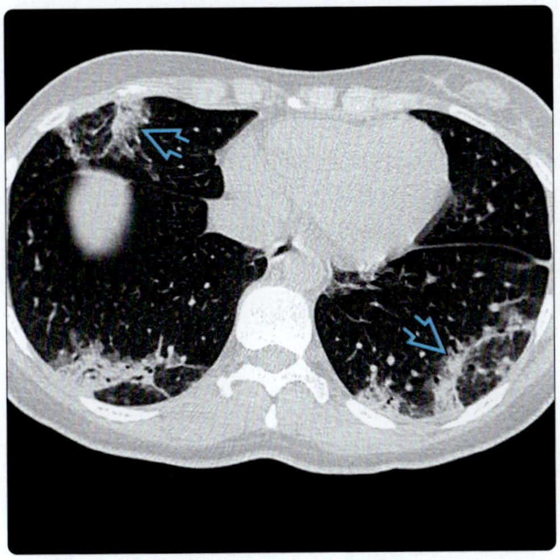

Nontuberculous Mycobacterial Infection

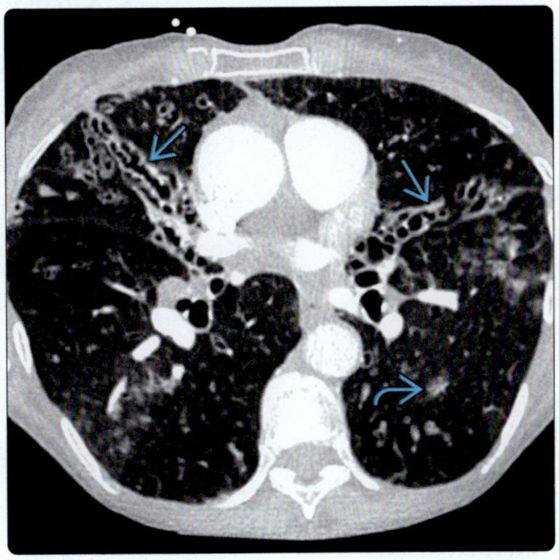

(Left) *Axial NECT of a patient with organizing pneumonia shows bilateral peripheral consolidations and ground-glass opacities that exhibit a perilobular distribution and the atoll or reversed halo sign, frequently seen in affected patients.* **(Right)** *Axial CECT of a patient with bronchiectatic nontuberculous mycobacterial infection shows severe middle lobe and lingular bronchiectasis with bronchial wall thickening, mucus plugs, and multifocal cellular bronchiolitis as well as acinar ground-glass opacities and consolidations.*

Pulmonary Vasculitis

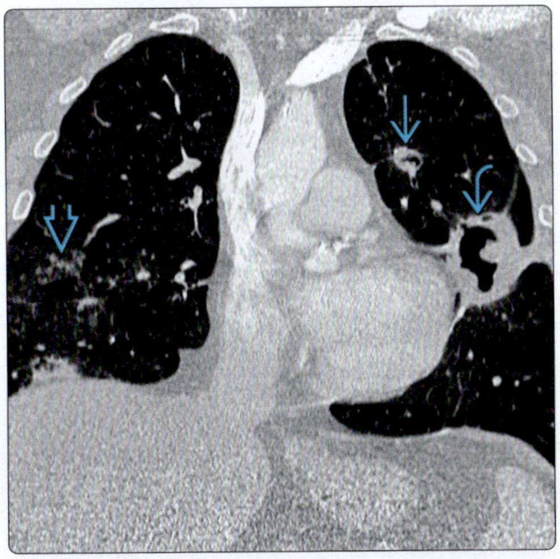

Pulmonary Hemorrhage

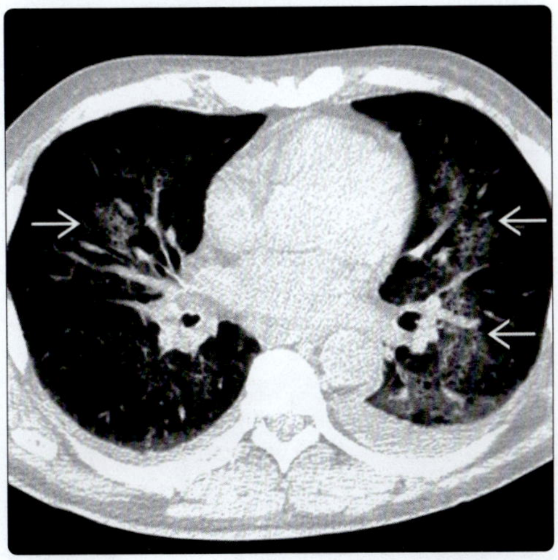

(Left) *Coronal CECT of a patient with granulomatosis with polyangiitis who presented with hemoptysis shows cavitary nodules and masses and patchy ground-glass attenuation centrilobular nodules.* **(Right)** *Axial NECT of a 59-year-old man with pulmonary hemorrhage secondary to Goodpasture syndrome shows bilateral patchy ground-glass opacities and a small left pleural effusion. Pulmonary opacities in patients with alveolar hemorrhage may exhibit a migratory pattern.*

DIFFERENTIAL DIAGNOSIS

Common

- Centrilobular
  - Infectious Bronchiolitis
    - Acute Bronchiolitis
    - Chronic Bronchiolitis
  - Aspiration Bronchiolitis
  - Respiratory Bronchiolitis
- Random
  - Hematogenous Dissemination of Infection
    - Miliary Tuberculosis
    - Miliary Histoplasmosis
- Perilymphatic
  - Sarcoidosis

Less Common

- Centrilobular
  - Other Cellular Bronchiolitis
    - Follicular Bronchiolitis
- Random
  - Metastatic Disease
- Perilymphatic
  - Silicosis

Rare but Important

- Centrilobular
  - Subacute or Cluster 1 Hypersensitivity Pneumonitis
  - Vascular
    - Excipient Lung Disease

ESSENTIAL INFORMATION

Key Differential Diagnosis Issues

- Micronodule: ≤ 3 mm in diameter
- **Centrilobular** micronodules do not involve pleura (i.e., subpleural sparing)
- **Perilymphatic** micronodules typically involve fissures and pleura
- **Miliary** micronodules exhibit diffuse and even distribution and reflect hematogenous dissemination

Helpful Clues for Common Diagnoses

- **Acute Infectious or Aspiration Bronchiolitis**
  - Cellular bronchiolitis: Scattered centrilobular micronodules
  - Aspiration should be considered in appropriate clinical context: Severe reflux, neurological condition, gastroparesis
- **Chronic Infectious Bronchiolitis**
  - Tuberculous and nontuberculous mycobacteria
  - Scattered centrilobular micronodules, cavitation, bronchiectasis, mosaic attenuation
- **Respiratory Bronchiolitis**
  - Upper lobe-predominant ground-glass centrilobular micronodules
- **Miliary Micronodules**
  - Miliary tuberculosis, miliary metastases
  - Diffuse and even micronodule distribution in central and peripheral interstitium
- **Sarcoidosis**
  - Perilymphatic micronodules, hilar and mediastinal lymphadenopathy

Helpful Clues for Rare Diagnoses

- **Subacute or Cluster 1 Hypersensitivity Pneumonitis**
  - Diffuse ground-glass centrilobular nodules with lobular mosaic attenuation and air-trapping
- **Excipient Lung Disease** (e.g., Cellulose Granulomatosis)
  - Diffuse and evenly distributed centrilobular nodules and tree-in-bud opacities
  - Cor pulmonale: Pulmonary hypertension and right ventricular strain

SELECTED REFERENCES

1. Winningham PJ et al: Bronchiolitis: a practical approach for the general radiologist. Radiographics. 37(3):777-94, 2017
2. Raoof S et al: Pictorial essay: multinodular disease: a high-resolution CT scan diagnostic algorithm. Chest. 129(3):805-15, 2006

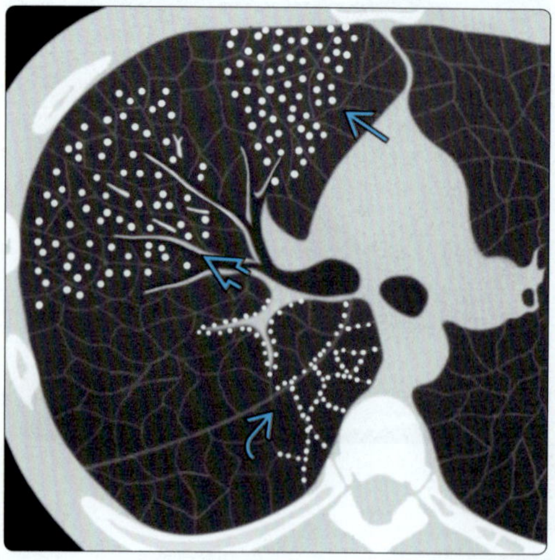

Acute Bronchiolitis

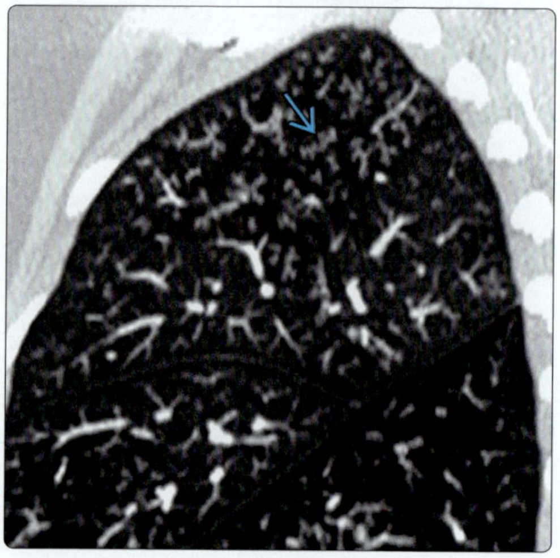

(Left) *Graphic shows the characteristic distribution of pulmonary micronodules, including random, centrilobular, and perilymphatic patterns.* **(Right)** *Sagittal NECT MIP image of a patient with infectious bronchiolitis shows upper lobe-predominant centrilobular and tree-in-bud micronodules. Note that the micronodules spare the subpleural lung and do not involve the interlobar fissures. These are classic and distinctive features of centrilobular micronodules.*

Micronodules

Aspiration Bronchiolitis

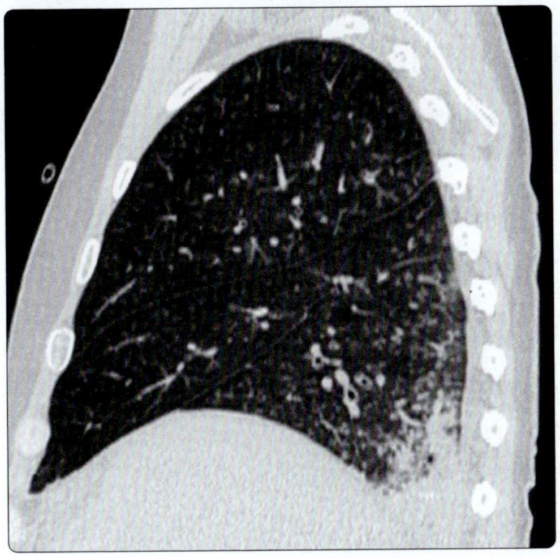

Respiratory Bronchiolitis

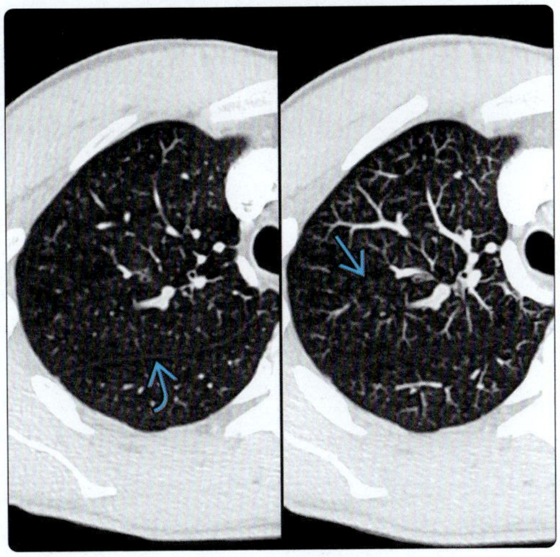

(Left) *Sagittal NECT MIP image of a patient with aspiration bronchiolitis in the setting of glottic carcinoma shows extensive centrilobular nodules and tree-in-bud opacities with coalescent consolidation in the right lower lobe. Note the absence of fissural involvement.* **(Right)** *Composite image with axial CECT (left) and axial CECT MIP image (right) of a patient with respiratory bronchiolitis shows centrilobular ground-glass nodules, more conspicuous on the MIP reformation. These nodules spare the subpleural lung.*

Miliary Histoplasmosis

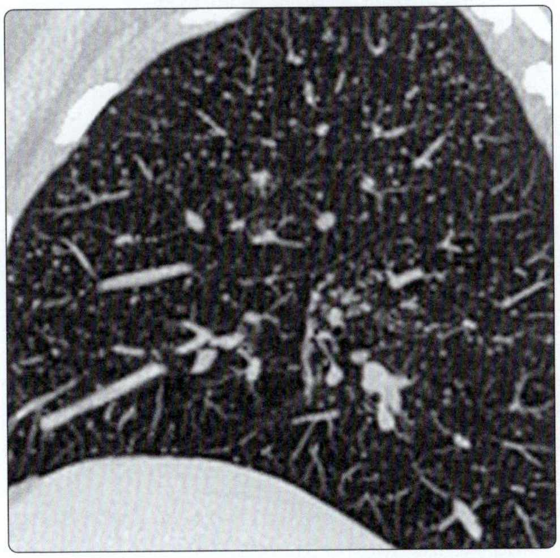

Sarcoidosis

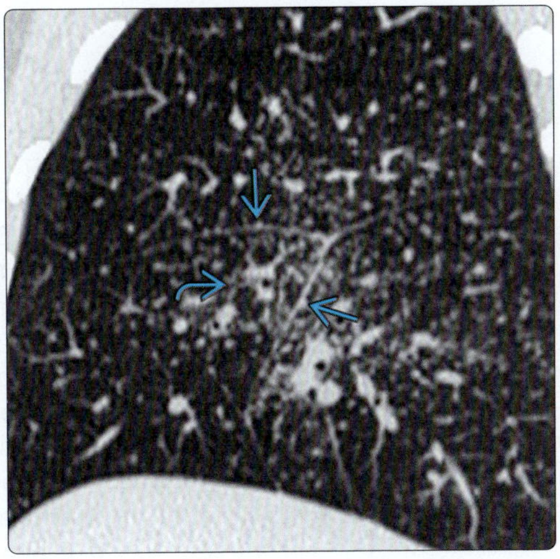

(Left) *Sagittal NECT MIP image of a patient with miliary histoplasmosis shows even and diffuse distribution of pulmonary micronodules, some of which abut the interlobar fissures. This is the so-called random distribution.* **(Right)** *Sagittal NECT MIP image of a patient with sarcoidosis shows multiple clustered micronodules that involve the bronchovascular bundles and interlobar fissures, which appear thick and nodular. This is the so-called perilymphatic distribution.*

Subacute or Cluster 1 Hypersensitivity Pneumonitis

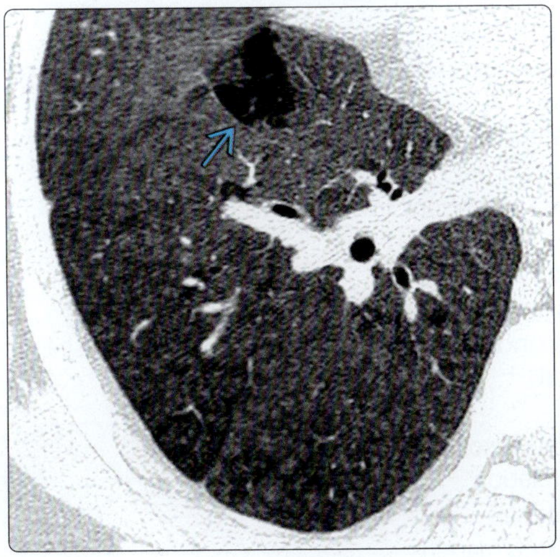

Excipient Lung Disease

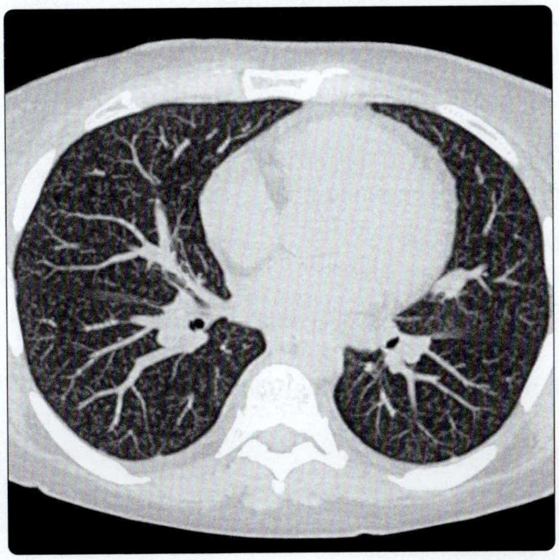

(Left) *Axial HRCT of a patient with cluster 1 hypersensitivity pneumonitis shows diffuse centrilobular ground-glass nodules and lobular air-trapping. Centrilobular ground-glass nodules are common in cluster 1 hypersensitivity pneumonitis.* **(Right)** *Axial NECT of a patient with excipient lung disease due to cellulose shows diffuse and evenly distributed centrilobular nodules and tree-in-bud opacities. This is commonly associated with findings of cor pulmonale (pulmonary hypertension and right ventricular strain).*

DIFFERENTIAL DIAGNOSIS

Common

- Pneumonia
- Organizing Pneumonia
- Pulmonary Contusion
- Lung Cancer

Less Common

- Pulmonary Infarct
- Rounded Atelectasis
- Septic Emboli

Rare but Important

- Chronic Eosinophilic Pneumonia

ESSENTIAL INFORMATION

Key Differential Diagnosis Issues

- Factors to consider in generating a differential diagnosis
  - Patient risk factors
  - Comorbidities
  - Medication use
  - Environmental exposures
  - Acuity or chronicity of findings on imaging
    - Acute abnormalities
      - Infection
      - Pulmonary infarct
      - Septic emboli
    - Chronic abnormalities
      - Lung cancer
      - Rounded atelectasis
      - Chronic eosinophilic pneumonia
- Imaging
  - Consolidation itself is nonspecific finding
    - Other imaging findings in combination with clinical information can assist in narrowing the differential diagnosis
  - Halo sign: Ground-glass opacity surrounding solid nodule or consolidation
    - Infection (angioinvasive aspergillosis and other fungi), septic emboli, organizing pneumonia, eosinophilic pneumonia, lung cancer, metastases
  - Reversed halo sign (atoll sign): Peripheral consolidation with central ground-glass opacity
    - Infection (mucormycosis and other fungi), organizing pneumonia, chronic eosinophilic pneumonia

Helpful Clues for Common Diagnoses

- **Pneumonia**
  - Correlation with sputum, WBC count, and clinical presentation paramount
  - Radiologic resolution after treatment lags behind clinical resolution of symptoms
  - Imaging
    - Airspace abnormality: Ground-glass opacities to dense consolidation
    - Focal, lobar, or multilobar consolidations
    - Associated with bacterial pneumonia: Centrilobular and tree-in-bud micronodules
    - Aspiration pneumonia commonly basal and peripheral (gravitational gradient)
    - Associated findings
      - Reactive lymphadenopathy
      - Parapneumonic pleural effusion or empyema
- **Organizing Pneumonia**
  - Entity associated with nonspecific clinical and imaging findings and pulmonary function test results
  - Histologic abnormalities
    - Granulation tissue polyps within alveolar ducts and alveoli
    - Chronic inflammation of adjacent lung parenchyma
  - Etiologies
    - Infection
    - Iatrogenic (medications, radiation therapy)
    - Illicit drugs
    - Autoimmune diseases
    - Idiopathic: Cryptogenic organizing pneumonia
  - Imaging
    - Most common findings
      - Ground-glass opacities
      - Consolidation
    - Reversed halo sign (atoll sign): Peripheral consolidation with central ground-glass opacity
    - Halo sign: Ground-glass opacity surrounding solid nodule or consolidation
    - Less common findings
      - Peribronchovascular opacities
      - Reticular opacities
      - Bronchiectasis
      - Interstitial nodules
      - Interlobular septal thickening
      - Airspace nodules
  - Distribution
    - Subpleural &/or bronchovascular
    - Middle and lower lobe predominance
    - Bilateral > unilateral
- **Pulmonary Contusion**
  - Clinical setting: Acute trauma to chest
  - Peripheral ground-glass opacity &/or consolidation
  - Under point of blunt kinetic energy absorption (coup-contrecoup injury)
  - Overlying rib fractures
    - Can occur without rib fractures in children and young adults
  - Appear at time of injury
  - Resolve in 3-5 days
  - Pulmonary lacerations ± air-fluid levels may also be present
- **Lung Cancer**
  - Smoking is major risk factor
  - Adenocarcinoma and squamous cell carcinoma can be peripheral
  - Imaging
    - Solid or subsolid nodule or mass; mass-like consolidation
    - Variable size
    - Spiculated margins
    - Thick-walled or nodular cavitation
    - Associated findings
      - Mediastinal &/or hilar lymphadenopathy
      - Concomitant emphysema if smoking history

Helpful Clues for Less Common Diagnoses

- **Pulmonary Infarct**
  - Typically results from pulmonary embolism (PE)
    - Complication of PE in 10-15% of cases
  - Often occurs in setting of superimposed cardiac dysfunction (cardiomyopathy, congestive heart failure)
    - Both pulmonary and bronchial arterial supply to lung are reduced
  - Independent risk factors
    - Greater patient height
    - Younger patients
    - Cigarette smokers
  - Higher likelihood of developing infarct with greater embolic burden
  - Imaging
    - Peripheral wedge-shaped consolidation
    - No air bronchograms
    - No enhancement
    - Internal lucencies due to noninfarcted aerated lung
    - Halo sign: Surrounding ground-glass opacities due to hemorrhage
    - Cavitation may be seen in septic emboli
    - Resolves over months (retains its original shape) rather than patchy resolution as in pneumonia
- **Rounded Atelectasis**
  - Associated with
    - Chronic pleural disease
    - Hemothorax
    - Empyema
    - Asbestos-related pleural disease
  - Definitive diagnosis on CT requires all 4 imaging findings
    - Pleural thickening, effusion, &/or pleural plaque
    - Broad-based intimate attachment of mass-like consolidation to pleural abnormality
    - Volume loss
    - Comet tail (or hurricane) sign: Swirling of bronchovascular structures into mass-like consolidation
- **Septic Emboli**
  - Risk factors
    - Indwelling catheters
    - IV drug users
  - Imaging
    - Multiple peripheral/subpleural nodules and wedge-shaped consolidation with rapid cavitation
    - Nodules/cavitary nodules are commonly more profuse in lower lobes due to hematogenous dissemination
    - Feeding vessel sign
      - Vessel leads directly to peripheral nodule or wedge-shaped consolidation
    - Associated findings
      - Exudative pleural effusion, often loculated

Helpful Clues for Rare Diagnoses

- **Chronic Eosinophilic Pneumonia**
  - Etiologies
    - Pulmonary toxicity (most common)
    - Idiopathic (rare)
  - Clinical symptoms are typically nonspecific
    - Chronic respiratory symptoms are most common
  - Imaging
    - Peripheral, upper lung predominant opacities
      - So-called 'photographic negative' of pulmonary edema
    - Consolidation along periphery of lung, usually subsegmental
      - Associated ground-glass is common
    - Waxing and waning opacities are characteristic
    - Tendency to resolve centripetally (from outer to inner)
    - Residual band of linear opacities parallels chest wall late in evolution of disease (subpleural bands)

Pneumonia

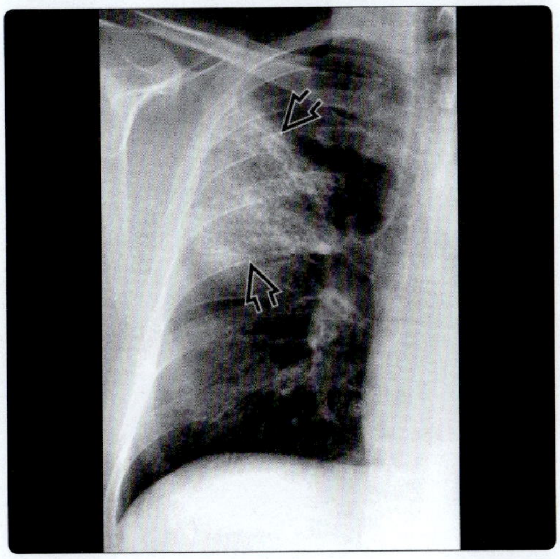

Pneumonia

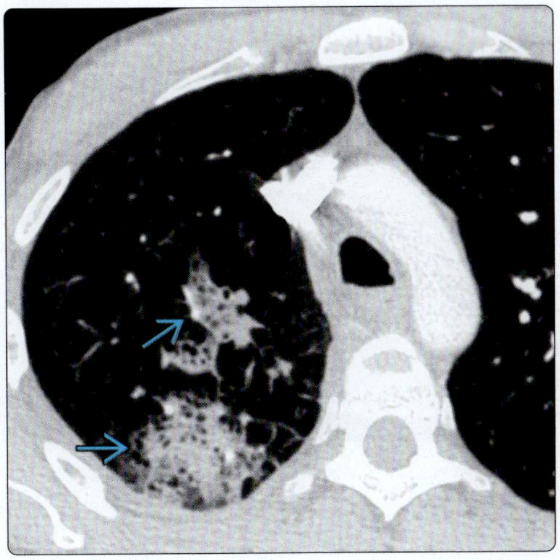

(Left) *Frontal chest radiograph shows peripheral consolidation ⇨ in the right upper lobe in a patient presenting with fever and chills. Consolidation resolved after treatment with antibiotics.* **(Right)** *Axial CECT of a different patient with hospital-acquired pneumonia shows multifocal consolidations with surrounding ground-glass opacity in the right upper lobe ⇨. In pneumonia, consolidations may be focal, lobar, or multilobar.*

(Left) *Frontal chest radiograph of a patient with recurrent aspiration pneumonia shows right basilar consolidation. The minor fissure is displaced inferiorly as a sign of middle lobe volume loss.* **(Right)** *Coronal CECT of the same patient shows sublobar consolidation and acinar nodules in this case of aspiration pneumonia. There is mucoid impaction of the the lower lobe bronchus. Aspiration pneumonia is typically basal and peripheral.*

Pneumonia

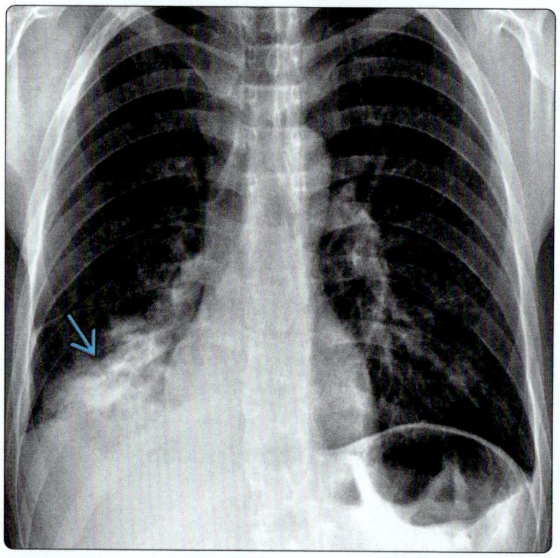

Pneumonia

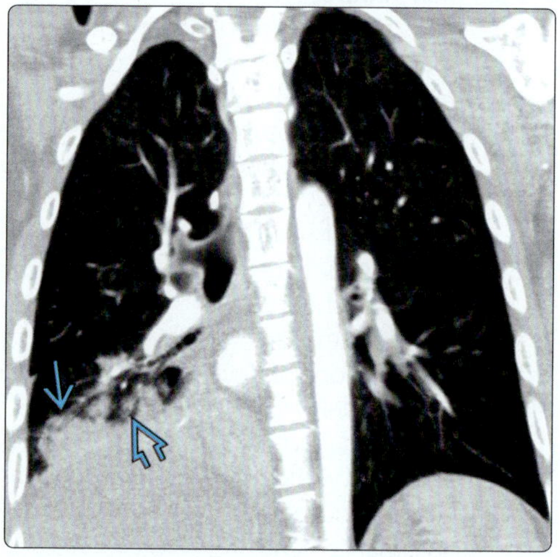

(Left) *Frontal chest radiograph of a patient following blunt trauma to the chest demonstrates homogeneous consolidation in the right upper lobe from lung contusion. Note the right chest tube.* **(Right)** *Axial CECT of the same patient shows focal consolidation in the posterior right hemithorax. Pulmonary contusion typically results from blunt trauma to the chest and manifests as peripheral consolidation &/or ground-glass opacities.*

Pulmonary Contusion

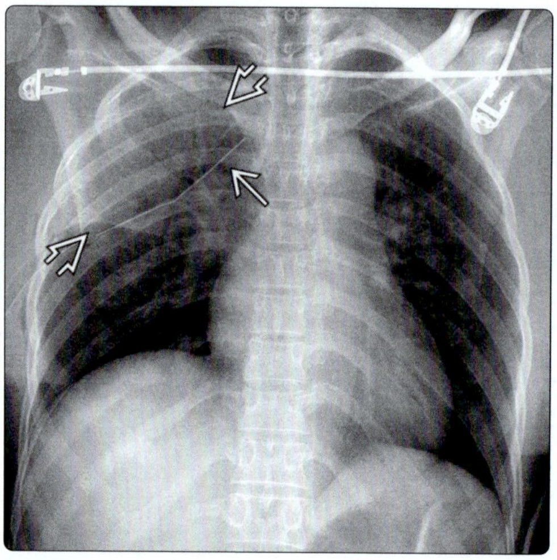

Pulmonary Contusion

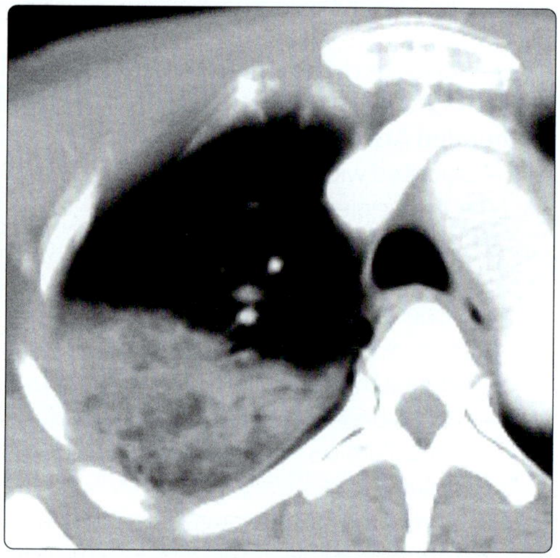

(Left) *Axial NECT shows small peripheral adenocarcinoma in the left upper lobe. Also note the fairly extensive paraseptal emphysema.* **(Right)** *Axial CECT of a different patient shows a necrotic and cavitary mass-like opacity in the periphery of the right lower lobe, which represents a primary lung cancer. Squamous cell carcinoma commonly but not exclusively manifests with cavitation.*

Lung Cancer

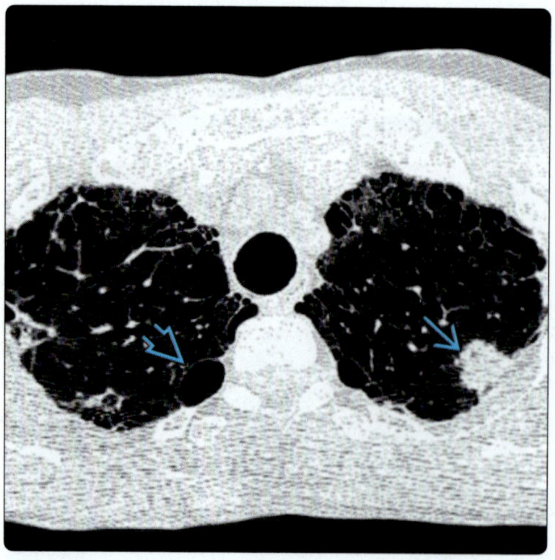

Lung Cancer

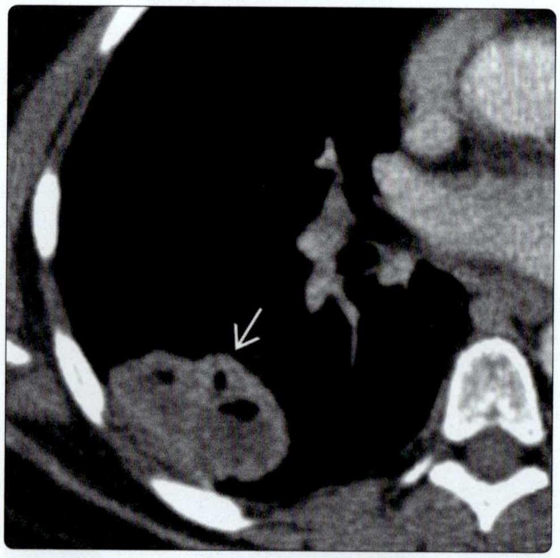

Pulmonary Infarct

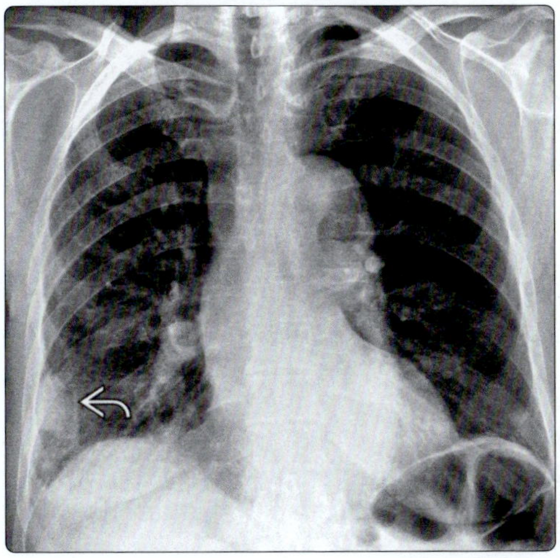

Pulmonary Infarct

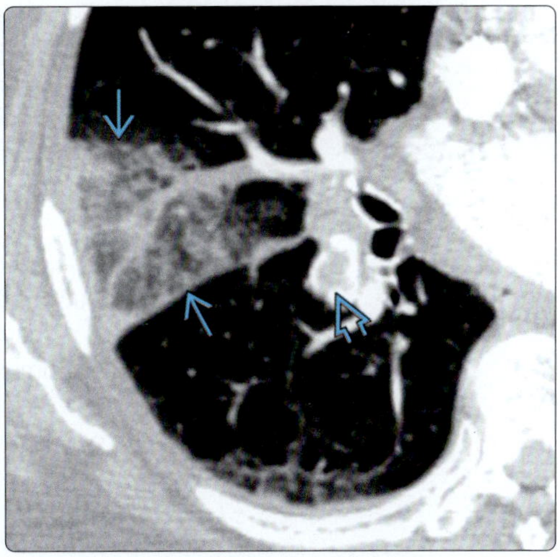

(Left) *Frontal chest radiograph of a patient with acute pulmonary embolism shows a basal peripheral focal consolidation, representing a pulmonary infarct.* **(Right)** *Axial CECT of a different patient with acute pulmonary embolism shows peripheral wedge-shaped ground-glass opacity and consolidation in the middle lobe, which represents the area of pulmonary ischemia. Multiple acute emboli are present in the pulmonary arteries.*

Rounded Atelectasis

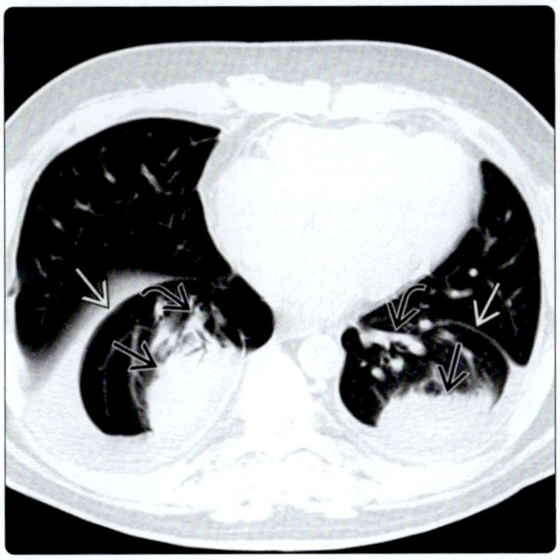

Rounded Atelectasis

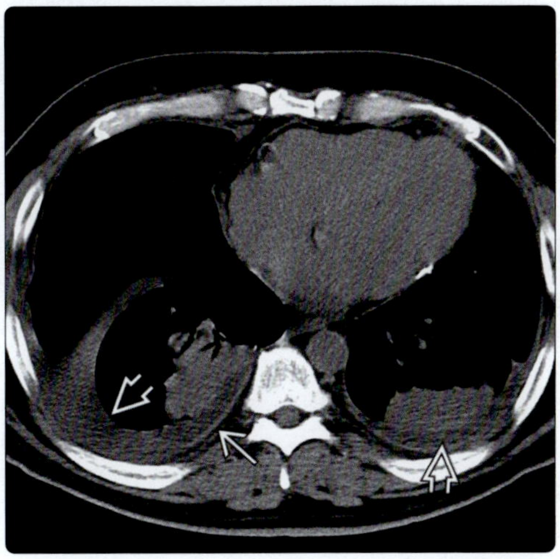

(Left) *Axial NECT (lung window) of a patient with rounded atelectasis shows bilateral lower lobe mass-like areas of consolidation into which curve pulmonary vessels. Note the posterior displacement and rotation of the major fissures.* **(Right)** *Axial NECT (soft tissue window) of the same patient shows small pleural effusions and associated smooth parietal pleural thickening associated with rounded atelectasis.*

Chronic Eosinophilic Pneumonia

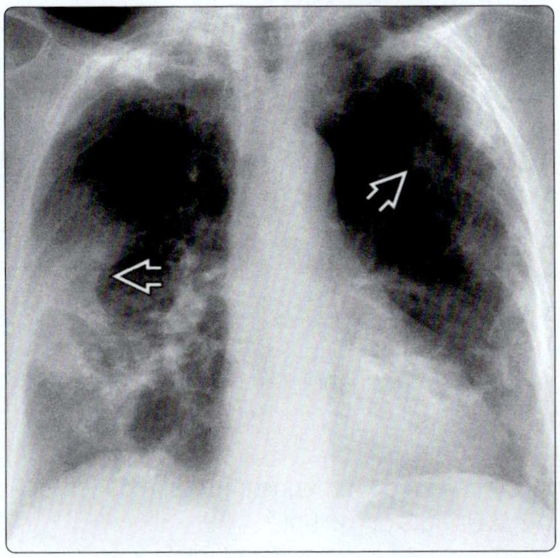

Chronic Eosinophilic Pneumonia

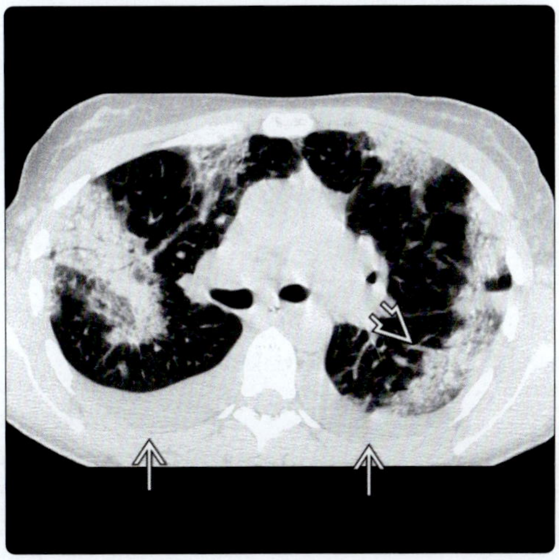

(Left) *Frontal chest radiograph of a patient with chronic eosinophilic pneumonia shows bilateral consolidations.* **(Right)** *Axial NECT of the same patient demonstrates multiple consolidations in the lungs bilaterally that are subpleural in location and small bilateral pleural effusions. These consolidations resolved completely after the administration of corticosteroids.*

DIFFERENTIAL DIAGNOSIS

Common

- Lung Cancer
- Lymphoma
- Pulmonary Abscess
- Pulmonary Infarct

Less Common

- Round Pneumonia
- Infection
  - Actinomycosis
  - Tuberculosis
  - Cryptococcosis
  - Coccidioidomycosis
  - Mucormycosis
- Sarcoidosis
- Silicosis
- Granulomatosis With Polyangiitis

Rare but Important

- Pulmonary Arteriovenous Malformation
- Behçet Disease
- Pulmonary Hamartoma
- Inflammatory Myofibroblastic Tumor
- Organizing Pneumonia
- Pulmonary Sequestration

ESSENTIAL INFORMATION

Key Differential Diagnosis Issues

- Mass: Opacity > 3 cm in diameter; regardless of contours, edges, and density
- Mass in patient older than 50 years is suspicious for neoplasm

Helpful Clues for Common Diagnoses

- **Lung Cancer**
  - Most common cause of cancer death
  - Smoking is main risk factor in 80-90% of cases
  - Asbestos exposure constitutes risk factor for lung cancer, can act synergistically with tobacco use
  - Other risk factors: Hereditary factors, genomic instability, preexisting lung disease and exposure (e.g., arsenic, radon, polycyclic aromatic hydrocarbons)
  - Most common imaging manifestation of lung cancer is pulmonary mass
    - Smooth, lobulated, or spiculated contours
    - Upper lobe predominance
    - Retraction of fissures
    - Pleural tagging
    - Cavitation (common in squamous cell carcinoma)
  - Associated findings
    - Atelectasis
    - Mediastinal lymphadenopathy
    - Pleural effusion
    - Bronchovascular and interlobular septal thickening (lymphangitic carcinomatosis)
- **Lymphoma**
  - Primary, secondary, or associated with immunosuppression
  - Pulmonary nodule/mass
    - Size variable
    - Well or ill-defined
    - Air bronchogram
    - "Halo sign" (surrounding ground-glass opacity) may be present
  - Other imaging findings
    - Consolidation (mass-like)
    - Bronchovascular and interlobular septal thickening
    - Mediastinal lymphadenopathy
- **Pulmonary Abscess**
  - Circumscribed area of necrosis in lung parenchyma
  - Primary
    - Aspiration pneumonia
  - Secondary
    - Bronchial obstruction (e.g., tumor, foreign body)
    - Coexisting lung diseases (e.g., bronchiectasis, bullous emphysema)
    - Hematogenous dissemination
  - Upper lobe predominance
  - Air-fluid level
  - Wall thickness (5-15 mm)
- **Pulmonary Infarct**
  - Ischemic lung injury
  - Basal (70%)
  - Cavitation (rare)
  - Wide pleural contact and vertex truncated towards hilum
  - Correspondent pulmonary arterial filling defect

Helpful Clues for Less Common Diagnoses

- **Round Pneumonia**
  - Children/young adults
  - Clinical manifestations of acute respiratory infection
  - Air bronchogram
- Infection
  - **Actinomycosis**
    - *Actinomyces* spp. infection
    - Subacute or chronic clinical manifestations
    - Alcoholism/poor dental hygiene
    - Upper lobe predominance
    - Cavitation
    - Pleural collection with extension to thoracic wall
  - **Tuberculosis**
    - *M. tuberculosis* infection
    - Epidemiologic background
    - Tuberculoma
      - Satellite nodules (80%)
      - Calcification (20-30%)
      - Cavitation (40-45%)
      - Upper lobe predominance
  - **Cryptococcosis**
    - *Cryptococcus* spp. infection
    - Immunocompetent or immunosuppressed patients
    - Nodule/mass, single or multiple
    - Cavitation (immunosuppressed patients)
  - **Coccidioidomycosis**
    - *Coccidioides* spp. infection
    - Deserts of Western hemisphere
    - Chronic coccidioidomycosis

- 5% of patients
- Symptoms > 6 weeks
- Coccidioidoma (5-7%)
- Cavitation

- **Mucormycosis**
  - Fungal infection due to Zygomycetes: *Mucor*, *Rhizopus*, and *Absidia*
  - Diabetes mellitus/immunosuppression
  - Halo and reversed halo sign
  - Cavitation

- **Sarcoidosis**
  - Multisystem granulomatous disease
  - Irregular contours with air bronchogram
  - Masses occur due to coalescence of perilymphatic nodules, often exhibit galaxy sign (distinct peripheral micronodules)
  - Bilateral hilar and right paratracheal lymphadenopathy
- **Silicosis**
  - Inhalation of silicon dioxide
  - Conglomerate or pseudotumoral silicosis
  - Progressive massive fibrosis: Relatively symmetric upper lobe peribronchovascular masses
  - Perilymphatic micronodularity
  - Eggshell calcification in lymph nodes
- **Granulomatosis With Polyangiitis**
  - Multisystem chronic granulomatous vasculitis
  - Upper respiratory tract and renal diseases
  - Cavitation and irregular thick wall

Helpful Clues for Rare Diagnoses

- **Pulmonary Arteriovenous Malformation**
  - Abnormal anatomic communication between branch of pulmonary artery and pulmonary vein
  - Associated with Rendu-Osler-Weber disease
  - Single or multiple
  - Basal predominance
  - Diagnosis requires identification of nidus and afferent/efferent vessels
- **Behçet Disease**
  - Chronic multisystem inflammatory disease
  - Aneurysms of pulmonary artery or its branches
  - Recurrent genital ulcers
  - Uveitis
  - Skin lesions
- **Pulmonary Hamartoma**
  - Benign neoplasm composed of mesenchymal tissues
  - 77% of benign lung tumors
  - Rounded soft tissue mass
  - Smooth or lobulated contours
  - Fat in 60% of tumors
  - Popcorn-like or central calcification in 25% of cases
- **Inflammatory Myofibroblastic Tumor**
  - Locally invasive low-grade neoplasm composed of myofibroblasts
  - Any age without sex predilection
  - 25% of cases occur under 18 years
  - Peripheral slow-growing mass of variable size
  - Lobulated or spiculated border
  - Cavitation uncommon
  - Calcification in tumors of children
  - Heterogeneous enhancement with contrast
- **Organizing Pneumonia**
  - Organizing pneumonia (OP) is pathologic pattern with buds of granulation tissue within lumen of distal pulmonary airspaces
  - Focal organizing pneumonia (FOP) is subset of OP
  - FOP represents 10-15% of all cases of OP
  - Peripheral predominance (86.7%)
  - Polygonal shape (perilobular pattern)
  - Air bronchogram or small bubble-like lucency (77.8%)
  - Halo sign (40%)
- **Pulmonary Sequestration**
  - Dysplastic nonfunctioning lung tissue communicated with bronchial tree with anomalous systemic irrigation
  - Children/young adults
  - Posterior basal segment of lower lobe, adjacent to hemidiaphragm
  - Demonstrate systemic blood loss

Lung Cancer

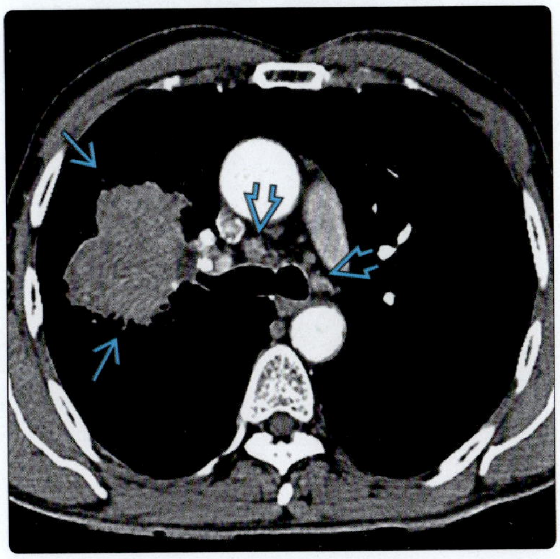

Lung Cancer

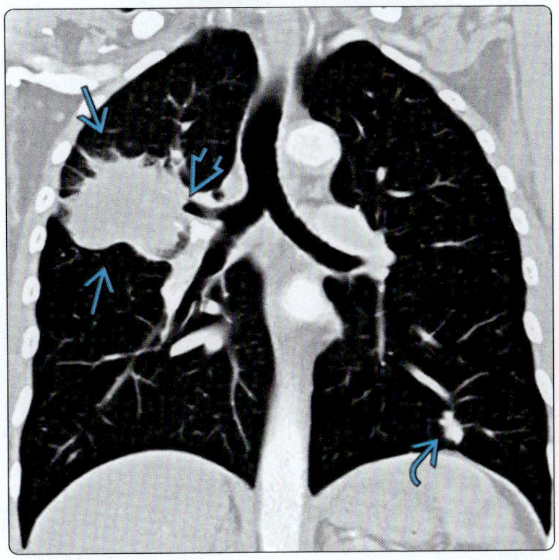

(Left) *Axial CECT of a 57-year-old male smoker with squamous cell carcinoma of the lung shows a large solid right upper lobe polylobulated mass ➡ with borderline-sized mediastinal lymph nodes ➡.* **(Right)** *Coronal CECT of the same patient shows a mass in the right upper lobe ➡, obstruction of the right upper lobe bronchus ➡, and a metastatic nodule in the left lower lobe ➡. Tobacco use is the most important risk factor for development of lung cancer.*

(Left) *Axial CECT of a 26-year-old woman with B-cell lymphoma shows multiple nodules and masses in the upper lobes, some of which are surrounded by ground-glass opacities, the so-called CT halo sign.* **(Right)** *Coronal CECT of the same patient shows multiple solid nodules and masses in the upper lobes, some of which exhibit surrounding ground-glass opacities. Lymphoma is a common cause of pulmonary mass though not as prevalent as lung cancer.*

Lymphoma

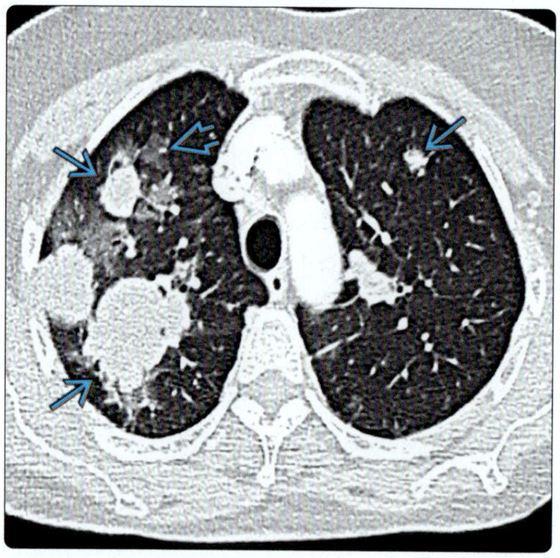

Lymphoma

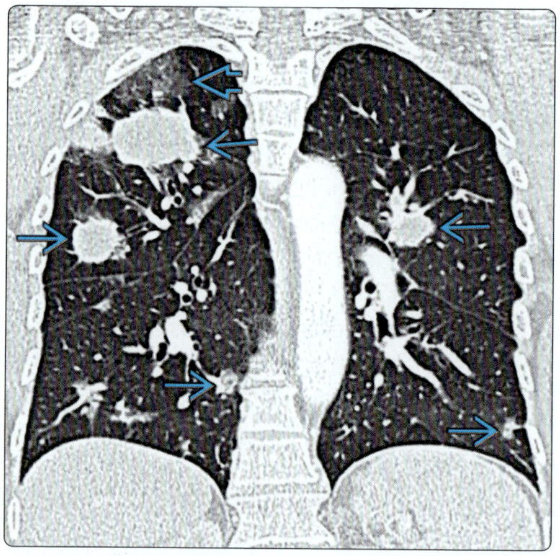

(Left) *Axial CECT of a 29-year-old man with pulmonary abscess shows a large right lower lobe mass with intrinsic hypodensity from necrosis and air. Pulmonary abscess is a common complication resulting from necrotizing pneumonia or aspiration.* **(Right)** *Coronal CECT of the same patient shows a right lower lobe cavitary mass. Pulmonary abscess is a complication that requires aggressive antibiotic treatment and occasionally surgical resection in unresponsive cases.*

Pulmonary Abscess

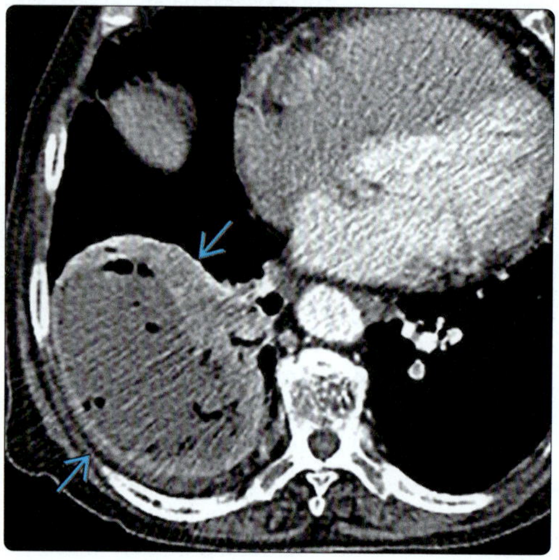

Pulmonary Abscess

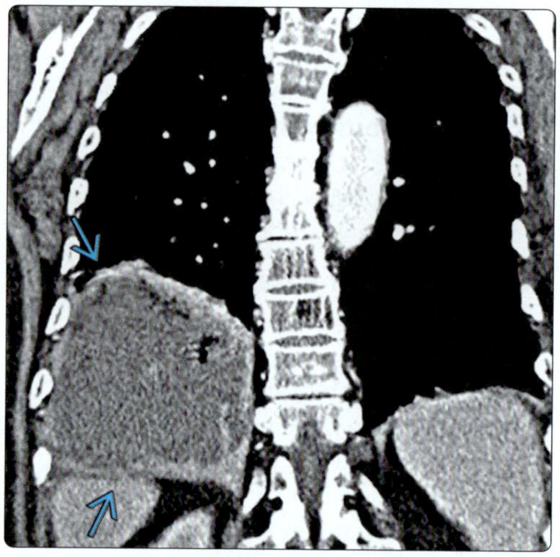

(Left) *PA chest radiograph of a 73-year-old man with pulmonary infarct shows a right basilar mass with intrinsic extensive cavitation.* **(Right)** *Coronal CT of the same patient shows a thick-walled cavitary mass in the right lower lobe. Note scattered areas of mosaic attenuation. Pulmonary infarcts are a common cause of pulmonary mass that typically will progressively decrease in size over time; however, infarcts can rarely undergo cavitation.*

Pulmonary Infarct

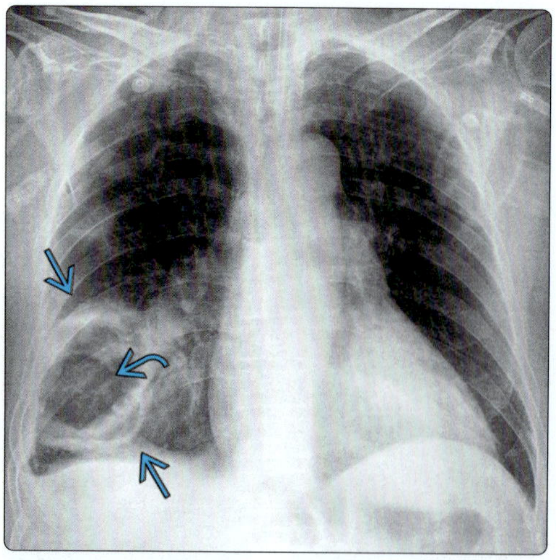

Pulmonary Infarct

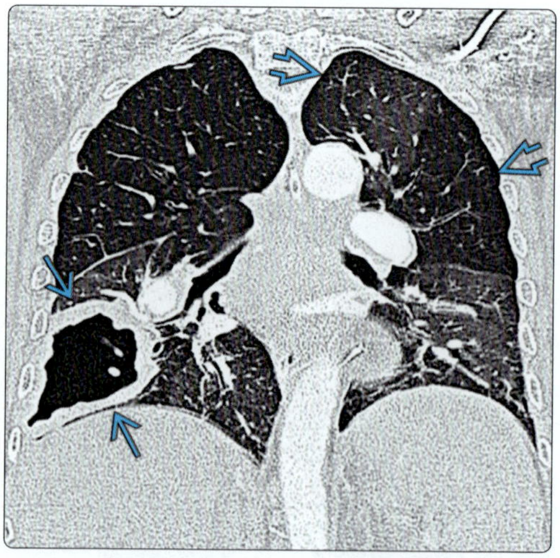

Round Pneumonia

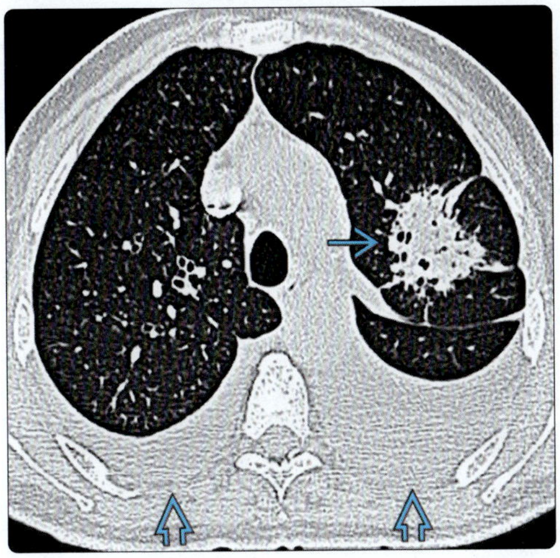

Round Pneumonia

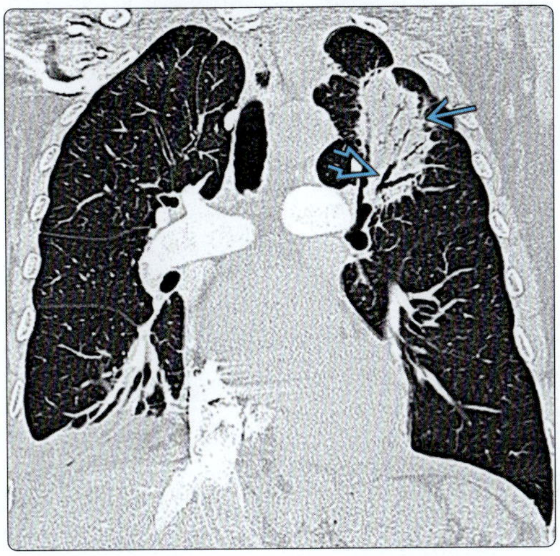

*(**Left**) Axial CECT of a 53-year-old man with pneumococcal pneumonia shows a spiculated left upper lobe mass →. Note bilateral pleural effusions →. (**Right**) Coronal CECT of the same patient shows a left upper lobe mass → with abundant air bronchograms →. Round pneumonia is more commonly seen in pediatric populations with Streptococcus pneumoniae infection. In adults it is a common mimic for lung cancer and a reason for close serial imaging follow-up.*

Tuberculosis

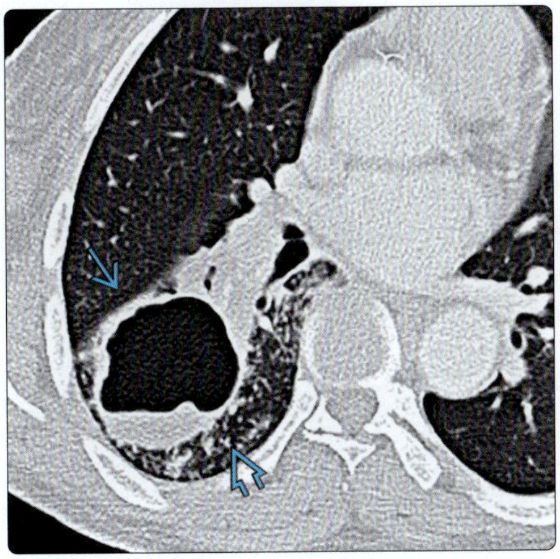

Tuberculosis

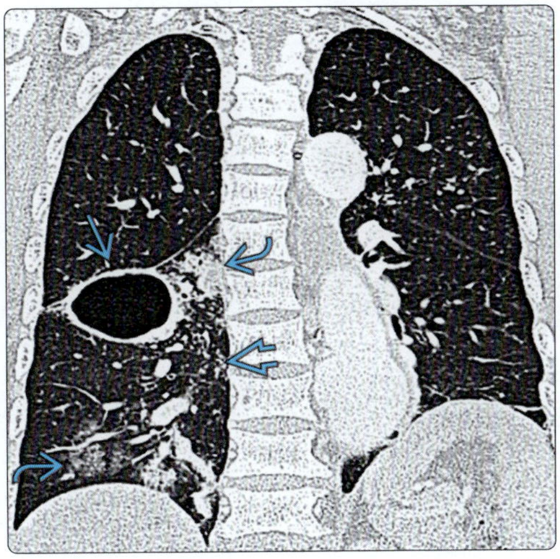

*(**Left**) Axial CECT of a 41-year-old man with tuberculosis shows a cavitary mass in the right lower lobe →. Note extensive tree-in-bud micronodules in the right lower lobe →. (**Right**) Coronal CECT of the same patient shows the cavitary mass in the right lower lobe → associated with tree-in-bud micronodules →. Peribronchovascular ground-glass and consolidation → are also seen. Tuberculosis is a common cause of upper lobe predominant pulmonary cavitary masses.*

Cryptococcosis

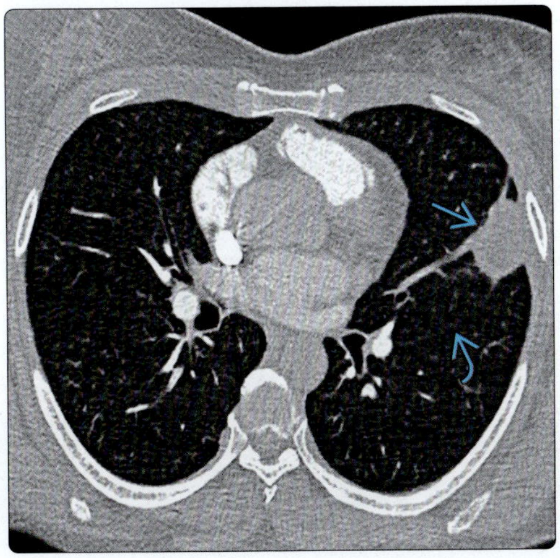

Cryptococcosis

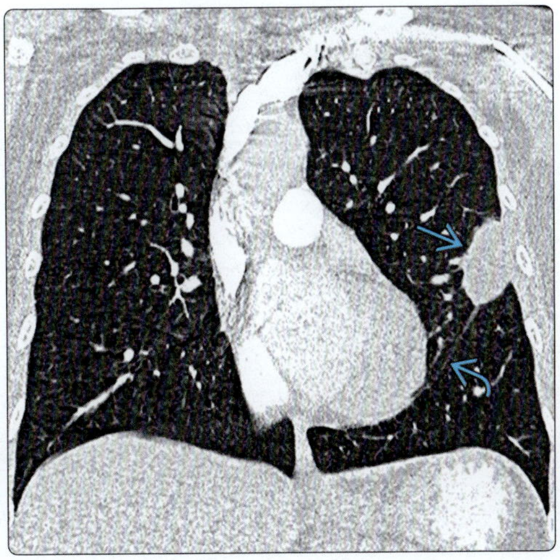

*(**Left**) Axial CECT of a 36-year-old woman with pulmonary cryptococcosis shows a subpleural solid ovoid mass in the left upper lobe → abutting the oblique fissure →. (**Right**) Coronal CECT of the same patient shows the subpleural solid ovoid mass in the left upper lobe → abutting the ipsilateral oblique fissure →. Pulmonary masses are often regarded as neoplastic; however, infectious masses are a common etiology to be considered. Among infections, fungal diseases are a common cause of pulmonary mass.*

(Left) *PA chest radiograph of a 49-year-old man with history of diabetes who developed pulmonary mucormycosis shows a left upper lobe cavitary mass with thick walls.* **(Right)** *Coronal CECT of the same patient shows the left upper lobe cavitary mass with thick walls. While rare, mucormycosis, often also referred as zygomycosis, is a life-threatening fungal infection that occurs more commonly in patients with history of diabetes.*

Mucormycosis

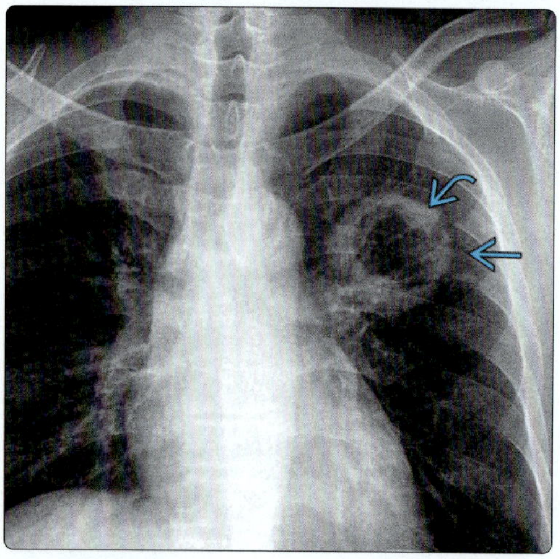

Mucormycosis

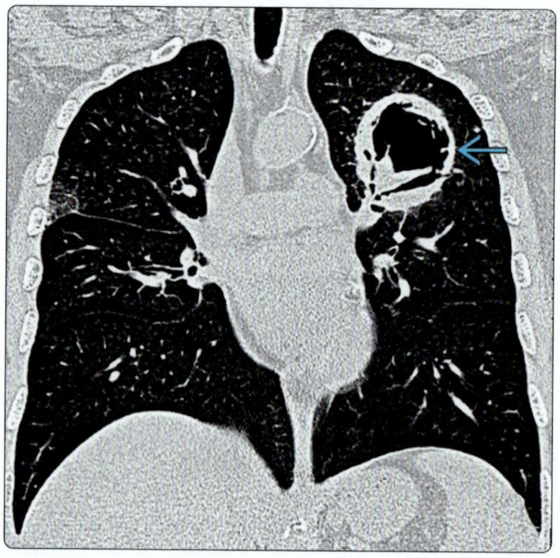

(Left) *PA chest radiograph of a 76-year-old man with conglomerate silicosis shows bilateral hilar masses and calcified lymph nodes, some of which demonstrate eggshell calcification.* **(Right)** *Coronal CECT of the same patient shows bilateral hilar masses and calcified lymph nodes. Masses occur in the context of complicated silicosis, a chronic form of the disease referred to as progressive massive fibrosis (PMF), occurring after years to decades of exposure.*

Silicosis

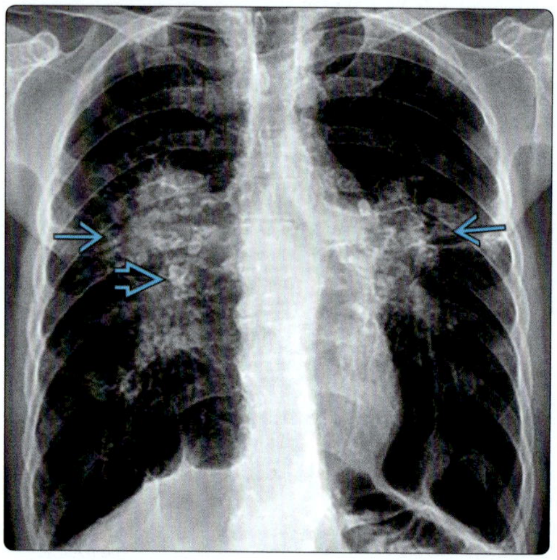

Silicosis

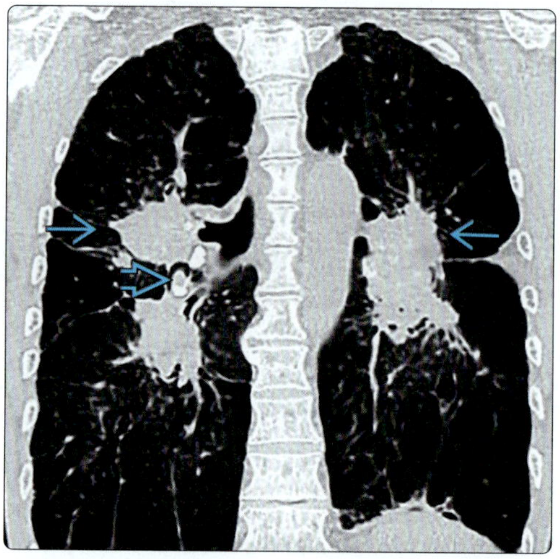

(Left) *PA chest radiograph of a 43-year-old man with granulomatosis with polyangiitis (GPA) shows right upper lobe-like mass consolidation.* **(Right)** *Axial CECT of the same patient shows mass-like consolidation with air bronchograms in the right upper lobe. Nodules, masses, and consolidations, which may be cavitary, are commonly seen in the setting of GPA. Patients with GPA can also present with hemoptysis and diffuse alveolar hemorrhage manifesting as bilateral opacities.*

Granulomatosis With Polyangiitis

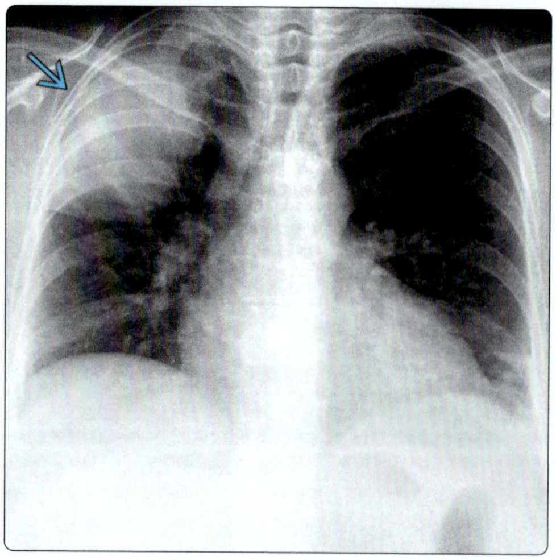

Granulomatosis With Polyangiitis

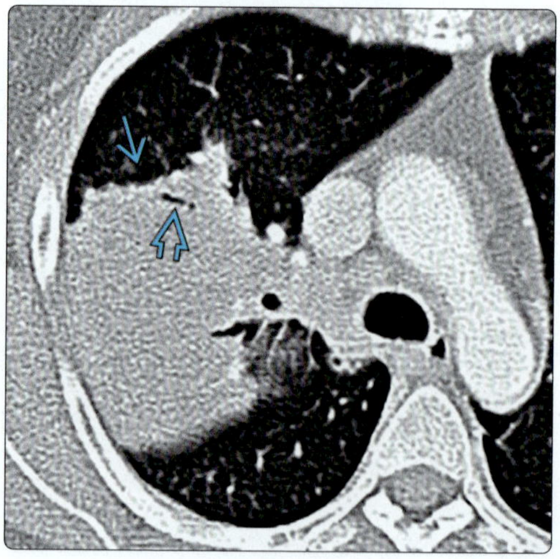

Pulmonary Arteriovenous Malformation

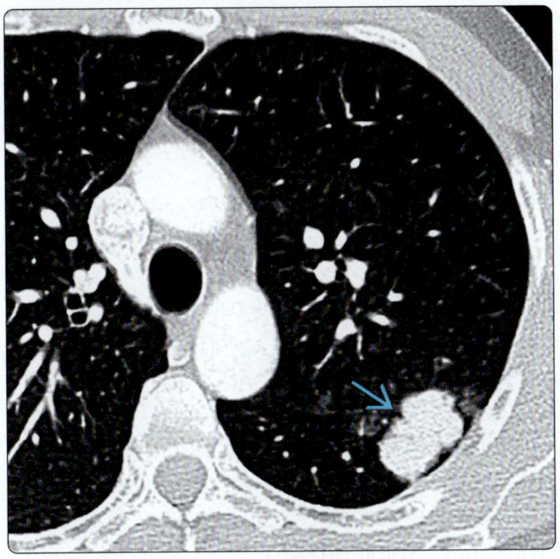

Pulmonary Arteriovenous Malformation

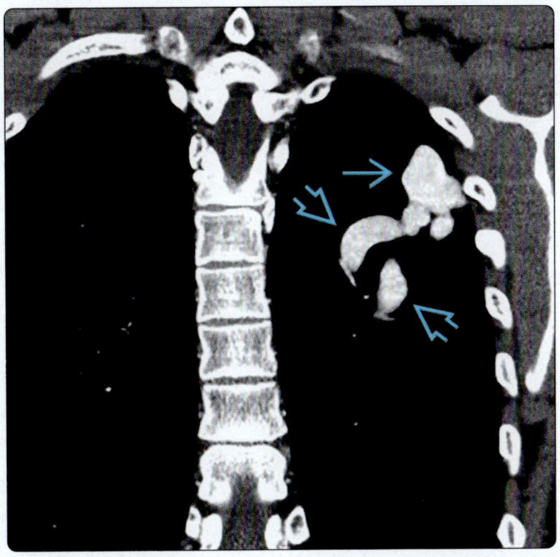

(Left) *Axial CT of a 35-year-old woman with pulmonary arteriovenous malformation (AVM) shows a markedly enhancing lobulated mass in the left upper lobe →.* **(Right)** *Coronal CECT of the same patient shows a lobulated markedly enhancing mass in the left upper lobe → that represents the AVM nidus with surrounding serpiginous tubular structures → that correspond to afferent and efferent vessels. AVM can be diagnosed with certainty when visualization of a nidus and afferent and efferent vessels is possible.*

Pulmonary Hamartoma

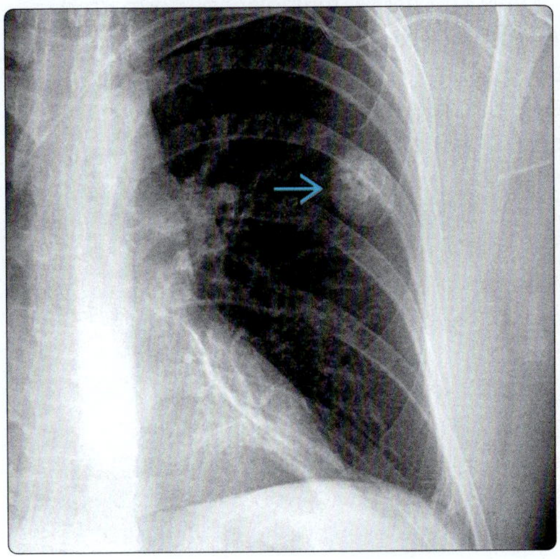

Pulmonary Hamartoma

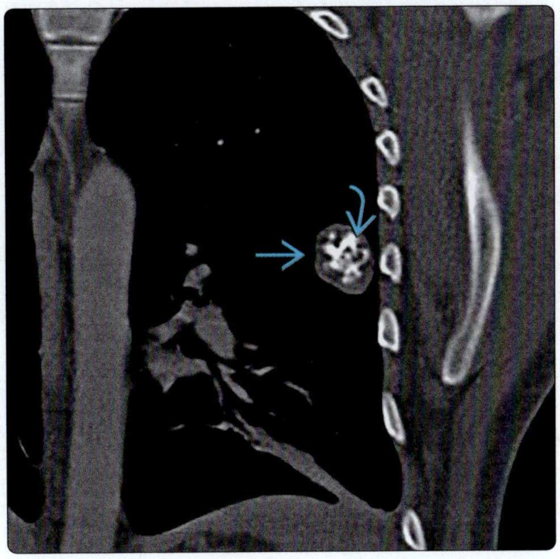

(Left) *PA chest radiograph of a 40-year-old man with pulmonary hamartoma shows a left upper lobe mass → with intrinsic calcifications.* **(Right)** *Coronal NECT of the same patient shows a left upper lobe solid mass → with the so-called popcorn pattern of intrinsic calcifications →. This pattern of calcification and the presence of macroscopic fat are pathognomonic of hamartomatous pulmonary lesions.*

Pulmonary Sequestration

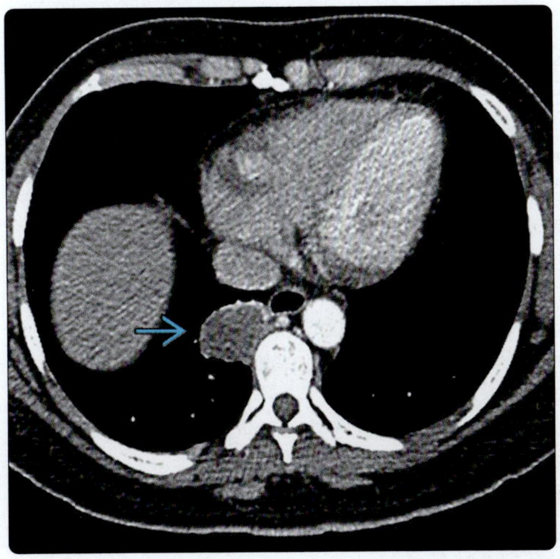

Pulmonary Sequestration

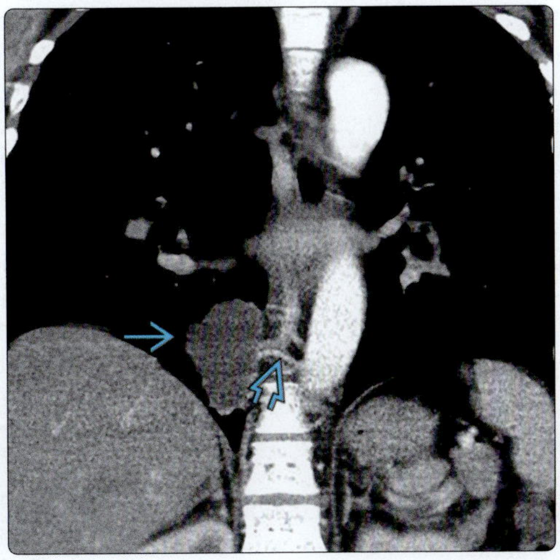

(Left) *Axial CT of a 39-year-old man with intralobar pulmonary sequestration shows a solid mass in the medial right lower lobe →.* **(Right)** *Coronal CECT of the same patient shows a lobulated solid mass in the right lower lobe →. Note arterial feeding vessel → arising directly from the aorta. The great majority of the intralobar sequestrations occur in the lower lobes. Demonstration of arterial systemic arterial supply is required for diagnosis with certainty and can often be identified on CECT.*

DIFFERENTIAL DIAGNOSIS

Common

- Granuloma
- Intrapulmonary Lymph Node
- Mucus Plug
- Lung Cancer
- Nodule Mimics

Less Common

- Atypical Adenomatous Hyperplasia
- Carcinoid
- Hamartoma
- Solitary Metastasis
- Infarct
- Laceration
- Abscess

Rare but Important

- Pulmonary Arteriovenous Malformation
- Amyloidoma
- Pulmonary Inflammatory Myofibroblastic Tumor

ESSENTIAL INFORMATION

Key Differential Diagnosis Issues

- **Solitary pulmonary nodule (SPN)**
  - Single focal rounded or ovoid opacity, ≤ 3 cm
- SPN detection
  - **Radiography**
    - SPN found in up to 2% of chest radiographs
    - Improved detection: Dual-energy radiography, bone suppression software, computer-aided detection
  - **CT**
    - Superior for SPN detection
    - Imaging study of choice for SPN characterization: Size, morphology, density (calcification, fat, air), attenuation (solid, subsolid), growth, enhancement, metabolic activity
    - Improved detection/characterization: Thin-section CT (1.0-1.5 mm), multiplanar reformations, maximum intensity projection (MIP), computer-aided detection
- General features
  - Size: 90% of nodules < 2 cm are benign
  - Spherical morphology is typical of benignity
  - Growth
    - 2-year stability implies benignity; but indolent lung cancer occurs
    - Doubling time < 30 days or > 465 days favors benignity
- SPN imaging assessment
  - Benign: No follow-up required
  - Indeterminate: Follow-up per published guidelines
    - Documentation of stability
    - Detection of growth
    - Detection of morphologic and attenuation changes
  - Possibly malignant
    - Short-term imaging follow-up to document growth
    - FDG PET/CT for assessment of metabolic activity
    - Tissue sampling: Image-guided biopsy, bronchoscopic biopsy, surgical resection

Helpful Clues for Common Diagnoses

- **Granuloma**
  - Solid nodule, stable size, typically small
  - Spherical, smooth or minimally lobular borders
  - Frequent calcification
    - SPN < 9 mm on radiography likely calcified granuloma
    - Complete or diffuse Ca++
    - Central Ca++, > 10% of nodule on cross section
    - Laminar or concentric Ca++
  - Satellite nodules
  - Histoplasmosis, coccidioidomycosis, tuberculosis
  - Asymptomatic adult
- **Intrapulmonary Lymph Node**
  - Frequent incidental finding on thin-section CT
    - 20% prevalence in lung screening population
  - Fissural or perifissural, juxtapleural; no pleural retraction
  - Within 20 mm of pleural surface, caudal to level of carina
  - Small, < 6 mm; may exhibit growth
  - Triangular or lentiform; smooth sharp margins
- **Mucus Plug**
  - May mimic SPN on axial CT; multiplanar reformatted images for differentiation
  - Identification of proximal and distal patent airway
  - Associated bronchial wall thickening, mucus plugs
- **Lung Cancer**
  - Risk factors
    - Exposure to cigarette smoke or other carcinogens
    - History of malignancy (pulmonary or extrapulmonary)
    - Pulmonary fibrosis
    - Lung cancer in 1st-degree relative
  - Most common in upper lobes
  - Increased risk of cancer in SPN > 1 cm
  - Doubling time 1-18 months; average: 100 days
  - Morphology: Irregular, spiculated, polylobular
    - Spiculation: Highly suggestive of malignancy
    - Pleural tags in 60-80% of peripheral lung cancers
    - Polylobular borders
      - Histologic heterogeneity
      - 40% of malignant nodules
  - Density
    - Air bronchograms/bronchiolograms and bubbly lucencies more common in malignant nodules
    - Calcification in 13%; eccentric, stippled
    - Cavitation: Irregular walls > 16 mm suggest malignancy
  - Attenuation
    - Solid (soft tissue): Most lung cancers, less likely to be malignant than part-solid or nonsolid nodules
    - Part-solid (soft tissue and ground-glass): 40-50% of part-solid SPNs < 1.5 cm are malignant; typically adenocarcinoma
    - Nonsolid (ground-glass): 34% malignant; particularly if > 1.5 cm; typically adenocarcinoma
  - Metabolic activity: FDG PET/CT
    - 90% likelihood of malignancy for FDG-avid SPNs in patients > 60 years
    - False-negative FDG PET/CT
      - Indolent and low-grade lung cancer
      - Malignant SPN < 1 cm

- **Nodule Mimic (Pseudonodule)**
  - Exclusion of underlying true SPN
  - **Nipple/skin lesion**
    - Nipples: Bilateral symmetric rounded opacities, mid to inferior hemithorax, midaxillary line, incomplete border sign
    - Radiography with metallic (nipple) markers
  - **Osseous lesion**
    - Asymmetric 1st costochondral articulation
    - Rib fracture, callus, bone island
  - **Dependent atelectasis**
    - May mimic nodule on CT; posterior subpleural, resolves on prone or follow-up imaging

Helpful Clues for Less Common Diagnoses

- **Atypical Adenomatous Hyperplasia**
  - Earliest preinvasive lesion of adenocarcinoma
  - Frequent incidental finding with adenocarcinoma
  - Pure ground-glass nodule, typically ≤ 5 mm
- **Carcinoid**
  - Well-defined lobular borders
  - Bronchus sign
    - Airway leads into or associated with SPN; "iceberg" lesion, endoluminal and dominant extraluminal SPN
    - Postobstructive effects: Atelectasis, bronchiectasis, mucus plugs
  - Contrast enhancement, tumor vascularity
  - Multifocal punctate or coarse calcification in 38%
    - More common in lesions adjacent to central airways
  - Somatostatin receptor PET (SSTR-PET) with Gallium-68 Dotatate (somatostatin analogue) PET/CT
    - Increased sensitivity and specificity for detection of neuroendocrine tumors
    - ↑ image resolution, faster image acquisition
  - False-negative on FDG PET/CT; low metabolic activity
- **Hamartoma**
  - Slow-growing benign neoplasm, well-defined lobular or notched borders
  - Intralesional fat on CT in > 50%; -40 to -120 HU
  - Popcorn calcification on CT in 10-15%
- **Solitary Metastasis**
  - Most common: Melanoma, sarcoma, testicular cancer
  - Also: Breast, prostate, colon, and renal cancers
  - Peripheral location
- **Infarct**
  - Lower lobe, peripheral, subpleural, wedge-shaped
  - Decreased contrast enhancement
  - Central lucency, cavitation, halo sign
  - Slow resolution (months); may heal with scar
  - 10-15% of patients with pulmonary embolism
- **Laceration**
  - Traumatic disruption of lung parenchyma ± adjacent rib fractures
  - Round or ovoid air-filled lesion on CT: Homogeneous or heterogeneous SPN when filled with blood &/or fluid
  - Surrounding ground-glass opacity from adjacent contusion
  - Slow resolution (months); may heal with scar
- **Abscess**
  - Spherical, thick-walled lesion with internal low attenuation or cavitation
  - Frequent associated pleural effusion
  - Signs and symptoms of infection, sequela of aspiration
  - Mixed aerobic/anaerobic polymicrobial infection

Helpful Clues for Rare Diagnoses

- **Pulmonary Arteriovenous Malformation**
  - Peripheral lower lobe predominant
  - Rounded, ovoid, 1- to 5-cm nidus; feeding and draining vessel(s)
  - Single in 2/3 of cases
  - Vascular enhancement
  - Right-to-left shunt; risk of peripheral abscess or infarct
- **Amyloidoma (Nodular Amyloidosis)**
  - Solitary nodule; variable border characteristics
  - May exhibit calcification
  - Older patient, male:female = 3:2
- **Inflammatory Myofibroblastic Tumor (Pseudotumor)**
  - Lung nodule or mass; well-defined borders
  - Young patient or child

Granuloma

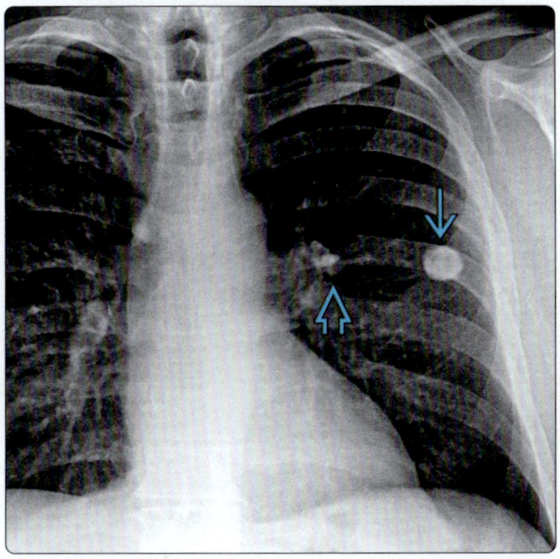

Granuloma

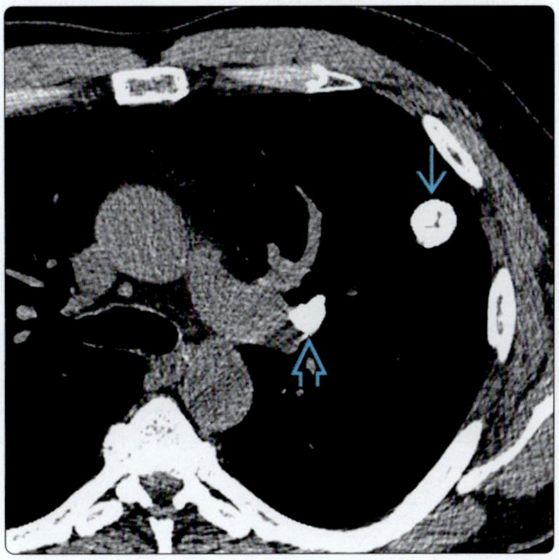

(Left) *Coned-down PA chest radiograph of an asymptomatic 71-year-old man shows a well-defined calcified left lung nodule ➔ and ipsilateral calcified nonenlarged left hilar lymph nodes ➱.* **(Right)** *Axial NECT of the same patient shows a mildly lobular left upper lobe nodule ➔ that demonstrates diffuse calcification, a benign pattern of calcification. Note associated calcified left hilar lymph node ➱. The findings are diagnostic of remote granulomatous disease secondary to histoplasmosis.*

(Left) *Coned-down PA chest radiograph of a 68-year-old woman shows a left mid lung zone nodule that exhibits central calcification, consistent with a granuloma. Calcification involves > 10% of the nodule diameter.* **(Right)** *Composite image with axial CECT in lung (left) and soft tissue (right) window of a 70-year-old woman shows a middle lobe granuloma with central calcification that involves > 10% of the cross section of this spherical nodule, a benign pattern of calcification for which no further imaging is warranted.*

Granuloma

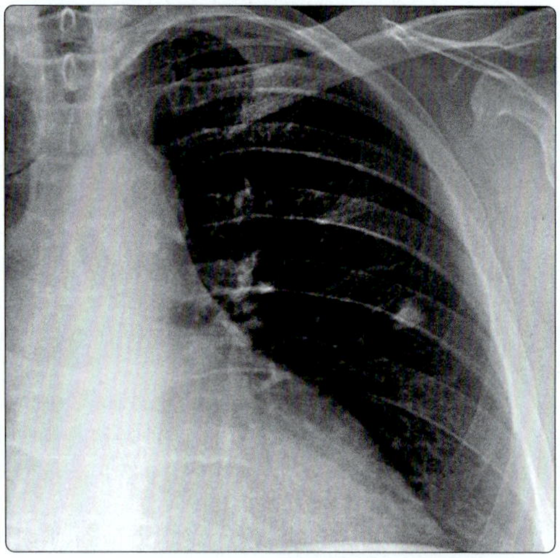

Granuloma

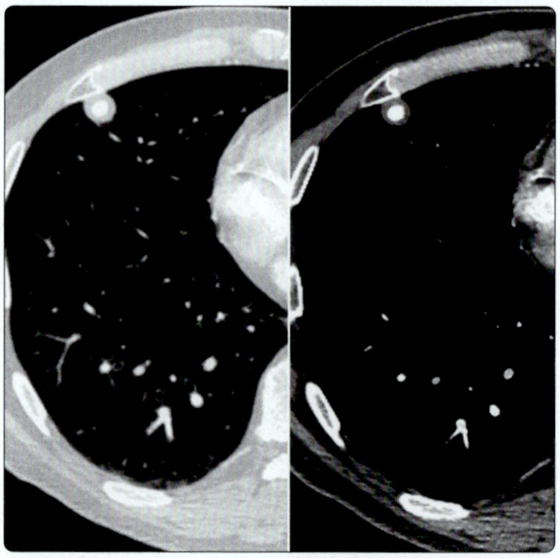

(Left) *Coronal CECT (bone window) of a 63-year-old woman with chest pain shows a left lower lobe nodule with central and laminar calcifications, both benign patterns of calcification typical of granuloma.* **(Right)** *Composite image with axial CECT MIP images in lung (left) and soft tissue (right) window of a 63-year-old woman with an abnormal radiograph shows a centrally calcified right lower lobe nodule with satellite micronodules and calcified right hilar lymph nodes, characteristic of remote histoplasmosis.*

Granuloma

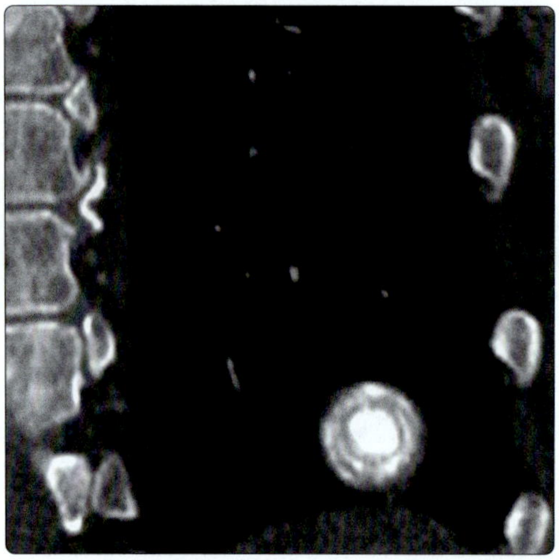

Granuloma

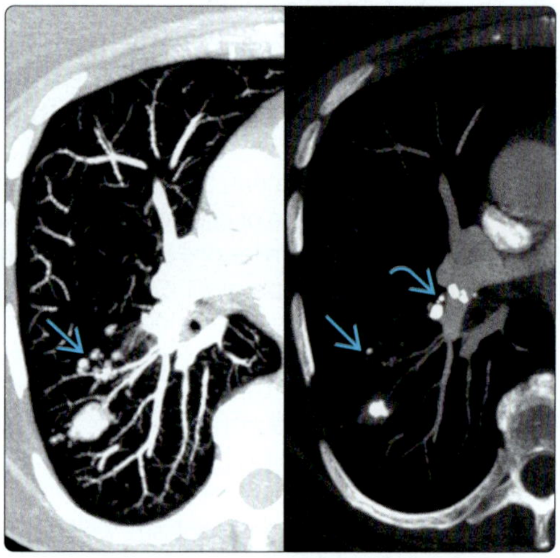

(Left) *Composite image with axial (left) and coronal (right) NECT shows an ovoid nodule adjacent to the minor fissure, which exhibits a lentiform morphology on coronal imaging, typical of intrapulmonary lymph node.* **(Right)** *Composite image with axial (left) and sagittal (right) NECT shows a right lower lobe nodular lesion and adjacent bronchial wall thickening. The nodule corresponds to an endobronchial mucus plug on sagittal imaging. Mucus plugs may mimic lung nodules on axial thin-section CT.*

Intrapulmonary Lymph Node

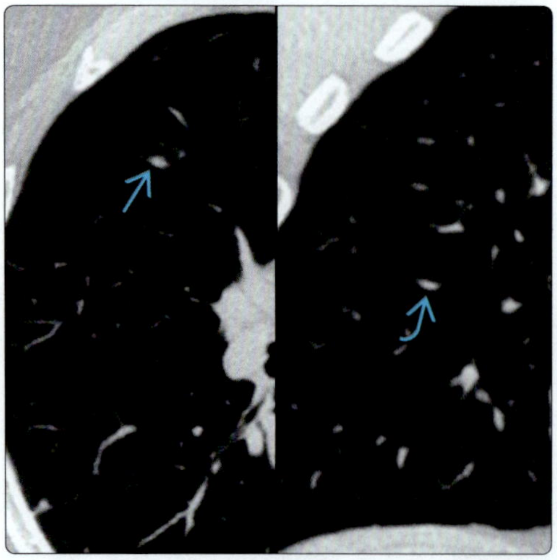

Mucus Plug

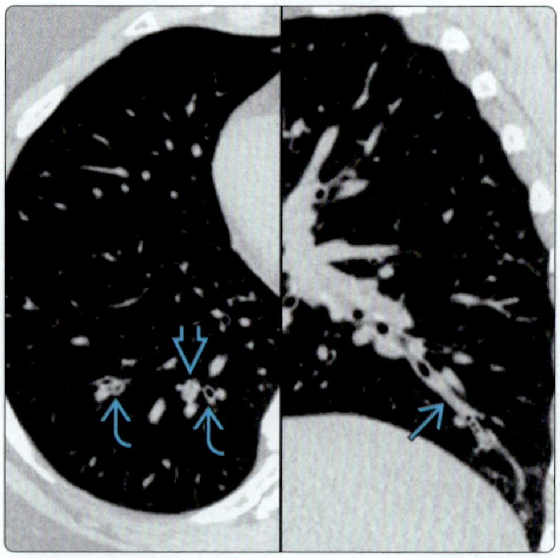

Lung Cancer

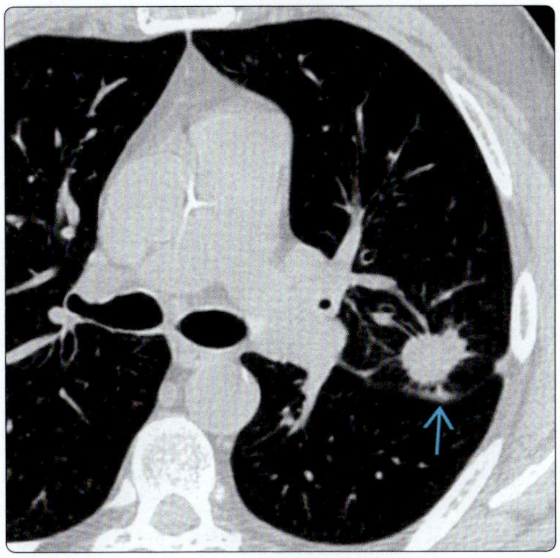

Lung Cancer

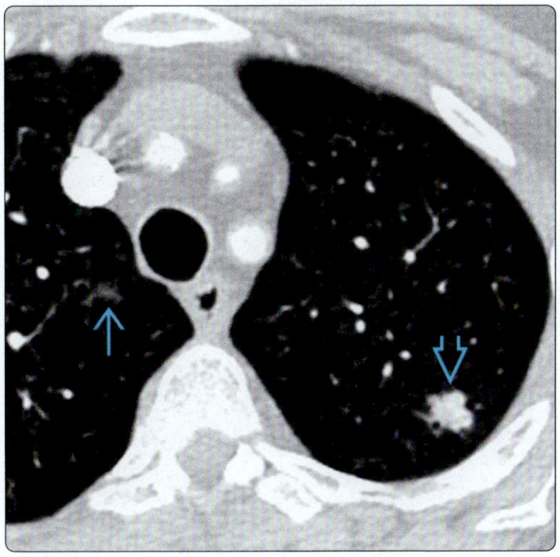

(Left) *Axial NECT of a 74-year-old smoker shows a left upper lobe lung cancer that manifests as a spiculated solid nodule with pleural tags* ⇒*. Spiculation and pleural tags are CT features suggestive of malignancy.* **(Right)** *Axial CECT of a 58-year-old woman shows a moderately differentiated left upper lobe adenocarcinoma manifesting as a solid nodule with polylobular borders* ⇒*. Note right upper lobe ground-glass nodule* → *that may represent atypical adenomatous hyperplasia, a preinvasive lesion of adenocarcinoma.*

Lung Cancer

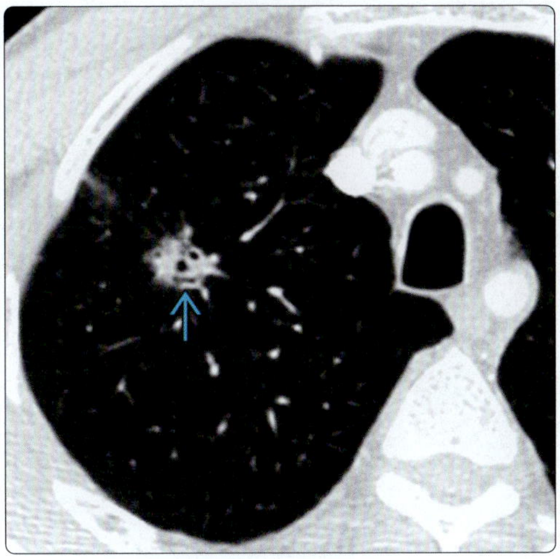

Lung Cancer

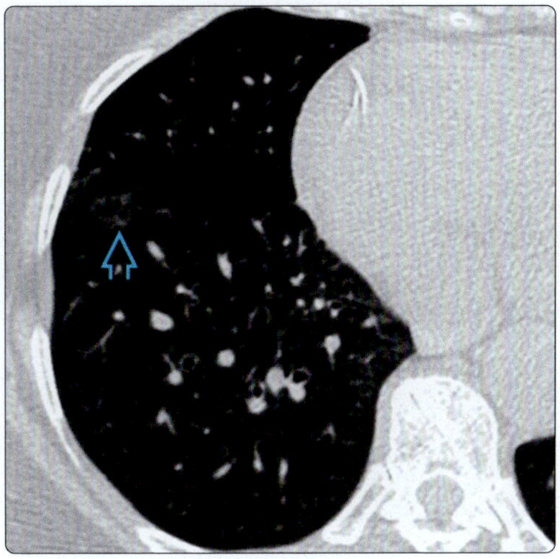

(Left) *Axial CECT of an asymptomatic 75-year-old man with a moderately differentiated right upper lobe adenocarcinoma shows a polylobular spiculated nodule* → *with intrinsic air bronchograms and small round "bubbly" lucencies.* **(Right)** *Axial NECT of an asymptomatic 79-year-old woman with a right lower lobe biopsy-proven minimally invasive adenocarcinoma that manifests as a right lower lobe ground-glass nodule* ⇒ *that abuts the adjacent right major fissure is shown.*

Nodule Mimics

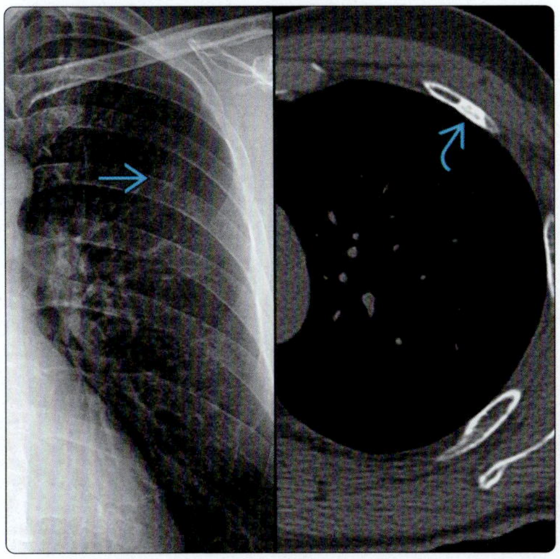

Nodule Mimics

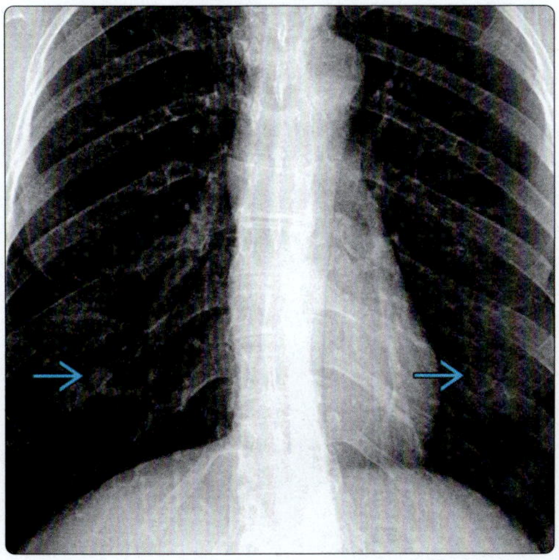

(Left) *Composite image with coned-down PA chest radiograph (left) and axial NECT (right) of a 63-year-old man shows an ill-defined left upper lung zone nodular opacity* → *that corresponded to a bone island* ↗ *on CT. Osseous lesions may mimic lung nodules.* **(Right)** *Coned-down PA chest radiograph of an asymptomatic adult shows bilateral symmetric nodular lesions* → *projecting over the lower lungs, typical of nipple shadows. The nodules exhibit the incomplete border sign, indicating that they are extrapulmonary.*

Carcinoid

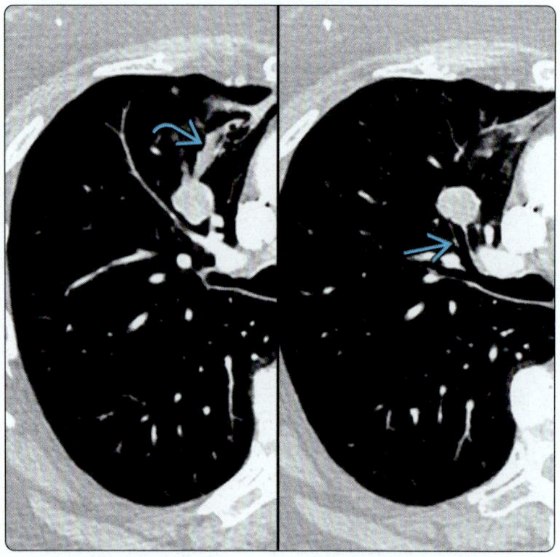

Carcinoid

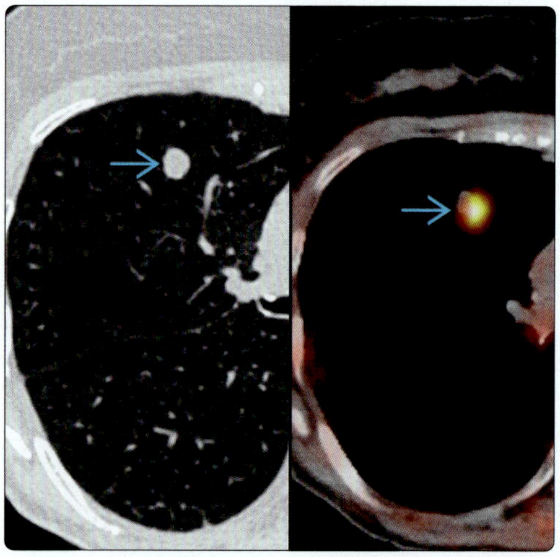

(Left) *Composite image with axial CECT of a 66-year-old woman with hemoptysis shows a right upper lobe solid nodule and a bronchus* *that courses into the lesion, the bronchus sign. Peripheral tubular opacities* *correspond to mucus plugs from bronchial obstruction.* **(Right)** *Composite image with axial NECT (left) and Gallium-68 Dotatate PET/CT (right) of a 59-year-old woman shows a right upper lobe solid nodule* *that exhibits Gallium-68 Dotatate avidity, consistent with a neuroendocrine tumor, in this case, a carcinoid tumor.*

Hamartoma

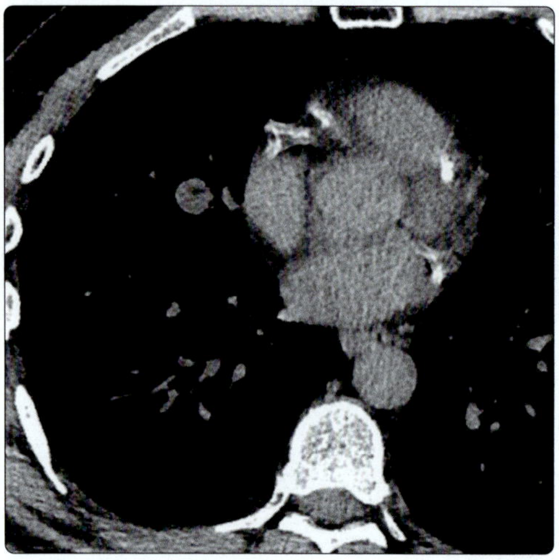

Solitary Metastasis

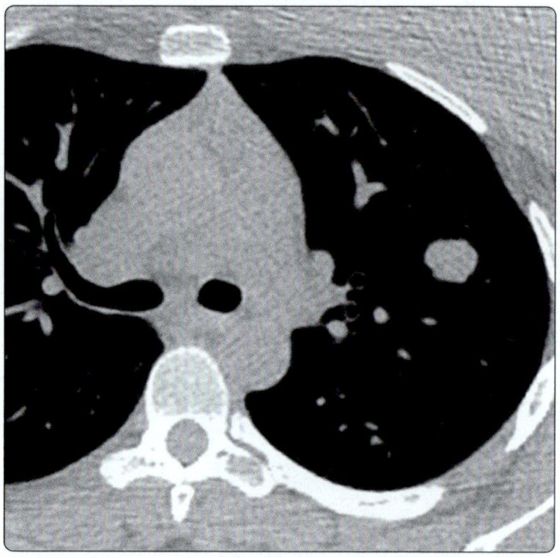

(Left) *Axial NECT of a 52-year-old man with a radiographic abnormality shows a middle lobe solid nodule with a small focus of internal macroscopic fat, an imaging finding diagnostic of hamartoma for which no further management is required.* **(Right)** *Axial NECT shows a 50-year-old woman smoker with breast cancer and a new left upper lobe nodule found on surveillance imaging, concerning for primary lung cancer. Biopsy demonstrated metastatic breast cancer. Solitary metastases are rare, but important, causes of solitary lung nodules.*

Infarct

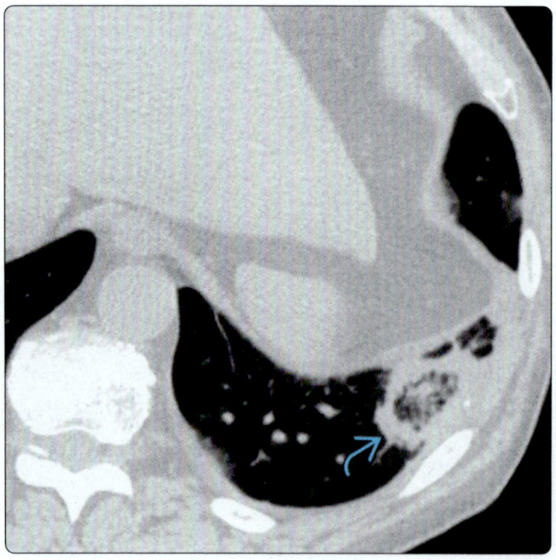

Infarct

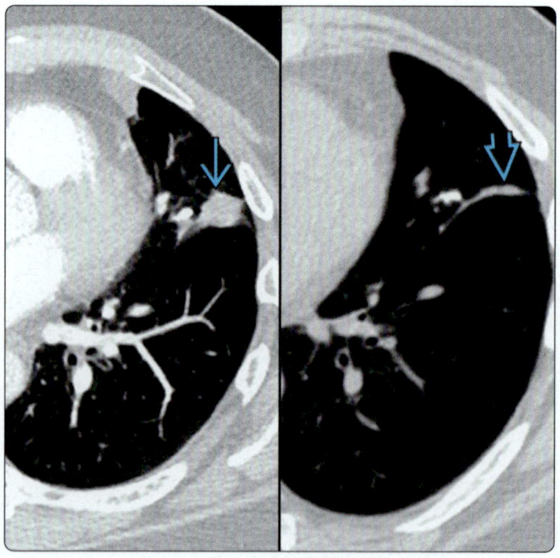

(Left) *Axial CECT of a 78-year-old man with chest pain secondary to pulmonary thromboembolism (not shown) shows a left lower lobe subpleural polylobular nodule with central lucency* *, characteristic of a pulmonary infarct.* **(Right)** *Composite image with axial CECT (left) and NECT obtained 8 months later (right) of a 63-year-old man with pulmonary thromboembolism (not shown) shows a lingular lung infarct that manifests as a solid lung nodule* *. Months later, the infarct demonstrates healing with linear scar formation* *.*

Laceration

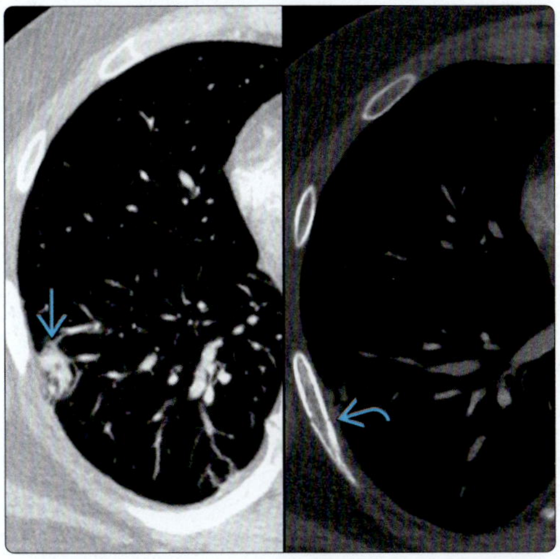

Abscess

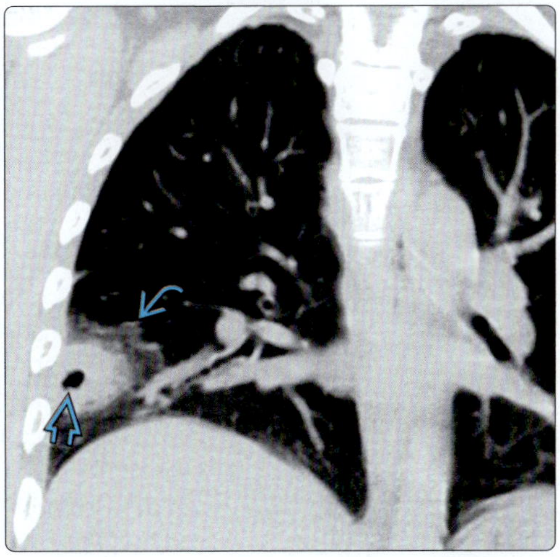

(Left) *Composite image with axial CECT in lung (left) and bone (right) window of a patient with chest trauma shows a heterogeneous right lower lobe subpleural nodule, characteristic of a pulmonary laceration. Note adjacent nondisplaced right rib fracture.* **(Right)** *Coronal NECT of a young man with fever, leukocytosis, and a peripheral right basilar nodule identified on radiography shows a right lower lobe subpleural nodule with cavitation and surrounding ground-glass opacity, consistent with a lung abscess.*

Pulmonary Arteriovenous Malformation

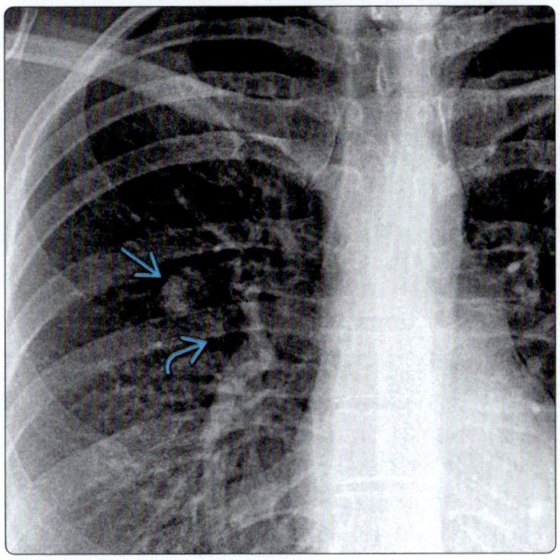

Pulmonary Arteriovenous Malformation

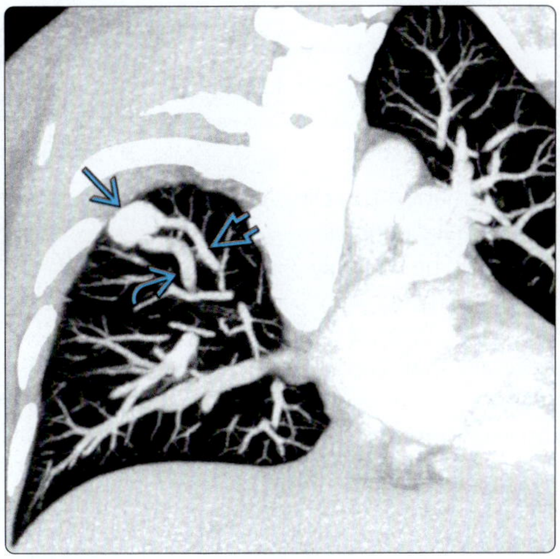

(Left) *Coned-down PA chest radiograph of an asymptomatic 38-year-old woman shows a well-defined right upper lobe nodule. Note the tubular opacity that courses from the nodule toward the ipsilateral right hilum.* **(Right)** *Coronal oblique CECT (MIP image) of the same patient confirms that the nodule represents a pulmonary arteriovenous malformation. Note the lesion's feeding artery and draining vein. The latter was visible on radiography and allowed the formulation of the correct diagnosis.*

Amyloidoma

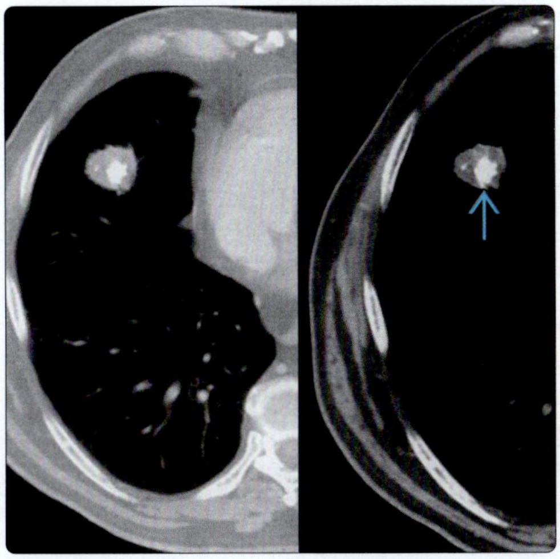

Pulmonary Inflammatory Myofibroblastic Tumor

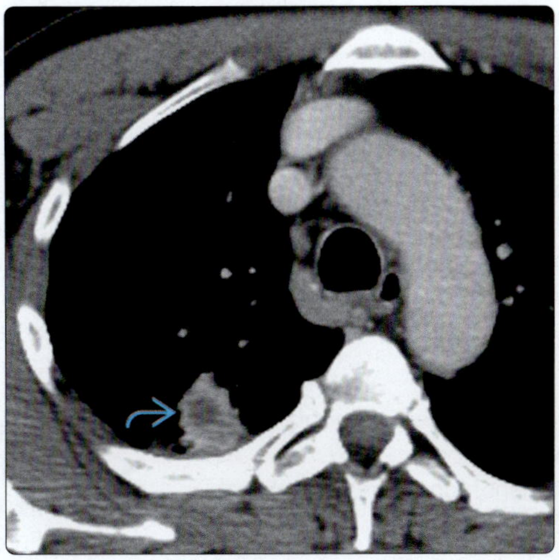

(Left) *Composite image with axial CECT in lung (left) and soft tissue (right) window of a 68-year-old man with prostate cancer and a radiographic abnormality shows a spiculated nodule with coarse eccentric calcification. Biopsy demonstrated an amyloidoma.* **(Right)** *Axial CECT of a 38-year-old man with an incidentally discovered radiographic abnormality shows a right upper lobe nodule with internal low attenuation suspicious for primary lung cancer. Biopsy demonstrated inflammatory myofibroblastic tumor.*

DIFFERENTIAL DIAGNOSIS

Common

- Metastases
- Granulomatous Infection
- Pneumonia
- Sarcoidosis

Less Common

- Septic Emboli
- Organizing Pneumonia
- Silicosis/Coal Workers' Pneumoconiosis
- Granulomatosis With Polyangiitis

Rare but Important

- Pulmonary Langerhans Cell Histiocytosis
- Angioinvasive Fungal Disease
- Diffuse Idiopathic Neuroendocrine Cell Hyperplasia
- Lung Cancer
- Lymphoma
- Kaposi Sarcoma
- Rheumatoid Nodules
- Nodular Amyloidosis

ESSENTIAL INFORMATION

Key Differential Diagnosis Issues

- Correlation with demographic information and clinical presentation helps narrow differential diagnosis
  - Hematogenous metastases should be strongly considered in patients with known malignancy
  - Multifocal calcified lung nodules associated with lymph node and splenic calcifications are characteristic of remote histoplasmosis infection
    - Frequent imaging finding in endemic areas
  - Multifocal pulmonary infection should be considered in patients with fever, leukocytosis, and elevated procalcitonin
    - Multifocal nodules in immunocompromised patient should suggest opportunistic infection
  - Upper lung-predominant nodules with associated symmetric lymphadenopathy should suggest sarcoidosis, diagnosis of exclusion
  - Multifocal primary lung cancer is typically adenocarcinoma
- CT imaging
  - Characterization of nodule morphology
  - Determination of nodule distribution
  - Correlation with clinical and demographic information for formulation of focused differential diagnosis

Helpful Clues for Common Diagnoses

- **Metastases**
  - Typically hematogenous dissemination of neoplasm
  - Patients with advanced malignancy
  - Basilar predominant (dominant blood flow), peripheral
  - Spherical nodules
    - Angiocentric distribution
    - Variable borders: Well-defined, smooth, spiculation, lobulation, halo sign (hemorrhagic metastases)
    - Cavitation
    - Calcification
- **Granulomatous Infection**
  - Histoplasmosis
    - Multifocal calcified lung nodules
    - Calcified intrathoracic lymph nodes
    - Frequent calcified splenic granulomas
  - Sequela of prior coccidioidomycosis and tuberculosis may also calcify
- **Pneumonia**
  - Acute clinical presentation
    - Cough, fever
    - Leukocytosis, ↑ procalcitonin
  - Imaging
    - Consolidation
    - Multifocal nodules of varying sizes ± associated consolidation, ground-glass opacity, cellular bronchiolitis
- **Sarcoidosis**
  - Mid and upper lung zone-predominant nodules
    - Peribronchovascular, septal, subpleural
    - Perilymphatic micronodules
  - Bilateral hilar and mediastinal lymphadenopathy
    - May exhibit calcification, including eggshell Ca++
  - Peribronchovascular nodular fibrosis

Helpful Clues for Less Common Diagnoses

- **Septic Emboli**
  - Fever, positive blood cultures, infective endocarditis in intravenous drug users
  - Multifocal bilateral peripheral pulmonary nodules
    - Intrinsic low attenuation
    - Cavitation
- **Organizing Pneumonia**
  - May be idiopathic; cryptogenic organizing pneumonia
  - Associated conditions: Connective tissue disease, drug reaction/toxicity, interstitial lung disease, malignancy
  - Chronic cough, dyspnea, fever, malaise
  - Multifocal bilateral pulmonary opacities, may be recurrent and migratory
  - Lower lobe predominant, peribronchovascular, perilobular
  - Characteristic reversed halo sign &/or atoll sign
- **Silicosis/Coal Workers' Pneumoconiosis**
  - Male patient, occupational exposure
  - Upper lobe-predominant micronodules; 1-3 mm, may calcify
  - Paracicatricial emphysema
  - Nodules > 1 cm indicate progressive massive fibrosis
  - Multiple nodules may aggregate as progressive massive fibrosis
  - May cavitate with mycetoma formation
  - Bilateral, R > L
  - Hilar/mediastinal lymphadenopathy; may calcify, including eggshell Ca++
- **Granulomatosis With Polyangiitis**
  - Multifocal pulmonary nodules
    - Frequent cavitation
    - Feeding vessel sign indicating angiocentric distribution
    - Halo sign indicating surrounding ground-glass opacity from pulmonary alveolar hemorrhage

- Other findings
  - Multifocal pulmonary masses &/or consolidations
  - May exhibit intrinsic cavitation; more common in large nodules and masses

Helpful Clues for Rare Diagnoses

- **Pulmonary Langerhans Cell Histiocytosis**
  - Young adults, both sexes, almost exclusively smokers
  - Centrilobular nodules 1-10 mm, stellate morphology
    - Nodules > 10 mm are uncommon
  - Cavitary nodules, cysts with nodular walls, bizarre shapes
  - Mid and upper lung zone predominance, lung bases spared
- **Angioinvasive Fungal Disease**
  - Febrile neutropenia, immunocompromised, high-dose steroids
  - Single or multiple nodules, masses, or consolidations
    - Nodules usually < 10 in number, 3 mm to 3 cm
  - May exhibit halo sign from surrounding hemorrhage
  - Cavitation and air-crescent sign with recovery of neutrophil function
  - Other signs
    - Occluded vessel sign: Interruption of pulmonary artery at lesion border
    - Hypodense sign: Central hypodensity within nodule
- **Diffuse Idiopathic Pulmonary Neuroendocrine Cell Hyperplasia**
  - Neuroendocrine cell (NEC) proliferations
    - Tumorlet: NEC proliferation that invades bronchiolar basement membrane
      - Small nodules: < 5 mm
    - Carcinoid tumor: Neoplasm, invades basement membrane
      - Nodules or masses: ≥ 5 mm
    - Constrictive bronchiolitis from NEC proliferations that produce peribronchiolar fibrosis
      - Mosaic attenuation
      - Expiratory air-trapping
  - Clinical
    - Female nonsmoker
    - 50-70 years
    - Cough, dyspnea, wheezing
- **Lung Cancer**
  - Synchronous lung cancers
  - Multicentric pulmonary adenocarcinoma
    - Multifocal part-solid nodules
    - Multifocal ground-glass nodules may represent preinvasive lesions: Atypical adenomatous hyperplasia
  - Invasive mucinous adenocarcinoma
    - Consolidation
    - May exhibit tracheobronchial dissemination with multifocal bilateral lung nodules
- **Lymphoma**
  - Non-Hodgkin lymphoma
    - Primary or secondary lung involvement
    - Extranodal marginal zone lymphoma, diffuse large B-cell lymphoma, lymphomatoid granulomatosis, posttransplantation lymphoproliferative disorder
  - Clinical: Asymptomatic; cough, fever, and weight loss; autoimmunity
  - Single or multiple nodules, masses, consolidations; may exhibit air bronchograms &/or cavitation
- **Kaposi Sarcoma**
  - Types: Kaposi sarcoma (KS), acquired immune deficiency syndrome with Kaposi sarcoma (AIDS-KS), iatrogenic Kaposi sarcoma (IKS)
  - Bilateral poorly marginated lung nodules, flame-shaped, peribronchovascular
    - May exhibit surrounding ground-glass opacity
  - Other findings: Lymphadenopathy, pleural effusion
- **Rheumatoid Nodules**
  - Rheumatoid arthritis; M > F; usually smokers
  - Single or multiple peripheral or subpleural nodules
    - Variable size
    - May exhibit cavitation
- **Nodular Amyloidosis**
  - Solitary or multiple well-defined nodules, often calcified
  - Associated lung cysts in patients with Sjögren syndrome

Metastases

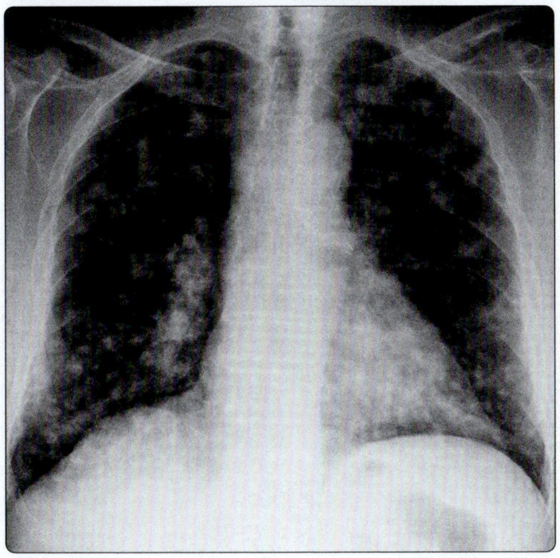

Metastases

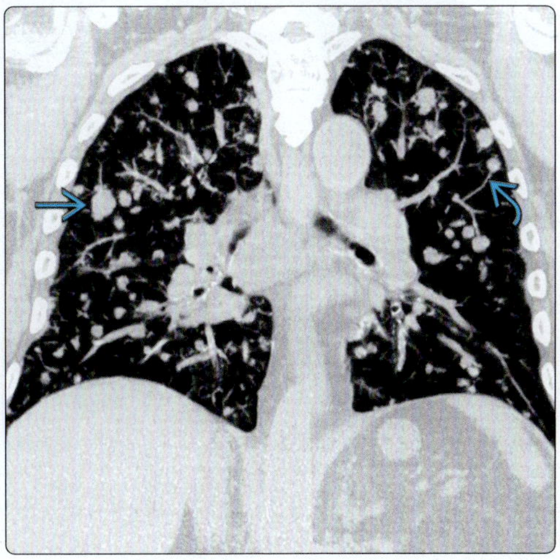

(Left) *PA chest radiograph of a 68-year-old man with metastatic bladder cancer shows numerous bilateral lung nodules of various sizes, consistent with pulmonary metastases.* **(Right)** *Coronal CECT (MIP image) of the same patient shows multifocal bilateral solid nodules, some with a polylobular morphology ➔ and some with an angiocentric distribution characterized by a vessel ➚ that courses into the nodule, consistent with hematogenous metastases. Metastases are a common cause of multifocal bilateral pulmonary nodules.*

Metastases

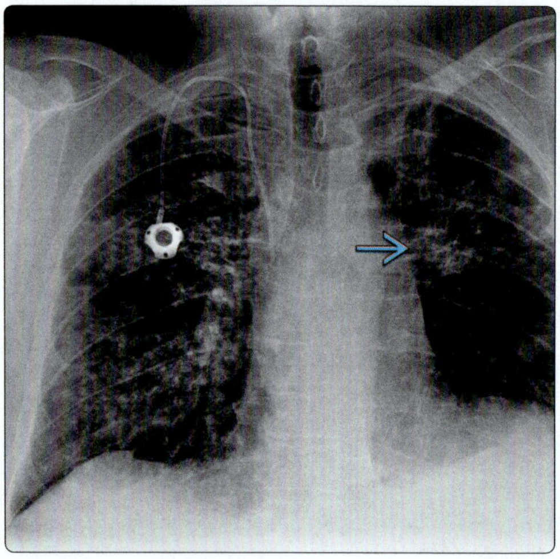

Metastases

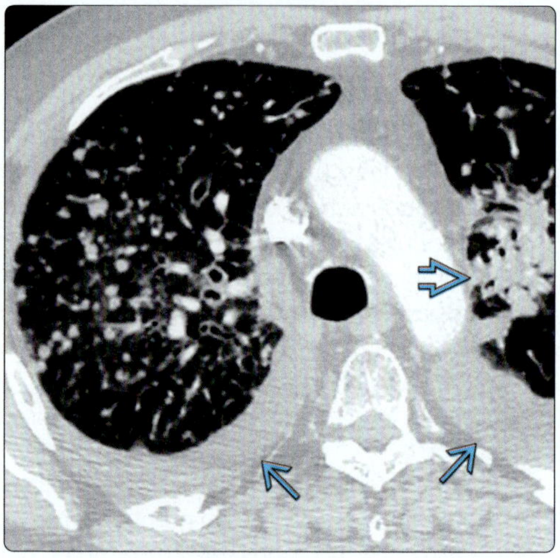

(Left) *PA chest radiograph of a 74-year-old man with metastatic lung cancer shows posttreatment changes in the left lung and innumerable small bilateral pulmonary nodules. The findings are consistent with disease progression secondary to hematogenous pulmonary metastases.* **(Right)** *Axial CECT of the same patient shows posttreatment changes in the left lung and multifocal bilateral small solid randomly distributed pulmonary nodules. Note associated small-to-moderate bilateral pleural effusions.*

Granulomatous Infection

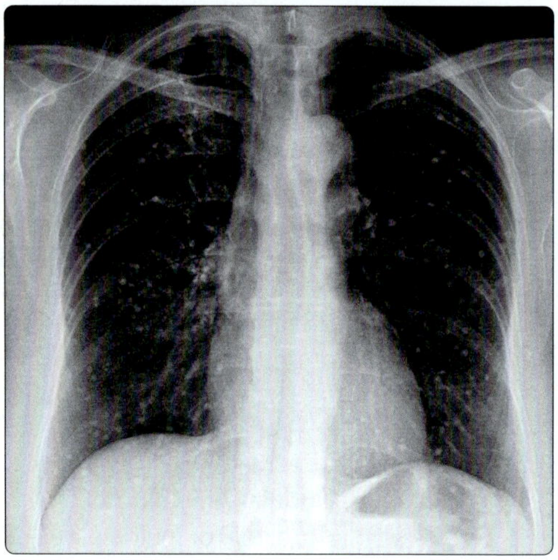

Granulomatous Infection

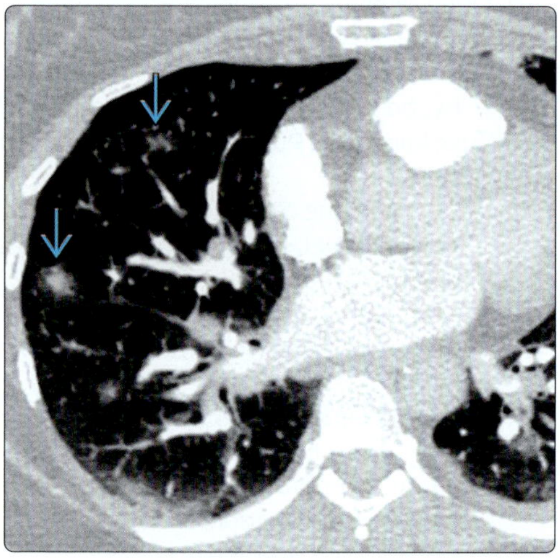

(Left) *PA chest radiograph of an asymptomatic 76-year-old woman shows multifocal bilateral small calcified pulmonary nodules, consistent with calcified granulomas presumably from remote histoplasmosis pulmonary infection.* **(Right)** *Axial CECT of a 45-year-old woman who presented acutely with fever and cough shows multifocal bilateral pulmonary nodules, some of which exhibit the CT halo sign, from surrounding alveolar hemorrhage. The diagnosis of acute histoplasmosis was confirmed on bronchoscopic biopsy.*

Granulomatous Infection

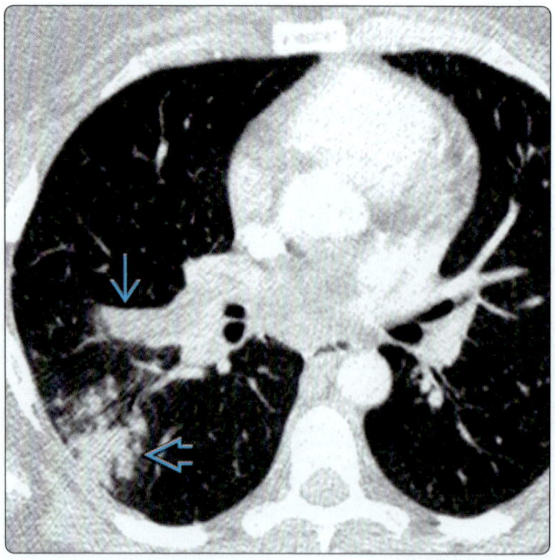

Granulomatous Infection

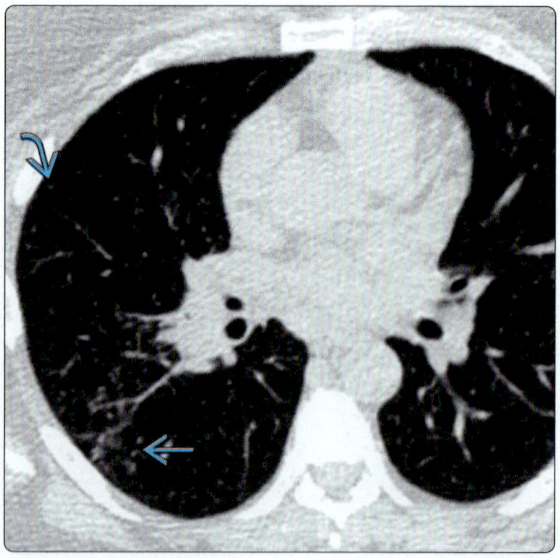

(Left) *Axial NECT of a 40-year-old woman with fever and cough from acute fungal pneumonia secondary to histoplasmosis shows multifocal clustered and coalescent right lower lobe nodules and an adjacent mass-like consolidation.* **(Right)** *Axial CECT of the same patient obtained 2 months after treatment shows marked improvement and decreased size of the right lower lobe nodules and multiple right lung micronodules not evident on the original study. Some of these nodules may later develop calcification.*

Pneumonia

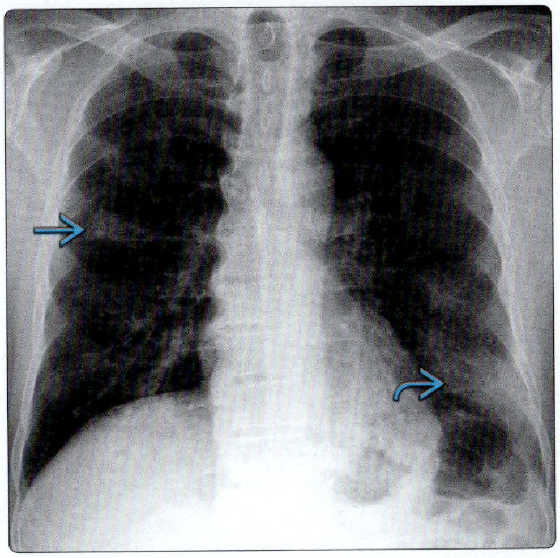

Pneumonia

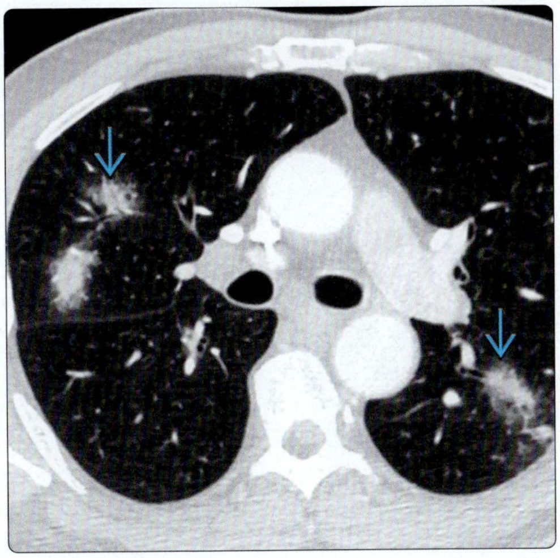

(Left) *PA chest radiograph of a 56-year-old man with cough, fever, and leukocytosis shows multiple bilateral nodules* → *and consolidations* ↗, *consistent with multifocal pneumonia, in this case, secondary to methicillin-sensitive Staphylococcus aureus.* **(Right)** *Axial CECT of the same patient shows that some of the radiographic abnormalities correspond to multifocal bilateral pulmonary nodules* → *with irregular margins and ground-glass opacity halos. Pneumonia may manifest with multifocal lung nodules and consolidations.*

Sarcoidosis

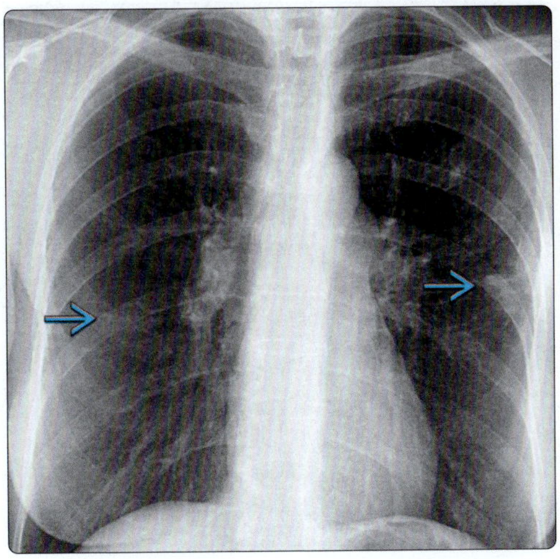

Sarcoidosis

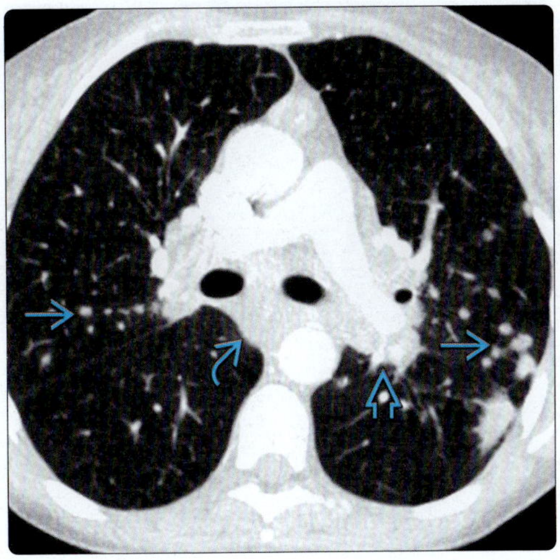

(Left) *PA chest radiograph of a 67-year-old woman who presented with dry cough and chest pain shows multifocal bilateral pulmonary nodules* →, *more numerous on the left, and bilateral hilar, right paratracheal and AP window lymphadenopathy.* **(Right)** *Axial NECT of the same patient shows multifocal bilateral clustered pulmonary nodules* → *and bilateral hilar* ⇒ *and subcarinal* ↗ *lymphadenopathy. Bronchoscopy and biopsy confirmed the suspected diagnosis of sarcoidosis.*

Sarcoidosis

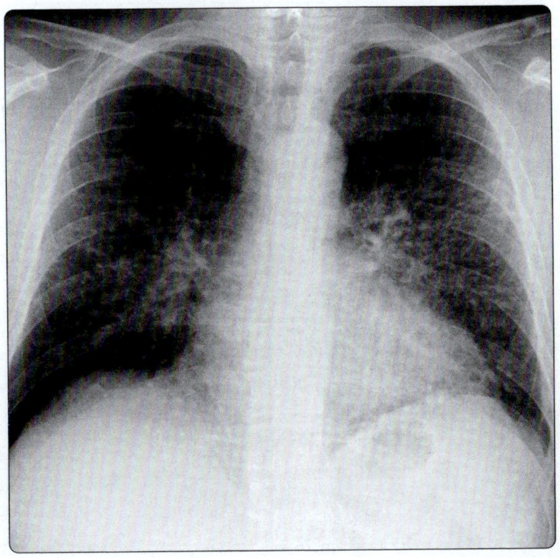

Sarcoidosis

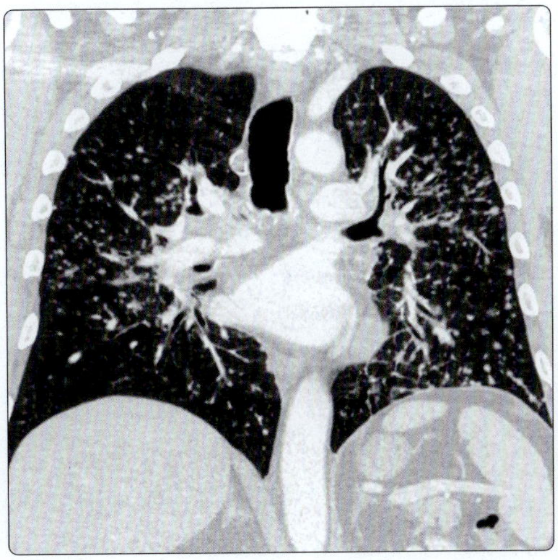

(Left) *PA chest radiograph of a 58-year-old man with chronic dyspnea shows multifocal bilateral small nodules clustered about the perihilar regions.* **(Right)** *Coronal NECT of the same patient shows multifocal bilateral small nodules clustered about the hila. The nodules are located about bronchovascular structures, interlobular septa, and subpleural regions, a perilymphatic distribution characteristic of sarcoidosis. Sarcoidosis is a diagnosis of exclusion, which was confirmed on bronchoscopic biopsy in this case.*

(Left) *Coronal NECT of a 56-year-old man with renal failure, an infected central line, fever, and positive blood cultures shows multifocal bilateral pulmonary nodules, one of which exhibits early cavitation, consistent with clinically suspected septic emboli.* **(Right)** *Coronal NECT of a 67-year-old man with an abnormal chest radiograph shows multifocal bilateral nodular opacities, one with a perilobular distribution and the reversed halo sign, consistent with clinically suspected organizing pneumonia.*

Septic Emboli

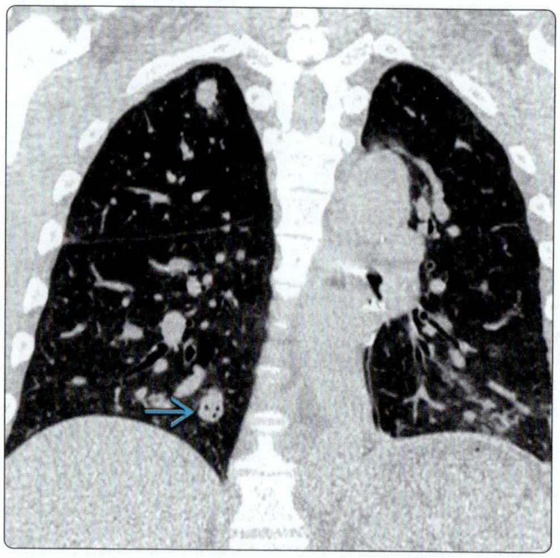

Organizing Pneumonia

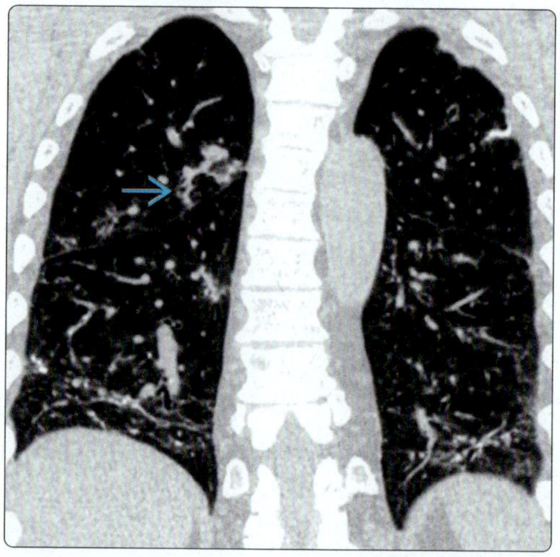

(Left) *Axial NECT of a 75-year-old retired sandblaster shows multiple bilateral upper lobe small nodules, some of which are calcified. Note areas of nodule coalescence and paracicatricial emphysema, characteristic of silicosis.* **(Right)** *Axial NECT of a 76-year-old man with granulomatosis with polyangiitis shows multiple bilateral pulmonary nodules, at least 2 of which exhibit early cavitation. Pulmonary vasculitis should be considered in the differential diagnosis of multifocal pulmonary nodules, with or without cavitation.*

Silicosis/Coal Workers' Pneumoconiosis

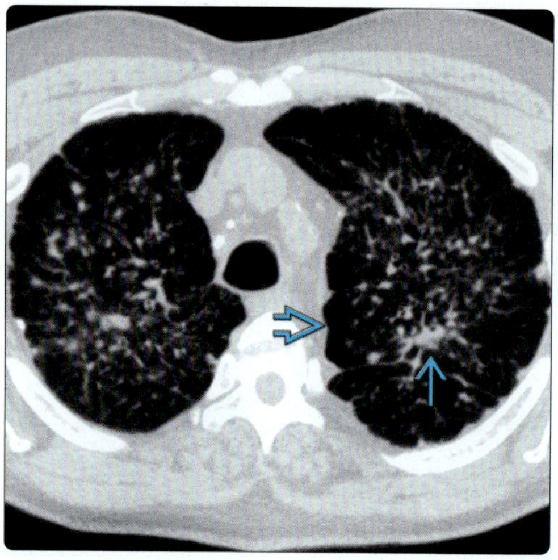

Granulomatosis With Polyangiitis

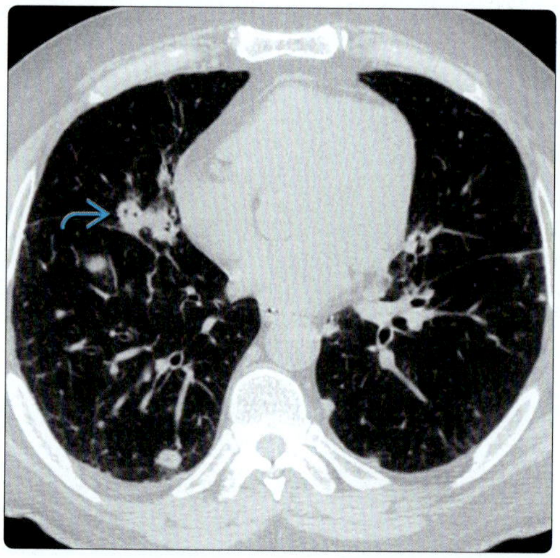

(Left) *Coronal NECT (MIP image) of a 45-year-old smoker shows mid and upper lung zone small pulmonary nodules that spare the lung bases. One of the nodules exhibits subtle intrinsic lucency. The findings are consistent with Langerhans cell histiocytosis.* **(Right)** *Composite image with axial (left) and coronal (right) NECT of a 55-year-old transplant recipient with neutropenic fever shows right upper lobe nodules with ground-glass opacity halos, diagnostic of invasive aspergillosis in this clinical setting.*

Pulmonary Langerhans Cell Histiocytosis

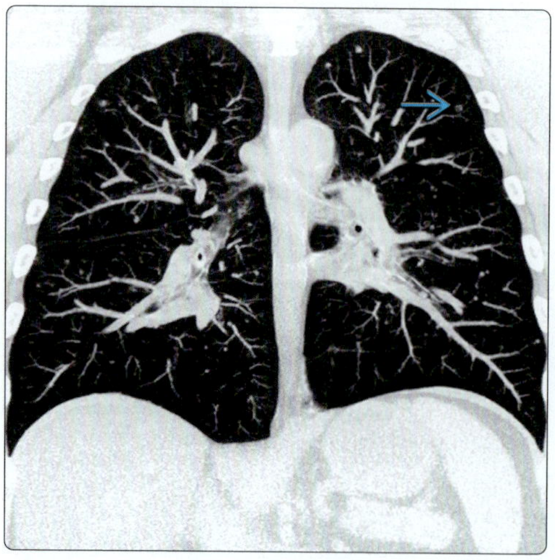

Angioinvasive Fungal Disease

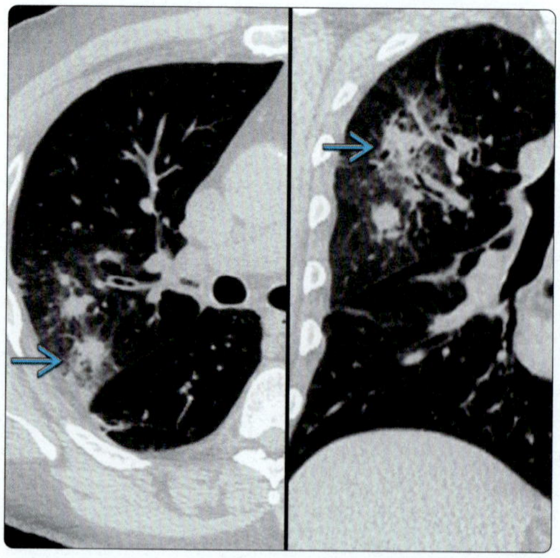

Diffuse Idiopathic Neuroendocrine Cell Hyperplasia

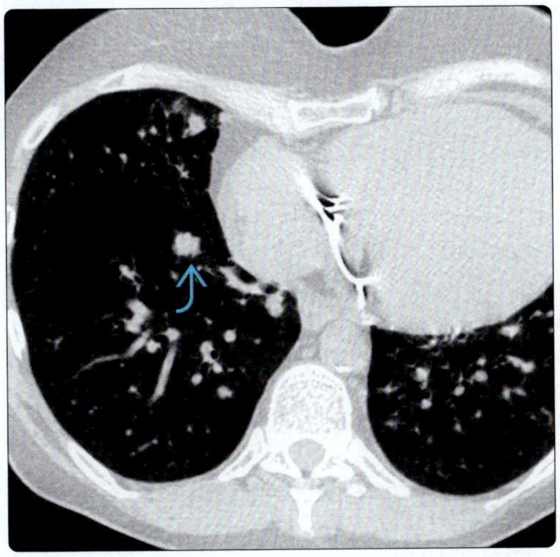

Lung Cancer

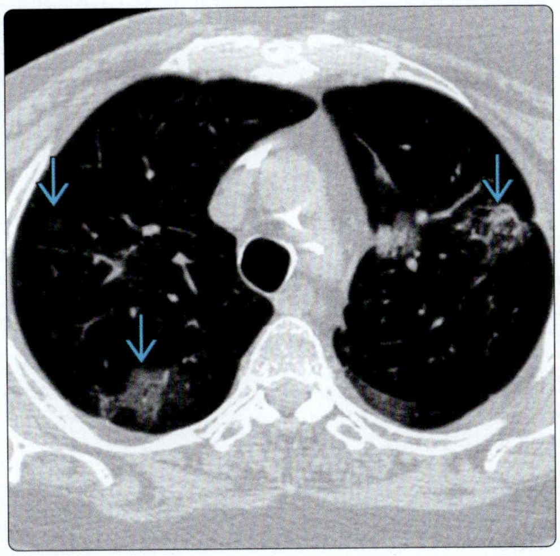

(Left) *Axial NECT (minIP image) of a 59-year-old woman with wheezing secondary to diffuse idiopathic neuroendocrine cell hyperplasia shows multifocal small nodules of varying sizes and mosaic attenuation, which represent neuroendocrine cell proliferations and constrictive bronchiolitis, respectively. The larger nodules are likely carcinoid tumors.* **(Right)** *Axial NECT of an asymptomatic 75-year-old woman demonstrates multifocal pulmonary adenocarcinomas that manifest with multiple bilateral subsolid nodules.*

Lymphoma

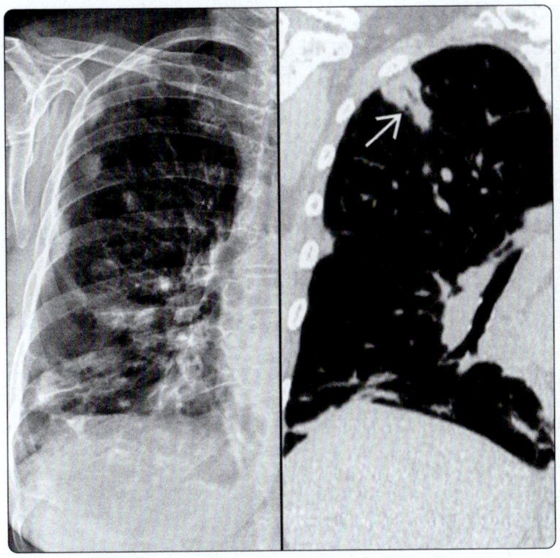

Kaposi Sarcoma

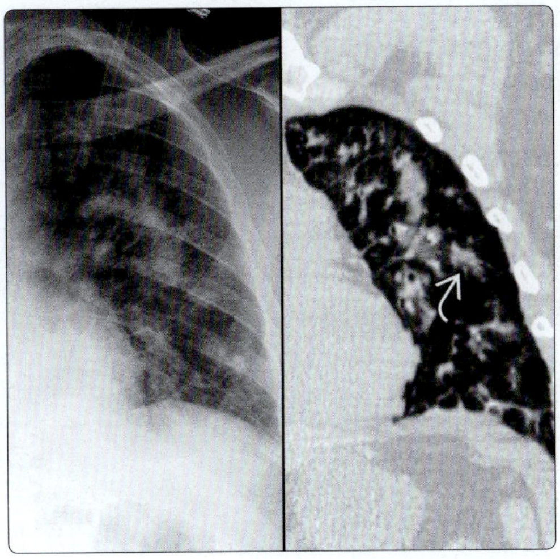

(Left) *Composite image with PA chest radiograph (left) and coronal NECT (right) of an asymptomatic 71-year-old woman with marginal zone primary pulmonary lymphoma that manifests with multifocal pulmonary nodules is shown. Note the air bronchogram in the right apical lung nodule.* **(Right)** *Composite image with PA chest radiograph (left) and coronal NECT (right) of a 49-year-old man with AIDS-Kaposi sarcoma shows multifocal irregular lung nodules, some of which exhibit a flame-shaped morphology on chest CT.*

Rheumatoid Nodules

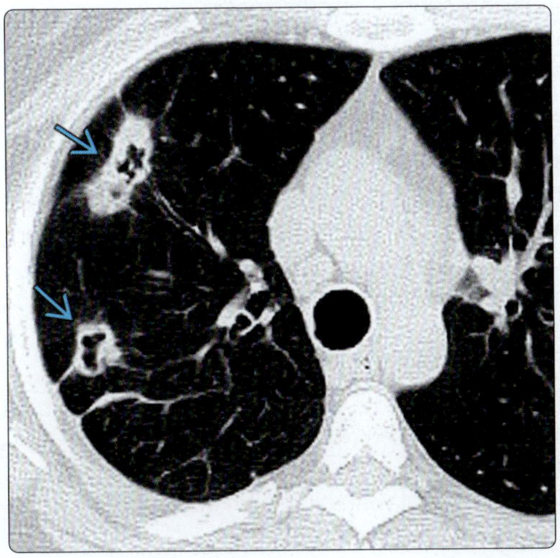

Nodular Amyloidosis

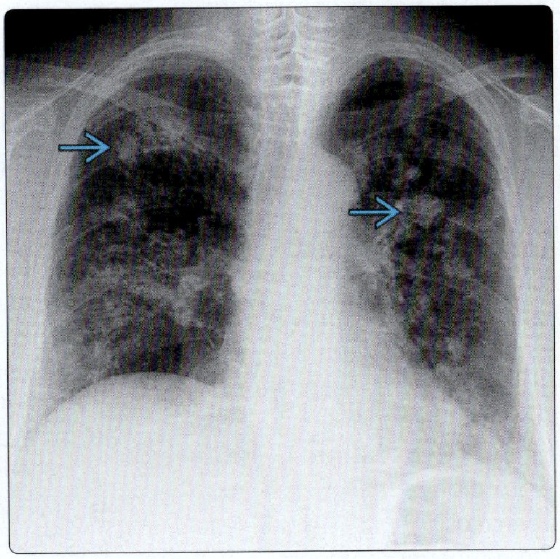

(Left) *Axial NECT of a 66-year-old man with rheumatoid arthritis shows multifocal rheumatoid nodules with polylobular morphologies and internal cavitation with variable thickness of the nodular cavity walls. Rheumatoid nodules are an unusual pulmonary manifestation of rheumatoid arthritis.* **(Right)** *PA chest radiograph of a 76-year-old woman with nodular amyloidosis and lymphoid interstitial pneumonia shows multifocal bilateral pulmonary nodules, many of which exhibit intrinsic calcification.*

DIFFERENTIAL DIAGNOSIS

Common

- Metastases
- Mycobacterial Infection
- Pulmonary Infarcts
- Septic Emboli
- Fungal Infection

Less Common

- Granulomatosis With Polyangiitis
- Pulmonary Langerhans Cell Histiocytosis
- Primary Lung Cancer
- Multifocal Pulmonary Lacerations

Rare but Important

- Lymphoma
- Rheumatoid Nodules
- Tracheobronchial Papillomatosis
- Sarcoidosis

ESSENTIAL INFORMATION

Key Differential Diagnosis Issues

- Identify primary source of malignancy if metastatic disease is suspected
- IV drug use and indwelling catheters should raise suspicion for septic emboli
- Opportunistic infections should be considered in immunocompromised patients

Helpful Clues for Common Diagnoses

- **Metastases**
    - Squamous cell carcinomas (e.g., head and neck cancer, cervical cancer)
    - Adenocarcinomas (e.g., gastrointestinal tract, breast) and sarcomas
    - Random distribution of lesions is helpful clue
    - Feeding vessel sign: Pulmonary artery branch leading into pulmonary lesion
- **Mycobacterial Infection**
    - Nontuberculous mycobacterial infection (bronchiectatic)
        - Middle lobe and lingular predominant distribution
        - Tree-in-bud opacities, waxing and waning nodules ± cavitation
        - Bronchiectasis and cicatricial atelectasis
    - Nontuberculous mycobacterial infection (classic fibrocavitary)
        - Upper lobe predominant fibrosis and cavitation
        - Typically thin cavity walls
            - Mild cavity wall thickening &/or nodular cavity walls may occur
            - Thick cavity walls are concerning for malignancy or superimposed/progressive infection
            - May develop intracavitary mycetomas
        - Frequently associated with emphysema
    - Post-primary pattern of tuberculosis
        - Upper lobes and lower lobe superior segments
        - Tree-in-bud opacities common in active disease
        - Cavitary nodules, masses, &/or consolidations
        - Intrathoracic lymphadenopathy may exhibit central low attenuation and peripheral enhancement
        - Pleural thickening, free or loculated pleural effusion
            - Hydropneumothorax should suggest bronchopleural fistula
        - Cavities may be complicated by acute infection or mycetoma
- **Pulmonary Infarcts**
    - Wedge-shaped peripheral subpleural consolidation(s) or nodule(s) with central lucency
    - Segmental or subsegmental pulmonary artery thromboembolism
    - Lower lobes > upper lobes
- **Septic Emboli**
    - History of IV drug use, endocarditis, indwelling vascular catheters, Lemierre syndrome
    - Peripheral distribution with mid and lower lung zone predominance
    - Small (< 3 cm), poorly-marginated thick or thin-walled nodules; rapid onset, various stages of cavitation
    - "Feeding vessel" sign
    - *Staphylococcus aureus* is commonly associated with indwelling catheters and IV drug use
- **Fungal Infection**
    - Immunocompromised patients are most susceptible
    - Chronic necrotizing pulmonary aspergillosis (formerly semi-invasive aspergillosis)
        - Rapidly progressive (< 3 months) in mildly to moderately immunocompromised patients
        - Upper lobes > lower lobes
        - Irregularly shaped nodules or consolidations with central necrosis and thick-walled cavities; may exhibit the air crescent sign
        - ± associated mycetoma
    - Angioinvasive aspergillosis
        - Profoundly immunocompromised patients with severe neutropenia
        - Solitary or multiple nodules, masses, or consolidations, ± cavitation
        - Halo sign: Ground-glass opacities surrounding dominant lesions, indicative of pulmonary hemorrhage from vascular invasion
    - Other fungal infections: Histoplasmosis, coccidioidomycosis, actinomycosis, nocardiosis, cryptococcosis

Helpful Clues for Less Common Diagnoses

- **Granulomatosis With Polyangiitis**
    - Multisystem necrotizing c-ANCA-associated granulomatous vasculitis of small to medium-sized blood vessels
    - Well-circumscribed nodules/masses ± cavitation; no zonal predilection
    - Ground-glass opacities and consolidations suggest hemorrhage
    - Intracavitary air-fluid levels suggests superimposed infection
    - Tracheal and bronchial wall thickening in 50-60% of affected patients, usually mild
    - Associated sinus and renal disease
- **Pulmonary Langerhans Cell Histiocytosis**
    - Almost exclusively smoking-related lung disease

- Upper and mid lung zone distribution, relative sparing of lung bases
- Multiple small nodules; size range from 0.1-1.0 cm, ± cavitation
  - "Cheerio sign": Nodules with central lucency
- Cysts with variable wall thickness and bizarre shapes; size range: 1.0-3.0 cm
- Cysts more common than nodules
- May be complicated by secondary spontaneous pneumothorax

- **Primary Lung Cancer**
  - Typically invasive mucinous adenocarcinoma
  - May involve single or multiple lung lobes
  - Persistent mass-like consolidation with surrounding nodules/small consolidations
  - May exhibit central lucency; so-called cheerio sign
- **Multifocal Pulmonary Lacerations**
  - Laceration of lung parenchyma following blunt or penetrating trauma
  - Areas of hemorrhage/contusion with associated laceration may exhibit cavitary nodular appearance
  - Typically identified at time of initial imaging following trauma
  - Rounded morphology of lacerations occurs due to pulmonary elastic recoil as surrounding lung tissue pulls back from laceration

Helpful Clues for Rare Diagnoses

- **Lymphoma**
  - MALToma
    - Most commonly solitary, well-defined soft tissue masses or nodules
    - Multiple unilateral or bilateral peribronchovascular nodules, ± cavitation
    - Extensive lobar consolidation with air bronchograms
  - High-grade B-cell, T-cell, and Hodgkin lymphoma
    - Consolidations, masses, nodules; ± cavitation
    - Mediastinal and hilar lymphadenopathy
  - Lymphomatoid granulomatosis
    - Small peribronchovascular nodules ± cavitation
    - Nodules often coalesce into larger nodules/masses with air bronchograms
    - Scattered thin-walled cysts
    - Interlobular septal thickening
    - Mediastinal and hilar lymphadenopathy
- **Rheumatoid Nodules**
  - Peripheral subpleural distribution
  - Single or multiple nodules; size range (0.5-5.0 cm)
  - May rarely calcify
  - May rupture into pleural space with resultant pneumothorax or empyema
  - Associated findings
    - Frequent pleural effusions ± thickening; unilateral > bilateral
    - Interstitial lung disease patterns: Usual interstitial pneumonia, nonspecific interstitial pneumonia, organizing pneumonia
    - Follicular bronchiolitis &/or constrictive bronchiolitis
    - Lower lobe predominant bronchiectasis
    - Cardiovascular: Pericardial effusion, myocarditis, pulmonary hypertension
- **Tracheobronchial Papillomatosis**
  - Airway papillomas secondary to human papilloma virus (HPV) infection
  - < 1% disseminate to lung
  - Airway and pulmonary nodules; 1-3 cm in diameter
  - Central perihilar and posterior dependent nodule distribution
  - Larger nodules more likely to cavitate; irregular thin or thick cavity walls
  - Complications: Squamous cell lung cancer, superimposed infection, atelectasis, post-obstructive pneumonia
- **Sarcoidosis**
  - Cavitary lesions are rare manifestation (< 1% of affected patients)
  - Perilymphatic nodules, masses, consolidations, ground-glass opacities
  - Symmetric mediastinal/hilar lymphadenopathy
  - Peribronchovascular mass-like fibrosis

Metastases

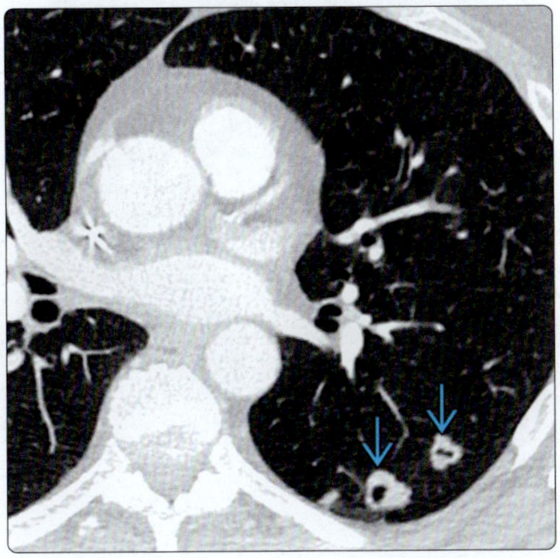

Mycobacterial Infection

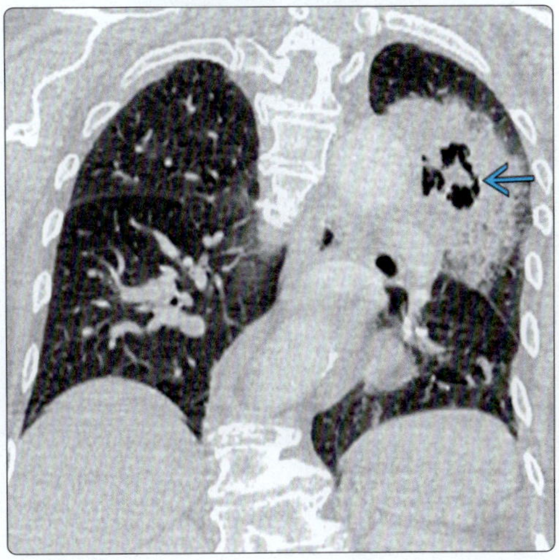

(Left) *Axial CECT of a patient with metastatic anal squamous cell carcinoma shows polylobular left lower lobe nodules with intrinsic cavitation ➡. Cavitary pulmonary metastases are characteristic of metastatic squamous cell cancers but may also occur in adenocarcinomas and sarcomas.* **(Right)** *Coronal NECT of a patient with post-primary pattern of tuberculosis shows a left upper lobe mass-like consolidation with intrinsic cavitation ➡. Tuberculosis must always be considered in patients with cavitary disease.*

(Left) *Composite image with PA chest radiograph (left) and coronal NECT (right) shows multiple left upper lobe clustered nodules and nodular consolidations, many with intrinsic cavitation secondary to multifocal Mycobacterium kansasii pulmonary infection.* **(Right)** *Axial CECT of a patient with prior pulmonary thromboembolism and pulmonary infarcts shows a right lower lobe subpleural nodule with central lucency and cavitation, consistent with evolution of prior lung infarct.*

Mycobacterial Infection

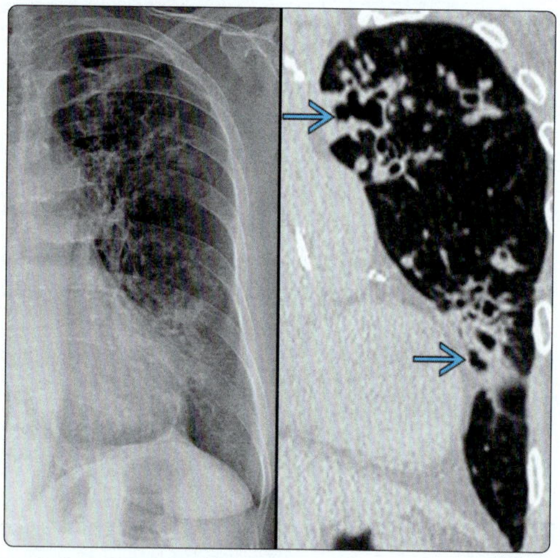

Pulmonary Infarcts

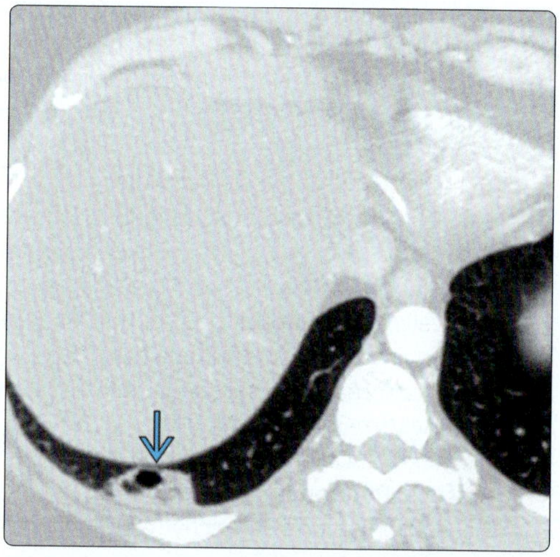

(Left) *Axial CECT of a patient with methicillin-resistant Staphylococcus aureus bacteremia secondary to intravenous drug use shows septic emboli manifesting as multifocal bilateral cavitary pulmonary nodules. Note small secondary spontaneous left pneumothorax due to rupture of a cavitary nodule into the adjacent left pleural space.* **(Right)** *Coronal CECT of an immunocompetent patient with acute histoplasmosis shows multiple small left upper lobe nodules adjacent to a dominant cavitary mass.*

Septic Emboli

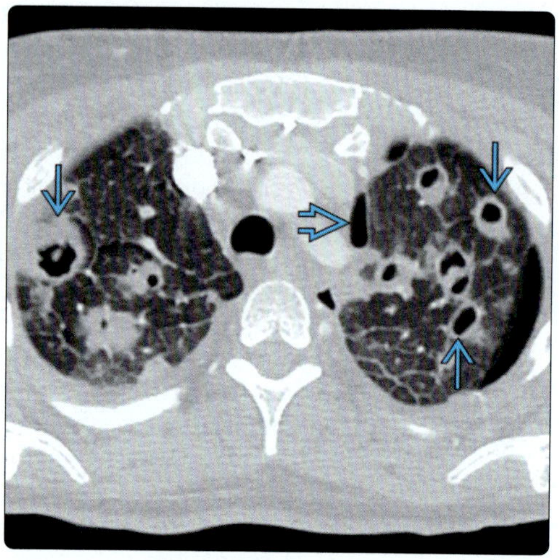

Fungal Infection

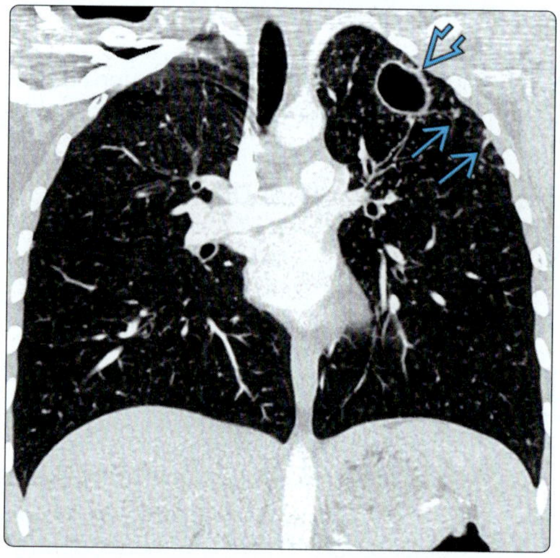

(Left) *Axial NECT of a patient with granulomatosis with polyangiitis shows a left upper lobe thick-walled cavitary nodule with surrounding ground-glass opacity secondary to hemorrhage. Note tracheal wall thickening, a characteristic ancillary finding in affected patients.* **(Right)** *Coronal NECT of a patient with pulmonary Langerhans cell histiocytosis shows multifocal mid and upper lung zone predominant small solid nodules and cystic or cavitary lesions, many with variable wall thickness and bizarre shapes.*

Granulomatosis With Polyangiitis

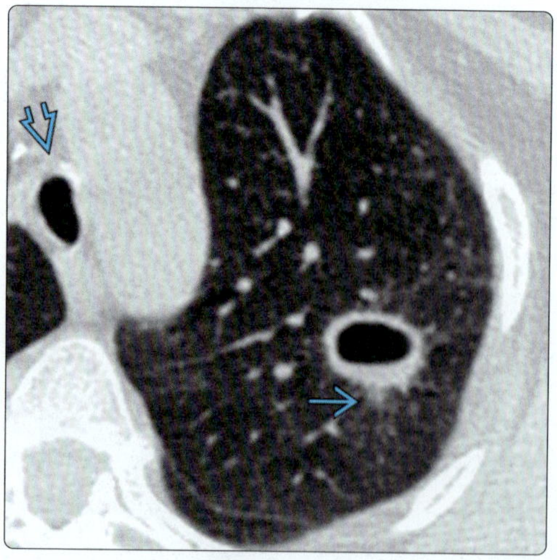

Pulmonary Langerhans Cell Histiocytosis

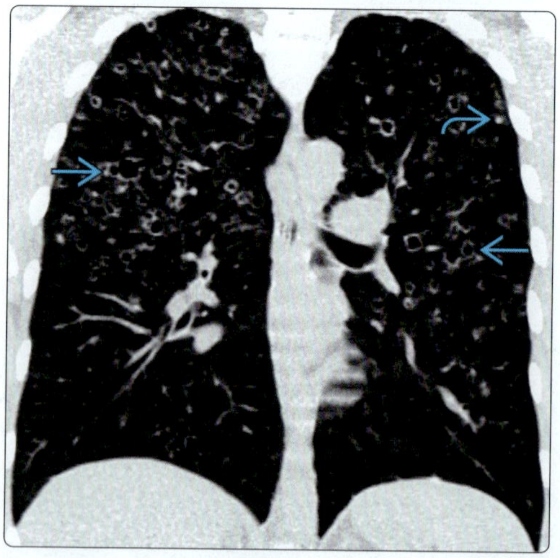

Primary Lung Cancer

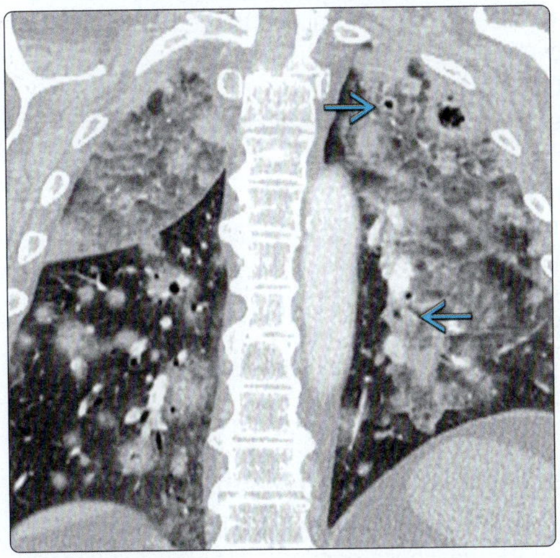

Multifocal Pulmonary Lacerations

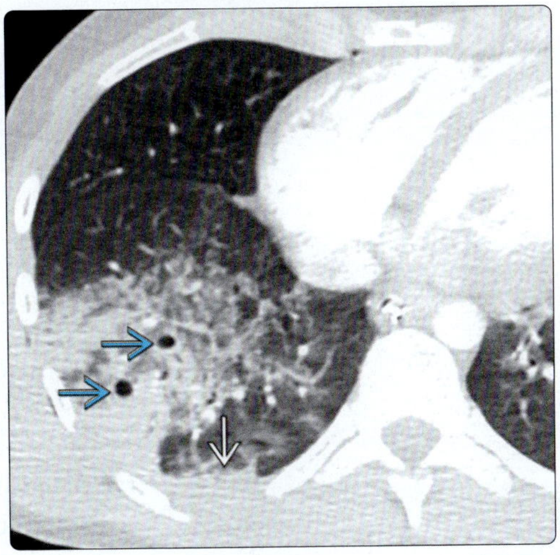

(Left) *Coronal CECT of a patient with multicentric invasive mucinous adenocarcinoma shows extensive ground-glass opacities and nodular consolidations with areas of intrinsic cavitation → that produce the so-called "Cheerio sign."* **(Right)** *Axial CECT of a patient who sustained blunt right chest trauma during a motor vehicle collision shows a right lower lobe consolidation with small intrinsic rounded lucencies → that represent pulmonary lacerations. Note small right hemothorax →.*

Lymphoma

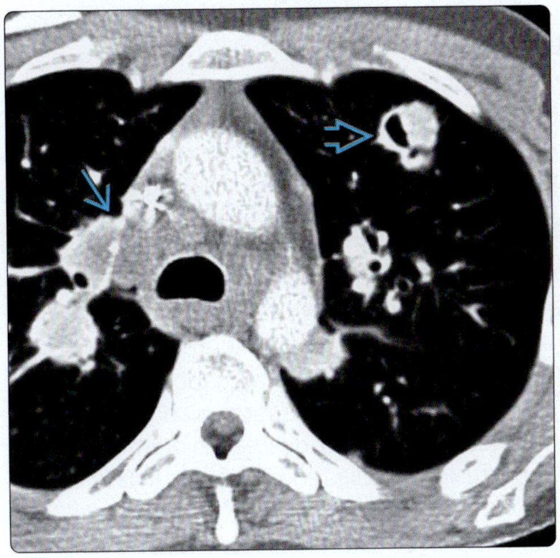

Rheumatoid Nodules

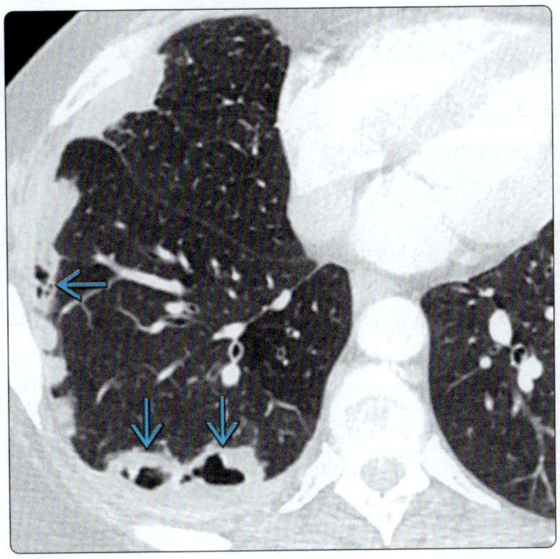

(Left) *Axial CECT of a patient with pulmonary Hodgkin lymphoma shows multifocal bilateral spiculated pulmonary nodules, some with intrinsic cavitation →. Note associated mediastinal and right hilar lymphadenopathy →.* **(Right)** *Axial CECT of a patient with pulmonary involvement by rheumatoid arthritis shows multifocal peripheral subpleural spiculated pulmonary nodules, some with intrinsic cavitation →, consistent with necrobiotic pulmonary nodules.*

Tracheobronchial Papillomatosis

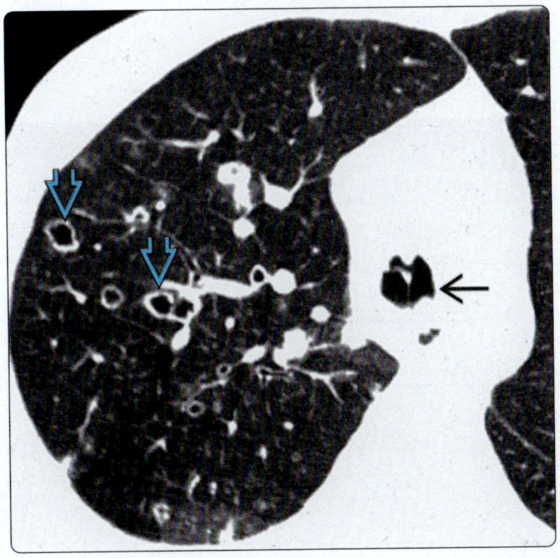

Sarcoidosis

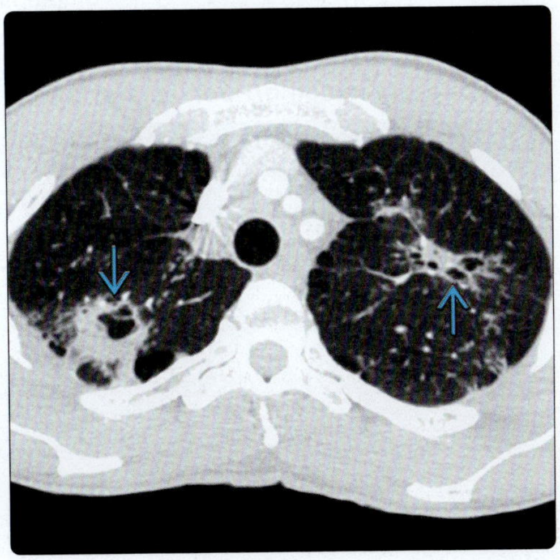

(Left) *Axial NECT of a patient with disseminated tracheobronchial papillomatosis shows multifocal cavitary pulmonary nodules →. Associated tracheal nodular mural thickening → helps suggest the correct diagnosis.* **(Right)** *Axial CECT of a patient with sarcoidosis shows multiple upper lobe peribronchovascular and perilymphatic nodules, with intrinsic cavitation →. Cavitary nodules are a rare manifestation of sarcoidosis, and other etiologies must be considered and excluded.*

Low Lung Volume

DIFFERENTIAL DIAGNOSIS

Common

- Expiratory Imaging/Poor Inspiration
- Atelectasis
- Lung Fibrosis
- Prior Surgery
- Pleural Disease
- Chest Wall Process
- Abdominal Process

Less Common

- Neuromuscular Disorder/Connective Tissue Disorder

Rare but Important

- Pulmonary Hypoplasia

ESSENTIAL INFORMATION

Key Differential Diagnosis Issues

- Inspiratory versus expiratory imaging
- Normal lungs versus fibrosis
- Assess for findings of prior surgery
- Identify pleural disease and diaphragmatic position

Helpful Clues for Common Diagnoses

- **Expiratory Imaging/Poor Inspiration**
  - Normal inspiration: Diaphragm intersected by 5th-7th anterior rib at midclavicular line
  - Expiration: Diaphragm elevation exaggerates heart size
- **Atelectasis**
  - Collapse of all or part of lung
  - Assessment of direct and indirect signs of atelectasis
- **Lung Fibrosis**
  - Idiopathic versus secondary/acquired etiologies
  - Reticulation, honeycombing, traction bronchiectasis, architectural distortion
- **Prior Surgery**
  - Surgical staple lines, surgical clips
  - Findings of lobectomy or sublobar resection
  - Chest wall surgical changes, rib resection, thoracoplasty
- **Pleural Disease**
  - Effusion, mass, pneumothorax: Relaxation atelectasis
  - Focal or diffuse (benign or malignant) pleural thickening with restrictive physiology
- **Chest Wall Process**
  - Decreased compliance with restrictive physiology
  - Kyphosis, scoliosis
  - Posttraumatic deformity
  - Congenital: Pectus excavatum and carinatum, Poland syndrome, skeletal dysplasias
  - Ankylosing spondylitis
- **Abdominal Process**
  - Obesity: Decreased chest wall compliance and restricted diaphragmatic motion
  - Ascites

Helpful Clues for Less Common Diagnoses

- **Neuromuscular Disorder/Connective Tissue Disorder**
  - Diaphragmatic weakness, paralysis, or hernia (unilateral or bilateral)
  - Myositis, muscular dystrophy
  - Myasthenia gravis
- **Shrinking Lung Syndrome**
  - Typically from systemic lupus erythematosus (SLE)
  - Also: Sjögren syndrome, scleroderma, rheumatoid arthritis, pleural disease, respiratory muscle weakness, diaphragm myopathy, phrenic nerve dysfunction

Helpful Clues for Rare Diagnoses

- **Pulmonary Hypoplasia**
  - Abnormal/incomplete lung development
  - Typically secondary causes that limit lung development
    - Intrathoracic: Congenital diaphragmatic hernia (most common), extralobar sequestration, diaphragmatic agenesis, mediastinal mass, decreased pulmonary vascular perfusion (cardiac anomalies or unilateral absence of pulmonary artery)
    - Extrathoracic: Oligohydramnios, skeletal dysplasia, abdominal mass with thoracic compression, neuromuscular conditions that affect fetal breathing
  - Idiopathic

Expiratory Imaging/Poor Inspiration

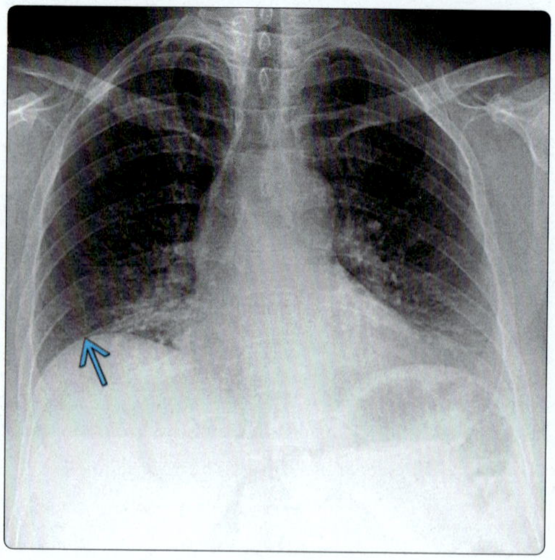

Atelectasis

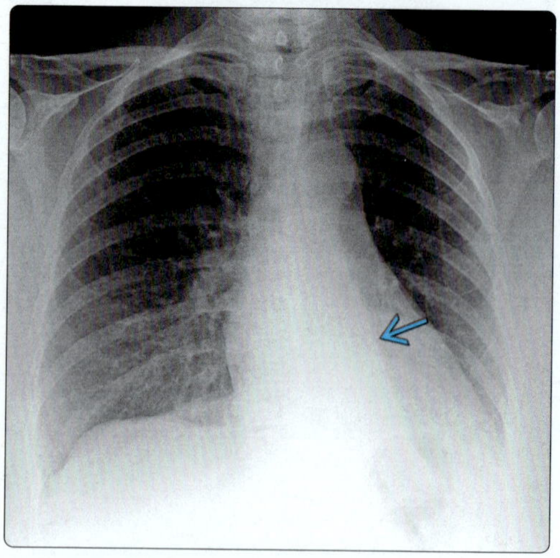

(Left) *PA chest radiograph shows low lung volume from expiratory imaging. The right hemidiaphragm intersects the right anterior 4th rib ➡. Note exaggerated heart size and basilar subsegmental atelectasis.* **(Right)** *AP chest radiograph shows low left lung volume from complete left lower lobe atelectasis that manifests with inferior displacement of the major fissure ➡. The opaque left lower lobe obliterates the left paraaortic interface and the medial left hemidiaphragm and results in inferior displacement of the left hilum.*

Lung Fibrosis

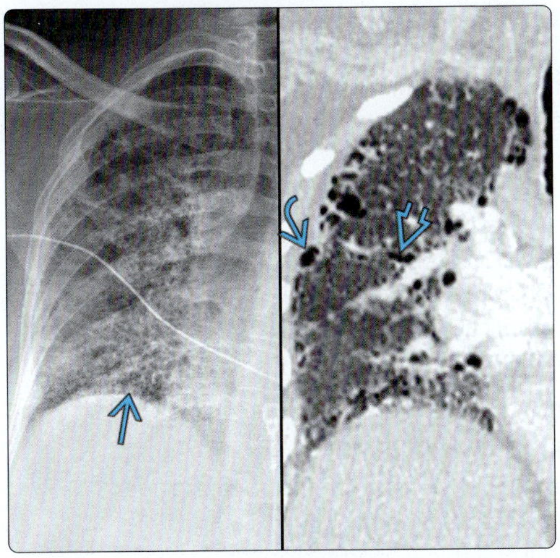

Prior Surgery

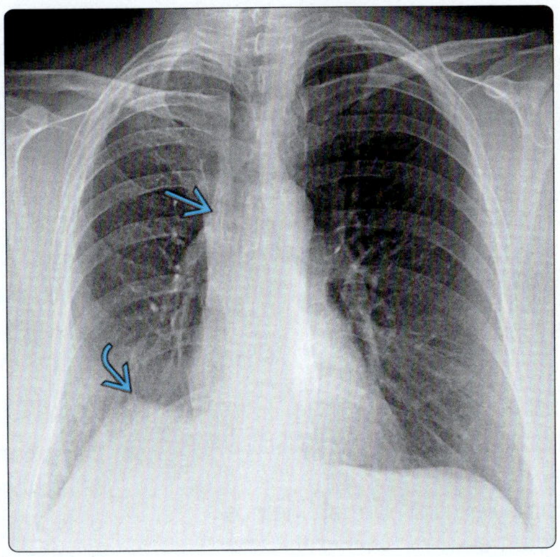

(Left) *Composite image with AP chest radiograph (left) and coronal NECT (right) of a patient with idiopathic pulmonary fibrosis shows low lung volume. Note diffuse basilar predominant reticulation, traction bronchiectasis, and subpleural honeycombing.* **(Right)** *PA chest radiograph shows low right lung volume secondary to prior right upper lobectomy. Note staple line adjacent to the right hilum and elevated right hemidiaphragm with a juxtaphrenic peak.*

Pleural Disease

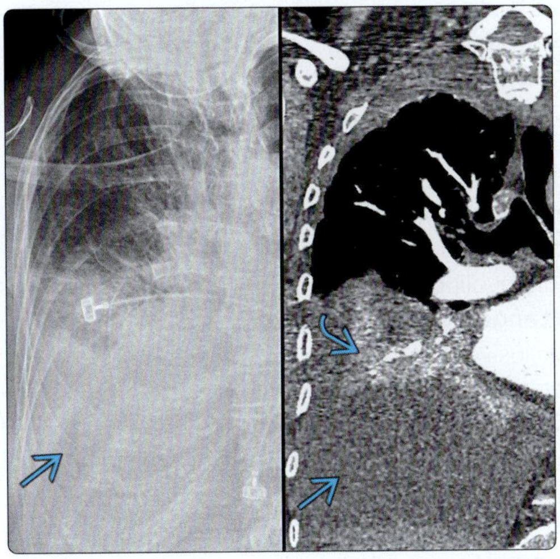

Pleural Disease

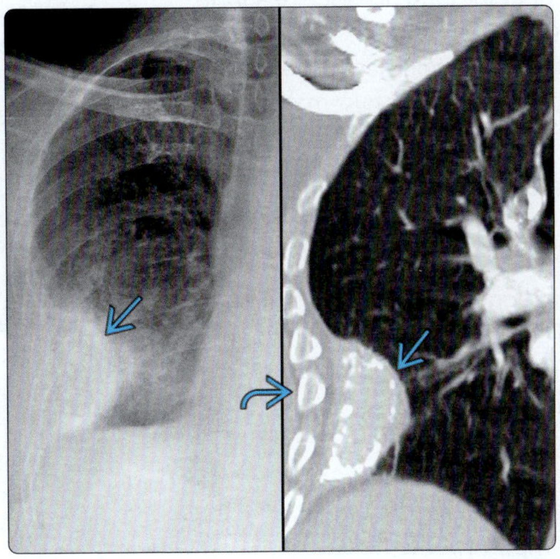

(Left) *Composite image with AP chest radiograph (left) and coronal CECT (right) demonstrates very low right lung volume secondary to a moderate right pleural effusion. Note resultant right basilar relaxation atelectasis.* **(Right)** *Composite image with PA chest radiograph (left) and coronal CECT (right) shows a calcified right basilar pleural mass secondary to fibrothorax. Note adjacent chest wall deformity and rib crowding due to retraction and restriction from adjacent fibrotic pleura.*

Chest Wall Process

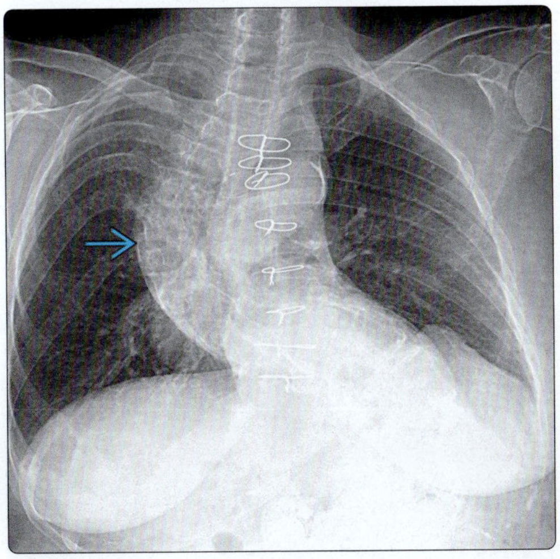

Pulmonary Hypoplasia

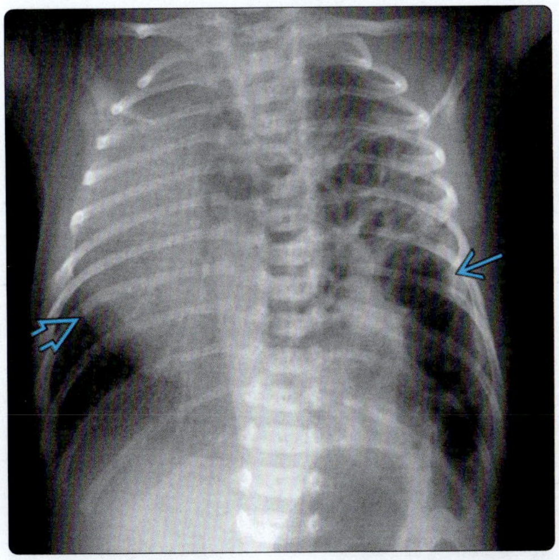

(Left) *PA chest radiograph shows bilateral low lung volume secondary to severe S-shaped thoracolumbar spine scoliosis. Chest wall deformities may produce low lung volume and restrictive lung physiology.* **(Right)** *AP chest radiograph of a newborn infant with severe respiratory distress shows very low left lung volume from pulmonary hypoplasia secondary to congenital diaphragmatic hernia. Note multiple intrathoracic gas-filled bowel loops, with mass effect on and leftward shift of the cardiothymic silhouette.*

Large Lung Volume

DIFFERENTIAL DIAGNOSIS

Common

- Emphysema
- Asthma

Less Common

- Lymphangioleiomyomatosis
- Pulmonary Langerhans Cell Histiocytosis

ESSENTIAL INFORMATION

Key Differential Diagnosis Issues

- Radiography
  - Normal lung volume on inspiration
    - Right hemidiaphragm intersected by anterior 5th-7th rib at midclavicular line
    - Young healthy subjects may exhibit normal findings that mimic large lung volume
  - May not reveal etiology of large lung volume
    - Low sensitivity for mild/moderate emphysema
    - Radiographic findings of cystic lung disease are subtle
  - Key radiographic findings
    - Pulmonary bullae (paraseptal emphysema)
    - Basilar hyperlucency (panlobular emphysema)
- CT: Optimal evaluation for etiology of large lung volume

Helpful Clues for Common Diagnoses

- **Emphysema**
  - Radiography
    - Low and flat hemidiaphragms
    - Increased retrosternal clear space
    - Blunt costophrenic angles
    - Paucity of vascular markings
  - Centrilobular
    - Smokers
    - Upper lobe predominant, may be confluent
    - Centrilobular lucency, imperceptible walls
  - Paraseptal
    - Subpleural cysts separated by interlobular septa
    - May give rise to giant bullous disease
  - Panlobular
    - Smokers with α-1-antitrypsin deficiency, IV crushed methylphenidate, HIV
    - Lower lobe predominant
    - ± bronchiectasis
- **Asthma**
  - Reversible airway obstruction, chronic inflammation of small and midsized airways
  - Bronchial wall thickening, mucus plugs, mosaic attenuation, expiratory air-trapping
  - May be complicated by spontaneous pneumomediastinum

Helpful Clues for Less Common Diagnoses

- **Lymphangioleiomyomatosis**
  - Almost exclusively women of child-bearing age
  - Normal or increased lung volume
  - Diffuse bilateral thin-walled cysts with normal intervening lung parenchyma
  - No zonal predominance
  - Associated findings
    - Patchy ground-glass opacity due to hemorrhage, multifocal micronodules
    - Interlobular septal thickening from lymphatic obstruction
  - Pneumothorax
  - Pleural effusion (chylous)
  - Lymphadenopathy
  - Renal angiomyolipomas
- **Pulmonary Langerhans Cell Histiocytosis**
  - Almost exclusively smokers; no sex predilection
  - Normal or increased lung volume
  - CT findings
    - Irregularly shaped cysts with thick &/or nodular walls
    - Centrilobular nodules with irregular margins, may cavitate and progress to cysts
    - Mid and upper lung zone predominant, spares lung bases
    - Coexistent centrilobular emphysema

Emphysema

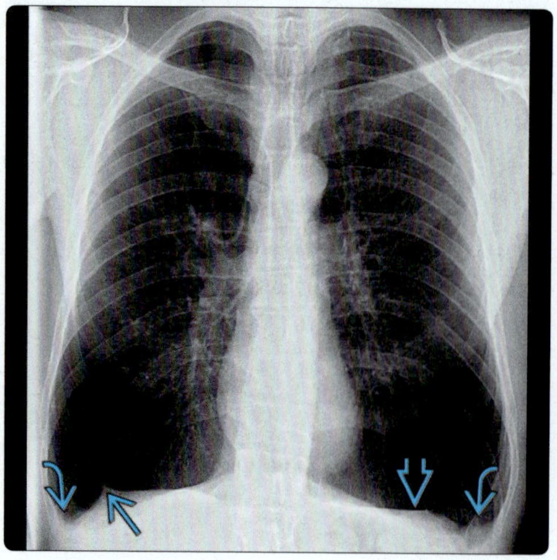

Emphysema

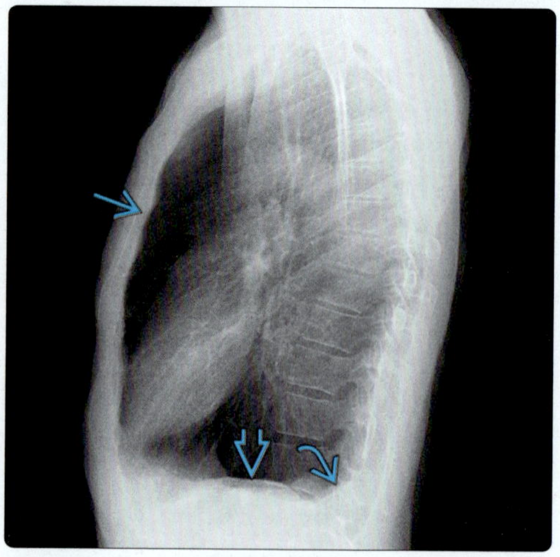

(Left) *PA chest radiograph of a patient with severe emphysema shows bilateral large lung volume, flat hemidiaphragms, blunt costophrenic angles, and paucity of peripheral pulmonary vascular markings. The right hemidiaphragm intersects the right anterior 8th rib at the midclavicular line.* **(Right)** *Lateral chest radiograph of the same patient shows an increased hyperlucent retrosternal clear space, flat bilateral hemidiaphragms, and blunt bilateral costophrenic angles.*

Emphysema

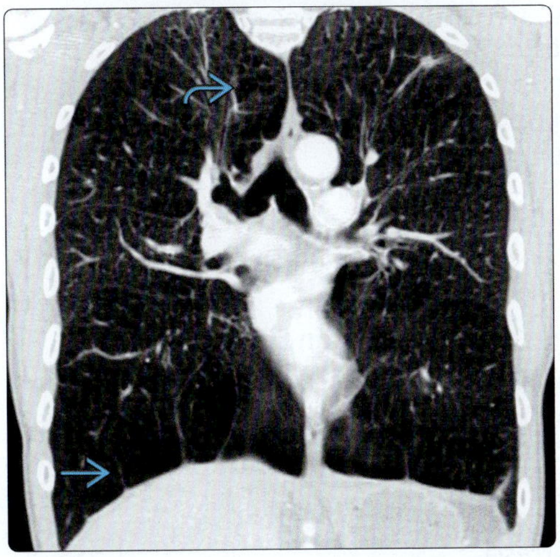

Asthma

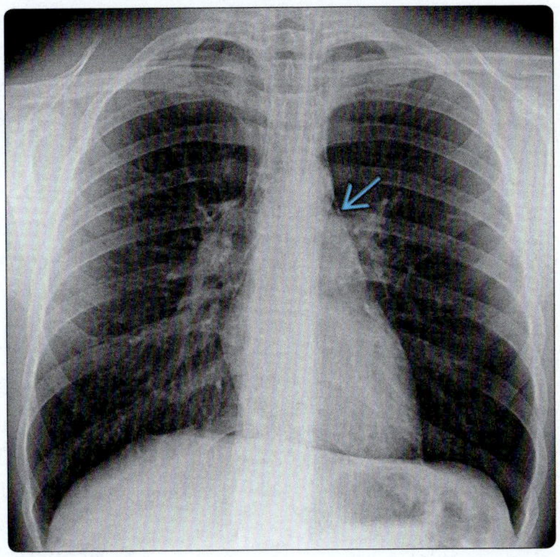

(Left) *Coronal CECT of a smoker with a-1 antitrypsin deficiency shows upper lung zone centrilobular emphysema and basilar panlobular emphysema. The former manifests as upper lung lucencies with imperceptible walls, the latter with basilar hyperlucent lung parenchyma and paucity of pulmonary vasculature.* **(Right)** *PA chest radiograph of a young patient with asthma and acute chest pain shows large lung volume and spontaneous pneumomediastinum, a complication of asthma.*

Lymphangioleiomyomatosis

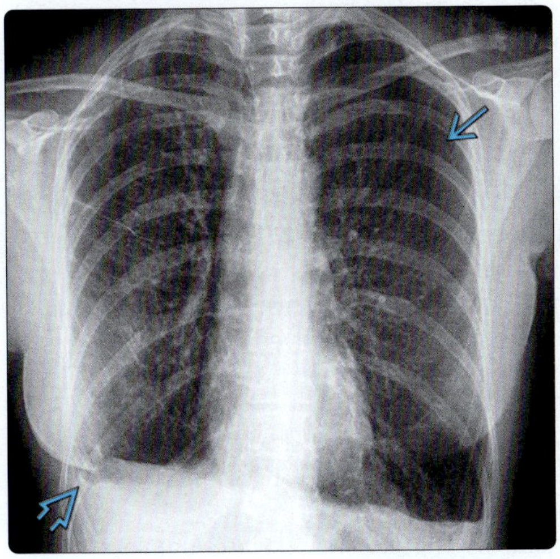

Lymphangioleiomyomatosis

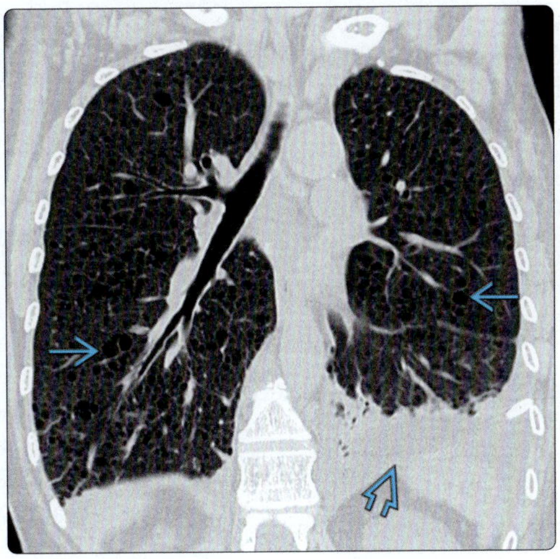

(Left) *PA chest radiograph of a woman with lymphangioleiomyomatosis who presented with dyspnea and chest pain shows large lung volume, fine linear opacities and cystic lucencies, and a left pneumothorax. Note the small right pleural effusion, which was proven to be chylous.* **(Right)** *Coronal NECT shows lymphangioleiomyomatosis manifesting with diffuse bilateral small thin-walled cysts, without apical or basilar predilection, and a small left pleural effusion, which was proven to be chylous.*

Pulmonary Langerhans Cell Histiocytosis

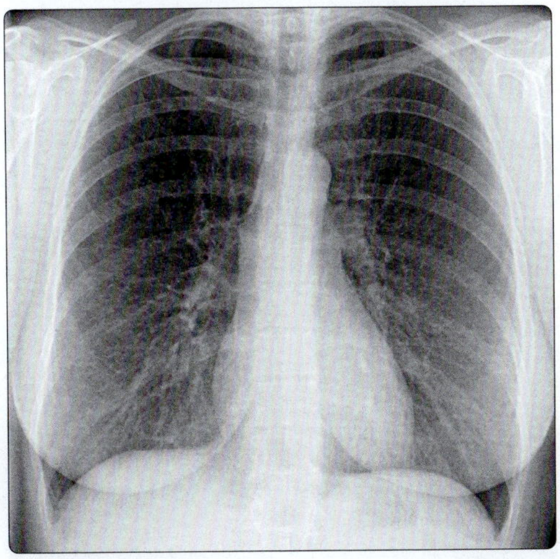

Pulmonary Langerhans Cell Histiocytosis

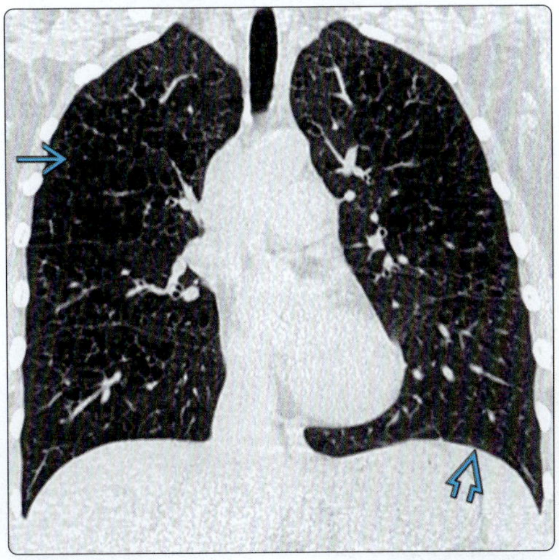

(Left) *PA chest radiograph of a smoker with pulmonary Langerhans cell histiocytosis shows normal lung volume, fine bilateral linear opacities, and the suggestion of upper lung zone predominant cystic lucencies.* **(Right)** *Coronal NECT of the same patient shows extensive bilateral thin-walled pulmonary cysts of varying shapes and sizes that exhibit an upper and mid lung zone predominance and spare the bilateral lung bases near the costophrenic angles, a characteristic finding of pulmonary Langerhans cell histiocytosis.*

DIFFERENTIAL DIAGNOSIS

Common

- Pneumothorax
- Emphysema
- Prior Surgery
  - Single Lung Transplant, Lobectomy
  - Mastectomy
- Bronchial Obstruction
- Pulmonary Thromboembolism

Less Common

- Swyer-James-McLeod Syndrome
- Bronchial Atresia

Rare but Important

- Congenital Lobar Emphysema
- Poland Syndrome

ESSENTIAL INFORMATION

Key Differential Diagnosis Issues

- Rotation may produce artifactual hyperlucency
- Unilateral airspace disease may produce artifactual hyperlucency of unaffected lung
- Assessment of whether hyperlucent lung volume increased or decreased

Helpful Clues for Common Diagnoses

- **Pneumothorax**
  - Visualization of pleural line; absence of lung markings
  - Deep sulcus sign on supine radiography
- **Emphysema**
  - ↑ lung volume; bullae, adjacent compressive atelectasis
- **Prior Surgery**
  - Single lung transplant: May be affected by constrictive bronchiolitis with air-trapping and oligemia
  - Lobectomy: Compensatory hyperexpansion of remaining ipsilateral lobe(s)
  - Mastectomy: Breast asymmetry, chest wall, &/or axillary surgical clips
- **Bronchial Obstruction**
  - Lobar atelectasis, hyperexpansion of ipsilateral lobe(s)
  - Ball-valve effect: Bronchial tumor, mucus plug, dynamic airway obstruction
    - Hyperlucency secondary to air-trapping
    - Obstructed lobe or segment may remain aerated through collateral air drift
    - Foreign body aspiration in children
- **Pulmonary Thromboembolism**
  - Westermark sign: Central embolism with peripheral oligemia

Helpful Clues for Less Common Diagnoses

- **Swyer-James-McLeod Syndrome**
  - Postinfectious; unilateral, focal, or diffuse involvement
  - Lung hyperlucency: Constructive bronchiolitis and air-trapping
    - ↓ volume of affected lung ± bronchiectasis
- **Bronchial Atresia**
  - Segmental or subsegmental lung hyperinflation (collateral air drift) distal to atretic bronchus
  - Left upper lobe typically affected
  - Mucocele (finger-in-glove sign) with surrounding hyperlucent oligemic lung
  - Mucocele may manifest as round, tubular, or branching opacity

Helpful Clues for Rare Diagnoses

- **Congenital Lobar Emphysema**
  - Typically affects neonates
  - Lobar hyperlucency and parenchymal hyperexpansion
  - Mass effect on adjacent uninvolved lung &/or mediastinum
  - Typically involves only 1 lobe
    - Frequency of involvement: Left upper lobe > middle lobe > right upper lobe
- **Poland Syndrome**
  - Hypoplasia/aplasia of pectoralis major &/or minor muscles
  - May affect 2nd-5th ribs and ipsilateral breast

Pneumothorax

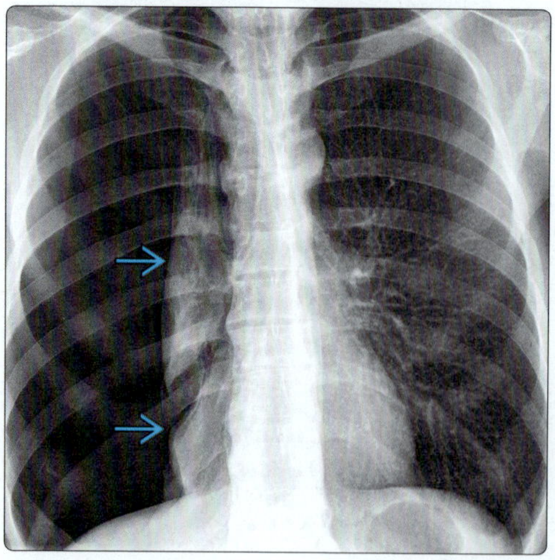

Emphysema

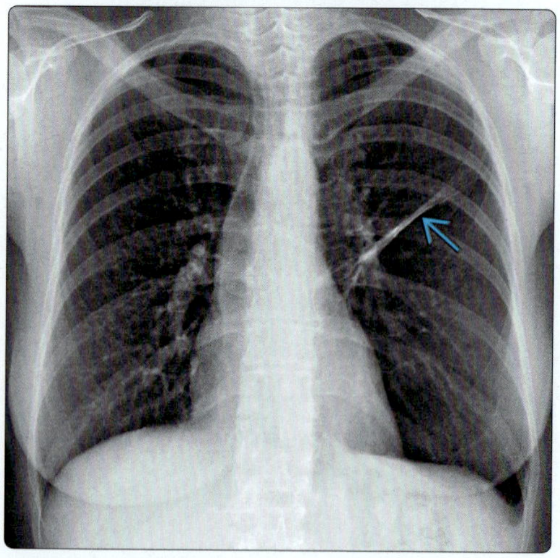

(Left) *PA chest radiograph of a young man who presented with acute onset of right chest pain shows a large right pneumothorax characterized by visualization of a pleural line* → *and absence of peripheral lung markings. Note mass effect on the mediastinum.* **(Right)** *PA chest radiograph of a patient with asymmetric bullous emphysema shows hyperlucency of the left mid and lower lung zones. Note compressive linear atelectasis* → *of the adjacent uninvolved lung and elevation of the left major fissure.*

Prior Surgery

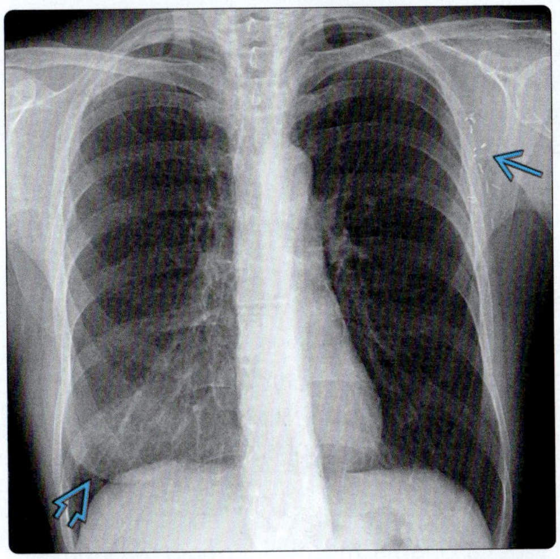

Bronchial Obstruction

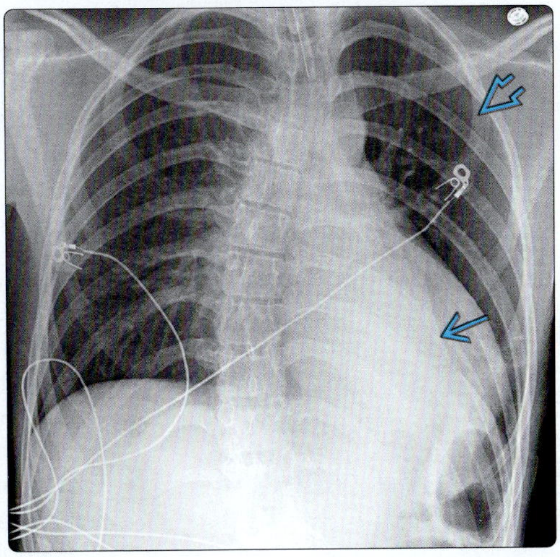

(Left) *PA chest radiograph of a patient with prior left mastectomy for breast cancer shows a hyperlucent left hemithorax. Note asymmetric visualization of the contralateral right breast tissue and left axillary surgical clips from an axillary lymph node dissection.* **(Right)** *AP supine chest radiograph of an intubated ICU patient shows complete left lower lobe atelectasis secondary to a centrally obstructing mucus plug and resultant left upper lobe hyperlucency and hyperexpansion.*

Pulmonary Thromboembolism

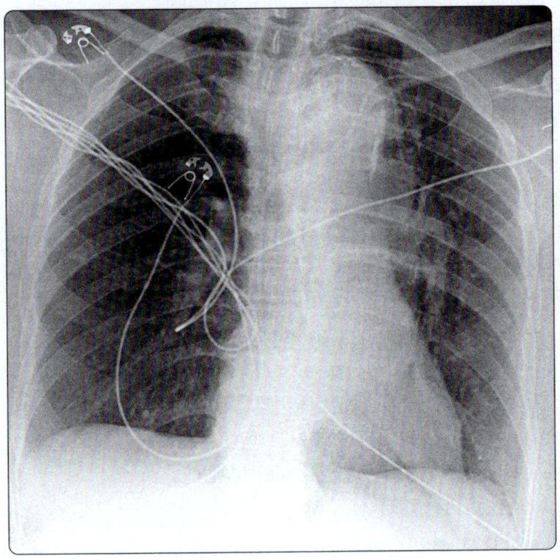

Swyer-James-McLeod Syndrome

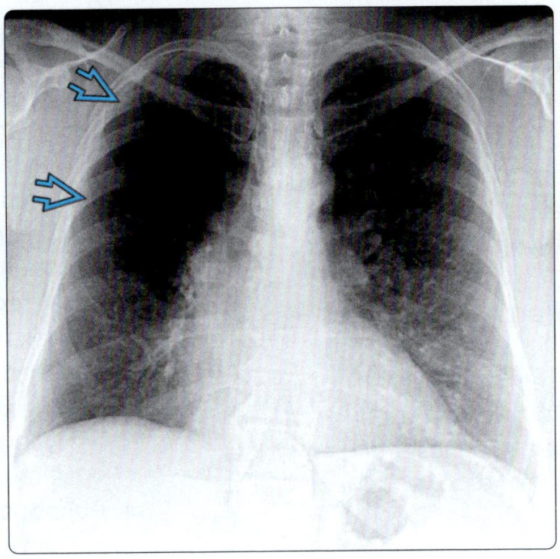

(Left) *AP chest radiograph of a patient with acute chest pain secondary to a large central right pulmonary thromboembolus shows the Westermark sign characterized by asymmetric right lung hyperlucency due to oligemia and diminutive peripheral vascular markings.* **(Right)** *PA chest radiograph of a patient with Swyer-James-McLeod syndrome secondary to childhood pulmonary infection shows low right lung volume and right upper lung zone asymmetric hyperlucency from postinfectious constrictive bronchiolitis.*

Bronchial Atresia

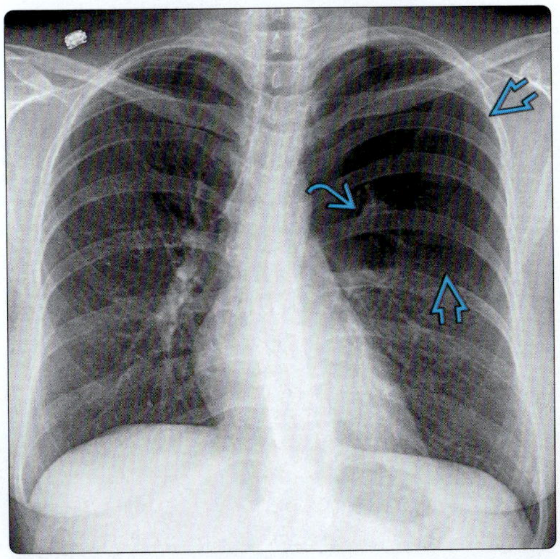

Congenital Lobar Emphysema

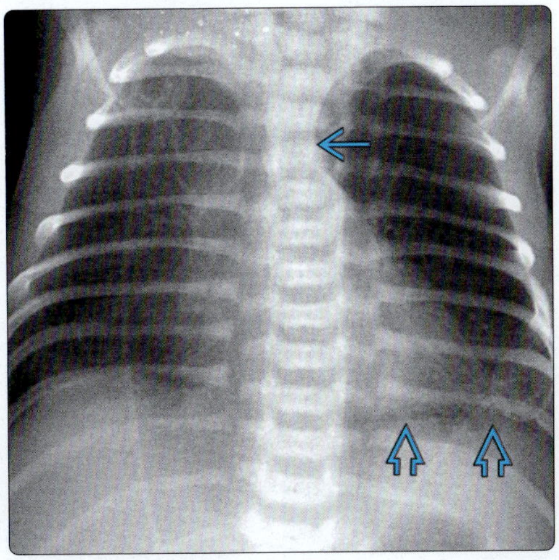

(Left) *PA chest radiograph of a patient with left upper lobe bronchial atresia shows a suprahilar tubular opacity representing a mucocele surrounded by pulmonary hyperlucency and oligemia. Although the bronchus is atretic, the surrounding lung becomes overinflated via collateral air drift.* **(Right)** *AP chest radiograph of a newborn with congenital lobar emphysema shows a hyperexpanded, hyperlucent left upper lobe with right-sided mediastinal shift and inferior displacement of the left hemidiaphragm.*

DIFFERENTIAL DIAGNOSIS

Common

- Pleural Effusion
- Pneumonectomy
- Pneumonia

Less Common

- Lung Cancer
- Endobronchial Lesion

Rare but Important

- Malignant Pleural Mesothelioma
- Localized Fibrous Tumor of Pleura
- Pulmonary Agenesis

ESSENTIAL INFORMATION

Key Differential Diagnosis Issues

- Massive pleural effusion: Increased volume of affected hemithorax, contralateral mediastinal shift
- Unilateral lung atelectasis: Decreased volume of affected hemithorax, ipsilateral mediastinal shift

Helpful Clues for Common Diagnoses

- **Pleural Effusion**
  - Massive pleural effusion
    - Malignant effusion more common than benign
    - Associated solid pleural nodules/masses on CT virtually diagnostic of malignancy
  - Empyema
    - Loculated fluid; may affect non-dependent pleural space
    - Split pleura sign: Fluid separates enhancing/high-attenuation visceral and parietal pleura
    - Gas in pleural space nearly diagnostic of bronchopleural fistula, in absence of prior pleural intervention
  - Hemothorax
    - Traumatic, iatrogenic, spontaneous
    - Hematocrit effect: High-attenuation fluid (> 50 HU)
- **Pneumonectomy**
  - Pneumonectomy space fills with fluid within 30 days
    - Persistent or increasing gas in pneumonectomy space should suggest infection or bronchial connection
    - Decreased volume of affected hemithorax, ipsilateral mediastinal shift
- **Pneumonia**
  - Extensive consolidation involving one or multiple lobes
  - Parapneumonic pleural effusion may be complicated by empyema

Helpful Clues for Less Common Diagnoses

- **Lung Cancer**
  - Mainstem bronchus compression/obstruction from surrounding mass or endoluminal lesion
  - Frequent mediastinal/hilar lymphadenopathy
- **Endobronchial Neoplasm**
  - Centrally obstructing neoplasm (lung cancer, carcinoid, adenoid cystic carcinoma, mucoepidermoid carcinoma, metastasis), mucus, broncholith, or foreign body
  - Lobar collapse more common than total lung collapse
  - Typically ipsilateral mediastinal shift, unless postobstructive pneumonia develops

Helpful Clues for Rare Diagnoses

- **Malignant Pleural Mesothelioma**
  - History of asbestos exposure
  - Circumferential nodular pleural thickening
  - May decrease or increase volume of affected hemithorax depending on size and extent of mass
- **Localized Fibrous Tumor of Pleura**
  - Typically benign; ~ 20% are malignant
  - Variable size; large tumors may occupy hemithorax
  - Rare association with paraneoplastic syndromes: Hypoglycemia, clubbing
  - Heterogeneous attenuation, ± calcification, necrosis
- **Pulmonary Agenesis**
  - Complete unilateral absence of one lung
  - Often associated with other congenital anomalies

Pleural Effusion

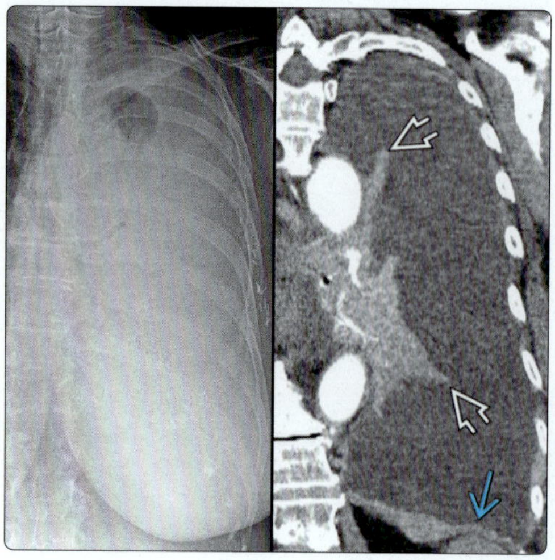

Pleural Effusion

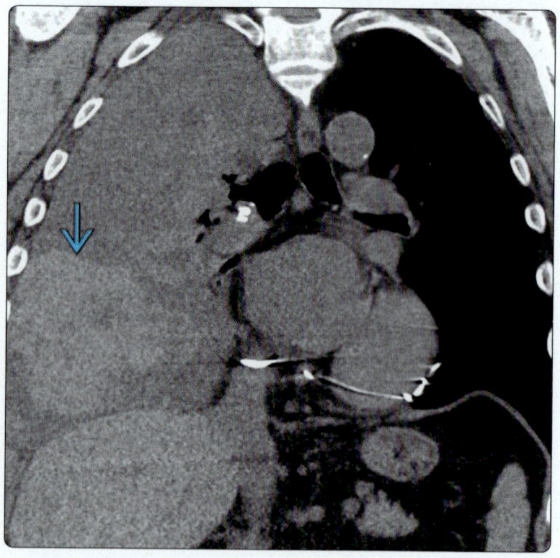

(Left) *Composite image with PA chest radiograph (left) and coronal CECT (right) shows an opaque left hemithorax with contralateral mediastinal shift due to a massive malignant pleural effusion from metastatic breast cancer. Note small solid pleural metastases ⇨ and left lung relaxation atelectasis ➡.* **(Right)** *Coronal NECT shows an opaque right hemithorax secondary to a large hemothorax caused by cardiac perforation by a pacemaker lead. High-attenuation content ⇨ in the right pleural space is diagnostic of hemothorax.*

Pneumonectomy

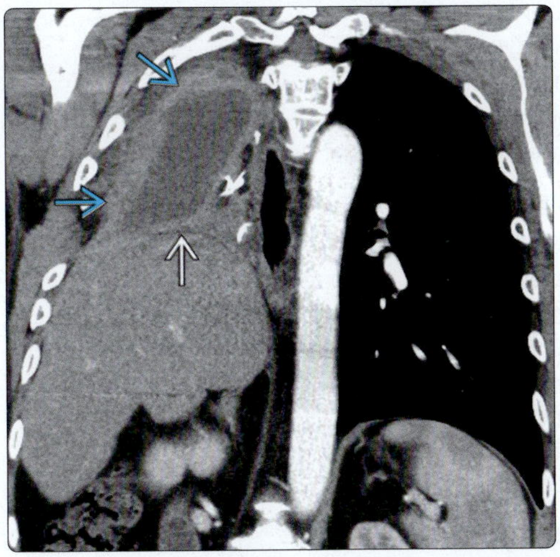

Pneumonia

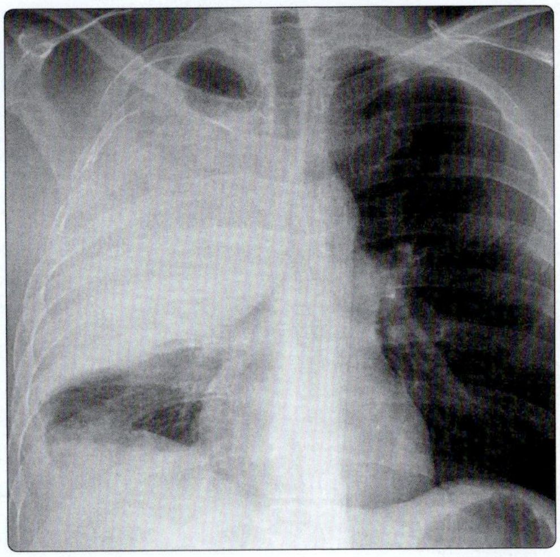

(Left) *Coronal CECT of a patient with an opaque right hemithorax on radiography (not shown) secondary to prior pneumonectomy shows a small right hemithorax, an elevated right hemidiaphragm, and fluid and soft tissue filling the right pneumonectomy space.* **(Right)** *PA chest radiograph of a patient with cough, fever, and leukocytosis shows a nearly opaque right hemithorax secondary to a large right upper lobe consolidation with lobar expansion and bulging fissures, consistent with Klebsiella pneumonia.*

Lung Cancer

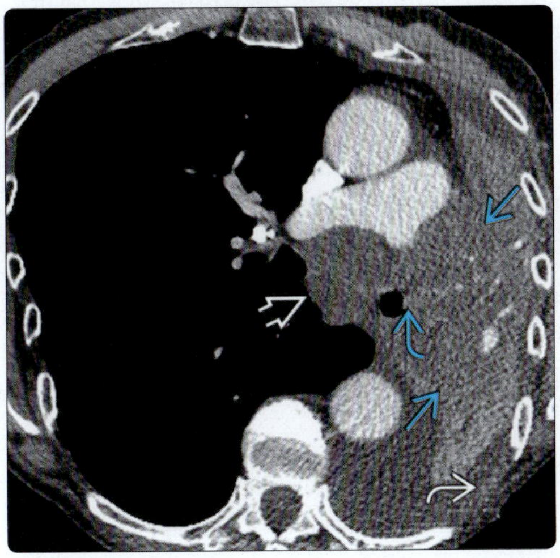

Endobronchial Lesion

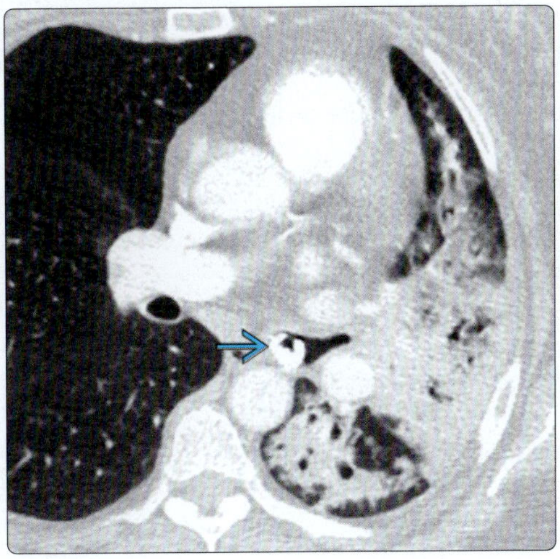

(Left) *Axial CECT shows a large centrally obstructing hypoenhancing left hilar mass with an endobronchial component that results in left lung post-obstructive atelectasis/pneumonia. Note metastatic subcarinal lymphadenopathy and a left malignant pleural effusion with solid pleural metastases.* **(Right)** *Axial CECT shows left lung post-obstructive pneumonia manifesting as an extensive left lung consolidation secondary to a centrally obstructing calcified broncholith in the left mainstem bronchus.*

Malignant Pleural Mesothelioma

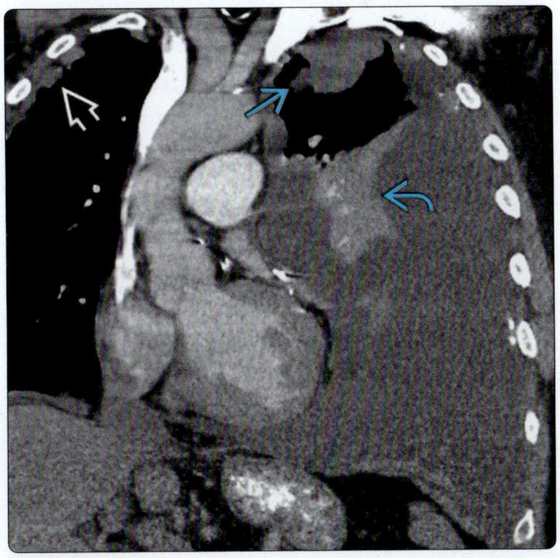

Localized Fibrous Tumor of Pleura

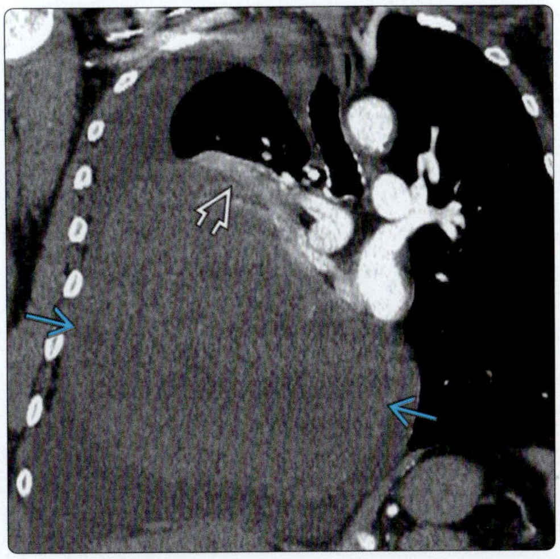

(Left) *Coronal CECT of a patient with malignant pleural mesothelioma shows a large left pleural effusion and 1 of several left pleural masses. Note near-complete left lung atelectasis, contralateral mediastinal shift, and contralateral pleural plaques from asbestos-related pleural disease.* **(Right)** *Coronal CECT shows a large right localized fibrous tumor of the pleura and a moderate ipsilateral right pleural effusion that result in middle and right lower lobe atelectasis and a nearly opaque right hemithorax.*

Luftsichel Sign

DIFFERENTIAL DIAGNOSIS

Common

- Central Obstructing Lesion

Less Common

- Endobronchial Plug

Rare but Important

- Bronchial Stenosis
- Mimics

ESSENTIAL INFORMATION

Key Differential Diagnosis Issues

- Luftsichel sign described in left upper lobe atelectasis
  - Luftsichel = air sickle
  - Crescentic lucency between mediastinum (aortic arch) and atelectatic left upper lobe, formed by hyperinflation of left lower lobe superior segment
    - Superior/anterior migration of atelectatic upper lobe
      - Anterior displacement of left major fissure on lateral chest radiography
    - Upward migration of hyperinflated left lower lobe superior segment
    - Anterior displacement of left major fissure on lateral chest radiography
    - ± juxtaphrenic peak sign or tenting/peaking of ipsilateral hemidiaphragm from upper lobe volume loss
  - Characteristically seen in left upper lobe atelectasis
    - Minor fissure prevents anteromedial displacement of major fissure in right upper lobe atelectasis
- Presence of luftsichel sign demands further evaluation with CT &/or bronchoscopy
- Absence of luftsichel sign does not exclude left upper lobe atelectasis

Helpful Clues for Common Diagnoses

- **Central Obstructing Lesion**
  - Lung cancer, carcinoid, metastasis
  - Extrinsic bronchial compression by lymphadenopathy
    - Small cell lung cancer
    - Lymphoma
    - Reactive lymphadenopathy
  - Benign neoplasms
    - Hamartoma, lipoma
      - May exhibit fat attenuation

Helpful Clues for Less Common Diagnoses

- **Endobronchial Plug**
  - Usually hospitalized or postoperative patients
  - Acute upper lobe collapse in patient with recently normal chest radiograph or associated with pneumonia
    - CT: Low-attenuation endoluminal content
    - ± intrinsic gas bubbles
  - Bedside bronchoscopy is both diagnostic and therapeutic

Helpful Clues for Rare Diagnoses

- **Bronchial Stenosis**
  - Most commonly secondary to *Mycobacterium tuberculosis*
    - Affects posterior walls of trachea and major bronchi
    - Necrosis and ulceration of bronchial mucosa → granulation tissue → scarring
      - May occur in active or treated tuberculosis
  - Other organisms: *Aspergillus fumigatus, Coccidioides immitis, Histoplasma capsulatum*, Mucormycosis
  - Other: Bronchial anthracosis, broncholithiasis
- **Mimics**
  - Nonobstructive pulmonary abnormalities may also mimic luftsichel sign
    - Right lung herniation
    - Pneumomediastinum
    - Left upper lobectomy

SELECTED REFERENCES

1. Day K et al: Signs in cardiopulmonary imaging: luftsichel sign. J Thorac Imaging. 30(3):W1, 2015

(Left) *PA chest radiograph of a 67-year-old woman shows left upper lobe atelectasis manifesting with the luftsichel sign. The left para-aortic hyperlucency represents the hyperinflated left upper lobe superior segment.* **(Right)** *Lateral chest radiograph of the same patient shows anterior displacement of the left major fissure due to left upper lobe atelectasis. Bronchoscopy and biopsy demonstrated squamous cell carcinoma. The luftsichel sign should suggest a centrally obstructing lesion.*

Central Obstructing Lesion

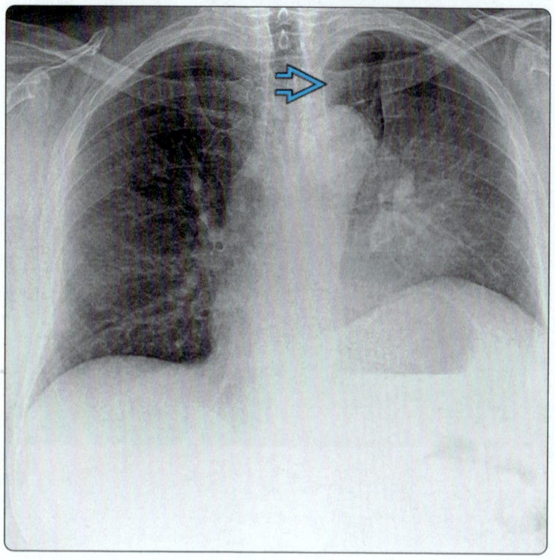

Central Obstructing Lesion

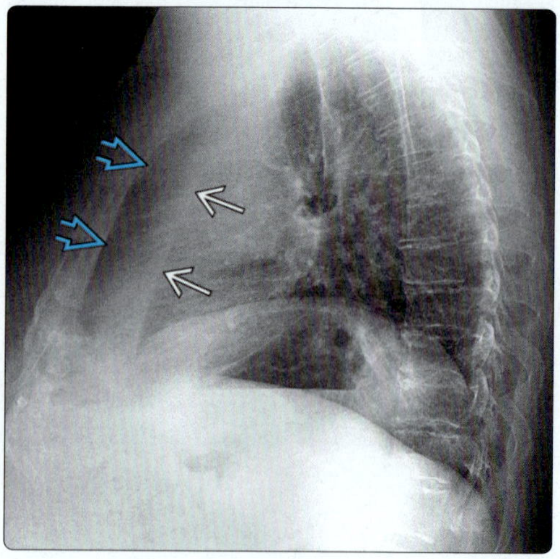

Central Obstructing Lesion

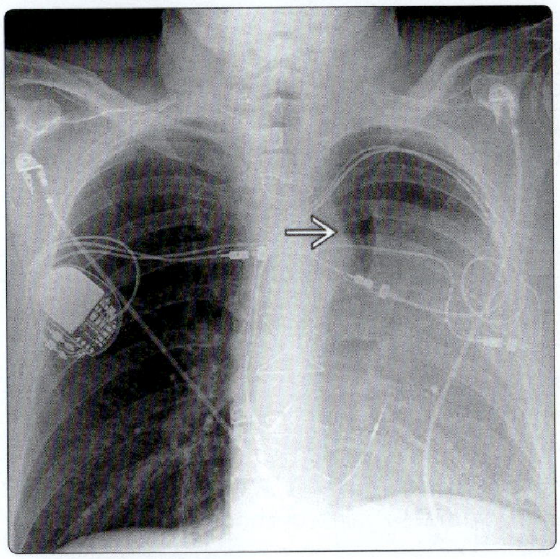

Central Obstructing Lesion

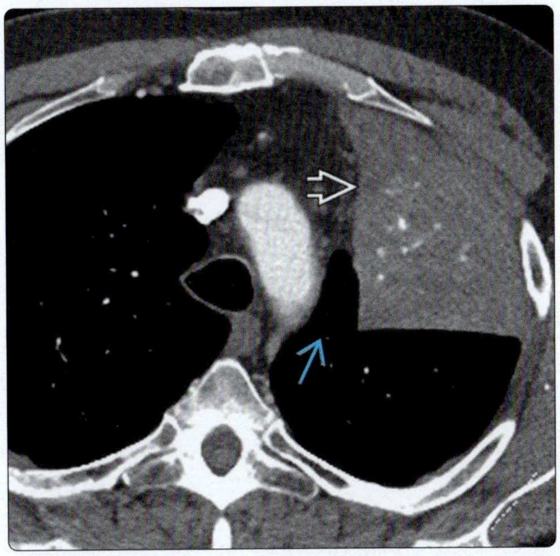

(Left) *AP chest radiograph of a 77-year-old man shows left upper lobe atelectasis manifesting with the luftsichel sign* ➔. **(Right)** *Axial CECT of the same patient shows post-obstructive atelectasis of the left upper lobe* ➔. *Note that the hyperinflated left upper lobe superior segment* ⇨ *migrates upward between the aortic arch and the atelectatic left upper lobe. Visualization of the luftsichel sign should prompt further assessment for exclusion of an endobronchial lesion, in this case, a squamous cell carcinoma.*

Bronchial Stenosis

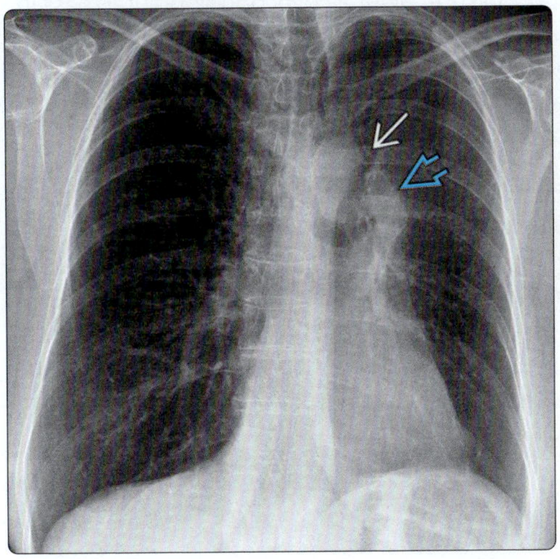

Bronchial Stenosis

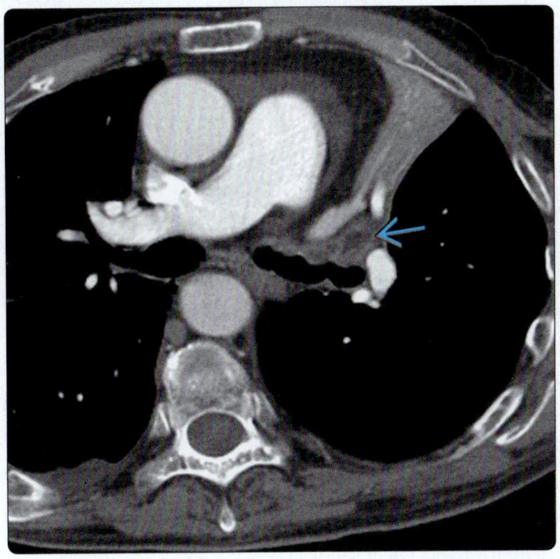

(Left) *PA chest radiograph of a patient with chronic leukemia shows left upper lobe atelectasis manifesting with the luftsichel sign* ➔. *Note the elevated left hilum* ⇨. **(Right)** *Axial CECT of the same patient shows low-attenuation content in the lumen of the left upper lobe bronchus* ⇨. *Bronchoalveolar lavage and culture demonstrated aspergillus. In addition to neoplasms, endobronchial plugs may produce lobar collapse, including infections and mucus plugs.*

Mimics

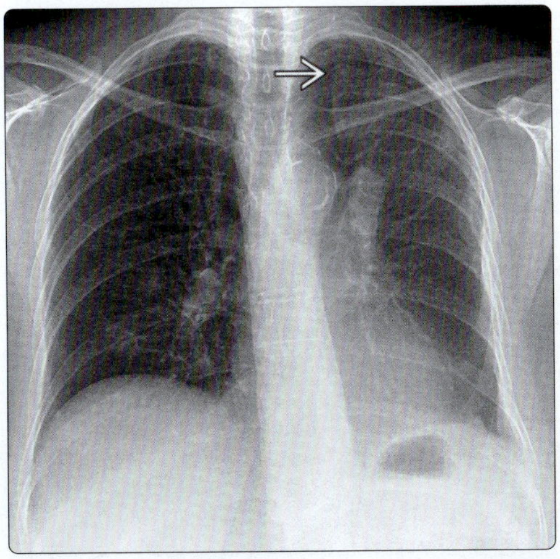

Mimics

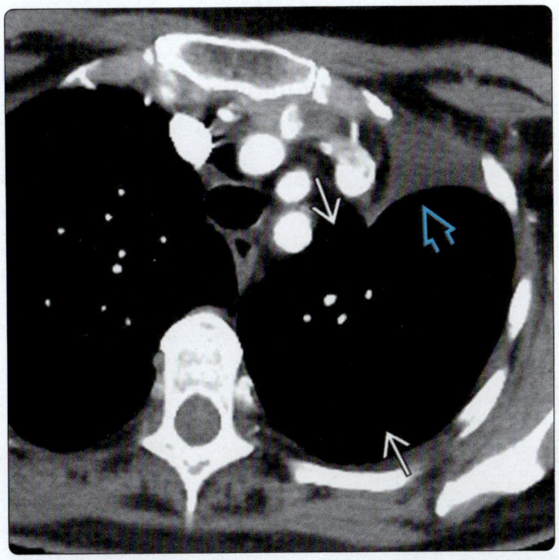

(Left) *PA chest radiograph of a patient with prior left upper lobectomy shows mildly increased density in the left upper hemithorax* ➔ *representing a loculated pleural effusion, which may mimic left upper lobe atelectasis. Left lower lobe hyperinflation compensates for the surgically absent left upper lobe.* **(Right)** *Axial CECT of the same patient confirms a small postsurgical loculated left pleural effusion* ⇨ *and a hyperinflated left lower lobe, which now occupies the entire left hemithorax* ➔.

DIFFERENTIAL DIAGNOSIS

Common

- Pneumonia
- Atelectasis
- Pleural Disease

Less Common

- Intrapulmonary Mass
- Mediastinal Mass
  - Lymphoma
  - Germ Cell Tumor
  - Thymic Epithelial Neoplasms
  - Morgagni Hernia

ESSENTIAL INFORMATION

Key Differential Diagnosis Issues

- Two structures in direct contact and of similar density cannot be distinguished from one another on radiography
  - Intrathoracic lesion anatomically contiguous with border of heart, aorta or diaphragm will obliterate that border
  - Loss of anatomic borders = "silhouette sign"
- Presence or absence of silhouette sign helps to localize lesion
- PA chest radiograph: Silhouette sign
  - Loss of right heart border: Middle lobe (medial segment)
  - Left heart border: Lingula (inferior segment)
  - Diaphragm: Lower lobes (basal segments), pleural effusion
  - Ascending aorta: Anterior segment of right upper lobe, right anterior mediastinum
  - Descending aorta: Left lower lobe (superior segment)
  - Aortic arch: Left upper lobe (apicoposterior segment)
- Lateral chest radiograph: Silhouette sign
  - Right hemidiaphragm: Right lower lobe (basal segments)
  - Left hemidiaphragm: Left lower lobe (basal segments)
- Silhouette sign can be used only if chest radiograph is technically adequate
- Pectus excavatum
  - Important mimic of silhouette sign
  - Congenital abnormality with abnormal appearance of ribs and sternum
  - Most are asymptomatic; male:female ratio 3:1
  - Depressed sternum leads to rotation of heart with loss air interface of adjacent lung
    - PA chest radiograph: Loss of right border of heart, leftward displacement of heart and apparent cardiomegaly
    - Lateral chest radiograph: Concave deformity of sternum

Helpful Clues for Common Diagnoses

- **Pneumonia**
  - Radiograph: Opacification + air bronchogram without volume loss
- **Atelectasis**
  - Radiograph: Volume loss, air bronchogram can be present
- **Pleural Disease**
  - Pleural effusion, empyema, pleural mass: Fluid in lower end of major fissure, pleural collection or pleural mass in anterior aspect of pleural space obliterates right or left border of heart
  - Radiography: Homogeneous increase in density, absence of air bronchogram

Helpful Clues for Less Common Diagnoses

- **Intrapulmonary Mass**
  - Primary lung malignancy, metastasis
- **Mediastinal Mass**
  - Anterior mediastinal mass: Increased mediastinal fat, Morgagni hernia, thymoma, lymphoma, germ cell tumor
    - Obliterates right or left border of heart &/or ascending aorta

Pneumonia

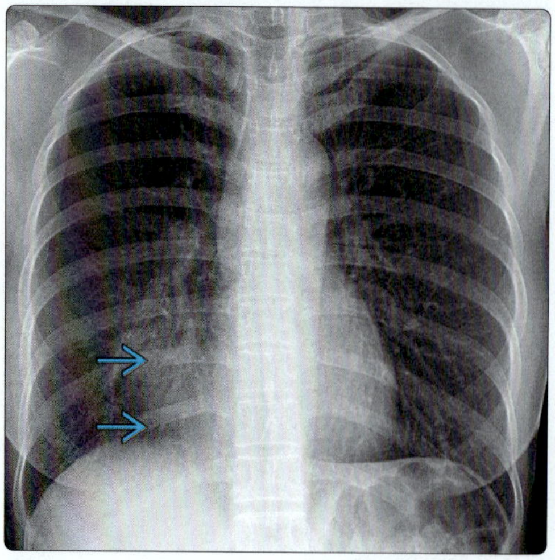

Pneumonia

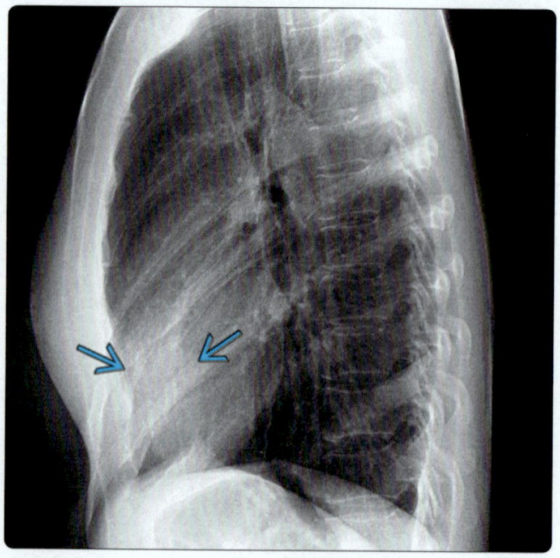

(Left) *PA chest radiograph of a 34-year-old woman with cough and fever shows an opacity along the right border of the heart ➔ representing middle lobe pneumonia obliterating the right border of the heart.* **(Right)** *Lateral chest radiograph of the same patient demonstrates the presence of middle lobe opacity consistent with pneumonia ➔. In order to have a silhouette sign, two structures must be in direct contact and share similar density.*

Atelectasis

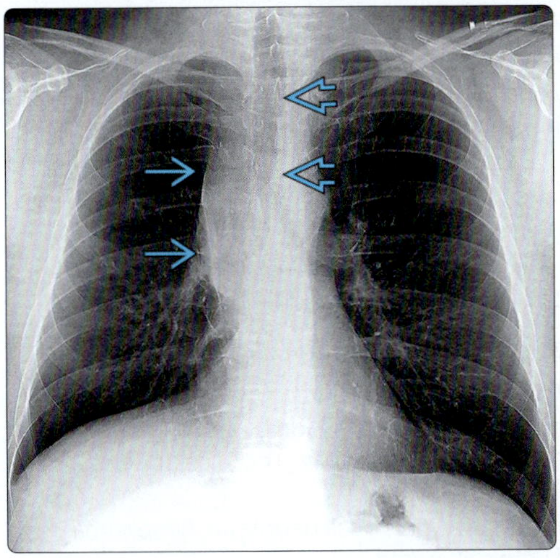

Atelectasis

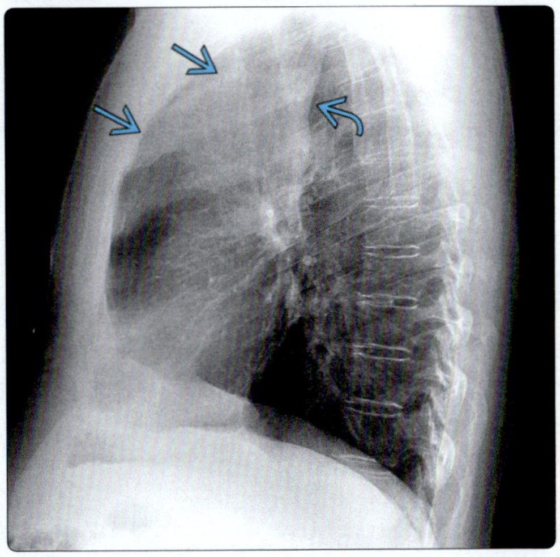

(Left) *PA chest radiograph of a 62-year-old man with squamous cell carcinoma shows an opacity in the right lung causing loss of the contour of the ascending aorta. There is displacement of the trachea to the right, consistent with volume loss.* **(Right)** *Lateral radiograph of the same patient shows right upper lobe atelectasis. The ascending aorta is not visible secondary to disease in the right upper lobe parenchyma contiguous with the aorta. Note anterior and superior displacement of the oblique fissure.*

Mediastinal Mass

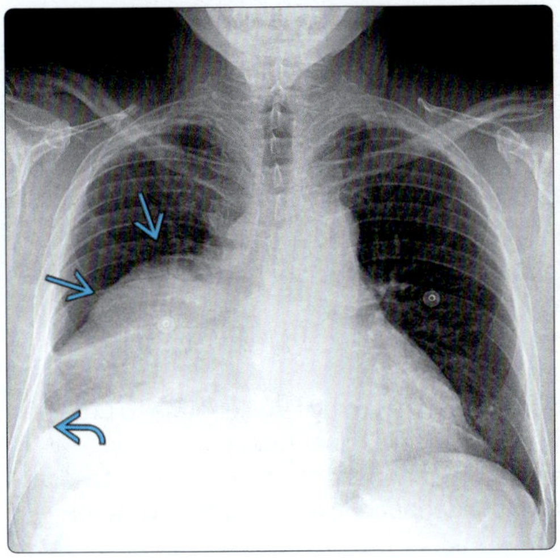

Mediastinal Mass

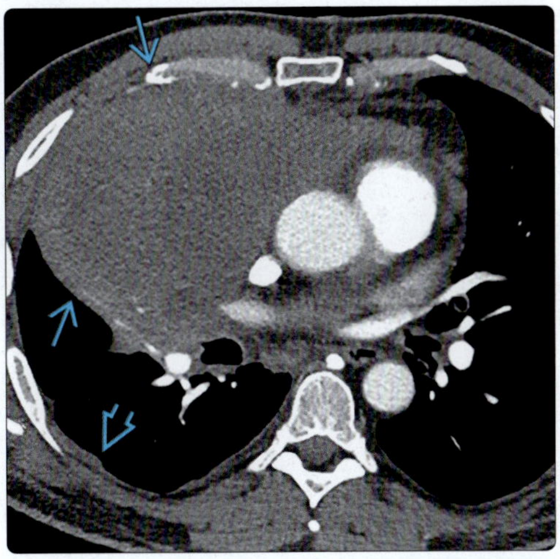

(Left) *PA chest radiograph of a 63-year-old woman with anterior mediastinal lymphoma shows dense homogeneous opacity in the right lower hemithorax with obscuration of the right heart border indicating that the lesion lies anteriorly. A small right pleural effusion is also noted.* **(Right)** *Axial CECT of the same patient shows a prevascular mediastinal mass. Note the presence of loculated ipsilateral effusion. The presence of the silhouette sign can be due to intrapulmonary, mediastinal, pleural or chest wall disease.*

Mediastinal Mass

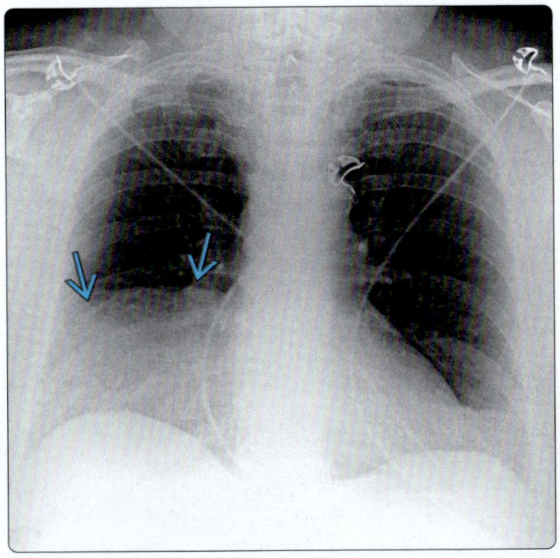

Mediastinal Mass

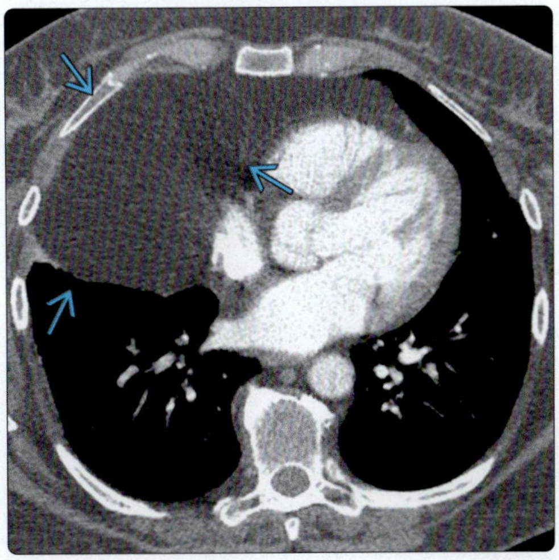

(Left) *Frontal chest radiograph of a young woman with Morgagni's hernia shows right basilar homogeneous opacity, which obscures the right heart border simulating a middle lobe pneumonia. Note the right hemidiaphragm is well identified, which indicates this abnormality is not located in the basilar region of the hemithorax.* **(Right)** *Axial CECT of the same patient shows a large fat attenuation mass occupying the right pericardiophrenic angle, consistent with large fat containing Morgagni's hernia.*

DIFFERENTIAL DIAGNOSIS

Common

- Lung Cancer

Less Common

- Mediastinal Malignancy

Rare but Important

- Endobronchial Metastasis

ESSENTIAL INFORMATION

Key Differential Diagnosis Issues

- S-sign of Golden indicates that lobar atelectasis is secondary to centrally obstructing mass
  - Typically described in right upper lobe collapse
  - Recognizable both on radiography and CT
- Frontal chest radiograph: Upper lung zone triangular opacity represents atelectatic lobe
  - Minor and major fissures migrate superiorly and medially toward mediastinum
    - Central mass produces convexity; prevents central lung from collapsing completely
      - Medial minor fissure outlines inferior margin of mass
      - Lateral minor fissure migrates superiorly and medially
- Lateral chest radiograph: Upward displacement of major and minor fissures
  - Ascending aorta obscured by atelectatic lobe
- Mimics: Mediastinal mass, right upper lobe mass
  - Additional signs of volume loss
    - Elevated right hilum, angulation of right mainstem and lower lobe bronchi
    - Juxtaphrenic peak
  - Hyperinflation of middle and lower lobes with resultant increased translucency of mid and lower lung
- Atelectasis may be due to bronchial stricture or mucus plug, but margin of atelectatic lung is straight
- FDG PET/CT: FDG avidity of central mass

Helpful Clues for Common Diagnoses

- **Lung Cancer**
  - Most common cause of right upper lobe atelectasis in adults
  - Centrally obstructing neoplasm with resultant atelectasis and retained endobronchial secretions
  - CT
    - NECT and CECT: Identification of central obstructive mass or irregular stenosis
    - Mucus-filled dilated bronchi within atelectatic lung
    - Hilar &/or mediastinal lymphadenopathy

Helpful Clues for Less Common Diagnoses

- **Mediastinal Malignancy**
  - Airway involvement/compression by large mediastinal tumor or lymphadenopathy may produce upper lobe collapse
  - Thymic malignancy, germ cell neoplasm, lymphoma, small cell lung carcinoma
  - CT
    - Prevascular or visceral mediastinal mass/lymphadenopathy: Compression &/or displacement of vessels and airways
    - Extrinsic compression of right upper lobe or right mainstem bronchi
    - Endobronchial involvement by primary malignancy

Helpful Clues for Rare Diagnoses

- **Endobronchial Metastases**
  - Unlike pulmonary metastases, endobronchial metastases are unusual
  - Most common primaries: Renal, breast, and colon cancers, melanoma
  - Endobronchial lesion has to be large enough to produce focal convexity of medial minor fissure
  - CECT: Identification of endobronchial mass, mediastinal &/or hilar lymphadenopathy, pulmonary metastases

SELECTED REFERENCES

1. Potdar PV et al: The Golden S sign. J Assoc Physicians India. 63(8):68, 2015

Lung Cancer

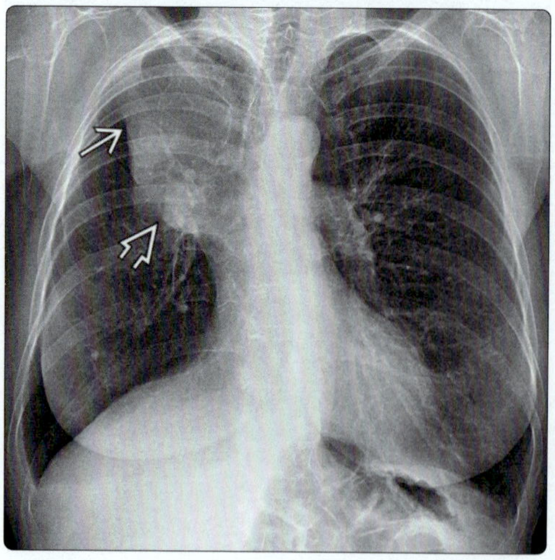

Lung Cancer

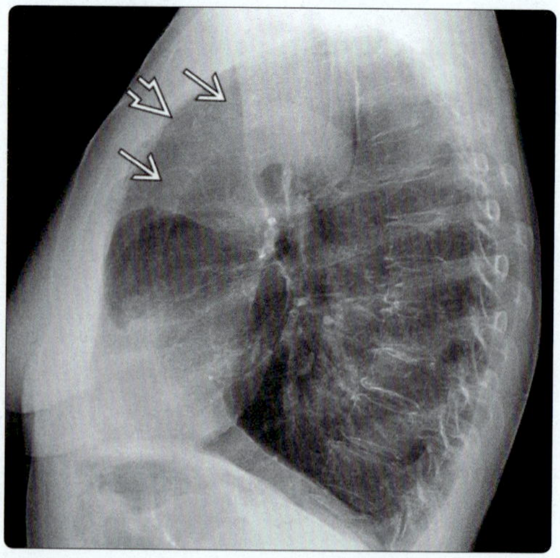

(Left) *PA chest radiograph of a 52-year-old woman shows the classic S-sign of Golden. The medial convexity represents the central mass. The lateral concavity represents the displaced minor fissure. Bronchoscopic biopsy showed non-small cell lung cancer.* **(Right)** *Lateral chest radiograph of the same patient shows right upper lobe atelectasis and obliteration of the retrosternal clear space. The ascending aorta is obscured by atelectasis. The S-sign of Golden is virtually diagnostic of a neoplastic etiology.*

S-Sign of Golden

Lung Cancer

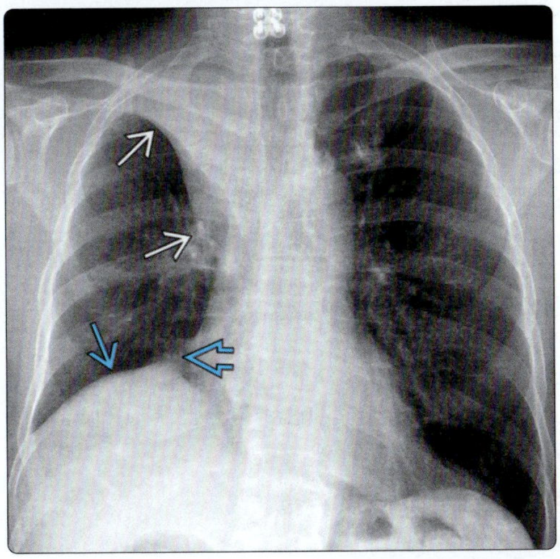

Lung Cancer

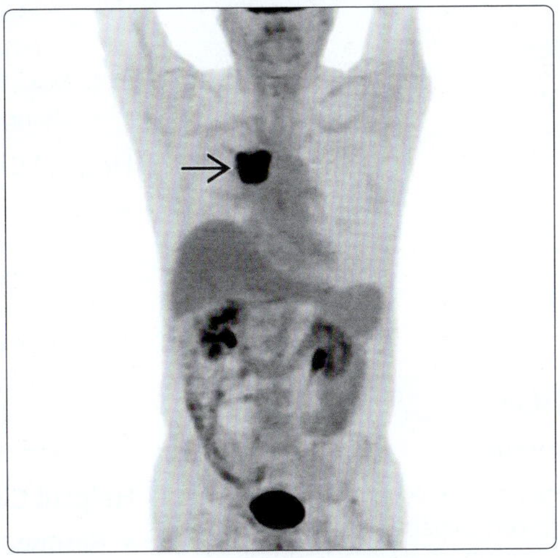

(Left) *PA chest radiograph of a 72-year-old man with non-small cell lung cancer demonstrates the S-sign of Golden. Elevation of the right hemidiaphragm and a juxtaphrenic peak are additional signs of right upper lobe volume loss.* **(Right)** *Coronal FDG PET of the same patient shows the central location of the mass that produces the right upper lobe atelectasis. Lobar collapse may also occur as a result of bronchial stricture or mucus plug, but in these cases, the margin of the collapsed lobe is straight.*

Mediastinal Malignancy

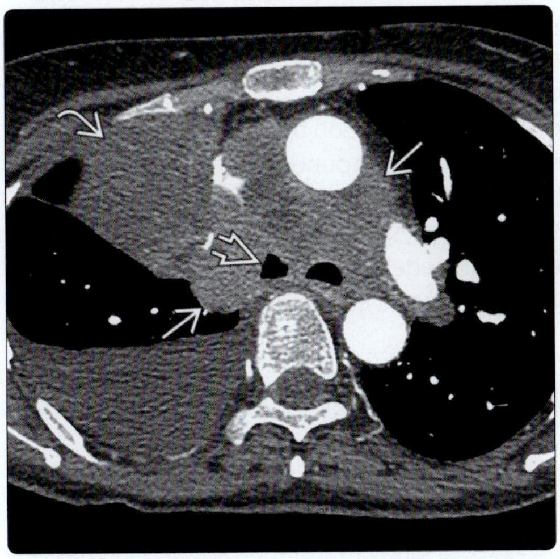

Mediastinal Malignancy

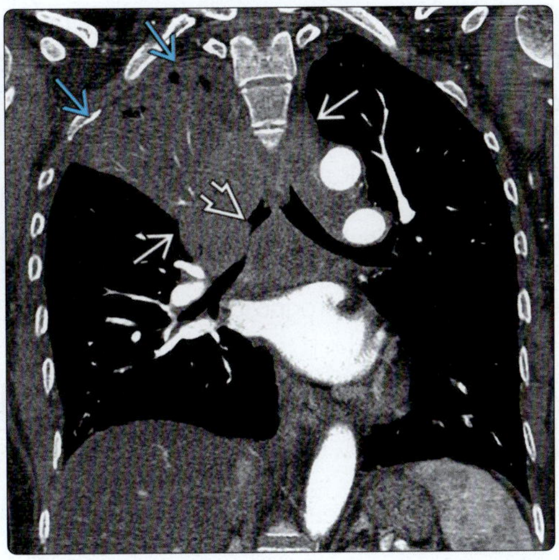

(Left) *Axial CECT of a 75-year-old man with small cell lung cancer shows coalescent mediastinal lymphadenopathy that obstructs the right mainstem bronchus and results in atelectasis of the right upper lobe.* **(Right)** *Coronal CECT of the same patient confirms obstruction of the right mainstem bronchus and right upper lobe atelectasis secondary to an endobronchial mass and extensive mediastinal lymphadenopathy. The S-sign of Golden is recognizable both on chest radiography and CT, as in this case.*

Endobronchial Metastasis

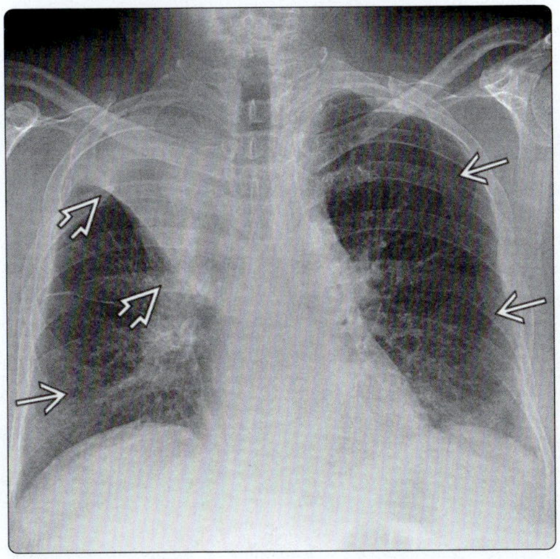

Endobronchial Metastasis

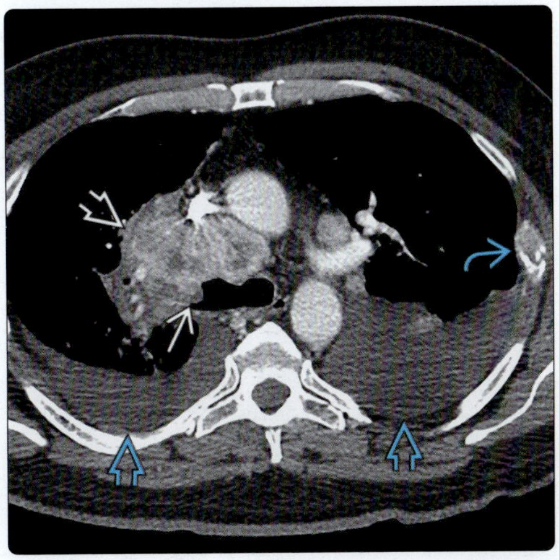

(Left) *PA chest radiograph of a 53-year-old man with metastatic renal cell carcinoma shows right upper lobe atelectasis that exhibits the S-sign of Golden. Interstitial opacities represent lymphangitic carcinomatosis.* **(Right)** *Axial CECT of the same patient shows a central obstructing endobronchial metastasis and mediastinal lymphadenopathy. Note left rib metastasis and bilateral pleural effusions. Extrinsic bronchial compression by mass or lymphadenopathy may produce the S-sign of Golden.*

DIFFERENTIAL DIAGNOSIS

Common

- Angioinvasive Fungal Infection
- Mycetoma

Less Common

- Lung Cancer
- Pulmonary Gangrene

Rare but Important

- Rasmussen Aneurysm
- Hydatid Cyst

ESSENTIAL INFORMATION

Key Differential Diagnosis Issues

- Air crescent sign: Complete or partial crescentic air around parenchymal nodule, mass, or consolidation
- Monod sign: Soft tissue mass surrounded by air within pre-existing lung cavity
- Development of air crescent sign in neutropenic patient strongly suggests angioinvasive fungal infection

Helpful Clues for Common Diagnoses

- **Angioinvasive Fungal Infection**
  - Aspergillosis, mucormycosis
  - Severely immunocompromised neutropenic patients: Hematologic malignancies (leukemia), allogeneic bone marrow and solid-organ transplant recipients, acquired immune deficiency syndrome (AIDS)
    - Development of air crescent sign is good prognostic indicator
  - Invasion of small arteries: Lung infarction and necrosis
  - Imaging
    - Single or multiple lung nodules or masses, may exhibit halo sign
    - Cavitation from tissue necrosis occurs 2 weeks later
- **Mycetoma**
  - Synonym: Aspergilloma
  - Typically *Aspergillus fumigatus*
  - Immunologically competent patient with pre-existent cavity
    - May be asymptomatic
    - Inflammation: Hemorrhage and hemoptysis
  - Mass (fungus ball) within cavity; may be mobile with change in patient position

Helpful Clues for Less Common Diagnoses

- **Lung Cancer**
  - Neoplasm may grow within pre-existing pulmonary cyst or cavity
  - Cavitary lung cancer may produce an air crescent sign
- **Pulmonary Gangrene**
  - Rare complication of severe pulmonary infection
  - Vascular thrombosis: Cavity formation with sloughing of devitalized lung tissue

Helpful Clues for Rare Diagnoses

- **Rasmussen Aneurysm**
  - Pulmonary artery pseudoaneurysm secondary to pulmonary tuberculosis
    - Thinned arterial wall and pseudoaneurysm formation
  - CECT: Vascular enhancement of "nodules" within walls of tuberculous cavities or consolidations
- **Hydatid Cyst**
  - Hydatid cyst: Human infection by canine tapeworm
    - Pericyst: Formed by surrounding compressed lung and fibrous tissue
    - Exocyst and endocyst: Parasite layers
  - Air crescent sign: Air between pericyst and exocyst
  - Water lily sign: Ruptured endocyst floats in fluid-filled exocyst

SELECTED REFERENCES

1. Shroff GS et al: CT signs in the lungs. Semin Ultrasound CT MR. 40(3):265-74, 2019
2. Sevilha JB et al: Infectious and non-infectious diseases causing the air crescent sign: A State-of-the-Art Review. Lung. 196(1):1-10, 2018
3. Hansell DM et al: Fleischner Society: glossary of terms for thoracic imaging. Radiology. 246(3):697-722, 2008
4. Franquet T et al: Spectrum of pulmonary aspergillosis: histologic, clinical, and radiologic findings. Radiographics. 21(4):825-37, 2001

Angioinvasive Fungal Infection

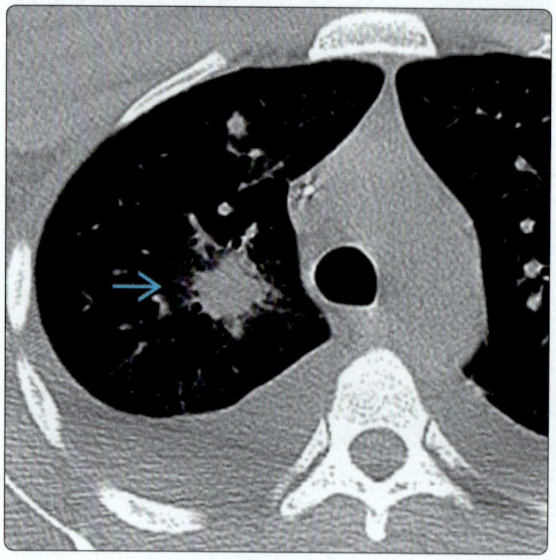

Angioinvasive Fungal Infection

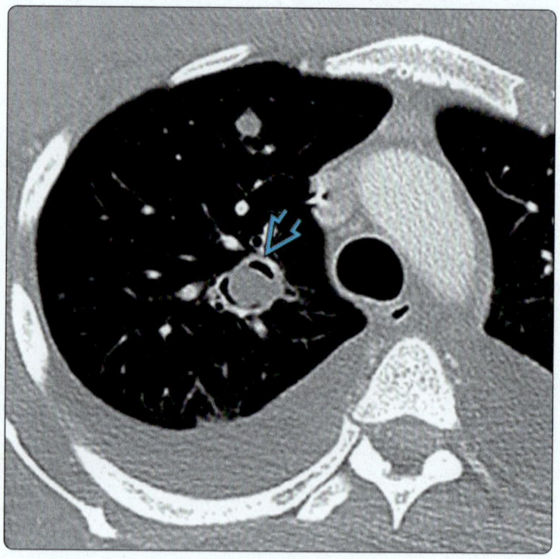

(Left) *Axial NECT of a patient with leukemia and febrile neutropenia shows a right upper lobe nodule with surrounding ground-glass opacity ➡, the so-called halo sign. In this clinical scenario, the findings are highly concerning for angioinvasive fungal infection.* **(Right)** *Axial CECT of the same patient obtained 2 weeks later shows resolution of the halo sign and a new air crescent sign ➡, caused by lung necrosis and tissue retraction. This is a good prognostic sign in this patient with angioinvasive aspergillosis.*

Mycetoma

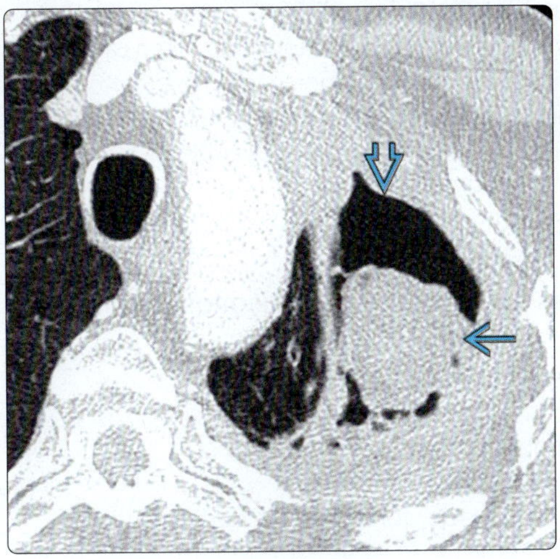

Mycetoma

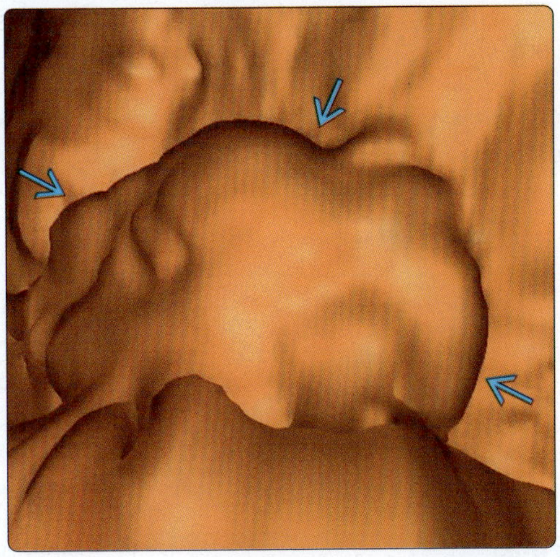

(Left) *Axial HRCT of a patient with prior cavitary tuberculosis shows a large left upper lobe cavity with a dependent lobular mass ➔ surrounded by an air crescent ➔. This is a typical appearance of an intracavitary mycetoma.* **(Right)** *3D surface shaded display of the same lesion shows the intracavitary lobular mass outlined by surrounding air within the cavity ➔. The intracavitary mass proved to represent a mycetoma related to saprophytic aspergillosis.*

Lung Cancer

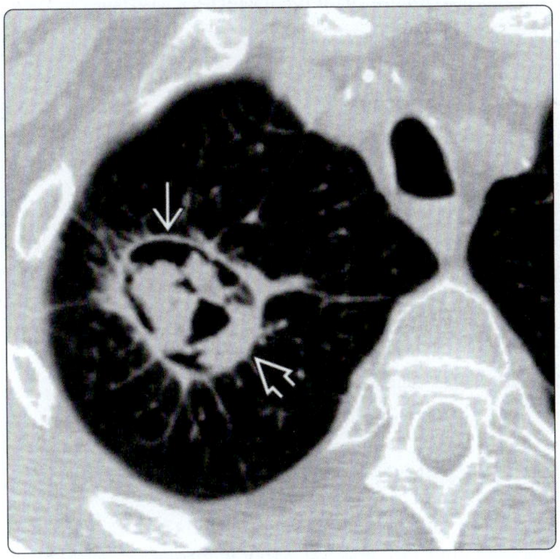

Pulmonary Gangrene

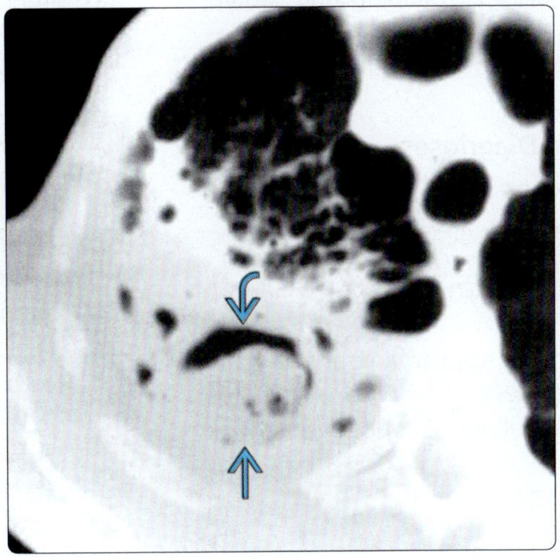

(Left) *Axial NECT of a patient with primary lung cancer shows a right upper lobe spiculated cavitary mass ➔. Tissue necrosis and retraction produce an air crescent sign ➔ that mimics the imaging findings of angioinvasive fungal infection.* **(Right)** *Axial NECT of a patient with severe necrotizing Klebsiella pneumonia shows a right upper lobe heterogeneous cavitary consolidation with an intracavitary mass ➔ that represents devitalized lung tissue. The necrotic lung is surrounded by an air crescent ➔.*

Rasmussen Aneurysm

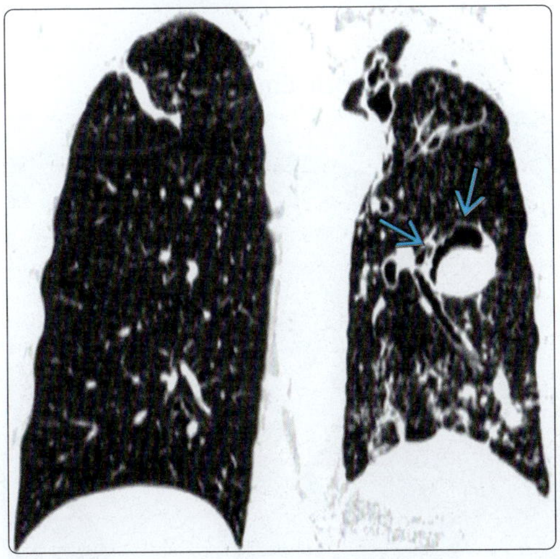

Rasmussen Aneurysm

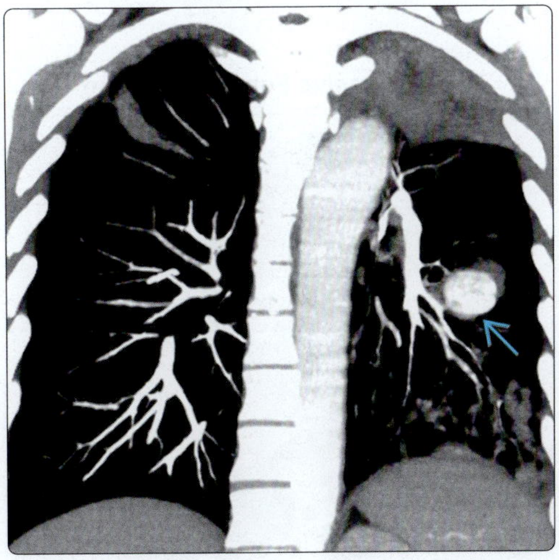

(Left) *Coronal NECT of a patient with tuberculosis who presented with hemoptysis shows marked left upper lobe volume loss, bronchiectasis, and cellular bronchiolitis. Note the dominant left lower lobe cavity with an intrinsic non-mobile nodule. The cavitary lesion exhibits the air crescent sign ➔.* **(Right)** *Coronal CECT MIP reformatted image of the same patient shows intense enhancement of the intracavitary nodule, which represented a Rasmussen aneurysm ➔. (Courtesy E. Marchiori, MD.)*

DIFFERENTIAL DIAGNOSIS

Common

- Angioinvasive Fungal Infection
- Septic Embolism
- Granulomatosis With Polyangiitis
- Cryptogenic Organizing Pneumonia

Less Common

- Infection
  - Histoplasmosis
  - Other Organisms
- Lepidic Lung Adenocarcinoma
- Metastases
  - Hemorrhagic Metastases
  - Lepidic Metastases
- Iatrogenic

ESSENTIAL INFORMATION

Key Differential Diagnosis Issues

- **Definition**: Ground-glass opacity surrounding lung nodule, mass, or consolidation
- Typically represents hemorrhage but also inflammation or neoplasm

Helpful Clues for Common Diagnoses

- **Angioinvasive Fungal Infection**
  - Angioinvasive aspergillosis (e.g., *Aspergillus fumigatus*); also *Candida* spp., *Mucor* spp.
  - Immunocompromised patient with severe/prolonged neutropenia
    - Early after bone marrow or solid organ transplant or prolonged steroid treatment
  - Rounded infarct with gray-yellow necrotic center and rim of peripheral hemorrhage
  - Cavitation occurs as immunity recovers
- **Septic Embolism**
  - Common with hematogenous dissemination of *Staphylococcus aureus* infection (e.g., endocarditis, infected central and peripheral lines)
  - Solid or cavitary nodules with surrounding ground-glass opacity
- **Granulomatosis With Polyangiitis**
  - Nodules, masses, or consolidations that often cavitate
  - May exhibit surrounding hemorrhage
- **Cryptogenic Organizing Pneumonia**
  - Idiopathic or associated numerous entities (e.g., autoimmunity, drugs, infection)
  - Subacute or chronic course; cough, dyspnea, fever, malaise, weight loss

Helpful Clues for Less Common Diagnoses

- **Infection**
  - Histoplasmosis and most endemic fungi
  - Mycobacteria, rickettsia, viruses (e.g.,Varicella zoster, herpes simplex, cytomegalovirus)
- **Lepidic Lung Adenocarcinoma**
  - Ground-glass opacity correlates with lepidic adenocarcinoma
    - Solid component correlates with invasive adenocarcinoma
  - ± metastatic hilar/mediastinal lymphadenopathy
- **Hemorrhagic Metastases**
  - Angiosarcoma, choriocarcinoma, osteosarcoma, renal cell carcinoma, melanoma
- **Lepidic Metastases**
  - Typically pancreatic adenocarcinoma, gastric adenocarcinoma, cholangiocarcinoma
  - Solitary metastasis may simulate primary lung adenocarcinoma
- **Iatrogenic**
  - Transbronchial or percutaneous lung biopsy
  - Postbiopsy hemorrhage manifests with ground-glass opacity surrounding target lesion

SELECTED REFERENCES

1. Algın O et al: Signs in chest imaging. Diagn Interv Radiol. 17(1):18-29, 2011
2. Marshall GB et al: Signs in thoracic imaging. J Thorac Imaging. 21(1):76-90, 2006
3. Lee YR, et al. CT halo sign: the spectrum of pulmonary diseases. Br J Radiol. 2005 Sep;78(933):862-5.

Angioinvasive Fungal Infection

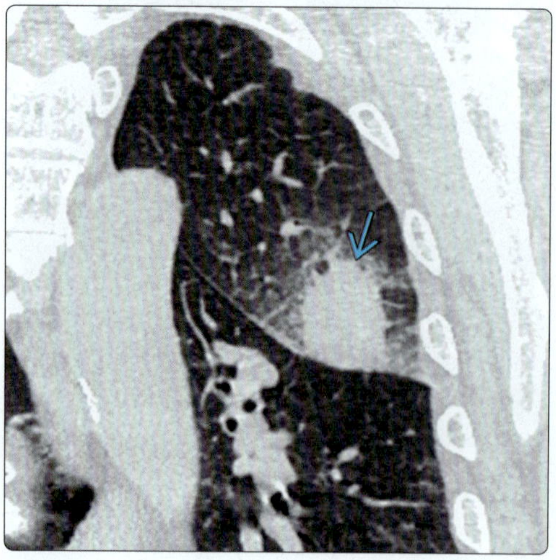

Septic Embolism

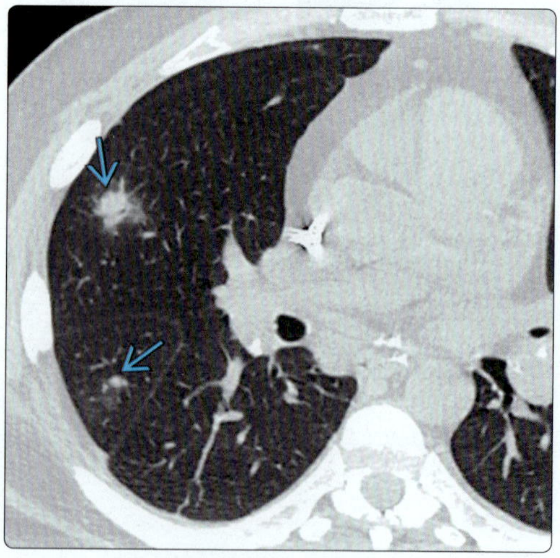

(Left) *Coronal NECT of a febrile neutropenic patient with angioinvasive aspergillosis shows a left upper lobe mass ⇨ with surrounding ground-glass opacity that corresponds to perilesional hemorrhage and produces the so-called halo sign. Angioinvasive fungal infection often occurs early after solid organ or bone marrow transplantation.* **(Right)** *Axial NECT of a patient with septic embolism shows multiple lung nodules ⇨ with surrounding ground-glass opacity. Septic emboli typically exhibit intrinsic cavitation.*

CT Halo Sign

Granulomatosis With Polyangiitis

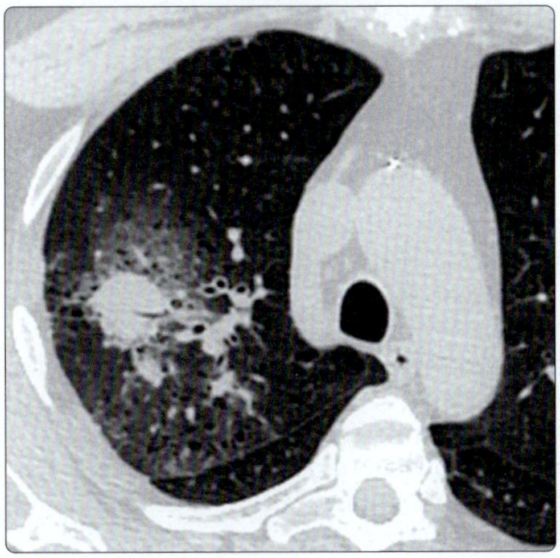

Cryptogenic Organizing Pneumonia

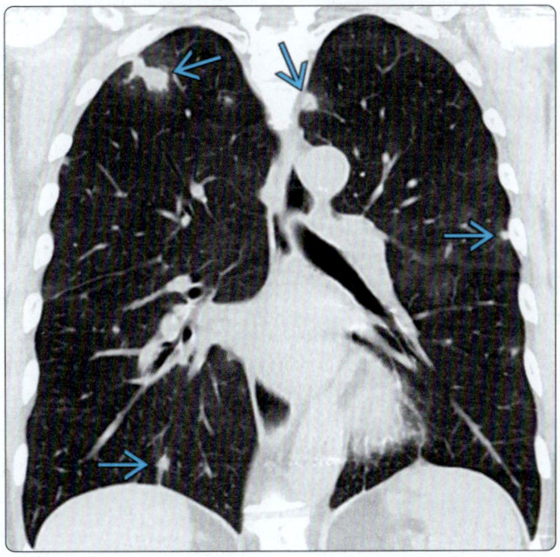

(Left) *Axial NECT of a patient with granulomatosis with polyangiitis shows right upper lobe clustered nodules with surrounding ground-glass opacity. Such ground-glass opacity halos often correlate with hemorrhage.* **(Right)** *Coronal NECT of a patient with cryptogenic organizing pneumonia shows multiple bilateral lung nodules → with surrounding ground-glass opacity halos. This is not a typical imaging feature of organizing pneumonia.*

Histoplasmosis

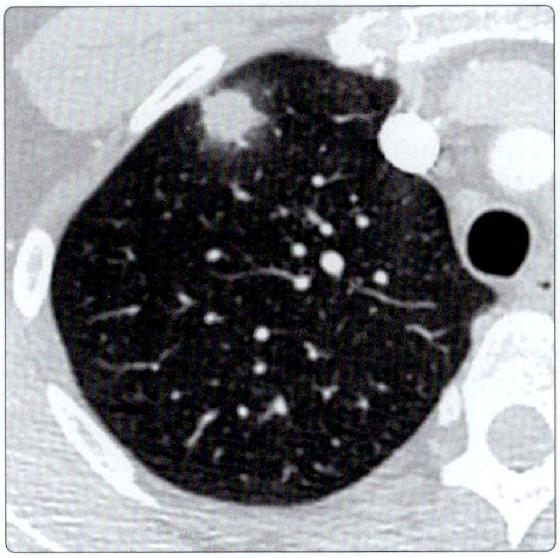

Lepidic Lung Adenocarcinoma

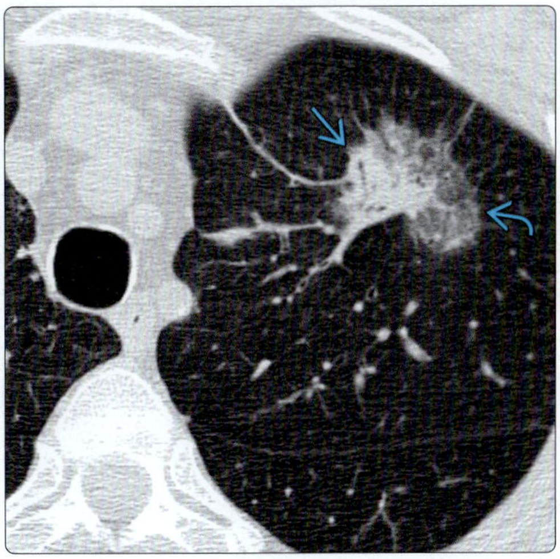

(Left) *Axial CECT of a patient with acute histoplasmosis shows a right upper lobe nodule with surrounding ground-glass opacity. In addition to angioinvasive fungi, endemic and other fungi may show the halo sign in patients without severe immunosuppression.* **(Right)** *Axial NECT of a patient with lung adenocarcinoma shows a part-solid nodule with solid → and ground-glass ↗ components. Indolent lung cancer should be considered in chronic solid lesions with surrounding ground-glass opacity.*

Lepidic Metastases

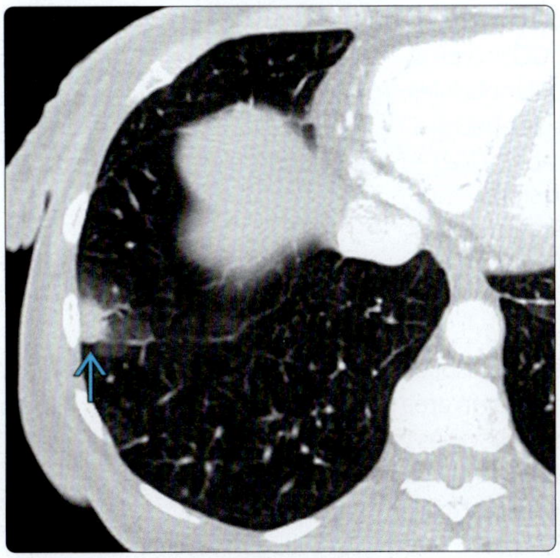

Iatrogenic

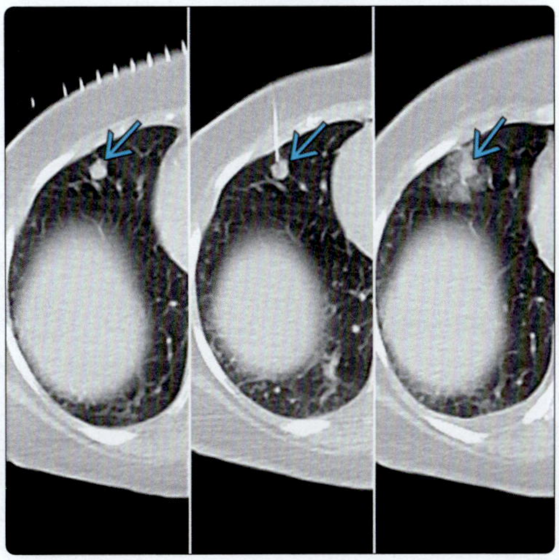

(Left) *Axial CECT of a patient with metastatic pancreatic adenocarcinoma shows a solid nodule → with surrounding ground-glass opacity. In such cases, the ground-glass component of the lesion correlates with lepidic tumor growth, commonly seen in pancreatic adenocarcinoma.* **(Right)** *Composite image with axial NECT of a patient with a middle lobe nodule → who underwent percutaneous biopsy shows development of postbiopsy perilesional ground-glass opacity secondary to postbiopsy hemorrhage.*

DIFFERENTIAL DIAGNOSIS

Common

- Acute
  - Pneumonia
  - Pulmonary Edema
  - Pulmonary Hemorrhage

Less Common

- Acute
  - Acute Interstitial Pneumonia
  - Hypersensitivity Pneumonitis
  - Radiation Pneumonitis
- Chronic
  - Nonspecific Interstitial Pneumonia
  - Smoking-Related Interstitial Lung Disease
    - Respiratory Bronchiolitis-Associated Interstitial Lung Disease
    - Desquamative Interstitial Pneumonia
- Lung Cancer
- Eosinophilic Pneumonia

Rare but Important

- Pulmonary Alveolar Proteinosis
- Drug Reaction
- Pulmonary Lymphoma

ESSENTIAL INFORMATION

Key Differential Diagnosis Issues

- Ground-glass opacity (GGO)
  - CT
    - Increased lung density or attenuation
    - Does not obscure underlying bronchovascular structures
  - Results from
    - Alveolar filling/collapse
    - Interstitial thickening
    - Increased blood volume
    - Combination of above mechanisms
  - Visualization on CT
    - Difficult if minimal or diffuse
    - Pitfalls
      - Normally seen with exhalation
      - Volume averaging with thick collimation (> 5 mm)
      - Window settings too narrow or too wide
      - Normal in dependent lung from atelectasis
  - Differential diagnosis depends in part on whether underlying etiology is acute or chronic

Helpful Clues for Common Diagnoses

- **Pneumonia**
  - Etiologies
    - Viruses
    - Mycoplasma
    - Pneumocystis jiroveci
  - Typically febrile immunocompromised patients
  - Presence of GGO should raise concern for opportunistic infection
- **Pulmonary Edema**
  - Cardiogenic
    - GGO is earliest parenchymal change
      - Usually gravity dependent
    - Increased severity leads to
      - Interlobular septal thickening
      - Consolidation
      - Pleural effusions
  - Noncardiogenic
    - Acute respiratory distress syndrome (ARDS)
    - GGO is predominant abnormality
    - Extent typically > 50% of lung
- **Pulmonary Hemorrhage**
  - Diffuse Alveolar Hemorrhage (DAH)
    - Lobular GGO often admixed with dense consolidation, gravity dependent
    - Hemorrhage may be associated with focal lesions, resulting in surrounding ground-glass (GG) 'halos'
      - Hemorrhagic metastases (e.g., renal cell carcinoma)
      - Invasive aspergillosis
      - Site of lung biopsy

Helpful Clues for Less Common Diagnoses

- **Acute Interstitial Pneumonia (AIP)**
  - Idiopathic interstitial pneumonia characterized by
    - Progressive respiratory failure of unknown etiology
    - Histologic features of diffuse alveolar damage (DAD)
  - Idiopathic form of ARDS; however, not all patients with ARDS have AIP
  - GGO and consolidations are predominant abnormalities
    - Extent
      - > 50% of lung
      - Patchy (2/3)
      - Diffuse (2/3)
    - Distribution
      - Lower lung zone (40%)
      - Upper lung zone (15%)
    - Patterns
      - Symmetric (common)
      - Often focal lobular sparing (geographic pattern)
    - More extensive GGO (without traction bronchiectasis) associated with better outcome
- **Hypersensitivity Pneumonitis**
  - Diffuse GGO is typical
  - Centrilobular nodules, 70%
  - Most specific pattern
    - Geographic GGO + normal lung + air trapping (head cheese sign)
- **Radiation Pneumonitis**
  - Typically occurs 1-6 months after completion of radiation therapy
  - Imaging
    - GGO &/or consolidations ± ipsilateral pleural effusion
      - Can occur in area of low dose exposure
      - Often obscures treated neoplasm
      - Imaging findings decrease over time
- **Nonspecific Interstitial Pneumonia**
  - Idiopathic or associated with collagen vascular diseases
  - GGO often basilar, follow bronchovascular pathways (fan- or wedge-shaped)
  - Traction bronchiectasis often out of proportion to severity of reticular opacities

- **Smoking-Related Interstitial Lung Disease**
  - Spectrum of cigarette-related injuries from respiratory bronchiolitis to desquamative interstitial pneumonia (DIP)
    - Generally dose related
    - More common with heavier cigarette smoking or use of unfiltered cigarettes
  - Respiratory bronchiolitis: Upper lobe centrilobular GGO
  - DIP: GGO in 100%
    - Often diffuse, symmetric, and panlobular
- **Lung Cancer**
  - Lesions in adenocarcinoma spectrum
  - Atypical adenomatous hyperplasia (AAH)
    - Preinvasive
    - GG nodule ≤ 0.5 cm
  - Adenocarcinoma in situ (AIS)
    - Malignant and preinvasive
    - GG nodule ≤ 3 cm
  - Minimally invasive adenocarcinoma (MIA)
    - GG nodule or part-solid nodule ≤ 3 cm (i.e., coexistent GG and solid components)
    - Solid component ≤ 0.5 cm
      - Correlates with invasive component at pathology
      - Often larger on imaging than on histology (adjacent atelectasis, inflammation, fibrosis)
    - GG component
      - Correlates with lepidic component
      - Invasive component can exist in GG nodule
  - Invasive adenocarcinoma
    - Lepidic-predominant adenocarcinoma (LPA)
      - Part-solid nodule or mass; GGO
      - Solid component > 0.5 cm
      - Intrinsic bubbly appearance
    - Acinar, papillary, micropapillary, or solid predominant with mucin production
      - Usually solid; may include GG component
  - Variants of invasive adenocarcinoma
    - Invasive mucinous adenocarcinoma
      - Formerly known as mucinous BAC
      - Variable appearance; focal or multifocal
      - Consolidations, air bronchogram
      - GG nodule, part-solid, or solid nodules or masses
      - Lower lobe predominance
- **Eosinophilic Pneumonia**
  - Acute
    - Pattern identical to pulmonary edema
    - GGO (100%) admixed with interlobular septal thickening, consolidation, random distribution
    - Pleural effusions common (80%)
  - Chronic
    - Typical distribution: Peripheral and upper lobes
    - Consolidation > GGO

Helpful Clues for Rare Diagnoses

- **Pulmonary Alveolar Proteinosis**
  - Disease characterized by abnormal intraalveolar accumulation of surfactant-derived lipoproteinaceous material
  - Typically admixed with interlobular septal thickening in "crazy-paving" pattern
- **Drug Reaction**
  - Histologic patterns
    - Diffuse alveolar damage
    - Hypersensitivity pneumonitis
    - Eosinophilic lung disease
    - DAH
  - Best diagnostic clue: High index of clinical suspicion
- **Pulmonary Lymphoma**
  - GGO is much more likely to be feature of pulmonary non-Hodgkin lymphoma than Hodgkin lymphoma
  - Airspace opacity: GGO ± interlobular septal thickening
  - Pulmonary intravascular lymphoma
    - Mild GG or reticular opacities
  - Peripheral T-cell lymphoma
    - GG centrilobular nodules

SELECTED REFERENCES

1. Miller WT Jr et al: Isolated diffuse ground-glass opacity in thoracic CT: causes and clinical presentations. AJR Am J Roentgenol. 184(2):613-22, 2005

Pneumonia

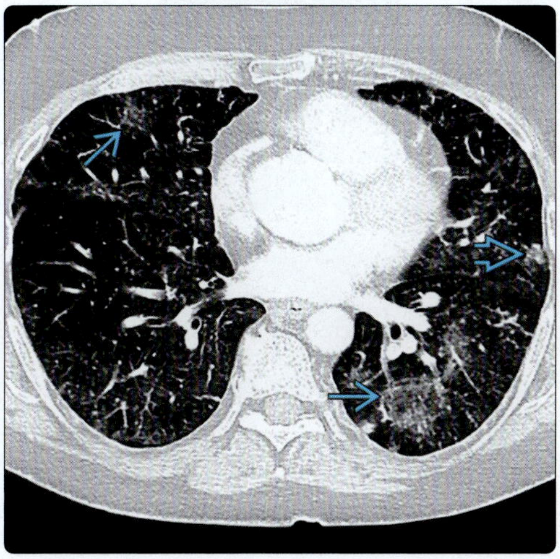

Pneumonia

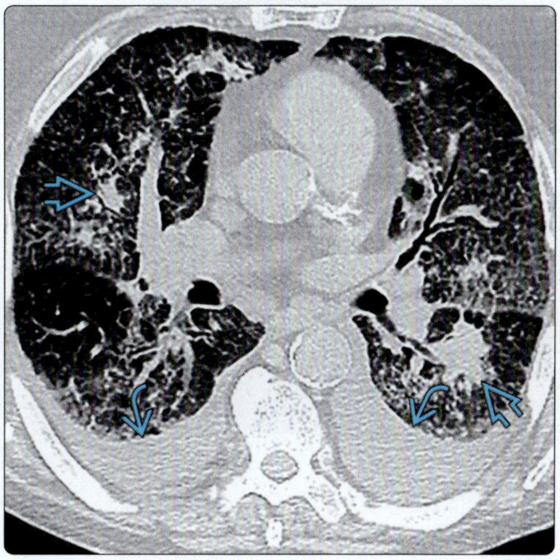

(Left) *Axial CECT of an immunocompromised patient with viral pneumonia demonstrates predominantly ground-glass opacities → bilaterally, although a few ill-defined nodular opacities → are also present.* **(Right)** *Axial NECT of an immunocompromised patient with pneumonia shows bilateral ground-glass opacities with coexistent interlobular septal thickening in a "crazy-paving" pattern. Several nodular opacities are also present →. Note the small bilateral pleural effusions →.*

(Left) *Axial CECT of a patient with congestive heart failure demonstrates ground-glass opacities bilaterally, representing pulmonary edema.* **(Right)** *Axial CECT of the same patient demonstrates enlargement of the cardiac chambers and bilateral pleural effusions →. Ground-glass opacities are the earliest parenchymal change of pulmonary edema. Interlobular septal thickening, consolidation, and pleural effusions may develop with increasing severity.*

Pulmonary Edema

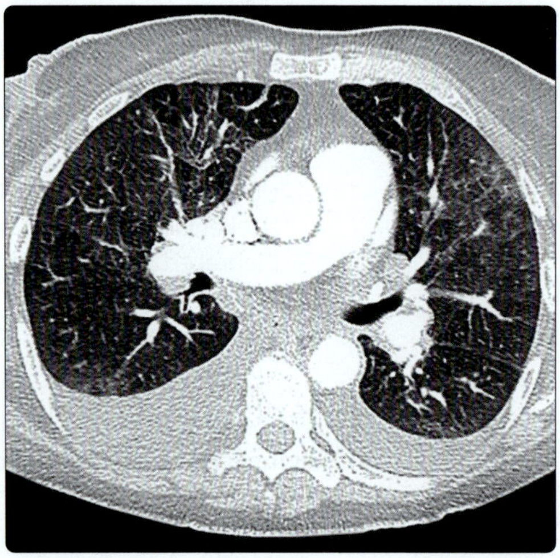

Pulmonary Edema

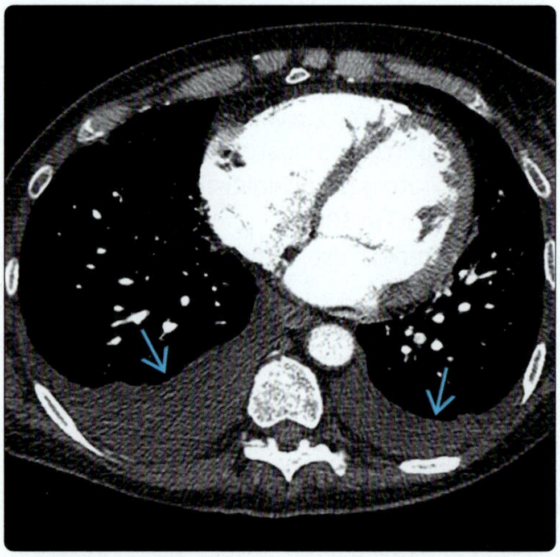

(Left) *Axial CECT of a patient presenting with hemoptysis demonstrates patchy ground-glass opacities bilaterally, representing pulmonary hemorrhage.* **(Right)** *Axial CECT of a patient with history of connective tissue disease shows more extensive ground-glass opacities bilaterally. Diffuse alveolar hemorrhage typically manifests as lobular ground-glass opacities often admixed with dense, gravity-dependent consolidation on CT.*

Pulmonary Hemorrhage

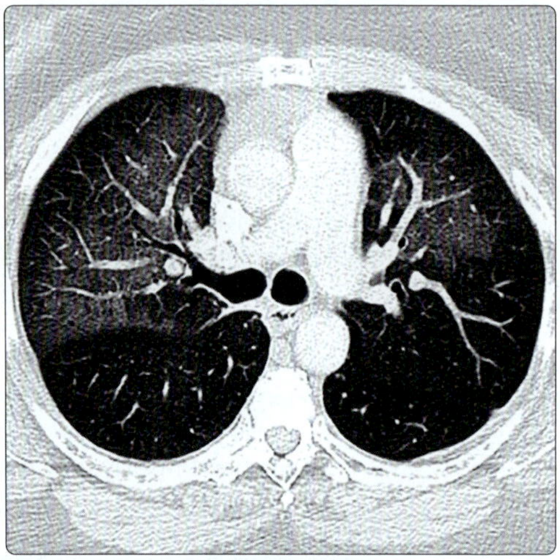

Pulmonary Hemorrhage

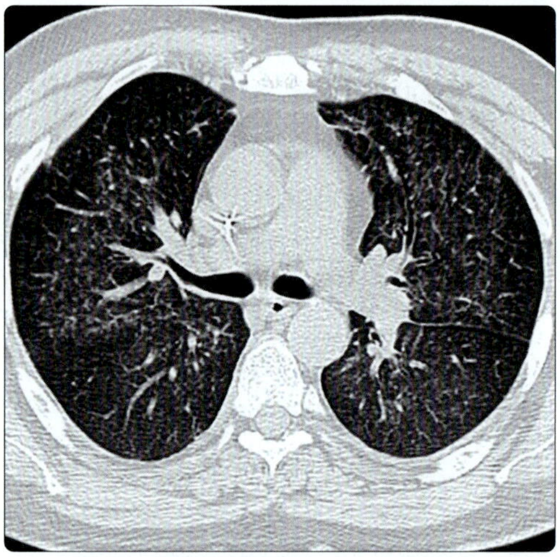

(Left) *Axial NECT demonstrates a focal ground-glass nodular opacity in the left upper lobe that did not resolve on subsequent CT →. Biopsy revealed adenocarcinoma in situ.* **(Right)** *Axial CECT of a patient with history of lung cancer shows a part-solid mass → in the left upper lobe composed of ground-glass opacity and a solid component →. Biopsy revealed minimally invasive adenocarcinoma. Adenocarcinoma of the lung must be considered when focal ground-glass opacities do not resolve on CT.*

Lung Cancer

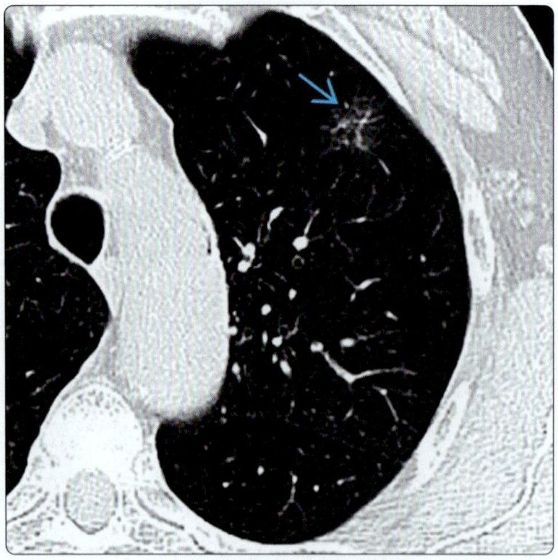

Lung Cancer

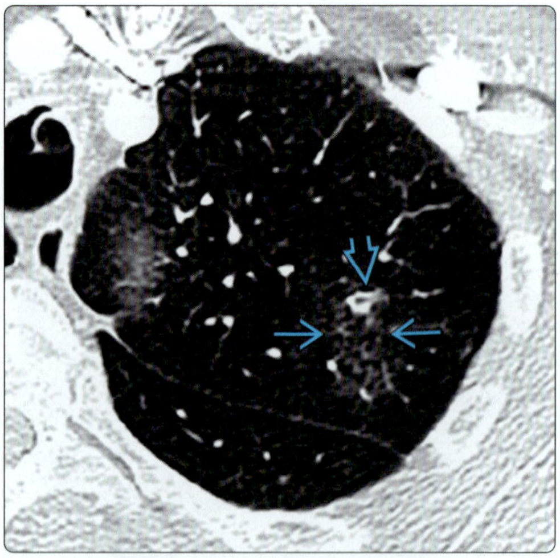

Lung Cancer

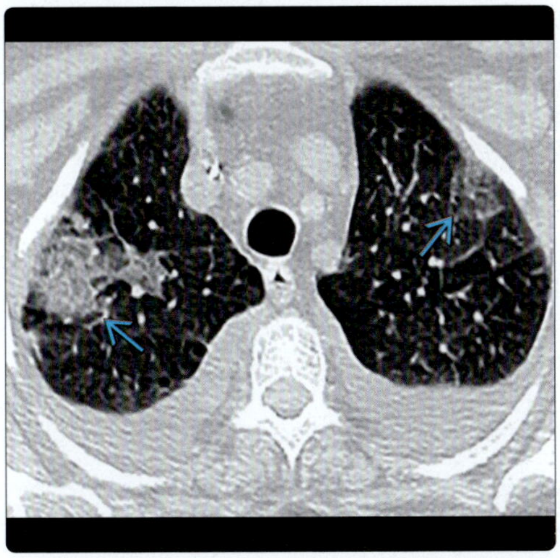

Lung Cancer

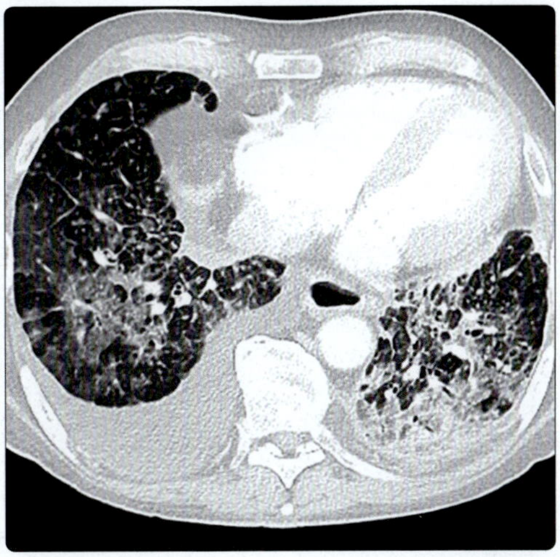

(Left) *Axial NECT of a patient with multifocal adenocarcinoma shows bilateral foci of ground-glass opacity with interlobular septal thickening →. Note bilateral pleural effusions.* **(Right)** *Axial CECT of a patient with diffuse adenocarcinoma of the lung demonstrates bilateral foci of ground-glass opacity with interlobular septal thickening in a "crazy-paving" pattern. Note the small right pleural effusion.*

Pulmonary Alveolar Proteinosis

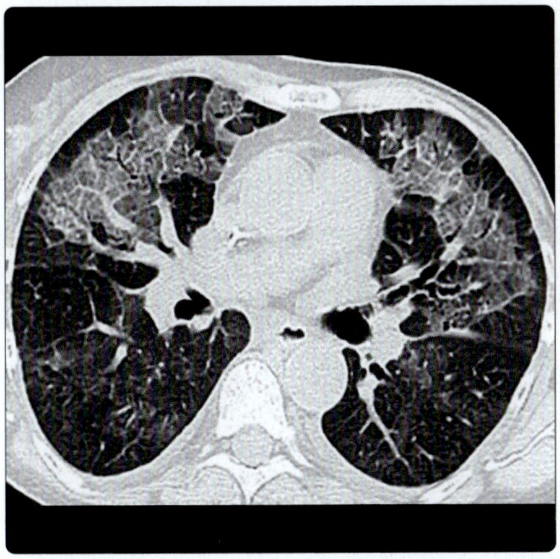

Pulmonary Alveolar Proteinosis

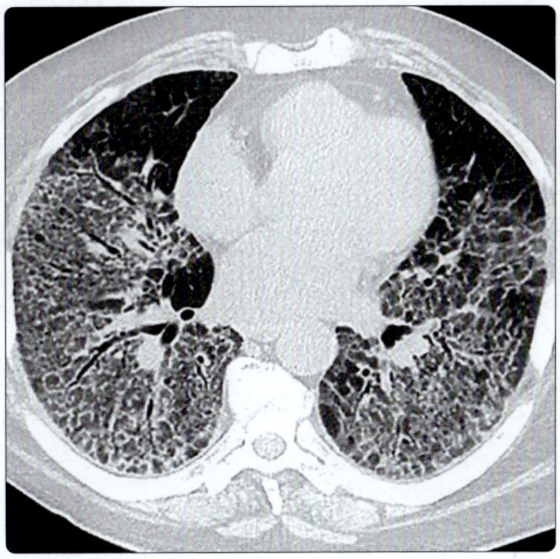

(Left) *Axial NECT of a patient with pulmonary alveolar proteinosis shows ground-glass opacities and interlobular septal thickening bilaterally. In this disease, ground-glass opacities are typically admixed with septal thickening in the "crazy-paving" pattern seen here.* **(Right)** *Axial CECT of a patient with long-standing pulmonary alveolar proteinosis demonstrates extensive "crazy paving" bilaterally. This disease is characterized by intraalveolar accumulation of surfactant-derived lipoproteinaceous material.*

Drug Reaction

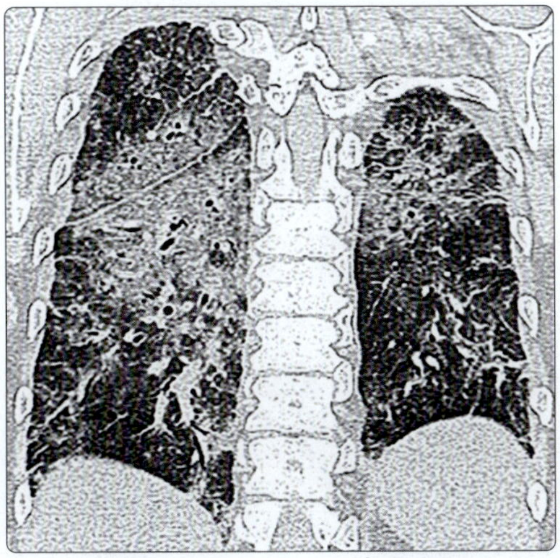

Drug Reaction

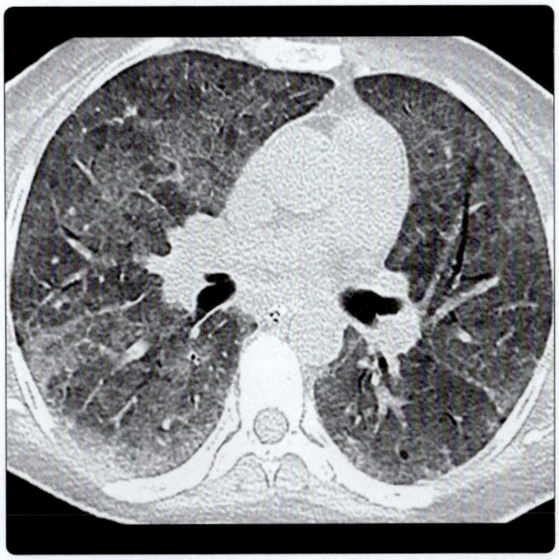

(Left) *Coronal NECT of a patient with lymphoma treated with chemotherapy shows diffuse ground-glass opacities bilaterally, representing drug reaction with a diffuse alveolar hemorrhage pattern. Other histologic patterns include diffuse alveolar damage, hypersensitivity pneumonitis, and eosinophilic lung disease.* **(Right)** *Axial NECT of a patient with melanoma treated with immunotherapy demonstrates diffuse ground-glass opacities representing pneumonitis, an immune-related adverse event.*

DIFFERENTIAL DIAGNOSIS

Common

- Organizing Pneumonia
- Fungal Infection
  - Angioinvasive Aspergillosis
  - Mucormycosis
  - *Pneumocystis jirovecii* Pneumonia
  - Other: Histoplasmosis, Cryptococcosis, Paracoccidioidomycosis
- Bacterial Infection
  - *Legionella pneumophila* Pneumonia
  - Tuberculosis
- Infarct
- Pulmonary Adenocarcinoma

Less Common

- Sarcoidosis
- Granulomatosis With Polyangiitis
- Lymphomatoid Granulomatosis
- Lipoid Pneumonia
- Chronic Eosinophilic Pneumonia

Rare but Important

- Radiofrequency Ablation

ESSENTIAL INFORMATION

Key Differential Diagnosis Issues

- Definition: Central ground-glass opacity surrounded by concentric or crescentic consolidation on CT
  - **Atoll sign**: Incomplete rim of consolidation

Helpful Clues for Common Diagnoses

- **Organizing Pneumonia**
  - Idiopathic (i.e., cryptogenic organizing pneumonia) or due to infection, autoimmunity, radiation, drug reaction
  - Subacute or chronic clinical presentation
- **Fungal Infection**
  - **Angioinvasive aspergillosis** typically seen in severe immunosuppression (e.g., post transplantation)
    - Internal reticulation, peripheral thickness > 1 cm, and pleural effusion
  - **Mucormycosis** typically seen diabetes and immunosuppression
  - **Other Fungi**: Nodular walls or internal nodules
- **Bacterial Infection**
  - *Legionella pneumophila* **Pneumonia**
    - Frequent cause of community acquired pneumonia
    - Multifocal consolidations + intrinsic ground-glass opacity
  - **Tuberculosis**
    - Nodular walls or internal nodules
    - Tree-in-bud opacities, cavitation
- **Infarct**
  - Consolidation with central lucency ± reticulation; single defect
  - Basilar predominance, pleural effusion
- **Pulmonary Adenocarcinoma**
  - Part-solid nodules; may exhibit reversed halo sign

Helpful Clues for Less Common Diagnoses

- **Sarcoidosis**
  - Nodular walls or internal nodules
  - Hilar and mediastinal lymphadenopathy ± perilymphatic nodules
- **Granulomatosis With Polyangiitis**
  - Multiple nodules or masses ± cavitation

Helpful Clues for Rare Diagnoses

- Radiofrequency Ablation
  - History of ablation for cancer or metastatic disease

SELECTED REFERENCES

1. Thomas R et al: Significance of the reverse halo sign in immunocompromised patients. AJR Am J Roentgenol. 1-6, 2019
2. Raju S et al: Chest CT signs in pulmonary disease: a pictorial review. Chest. 151(6):1356-74, 2017
3. Walsh S et al: Importance of the reversed halo sign for the diagnosis of angioinvasive pulmonary aspergillosis. Respir Med. 108(8):1240, 2014
4. Marchiori E et al: Reversed halo sign on computed tomography: state-of-the-art review. Lung. 190(4):389-94, 2012

Organizing Pneumonia

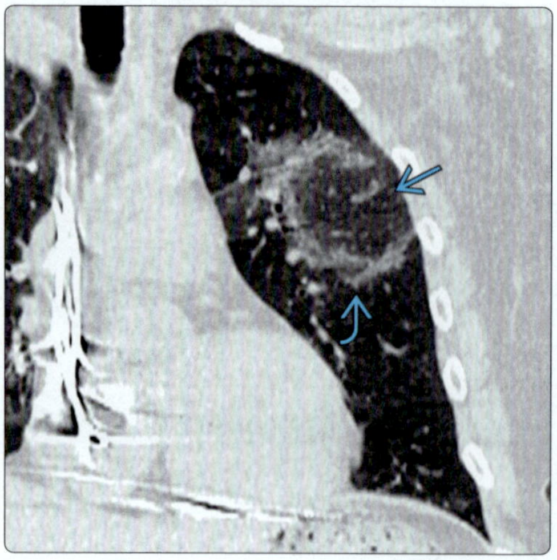

Organizing Pneumonia

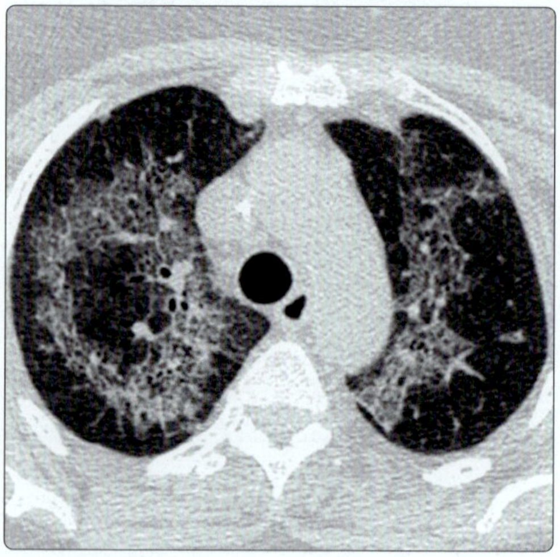

(Left) *Coronal NECT shows left upper lobe cryptogenic organizing pneumonia with the classic reversed halo sign characterized by central ground-glass opacity ➔ with a peripheral rim of consolidation ➔. Originally thought to be a specific finding of organizing pneumonia, the reversed halo sign has been described in other diseases.* **(Right)** *Axial NECT of a patient with Crohn disease and organizing pneumonia shows bilateral upper lobe ground-glass opacities. The right upper lobe lesion exhibits the reversed halo sign.*

Mucormycosis

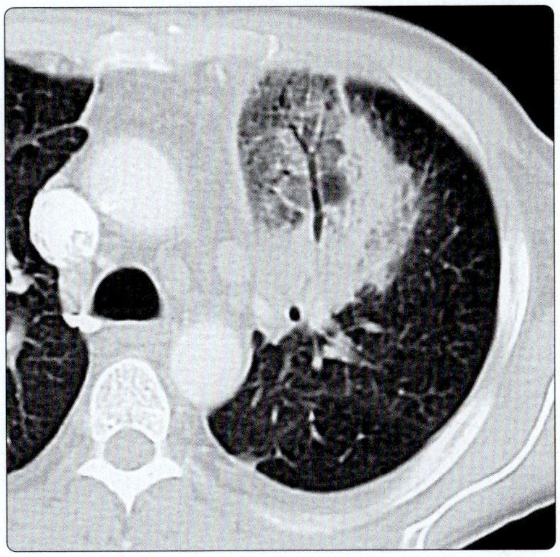

Tuberculosis

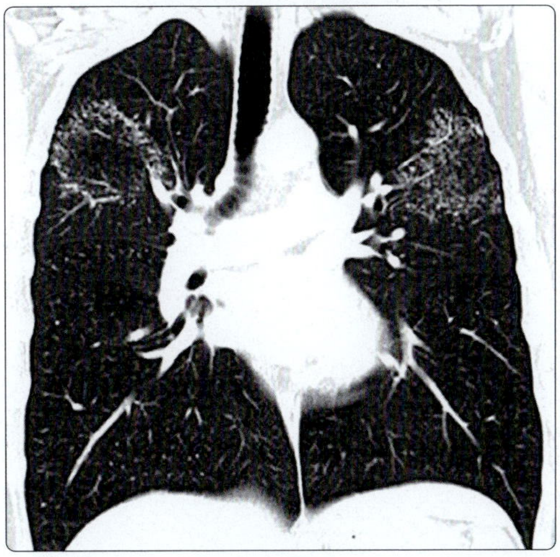

(Left) *Axial CECT of a patient with diabetes and left upper lobe mucormycosis exhibits the reversed halo sign. Mucormycosis is particularly common in patients with uncontrolled diabetes or immunosuppression.* **(Right)** *Coronal HRCT of a patient with tuberculosis shows bilateral upper lobe airspace disease that exhibits the reversed halo sign. Note micronodularity along the peripheral rim of consolidation, which is more common in granulomatous infections. (Courtesy K. S. Lee, MD.)*

Infarct

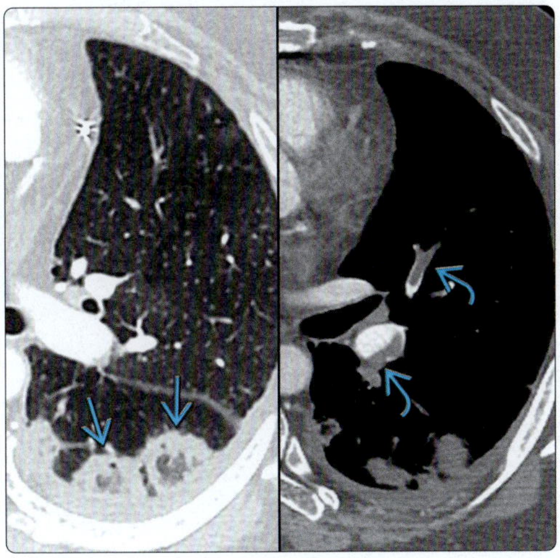

Pulmonary Adenocarcinoma

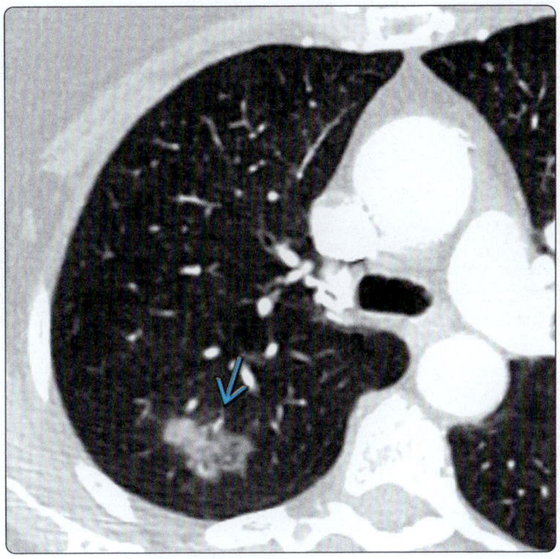

(Left) *Composite image with axial CECT in lung (left) and soft tissue (right) window of a patient with acute pulmonary thromboembolism shows peripheral nodules exhibiting the reversed halo sign ➔. Note arterial filling defects ➔, consistent with acute pulmonary emboli.* **(Right)** *Axial CECT of a patient with lung adenocarcinoma shows a spiculated part-solid nodule ➔ exhibiting the reversed halo sign with ground-glass opacity surrounded by consolidation. Such cancers are typically indolent slow-growing malignancies.*

Sarcoidosis

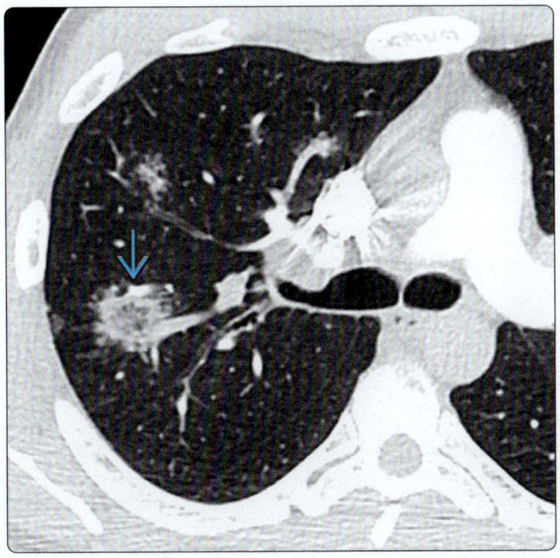

Granulomatosis With Polyangiitis

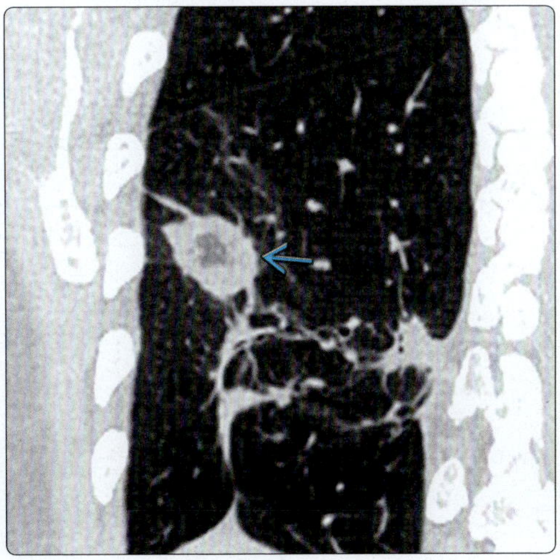

(Left) *Axial CECT of a patient with sarcoidosis shows multiple pulmonary nodules, one of which exhibits the reversed halo sign ➔. Micronodularity along the nodule periphery suggests the galaxy sign often seen in sarcoidosis.* **(Right)** *Coronal NECT of a patient with granulomatosis with polyangiitis shows right lower lobe pulmonary nodules, one of which exhibits the reversed halo sign ➔. These nodules may later develop central necrosis and cavitation.*

SECTION 3

Interstitium

Approach to Interstitium

General Imaging Patterns

Modality-Specific Imaging Findings: Computed Tomography

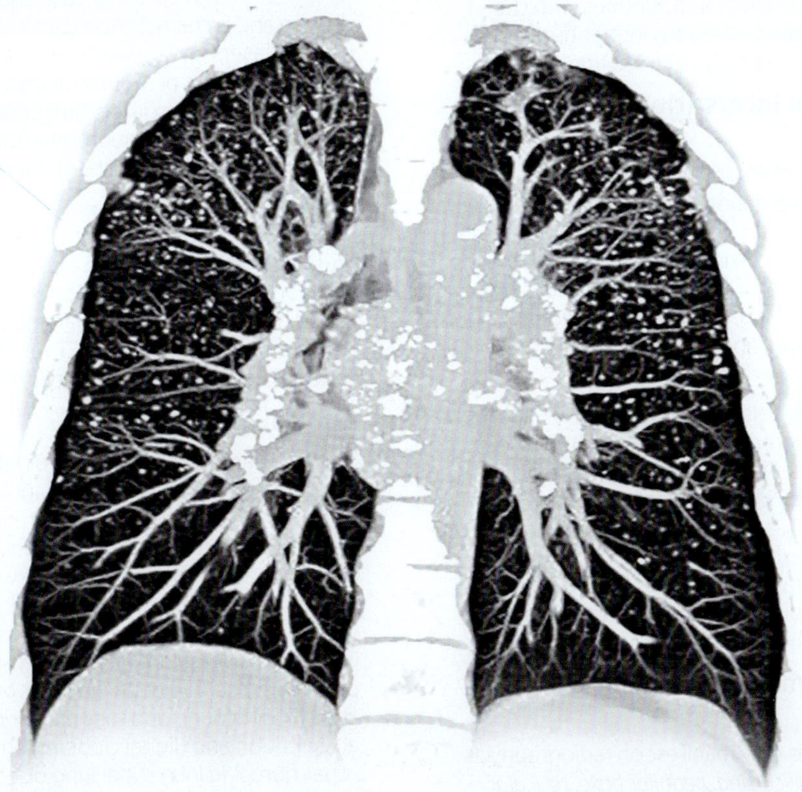

Introduction

The interstitial network of the lung is a continuum of loose connective tissue that is anchored at the hila and extends peripherally to the visceral pleura. Microscopically, the interstitial network is composed of fine reticulin and elastin fibers as well as coarser collagen fibers. In addition to the matrix components of the interstitium, there are also cellular components that include fibroblasts, mast cells, tissue macrophages, and lymphocytes. The interstitial network is continuous with the epithelial and endothelial basement membranes. The pulmonary interstitium is thus found throughout the lung, provides structural support for all the pulmonary anatomic components, and allows the changes in lung morphology that occur with respiration.

Interstitial Anatomy

The interstitial network is a continuum that can be divided into three subdivisions depending on its anatomic location.

Axial or Bronchoarterial Interstitium

The axial interstitium surrounds the bronchoarterial bundles and extends from the hila to the respiratory bronchioles in the lung periphery.

Parenchymal or Intralobular Interstitium

The parenchymal interstitium is a fine network of connective tissue fibers within the alveolar walls located between the alveolar and capillary basement membranes and supports the structures of the secondary pulmonary lobule.

Peripheral or Subpleural Interstitium

The peripheral interstitium is located between the pleura and the adjacent lung parenchyma, is continuous with the interlobular septa and the perivenous interstitium, and extends from the lung periphery to the pulmonary hila.

Imaging of Normal Interstitium

Radiography

The normal pulmonary interstitium is not visible on radiography. In fact, visualization of interstitial markings on radiography should suggest the presence of interstitial lung disease. The location of the axial interstitium is inferred by the radiographic identification of the bronchoarterial bundles. The location of the peripheral interstitium is inferred by identification of the pleura and the interlobar fissures.

CT/HRCT

The normal interstitium is also invisible on CT. The location of the axial interstitium is inferred by visualization of the bronchoarterial bundles. The location of the parenchymal interstitium is inferred by identification of the secondary pulmonary lobule, which is bound by pulmonary veins in the interlobular septa and exhibits a central lobular artery. The location of the peripheral interstitium is inferred by visualization of the subpleural regions and the pulmonary veins, which course in the interlobular septa.

Imaging of Abnormal Interstitium

Radiography

Interstitial abnormalities may manifest on radiography as *septal lines*, *peribronchial cuffing*, *perihilar haze*, *reticular opacities*, *nodular opacities*, and *reticulonodular opacities*. *Septal lines* are characterized by thickening of the interlobular septa. *Peribronchial cuffing* is characterized by end-on visualization of bronchi with conspicuous or thick walls. *Perihilar haze* manifests as blurring of central vascular borders. *Reticular opacities* manifest as multiple intersecting irregular lines that collectively resemble the morphology of a net. *Interstitial nodules* or *nodular opacities* are typically small, measure 1-2 mm, and exhibit well-defined borders. *Reticulonodular opacities* result from a combination of interstitial reticular and nodular opacities.

CT/HRCT

Thin-section CT and HRCT are the modalities of choice for the evaluation of the abnormal interstitium, as they allow identification and characterization of the various manifestations of interstitial lung disease. *Peribronchovascular interstitial thickening* manifests as apparent thickening of bronchial walls and may be smooth, nodular, or irregular. It may be associated with dilatation of adjacent bronchi or traction bronchiectasis/bronchiolectasis. Although a few interlobular septa may be normally visible on thin-section CT or HRCT, visualization of frank *interlobular septal thickening* indicates an abnormal interstitium. Etiologies of septal thickening include interstitial fluid, fibrosis, and cellular infiltration. Septal thickening may be smooth (e.g., interstitial edema), nodular (e.g., lymphangitic carcinomatosis), or irregular (e.g., interstitial fibrosis). Ground-glass opacity on a background of septal thickening is known as the *crazy-paving pattern* and is characteristic of alveolar proteinosis. *Parenchymal bands* represent linear interstitial opacities that are 2-5 cm long, 1-3 mm thick, typically contact the pleura, and are characteristic of asbestosis. *Intralobular lines* are often indicative of fibrosis and produce a fine reticular pattern that may be seen in association with interlobular septal thickening and traction bronchiectasis/bronchiolectasis. *Honeycombing* or *honeycomb lung* represents the end-stage of fibrotic lung disease and is characterized by clustered cystic spaces that occur in layers and measure 3-10 mm in diameter with intervening walls of 1-3 mm in thickness. The presence of honeycombing is an important criterion for the diagnosis of the usual interstitial pneumonia (UIP) pattern of interstitial fibrosis and is characteristic of idiopathic pulmonary fibrosis (IPF).

The reticular pattern is optimally evaluated on thin-section CT and HRCT and results from a combination of several components of interstitial fibrosis, including interlobular septal thickening, intralobular lines, &/or honeycombing. The reticulonodular pattern on CT results from a combination of reticular opacities and pulmonary micronodules.

Clinical Presentation

The approach to the diagnosis of interstitial lung disease requires correlation of demographic information, clinical presentation, imaging features, functional abnormalities, and histologic findings. For example, interstitial edema typically affects patients with heart failure who present acutely with dyspnea. The interstitial abnormalities are usually associated with cardiomegaly and pleural effusion. IPF demonstrates an increasing disease prevalence with increasing age. Affected patients present with an insidious onset of exertional dyspnea and chronic cough and may exhibit fine basilar crackles on auscultation and digital clubbing on physical examination. Like other fibrosing interstitial lung diseases, multidisciplinary discussion is of paramount importance in establishing the diagnosis.

Selected References

1. Hansell DM et al: Fleischner Society: glossary of terms for thoracic imaging. Radiology. 246(3):697-722, 2008

Interlobular Septal Thickening

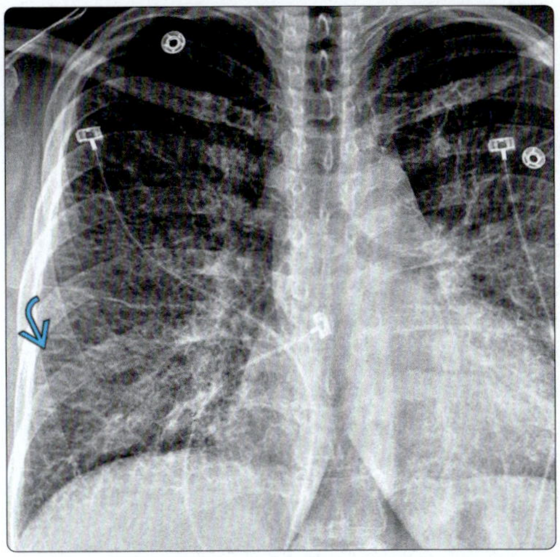

Interlobular Septal Thickening

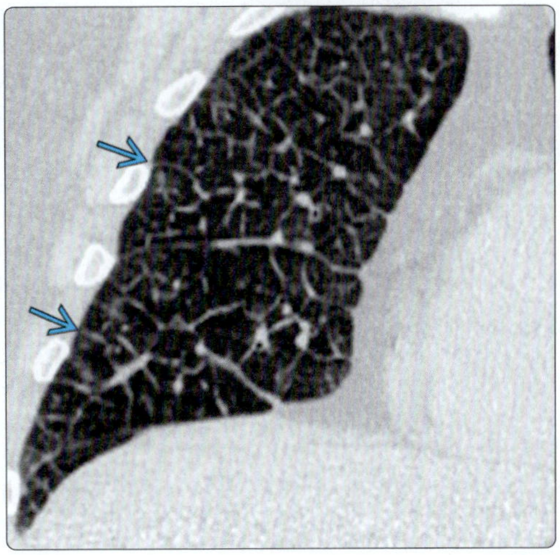

(Left) *PA chest radiograph of a patient with heart failure who presented acutely with dyspnea and chest pain shows profuse bilateral septal lines that represent thick interlobular septa. The thin linear opacities that occur at right angles with the pleura are known as Kerley B lines .* **(Right)** *Coronal NECT of the same patient shows septal lines that outline multiple secondary pulmonary lobules and correspond to the radiographic Kerley B lines. Interstitial edema is characterized by smooth interlobular septal thickening.*

Reticular Opacities

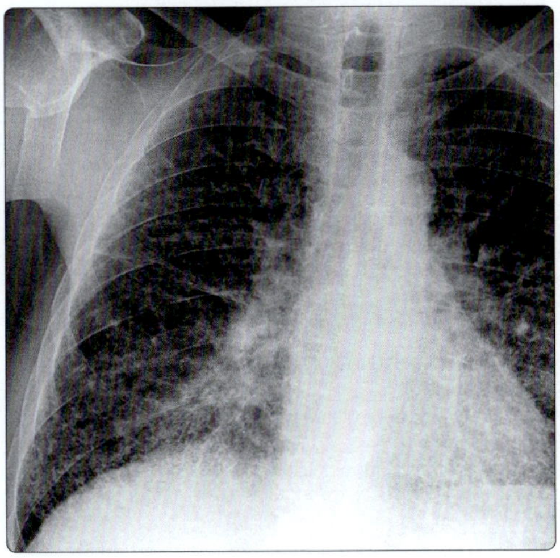

Reticular Opacities

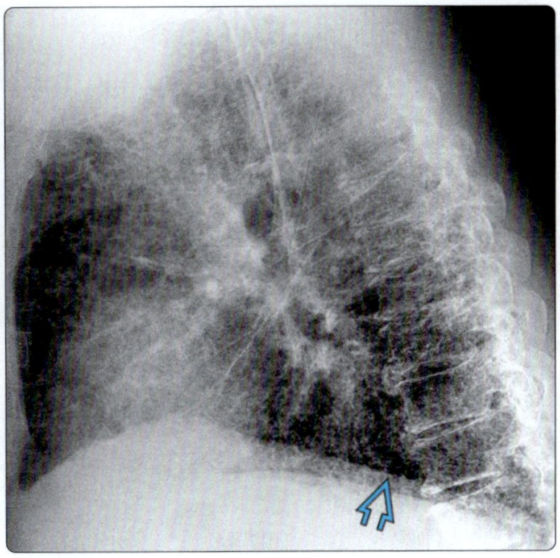

(Left) *Coned-down PA chest radiograph of a patient with idiopathic pulmonary fibrosis (IPF) who presented with an insidious onset of exertional dyspnea and chronic cough shows basilar predominant profuse bilateral reticular opacities that manifest as multiple intersecting fine lines.* **(Right)** *Lateral chest radiograph of the same patient shows diffuse basilar predominant reticular opacities where summation of these fine lines produces a net-like appearance.*

Honeycombing

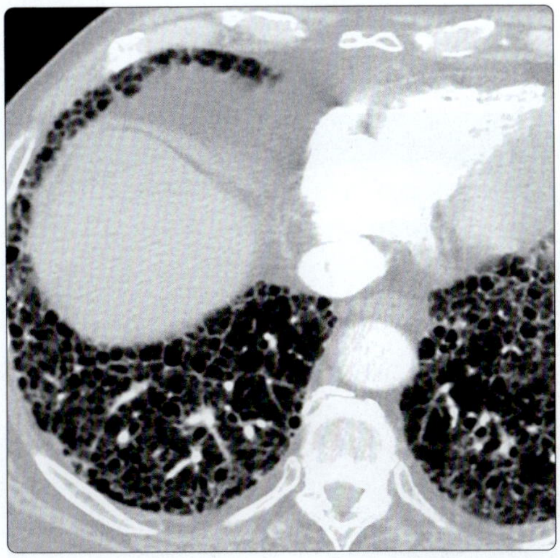

Honeycombing

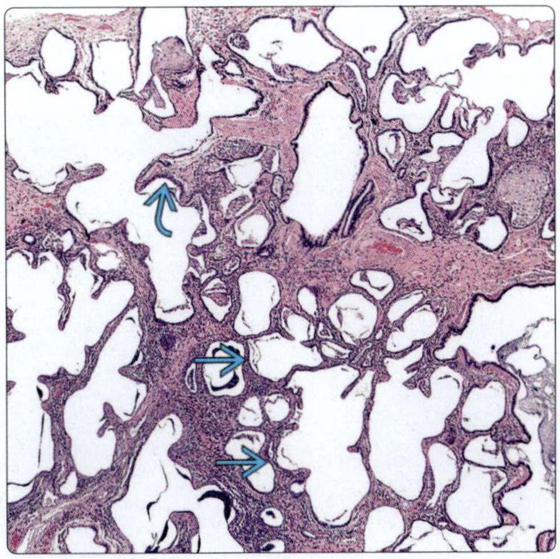

(Left) *Axial CECT of the same patient shows basilar-predominant clustered subpleural honeycomb cysts in layers, a pattern best characterized as typical usual interstitial pneumonia (UIP) CT pattern and consistent with the diagnosis of IPF in this case.* **(Right)** *Low-power photomicrograph (H&E stain) of a specimen from a patient with IPF shows numerous clustered honeycomb cysts lined by columnar respiratory-type epithelium .*

DIFFERENTIAL DIAGNOSIS

Common

- Fibrosing Interstitial Lung Disease (ILD)
  - Subpleural
    - Usual Interstitial Pneumonia
    - Nonspecific Interstitial Pneumonia
      - Idiopathic
      - Connective Tissue Disease-Associated ILD
    - Asbestosis
  - Peribronchovascular
    - Chronic or Cluster 2 Hypersensitivity Pneumonitis
    - Sarcoidosis

Less Common

- Mimics
  - Pulmonary Edema Superimposed on Emphysema
  - Cystic Diseases
    - Lymphangioleiomyomatosis
    - Pulmonary Langerhans Histiocytosis
  - Artifact

ESSENTIAL INFORMATION

Key Differential Diagnosis Issues

- **Reticular opacities**
  - Radiographic and CT descriptor or finding
    - CT: Interlobular septal thickening, intralobular lines, honeycombing, or combination
    - Reticular opacities optimally ascertained with thin-section CT/HRCT
  - **Radiographic reticular opacities may be due to reticulation from ILD or mimics**

Helpful Clues for Common Diagnoses

- **Usual Interstitial Pneumonia (UIP)**
  - Defined by presence of honeycombing; absence of subpleural honeycombing suggests other fibrosing ILDs [e.g., nonspecific interstitial pneumonia (NSIP), hypersensitivity, sarcoidosis]
- **Nonspecific Interstitial Pneumonia (NSIP)**
  - Idiopathic or most commonly connective tissue disease-associated ILD
  - Reticulation is principal radiographic or CT abnormality
    - Typically exhibits apicobasilar gradient and traction bronchiectasis/bronchiolectasis
    - Peribronchovascular predominance with subpleural sparing is specific for NSIP but not always present
  - **Connective Tissue Disease-Associated ILD**
    - History of connective tissue disease is principal differentiator from idiopathic NSIP or UIP
    - NSIP is typical and more common than UIP
    - UIP is more common in rheumatoid arthritis
  - **Asbestosis**
    - Reticulation and honeycombing identical to UIP
    - Coexistent asbestos-related pleural disease or pleural plaques
  - **Chronic or Cluster 2 Hypersensitivity Pneumonitis**
    - Reticulation, honeycombing, and traction bronchiectasis/bronchiolectasis
      - Mid and upper lobe predominant (common); may be subpleural and lower lobe predominant
      - Ancillary findings: Air-trapping (lobular pattern), ground-glass centrilobular nodules
  - **Sarcoidosis**
    - Mid and upper lobe predominant reticulation, honeycombing and traction bronchiectasis/bronchiolectasis
    - Ancillary findings: Lymphadenopathy, calcified lymph nodes (central or egg-shell calcification)

SELECTED REFERENCES

1. Capobianco J et al: Thoracic manifestations of collagen vascular diseases. Radiographics. 32(1):33-50, 2012
2. Hansell DM et al: Fleischner Society: glossary of terms for thoracic imaging. Radiology. 246(3):697-722, 2008
3. Screaton NJ et al: Differential diagnosis in chronic diffuse infiltrative lung disease on high-resolution computed tomography. Semin Roentgenol. 37(1):17-24, 2002

Usual Interstitial Pneumonia

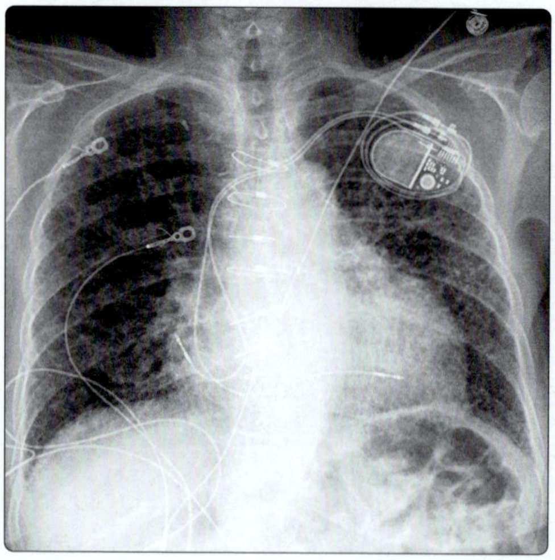

Usual Interstitial Pneumonia

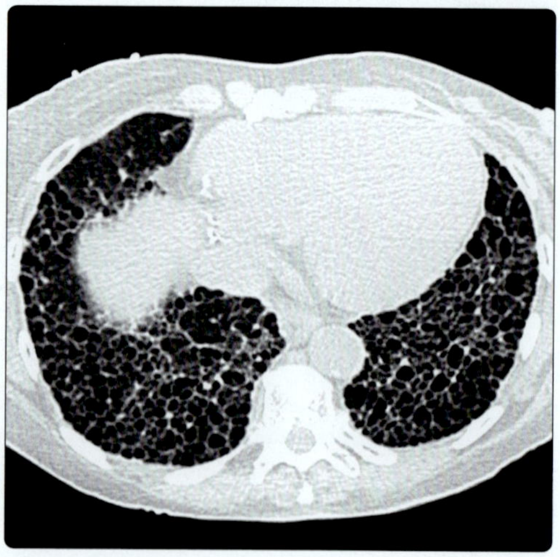

(Left) *PA chest radiograph of a patient with idiopathic pulmonary fibrosis shows low lung volume and diffuse bilateral reticular opacities. Note that the reticulation is more conspicuous in the lower lobes.* **(Right)** *Axial HRCT of the same patient shows extensive basilar-predominant subpleural honeycombing, consistent with usual interstitial pneumonia. When this pattern of interstitial lung disease is present, the diagnosis of usual interstitial pneumonia can be made with confidence, and lung biopsy confirmation is not needed.*

Nonspecific Interstitial Pneumonia

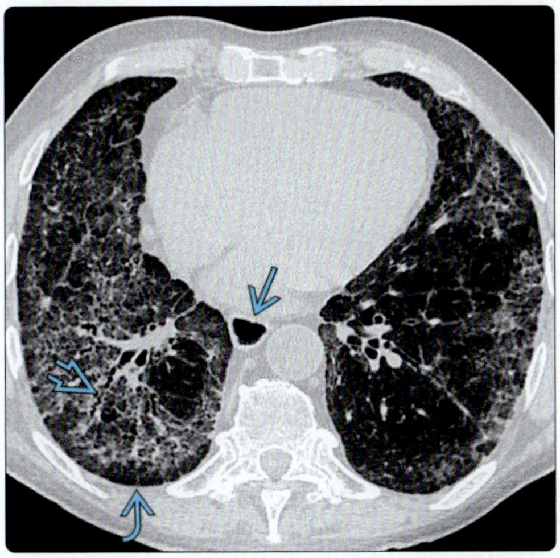

Chronic or Cluster 2 Hypersensitivity Pneumonitis

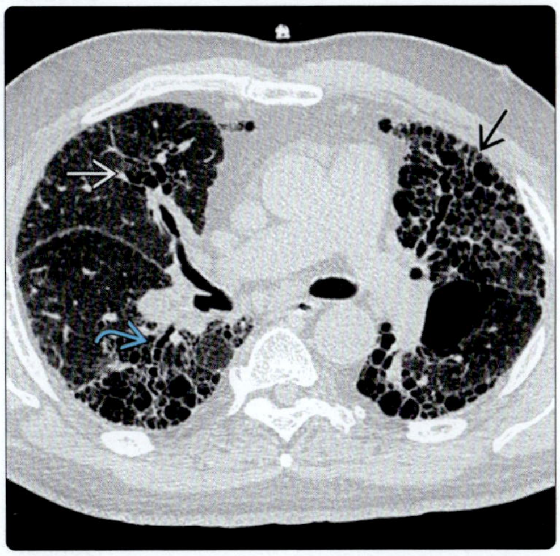

(Left) *Axial HRCT of a patient with scleroderma and associated nonspecific interstitial pneumonia (NSIP) shows basilar reticulation without honeycombing and traction bronchiectasis . Note dilated esophagus and subpleural sparing , the latter a specific imaging finding of NSIP.* **(Right)** *Axial HRCT of a patient with chronic or cluster 2 hypersensitivity pneumonitis shows peribronchovascular and subpleural reticulation and honeycombing with associated traction bronchiectasis .*

Pulmonary Edema Superimposed on Emphysema

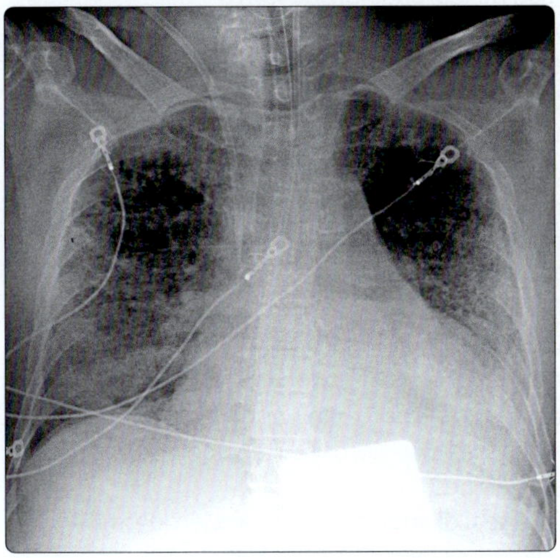

Pulmonary Edema Superimposed on Emphysema

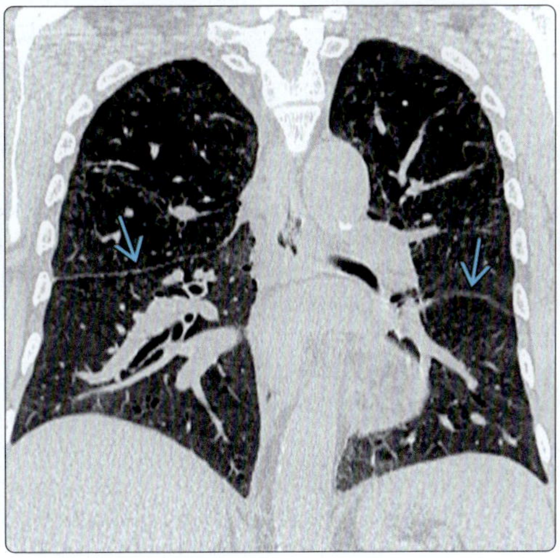

(Left) *PA chest radiograph of a patient with emphysema and pulmonary edema shows diffuse bilateral reticular opacities that are difficult to differentiate from diffuse fibrosing interstitial lung disease on radiography.* **(Right)** *Coronal NECT of the same patient obtained a few hours after the chest radiograph and following treatment with diuretics shows upper lobe predominant centrilobular emphysema and scattered ground-glass opacities. Thick interlobar fissures are related to residual subpleural edema.*

Lymphangioleiomyomatosis

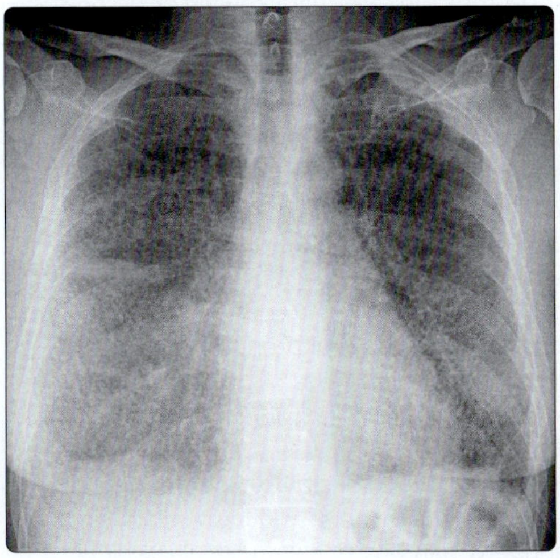

Lymphangioleiomyomatosis

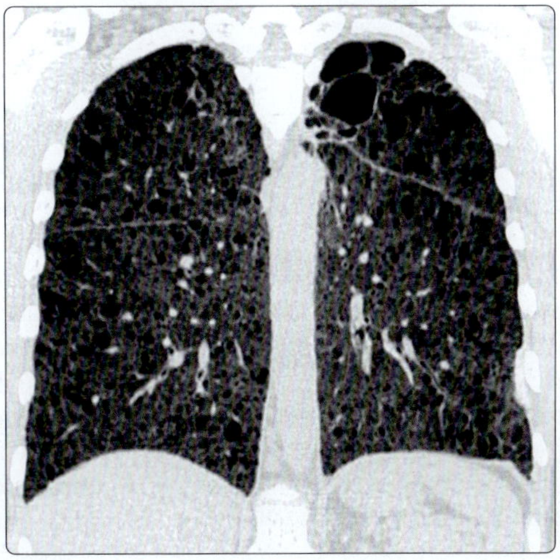

(Left) *PA chest radiograph of a woman with lymphangioleiomyomatosis shows diffuse bilateral pulmonary reticulation, which is difficult to differentiate from diffuse fibrosing interstitial lung disease on radiography.* **(Right)** *Coronal HRCT of the same patient shows diffuse bilateral thin-walled cysts with normal intervening lung parenchyma. Cystic lung disease may mimic fibrosing interstitial lung disease on radiography. CT is the imaging study of choice for evaluation of diffuse lung disease.*

DIFFERENTIAL DIAGNOSIS

Common

- Subpleural
  - Usual Interstitial Pneumonia
  - Nonspecific Interstitial Pneumonia
  - Combined Pulmonary Fibrosis and Emphysema
- Peribronchovascular
  - Chronic or Cluster 2 Hypersensitivity Pneumonitis
  - Sarcoidosis

Less Common

- Subpleural
  - Asbestosis
- Anterior
  - Acute Respiratory Distress Syndrome Related
  - Unilateral Absence of Pulmonary Artery

Rare but Important

- Peribronchovascular
  - Hemosiderosis
- Hermansky-Pudlak Syndrome
- Sickle Cell Disease

ESSENTIAL INFORMATION

Key Differential Diagnosis Issues

- Honeycombing
  - Implies mature, end-stage, and irreversible pulmonary fibrosis
  - May be microscopic on histology and not appreciable on imaging
  - Term preferably used to refer to CT findings and only when manifestations are characteristic given prognostic implications
  - Poor prognostic indicator
- Radiography
  - Closely approximated ring shadows
  - Size: 3-10 mm
  - Wall thickness: 1-3 mm
- CT
  - Clustered cysts that share well-defined walls
  - Cyst size: Average 3-10 mm; as large as 2.5 cm
  - Wall thickness 1-3 mm
  - Stacked rows of cysts
  - Ancillary findings
    - Bronchiectasis &/or bronchiolectasis
    - Reticulation
    - Ground-glass opacities
  - Differentiation from paraseptal emphysema
    - 1 layer of cyst-like structures (as opposed to stacked cysts)
  - Differentiation from bronchiectasis in scleroderma
    - Scleroderma + NSIP often manifests with traction bronchiectasis that is out of proportion to pulmonary involvement and may simulate honeycombing on axial imaging
    - Differentiation relies on multiplanar CT demonstrating that cyst-like structures on axial imaging exhibit tubular or branching morphology on sagittal or coronal imaging

Helpful Clues for Common Diagnoses

- **Usual Interstitial Pneumonia (UIP)**
  - Histologic pattern of pulmonary fibrosis
  - Specific imaging findings
    - Subpleural and basilar honeycombing &/or reticulation
    - Apicobasilar gradient (i.e., lower lobe predominant)
    - Lower lobe subpleural honeycombing is diagnostic of UIP, and biopsy is not required
  - Other causes of UIP pattern
    - Autoimmune diseases (e.g., rheumatoid arthritis, systemic lupus erythematosus)
    - Pneumoconiosis (e.g., asbestosis)
    - Allergic alveolitis (i.e., hypersensitivity pneumonitis)
    - Drug toxicity
    - Familial pulmonary fibrosis
  - UIP is most common cause of honeycombing
- **Nonspecific Interstitial Pneumonia (NSIP)**
  - Histologic pattern of interstitial fibrosis characterized by variable amounts of interstitial inflammation and fibrosis with cellular, mixed, and fibrotic forms
  - History of autoimmune disease
    - Progressive systemic sclerosis (scleroderma)
    - Mixed connective tissue disease
    - Polymyositis
  - Other causes of NSIP pattern
    - Idiopathic
    - Drug toxicity
    - Familial
  - Specific findings
    - Subpleural and basilar reticulation; absent or sparse honeycombing
    - Apicobasilar gradient (i.e., lower lobe predominant)
    - Peribronchovascular fibrosis with subpleural sparing
    - Ancillary findings
      - Esophageal dilation common in scleroderma and mixed connective tissue disease
- **Combined Pulmonary Fibrosis and Emphysema**
  - Coexistence of upper lobe emphysema and lower lobe pulmonary fibrosis clinically characterized by dyspnea and abnormalities of gas exchange
  - CT
    - Upper lobe predominant centrilobular, paraseptal, &/or panlobular emphysema
    - Decreased lung attenuation ± bullae
    - Subpleural reticulation &/or honeycombing with apicobasilar gradient
    - Subpleural ground-glass opacities with apicobasilar gradient
    - Traction bronchiectasis &/or bronchiolectasis
    - Architectural distortion
    - Dilated pulmonary trunk indicating pulmonary hypertension
- **Chronic or Cluster 2 Hypersensitivity Pneumonitis**
  - Fibrosis resulting from hypersensitivity reaction to organic antigens, haptens, or low-molecular-weight inorganic compounds
    - Mold and avian antigens most common causes
    - Inorganic compounds include isocyanate (industrial paints)

- Specific findings
  - Mid and upper lung zone peribronchovascular fibrosis (i.e., reticulation &/or honeycombing, traction bronchiectasis/bronchiolectasis, architectural distortion)
    - Identical findings may occur in chronic/end-stage sarcoidosis (i.e., subpleural reticular opacities &/or honeycombing with traction bronchiectasis/bronchiolectasis)
  - Findings identical to those of UIP and NSIP are also common
- Ancillary findings
  - Lobular foci of air-trapping
  - Centrilobular ground-glass micronodules

- **Sarcoidosis**
  - Honeycombing may occur with end-stage pulmonary involvement
  - Honeycombing tends to be peribronchovascular and involve mid and upper lung zones
    - May be associated with upper lobe peribronchovascular nodules or masses (i.e., progressive massive fibrosis) ± calcification
  - Subpleural honeycombing may coexist
  - Perilymphatic micronodules
  - Lymphadenopathy or calcified lymph nodes (diffuse, central, or eggshell calcification)

Helpful Clues for Less Common Diagnoses

- **Asbestosis**
  - Interstitial fibrosis secondary to asbestos exposure; identical to UIP
  - CT
    - Early fibrosis may appear as subpleural curvilinear opacities; may progress to classic findings of UIP
    - Asbestos-related pleural disease
      - Discontinuous partially calcified pleural plaques
      - Pleural effusion &/or thickening
    - Rounded atelectasis
- **Acute Respiratory Distress Syndrome (ARDS) Related**
  - Remote history of ARDS
  - CT
    - Subpleural honeycombing involving anterior mid and upper lung zones
- **Unilateral Absence of Pulmonary Artery (UAPA)**
  - CT
    - Abrupt cut-off of pulmonary artery
    - Small affected lung with diffuse areas of fibrosis &/or honeycombing
    - Bronchiectasis
    - Abundant arterial collaterals from adjacent sources (e.g., internal mammary and subclavian arteries)

Helpful Clues for Rare Diagnoses

- **Hermansky-Pudlak Syndrome**
  - Autosomal recessive disorder
    - Oculocutaneous albinism
    - Platelet dysfunction
    - Granulomatous colitis
  - Largest patient cohort in Puerto Rico
  - CT
    - Early
      - Ground-glass opacities
      - Interlobular septal thickening
      - Reticular opacities
      - Perihilar fibrosis
    - Advanced
      - Subpleural cysts
      - Peribronchial thickening
      - Traction bronchiectasis/bronchiolectasis
      - Honeycombing
- **Sickle Cell Disease**
  - History of sickle cell disease with recurrent episodes of acute chest pain
  - CT
    - Basilar predominant reticular opacities
    - Honeycombing (uncommon)
    - Osseous abnormalities (e.g., H-shaped vertebrae)

Usual Interstitial Pneumonia

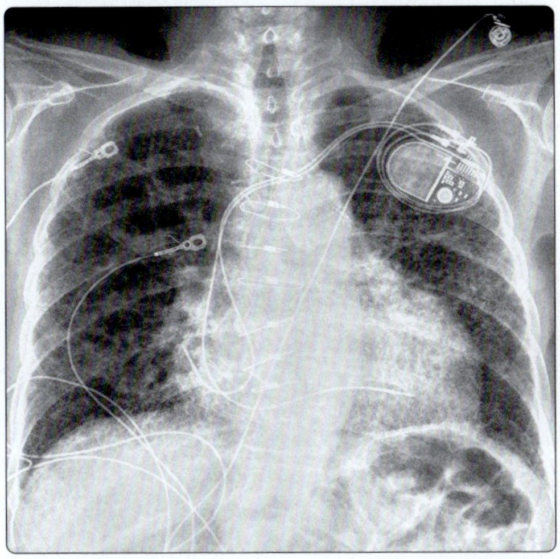

Usual Interstitial Pneumonia

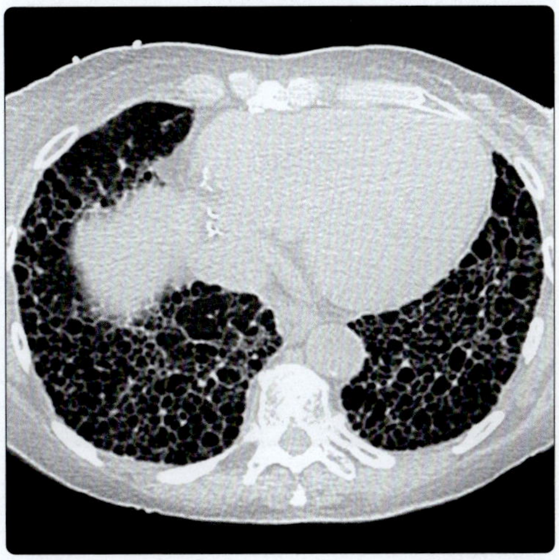

(Left) *PA chest radiograph of a patient with idiopathic pulmonary fibrosis shows low lung volume and diffuse lower lung zone predominant reticular opacities.* **(Right)** *Axial HRCT of the same patient shows subpleural and lower lobe predominant profuse honeycombing. These imaging findings suffice to establish the diagnosis of usual interstitial pneumonia (UIP) without the need for a pulmonary biopsy. Idiopathic pulmonary fibrosis carries a poor prognosis.*

(**Left**) *Sagittal HRCT of the same patient highlights the characteristic apicobasilar gradient of honeycombing, a finding required for the imaging diagnosis of UIP. Note that the most severe involvement is in the subpleural lower lobes.* (**Right**) *Axial prone HRCT of the same patient shows persistent basilar honeycombing. Prone imaging is important for differentiation of dependent atelectasis from basilar interstitial lung disease, as the former typically resolves on prone imaging.*

Usual Interstitial Pneumonia

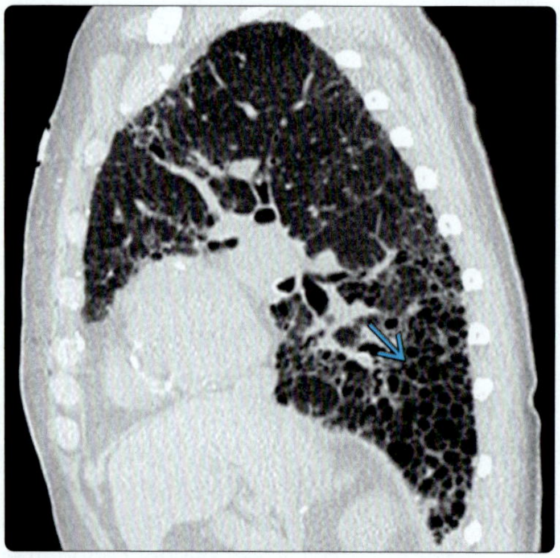

Usual Interstitial Pneumonia

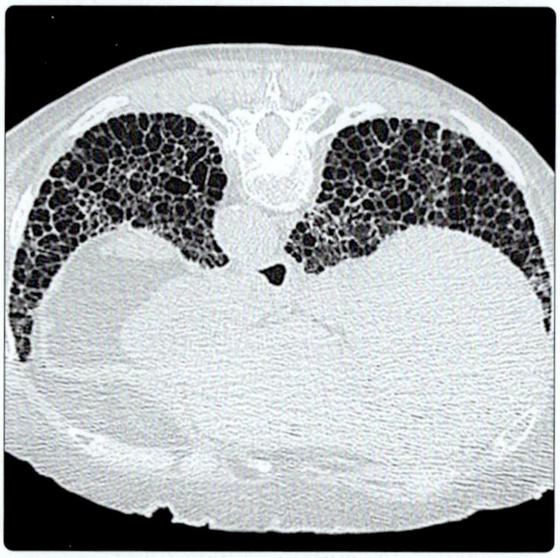

(**Left**) *Axial HRCT of a patient with combined pulmonary fibrosis and emphysema shows multifocal subpleural reticulation and honeycombing. Note the right pneumothorax with a right chest tube in place. The pneumothorax resulted from spontaneous rupture of a peripheral pulmonary bulla.* (**Right**) *Sagittal HRCT of the same patient shows lower lobe predominant subpleural reticulation and honeycombing and upper lobe predominant emphysema.*

Combined Pulmonary Fibrosis and Emphysema

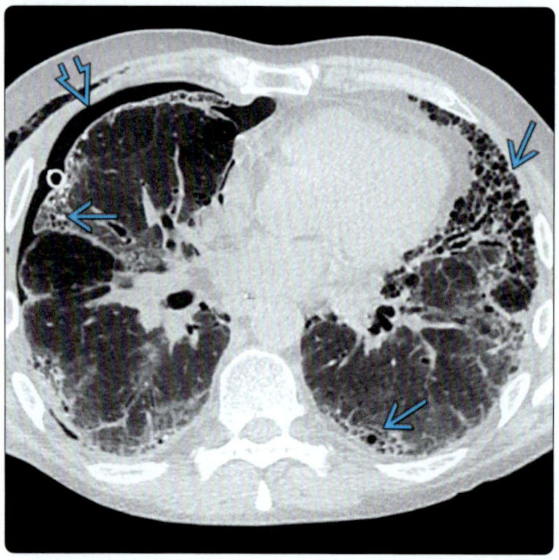

Combined Pulmonary Fibrosis and Emphysema

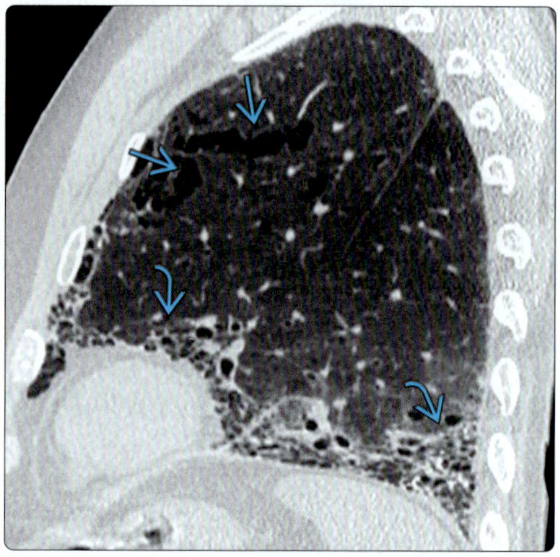

(**Left**) *Axial HRCT of a patient with chronic or cluster 2 hypersensitivity pneumonitis shows extensive subpleural and peribronchovascular honeycombing and traction bronchiectasis, which is most pronounced in the upper lobes.* (**Right**) *Axial prone HRCT of a patient with end-stage sarcoidosis shows exuberant peribronchovascular honeycombing and traction bronchiectasis. Note that while the areas of fibrosis extend to the pleura, they are more prominent along the peribronchovascular interstitium.*

Chronic or Cluster 2 Hypersensitivity Pneumonitis

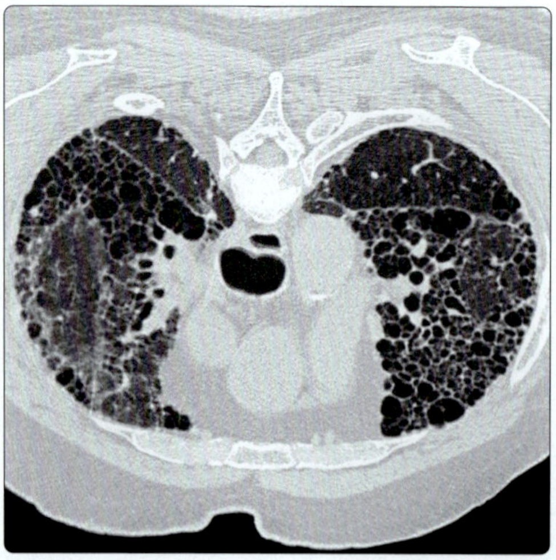

Sarcoidosis

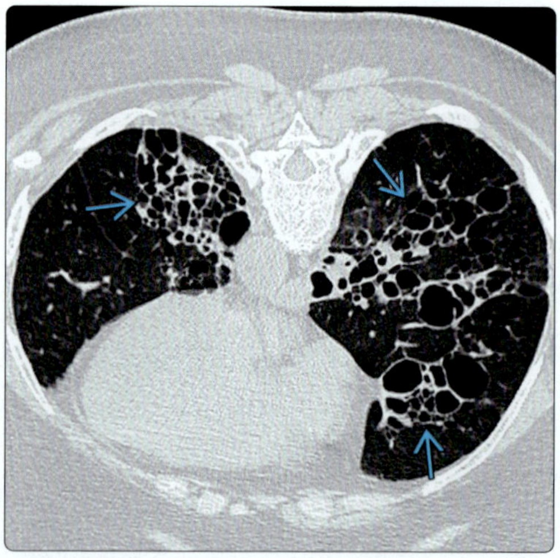

Asbestosis

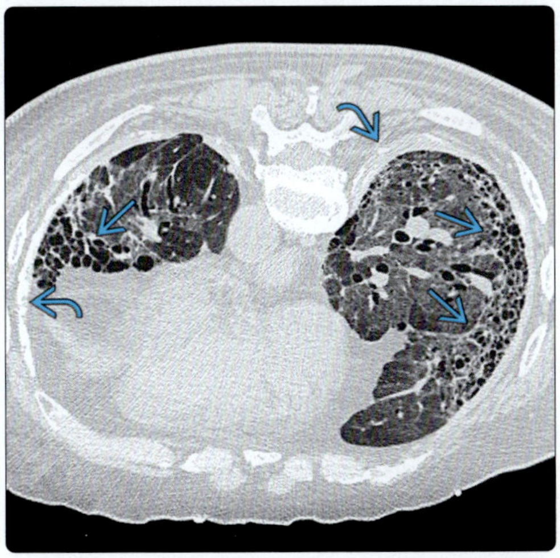

Acute Respiratory Distress Syndrome Related

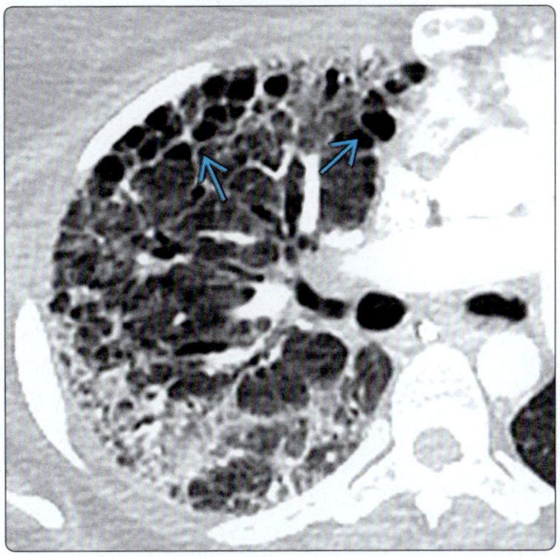

(Left) *Axial prone HRCT shows findings of asbestosis characterized by lower lobe ground-glass opacities, honeycombing ➔, and traction bronchiectasis. Note bilateral calcified pleural plaques ➔.* **(Right)** *Axial CECT of a patient with late-stage adult respiratory distress syndrome shows anterior upper lobe subpleural honeycombing ➔. This distribution of honeycombing is postulated to result from oxygen toxicity in the nondependent lung, which is preferentially ventilated in the supine position.*

Unilateral Absence of Pulmonary Artery

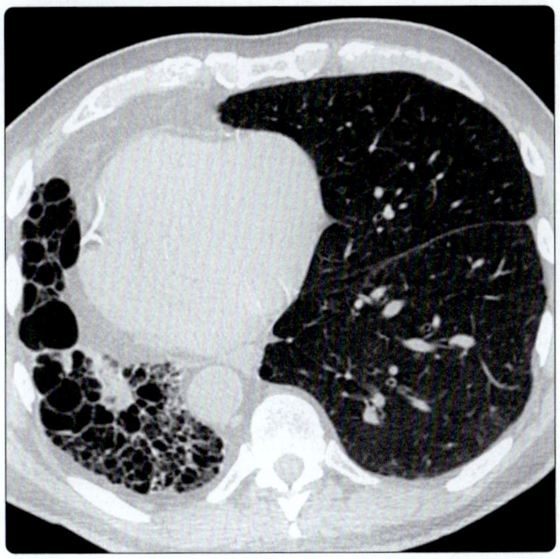

Unilateral Absence of Pulmonary Artery

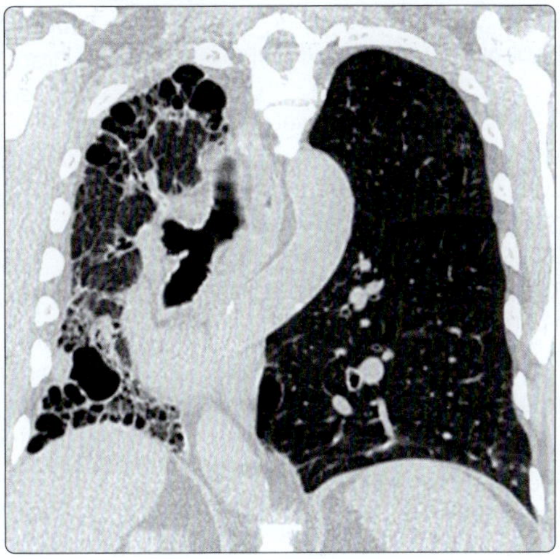

(Left) *Axial NECT of a patient with unilateral absence of the right pulmonary artery shows extensive honeycombing involving the right lung. This is a common ancillary finding that often occurs in the setting of unilateral absence of the pulmonary artery.* **(Right)** *Coronal HRCT of the same patient shows extensive right lung subpleural honeycombing. It is postulated that resultant pulmonary hypoperfusion results in abnormal lung growth and eventually leads to pulmonary fibrosis and honeycombing.*

Hermansky-Pudlak Syndrome

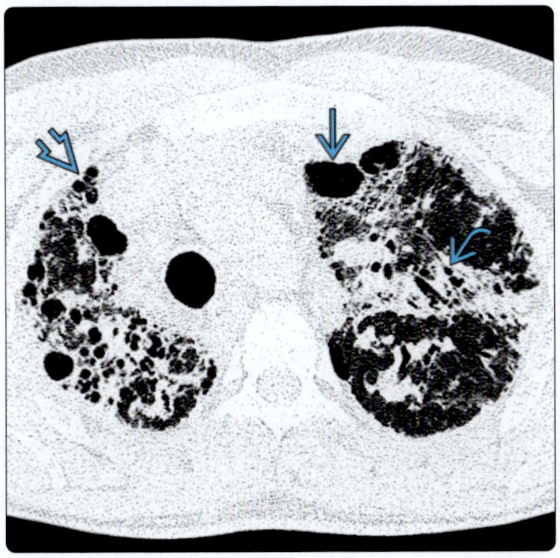

Sickle Cell Disease

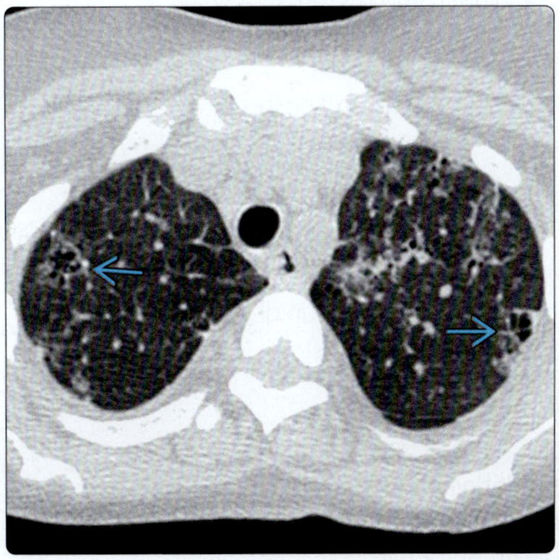

(Left) *Axial HRCT of a 43-year-old man with oculocutaneous albinism and chronic progressive dyspnea secondary to Hermansky-Pudlak syndrome shows advanced bilateral upper lobe pulmonary fibrosis characterized by architectural distortion, subpleural cysts ➔, honeycombing ➔, and traction bronchiectasis ➔.* **(Right)** *Axial NECT of a patient with sickle cell disease shows multifocal areas of bilateral honeycombing ➔. This is a relatively uncommon complication in patients with sickle cell disease.*

Upper Lung Zone Predominant Lung Disease

DIFFERENTIAL DIAGNOSIS

Common

- Silicosis
- Sarcoidosis
- Tuberculosis
- Hypersensitivity Pneumonitis
- Centrilobular Emphysema

Less Common

- Allergic Bronchopulmonary Aspergillosis
- Pulmonary Langerhans Cell Histiocytosis
- Neurogenic Pulmonary Edema

Rare but Important

- Chronic Eosinophilic Pneumonia
- Pleuropulmonary Fibroelastosis

ESSENTIAL INFORMATION

Key Differential Diagnosis Issues

- Lung presents disparities between apex and bases in its ventilatory:perfusion ratio and in lymphatic flow that explains greater involvement of upper versus lower lung zones
- In erect individual, lung apex is relatively overventilated and base is relatively overperfused
- Lymphatic clearance is relatively lower in pulmonary apices, which explains prevalence of alterations in upper lobes in patients with granulomatous diseases
- Greater relative ventilation of apices explains prevalence of alterations in upper lobes in patients with diseases of inhalation nature

Helpful Clues for Common Diagnoses

- **Silicosis**
  - Results from inhalation of crystalline silicon dioxide (silica) and its accumulation in lungs
  - Simple silicosis
    - Silicotic nodules in lungs
    - Abnormalities develop 10-20 years after exposure
    - Multiple small nodules ranging from 1-10 mm (typically 2-5 mm)
    - Centrilobular and perilymphatic distribution
    - Upper lung zone predominance (apical and posterior segments)
    - Subpleural nodularity
    - Hilar and mediastinal lymphadenopathy (eggshell calcification in 5%)
  - Complicated silicosis
    - Coalescence of silicotic nodules and distortion of pulmonary architecture
    - Nodule > 10 mm
    - Conglomerate masses
      - Typically symmetric
      - Lateral margin sharply defined and medial inner edge less well defined
    - Associated paracicatricial emphysema
- **Sarcoidosis**
  - Systemic chronic granulomatous disease characterized by noncaseating granulomas
  - Perilymphatic micronodules (75-90%)
    - Peribronchovascular, subpleural, and interlobular septa
    - Rounded, 2-4 mm
    - Upper and mid lung zone predominance
  - Fibrosis (20%)
    - Linear opacities, parenchymal bands, traction bronchiectasis, and architectural distortion
  - Large nodules and masses
    - Related to coalescence of granulomas
    - Diameter 1-4 cm
    - Perihilar and peripheral distribution
    - Surrounded by small satellite nodules (galaxy sign)
  - Consolidation (10-20%)
    - Secondary to confluent micronodules compressing alveoli
    - Blurred margins radiating from hilum toward periphery
    - Bilateral and symmetric, often with air bronchogram
  - Lymphadenopathy
    - Bilateral, symmetric hilar and right paratracheal
    - Calcification (20% at diagnosis)
- **Tuberculosis**
  - Granulomatous disease caused by *Mycobacterium tuberculosis*
  - Clinical course often chronic with symptoms
    - Productive cough
    - Hemoptysis
    - Weight loss
    - Fever
    - Night sweats
  - Epidemiologic studies have shown that radiologic manifestations are related to patient's immune status rather than time of acquisition of infection
  - Immunocompetent adults with tuberculosis due to reactivation or reinfection, alterations in upper lobes are predominant
  - According to time of disease, changes evolve from areas of consolidation (exudative form) to destruction of parenchyma with nodules, bronchiectasis, and cavitation (fibrotic form)
    - Upper lobe apical and posterior segments and lower lobe superior segment predominance
    - Small centrilobular micronodules and branching opacities (tree-in-bud pattern)
    - Bronchial wall thickening
    - Tuberculoma (focal nodule/mass)
- **Hypersensitivity Pneumonitis**
  - Immunologically mediated lung disease resulting from response to inhaled antigen to which patient has been previously sensitized
  - Acute/cluster 1 HP (duration of symptoms usually < 6 months)
    - Upper and mid lung zone predominance
    - Ground-glass opacities
    - Poorly defined centrilobular nodules
    - Mosaic attenuation/air-trapping
  - Chronic/cluster 2 HP (duration of symptoms usually > 6 months)
    - Upper and mid lung zone predominant fibrosis

- Reticular opacities, architectural distortion, and traction bronchiectasis ± honeycombing
  - Peribronchovascular or subpleural distribution
- Centrilobular nodules
- Mosaic attenuation/air-trapping
- Relative sparing of bases

- **Centrilobular Emphysema**
  - Loss of septa around respiratory bronchioles (middle of secondary pulmonary lobule)
  - Destruction of respiratory bronchioles progresses distally and extends to nearby alveoli with relative respect for alveolar sacs and peripheral alveoli (adjacent to septa)
  - Strongly associated with cigarette smoking
  - Hyperlucent foci without well-defined walls, surrounded by normal lung
  - Upper lung zone predominance
  - Early centrilobular emphysema
    - Central punctate density representing centrilobular arteriole ("central dot" sign)
  - Advanced centrilobular emphysema
    - Destruction extends to entire pulmonary lobule with fusion of several lobules, which can coalesce with bullous formation

Helpful Clues for Less Common Diagnoses

- **Allergic Bronchopulmonary Aspergillosis**
  - Immunologic pulmonary disorder caused by hypersensitivity to *Aspergillus fumigatus*
  - Predisposing conditions
    - Asthma, cystic fibrosis
  - Aspergillus skin test positive
  - Elevated total IgE levels (> 1000 IU/mL)
  - IgG antibodies against *A. fumigatus* in serum
  - Total eosinophil count > 500 cells/μL
  - Central bronchiectasis
    - Upper lung zone predominance
    - Mucoid impaction (finger-in-glove sign)
      - Secretions may be hyperattenuating on CT due to presence of calcium oxalate

- **Pulmonary Langerhans Cell Histiocytosis**
  - Isolated form of Langerhans cell histiocytosis occurring in smokers characterized by granulomatous infiltration of distal bronchial walls with cells derived from myeloid dendritic cells (i.e., Langerhans cells)
  - Early-stage disease
    - Nodules (upper lung zone predominance, centrilobular, 1-10 mm, stellate morphology, ± cavitation)
  - Late-stage disease
    - Cysts (upper lung zone predominance, thin or thick nodular walls, bizarre or irregular shapes, variable sizes)
- **Neurogenic Pulmonary Edema**
  - Pulmonary edema in setting of sudden neurologic event (e.g., subarachnoid hemorrhage, intracranial hemorrhage, head injury, stroke, and seizure)
  - Although traditionally it was considered mixed edema, in most patients main mechanism is hydrostatic
  - Multilobar consolidation with upper lung zone predominance

Helpful Clues for Rare Diagnoses

- **Chronic Eosinophilic Pneumonia**
  - Respiratory symptoms > 2 weeks
  - Lung and blood eosinophilia
  - Ground-glass opacities/consolidation
    - Bilateral, nonsegmental, symmetric
    - Peripheral and upper lung zone predominance (photographic negative of pulmonary edema)
  - Parenchymal bands parallel to pleura
- **Pleuropulmonary Fibroelastosis**
  - Rare entity characterized by upper lung zone predominant elastotic fibrosis involving pleura and subpleural lung parenchyma
  - Idiopathic or associated with lung transplantation, bone marrow transplantation, chemotherapy, occupational dust exposure, infection, and autoimmune disease
  - Upper lung zone predominant pleuroparenchymal thickening (4-15 mm)
  - Upper lung zone volume loss; dense subpleural opacities

Silicosis

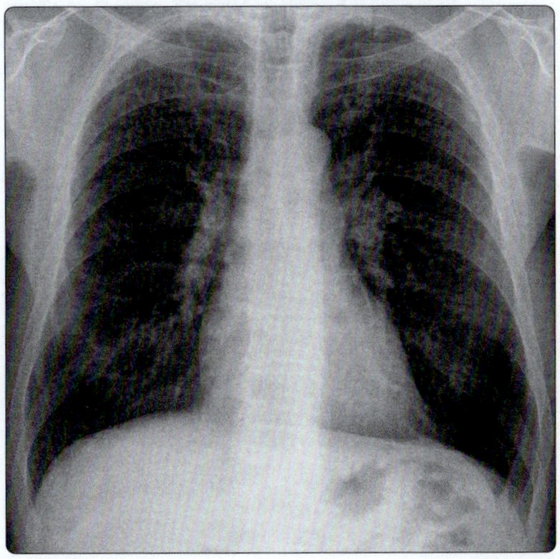

Silicosis

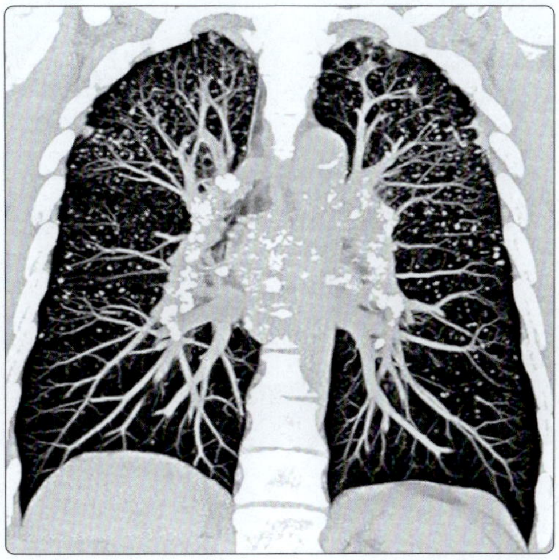

(Left) *Frontal chest radiograph of a 72-year-old man with simple silicosis shows bilateral upper lung zone predominant micronodules.* **(Right)** *Coronal MIP of the same patient shows bilateral upper lobe predominant centrilobular and perilymphatic small nodules, many of which appear calcified. Note also extensive calcified bilateral hilar and mediastinal lymph nodes. Silicosis is a predominantly upper lobe disease initially presenting with micronodules and eventually complicating into progressive massive fibrosis.*

(Left) *Axial NECT of a 42-year-old woman with sarcoidosis shows perilymphatic micronodules and beaded interlobular septal thickening .* **(Right)** *Coronal NECT of the same patient shows upper lobe predominant perilymphatic micronodules and beaded interlobular septal thickening. Sarcoidosis is an inflammatory granulomatous disease and a classic example of a disease with perilymphatic distribution (i.e., both peribronchovascular and peripheral interstitium).*

Sarcoidosis

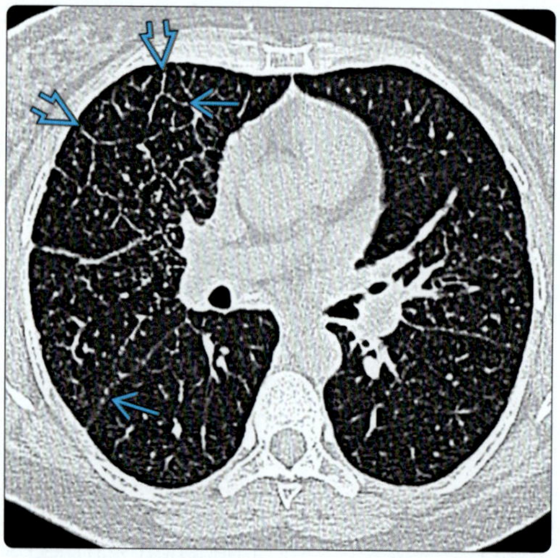

Sarcoidosis

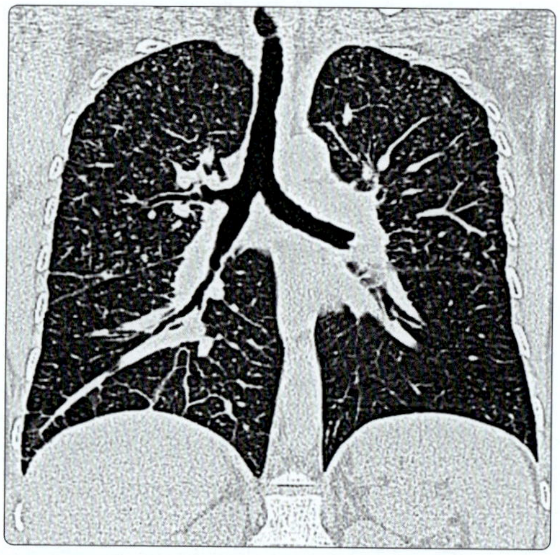

(Left) *PA chest radiograph of a 41-year-old man with the postprimary pattern of tuberculosis shows upper lung zone predominant opacities, small nodules, and cavitation .* **(Right)** *Coronal NECT of the same patient shows upper lobe predominant centrilobular micronodules with discrete tree-in-bud opacities , bronchiectasis , and cavitary nodules . The postprimary pattern of tuberculosis tends to occur in patients with relatively preserved immunity.*

Tuberculosis

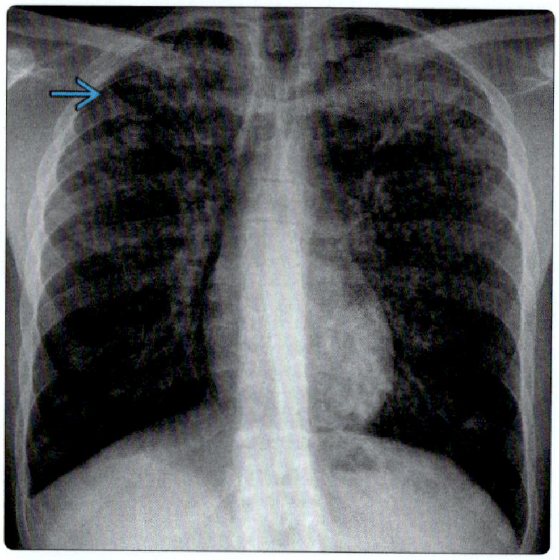

Tuberculosis

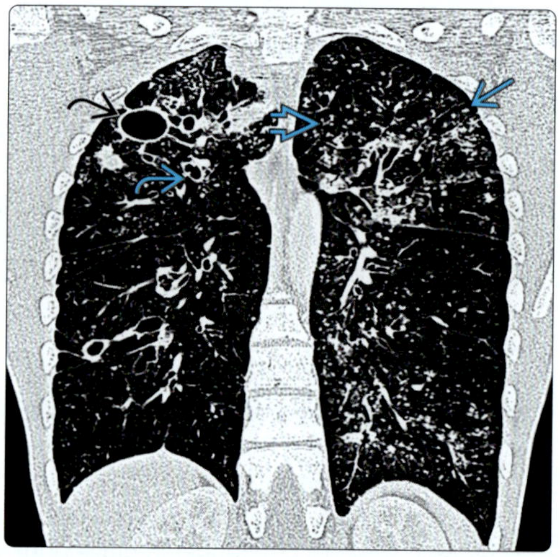

(Left) *Axial HRCT of a 66-year-old man with hypersensitivity pneumonitis chronic/cluster 2 shows upper lobe predominant traction bronchiectasis and honeycombing . This distribution of honeycombing should be contrasted with UIP, which involves the subpleural lower lobes predominantly.* **(Right)** *Coronal HRCT of the same patient shows upper lobe predominant traction bronchiectasis and honeycombing . Oftentimes, HP is indistinguishable from UIP based on imaging abnormalities.*

Hypersensitivity Pneumonitis

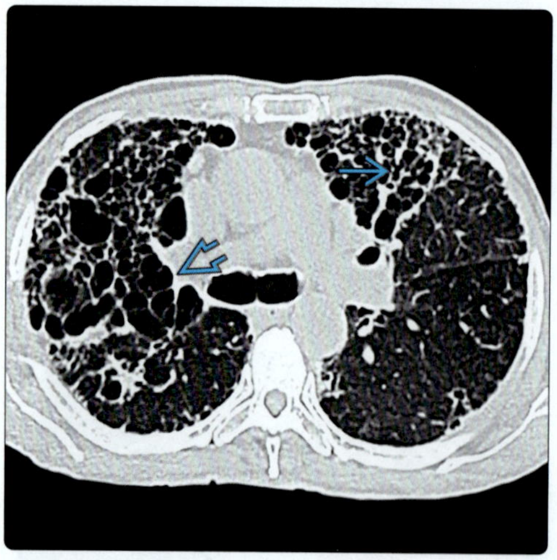

Hypersensitivity Pneumonitis

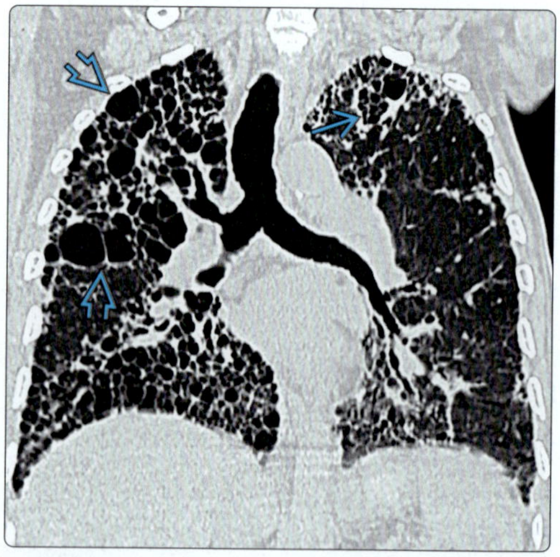

Centrilobular Emphysema

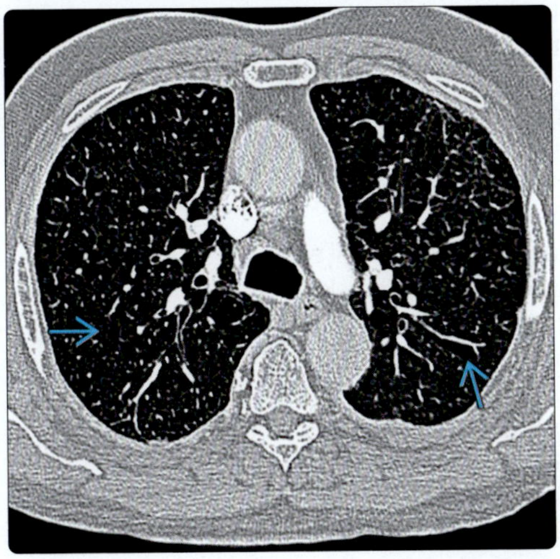

Centrilobular Emphysema

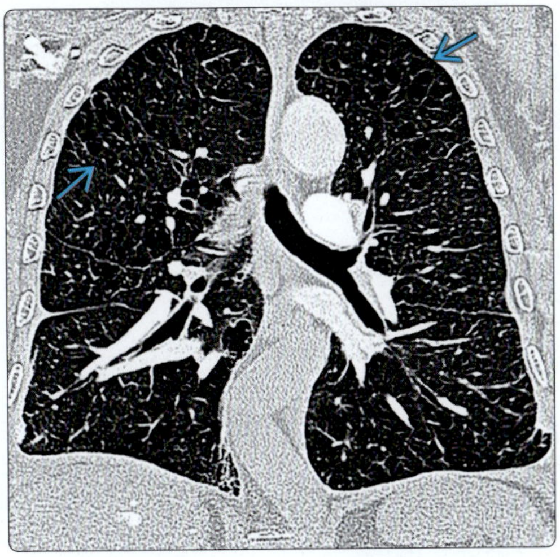

(Left) *Axial CECT of a patient with centrilobular emphysema shows bilateral upper lobe lucencies without perceptible walls →, characteristic of emphysema and a feature that allows differentiation from cysts.* **(Right)** *Coronal CECT of the same patient shows upper lobe predominant lucencies from emphysema without perceptible walls →. These lucencies often exhibit a central nodule (i.e., central dot sign) from centrilobular arteries, another useful sign to differentiate from cysts.*

Pulmonary Langerhans Cell Histiocytosis

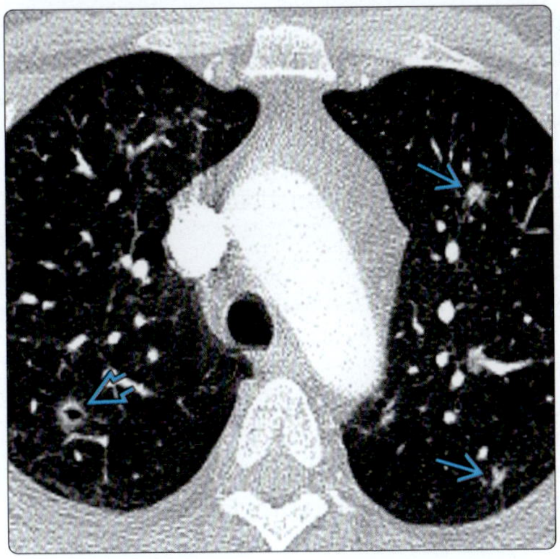

Pulmonary Langerhans Cell Histiocytosis

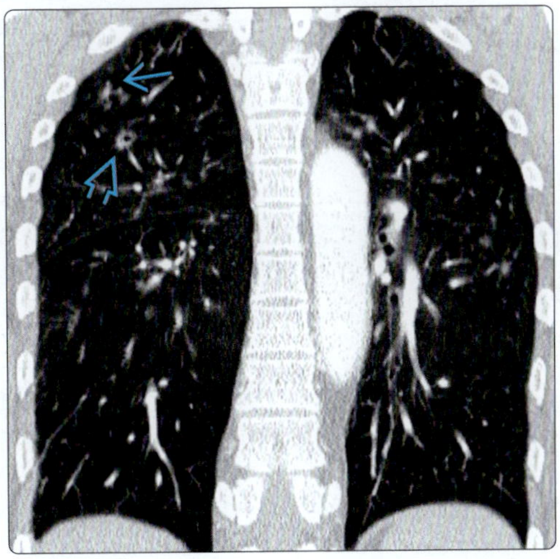

(Left) *Axial NECT of a patient with pulmonary Langerhans cell histiocytosis shows left upper lobe stellate nodules →, at least 1 of which appears cavitary in nature ⇒.* **(Right)** *Coronal CECT of the same patient shows upper lobe predominant stellate → and cavitary ⇒ nodules. Pulmonary Langerhans cell histiocytosis is a smoking-related disease with predominantly upper lobe centrilobular nodules classically exhibiting bizarre shapes and cavitation.*

Chronic Eosinophilic Pneumonia

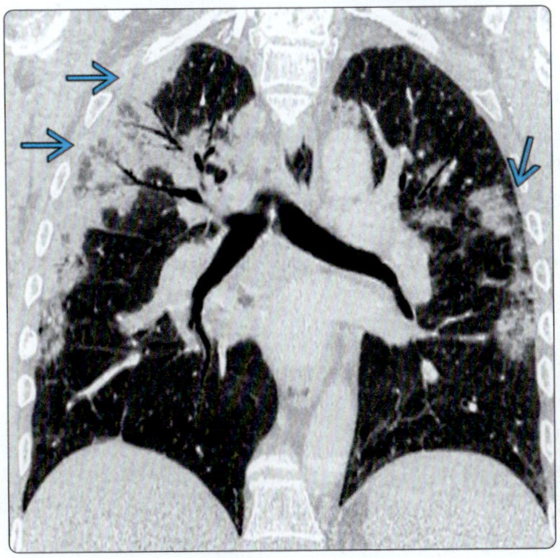

Pleuropulmonary Fibroelastosis

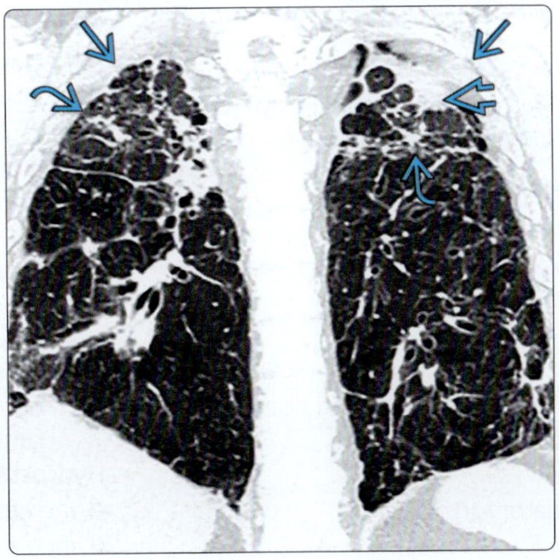

(Left) *Coronal NECT of a patient with chronic eosinophilic pneumonia shows upper lobe predominant subpleural consolidation → with a pattern often referred to as the photographic negative of pulmonary edema.* **(Right)** *Coronal NECT of a patient with pleuropulmonary fibroelastosis shows upper lobe pleuroparenchymal thickening → and upper lobe predominant subpleural consolidation ⇒, parenchymal bands, and traction bronchiectasis ↷.*

DIFFERENTIAL DIAGNOSIS

Common

- Usual Interstitial Pneumonia
  - Idiopathic Pulmonary Fibrosis
  - Connective Tissue Disease Related
  - Drug-Induced Lung Disease
  - Asbestosis
- Nonspecific Interstitial Pneumonia
  - Idiopathic Nonspecific Interstitial Pneumonia
  - Connective Tissue Disease
  - Drug-Induced Lung Disease
- Hydrostatic Pulmonary Edema
- Aspiration
- Hematogenous Dissemination
  - Hematogenous Metastases
  - Septic Embolism
- Bronchiectasis

Less Common

- Hypersensitivity Pneumonitis
- Organizing Pneumonia

Rare but Important

- Lymphoid Interstitial Pneumonia
- Acute Interstitial Pneumonia
- Desquamative Interstitial Pneumonia

ESSENTIAL INFORMATION

Key Differential Diagnosis Issues

- Usual interstitial pneumonia (UIP) pattern
  - Honeycombing
  - Traction bronchiectasis/bronchiolectasis
  - Fine reticulation/ground-glass opacities
  - Subpleural and basilar predominance
- Nonspecific interstitial pneumonia (NSIP) pattern
  - Reticular &/or ground-glass opacities
    - Basilar predominance
  - Traction bronchiectasis
    - Central predominance
  - Subpleural sparing
  - Lower lobe volume loss
  - Most common histologic pattern of interstitial lung disease in patients with connective tissue disease

Helpful Clues for Common Diagnoses

- **Usual Interstitial Pneumonia**
  - Idiopathic pulmonary fibrosis
    - 6th-7th decades of life
    - Chronic dyspnea
    - UIP pattern on HRCT
    - Exclusion of other causes of interstitial lung disease
  - Connective tissue disease related
    - Rheumatoid arthritis
      - □ Destructive inflammatory arthritis
      - □ 25-50 years of age
      - □ Female predominance; F:M = 3:1
      - □ + anticyclic citrullinated peptide (CCP) antibody
      - □ UIP: Most frequent pattern of interstitial disease in patients with rheumatoid arthritis
  - Drug-induced lung disease
    - UIP: Uncommon manifestation of drug toxicity
    - Drug-induced UIP-like pattern most commonly reported with nitrofurantoin
    - Other drugs that cause UIP-like pattern: Cyclophosphamide, chlorambucil, pindolol
  - Asbestosis
    - Fibrotic pulmonary disease secondary to asbestos exposure
    - ≥ 20 years following initial exposure
    - UIP pattern of lung fibrosis
    - Other manifestations
      - □ Pleural plaques
      - □ Subpleural curvilinear opacities
      - □ Poorly defined centrilobular nodules
- **Nonspecific Interstitial Pneumonia**
  - Idiopathic
    - Average age of onset is 50 years
    - Breathlessness and cough (6-7 months)
    - Female predominance
  - Connective tissue diseases-related
    - Systemic sclerosis
      - □ Inflammation, vascular damage, fibrosis
      - □ 5th-7th decades of life
      - □ Female predominance; F:M = 3-8:1
      - □ Prevalence of interstitial lung disease: 25-90%
      - □ NSIP is most frequent interstitial lung disease pattern
    - Sjögren syndrome
      - □ Lymphocytic infiltration of exocrine glands with xerophthalmia (dry eyes) and xerostomia (dry mouth)
      - □ 4th-5th decades of life
      - □ Female predominance; F:M = 9:1
      - □ Prevalence of interstitial lung disease: 9-60%
      - □ NSIP: Most frequent pattern of interstitial lung disease
    - Idiopathic inflammatory myopathies
      - □ Progressive myalgias, arthralgias, and proximal muscle weakness
      - □ 5th-6th decades of life
      - □ Female predominance; F:M = 2:1
      - □ + anti-Jo-1, anti-PL-7, and anti-PL-12
      - □ Prevalence of interstitial lung disease: 40-65%
      - □ NSIP is most frequent pattern of interstitial lung disease (80%)
  - Drug-induced lung disease
    - NSIP pattern frequently described in association with drug toxicity
    - Drug-induced NSIP-like pattern most commonly reported with amiodarone, methotrexate, nitrofurantoin, bleomycin, hydrochlorothiazide, and carmustine
- **Hydrostatic Pulmonary Edema**
  - Increased pulmonary capillary hydrostatic pressure
  - Increased left ventricular end-diastolic pressure
  - Increased left atrial pressure
  - Gravity-dependent involvement
    - Ground-glass opacities
    - Consolidations

- Associated findings
  - Cardiomegaly
  - Wide vascular pedicle (> 70 mm)
  - Interlobular septal thickening
  - Pleural effusion
- **Aspiration**
  - Foreign body
    - Most common in childhood
    - Often clinically silent in adults
    - Atelectasis, recurrent pneumonia, bronchiectasis
  - Gastric contents
    - Lung injury depends on volume, pH, and particulate material in aspirate
    - Ground-glass opacities &/or consolidations in 1 or both lung bases
  - Chronic exogenous lipoid pneumonia
    - Repeated aspiration or inhalation of mineral oil or related substance
    - Treatment of constipation with mineral oil or oily nose drop use
    - Mass or consolidation with attenuation values approaching those of fat
- **Hematogenous Dissemination**
  - Septic embolism
    - Dislodged thrombus containing microorganisms (bacteria, fungi, parasites) that reaches pulmonary arteries
    - Parenchymal nodules in different stages of cavitation
    - Feeding vessels coursing into nodules (60-70%)
  - Hematogenous metastases
    - Most lung metastases reach lungs via pulmonary arteries
    - Multiple subpleural and basilar nodules
    - Peripheral and basilar predominance
- **Bronchiectasis**
  - Permanent irreversible airway dilatation
  - Bronchiectasis with lower lung zone predominance
    - Primary ciliary dyskinesia
      - Kartagener syndrome
    - Chronic aspiration

Helpful Clues for Less Common Diagnoses

- **Hypersensitivity Pneumonitis**
  - Immune-mediated response to inhaled antigen that produces pulmonary inflammation &/or fibrosis
  - Chronic hypersensitivity pneumonitis may manifest as UIP-like pattern (5.9%)
  - Mosaic attenuation (80%)
- **Organizing Pneumonia**
  - Nonspecific response to lung injury characterized by intraluminal organizing fibroblastic tissue in distal air spaces
  - Idiopathic: Cryptogenic organizing pneumonia
  - Secondary: Connective tissue disease, infection, drugs, radiation
  - Subpleural peripheral consolidation with basilar predominance

Helpful Clues for Rare Diagnoses

- **Lymphoid Interstitial Pneumonia**
  - Idiopathic or associated with Sjögren syndrome, dysgammaglobulinemia, AIDS
  - 5th decade of life
  - Female predominance
  - Centrilobular nodules, ground-glass opacities, lung cysts
- **Acute Interstitial Pneumonia**
  - Idiopathic form of acute lung injury characterized by acute respiratory failure, bilateral parenchymal opacities, and diffuse alveolar damage on histology
  - Diagnosis requires absence of identifiable etiology or predisposing condition
  - Ground-glass opacities &/or consolidations in dependent lung
- **Desquamative Interstitial Pneumonia**
  - Smokers (58-91%)
  - Ground-glass opacities (lower lung zone predominance)
  - Subpleural reticular opacities

Idiopathic Pulmonary Fibrosis

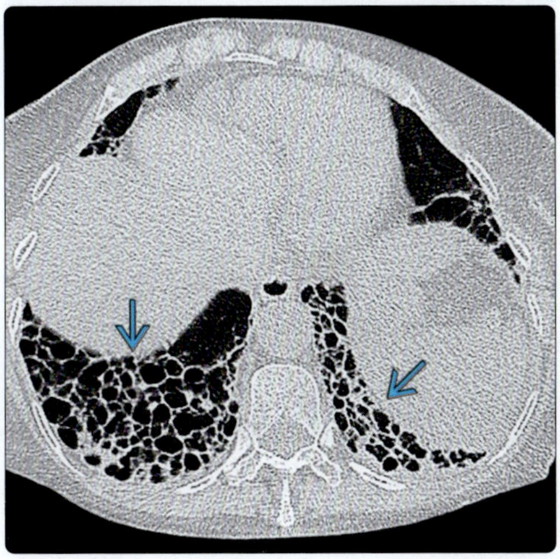

Idiopathic Pulmonary Fibrosis

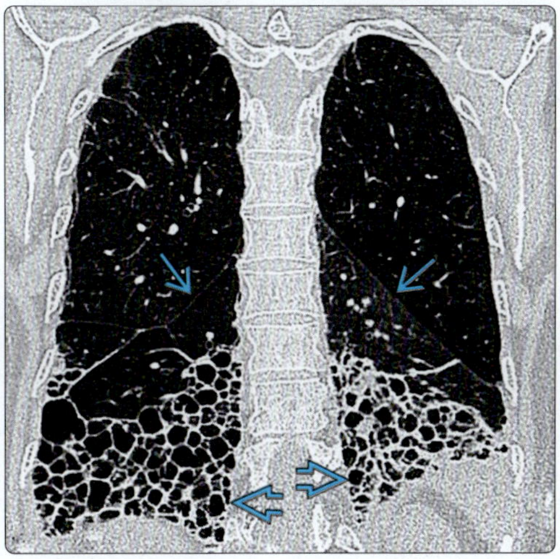

(Left) *Axial HRCT of a 65-year-old man with chronic cough and dyspnea secondary to idiopathic pulmonary fibrosis shows extensive basilar honeycombing ➡ and a typical usual interstitial pneumonia (UIP) pattern characterized by layers of basilar subpleural cysts.* **(Right)** *Coronal HRCT of the same patient shows lower lobe volume loss with resultant inferomedial displacement of the bilateral major fissures ➡ and extensive honeycombing ➡ that exhibits an apical-basilar gradient.*

(Left) *Axial NECT of a 69-year-old man with a history of occupational exposure to asbestos shows bilateral discontinuous foci of pleural thickening with calcification consistent with pleural plaques → typical of asbestos-related pleural disease.* **(Right)** *Axial HRCT of the same patient shows basilar predominant subpleural reticular opacities → and traction bronchiolectasis → consistent with pulmonary fibrosis secondary to asbestosis. The diagnosis is supported by the occupational exposure history.*

Asbestosis

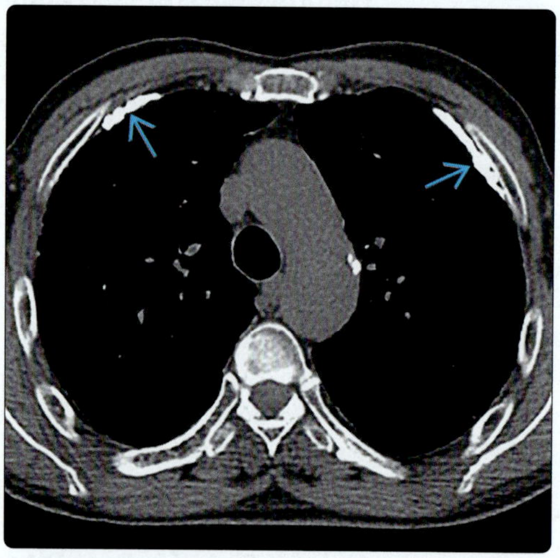

Asbestosis

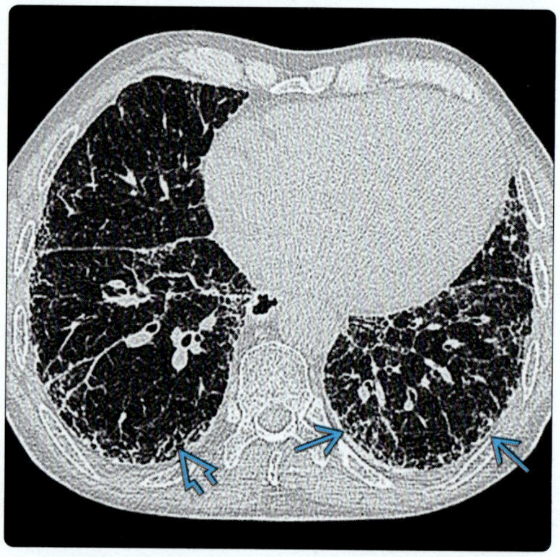

(Left) *Axial HRCT of a 67-year-old man with rheumatoid arthritis and a nonspecific interstitial pneumonia pattern of pulmonary fibrosis shows extensive basilar predominant reticulation →, ground-glass opacities →, and traction bronchiectasis →.* **(Right)** *Coronal HRCT of the same patient shows basilar predominant subpleural reticular opacities → and associated traction bronchiectasis → indicative of fibrosing interstitial lung disease.*

Connective Tissue Disease

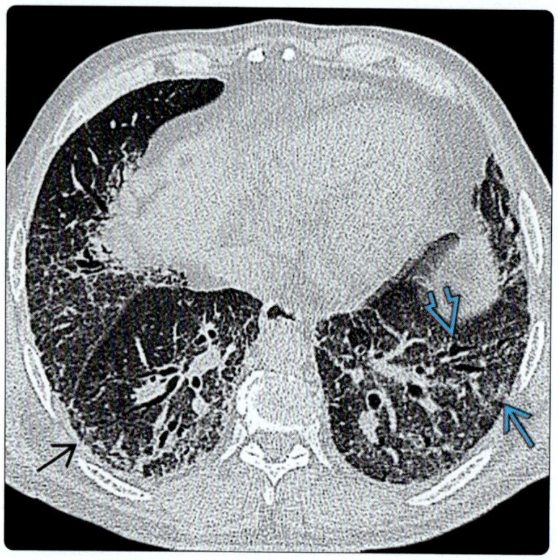

Connective Tissue Disease Related

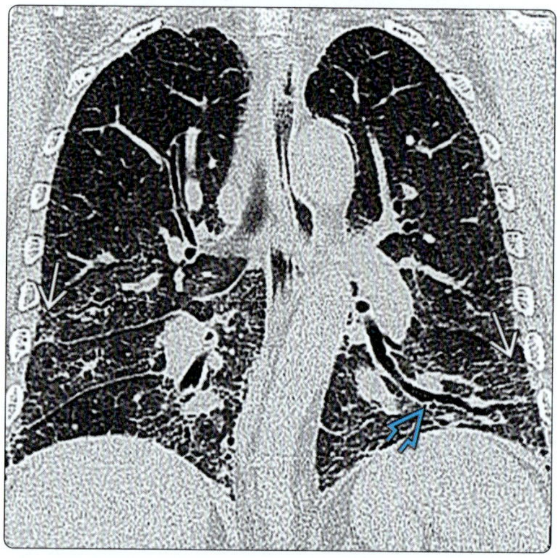

(Left) *PA chest radiograph of a 65-year-old man with pulmonary edema secondary to acute myocardial infarction shows central and basilar predominant ill-defined pulmonary opacities →.* **(Right)** *Axial CT of the same patient shows extensive basilar predominant ground-glass opacities → that correspond to pulmonary alveolar edema. Hydrostatic alveolar edema often manifests with gravity-dependent ground-glass opacities and consolidations.*

Hydrostatic Pulmonary Edema

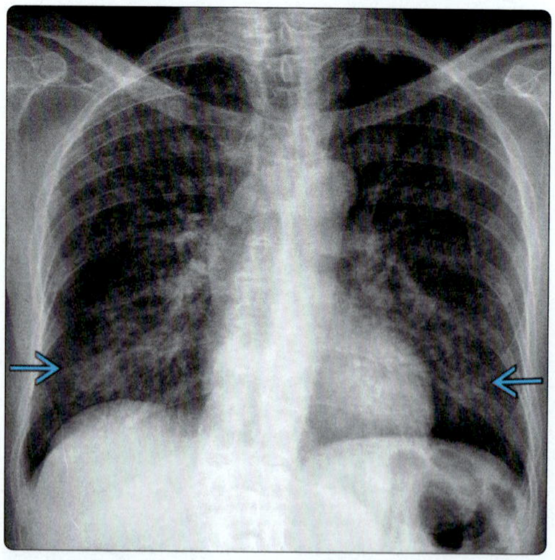

Hydrostatic Pulmonary Edema

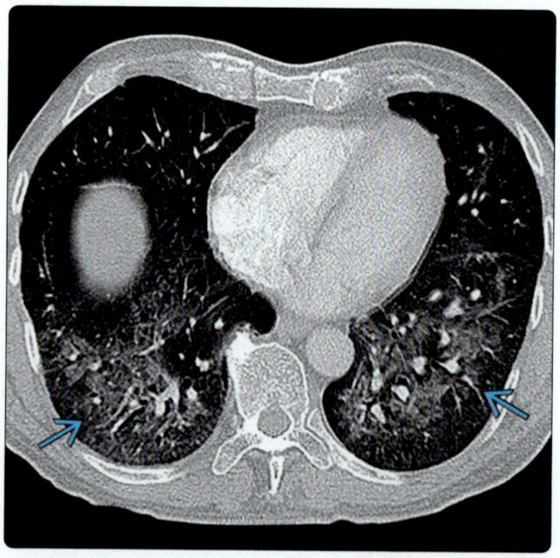

Pulmonary Alveolar Proteinosis

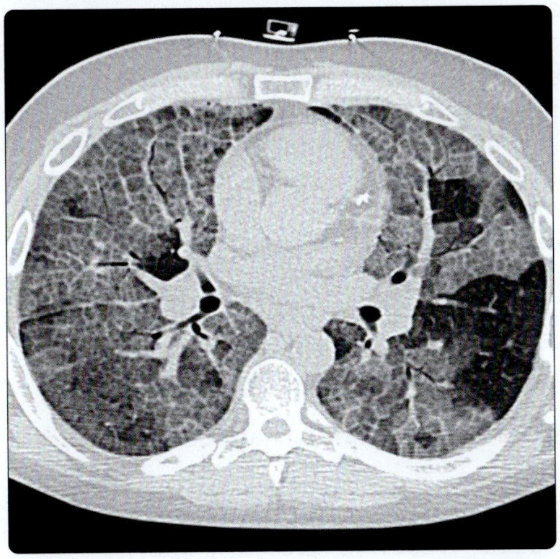

Pulmonary Venoocclusive Disease

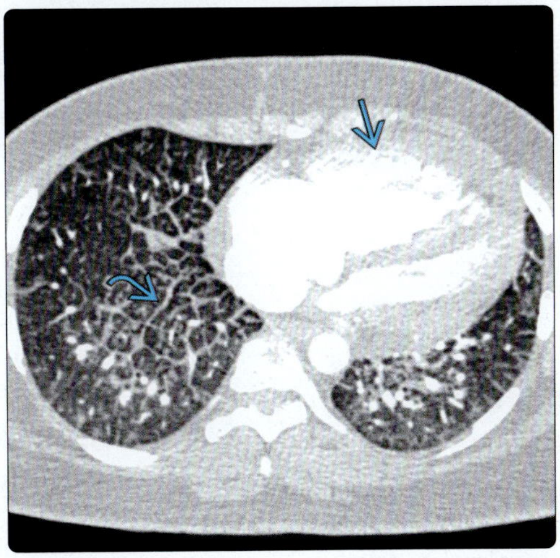

(Left) *Axial HRCT of a patient with pulmonary alveolar proteinosis shows bilateral geographic crazy paving. This finding was originally thought to be specific for alveolar proteinosis, but is now known to be nonspecific with an extensive differential diagnosis.* **(Right)** *Axial CECT of a 27-year-old woman with pulmonary venoocclusive disease shows smooth interlobular septal thickening → and an enlarged right heart →. The constellation of imaging findings is considered characteristic of pulmonary venoocclusive disease.*

Invasive Mucinous Lung Adenocarcinoma

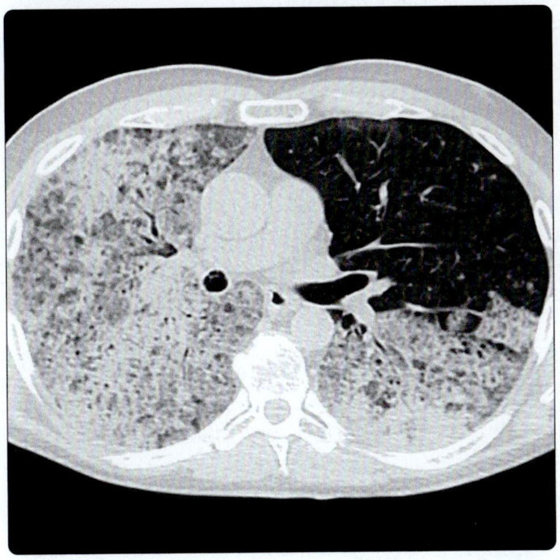

Erdheim-Chester Disease

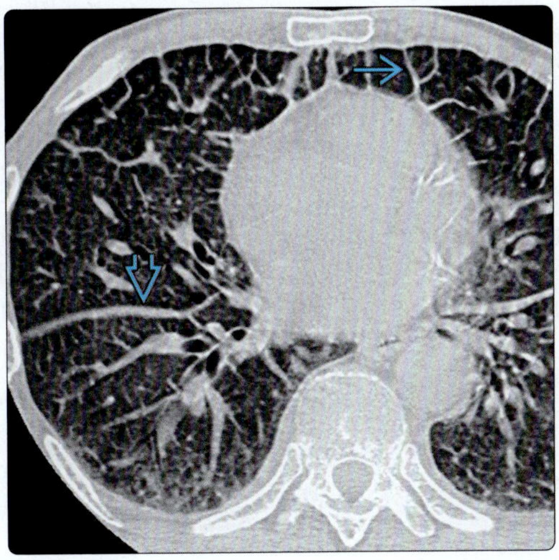

(Left) *Axial NECT of a patient with invasive mucinous lung adenocarcinoma shows diffuse bilateral airspace disease that exhibits the crazy-paving pattern. The diagnosis is usually only suspected when consolidations do not resolve after appropriate treatment.* **(Right)** *Axial chest NECT of a patient with Erdheim-Chester disease shows marked bilateral interlobular septal →, fissural →, and pleural thickening. Erdheim-Chester disease is a histiocytosis that frequently exhibits osseous involvement and may occasionally affect the thorax.*

Lipoid Pneumonia

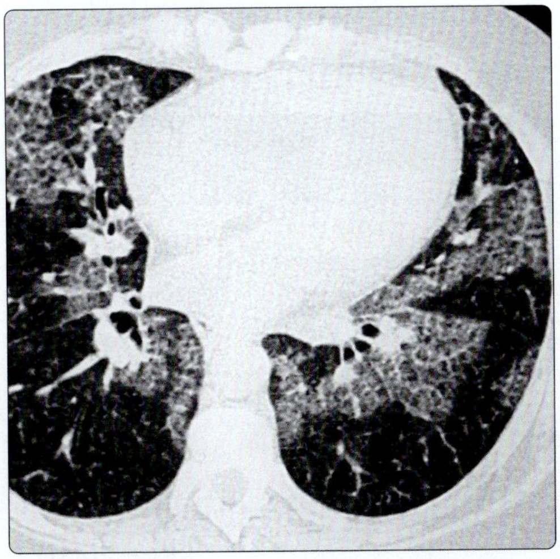

Acute Eosinophilic Pneumonia

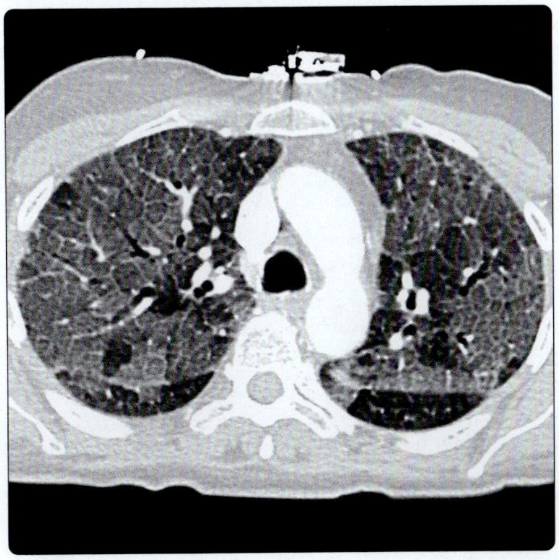

(Left) *Axial HRCT of a patient with lipoid pneumonia shows geographic areas of crazy paving bilaterally. Lipoid pneumonia typically manifests with fat attenuation consolidations but may also exhibit the crazy-paving pattern.* **(Right)** *Axial CECT of a patient with acute eosinophilic pneumonia shows diffuse crazy paving bilaterally. The clinical presentation (e.g., recent onset of smoking initiation) and the presence of peripheral eosinophilia are helpful clues to the diagnosis.*

DIFFERENTIAL DIAGNOSIS

Common

- Sarcoidosis
- Silicosis and Coal Workers' Pneumoconiosis

Less Common

- Berylliosis
- Radiation Fibrosis
- Hemosiderosis

Rare but Important

- Pulmonary Talcosis

ESSENTIAL INFORMATION

Key Differential Diagnosis Issues

- Progressive massive fibrosis (PMF): Fibrotic often bilateral upper lobe peribronchovascular masses
    - PMF typically linked to silicosis/coal workers' pneumoconiosis and sarcoidosis
    - **Classic imaging findings of PMF**
        - Upper lobe, bilateral, relatively symmetric, peribronchovascular ovoid nodule(s) or mass(es)
            - Outer lesion margin parallels adjacent chest wall
        - Air bronchograms ± volume loss (i.e., fissural displacement) and traction bronchiectasis
        - ± calcification

Helpful Clues for Common Diagnoses

- **Sarcoidosis**
    - PMF due to sarcoidosis, silicosis, or CWP are indistinguishable
        - Perilymphatic micronodules
        - Paracicatricial emphysema
    - Mediastinal and bilateral hilar lymphadenopathy ± calcification or egg-shell calcification
- **Silicosis and CWP**
    - Exposure to coal dust or free silica
    - Develops after 20 years of exposure, earlier if exposure to high concentrations; may progress after cessation of exposure
    - Lesion originates in peribronchovascular location and retracts toward hila as it progresses
        - Bilateral posterior upper lobe rounded or ovoid nodule or mass with well-defined margins
            - May involve lower lobe superior segments on FDG PET/CT
        - Exhibits FDG avidity
    - Cavitation implies necrosis or infection
        - Tuberculosis (i.e., silicotuberculosis)
    - Common mediastinal and hilar lymphadenopathy with diffuse, central, eccentric, or egg-shell calcifications

Helpful Clues for Less Common Diagnoses

- **Berylliosis**
    - Occupational exposure: Dentistry and aerospace, ceramic, nuclear weapons, and reactor industries
    - Indistinguishable from sarcoidosis: Perilymphatic micronodules and lymphadenopathy
    - PMF is uncommon manifestation
- **Radiation Fibrosis**
    - Not cause of classic PMF; may exhibit mass-like morphology
    - History of thoracic irradiation
    - Opacity with linear interface between fibrotic radiated and normal lung; crosses fissural boundaries, intrinsic air bronchograms, volume loss
- **Hemosiderosis**
    - Recurrent alveolar hemorrhage

Helpful Clues for Rare Diagnoses

- **Pulmonary Talcosis**
    - PMF can result from intravenous or inhaled talc
    - Conglomerate masses develop with progressive disease
        - Similar to silicosis and CWP on imaging

SELECTED REFERENCES

1. Cox CW et al: State of the art: imaging of occupational lung disease. Radiology. 270(3):681-96, 2014

Sarcoidosis

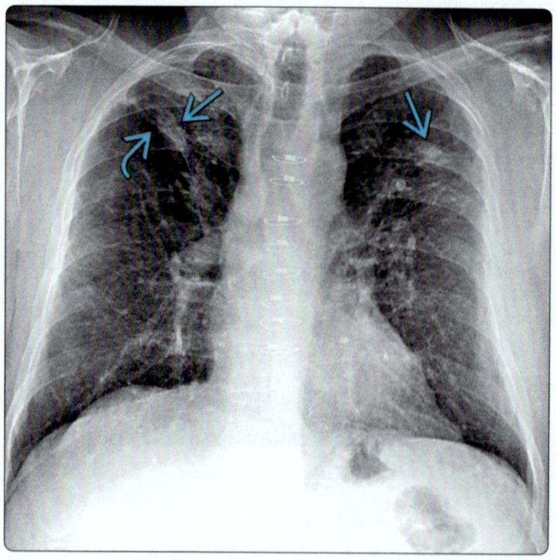

Sarcoidosis

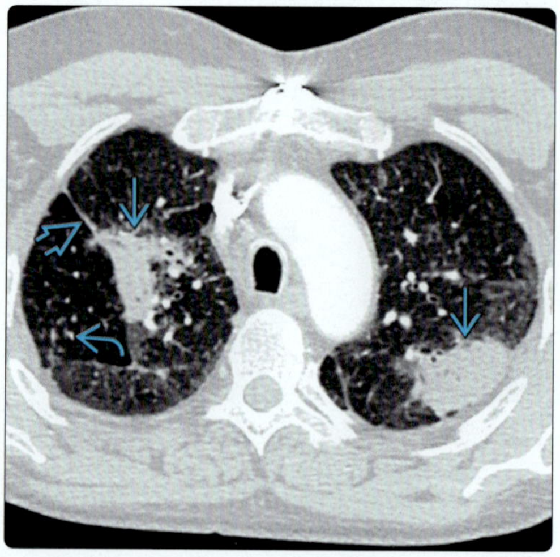

(Left) *PA chest radiograph of a patient with longstanding sarcoidosis and progressive massive fibrosis shows bilateral ill-defined upper lobe masses with volume loss. Note marked displacement of the minor fissure.* **(Right)** *Axial CECT of the same patient shows bilateral upper lobe peribronchovascular well-defined masses and marked upward displacement of the oblique fissure. Note perilymphatic micronodules and ground-glass opacities, which are common ancillary findings of pulmonary sarcoidosis.*

Silicosis and Coal Workers' Pneumoconiosis

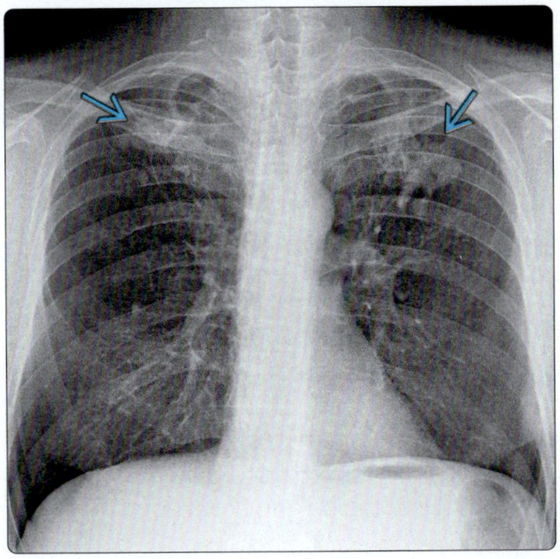

Silicosis and Coal Workers' Pneumoconiosis

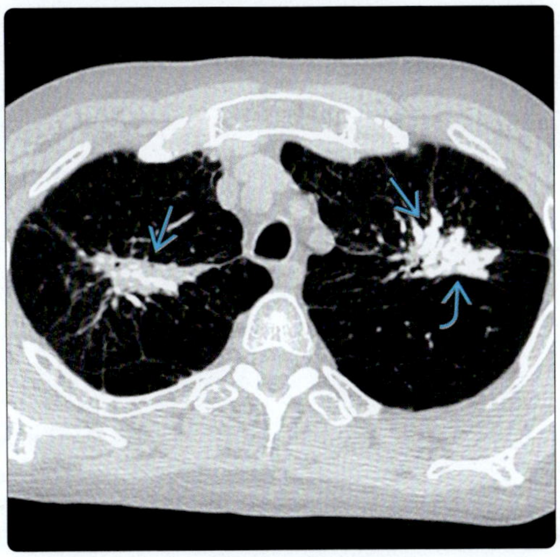

(Left) *PA chest radiograph of a patient with silicosis and progressive massive fibrosis shows bilateral upper lobe masses* ➔ *and volume loss.* **(Right)** *Axial NECT of the same patient shows peribronchovascular masses* ➔ *with irregular borders and intrinsic coarse calcifications. Note displaced and retracted left oblique fissure* ➚ *secondary to volume loss. These lesions are often bilateral, relatively symmetrical, and typically originate in the periphery and migrate centrally with progression of fibrosis.*

Silicosis and Coal Workers' Pneumoconiosis

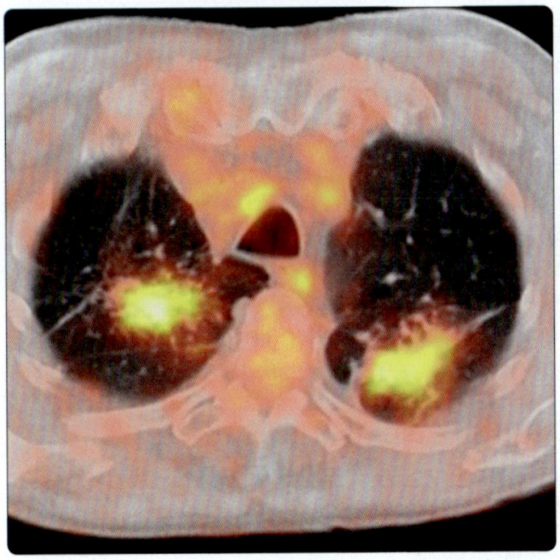

Radiation Fibrosis

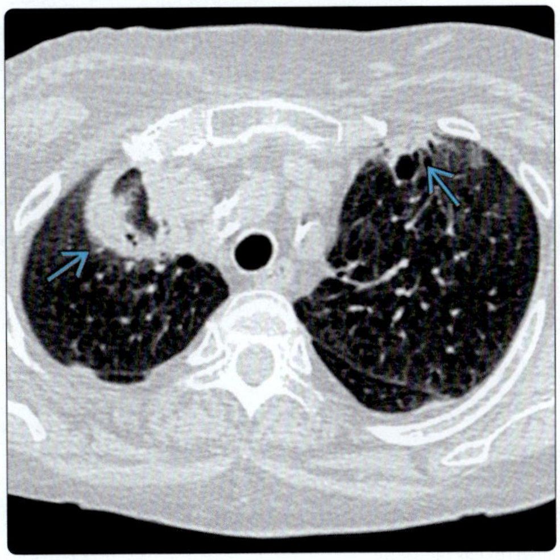

(Left) *Fused axial FDG PET/CT of a patient with silicosis and progressive massive fibrosis shows bilateral upper lobe peribronchovascular masses that exhibit marked FDG avidity. Similar findings may occur in patients with progressive massive fibrosis secondary to sarcoidosis.* **(Right)** *Axial NECT of a patient with lung cancer who was treated with radiation shows bilateral right larger than left mass-like opacities* ➔ *within the radiated field, consistent with radiation fibrosis. These abnormalities remained unchanged on serial imaging.*

Hemosiderosis

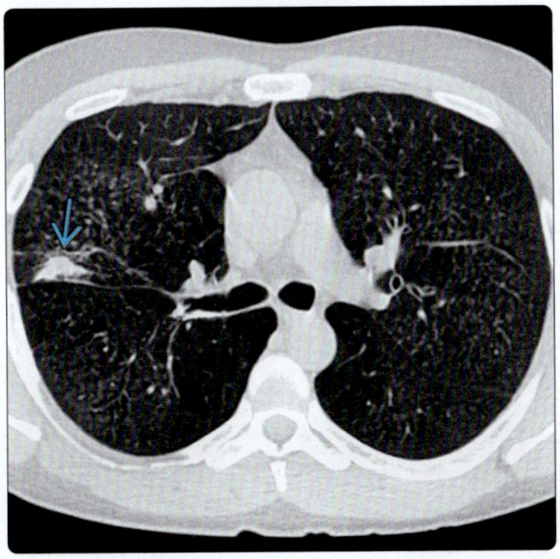

Hemosiderosis

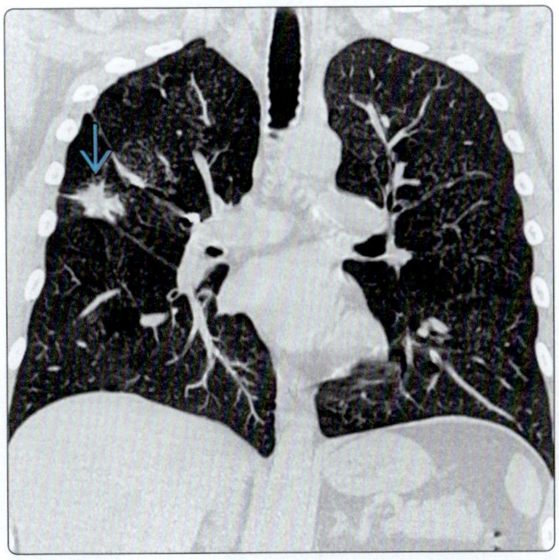

(Left) *Axial NECT of a patient with history of granulomatosis with polyangiitis and recurrent episodes of diffuse alveolar hemorrhage shows a dominant irregular right upper lobe peribronchovascular nodule* ➔ *that represented focal mass-like fibrosis. Note diffuse bilateral centrilobular micronodules secondary to recurrent remote episodes of hemorrhage.* **(Right)** *Coronal NECT of the same patient shows a right upper lobe spiculated soft tissue nodule* ➔ *due mass-like fibrosis. The lesion remained stable over serial annual surveillance.*

Miliary Nodules

DIFFERENTIAL DIAGNOSIS

Common

- Tuberculosis
- Fungal Infection
  - *Histoplasma capsulatum*, *Blastomyces dermatitidis*, *Coccidioides immitis*, and *Coccidioides posadasii*

Less Common

- Hematogenous Metastases
  - Lung Cancer
  - Thyroid Cancer

Rare but Important

- Benign Metastasizing Leiomyomatosis
- BCG *Mycobacterium bovis* Infection
- Sarcoidosis

ESSENTIAL INFORMATION

Key Differential Diagnosis Issues

- Miliary: Implies random or hematogenous distribution
- Assessment of micronodule distribution essential for formulation of differential diagnosis
- Micronodule distribution: Miliary (hematogenous), centrilobular (small airways or vascular), and perilymphatic
  - Centrilobular: No fissural or pleural involvement
  - Perilymphatic: Tend to conglomerate along fissures and bronchovascular bundles
  - Random (miliary): Even distribution throughout lung
    - Fissural nodularity is not as conspicuous as with perilymphatic micronodules

Helpful Clues for Common Diagnoses

- **Tuberculosis**
  - Miliary micronodules should always raise concern for miliary tuberculosis
    - Initiation of empiric treatment before confirmation may be justified given high mortality
  - Occasionally associated with necrotic mediastinal lymphadenopathy
- **Fungal Infection**
  - Histoplasmosis: Most common fungal infection
  - Miliary dissemination in immunocompromised patients
  - Remote infection may manifest with calcified miliary micronodules

Helpful Clues for Less Common Diagnoses

- **Hematogenous Metastases**
  - History of known malignancy
    - Lung cancer: Particularly if *EGFR* mutation present
    - Papillary thyroid carcinoma

Helpful Clues for Rare Diagnoses

- Rare causes of miliary micronodules are often diagnosis of exclusion
- **Benign Metastasizing Leiomyomatosis**
  - More commonly manifests with discrete hematogenous pulmonary nodules (i.e., typical hematogenous metastases)
  - Miliary pattern rare but reported
- **BCG *Mycobacterium bovis* Infection**
  - Treatment of bladder cancer with intravesical bacillus Calmette-Guérin (BCG: *Mycobacterium bovis*)
    - Miliary pattern in treated patients; occurs in ~ 4% of all subjects treated with intravesical BCG
    - Often requires open lung biopsy for confirmation
- **Sarcoidosis**
  - Sarcoidosis may mimic miliary pattern, referred to as miliary sarcoidosis
    - Absence of fissural nodularity due to inconspicuous involvement of subpleural interstitium
    - Differentiation may be challenging and often requires open lung biopsy

SELECTED REFERENCES

1. Kimmig L et al: Miliary nodules: not always tuberculosis. Ann Am Thorac Soc. 14(12):1858-60, 2017
2. Taki M et al: Pulmonary sarcoidosis presenting with miliary opacities. Intern Med. 54(19):2483-6, 2015
3. Furqan M et al: Miliary pattern on chest radiography: TB or not TB? Mayo Clin Proc. 85(2):108, 2010

Tuberculosis

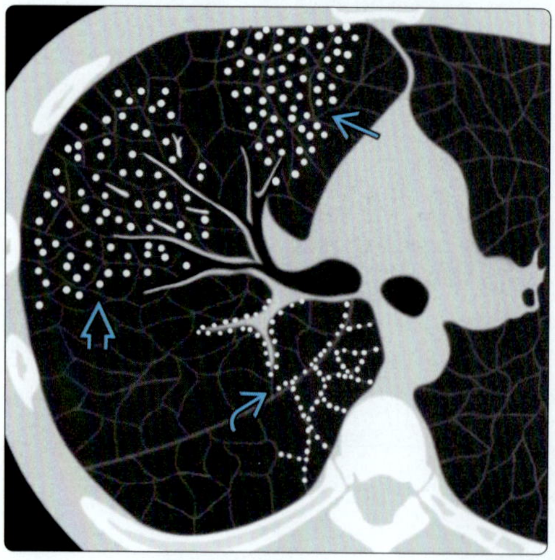

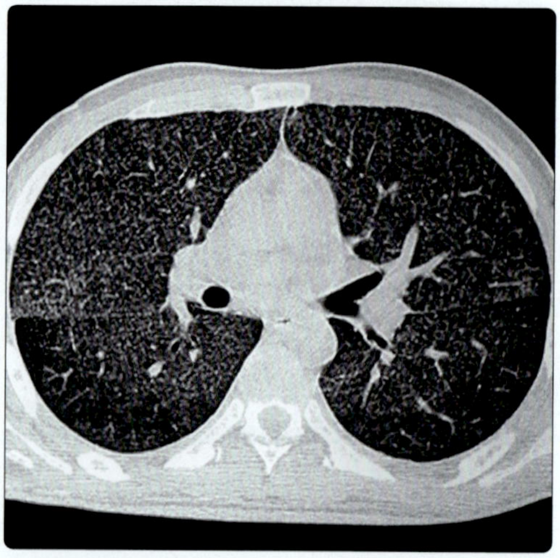

(Left) *Graphic shows the classic distribution of micronodules, including random or miliary ➔, centrilobular ➔, and perilymphatic ➔.* **(Right)** *Axial NECT of a patient with miliary tuberculosis shows profuse bilateral random pulmonary micronodules. The nodules are evenly distributed and involve all interstitial compartments. The miliary pattern should always raise suspicion for miliary tuberculosis, and treatment should be initiated promptly, often before confirmation, given high risk of mortality.*

Fungal Infection

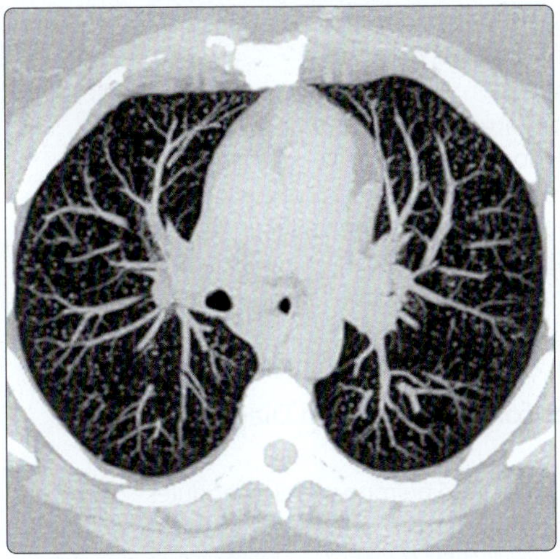

Hematogenous Metastases

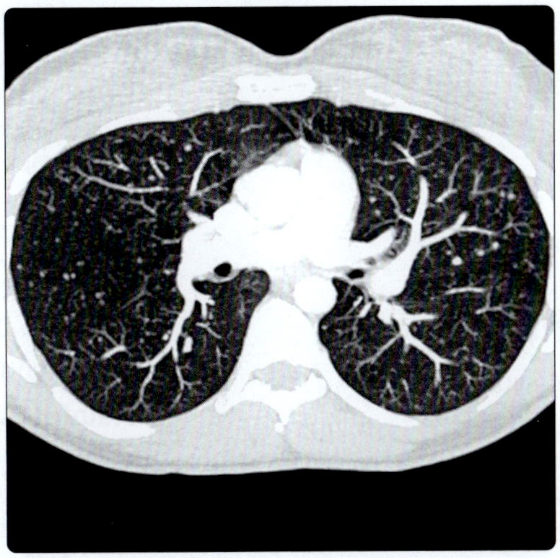

(Left) *Axial NECT MIP reformatted image of a patient with miliary histoplasmosis shows diffuse bilateral random micronodules, the so-called miliary pattern. Miliary micronodules should raise concern for miliary tuberculosis, but disseminated fungal infection, specifically histoplasmosis, is a common cause of miliary micronodules.* **(Right)** *Axial CECT (MIP reformatted image) of a patient with metastatic papillary thyroid carcinoma shows diffuse random micronodules.*

Hematogenous Metastases

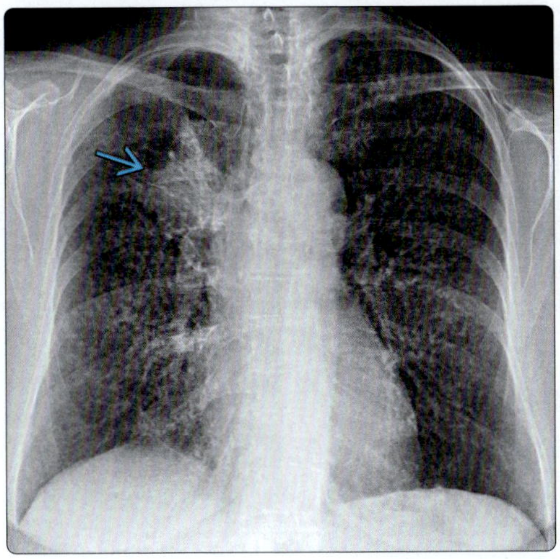

Hematogenous Metastases

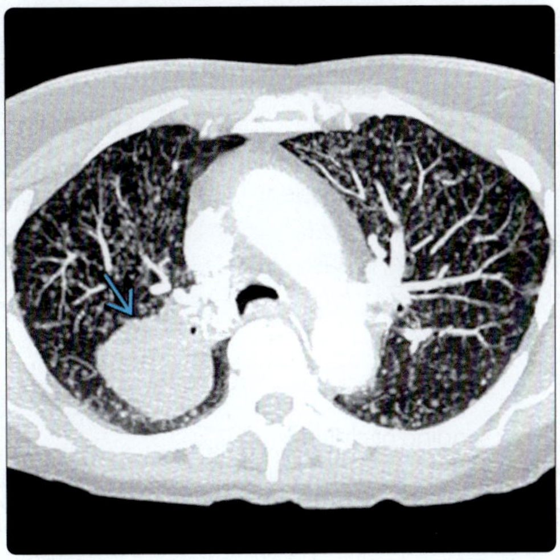

(Left) *PA chest radiograph of a patient with metastatic lung adenocarcinoma shows a dominant right upper lobe mass ➙ that represents the primary malignancy. Note profuse bilateral evenly distributed miliary micronodules from hematogenous metastases.* **(Right)** *Axial CECT (MIP reformatted image) of the same patient shows the right upper lobe adenocarcinoma ➙ and profuse bilateral miliary micronodules. Micronodular metastases are also common in metastatic papillary thyroid carcinoma.*

Benign Metastasizing Leiomyomatosis

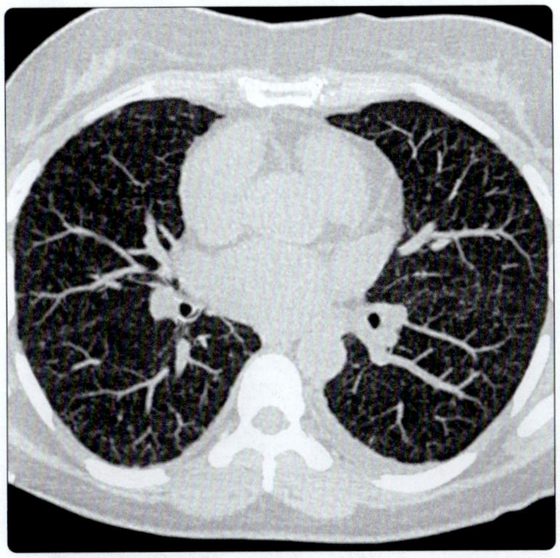

BCG *Mycobacterium bovis* Infection

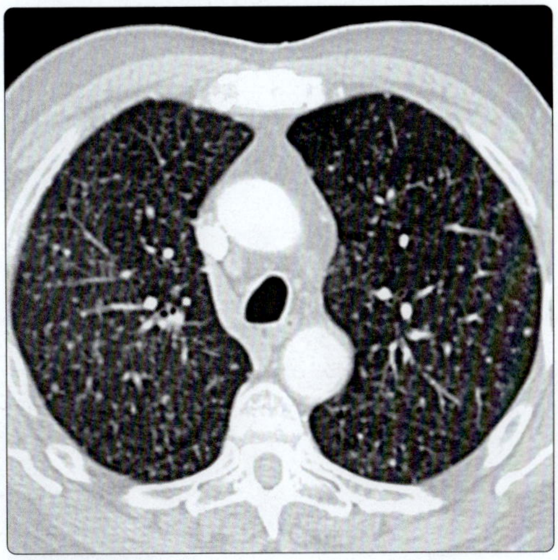

(Left) *Axial NECT (MIP reformatted image) of a patient who underwent hysterectomy for uterine leiomyoma shows diffuse bilateral miliary micronodules. A lung biopsy demonstrated benign metastatic leiomyomatosis.* **(Right)** *Axial CECT of a patient recently diagnosed with bladder carcinoma treated with intravesical BCG (Mycobacterium bovis) shows miliary micronodules secondary to mycobacterial infection, a rare complication of intravesical bladder cancer treatment.*

Perilymphatic Nodules

DIFFERENTIAL DIAGNOSIS

Common

- Sarcoidosis
- Lymphangitic Carcinomatosis

Less Common

- Silicosis

Rare but Important

- Amyloidosis

ESSENTIAL INFORMATION

Key Differential Diagnosis Issues

- Perilymphatic micronodules
  - Involve both peripheral and central interstitium
  - Peribronchovascular, septal, fissural, subpleural
- Differentiation from centrilobular and random micronodules
  - Centrilobular
    - Spare fissures and pleura
  - Random (miliary)
    - Even distribution, no coalescence
    - Sporadic involvement of fissures and pleura
- Importance of clinical data
  - Sarcoidosis
    - Often incidental finding in asymptomatic patient
  - Lymphangitic carcinomatosis
    - History of adenocarcinoma (e.g., lung, breast, stomach, colon, prostate)
  - Silicosis
    - Exposure to silica or coal
      - Industrial sanding
      - Sawing brick or concrete; sanding or drilling concrete walls; grinding mortar; manufacturing brick, concrete blocks, or ceramic products
      - Cutting or crushing stone generates respirable dust
  - Amyloidosis
    - Progressive dyspnea, respiratory failure, pulmonary hypertension

Helpful Clues for Common Diagnoses

- **Sarcoidosis**
  - Perilymphatic micronodules may exhibit coalescence, often referred to as galaxy sign
  - Pipe-cleaner sign: Beaded bronchovascular bundles
  - Frequent bilateral hilar and mediastinal lymphadenopathy; egg-shell calcification may occur
  - Nodular septal thickening may occur but not as conspicuous as in lymphangitic carcinomatosis
- **Lymphangitic Carcinomatosis**
  - Exuberant beaded &/or smooth interlobular septal thickening
  - Bronchial wall thickening (common), pleural effusion

Helpful Clues for Less Common Diagnoses

- **Silicosis**
  - Numerous calcified pulmonary micronodules
  - Late-stage disease may be associated with upper lobe peribronchovascular masses (i.e., progressive massive fibrosis)
  - Aggregates of subpleural micronodules may produce pseudoplaques
  - Hilar and mediastinal lymphadenopathy; characteristic egg-shell calcification

Helpful Clues for Rare Diagnoses

- **Amyloidosis**
  - Pulmonary involvement
    - Diffuse alveolar septal amyloidosis: Interlobular septal thickening, perilymphatic nodules, consolidation
    - Nodular pulmonary amyloidosis: Well-circumscribed, solitary or multiple lung nodules; often calcified

SELECTED REFERENCES

1. Shroff GS et al: Beyond metastatic disease: a pictorial review of multinodular lung disease with computed tomographic pathologic correlation. Can Assoc Radiol J. 66(1):16-23, 2015
2. Marchiori E et al: Atypical distribution of small nodules on high resolution CT studies: patterns and differentials. Respir Med. 105(9):1263-7, 2011
3. Raoof S et al: Pictorial essay: multinodular disease: a high-resolution CT scan diagnostic algorithm. Chest. 129(3):805-15, 2006

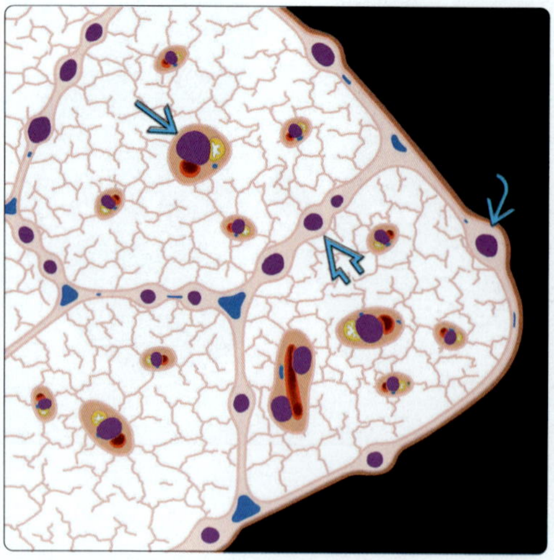

Sarcoidosis

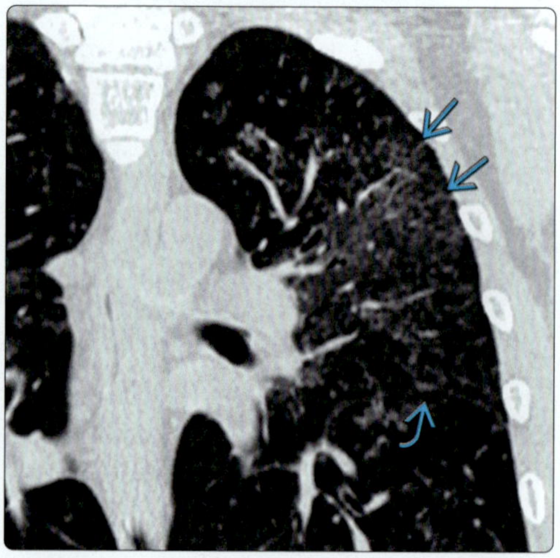

(Left) *Graphic shows the distribution of perilymphatic micronodules in reference to the anatomy of the secondary pulmonary lobule. The pulmonary lymphatics are located along bronchovascular bundles (i.e., axial interstitium), interlobular septa, and subpleural regions (i.e., peripheral interstitium).* **(Right)** *Coronal NECT of a patient with sarcoidosis shows clustered perilymphatic micronodules involving the interlobular interstitium (i.e., interlobular septa) and the fissures.*

Sarcoidosis

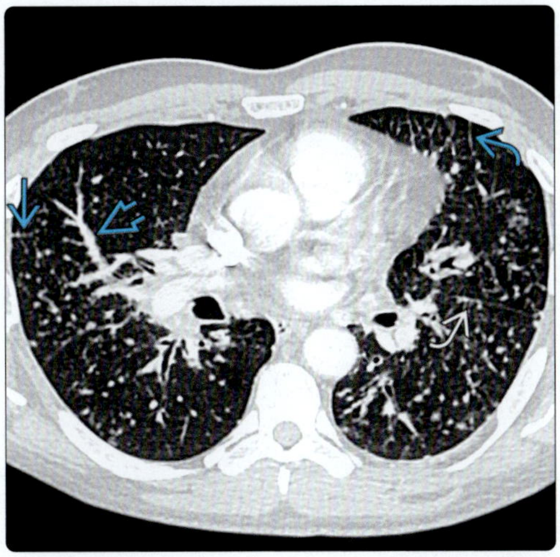

Sarcoidosis

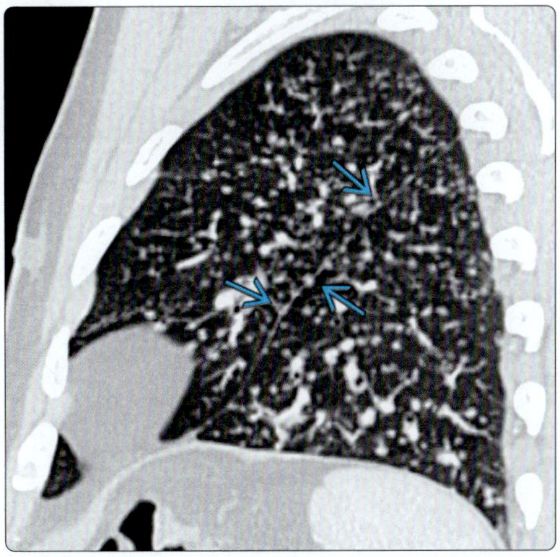

(Left) *Axial CECT of a patient with sarcoidosis shows diffuse bilateral perilymphatic micronodules that manifest with nodular and smooth septal lines, the pipe-cleaner sign (peribronchovascular thickening and nodularity), and fissural nodularity.* **(Right)** *Sagittal CECT of the same patient shows perilymphatic micronodules that manifest with fissural nodularity. Miliary nodules may exhibit fissural involvement, but it is not as profuse as in perilymphatic micronodules.*

Lymphangitic Carcinomatosis

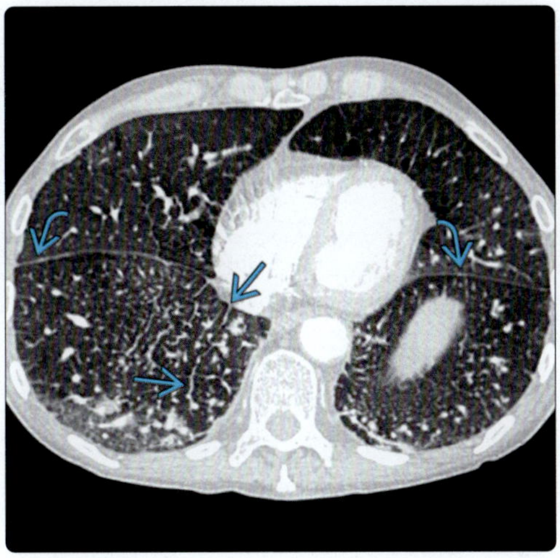

Lymphangitic Carcinomatosis

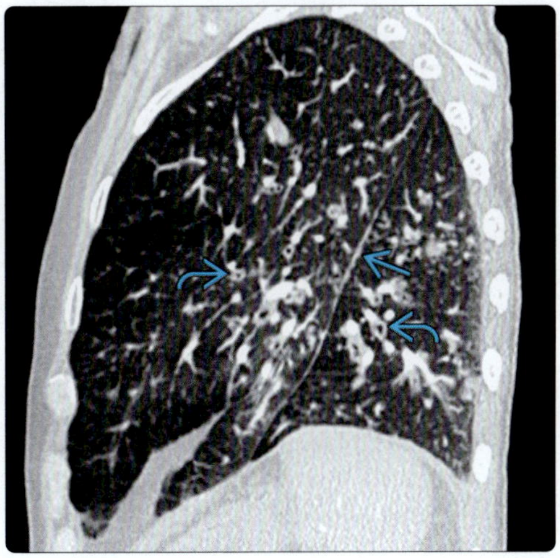

(Left) *Axial CECT of a patient with colon cancer and lymphangitic carcinomatosis shows extensive nodular and smooth interlobular septal thickening and perilymphatic micronodules. Note associated fissural nodularity.* **(Right)** *Sagittal CECT of the same patient shows fissural nodularity and marked bronchial wall thickening, which constitutes a characteristic perilymphatic distribution. Adenocarcinoma is the most common histologic type associated with lymphangitic carcinomatosis.*

Silicosis

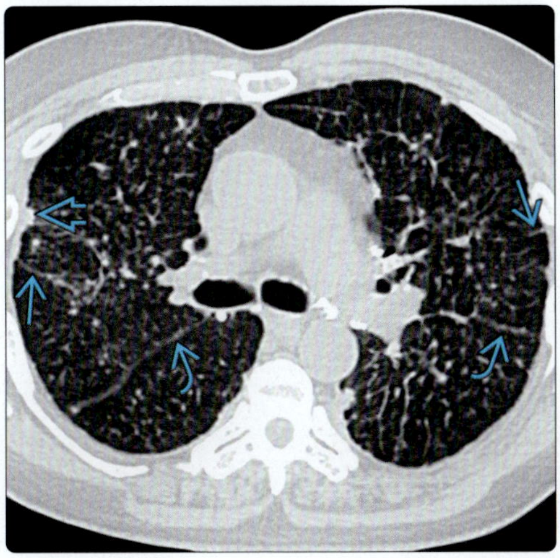

Silicosis

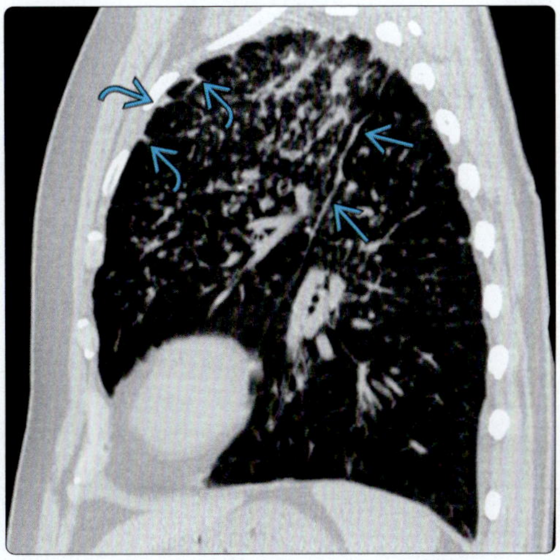

(Left) *Axial NECT of a patient with silicosis shows diffuse bilateral pulmonary micronodules, beaded interlobular septa, and nodular interlobar fissures. Note coalescent micronodules that form pseudoplaques.* **(Right)** *Sagittal NECT of the same patient shows nodularity along the left oblique fissure and extensive subpleural and peribronchovascular micronodules. Silicosis may progress to progressive massive fibrosis, which manifests as discrete upper lobe peribronchovascular masses.*

SECTION 4

Airways

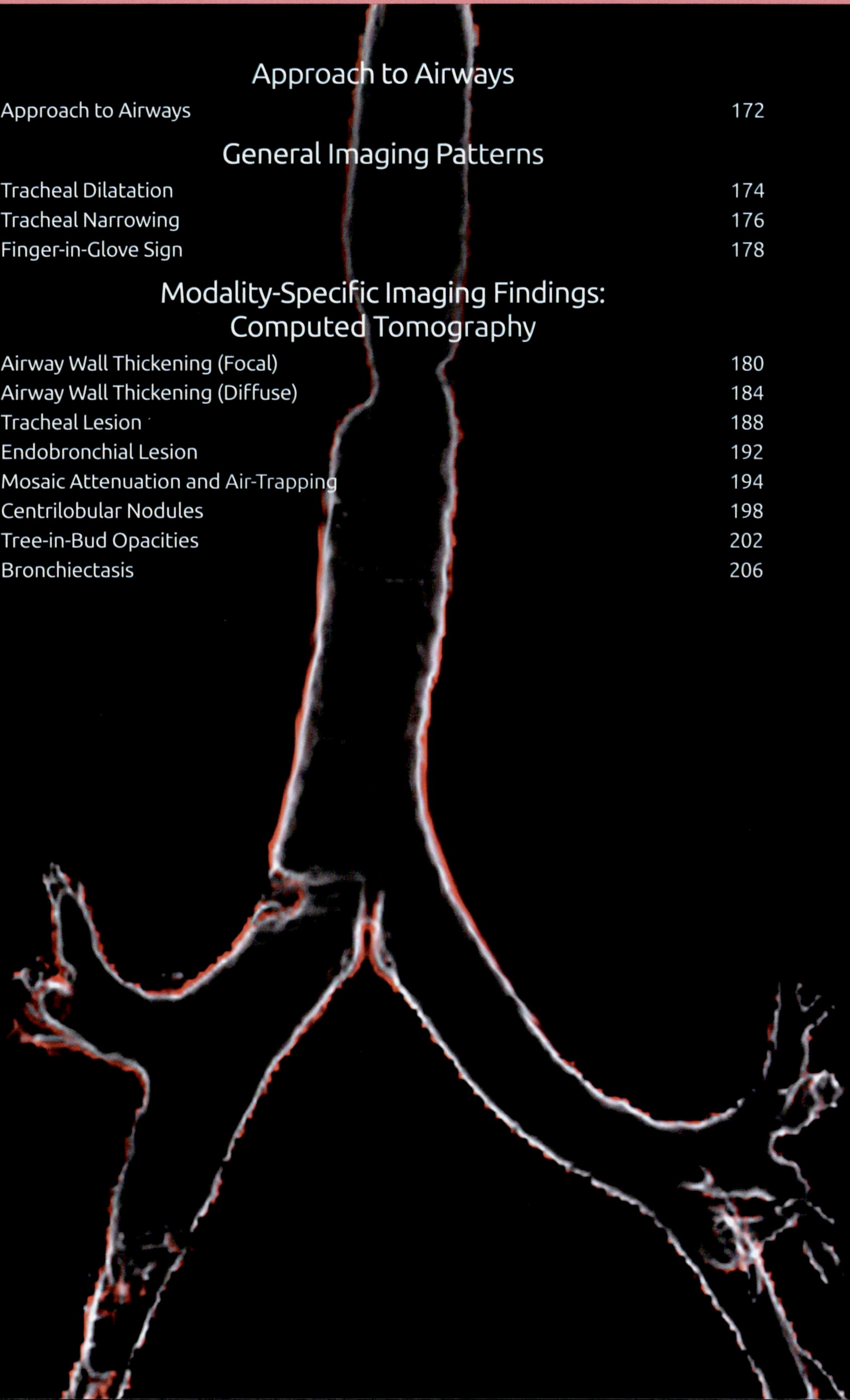

Approach to Airways

General Imaging Patterns

Modality-Specific Imaging Findings: Computed Tomography

Anatomic Considerations

The airways are tubular branching structures that conduct air to and from the lungs. They are classified as *large airways* (trachea and bronchi) and *small airways* (bronchioles, terminal bronchioles, respiratory bronchioles, and alveolar ducts). The trachea and bronchi are characterized by cartilage in their walls, whereas the bronchioles and more peripheral airways lack mural cartilage. Functionally, the airways can be classified into three zones with overlapping features: (1) *Conductive zone* (air conduction only) consisting of the trachea, bronchi, and membranous bronchioles, (2) *Transitional zone* (air conduction and respiration) comprised of respiratory bronchioles and alveolar ducts, and (3) *Respiratory zone* (respiration only) consisting of alveolar sacs and alveoli.

A variety of diseases and disorders may affect the airways, including congenital, neoplastic, infectious, and inflammatory conditions. For practical purposes, airway diseases can be classified as those involving the large airways and those involving the small airways.

Large Airways Diseases

Neoplasms

Benign and malignant neoplasms may affect the large airways either primarily or by secondary involvement of the airway wall &/or lumen. Malignant neoplasms that involve the airways include primary lung cancer, carcinoid tumor, adenoid cystic carcinoma, mucoepidermoid carcinoma, and metastatic disease. In the case of primary lung cancer, there may be invasion of the adjacent airways resulting in luminal obstruction with resultant atelectasis &/or consolidation. Such secondary effects of the centrally obstructing neoplasm may obscure visualization of the mass, but its presence may be inferred by identification of classic signs of neoplastic volume loss, such as the *S sign of Golden* and the *Luftsichel sign*. Primary neoplasms of the airway may manifest as an endoluminal nodule or mass or as circumferential airway stenosis that may be focal or diffuse. In general, patients with central neoplasms that produce airway obstruction present with symptoms that may include cough, wheezing, and hemoptysis. Stridor is a high-pitched sound produced by disruption of airway flow by stenosis or partial obstruction of the trachea or larynx. However, it should be noted that central tracheal tumors may obliterate up to 75% of the tracheal lumen before producing symptoms. Benign neoplasms may also affect the airways and include papilloma, lipoma, hamartoma, and neurogenic tumor. Although the presence of an airway neoplasm may be suspected because of a central airway abnormality identified on radiography, CT is the imaging modality of choice for the initial characterization and staging of these lesions.

Morphologic Alterations of Airway Lumen

A variety of non-neoplastic conditions may produce airway narrowing or stenosis. Most cases of acquired tracheal stenosis are a complication of prolonged endotracheal intubation. Tracheal narrowing may manifest as *saber-sheath trachea*, characterized by decreased coronal and increased sagittal tracheal diameters in association with chronic obstructive airway disease. *Tracheomalacia* and *tracheobronchomalacia* may produce functional airway stenosis due to weakness of the airway cartilages that results in expiratory airway collapse. Inflammatory conditions such as *granulomatosis with polyangiitis*, *amyloidosis*, and *relapsing polychondritis* may also produce airway stenosis.

Abnormal airway dilatation may affect the trachea &/or bronchi. *Mounier-Kuhn syndrome* typically affects only the trachea but may also affect the central bronchi. *Bronchiectasis* refers to irreversible bronchial dilatation and may be classified as cylindrical, varicose, or cystic in increasing order of severity. A large number of conditions may result in bronchiectasis. CT imaging of the airways allows detection of bronchiectasis and assessment of its distribution and severity. An understanding of the many causes of bronchiectasis allows the radiologist to provide a focused differential diagnosis and suggest specific etiologies of bronchiectasis, thus impacting patient management.

Small Airways Diseases

The normal small airways are not visible on radiography or CT. However, disorders of the small airways are readily evaluated on thin-section chest CT and high-resolution CT (HRCT).

Emphysema

In spite of the decline in tobacco use in the United States of America, emphysema remains a prevalent disease and is frequently identified as an incidental finding on chest CT. CT allows identification and characterization of emphysema as centrilobular, paraseptal, or panlobular subtypes and helps provide both visual and computer assisted quantification of its severity.

Cellular Bronchiolitis

Cellular bronchiolitis comprises diseases characterized by inflammatory cellular infiltration of the airway lumen and wall and manifests as centrilobular nodules that characteristically spare the adjacent pleural surfaces and interlobular septa. Centrilobular nodules may be of soft tissue or ground-glass attenuation and may be associated with branching tree-in-bud opacities. The linear component of the tree-in-bud opacity corresponds to the dilated centrilobular bronchiole impacted with mucus, fluid, or pus, and the nodular component corresponds to peribronchiolar inflammation. Cellular bronchiolitis typically implies *pulmonary infection* but can also be seen in cases of *aspiration*. Other types of cellular bronchiolitis include *respiratory and follicular bronchiolitis*, *panbronchiolitis*, bronchiolitis associated with *hypersensitivity pneumonitis* and *asthma*.

Constrictive Bronchiolitis

Constrictive bronchiolitis is characterized by concentric peribronchiolar fibrosis in the absence of surrounding inflammation or endoluminal involvement with resultant bronchiolar narrowing &/or luminal obliteration. The disease demonstrates a patchy distribution in the lung that leads to multifocal areas of airflow obstruction. Radiographs of affected patients may be entirely normal. Thin-section CT and HRCT may demonstrate patchy mosaic attenuation and air-trapping on expiratory imaging. Expiratory air-trapping may also occur in the setting of completely normal inspiratory CT. In some cases, bronchiectasis may also be present. Constrictive bronchiolitis may be seen as an *idiopathic* condition, in association with *rheumatoid arthritis*, as a complication of *heart-lung, lung or bone marrow transplantation*, or as the sequela of *smoke inhalation injury*. It may also occur as a sequela of *remote infection* (*Swyer-James-McLeod syndrome*) or in association with *diffuse idiopathic pulmonary neuroendocrine cell hyperplasia* (DIPNECH).

Secondary Tracheal Neoplasm

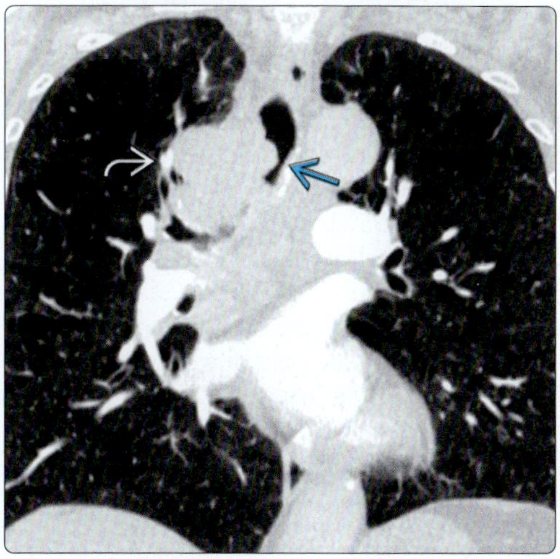

Primary Tracheal Neoplasm

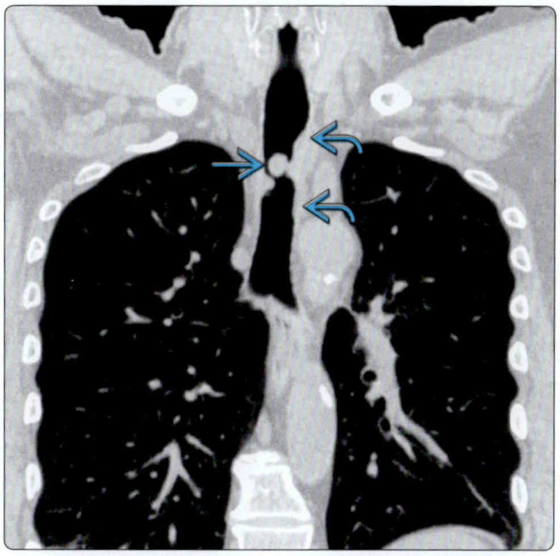

(Left) *Coronal CECT of a 77-year-old woman who presented with stridor shows a right upper lobe lung cancer that manifests as a large polylobular soft tissue mass that directly invades the trachea and produces severe stenosis of the tracheal lumen.* **(Right)** *Coronal NECT of a 35-year-old man with stridor and adenoid cystic carcinoma shows that the tumor produces long-segment tracheal stenosis and an endoluminal nodule. The tracheal lumen may be narrowed by up to 75% before the onset of symptoms.*

Tracheal Dilatation

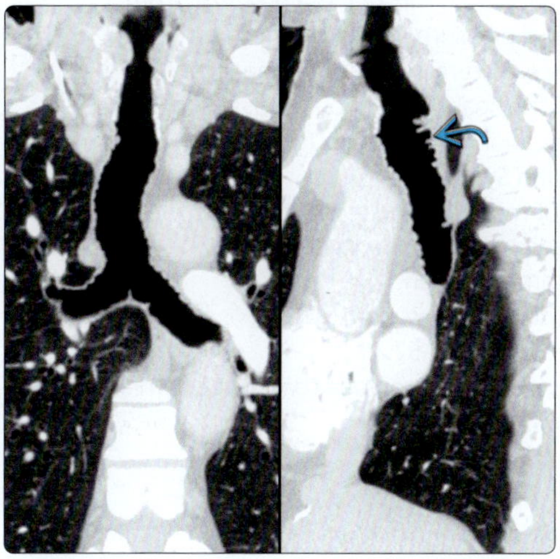

Bronchiectasis

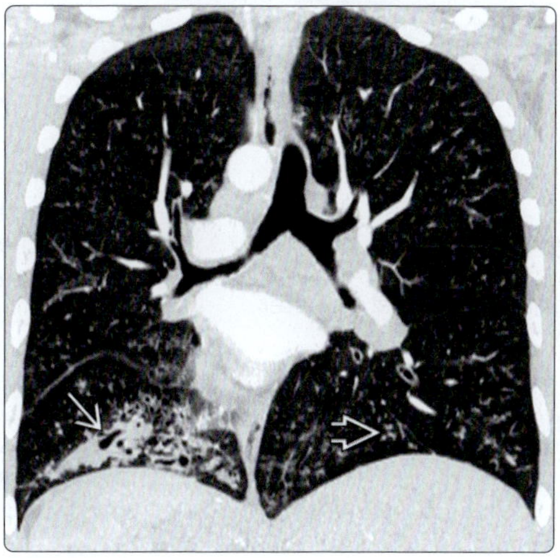

(Left) *Composite image with coronal (left) and sagittal (right) CECT of an asymptomatic 79-year-old man shows marked tracheal dilatation and a "corrugated" tracheal wall morphology secondary to so-called tracheal diverticulosis as mucosa protrudes between adjacent tracheal cartilages, typical of Mounier-Kuhn syndrome.* **(Right)** *Coronal CECT of a 31-year-old man with Kartagener syndrome and recurrent pulmonary infections shows situs inversus, bronchiectasis, and cellular bronchiolitis.*

Cellular Bronchiolitis

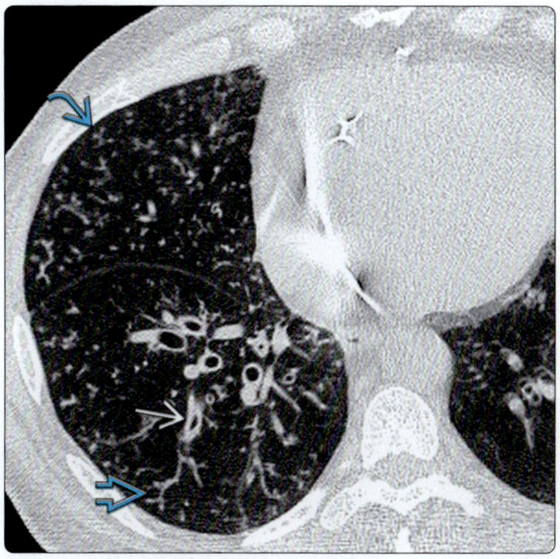

Constrictive Bronchiolitis

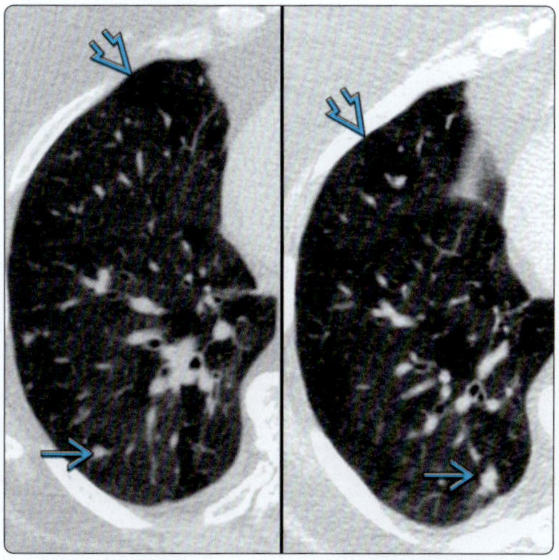

(Left) *Axial NECT of a 68-year-old man with Pseudomonas pulmonary infection shows profuse cellular bronchiolitis manifesting with multifocal centrilobular nodules, tree-in-bud opacities, and bronchial wall thickening.* **(Right)** *Axial NECT of a 68-year-old woman with diffuse idiopathic pulmonary neuroendocrine cell hyperplasia who presented with wheezing shows mosaic attenuation secondary to constrictive bronchiolitis. Note multifocal solid nodules, some of which represent carcinoid tumors.*

Tracheal Dilatation

DIFFERENTIAL DIAGNOSIS

Common

- Upper Lobe Fibrosis
- Overdistention of Endotracheal Tube Cuff
- Saber-Sheath Trachea
- Tracheobronchomalacia

Less Common

- Tracheal Diverticulum
- Mounier-Kuhn Syndrome

ESSENTIAL INFORMATION

Key Differential Diagnosis Issues

- Tracheal wall composed of several layers: Mucosa, submucosa, cartilage or muscle, and adventitia
- Horseshoe-shaped bands of hyaline cartilage support anterior and lateral tracheal walls
- Posterior tracheal wall lacks cartilage and is supported by band of smooth muscle
- During expiration: Anterior bulging of posterior wall of intrathoracic trachea and ↓ of tracheal AP diameter by 32%
- Tracheal dilatation
  - Women
    - Tracheal transverse diameter > 21 mm, sagittal diameter > 23 mm
  - Men
    - Tracheal transverse diameter > 25 mm, sagittal diameter > 27 mm
  - Tracheal index: Coronal diameter/sagittal diameter measured 1 cm above aortic arch
    - Normal index ~ 1

Helpful Clues for Common Diagnoses

- **Upper Lobe Fibrosis**
  - Retraction of tracheobronchial walls
    - Tuberculosis
    - Sarcoidosis
    - Hypersensitivity pneumonitis
- **Overdistention of Endotracheal Tube Cuff**
  - Endotracheal tube or tracheostomy cannula cuff should not result in tracheal wall bulging
  - Endotracheal cuff located 2 cm from distal end
  - Overinflation of balloon to 1.5x diameter of normal trachea is associated with tracheal injury
- **Saber-Sheath Trachea**
  - ↓ in coronal diameter of intrathoracic trachea associated with ↑ in sagittal diameter
  - Associated with COPD (95%)
  - Likely related to abnormal intrathoracic pressure
- **Tracheobronchomalacia**
  - Condition characterized by excessive airway collapsibility caused by weakness of airway walls due to softening or destruction of supporting cartilage
  - Tracheomalacia patients have dilated and flaccid airway
  - ↓ in cross-sectional area > 70% during expiration compared with inspiration is generally considered diagnostic

Helpful Clues for Less Common Diagnoses

- **Tracheal Diverticulum**
  - Mucosal herniation through tracheal wall from ↑ intraluminal pressure
  - Right posterolateral tracheal wall near thoracic inlet
  - Between tracheal cartilaginous and muscular portions
  - Communication with tracheal lumen rarely identified
- **Mounier-Kuhn Syndrome**
  - Atrophy of muscular and elastic tissues in walls of trachea and mainstem bronchi
  - More common in men
  - Tracheal diameter > 30 mm (81.2%)
  - Bronchiectasis (48.6-57.6%)
  - Tracheal wall corrugated due to mucosa herniating between tracheal rings

SELECTED REFERENCES

1. Gayer G: Tracheal diverticula. Semin Ultrasound CT MR. 37(3):190-5, 2016
2. Chung JH et al: CT of diffuse tracheal diseases. AJR Am J Roentgenol. 196(3):W240-6, 2011

Upper Lobe Fibrosis

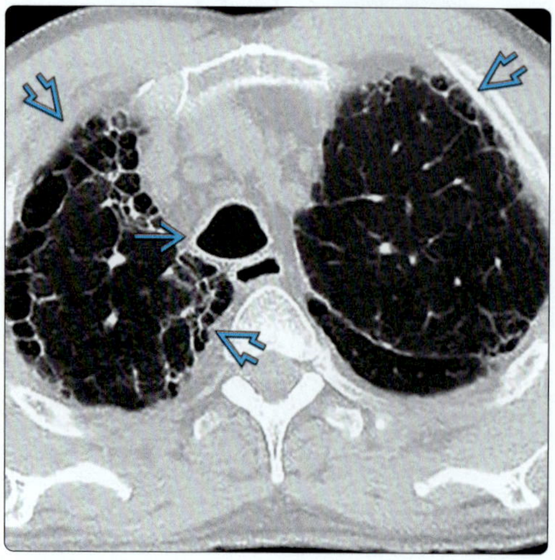

Upper Lobe Fibrosis

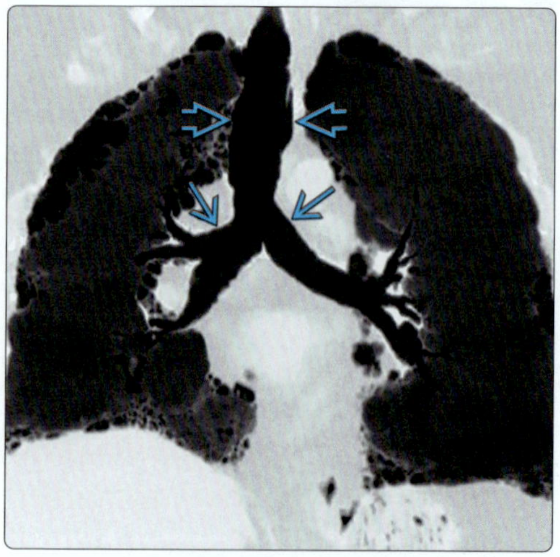

(Left) *Axial HRCT of a 62-year-old man with upper lobe-predominant fibrosis from chronic hypersensitivity pneumonitis shows tracheal dilatation* ➔ *and upper lobe predominant honeycombing* ➔. **(Right)** *Coronal CT (minIP reformation) of the same patient shows dilatation of the trachea* ➔ *and mainstem bronchi* ➔. *This phenomenon is thought to be related to traction exerted by surrounding pulmonary fibrosis similar to traction bronchiectasis and bronchiolectasis seen in the same process.*

Overdistention of Endotracheal Tube Cuff

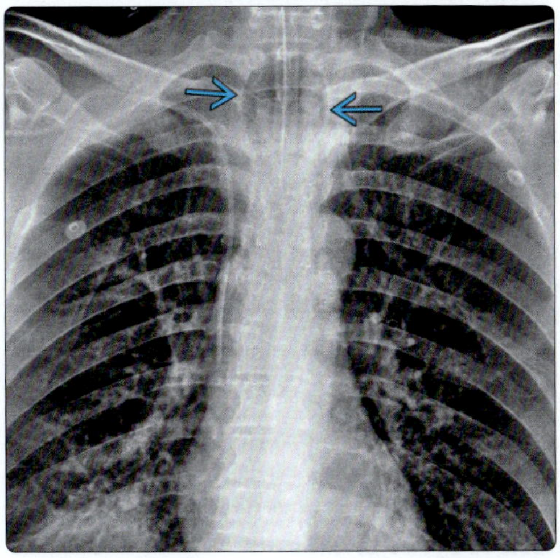

Overdistention of Endotracheal Tube Cuff

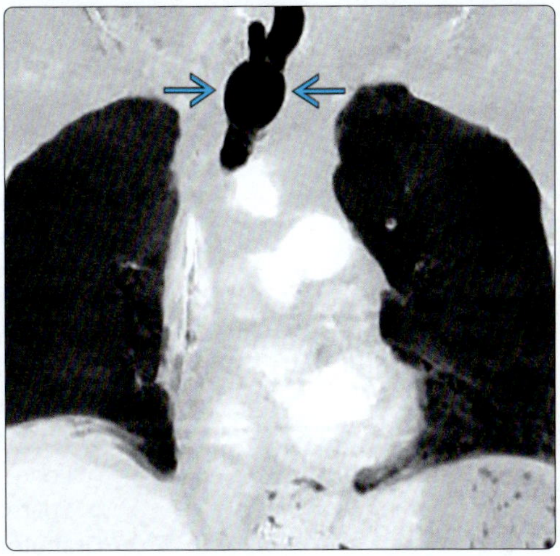

(Left) *Frontal chest radiograph of an intubated patient demonstrates bulging of the tracheal wall → secondary to overdistension of the endotracheal tube cuff.* **(Right)** *Coronal CT (minIP reformation) of a patient with tracheostomy cannula shows bulging of the tracheal wall → by overdistension of the endotracheal tube cuff. Dilatation of the trachea from overdistention of an endotracheal tube cuff or tracheostomy cannula often results in tracheal injury with increased risk of subsequent tracheal stenosis.*

Saber-Sheath Trachea

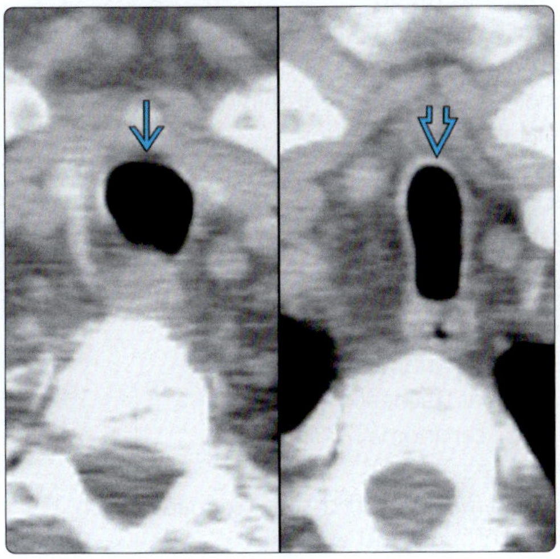

Tracheal Diverticulum

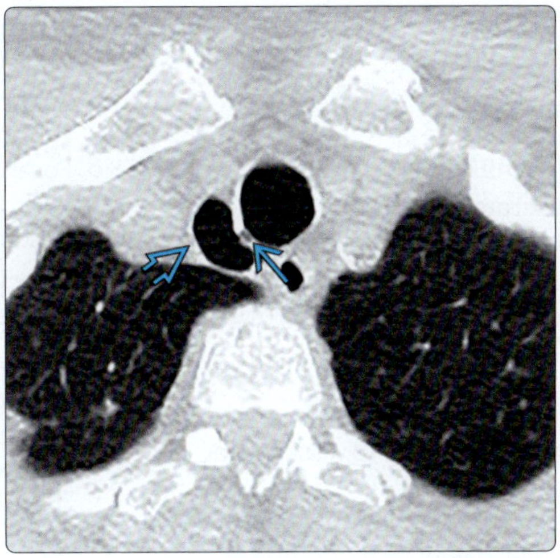

(Left) *Composite image with axial NECT at the thoracic inlet (left) and axial NECT at a lower level (right) of a patient with COPD shows the normal shape of the extrathoracic trachea → and the saber-sheath configuration ⇨ of the intrathoracic trachea.* **(Right)** *Axial NECT of a 59-year-old woman with tracheal diverticulum demonstrates a right paratracheal air collection ⇨. Note the diminutive and subtle connection with the trachea →.*

Mounier-Kuhn Syndrome

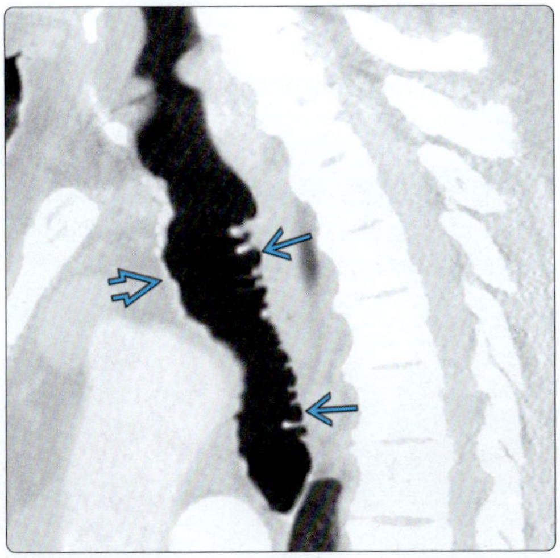

Mounier-Kuhn Syndrome

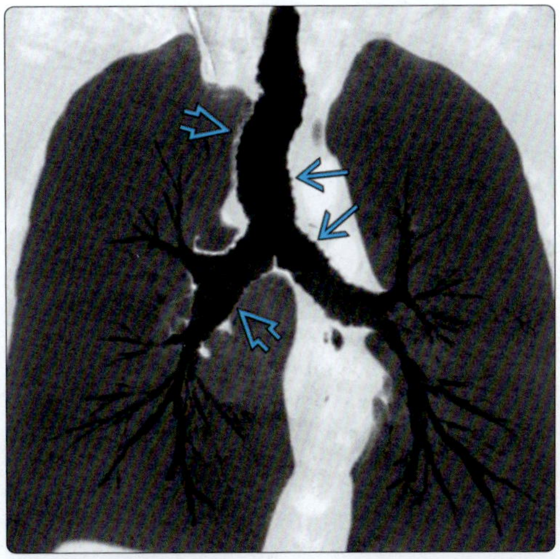

(Left) *Sagittal NECT (MIP reformation) of a patient with Mounier-Kuhn syndrome shows tracheal dilatation ⇨ with abundant characteristic tracheobronchial diverticula →. Tracheobronchial dilatation leads to impaired airway secretion clearance associated with recurrent infection and cough.* **(Right)** *Coronal CECT minIP reformation of the same patient shows airway dilatation ⇨ and the corrugated appearance → due to mucosa herniating between tracheal rings.*

DIFFERENTIAL DIAGNOSIS

Common

- Postintubation/Posttracheostomy Stenosis
- Tracheobronchomalacia

Less Common

- Tracheobronchopathia Osteochondroplastica
- Relapsing Polychondritis
- Granulomatosis With Polyangiitis
- Amyloidosis

Rare but Important

- Tracheal Neoplasm

ESSENTIAL INFORMATION

Key Differential Diagnosis Issues

- Symptoms usually do not develop until tracheal lumen reduced > 50%
- Differentiation between focal or diffuse narrowing is helpful
- Some diseases can cause either focal or diffuse airway narrowing
- In patients with long segment narrowing, identification of posterior wall involvement is important

Helpful Clues for Common Diagnoses

- **Postintubation/Posttracheostomy Stenosis**
  - Complication of endotracheal intubation or placement of tracheostomy tube
  - Location either at tracheal stoma or level of tube balloon
  - Symmetric narrowing < 2 cm in length
  - Hourglass shape
- **Tracheobronchomalacia**
  - Excessive expiratory airway collapse due to weakness of airway walls (> 70%)
  - Present in 23% of patients with COPD
  - Dynamic expiratory CT is highly sensitive for detecting airway malacia

Helpful Clues for Less Common Diagnoses

- **Tracheobronchopathia Osteochondroplastica**
  - Idiopathic
  - Elderly patients
  - Usually incidental finding at autopsy
  - Multiple calcified tracheal nodules
  - Long segment tracheal narrowing
  - Spares posterior membrane
- **Relapsing Polychondritis**
  - Systemic autoimmune disorder characterized by degeneration and deformation involving cartilage of ears, nose, larynx, and tracheobronchial tree
  - Diffuse or localized tracheobronchial involvement (20-50% of patients)
  - Tracheal wall thickening > 2 mm (40%)
  - Long segment tracheobronchial strictures
  - Spares posterior membrane
- **Granulomatosis With Polyangiitis**
  - Systemic necrotizing granulomatous vasculitis
  - Circumferential, focal or diffuse mucous thickening, irregular, with ulceration
  - Tracheal strictures (7% of patients)
- **Amyloidosis**
  - Spectrum of disease characterized by abnormal extracellular protein deposition
  - Focal or diffuse nodular soft tissue thickening of airway wall ± calcification/ossification
  - Posterior membrane involvement

Helpful Clues for Rare Diagnoses

- **Tracheal Neoplasm**
  - Squamous cell carcinoma (50%)
    - Large irregular tracheal mass
  - Adenoid cystic carcinoma (33%)
    - Lower trachea
    - Intraluminal mass of soft tissue attenuation with extension through tracheal wall
    - Homogeneous mass encircling trachea with wall thickening

Postintubation/Posttracheostomy Stenosis

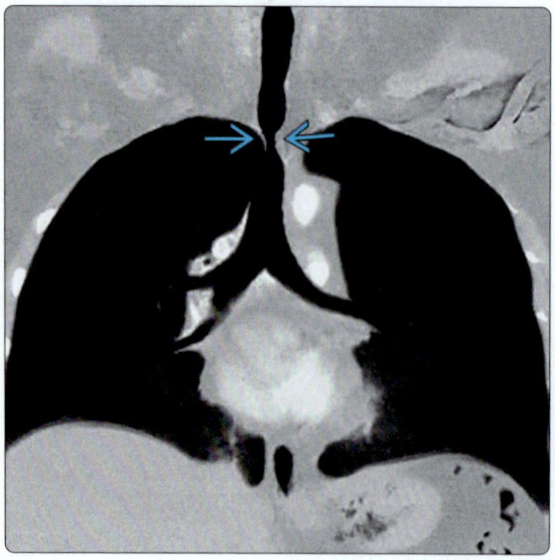

Tracheobronchomalacia

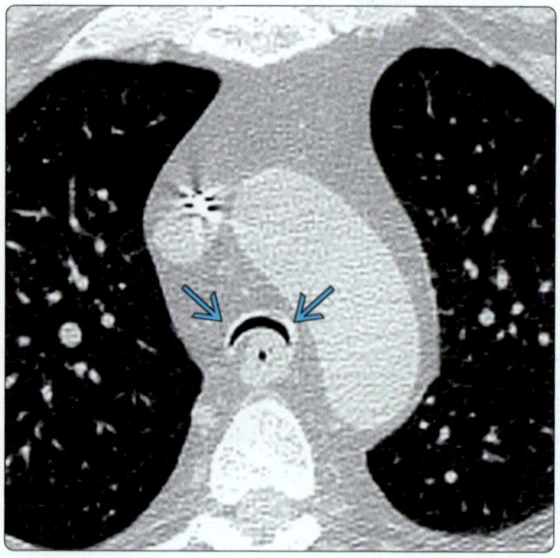

(Left) *Coronal CT (minIP reformation) of a 26-year-old woman with tracheal narrowing following intubation demonstrates an hourglass shape of the trachea near the thoracic inlet ➔.* **(Right)** *Axial expiratory NECT of a patient with tracheobronchomalacia shows expiratory collapse of the distal tracheal ➔. The diagnosis of tracheobronchomalacia requires further evaluation with expiratory CT as areas of collapse are often not noticeable during inspiration.*

Tracheobronchopathia Osteochondroplastica

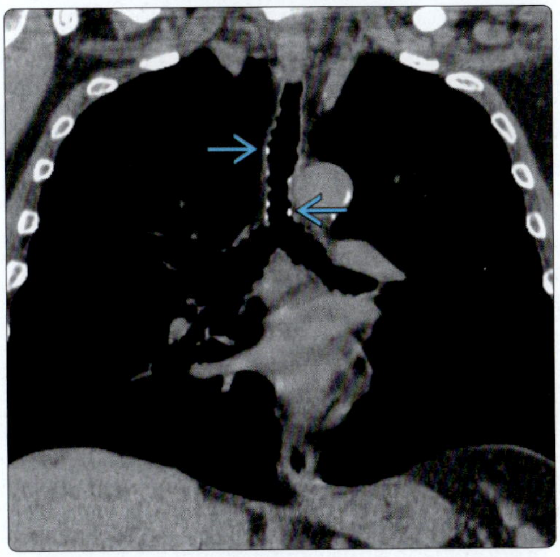

Relapsing Polychondritis

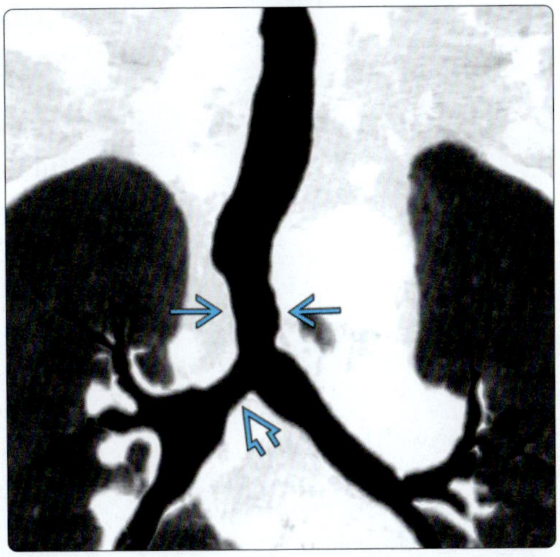

(Left) *Coronal NECT of a patient with tracheobronchopathia osteochondroplastica shows calcified small nodules protruding into the tracheal lumen. This diagnosis is often an incidental finding although it can be associated with chronic cough and wheezing.* **(Right)** *Coronal CECT (minIP reformation) of a patient with relapsing polychondritis shows narrowing of the distal trachea and right mainstem bronchus.*

Granulomatosis With Polyangiitis

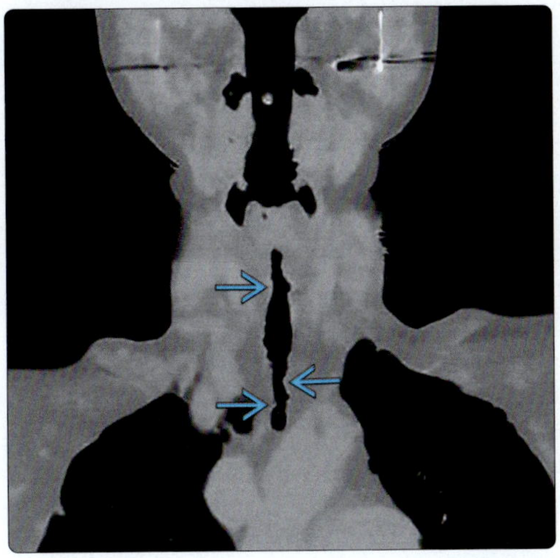

Amyloidosis

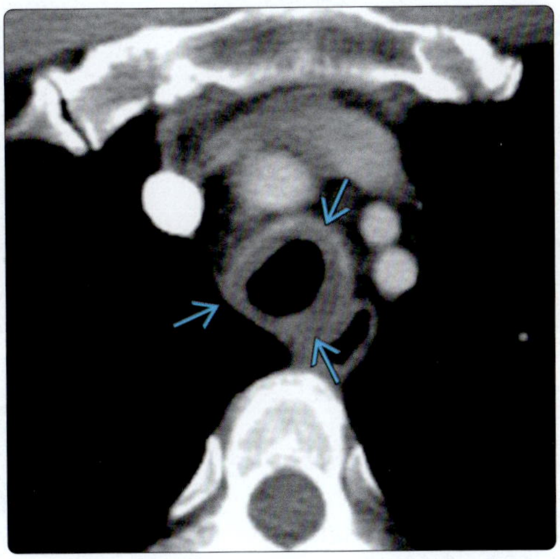

(Left) *Coronal CECT minIP reformation of a patient with granulomatosis with polyangiitis shows diffuse mucosal nodularity with segmental tracheal narrowing.* **(Right)** *Axial CECT of a patient with amyloidosis shows concentric tracheal thickening. Note involvement of the posterior tracheal membrane which is an important clue in the differential diagnosis. Tracheobronchopathia osteochondroplastica and relapsing polychondritis spare the posterior tracheal membrane.*

Tracheal Neoplasm

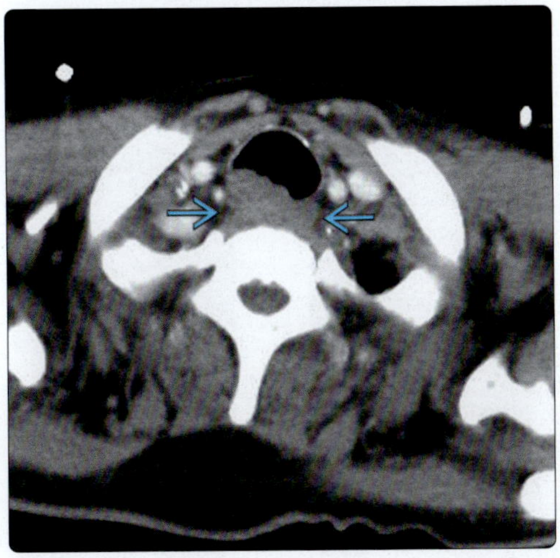

Tracheal Neoplasm

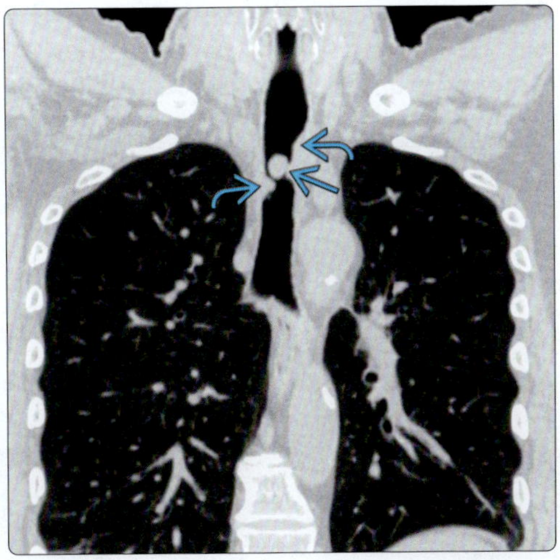

(Left) *Axial CECT of a patient with squamous cell carcinoma of the trachea shows a lobulated homogeneous mass involving the posterior tracheal wall.* **(Right)** *Coronal NECT of a patient with adenoid cystic carcinoma shows thickening of the tracheal wall and a large endoluminal nodule. Focal endoluminal tracheal lesion should always be further evaluated with bronchoscopy and biopsy to assess for the possibility of tracheal malignancy.*

DIFFERENTIAL DIAGNOSIS

Common

- Allergic Bronchopulmonary Aspergillosis
- Congenital Bronchial Atresia

Less Common

- Bronchiectasis
- Benign Airway Neoplasm
- Malignant Airway Neoplasm
- Foreign Body

ESSENTIAL INFORMATION

Key Differential Diagnosis Issues

- Finger-in-glove sign: Mucoid impaction with resultant dilated or impacted bronchi
  - Bronchial obstruction: Atresia, foreign body, neoplasm
  - Nonobstructive entities: Allergic bronchopulmonary aspergillosis, cystic fibrosis
- Radiography/CT: Branching tubular opacities that typically radiate from hilum toward lung periphery
- Differential diagnosis of bronchial branching tubular opacities
  - Arteriovenous malformation
    - Exhibits contrast enhancement
    - Demonstrates afferent and efferent vessels: Feeding artery(ies) and draining vein(s)

Helpful Clues for Common Diagnoses

- **Allergic Bronchopulmonary Aspergillosis**
  - Immunologic disorder caused by hypersensitivity to *Aspergillus fumigatus*
  - Predisposing conditions: Asthma, cystic fibrosis
  - Laboratory findings: Positive aspergillus skin test, elevated IgE levels against *Aspergillus fumigatus*
    - Total IgE levels > 1,000 IU/mL
    - IgG antibodies against *A. fumigatus* in serum
    - Total eosinophil count > 500 cells/mL
  - Imaging: Branching tubular opacities, high attenuation on CT due to intrinsic calcium oxalate
- **Congenital Bronchial Atresia**
  - Focal atresia of segmental bronchus
  - Typically affects left upper lobe apicoposterior segment
  - Recurrent infection in 20% of patients
  - CT: Tubular or branching opacity surrounded by hyperlucent lung due to air-trapping and oligemia

Helpful Clues for Less Common Diagnoses

- **Bronchiectasis**
  - Cystic fibrosis
    - Autosomal recessive disorder that affects regulation of chloride transport
    - Recurrent infection, progressive bronchial wall injury
    - Diffuse bronchiectasis (upper lobe predominant); central and peripheral airways affected
  - Primary ciliary dyskinesia
    - Structural abnormality that affects ciliary motion
    - Bronchiectasis, sinusitis, infertility
    - Basilar predominant airway involvement
- **Benign Airway Neoplasm**
  - Hamartoma
    - Endobronchial (1.4% of cases)
    - Fat &/or calcification in endobronchial lesion supports diagnosis
  - Lipoma
    - Endobronchial lipoma (0.1-0.5% of lung tumors)
    - Nonenhancing homogeneous fat attenuation lesion
- **Malignant Airway Neoplasm**
  - Carcinoid tumor
    - Low-grade neuroendocrine neoplasm
    - Intrinsic calcification; may be eccentric
    - Marked contrast enhancement
  - Lung cancer
    - Centrally obstructing mass
    - Mucoid impaction uncommon
- **Foreign Body**
  - Patients < 15 years of age (70%)
  - Most frequent location: Right lower lobe bronchus and bronchus intermedius
  - Adults: Chronic clinical course, recurrent pneumonia

Allergic Bronchopulmonary Aspergillosis

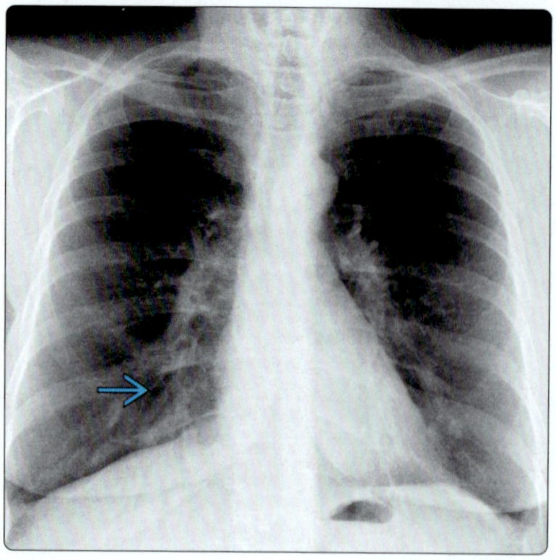

Allergic Bronchopulmonary Aspergillosis

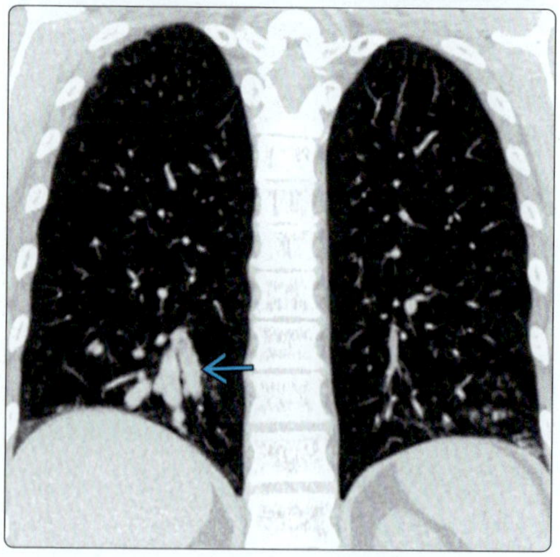

(Left) *PA chest radiograph of a patient with asthma and allergic bronchopulmonary aspergillosis shows right basilar tubular opacities* ➡ *corresponding to mucoid impaction in dilated airways.* **(Right)** *Coronal NECT of the same patient shows right basilar branching tubular opacities that correspond to right lower lobe bronchiectasis with intrinsic mucus plugs* ➡*. Impacted mucus may exhibit high attenuation. Allergic bronchopulmonary aspergillosis is due to hypersensitivity to fungal antigens.*

Congenital Bronchial Atresia

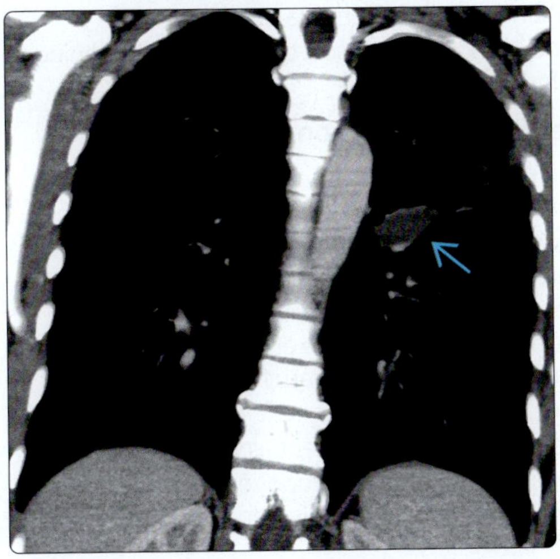

Congenital Bronchial Atresia

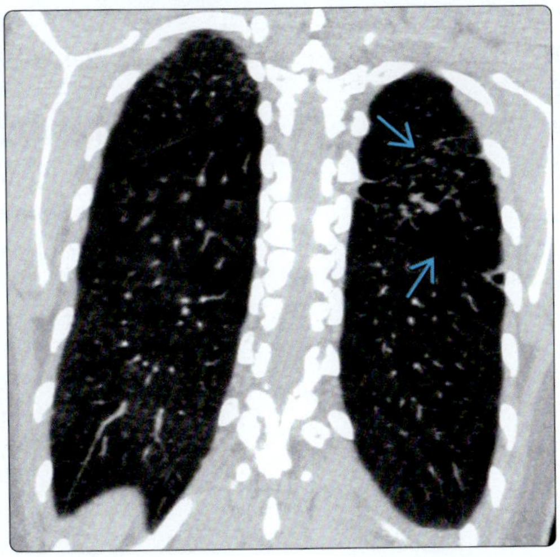

(Left) *Coronal CECT of a 27-year-old man with bronchial atresia shows a nonenhancing left upper lobe tubular opacity that corresponds to an atretic bronchus impacted with mucus →.* **(Right)** *Coronal CECT of the same patient shows focal air-trapping → in the left upper lobe distal to the impacted atretic bronchus and mucocele. Bronchial atresia most frequently affects the left upper lobe apicoposterior bronchus. Affected patients are typically asymptomatic.*

Bronchiectasis

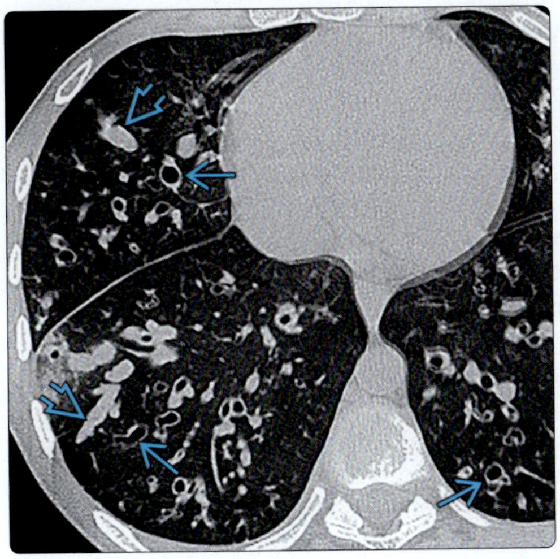

Bronchiectasis

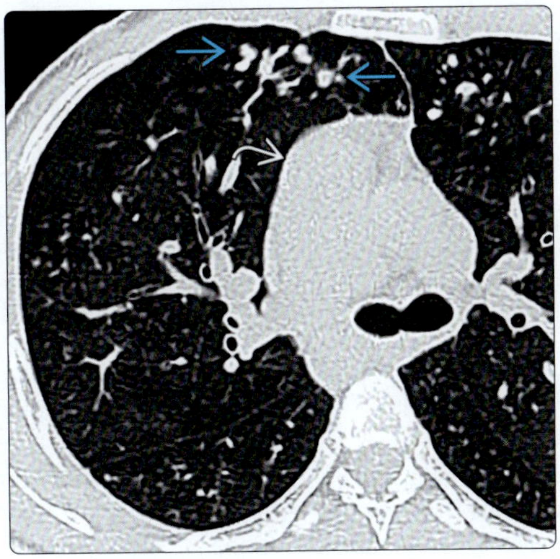

(Left) *Axial NECT of a 20-year-old man with cystic fibrosis shows multifocal bronchiectasis →, bronchial wall thickening, and soft tissue tubular opacities that correspond to impacted mucus → within dilated peripheral airways.* **(Right)** *Axial NECT of a 34-year-old-man with primary ciliary dyskinesia and Kartagener syndrome shows bilateral upper lobe branching tubular opacities → that correspond to impacted mucus within bronchiectatic airways. Note coexistent situs inversus and right aortic arch →.*

Malignant Airway Neoplasm

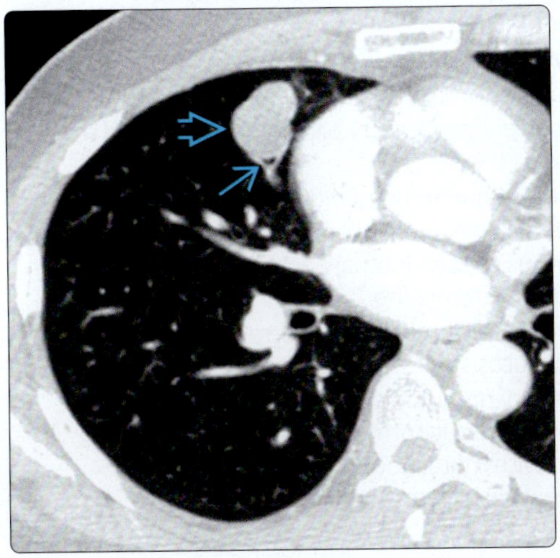

Malignant Airway Neoplasm

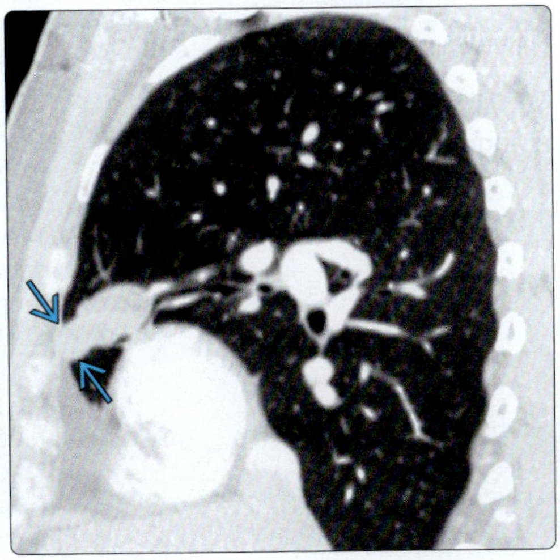

(Left) *Axial CECT of a patient with a history of chronic cough and blood-tinged sputum shows a polylobular middle lobe soft tissue mass → that exhibits an endobronchial component → and obstructs a small airway in the middle lobe. Carcinoid tumor was diagnosed at surgery.* **(Right)** *Sagittal CECT of the same patient shows the centrally obstructing carcinoid tumor and peripheral mucoid impaction →. Carcinoid tumor is a low-grade malignant neoplasm with frequent endobronchial involvement.*

DIFFERENTIAL DIAGNOSIS

Common

- Tracheobronchial Secretions
- Postintubation Tracheal Stenosis

Less Common

- Malignant Neoplasm
  - Squamous Cell Carcinoma
  - Carcinoid
  - Adenoid Cystic Carcinoma
  - Mucoepidermoid Carcinoma
  - Metastasis
- Benign Neoplasm
  - Papilloma
  - Lipoma
  - Leiomyoma
  - Hamartoma
  - Pulmonary Pleomorphic Adenoma
  - Paraganglioma
- Infection
  - Tuberculosis
  - Rhinoscleroma
- Amyloidosis
- Granulomatosis With Polyangiitis
- Tracheobronchopathia Osteochondroplastica
- Bronchial Anthracofibrosis
- Foreign Body

Rare but Important

- Broncholithiasis

ESSENTIAL INFORMATION

Key Differential Diagnosis Issues

- Airway narrowing, airway wall thickening, and endoluminal secretions may be indistinguishable from each other on imaging (e.g., mucus plugs may mimic endoluminal lesions and may appear as focal mural thickening &/or narrowing)
- Chest radiography is insensitive for identification &/or characterization of focal airway narrowing
- CT is modality of choice for assessment of tracheobronchial thickening &/or narrowing
- 90% of tracheal neoplasms are malignant

Helpful Clues for Common Diagnoses

- **Tracheobronchial Secretions**
  - Often referred to as mucus plugs
  - CT
    - Focal or multifocal endoluminal filling defects often containing intrinsic air
    - Dependent location (i.e., posterior)
    - Mucus plugs
      - ▫ Common in patients with chronic obstructive pulmonary disease (COPD) and aspiration
      - ▫ Nodular endoluminal plugs may be indistinguishable from early benign or malignant neoplasms
      - ▫ May require follow-up imaging or bronchoscopy to document resolution
  - Aspirated material (e.g., esophageal or gastric secretions, blood)
- **Postintubation Tracheal Stenosis**
  - Chronic sequela of intubation (common) versus acute and transient airway wall edema (rare)
  - CT: Eccentric or concentric soft tissue mural thickening, normal underlying cartilage

Helpful Clues for Less Common Diagnoses

- **Malignant Neoplasm**
  - **Squamous Cell Carcinoma**
    - Pulmonary squamous cell carcinoma tends to be central; may also be primary tracheal malignancy
    - CT: Central nodule or mass with endoluminal component; postobstructive atelectasis or pneumonitis; lymphadenopathy
  - **Carcinoid**
    - Central or peripheral, frequent airway relationship
    - CT: Smaller endoluminal component with larger component outside bronchus ("tip of the iceberg" sign)
  - **Adenoid Cystic Carcinoma**
    - Low-grade malignancy
    - Primary tracheal neoplasm
    - CT: Endoluminal tracheal nodule/mass with focal, circumferential, or diffuse mural thickening
  - **Mucoepidermoid Carcinoma**
    - Histologically identical to primary salivary gland neoplasms of same name; neoplasms of bronchial wall origin may involve airways &/or lung
    - CT: Endobronchial mass/nodule; may exhibit calcification; heterogeneous contrast enhancement
  - **Metastasis**
    - Contiguous airway involvement (e.g., lung cancer) versus hematogenous metastasis(es)
    - Primary cancers that may cause hematogenous airway metastases: Renal cell carcinoma, melanoma, breast cancer, thyroid cancer, colon cancer, cervical cancer, gastric cancer, ovarian cancer, endometrial carcinoma, prostate cancer, testicular cancer, and adrenal carcinoma
    - CT: Endoluminal nodule ± postobstructive atelectasis/pneumonitis, lymphadenopathy
- **Benign Neoplasm**
  - **Papilloma**
    - Typically secondary to human papilloma virus (HPV)
      - ▫ Recurrent respiratory papillomatosis linked to HPV 6 and 11
    - Histology: Squamous, glandular, or mixed
    - May undergo malignant transformation into squamous cell carcinoma; postulated to relate to HPV infection and smoking
    - Solitary (rare) or multiple (recurrent respiratory papillomatosis)
    - CT: Solitary or multiple tracheobronchial nodules, often with verruciform morphology; cystic lung lesions with mural nodularity in patients with recurrent respiratory papillomatosis
  - **Lipoma**
    - Benign endoluminal fatty neoplasm
    - CT: Endobronchial nodule of fat or soft tissue attenuation
  - **Leiomyoma**

- Tumor of smooth muscle origin
- CT: Smooth or lobular soft tissue mass ± postobstructive atelectasis/pneumonitis; homogeneous enhancement; may exhibit intrinsic calcification; "tip of the iceberg" sign in 15% of cases

- **Hamartoma**
  - May contain cartilage, bone, fat, muscle, and respiratory epithelium; rarely endoluminal
  - CT: Smoothly marginated endobronchial polypoid or sessile nodule
- **Pulmonary Pleomorphic Adenoma**
  - Originates from tracheal and bronchial glands
  - CT: Homogenous polypoid endobronchial nodule
- **Paraganglioma**
  - Exceedingly rare
  - Origin from extraadrenal chromaffin cells
  - CT: Endoluminal lesion with marked contrast enhancement

- **Infection**
  - **Tuberculosis**
    - Active disease: Irregular, circumferential luminal narrowing ± mediastinitis
    - Fibrotic disease: Bronchial narrowing with smooth lumen
  - **Rhinoscleroma**
    - Etiology: *Klebsiella rhinoscleromatis*
    - CT: Focal or diffuse tracheal wall thickening ± nodularity
- **Amyloidosis**
  - Idiopathic deposition of fibrillar proteins along tracheobronchial tree
  - CT: Endobronchial irregularity/nodularity; focal or diffuse circumferential mural thickening; ± calcification; involvement of posterior tracheal wall
- **Granulomatosis With Polyangiitis**
  - Chronic granulomatous vasculitis involving small and medium-sized vessels
  - CT: Focal or diffuse smooth or nodular circumferential tracheal wall thickening with posterior tracheal wall involvement; may produce tracheal stenosis
- **Tracheobronchopathia Osteochondroplastica**
  - Idiopathic development of tracheal osseous &/or cartilaginous small submucosal nodules (1-8 mm)
  - CT: Focal or diffuse soft tissue submucosal nodules ± calcification; sparing of posterior tracheal wall
- **Bronchial Anthracofibrosis**
  - Bronchial narrowing with anthracotic pigmentation on bronchoscopy; unknown etiology
  - Association with tuberculosis
  - CT: Focal bronchial narrowing adjacent to calcified lymph nodes; may cause middle lobe syndrome/atelectasis
- **Foreign Body**
  - Various foreign bodies may cause airway obstruction and mural thickening often with postobstructive atelectasis/pneumonitis
  - CT: Bronchial obstruction; foreign body may exhibit high or low attenuation

Helpful Clues for Rare Diagnoses

- **Broncholithiasis**
  - Erosion of calcified lymph node into adjacent airway causing partial or complete obstruction
  - CT: Rounded calcified endoluminal nodule; postobstructive pneumonitis or atelectasis

SELECTED REFERENCES

1. Dimachkieh AL et al: Tracheal paraganglioma presenting as stridor in a pediatric patient, case report and literature review. Int J Pediatr Otorhinolaryngol. 107:145-9, 2018
2. Theriault MM et al: Diseases involving the central bronchi: multidetector CT for detection, characterization, and differential diagnosis. Radiographics. 38(1):58-9, 2018
3. Fortes HR et al: Laryngotracheobronchial papillomatosis: chest CT findings. J Bras Pneumol. 43(4):259-63, 2017
4. Silveira MGM et al: Tracheobronchopathia osteochondroplastica. J Bras Pneumol. 43(2):151-3, 2017
5. Kim YK et al: Airway leiomyoma: imaging findings and histopathologic comparisons in 13 patients. AJR Am J Roentgenol. 189(2):393-9, 2007
6. O'Regan A et al: Tracheobronchial amyloidosis. the Boston University experience from 1984 to 1999. Medicine (Baltimore). 79(2):69-79, 2000

Tracheobronchial Secretions

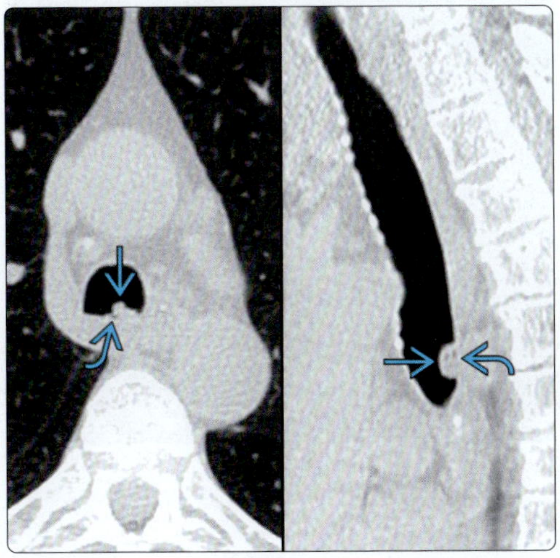

Postintubation Tracheal Stenosis

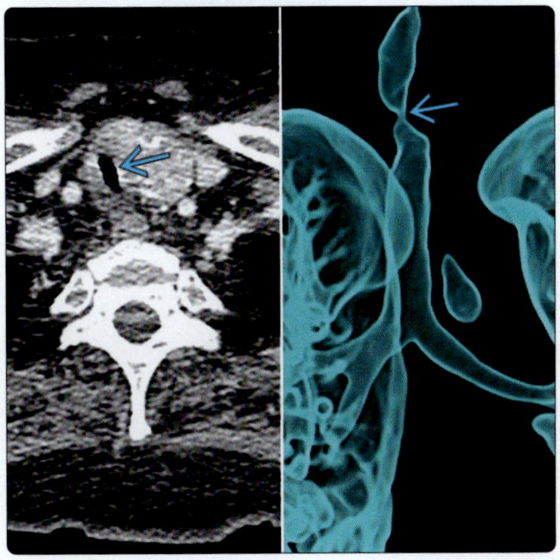

(Left) *Composite image with axial (left) and coronal (right) NECT shows tracheal secretions that manifest as a posterior endoluminal polypoid lesion ⇒ that mimics an airway neoplasm. Intrinsic air within the lesion ⇒ helps exclude a neoplastic etiology.* **(Right)** *Composite image with axial CECT (left) and volume-rendered reformatted image (right) of a patient with multiple prior intubations and tracheostomy shows marked focal tracheal stenosis ⇒, consistent with postintubation stenosis.*

(Left) *Composite image with axial NECT (left) and FDG PET (right) of a patient with primary tracheal squamous cell carcinoma shows a well-marginated small anterior tracheal nodule → with intense FDG avidity ↪.* **(Right)** *Composite image with axial CECT of a patient with lung cancer shows a spiculated right lower lobe nodule → with extensive mediastinal lymphadenopathy and secondary invasion and mural thickening of the trachea ↪.*

Squamous Cell Carcinoma

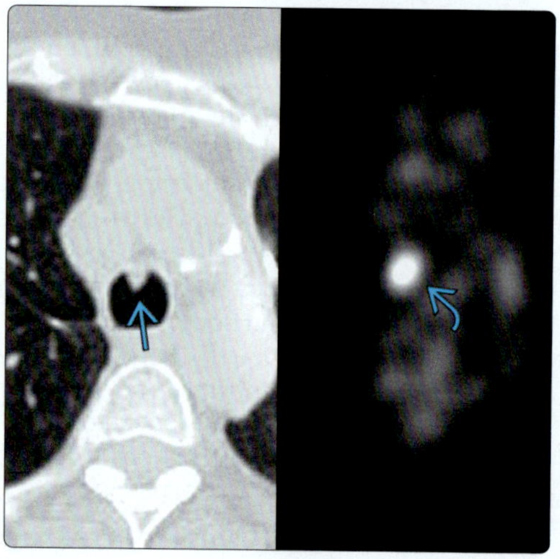

Squamous Cell Carcinoma

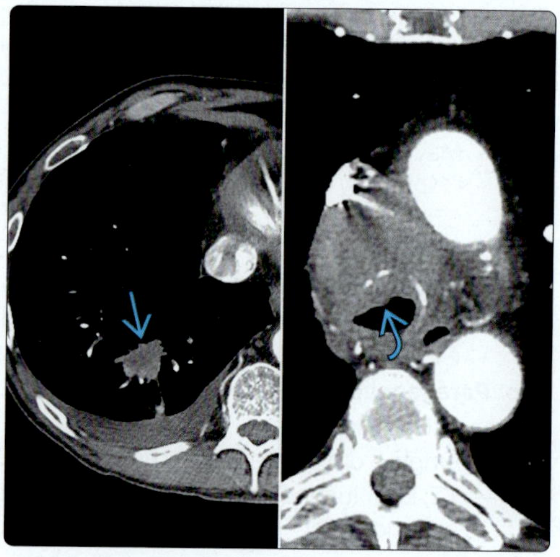

(Left) *Axial NECT shows a bronchial carcinoid that obstructs the right upper lobe posterior segmental bronchus → and associated postobstructive pneumonia ↪. While the lesion has a discrete endoluminal component, a significant portion is extraluminal ("tip of the iceberg" sign).* **(Right)** *Composite image with axial (left) and coronal (right) NECT shows an adenoid cystic carcinoma that exhibits concentric mural thickening of the trachea → and a focal polypoid endoluminal lesion ↪.*

Carcinoid

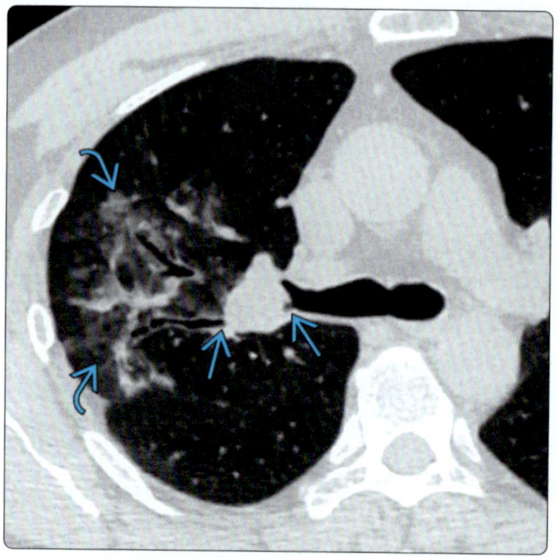

Adenoid Cystic Carcinoma

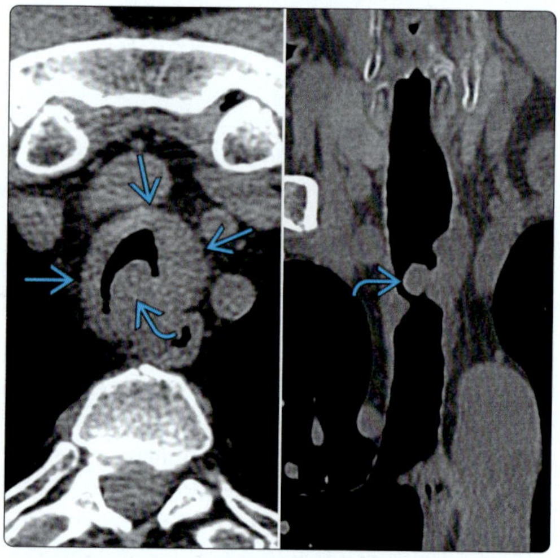

(Left) *Axial oblique CECT of a patient with mucoepidermoid carcinoma involving the middle lobe shows a focal endoluminal neoplasm → at the origin of the middle lobe bronchus and extensive middle lobe postobstructive pneumonitis and tumor involvement ↪.* **(Right)** *Axial CECT of a patient with metastatic renal clear cell carcinoma shows an obstructive endobronchial metastasis → with an enhancing endobronchial component ↪ and surrounding postobstructive atelectasis and pneumonia.*

Mucoepidermoid Carcinoma

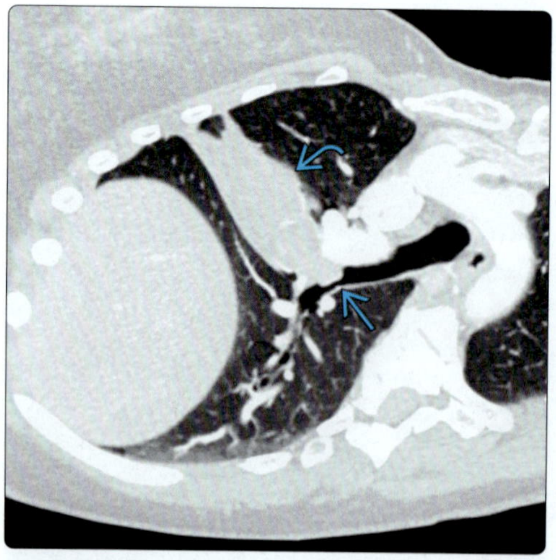

Metastasis

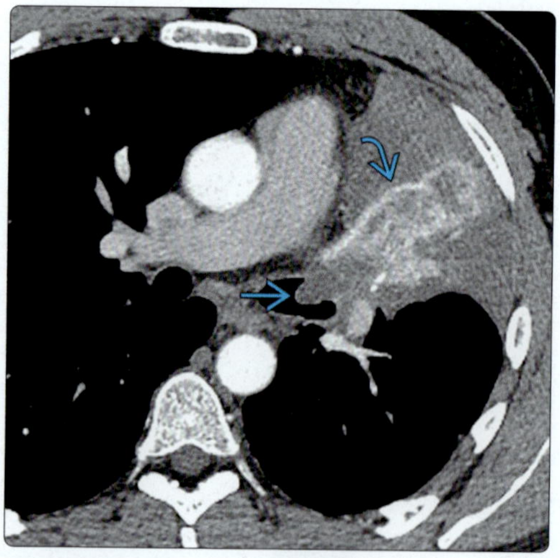

Papilloma

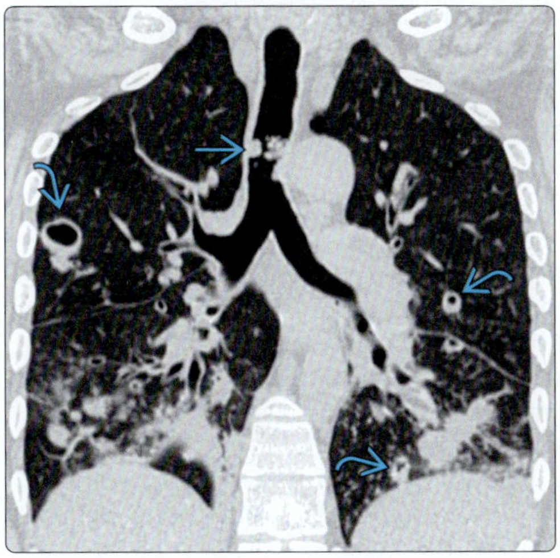

Papilloma

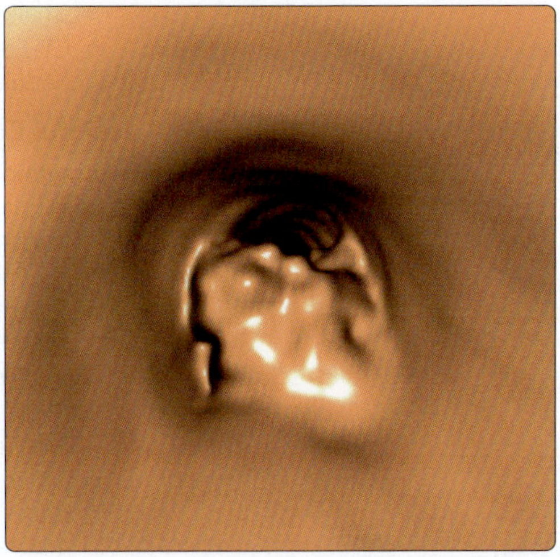

(Left) *Coronal CECT of a patient with recurrent respiratory papillomatosis shows cauliflower-like endoluminal tracheal lesions* → *and multiple solid and cavitary nodules* ↗ *and tree-in-bud opacities, which are classic associated findings.* **(Right)** *Virtual bronchoscopy of the same patient shows a verruciform appearance of a tracheal nodule. Recurrent respiratory papillomatosis has been linked with human papillomavirus (HPV) subtypes 6 and 11. Pulmonary papillomas often exhibit cavitation.*

Amyloidosis

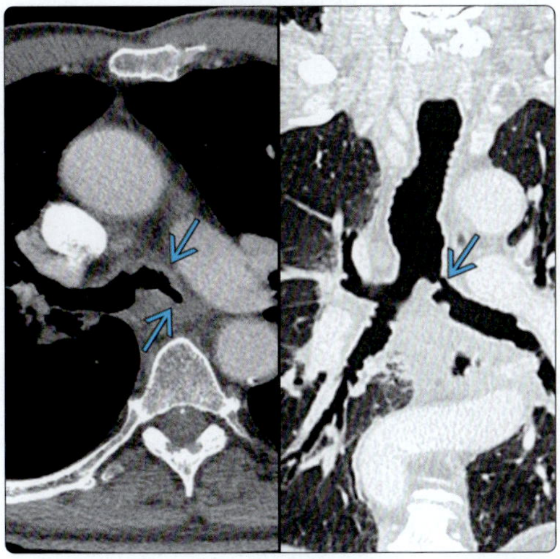

Granulomatosis With Polyangiitis

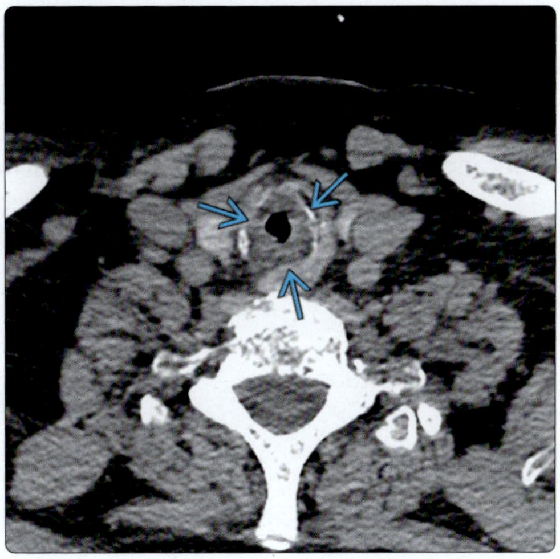

(Left) *Axial (left) and coronal (right) CECTs of amyloidosis and marginal zone lymphoma show irregular nodular thickening involving proximal left mainstem bronchus* →*. Biopsy confirmed tracheobronchial amyloidosis.* **(Right)** *Axial NECT of a patient with granulomatosis and polyangiitis shows focal concentric thickening and narrowing of upper trachea* →*. Involvement of posterior tracheal wall is helpful for differentiating from amyloidosis or tracheobronchopathia osteochondroplastica.*

Granulomatosis With Polyangiitis

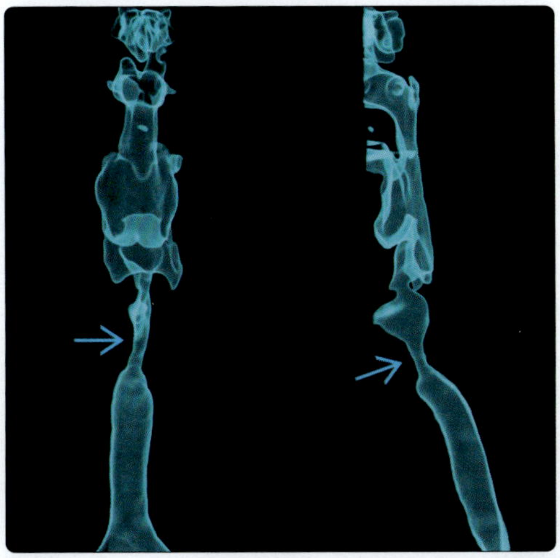

Tracheobronchopathia Osteochondroplastica

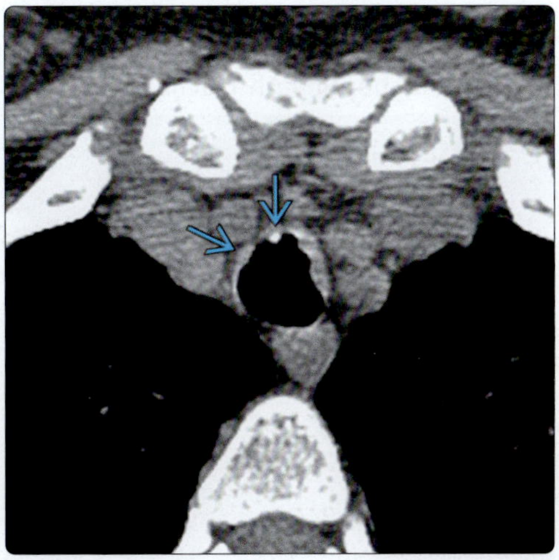

(Left) *Composite image with coronal (left) and sagittal (right) 3D surface rendered reformation of the same patient shows short segment stenosis of the upper trachea* →*.* **(Right)** *Axial NECT of a patient with tracheobronchopathia osteochondroplastica shows multiple soft tissue and calcified nodules* → *affecting anterolateral tracheal wall. Note sparing of posterior membranous tracheal wall.*

Airway Wall Thickening (Diffuse)

DIFFERENTIAL DIAGNOSIS

Common

- Saber-Sheath Trachea
- Bronchitis
- Pulmonary Edema
- Tracheobronchopathia Osteochondroplastica

Less Common

- Amyloidosis
- Granulomatosis With Polyangiitis
- Relapsing Polychondritis
- Infection
  - Tracheobronchial Papillomatosis
  - Rhinoscleroma
  - Other: Tuberculosis, histoplasmosis, coccidioidomycosis, mucormycosis, aspergillosis (airway-invasive aspergillosis)

ESSENTIAL INFORMATION

Helpful Clues for Common Diagnoses

- **Saber-Sheath Trachea**
  - May mimic diffuse tracheal narrowing; common in chronic obstructive pulmonary disease (COPD)
  - CT: Medial displacement of lateral tracheal walls with ↓ coronal and ↑ sagittal diameters; mild tracheal wall thickening; tracheal ring calcification
- **Bronchitis**
  - Chronic bronchitis is part of COPD spectrum
    - May also occur in asthma or acute infection
  - Bronchial wall thickening is nonspecific
  - Radiography: Peribronchial cuffing
  - CT: Bronchial wall thickening; bronchial pitting
- **Pulmonary Edema**
  - Cardiogenic pulmonary edema
  - Diffuse bronchial wall thickening secondary to extravascular water in axial or peribronchovascular interstitium
  - Ancillary findings: Peribronchovascular opacities, septal thickening, pleural effusions, cardiomegaly
- **Tracheobronchopathia Osteochondroplastica**
  - Idiopathic; development of osseous &/or cartilaginous small submucosal tracheal wall nodules (1-8 mm)
  - CT: Focal or diffuse soft tissue &/or calcified mural nodules; spare posterior tracheal wall

Helpful Clues for Less Common Diagnoses

- **Amyloidosis**
  - Idiopathic; deposition of fibrillar proteins along tracheobronchial tree
  - CT: Endobronchial irregularity/nodularity; focal or diffuse circumferential wall thickening; mural calcification; posterior tracheal wall involvement
- **Granulomatosis With Polyangiitis**
  - Chronic granulomatous vasculitis involving small and medium-sized vessels
  - CT: Focal or diffuse smooth or nodular circumferential tracheal wall thickening; posterior tracheal involvement; may result in tracheal stenosis
- **Relapsing Polychondritis**
  - Autoimmune disease with recurrent inflammation of cartilage in trachea and in other organs
  - CT: Long-segment tracheobronchial narrowing with mural thickening ± calcification; posterior tracheal sparing; tracheobronchial collapse on expiratory imaging
- **Infection**
  - **Tracheobronchial Papillomatosis**
    - Recurrent respiratory papillomatosis linked to HPV 6 and 11
    - CT: Solitary or multiple tracheobronchial nodules, often with verruciform morphology; thin-walled cysts with mural nodularity

SELECTED REFERENCES

1. Shepard JO et al: Imaging of the trachea. Ann Cardiothorac Surg. 7(2):197-209, 2018
2. Shroff GS et al: Pathology of the trachea and central bronchi. Semin Ultrasound CT MR. 37(3):177-89, 2016
3. Marom EM et al: Diffuse abnormalities of the trachea and main bronchi. AJR 2001;176;(3):713-7

Saber-Sheath Trachea

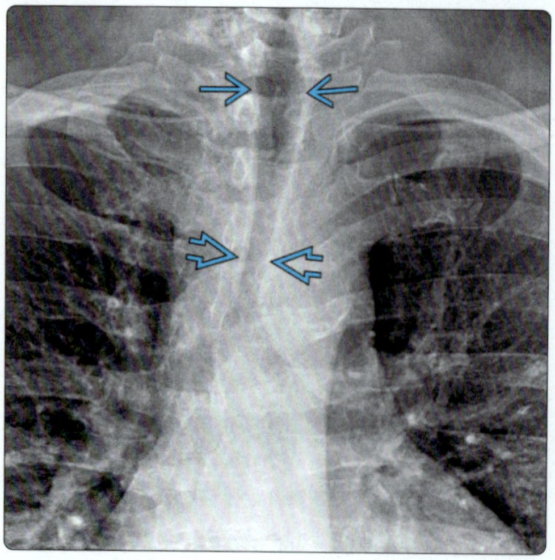

Saber-Sheath Trachea

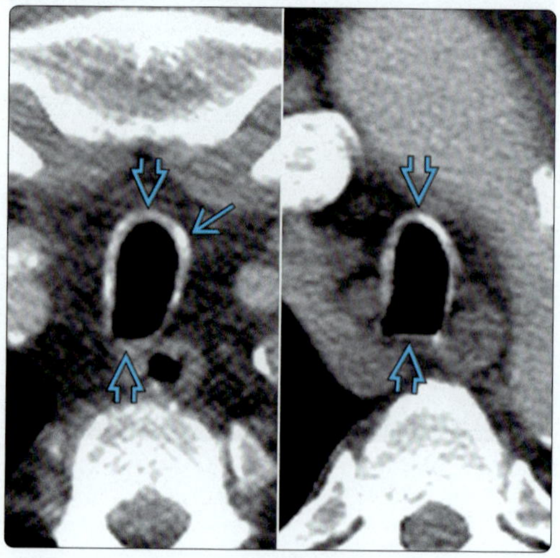

(Left) *PA chest radiograph of a patient with chronic obstructive pulmonary disease (COPD) and saber-sheath trachea shows marked narrowing of the distal trachea* ➡ *as compared to the normal caliber of the upper trachea* ➡. **(Right)** *Composite image with axial CECT of the same patient shows an abnormal tracheal morphology in which the AP tracheal diameter* ➡ *exceeds its transverse diameter. Note mild thickening of the tracheal wall* ➡. *Saber-sheath trachea is commonly seen in the setting of COPD.*

Bronchitis

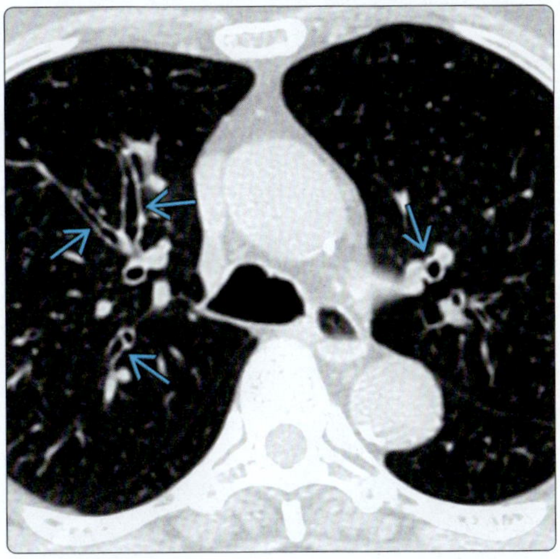

Bronchitis

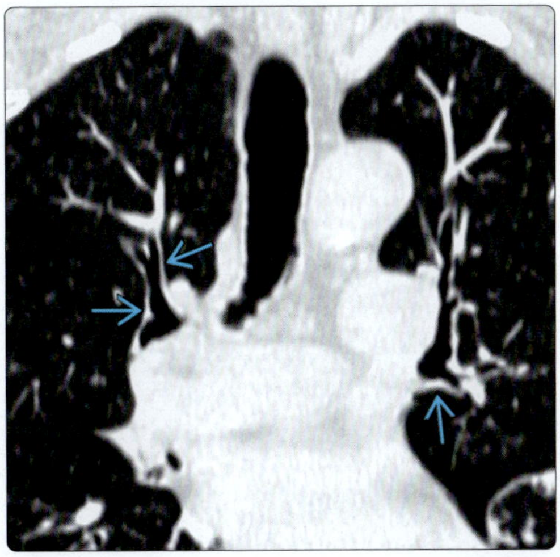

(Left) *Axial NECT of a patient with chronic bronchitis shows diffuse bronchial wall thickening bilaterally* → *. This is a nonspecific imaging finding, which may be seen in acute and chronic bronchitis of either infectious or inflammatory (e.g., asthma) etiology, as well as in pulmonary edema. While the diagnosis of chronic bronchitis is made clinically, bronchial wall thickening is a commonly associated CT finding.* **(Right)** *Coronal NECT of the same patient shows diffuse bilateral mild bronchial wall thickening* → *.*

Bronchitis

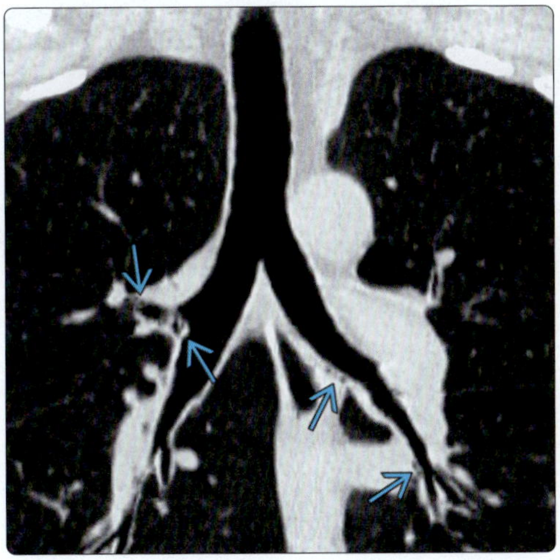

Pulmonary Edema

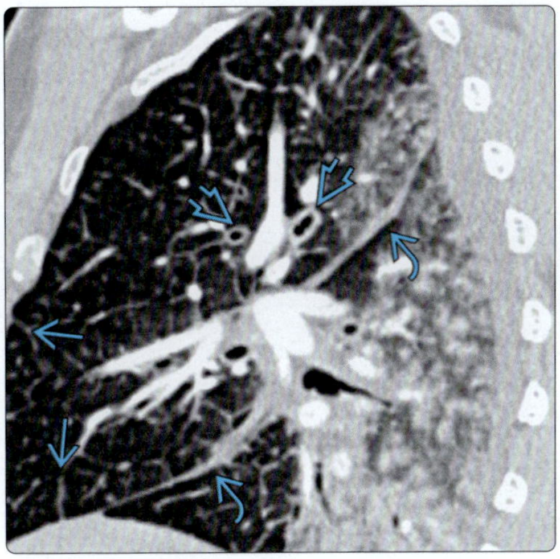

(Left) *Coronal NECT (minIP reformation) of a patient with chronic bronchitis shows central airway bronchial pitting* → *, which results from increased submucosal glands. While not always present, this finding is specific for chronic bronchitis.* **(Right)** *Sagittal CECT of a patient with interstitial and alveolar cardiogenic pulmonary edema shows diffuse bronchial wall thickening* → *. Note thick interlobar fissures* → *, septal thickening* → *, and lower lobe predominant acinar opacities, the latter from alveolar edema.*

Tracheobronchopathia Osteochondroplastica

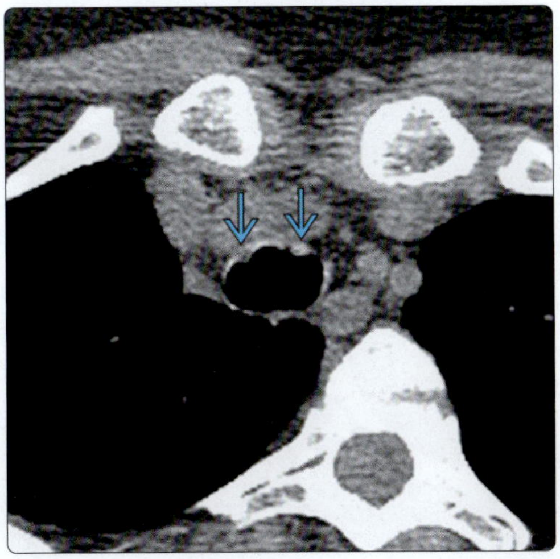

Tracheobronchopathia Osteochondroplastica

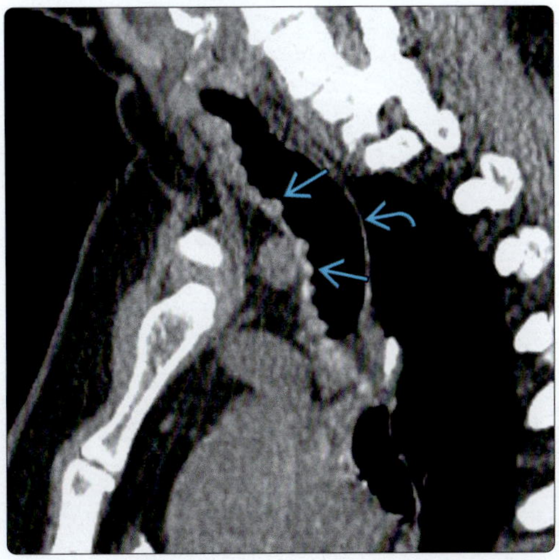

(Left) *Axial NECT of an asymptomatic patient with tracheobronchopathia osteochondroplastica shows mural nodularity* → *of the anterior trachea with characteristic sparing of the membranous posterior tracheal wall.* **(Right)** *Sagittal NECT of the same patient shows mural nodularity of the anterior trachea* → *. Note sparing of the posterior (membranous) tracheal wall* → *. Tracheobronchopathia osteochondroplastica is commonly asymptomatic but may manifest with cough and wheezing.*

(Left) *Axial CECT of a patient with tracheal amyloidosis shows marked concentric mural thickening of trachea → with resultant luminal narrowing. Note involvement of posterior tracheal wall ↷.* **(Right)** *Coronal CECT of the same patient shows diffuse mural thickening with intrinsic ill-defined calcifications of trachea and central bronchi. While rare, amyloidosis is well recognized cause of diffuse tracheal wall thickening. Involvement of posterior membranous tracheal wall is typical. (Courtesy L. Arias, MD.)*

Amyloidosis

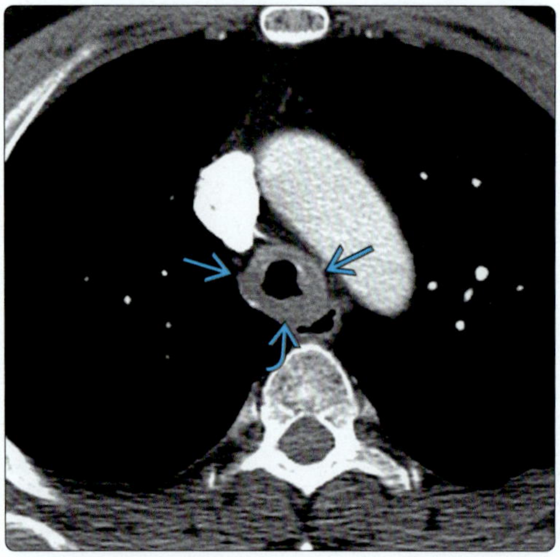

Amyloidosis

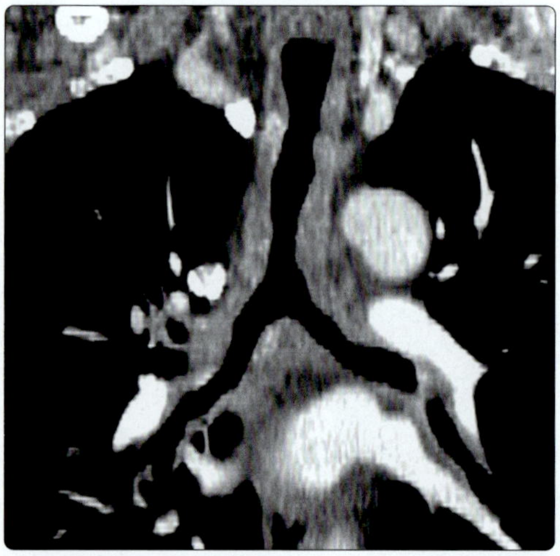

(Left) *Axial CECT of a patient with tracheobronchial amyloidosis shows concentric thickening of the trachea → with involvement of the posterior membranous tracheal wall ↷. The latter is a helpful finding for differential diagnosis, as other diseases do not typically involve this area (e.g., tracheobronchopathia osteochondroplastica, relapsing polychondritis).* **(Right)** *Axial CECT of the same patient shows concentric mural thickening → of the central bronchi bilaterally, also a characteristic finding.*

Amyloidosis

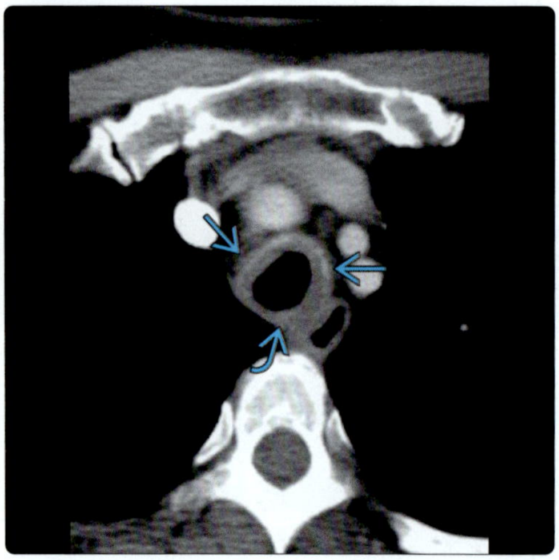

Amyloidosis

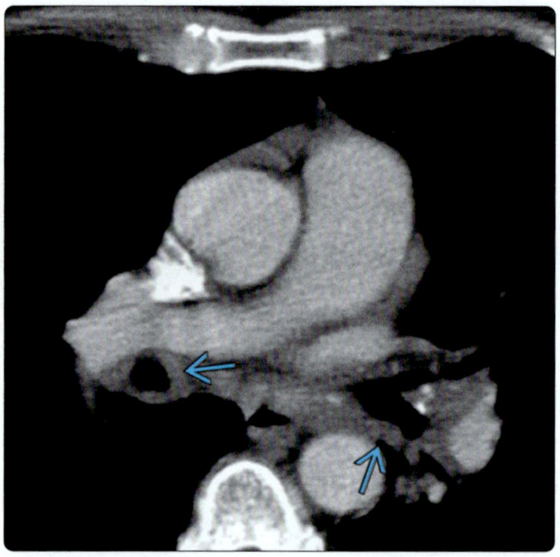

(Left) *Axial CECT of a patient with granulomatosis with polyangiitis shows circumferential thickening and narrowing of the left mainstem bronchus →. Airway involvement may be focal or diffuse and often involves the posterior tracheal wall. Note left upper lobe airspace disease ↷ from pulmonary vasculitis.* **(Right)** *Axial CECT of the same patient shows a large left upper lobe consolidation ↷ and associated circumferential thickening and narrowing of the left mainstem bronchus →.*

Granulomatosis With Polyangiitis

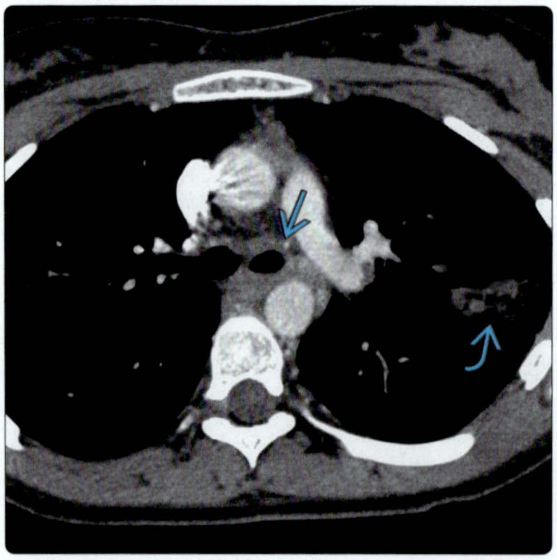

Granulomatosis With Polyangiitis

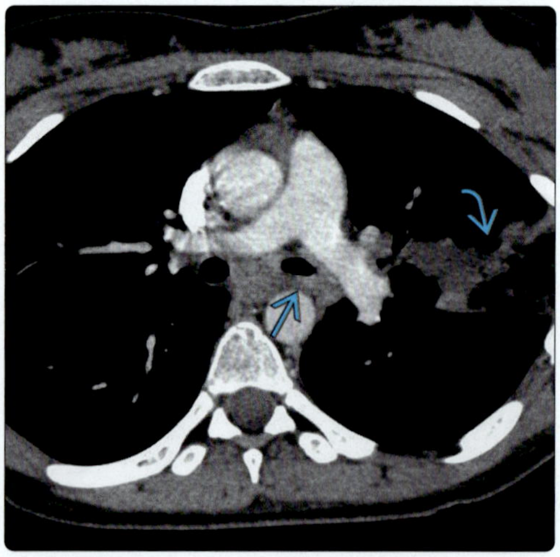

Relapsing Polychondritis

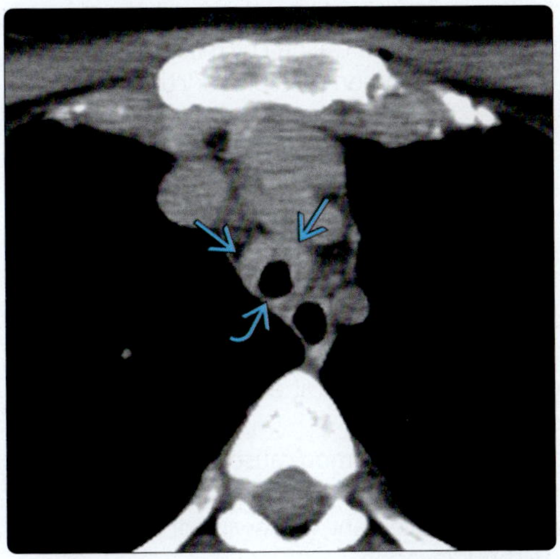

Relapsing Polychondritis

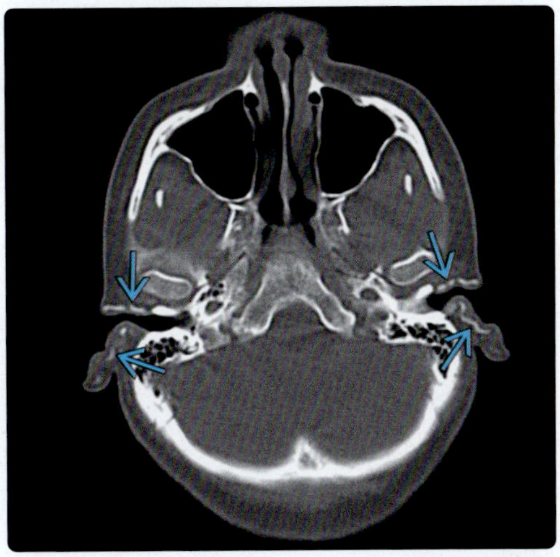

(Left) *Axial NECT of a patient with relapsing polychondritis shows marked thickening and narrowing of the trachea →. Note sparing of the posterior tracheal wall →. While tracheobronchial involvement by relapsing polychondritis is often diffuse, it may occasionally be focal.* **(Right)** *Axial NECT of the head of the same patient shows numerous linear calcifications along the bilateral external ear cartilages →, a known sequela of relapsing polychondritis.*

Relapsing Polychondritis

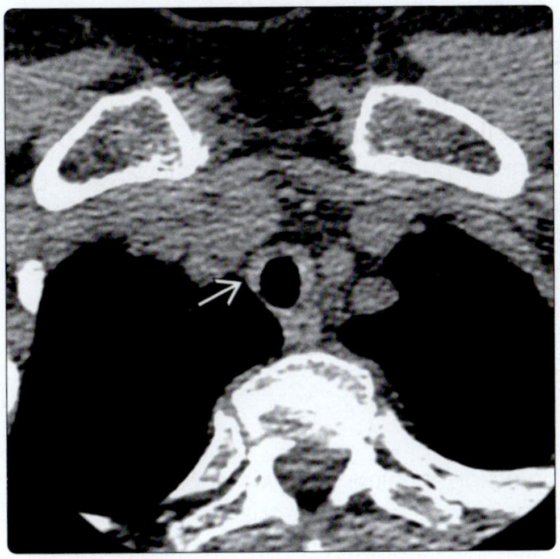

Relapsing Polychondritis

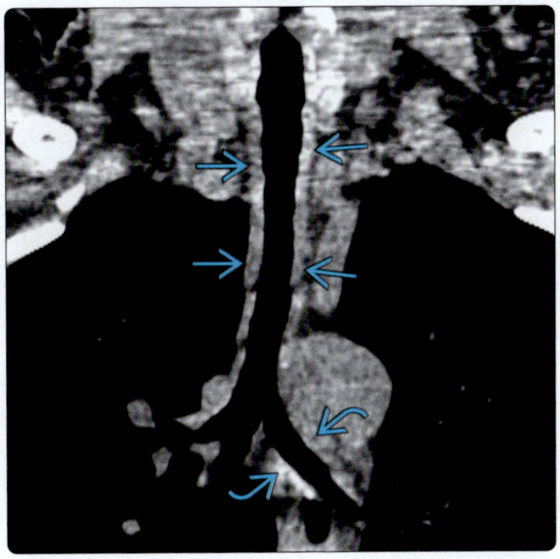

(Left) *Axial NECT of a patient with tracheobronchial relapsing polychondritis shows anterolateral mural thickening of the trachea → with sparing of the posterior tracheal wall or membranous trachea.* **(Right)** *Coronal NECT of the same patient shows diffuse tracheal wall thickening → with mild luminal narrowing as well as mild bronchial wall thickening →. Relapsing polychondritis and tracheobronchopathia osteochondroplastica are disease entities that typically spare the posterior tracheal wall.*

Tracheobronchial Papillomatosis

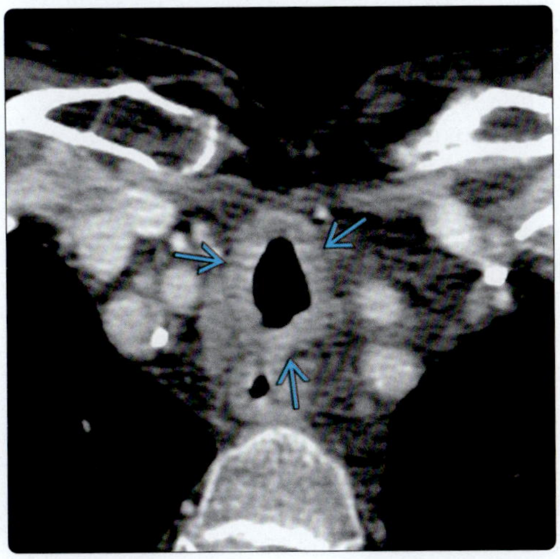

Tracheobronchial Papillomatosis

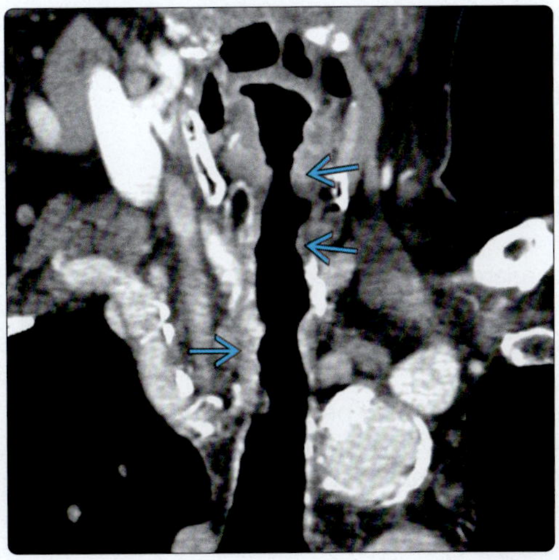

(Left) *Axial CECT of a patient with recurrent tracheobronchial papillomatosis shows marked concentric nodular mural thickening → of the upper trachea with involvement of the posterior tracheal wall.* **(Right)** *Coronal CECT of the same patient shows a long segment of mural thickening → and narrowing of the upper trachea. Papillomatosis is typically associated with focal verruciform lesions that result in tracheobronchial mural thickening and luminal narrowing, but diffuse airway involvement may also occur.*

DIFFERENTIAL DIAGNOSIS

Common

- Tracheal Stenosis
- Secondary Malignant Tracheal Neoplasm
- Extrinsic Compression

Less Common

- Primary Malignant Tracheal Neoplasm
  - Squamous Cell Carcinoma
  - Adenoid Cystic Carcinoma
  - Mucoepidermoid Carcinoma

Rare but Important

- Amyloidosis
- Tracheobronchopathia Osteochondroplastica
- Relapsing Polychondritis
- Tracheal Papillomatosis
- Granulomatosis With Polyangiitis
- Benign Tracheal Neoplasm

ESSENTIAL INFORMATION

Key Differential Diagnosis Issues

- Most common cause of tracheal stenosis is iatrogenic injury after endotracheal intubation and tracheostomy
- Tracheal involvement by extratracheal neoplasm is more common than primary tracheal neoplasms
  - Most common cause of extrinsic tracheal compression is goiter
- Primary malignant neoplasms are more common than primary benign neoplasms
  - Squamous cell carcinoma and adenoid cystic carcinoma are most common primary tracheal malignancies
    - Squamous cell carcinoma is smoking-related tumor, and patients are usually older than 50 years
- Extensive smooth or nodular thickening or multiple tracheal nodules suggests benign etiology
  - Tracheobronchopathia osteochondroplastica and relapsing polychondritis spare posterior membrane
- Multiplanar reformatted images, 3D reconstruction, and virtual bronchoscopy are accurate for assessing length and severity of tracheal narrowing

Helpful Clues for Common Diagnoses

- **Tracheal Stenosis**
  - Common after tracheostomy and intubation
  - Most common at site of balloon cuff and at tracheostomy opening
    - Length and severity are related to duration of intubation, size of cuff, and cuff pressure
      - Stenosis can develop after intubation, lasting as short as 24 hours
    - Ischemia of mucosa develops when cuff pressure is higher than capillary arterial pressure, ischemia results in ulceration and formation of granulation tissue and stenosis
  - Multiplanar reformatted images and virtual bronchoscopy are accurate for assessing length and severity of stenosis
  - CT: Focal, proximal tracheal narrowing with eccentric or concentric soft tissue thickening
    - Narrowing of lumen: "Hourglass" appearance, 1-4 cm in length
- **Secondary Malignant Tracheal Neoplasm**
  - Secondary involvement of trachea by malignant neoplasms is more common than primary tracheal malignancies
    - Direct invasion, hematogeneous or lymphatic dissemination
  - Direct invasion by adjacent neoplasm is most common cause of malignant tracheal narrowing
    - Lung, thyroid, and esophageal carcinoma
  - Hematogeneous and lymphatic metastases are less frequent
    - Melanoma, breast, colorectal, and renal carcinoma
- **Extrinsic Compression**
  - Thyroid goiter is most common cause of extrinsic tracheal compression
    - CT: Tracheal displacement, narrowing of tracheal lumen without invasion
      - Loss of mediastinal tissue planes, cervical or mediastinal lymphadenopathy, and endoluminal mass suggest thyroid malignancy

Helpful Clues for Less Common Diagnoses

- Primary Malignant Tracheal Neoplasm
  - **Squamous Cell Carcinoma**
    - Most common primary tracheal malignancy
    - Adults (50-60 years), male predominance
    - Smoking-related tumor
      - Can present as synchronous or metachronous neoplasm (head and neck or lung)
    - Most common in distal two-thirds of trachea and posterior wall
    - Multifocal in 10% of cases
    - CT
      - Polypoid intraluminal mass with lobular or irregular margins or focal circumferential thickening
      - Extraluminal component, invasion of adjacent structures
      - Metastatic lymphadenopathy &/or lung metastases present in 30%
    - FDG PET/CT: Increased FDG uptake
  - **Adenoid Cystic Carcinoma**
    - Second most common primary tracheal malignancy after squamous cell carcinoma
    - Adults (30-40 years), men and women are equally affected
    - Not smoking related
    - Most common in proximal half of trachea and posterolateral wall
    - Neoplasm originates in submucosa; mucosa is frequently intact
    - CT
      - Circumferential thickening of tracheal wall or intraluminal focal nodule or mass with smooth contour
      - Extensive submucosal and transmural spread
      - Lymph node and distant metastases are uncommon and occur late in disease course
    - FDG PET/CT: Variable metabolic activity depending on differentiation

- Mucoepidermoid Carcinoma
  - Majority of patients are less than 30 years of age
  - Imaging features similar to other primary tracheal neoplasms
    - CT: Focal soft tissue endoluminal mass
  - FDG PET/CT: Increased FDG uptake

Helpful Clues for Rare Diagnoses

- **Amyloidosis**
  - Deposition of amyloid protein in extracellular tissue in various organs
    - Tracheobronchial amyloidosis is most common manifestation of thoracic amyloidosis
  - Concentric or focal involvement of trachea with posterior membrane involvement
    - Mainstem bronchi can be affected
  - Amyloid deposits may calcified
  - CT
    - Focal or diffuse smooth wall thickening &/or nodules with or without calcification
- **Tracheobronchopathia Osteochondroplastica (TBO)**
  - Idiopathic benign condition, incidental finding
  - Numerous osteocartilaginous nodules in submucosa of lower trachea and proximal mainstem bronchi
  - Spares posterior tracheal membrane
  - Men > 50 years, asymptomatic
  - Cartilaginous and osseous nodules with "cobblestone" appearance
  - CT
    - 1- to 5-mm calcified and non-calcified nodules protruding into lumen
- **Relapsing Polychondritis**
  - Systemic disease of unknown etiology characterized by inflammation of cartilaginous structures
    - Clinical findings include pain and swelling of ears, nose, and costochondral junctions
  - Airways are involved in 50% of cases
  - Adults 50-60 years of age; men and women are equally affected
  - Most commonly affects larynx and upper trachea
  - Typically posterior tracheal membrane
  - Short or long segment of narrowing of lumen
  - CT
    - Smooth diffuse thickening of trachea and mainstem bronchi sparing posterior membranae
- **Tracheal Papillomatosis**
  - Infection secondary to HPV that occurs during birth
  - Children and young adults are most commonly affected
  - Involves predominantly larynx but can spread into trachea and distal bronchi in 5% of cases
    - Lung can be affected in 1% of cases
  - Malignant transformation into squamous cell carcinoma in 2%, associated with smoking and HPV 11 subtype
  - CT
    - Multiple intraluminal nodules of varying size affecting trachea and bronchi causing narrowing of lumen
      - Lungs: Bilateral thin-walled cysts and nodules
- **Granulomatosis With Polyangiitis**
  - Upper airways are nearly always involved
    - Lungs and kidneys are involved in 80% and 90%, respectively
  - Subglottic trachea is frequently affected
  - CT
    - Circumferential wall thickening, smooth or nodular
      - Nodular thickening may have calcification resembling relapsing polychondritis
      - Posterior tracheal membrane is involved
    - Pulmonary findings: Nodules that can be cavitary, consolidation, and ground-glass opacities
- **Benign Tumors**
  - Hamartoma
    - Adults 50-60 years of age
    - Smooth endoluminal nodule, fat, and cartilaginous calcification present in 25%
  - Chondroma
    - Well-defined mass with mottled cartilaginous calcification

Tracheal Stenosis

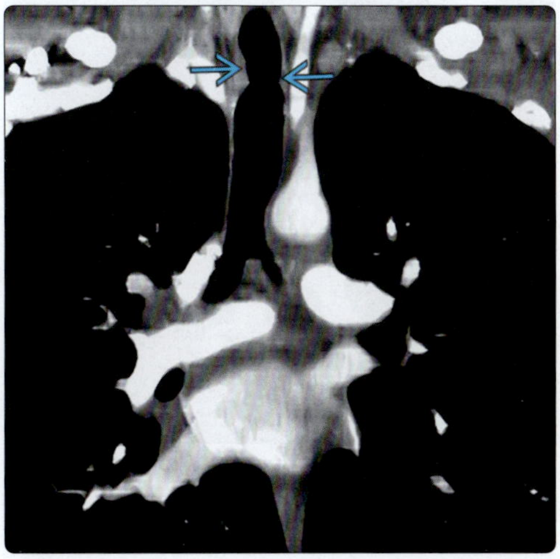

Tracheal Stenosis

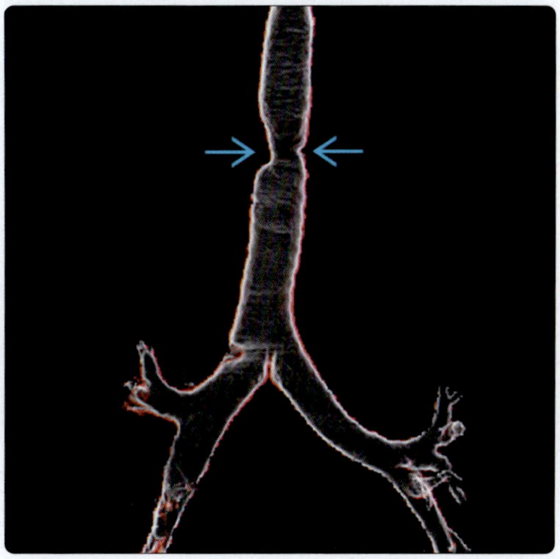

(Left) *Coronal CECT of a 37-year-old woman with history of endotracheal intubation shows an area of tracheal stenosis at the level of the thoracic inlet ➡. Tracheal stenosis is common following intubation, regardless of duration.* **(Right)** *3D surface rendering of the same patient confirms the presence of asymmetric short segment stenosis ➡. Reformatted images, 3D reconstruction, and virtual bronchoscopy provide precise information regarding exact location and extent of stenosis.*

(Left) *Axial CECT of 64-year-old man with papillary thyroid carcinoma shows a heterogeneous mass invading the trachea. Direct invasion by adjacent neoplasms is the most common cause of malignant tracheal narrowing.* **(Right)** *Axial CECT of a 70-year-old man with goiter shows extrinsic compression of the trachea with marked narrowing of the lumen. Loss of mediastinal tissue planes, tracheal invasion, or lymphadenopathy in a patient with goiter is concerning for malignancy.*

Secondary Malignant Tracheal Neoplasm

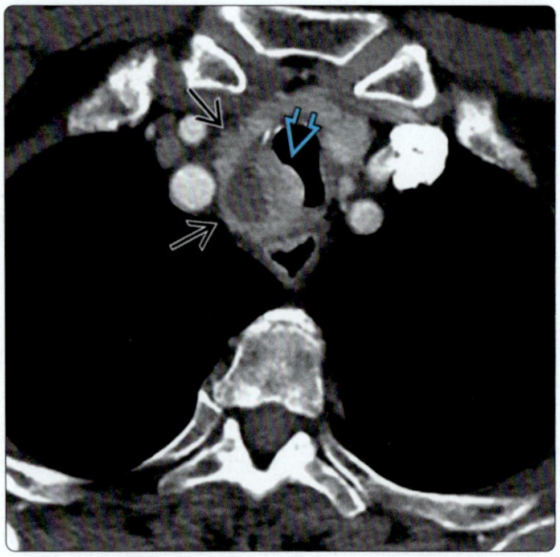

Secondary Malignant Tracheal Neoplasm

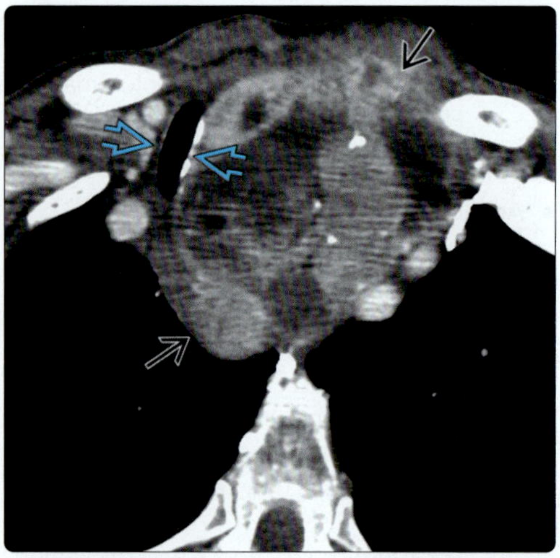

(Left) *Axial CECT of a 67-year-old man shows a soft tissue nodule involving the tracheal wall and adjacent mediastinal fat. Biopsy demonstrated squamous cell carcinoma. Squamous cell carcinoma is an aggressive neoplasm associated with smoking with a peak incidence between the ages of 50 and 70 years.* **(Right)** *Fused axial FDG PET/CT of the same patient shows intense metabolic activity within the lesion, which is a characteristic finding of this type of neoplasm.*

Squamous Cell Carcinoma

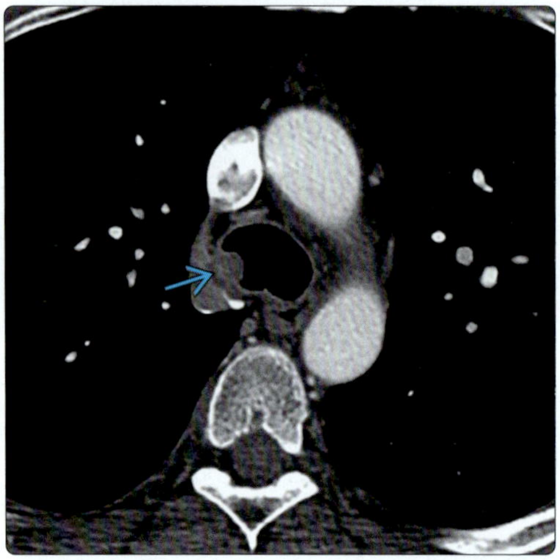

Squamous Cell Carcinoma

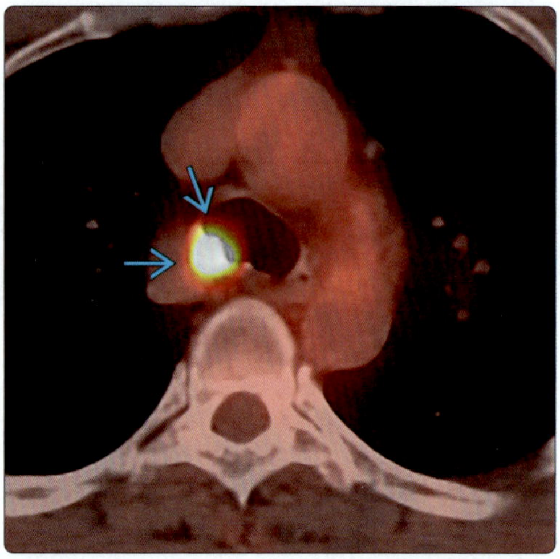

(Left) *Axial CECT of a 33-year-old woman shows circumferential thickening of the tracheal wall with narrowing of the lumen. Biopsy showed adenoid cystic carcinoma. This neoplasm should be considered in the differential diagnosis of a tracheal mass in young people.* **(Right)** *Axial CECT of a 46-year-old woman with biopsy-proven adenoid cystic carcinoma shows a focal mass in the trachea with a smooth border. The lesion may present as circumferential tracheal thickening or as a focal mass.*

Adenoid Cystic Carcinoma

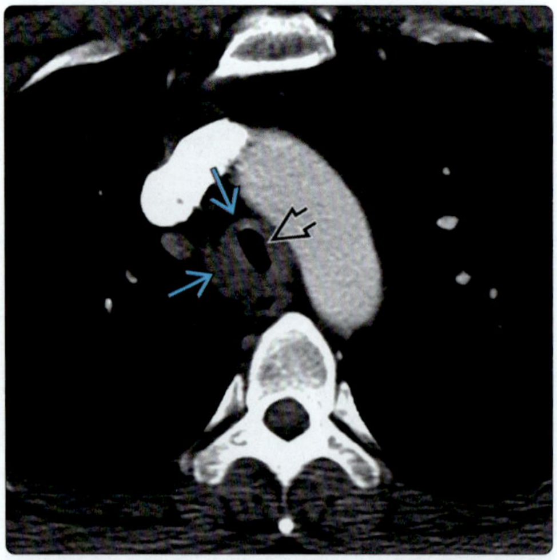

Adenoid Cystic Carcinoma

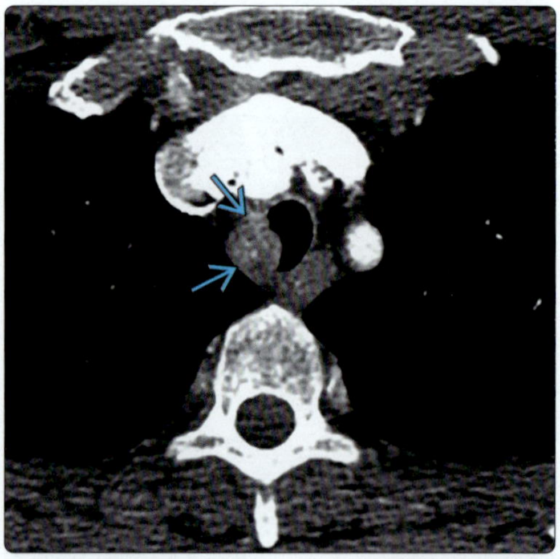

Amyloidosis

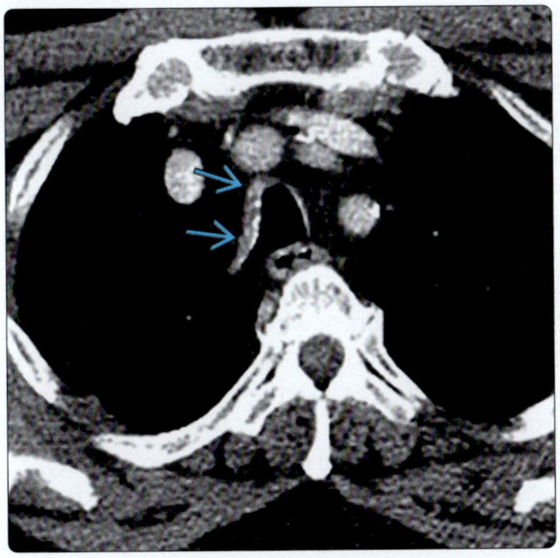

Amyloidosis

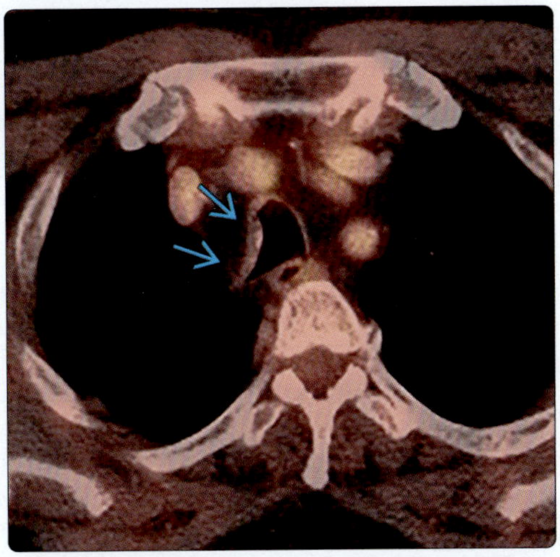

(Left) *Axial CECT of a 59-year-old man with history of myeloma and primary amyloidosis shows partially calcified plaque-like thickening → along the tracheal wall, consistent with an amyloid deposit. Tracheobronchial amyloidosis may present as concentric or focal thickening of the tracheal wall with involvement of the posterior membrane.* **(Right)** *Fused axial FDG PET/CT of the same patient shows no evidence of metabolic activity along the tracheal wall →, consistent with a benign process.*

Tracheobronchopathia Osteochondroplastica

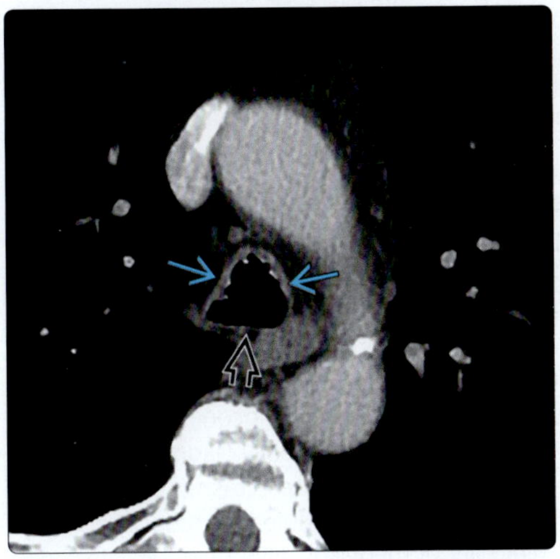

Tracheal Papillomatosis

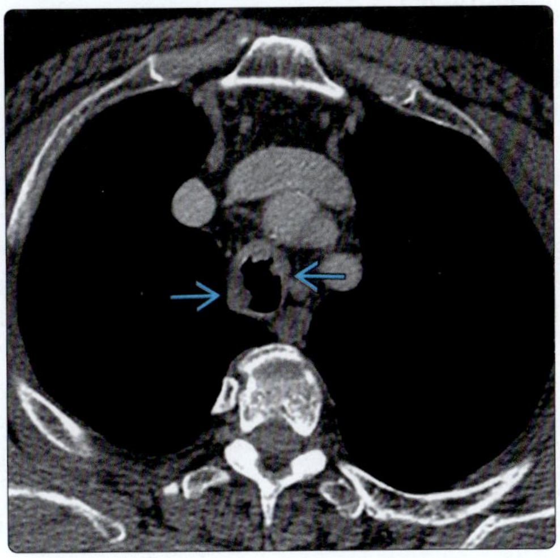

(Left) *Axial CECT of a 72-year-old man shows several calcified and noncalcified tracheal nodules → sparing the posterior membrane ⇨, consistent with tracheobronchopathia osteochondroplastica, an entity that is usually asymptomatic and often found incidentally.* **(Right)** *Axial CECT of a 64-year-old man with history of papillomatosis shows multiple endoluminal nodules → with narrowing of the tracheal lumen. The patient was periodically treated with laser ablation to keep the airway patent.*

Benign Tracheal Neoplasm

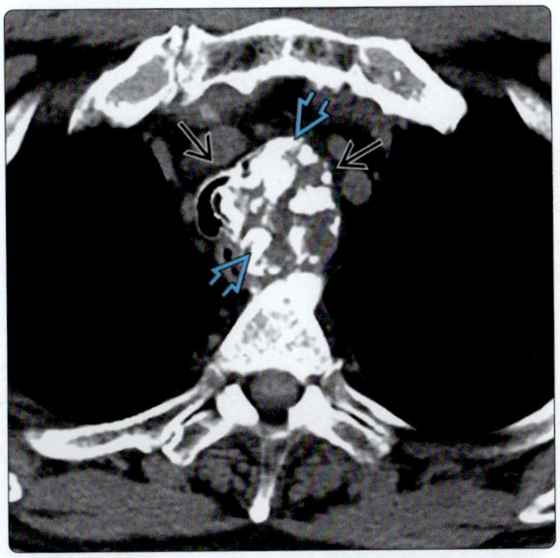

Benign Tracheal Neoplasm

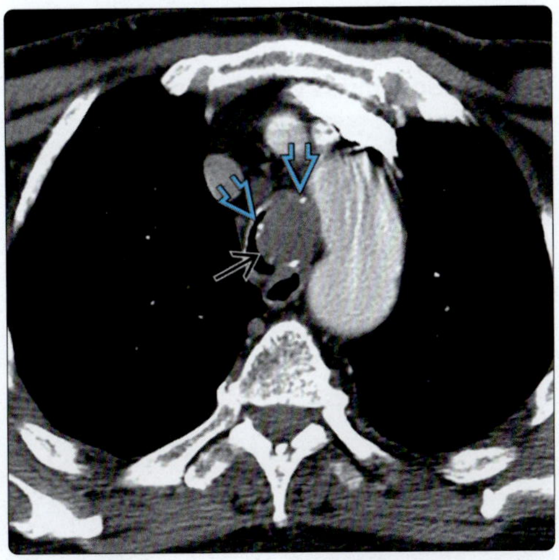

(Left) *Axial CECT of a 62-year-old man shows a large tracheal mass → with popcorn-like calcifications ⇒. Hamartoma was confirmed after surgical resection. Macroscopic fat and chondroid calcification are identified in 25% of cases.* **(Right)** *Axial CECT of a 77-year-old man shows a large intraluminal mass → with focal calcifications ⇒. Biopsy demonstrated chondroma. If chondroid calcification is present within a mass, the differential diagnosis includes hamartoma and chondroma.*

DIFFERENTIAL DIAGNOSIS

Common

- Squamous Cell Carcinoma
- Small Cell Carcinoma

Less Common

- Carcinoid Tumor
- Metastasis

Rare but Important

- Broncholith

ESSENTIAL INFORMATION

Key Differential Diagnosis Issues

- Symptoms and signs primarily depend on size rather than pathologic features
- Findings
  - Postobstructive atelectasis or recurrent pneumonia
- Most endobronchial neoplasms are malignant

Helpful Clues for Common Diagnoses

- **Squamous Cell Carcinoma**
  - > 90% of malignant endobronchial neoplasms
  - More common in men, peak of incidence 50-70 years
  - Imaging
    - Sessile or polypoid lesion, eccentric luminal narrowing, circumferential wall thickening
    - Lobar collapse: Primary malignancy differentiated from adjacent atelectasis by presence/extent of contrast enhancement
    - Air-trapping, obstructive pneumonia, mucoid impaction
- **Small Cell Carcinoma**
  - Peribronchial with submucosal extension; primary malignancy may not be visible on imaging
  - Marked hilar and mediastinal lymphadenopathy at presentation

Helpful Clues for Less Common Diagnoses

- **Carcinoid Tumor**
  - Bronchial carcinoid: Up to 25% of all carcinoids
    - Typical (low grade) carcinoid: 80-90%
    - Atypical (higher grade) carcinoid: 10-20%
  - Imaging
    - Homogeneous well-defined spherical or ovoid endobronchial nodule
    - Intense enhancement, eccentric calcification (26% on CT, 5% on radiography)
    - Postobstructive atelectasis or pneumonitis; air-trapping
  - Rare paraneoplastic syndromes: 3-5% of cases reported with large carcinoid tumors or with metastatic disease
    - Somatostatin receptors in up to 80% of carcinoids
      - May be targeted by radioactive octreotide or pentetreotide
      - Indium-111-radiolabeled octreotide scintigraphy valuable for detection of early recurrence and metastases
- **Metastasis**
  - Hematogenous dissemination
    - Adenocarcinoma (breast, colon, kidney), melanoma
  - Direct invasion
    - Lung, esophagus, thyroid
  - Frequent contrast enhancement (renal cell carcinoma, melanoma)
  - Lobar or segmental atelectasis

Helpful Clues for Rare Diagnoses

- **Broncholith**
  - Calcified material within tracheobronchial tree
    - Frequently secondary to erosion and extrusion of adjacent calcified lymph node
    - Tuberculosis and histoplasmosis most common causes, may also occur in pneumoconiosis
  - Lithoptysis very uncommon; virtually diagnostic
  - Radiography: Postobstructive atelectasis or pneumonitis
  - CT: Calcified endobronchial nodule with associate peribronchial, hilar or mediastinal lymph nodes

Squamous Cell Carcinoma

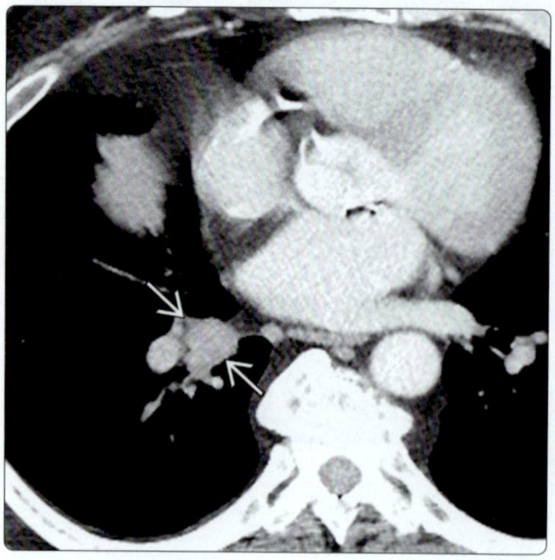

Squamous Cell Carcinoma

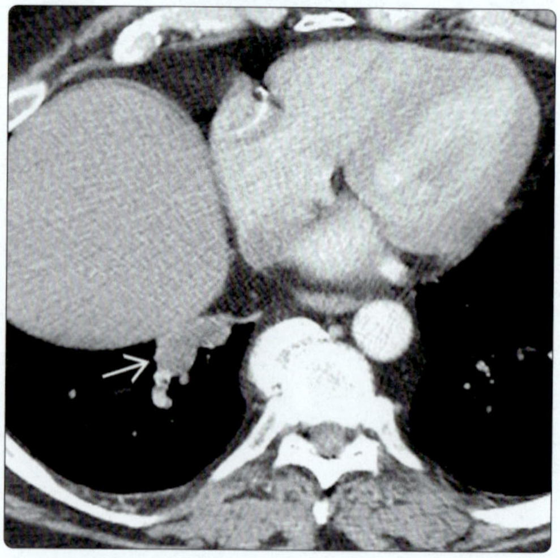

(Left) *Axial CECT of a 65-year-old man shows an enhancing polylobular soft tissue lesion that obstructs the lumen of the right lower lobe bronchus* ➡. **(Right)** *Axial CECT of the same patient shows a mucus-filled branching bronchus* ➡ *distal to the obstructing lesion. Biopsy showed squamous cell carcinoma which accounts for over 90% of malignant endobronchial neoplasms. Endobronchial tumors may be associated with postobstructive atelectasis or pneumonitis, air-trapping, and peripheral mucoid impaction.*

Small Cell Carcinoma

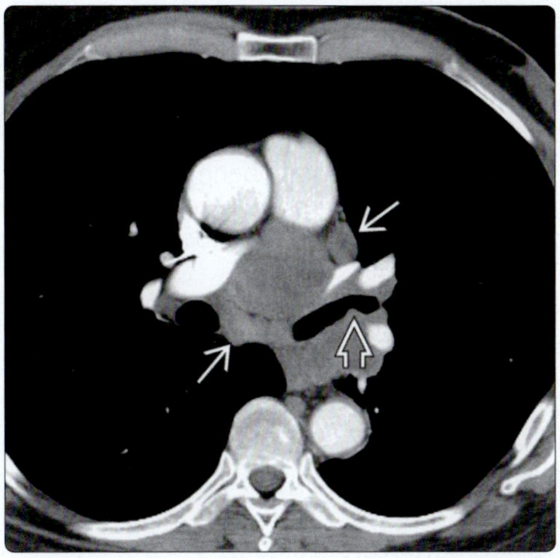

Carcinoid Tumor

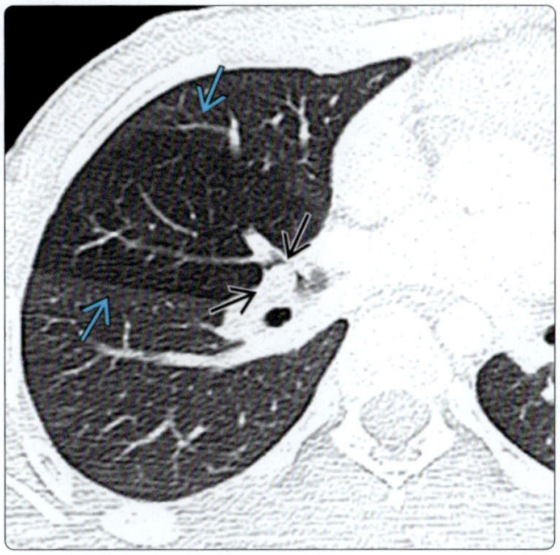

(Left) *Axial CECT of a patient with biopsy-proven small cell carcinoma shows a small endoluminal lesion in the distal left mainstem bronchus →. Note extensive mediastinal lymphadenopathy →. Extensive metastatic lymphadenopathy at presentation is very common in affected patients.* **(Right)** *Axial CECT of a patient with persistent cough for 6 months shows an obstructing soft tissue nodule in the middle lobe bronchus → and peripheral air-trapping →. Bronchial carcinoid accounts for up to 25% of all carcinoids.*

Carcinoid Tumor

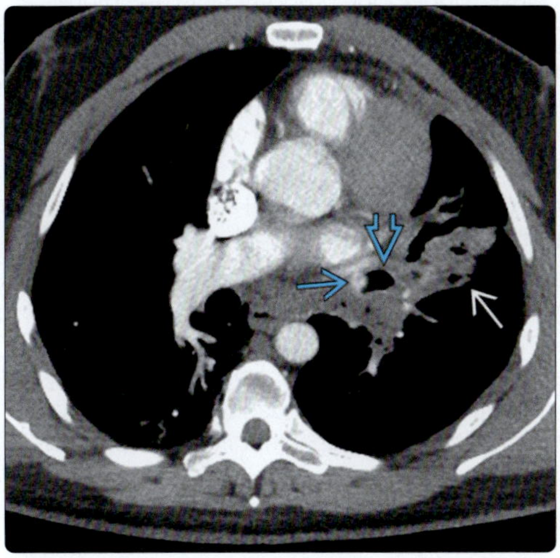

Metastasis

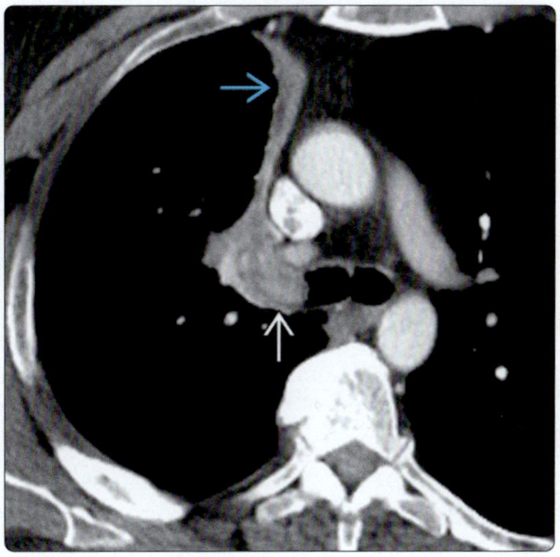

(Left) *Axial CECT shows an intensely enhancing endobronchial nodule in the left lower lobe bronchus →, dilatation of the left lower lobe bronchus →, and peripheral postobstructive pneumonitis →. Carcinoid tumor frequently exhibits intense enhancement on CECT.* **(Right)** *Axial CECT of a patient with renal cell carcinoma shows an enhancing endoluminal right mainstem bronchus lesion → and right upper lobe atelectasis →. Metastatic disease was confirmed on biopsy.*

Broncholith

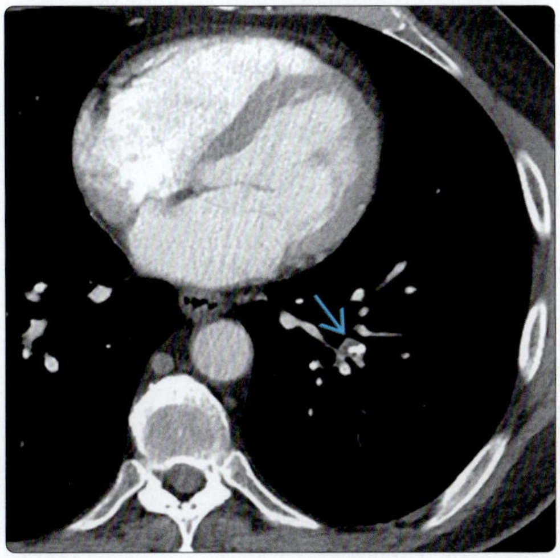

Broncholith

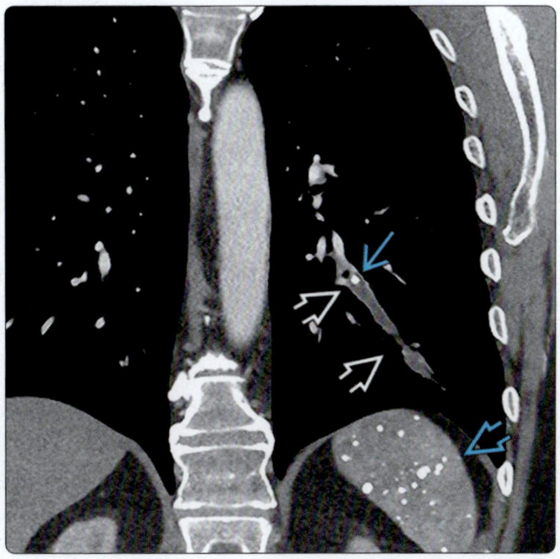

(Left) *Axial CECT of a patient with a history of chronic productive cough shows a dilated left lower lobe bronchus that contains an endoluminal calcified nodule →.* **(Right)** *Coronal CECT of the same patient shows the dilated mucus-filled bronchus → and the endoluminal broncholith →. Note multiple calcified granulomas in the spleen →. Tuberculosis and histoplasmosis are the most common causes of broncholithiasis.*

DIFFERENTIAL DIAGNOSIS

Common

- Small Airways Disease
  - Constrictive Bronchiolitis
  - Cellular Bronchiolitis
    - Infectious Bronchiolitis
    - Aspiration Bronchiolitis
    - Respiratory Bronchiolitis
  - Asthma
  - Bronchiectasis
- Ground-Glass Opacities
  - Infection
    - *Pneumocystis jirovecii, Mycoplasma pneumoniae*
  - Pulmonary Edema

Less Common

- Small Airways Disease
  - Cellular Bronchiolitis
    - Hypersensitivity Pneumonitis
- Ground-Glass Opacities
  - Acute
    - Diffuse Alveolar Hemorrhage
- Chronic Vascular Obstruction
  - Chronic Thromboembolic Disease
  - Pulmonary Hypertension
  - Obesity Hypoventilation Syndrome

Rare but Important

- Small Airways Disease
  - Sarcoidosis

ESSENTIAL INFORMATION

Key Differential Diagnosis Issues

- Mosaic attenuation
  - Patchwork of areas of different attenuation on inspiratory CT
  - Most cases are related to small-airways disease
  - Differentiation between small airways disease and ground-glass opacities
    - Ground-glass opacities: Similar diameter of vessels coursing into areas of different attenuation
    - Small airways disease, chronic vascular obstruction: Different diameter of vessels coursing into areas of different attenuation
  - Difficult if not impossible differentiation between small airways disease and chronic vascular obstruction
    - Small airways disease
      - Subtle mosaic attenuation on inspiration, air-trapping on expiration
      - Ancillary findings: Bronchial wall thickening, bronchiectasis, mucous plugging
    - Chronic vascular obstruction
      - Mosaic attenuation very evident on inspiration, air-trapping on expiration
      - Ancillary findings: Dilated pulmonary trunk, web-like or peripheral pulmonary artery filling defects on CECT
- Air-trapping: Finding on expiratory CT
  - Absence of increased attenuation on expiration
  - Seen in small airways disease and chronic vascular obstruction

Helpful Clues for Common Diagnoses

- **Constrictive Bronchiolitis**
  - Bronchiolar luminal narrowing from scarring
  - Etiology: Postinfectious (i.e., Swyer-James syndrome), posttransplantation (e.g., lung and bone marrow), autoimmunity, toxic/fume exposure, drug reaction, diffuse idiopathic pulmonary neuroendocrine cell hyperplasia, idiopathic
  - CT
    - Expiratory air-trapping
    - Bronchiectasis, bronchial wall thickening, centrilobular nodules, mucous plugs (may be present but not salient feature)
- **Infectious Bronchiolitis**
  - Acute
    - Bacterial or viral; clinical pneumonia
    - CT: Scattered tree-in-bud opacities
  - Chronic
    - Tuberculosis: Upper lobe predominant tree-in-bud opacities, cavities, discrete nodules
    - Nontuberculous mycobacteria
      - Preexistent lung disease (e.g., COPD, pulmonary fibrosis), white elderly women without preexistent lung disease
      - Cavitary form: May be identical to tuberculosis
      - Bronchiectatic form: Bronchiectasis, tree-in-bud opacities, mucous plugs, more severe in middle lobe and lingula; mosaic attenuation, air-trapping
- **Aspiration Bronchiolitis**
  - Chronic aspiration: Achalasia, esophageal cancer, gastroesophageal reflux, gastric banding, neurologic conditions involving esophageal motility, gastroparesis
  - CT
    - Tree-in-bud opacities, often indistinguishable from infectious bronchiolitis
    - Mosaic attenuation, air-trapping
- **Respiratory Bronchiolitis**
  - Spectrum of tobacco-related diseases: Respiratory bronchiolitis-interstitial lung disease, desquamative interstitial pneumonia
  - CT
    - Upper lobe predominant ground-glass centrilobular micronodules
    - Mosaic attenuation, air-trapping
- **Asthma**
  - Bronchial hyperreactivity associated with allergic reaction or other forms of hypersensitivity
  - CT
    - Mosaic attenuation, air-trapping
    - Mucous plugs, bronchial wall thickening, bronchiectasis
- **Bronchiectasis**
  - Wide variety of causes (e.g., postinfectious, postinhalation injury, cystic fibrosis)
  - Radiography: Tram-track opacities
  - CT
    - ↑ bronchoarterial ratio: > 1.5 indicative of bronchiectasis

- Absence of bronchial tapering
- Mosaic perfusion, air-trapping
- **Infection**
  - *Pneumocystis jirovecii*, *Mycoplasma pneumoniae*,
  - CT: Ground-glass opacities alternating with normal lung; air-trapping not typical component
- **Pulmonary Edema**
  - Cardiogenic or non-cardiogenic
  - CT
    - Interlobular septal thickening
    - Bronchial wall thickening
    - Mosaic attenuation due to ground-glass opacities (alveolar edema)

Helpful Clues for Less Common Diagnoses

- **Hypersensitivity Pneumonitis**
  - Allergic inflammatory response to inhaled organic antigens or haptens (low molecular weight inorganic molecules)
  - CT
    - Cluster 1 (subacute): Coexistence of ground-glass opacities, normal lung, and lobular mosaic attenuation/air-trapping
    - Mosaic attenuation; often exhibits lobular pattern
- **Diffuse Alveolar Hemorrhage**
  - Idiopathic or associated with autoimmunity (e.g., systemic lupus erythematosus, Goodpasture syndrome, granulomatosis with polyangiitis)
  - Hemoptysis common but may be absent
  - ↓ hemoglobin and hematocrit
  - CT
    - Mosaic attenuation from ground-glass opacities
    - Crazy-paving pattern may occur in subacute stages
- **Chronic Thromboembolic Disease**
  - Recurrent episodes of pulmonary embolism resulting in pulmonary hypertension, right ventricular strain, and mosaic attenuation
  - CT
    - Linear (web-like), eccentric or peripheral pulmonary artery filling defects often with remodeling of vessels
    - Abrupt vascular tapering or amputation
    - Mosaic attenuation from decreased vascularity on inspiration and expiration; difficult differentiation from small airways disease
    - Dilated pulmonary trunk, right ventricular dilatation (strain)
    - Hypertrophied bronchial arteries
- **Pulmonary Hypertension**
  - Multiple etiologies: Idiopathic, chronic thromboembolic disease, COPD/small airways disease, valvular heart disease, congenital heart disease
  - CT
    - Dilated pulmonary artery ± right ventricular dilatation (strain)
    - Ancillary findings: Emphysema, mitral valve disease, web-like pulmonary artery filling defects
- **Obesity Hypoventilation Syndrome**
  - Pulmonary hypertension due to various factors
    - Chronic hypoxia
    - Restrictive lung disease from severe obesity, high intrathoracic pressure from increased upper airway resistance
  - CT
    - Large body habitus
    - Pulmonary hypertension + mosaic attenuation

Helpful Clues for Rare Diagnoses

- **Sarcoidosis**
  - May rarely involve medium &/or small airways
  - CT
    - Mosaic attenuation
    - Hilar/mediastinal lymphadenopathy
    - Perilymphatic nodules

SELECTED REFERENCES

1. Almeneessier AS et al: The prevalence of pulmonary hypertension in patients with obesity hypoventilation syndrome: a prospective observational study. J Thorac Dis. 9(3):779-88, 2017
2. Kligerman SJ et al: Mosaic attenuation: etiology, methods of differentiation, and pitfalls. Radiographics. 35(5):1360-80, 2015

Constrictive Bronchiolitis

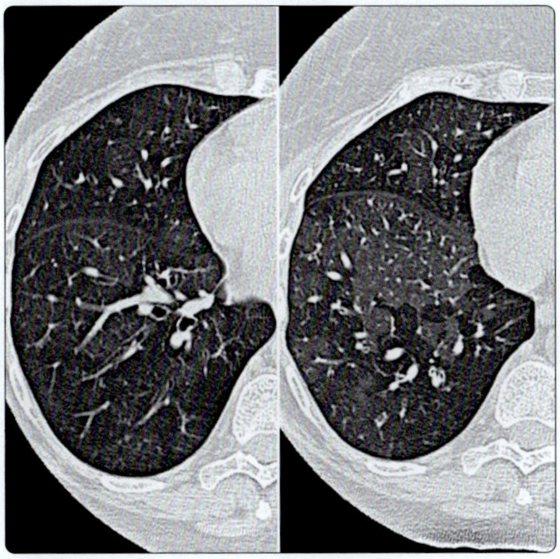

Constrictive Bronchiolitis

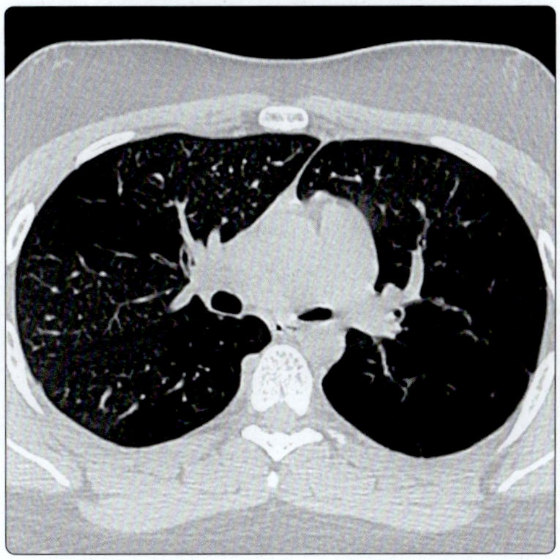

(Left) *Composite image with inspiratory (left) and expiratory (right) axial HRCT of a patient with constrictive bronchiolitis shows subtle mosaic attenuation on inspiration and frank air-trapping on expiration.* **(Right)** *Axial NECT of a patient with Swyer-James syndrome due to Adenovirus infection in childhood shows extensive mosaic attenuation. Note the changing caliber of vessels coursing into areas of different attenuation, which is helpful in differentiating mosaic attenuation from ground-glass opacities.*

(**Left**) *Axial NECT of a patient with aspiration bronchiolitis due to a large hiatus hernia (not shown) and gastroesophageal reflux shows clustered pulmonary micronodules* ➡ *on a background of mosaic attenuation.* (**Right**) *Axial HRCT of a smoker with respiratory bronchiolitis shows bilateral mosaic attenuation, consistent with small airways disease. Mosaic attenuation and air-trapping are common ancillary CT findings seen not only in the setting of constrictive bronchiolitis but in all cellular bronchiolitides.*

Aspiration Bronchiolitis

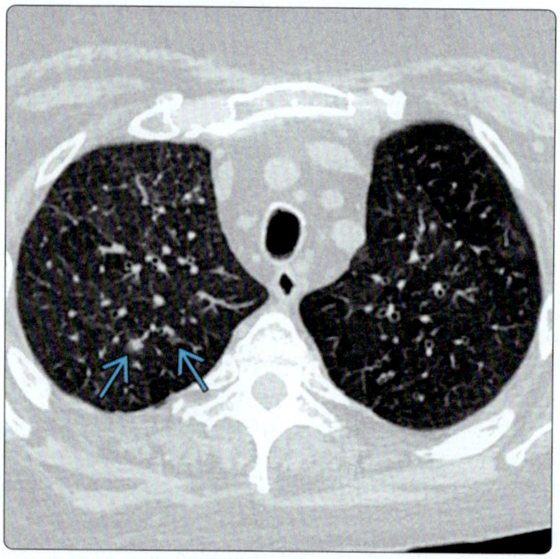

Respiratory Bronchiolitis

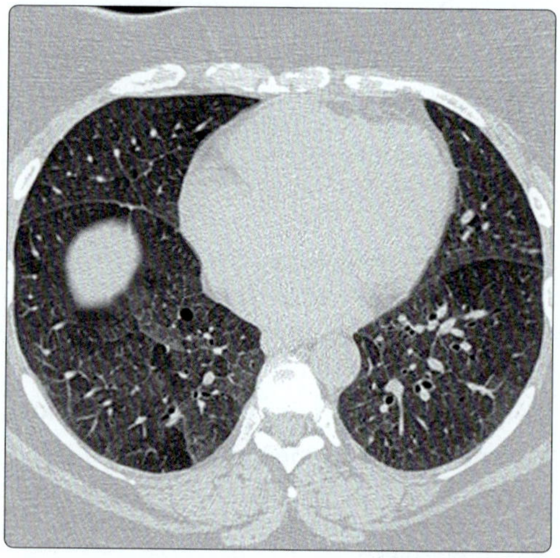

(**Left**) *Axial HRCT of a patient with asthma shows diffuse bilateral mosaic attenuation. In asthma, air-trapping may be related to bronchial narrowing that initially results from hypertrophy, hyperplasia, epithelial sloughing, and inflammatory infiltration, and later from the development of constrictive bronchiolitis.* (**Right**) *Coronal NECT of a patient with Kartagener syndrome shows diffuse bronchial thickening* ➡ *and bronchiectasis on a background of mosaic attenuation secondary to constrictive bronchiolitis.*

Asthma

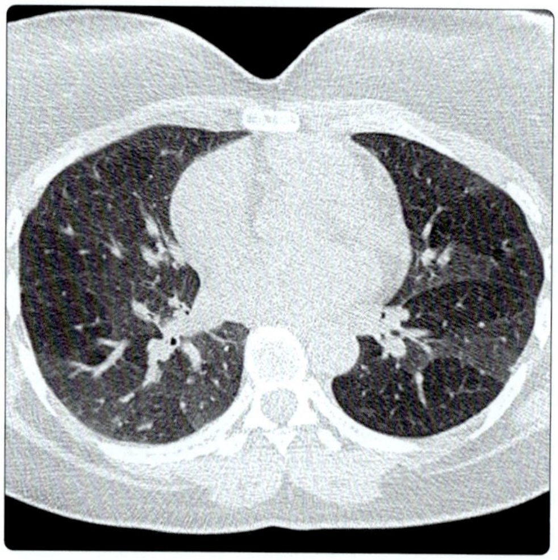

Bronchiectasis

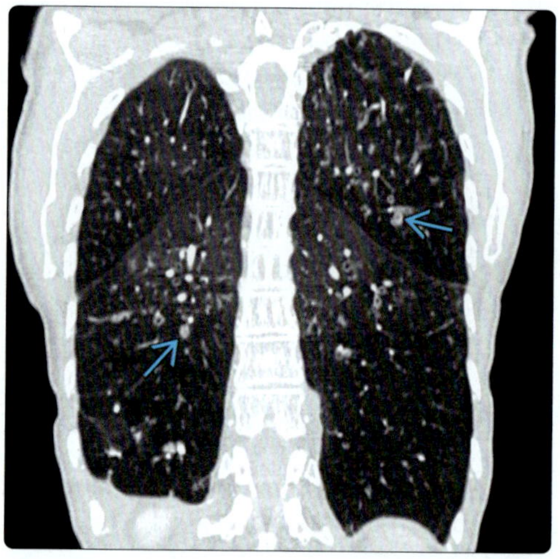

(**Left**) *Coronal NECT of a patient with acquired immune deficiency syndrome (AIDS) and Pneumocystis jirovecii pneumonia shows diffuse upper lobe predominant ground-glass opacities alternating with areas of normal lung.* (**Right**) *Axial CECT of a patient with cardiogenic pulmonary edema shows scattered geographic ground-glass opacities alternating with normal lung (i.e., mosaic attenuation) and small bilateral pleural effusions* ➡*. Ground-glass opacities may produce a pattern of mosaic attenuation.*

Infection

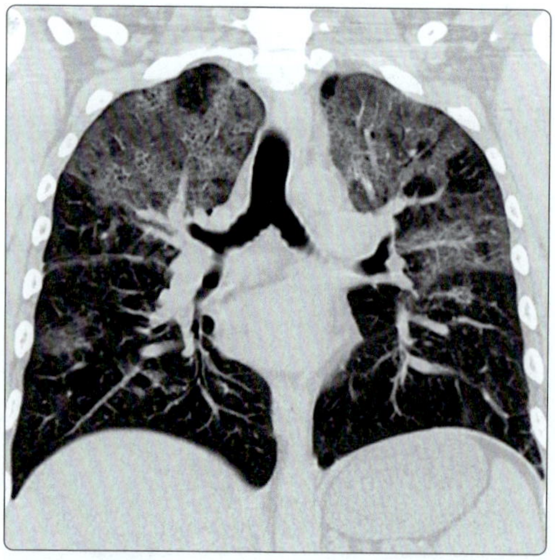

Pulmonary Edema

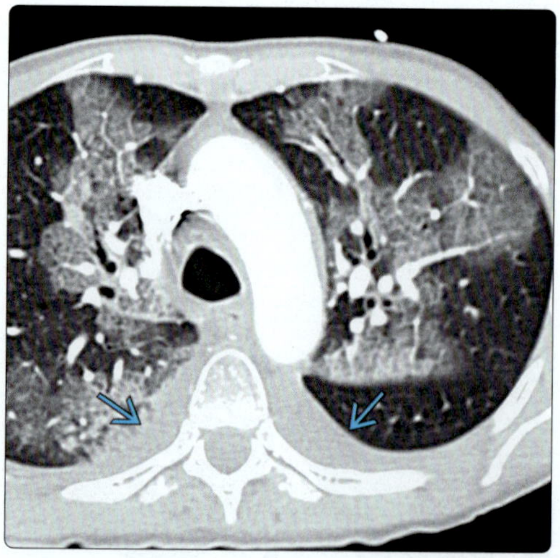

Hypersensitivity Pneumonitis

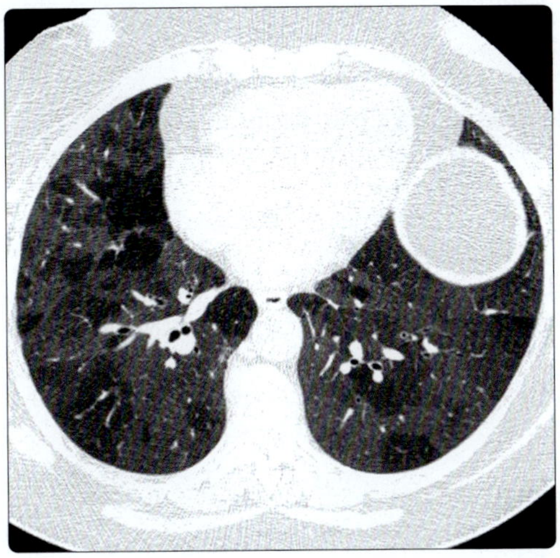

Diffuse Alveolar Hemorrhage

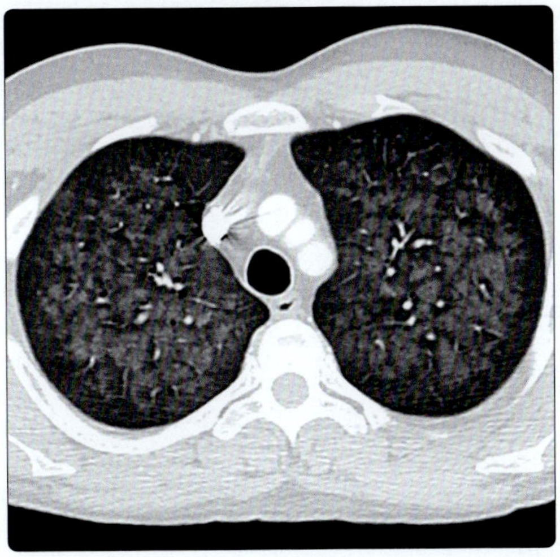

(Left) *Axial HRCT of a patient with hypersensitivity pneumonitis shows mosaic attenuation in a subsegmental and lobular pattern. The lobular pattern is not a specific finding but is commonly seen in hypersensitivity pneumonitis and is often associated with ground-glass opacities and ground-glass centrilobular nodules.* **(Right)** *Axial CECT of a patient with diffuse alveolar hemorrhage who presented with hemoptysis shows patchy peribronchovascular ground-glass opacities alternating with normal lung.*

Chronic Thromboembolic Disease

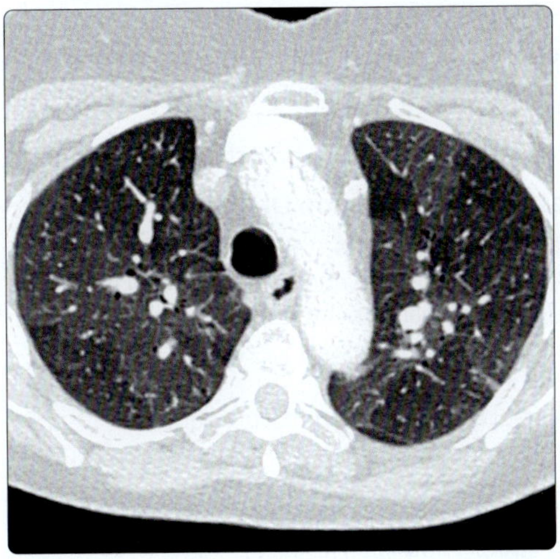

Pulmonary Hypertension

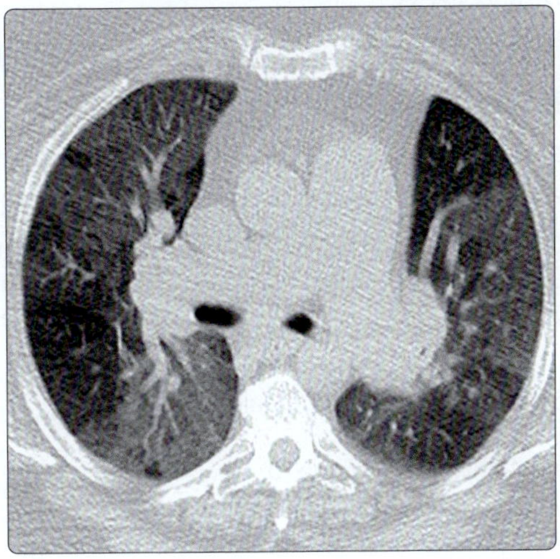

(Left) *Axial CECT of a patient with chronic pulmonary thromboembolic disease shows bilateral mosaic attenuation. Chronic linear pulmonary artery filling defects, pulmonary hypertension, and dilated right heart chambers were also noted (not shown).* **(Right)** *Axial NECT of a patient with pulmonary hypertension from remote use of fenfluramine shows bilateral mosaic attenuation. This drug is no longer available in the market due to its association with the development of primary pulmonary hypertension.*

Obesity Hypoventilation Syndrome

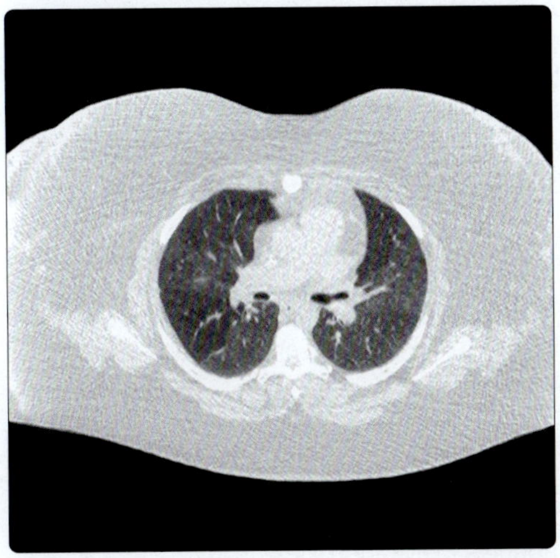

Sarcoidosis

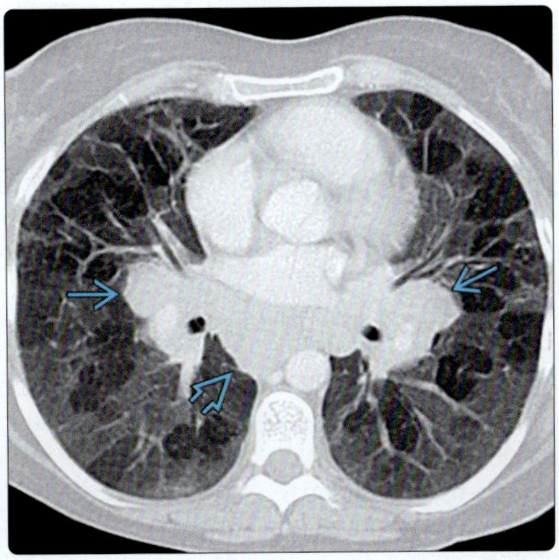

(Left) *Axial CECT of a patient with large body habitus and secondary obesity hypoventilation syndrome shows bilateral mosaic attenuation. This finding is related to pulmonary hypertension resulting from chronic hypoxia, restriction, and increased upper airway resistance due to obesity.* **(Right)** *Axial HRCT of a patient with sarcoidosis shows extensive bilateral mosaic attenuation. Note bilateral hilar → and mediastinal ⇨ lymphadenopathy.*

DIFFERENTIAL DIAGNOSIS

Common

- Respiratory Bronchiolitis
- Viral Pneumonia
- Bacterial Pneumonia
- Tuberculosis
- Aspiration

Less Common

- Hypersensitivity Pneumonitis
- Pulmonary Langerhans Cell Histiocytosis
- Vasculitis
- Silicosis

Rare but Important

- Follicular Bronchiolitis
- Diffuse Panbronchiolitis
- Organizing Pneumonia Pattern
- Lymphoid Interstitial Pneumonia
- Fat Embolism Syndrome
- Allergic Bronchopulmonary Aspergillosis
- Invasive Tracheobronchial Aspergillosis

ESSENTIAL INFORMATION

Key Differential Diagnosis Issues

- Centrilobular nodules: Diseases with lesions anatomically related to bronchioles; less frequently arteriolar diseases
- Imaging
  - Bronchiolar disease
    - Centrilobular nodules do not contact pleura, fissures, or interlobular septa
    - Distance of 5-10 mm between centrilobular nodule and pleura
    - Nodules may exhibit central hypodensity due to endoluminal bronchiolar air
    - Isolated nodules versus rosettes, variable attenuation (solid or ground-glass), well- or ill-defined borders, size of 2-3 mm to 1 cm
    - Infection: Frequent tree-in-bud opacities
  - Arteriolar disease: Frequent loss of arteriolar contours

Helpful Clues for Common Diagnoses

- **Respiratory Bronchiolitis**
  - Asymptomatic, 3rd-5th decades of life
  - History of cigarette smoking
  - Imaging
    - Nodules: Respiratory bronchiole inflammation and luminal pigmented macrophages
    - Upper lung zone: Ground-glass opacities, central and peripheral bronchial wall thickening
- **Viral Pneumonia**
  - Frequent etiology of pneumonia in immunocompetent and immunocompromised adults
  - Immunocompetent: Influenza virus types A and B, hantaviruses, Epstein-Barr virus, and adenoviruses
  - Immunocompromised: Cytomegalovirus, herpesviruses, measles virus, and adenoviruses
  - Imaging
    - Ground-glass opacities, consolidation
    - Tree-in-bud opacities
    - Interlobular septal thickening
- **Bacterial Pneumonia**
  - *S. aureus*, *S. pyogenes*, *P. aeruginosa*, *H. influenzae*, and *M. pneumoniae*
  - Imaging
    - Bronchopneumonia: Centrilobular nodules and peribronchiolar inflammation involving adjacent alveoli
    - Patchy consolidation, multisegmental distribution
    - Bronchial wall thickening
- **Tuberculosis**
  - Exposed individuals and those at risk for active disease
  - Imaging
    - Centrilobular nodules + bronchogenic dissemination; 95% of patients with active tuberculosis
    - Cavitation
    - Tree-in-bud opacities
    - Consolidation and parenchymal bands
    - Bronchiectasis
- **Aspiration**
  - Chronic bronchiolar inflammatory reaction to repeated foreign body aspiration
  - Risk factors: Esophageal disease, esophagectomy with gastric pull-up or colonic interposition, neurologic disease
  - Imaging: Tree-in-bud opacities, bronchial wall thickening

Helpful Clues for Less Common Diagnoses

- **Hypersensitivity Pneumonitis**
  - Immune-mediated disease due to inhalation of specific antigens (usually organic) by susceptible individuals
  - History of environmental exposure &/or specific inhalation challenge testing
  - Bronchoalveolar lavage: Inflammatory pattern
  - Imaging
    - Ground-glass opacities (acute)
    - Upper and mid lung zone or peribronchovascular fibrosis, honeycombing (chronic)
- **Pulmonary Langerhans Cell Histiocytosis**
  - 20-40 years of age
  - History of cigarette smoking
  - Imaging
    - Nodules: Langerhans cells and eosinophils in respiratory bronchioles and adjacent interstitium
    - Upper/mid lung zone cavitary nodules and bizarre-shaped cysts
- **Vasculitis**
  - Systemic disease: Lung, skin, kidney, gastrointestinal tract
  - Granulomatosis with polyangiitis (GPA), microscopic polyangiitis (MPA), eosinophilic granulomatosis with polyangiitis (EGPA)
  - Imaging
    - Centrilobular nodules with bronchiolar inflammation (GPA), periarteriolar alveolar hemorrhage (MPA), eosinophilic bronchiolitis (EPGA)
    - Large nodules ± cavitation (GPA)
    - Ground-glass opacities &/or consolidations due to diffuse alveolar hemorrhage (MPA)
    - Migratory ground-glass opacities (EPGA)
- **Silicosis**

Helpful Clues for Less Common Diagnoses

- **Follicular Bronchiolitis**
  - Proliferation of bronchus-associated lymphoid tissue (BALT) with reactive germinal centers distributed along bronchioles
    - Associated with immunologic conditions and collagen vascular diseases (rheumatoid arthritis, Sjögren syndrome)
  - CT
    - Bilateral centrilobular and peribronchial nodules (< 3 mm), ground-glass opacities, mild bronchial dilatation, bronchial wall thickening

Helpful Clues for Rare Diagnoses

- **Diffuse Panbronchiolitis**
  - Idiopathic chronic inflammation of respiratory bronchioles
    - Primarily seen in Japan and Eastern Asia
    - Middle-aged men (most patients over 40 years)
      - Pansinusitis in > 80% of patients
  - CT
    - Combination of bronchial wall thickening, centrilobular nodules, TIB opacities, bronchiectasis, bronchiolectasis, and air-trapping
- **Laryngeal Papillomatosis**
  - Human papilloma virus (HPV) types 6 and 11
  - May affect any site on laryngeal mucosa not covered by stratified squamous epithelium
  - Bimodal age distribution
    - Juvenile laryngeal papillomatosis: < 5 years
    - Adult laryngeal papillomatosis: 4th decade
  - Airway solid and cystic nodules in trachea and about central airways
    - Gravity-dependent distribution in dorsal lung
- **Intravascular Metastases**
  - Rare cause of TIB
    - Hepatocellular carcinoma
    - Breast cancer
    - Renal cell carcinoma
    - Gastric carcinoma
    - Prostate cancer
    - Choriocarcinoma
    - Angiosarcoma
  - Dilated and beaded peripheral pulmonary arteries
  - Enlarged central pulmonary arteries: Pulmonary arterial hypertension
- **Foreign Body (Cellulose) Granulomatosis**
  - Granulomatous reaction to injected cocaine cut with talc, crushed oral medications, cellulose often used as filler (cellulose granulomatosis)
    - Perivascular foci of foreign body reaction and fibrosis
    - Differential diagnosis
      - Talc pneumoconiosis due to inhalation of microscopic dust particles
  - Underrecognized cause of pulmonary hypertension
- **Fibrosing Bronchiolitis**
  - Rare pattern due to infectious or inhalational acute bronchiolitis
    - Pathologic bronchiolar abnormalities
      - Overlapping features with organizing pneumonia
      - Reversible polypoid plugs of granulation tissue
  - CT
    - Centrilobular nodules and variable TIB opacities

SELECTED REFERENCES

1. Im JG et al: Tree-in-bud pattern of pulmonary tuberculosis on thin-section ct: pathological implications. Korean J Radiol. 19(5):859-65, 2018
2. Cordier JF et al: Many faces of bronchiolitis and organizing pneumonia. Semin Respir Crit Care Med. 37(3):421-40, 2016
3. Ryerson CJ et al: Fibrosing bronchiolitis evolving from infectious or inhalational acute bronchiolitis. a reversible lesion. Ann Am Thorac Soc. 12(9):1323-7, 2015
4. Griffith CC et al: Intravascular talcosis due to intravenous drug use is an underrecognized cause of pulmonary hypertension. Pulm Med. 2012:617531, 2012
5. Rossi SE et al: Tree-in-bud pattern at thin-section CT of the lungs: radiologic-pathologic overview. Radiographics. 25(3):789-801, 2005
6. Franquet T et al: Thrombotic microangiopathy of pulmonary tumors: a vascular cause of tree-in-bud pattern on CT. AJR Am J Roentgenol. 179(4):897-9, 2002

Infectious Bronchiolitis

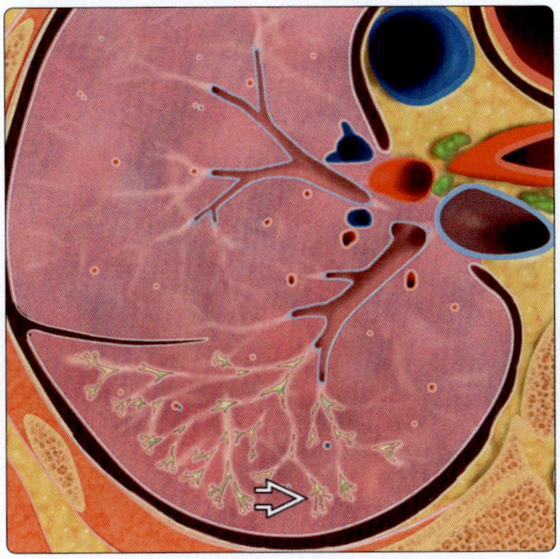

Infectious Bronchiolitis

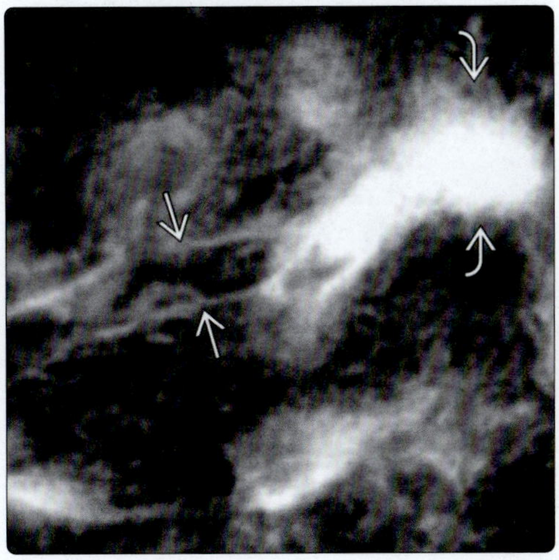

(Left) *Graphic shows branching centrilobular nodules that correlate with tree-in-bud opacities caused by luminal impaction by mucoid material* ➡. **(Right)** *Postmortem radiograph shows tuberculosis manifesting with a tree-in-bud lesion. The smoothly marginated bronchiole* ➡ *corresponds to the tree and the distal clubbed end* ➡ *to the bud (alveolar ducts filled with inflammatory substances). The bud measures 1-2 mm in diameter and is larger than the parent bronchiole. (Courtesy J. G. Im, MD.)*

(Left) *Axial CECT of a patient with infectious cellular bronchiolitis shows left lower lobe clustered centrilobular nodules and tree-in-bud opacities ➡. Note associated bronchiolar and peribronchiolar inflammation manifesting with bronchial wall thickening ➡.* (Right) *Axial NECT (MIP reformatted image) of a patient with infectious bronchiolitis shows multifocal right lower lobe tree-in-bud opacities ➡ and a peripheral lobular consolidation that represented associated bronchopneumonia ➡.*

Infectious Bronchiolitis

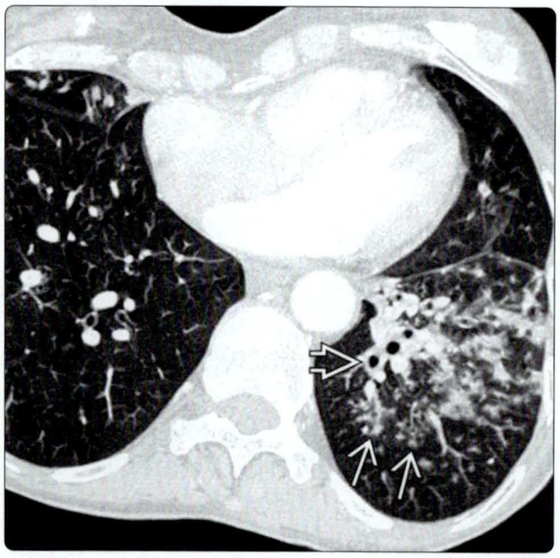

Infectious Bronchiolitis

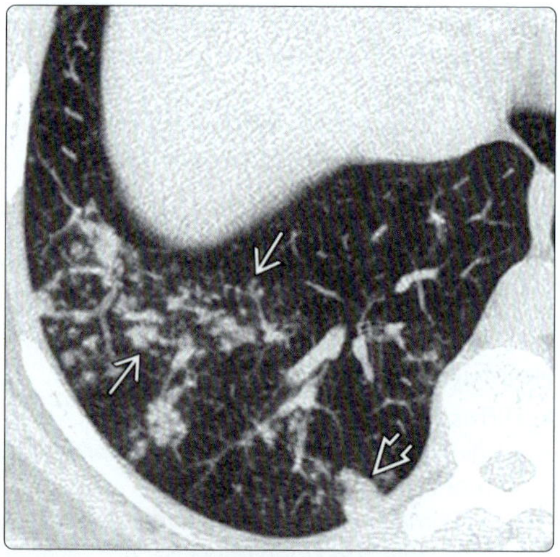

(Left) *Axial CECT (MIP reformatted image) of a patient with infectious viral bronchiolitis shows multifocal bilateral centrilobular tree-in-bud opacities ➡. MIP reformatted images help increase the conspicuity of pulmonary nodules and micronodules.* (Right) *Axial NECT of a patient with pulmonary tuberculosis shows multifocal right lower lobe centrilobular micronodules ➡ and tree-in-bud opacities ➡. Note that the micronodules spare the subpleural lung parenchyma given their centrilobular location.*

Infectious Bronchiolitis

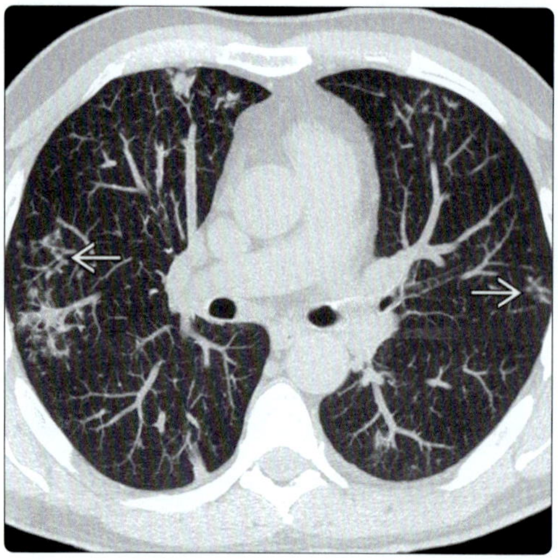

Infectious Bronchiolitis

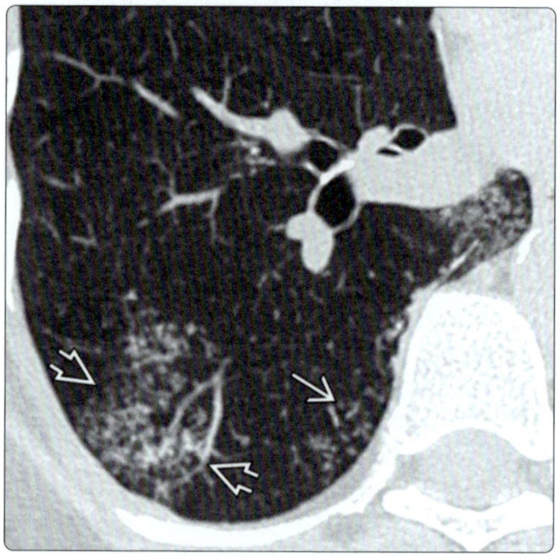

(Left) *Axial CECT of an HIV-infected patient with Mycobacterium abscessus pulmonary infection shows multiple bilateral cavitary nodules ➡ and nodular consolidations as well as scattered centrilobular micronodules and tree-in-bud opacities ➡.* (Right) *Coronal NECT of a 77-year-old man with head and neck cancer and a history of chronic aspiration shows bibasilar consolidations and profuse surrounding centrilobular nodules and tree-in-bud opacities ➡ consistent with aspiration bronchiolitis.*

Infectious Bronchiolitis

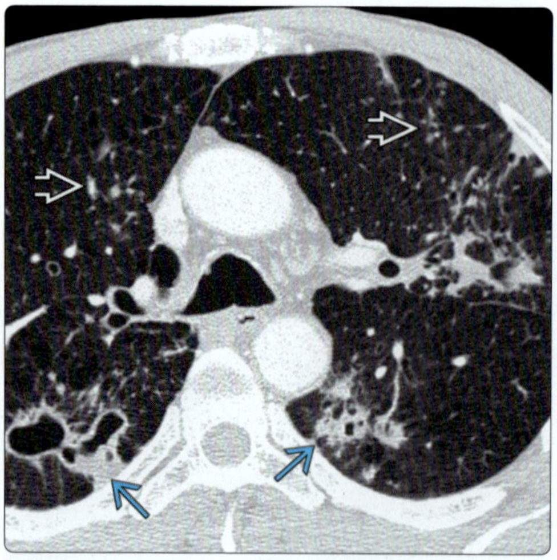

Aspiration Bronchiolitis

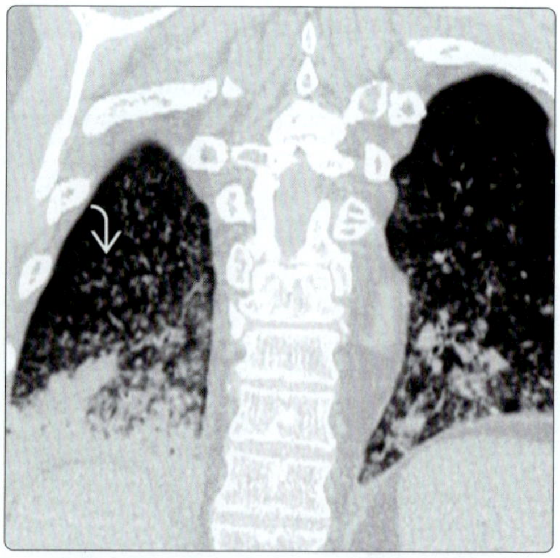

Tree-in-Bud Opacities

Bronchiectasis

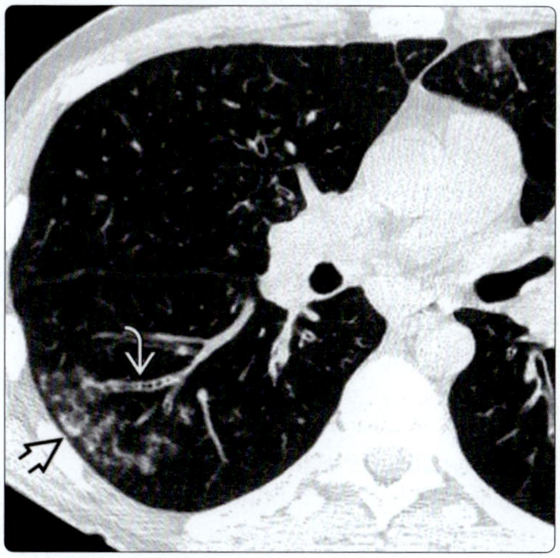

Bronchiectasis

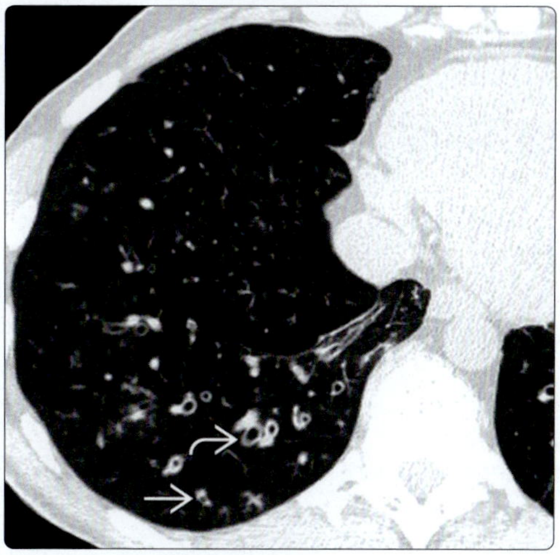

(Left) *Axial NECT of a 44-year-old man with bronchiectasis secondary to primary ciliary dyskinesia shows cylindrical bronchiectasis* → *with bronchial wall thickening and endoluminal mucus plugs, as well as scattered centrilobular micronodules and tree-in-bud opacities* →*.* **(Right)** *Axial NECT of the same patient shows lower lobe predominant bronchiectasis and bronchial wall thickening* → *and adjacent subtle centrilobular micronodules and tree-in-bud opacities* →*.*

Follicular Bronchiolitis

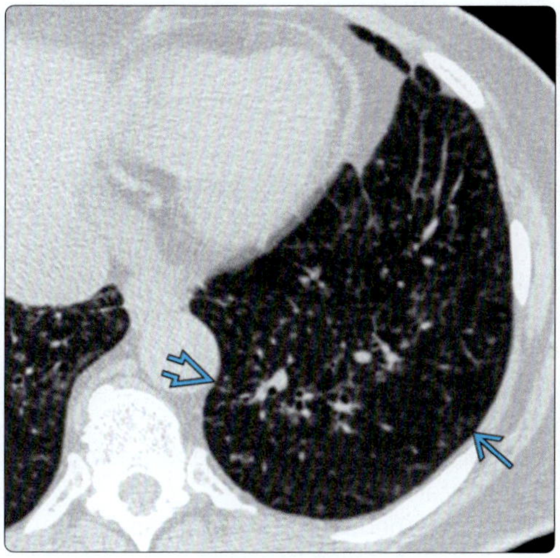

Diffuse Panbronchiolitis

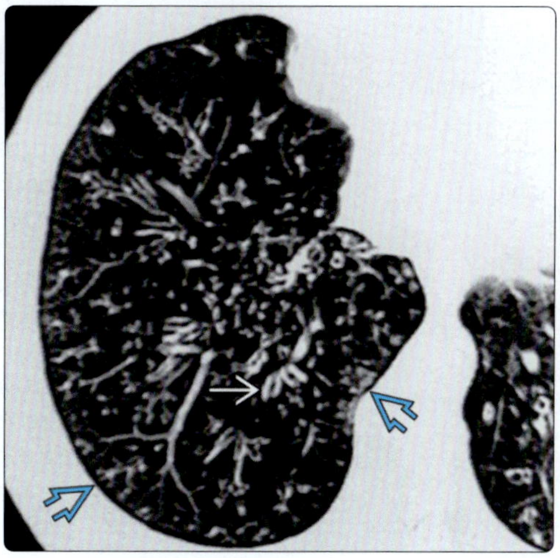

(Left) *Axial NECT of a patient with rheumatoid arthritis shows multifocal bilateral lower lobe centrilobular micronodules* → *and tree-in-bud opacities* → *secondary to follicular bronchiolitis, which may occur in association with rheumatoid arthritis &/or its drug therapy.* **(Right)** *Axial HRCT of a Japanese man with diffuse panbronchiolitis shows multifocal bilateral centrilobular micronodules and tree-in-bud opacities* → *and diffuse bronchial wall thickening* →*. In this disease, the bronchiolitis is very extensive and chronic.*

Intravascular Metastases

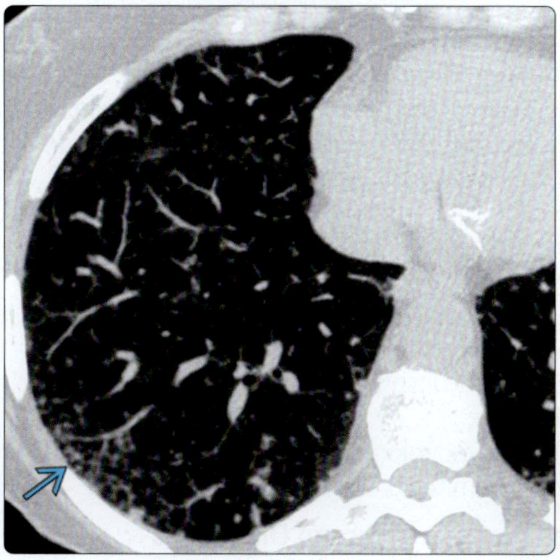

Foreign Body (Cellulose) Granulomatosis

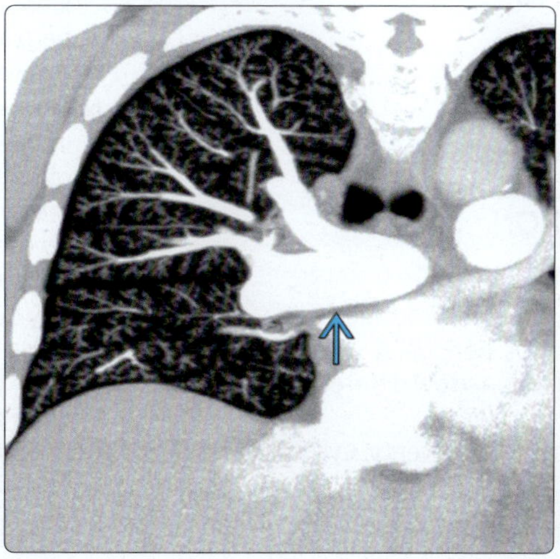

(Left) *Axial NECT of a patient with pancreatic carcinoma and progressive dyspnea shows basilar centrilobular micronodules and tree-in-bud opacities* → *representing intravascular metastases that were confirmed at open lung biopsy.* **(Right)** *Coronal CECT (MIP reformatted image) of a patient with cellulose granulomatosis due to crushed injected tablets shows a profuse vascular tree-in-bud pattern that characteristically spares the subpleural regions. Note enlarged pulmonary arteries* → *due to coexistent pulmonary hypertension.*

DIFFERENTIAL DIAGNOSIS

Common

- Diffuse Peripheral
  - Upper Lobe Predominant
    - Sarcoidosis
    - Cystic Fibrosis
    - Tuberculosis
    - Nontuberculous Mycobacterial Infection (Cavitary)
  - Lower Lobe Predominant
    - Idiopathic Diffuse Fibrosing Lung Disease
    - Connective Tissue Disease-Related Interstitial Lung Disease
    - Aspiration Bronchiolitis
  - Middle Lobe/Lingular Predominant
    - Nontuberculous Mycobacterial Infection (Bronchiectatic)
- Focal
  - Endobronchial Neoplasm
  - Post Radiation

Less Common

- Diffuse Central
  - Allergic Bronchopulmonary Aspergillosis
- Diffuse Peripheral
  - Upper Lobe Predominant
    - Hypersensitivity Pneumonitis
  - Lower Lobe Predominant
    - Alpha-1-Antitrypsin Deficiency
    - Immunodeficiency
  - Middle Lobe/Lingular Predominant
    - Primary Ciliary Dyskinesia
    - Acute Respiratory Distress Syndrome
- Diffuse
  - Constrictive Bronchiolitis
- Focal
  - Bronchial Obstruction
    - Broncholithiasis
    - Foreign Body
  - Congenital Bronchial Atresia

Rare but Important

- Diffuse Central
  - Mounier-Kuhn Syndrome
  - Williams-Campbell Syndrome

ESSENTIAL INFORMATION

Key Differential Diagnosis Issues

- Wide variety of entities may produce bronchiectasis
- Anatomic localization (central vs. peripheral, upper lobe vs. lower lobe predominance) helps narrow differential diagnosis
- Morphologic classification based on severity: Cylindrical, varicose, cystic/saccular

Helpful Clues for Common Diagnoses

- **Sarcoidosis**
  - Idiopathic granulomatous inflammatory disease with perilymphatic distribution
  - Chronic disease: Upper lobe peripheral bronchiectasis ± peribronchovascular reticulation and honeycombing
- **Cystic Fibrosis**
  - Autosomal recessive disorder
  - Often diagnosed in childhood
  - Thick mucus secretions, inefficient mucociliary clearance, predisposition to infection and bronchiectasis
  - Bronchiectasis is typically diffuse
    - Most severe in upper lobes, central lungs, and apical segments of lower lobes
- **Tuberculosis**
  - Fibrocavitary disease and bronchiectasis; asymmetric upper lobe involvement
  - Imaging: Upper lobe cavitation + tree-in-bud nodules and bronchiectasis
- **Nontuberculous Mycobacterial Infection (Cavitary)**
  - Upper lobe cavitary disease indistinguishable from tuberculosis
  - Imaging: Upper lobe cavitation with tree-in-bud nodules and bronchiectasis
- **Idiopathic Diffuse Fibrosing Lung Disease**
  - Traction bronchiectasis common in usual interstitial pneumonia (UIP) and nonspecific interstitial pneumonia (NSIP)
  - Lower lobe subpleural predominance, associated reticulation &/or honeycombing
- **Connective Tissue Disease-Related Interstitial Lung Disease**
  - Diffuse fibrosing lung disease associated with autoimmunity (e.g., scleroderma, lupus, rheumatoid arthritis)
  - Imaging features identical to those of other diffuse fibrosing lung diseases
- **Aspiration Bronchiolitis**
  - a.k.a. diffuse aspiration bronchiolitis or lentil pneumonia
  - Recurrent subclinical microaspiration
    - Risk factors: Hiatus hernia, reflux, esophageal dysmotility, gastric banding, achalasia, scleroderma, neurologic conditions involving esophagus
  - Bronchiectasis + scattered tree-in-bud opacities; identification of associated causative findings (hiatus hernia, dilated esophagus)
  - ↑ awareness and clinical suspicion required for diagnosis
- **Nontuberculous Mycobacterial Infection (Bronchiectatic)**
  - Indolent infectious bronchiolitis due to *Mycobacterium avium-intracellulare, Mycobacterium gordonae*
  - Tree-in-bud opacities and bronchiectasis, often more severe in middle lobe and lingula
- **Endobronchial Neoplasm**
  - Any benign or malignant endobronchial tumor may cause obstruction, distal postobstructive pneumonia ± bronchiectasis and inspissated mucus
- **Post Radiation**
  - Consolidation &/or volume loss with traction bronchiectasis limited to radiation field

Helpful Clues for Less Common Diagnoses

- **Allergic Bronchopulmonary Aspergillosis**
  - Hypersensitivity to *Aspergillus* antigens leads to chronic inflammation/airway damage and bronchiectasis

- High-attenuation or calcified inspissated mucus in dilated bronchi
- **Hypersensitivity Pneumonitis**
  - Inflammatory disease due to allergic reaction to various antigens (animal proteins, bacteria, mold) or haptens (e.g., isocyanate, zinc, inks, and dyes)
  - Chronic disease may lead to fibrosis
  - CT: Honeycombing and traction bronchiectasis/bronchiolectasis
    - Mid and lower lobe predominant, peribronchovascular, or lower lobe predominant (similar to UIP or NSIP)
- **Alpha-1-Antitrypsin Deficiency**
  - Autosomal codominant genetic disorder: ↓ production of alpha-1-antitrypsin leads to pulmonary (i.e., emphysema) and liver (i.e., cirrhosis) disease
  - Imaging: Lower lobe predominant panlobular emphysema, bronchial wall thickening, bronchiectasis
- **Immunodeficiency**
  - Congenital or acquired (i.e., HIV) immunodeficiency, ↑ risk of infection with resultant bronchiectasis
- **Primary Ciliary Dyskinesia**
  - Autosomal recessive defect of ciliary structure/function with impaired mucociliary clearance
  - Kartagener syndrome: Bronchiectasis, situs inversus, chronic sinusitis
- **Acute Respiratory Distress Syndrome**
  - Acute and rapidly progressive lung damage due to variety of pulmonary and nonpulmonary infections or inflammatory processes, aspiration, inhalational injury
  - Chronic stage: Anterior nondependent fibrosis and bronchiectasis
- **Constrictive Bronchiolitis**
  - Bronchiolar narrowing caused by submucosal scarring and chronic inflammatory changes
  - Various etiologies: Idiopathic, post bone marrow or lung transplant, Swyer-James syndrome, autoimmunity, diffuse idiopathic neuroendocrine cell hyperplasia
  - Imaging: Mosaic attenuation and expiratory air-trapping are typical findings; bronchiectasis and bronchial wall thickening often identified
- **Constrictive Broncholithiasis**
  - Endobronchial calcified nodule commonly related to calcified lymph node erosion and extrusion into bronchial lumen
  - CT is imaging modality of choice: Endobronchial calcification ± postobstructive pneumonitis
- **Foreign Body**
  - Aspiration and endobronchial lodging of foreign body
  - CT is most sensitive imaging modality: Foreign body may be high or low attenuation, often associated with postobstructive pneumonitis
- **Congenital Bronchial Atresia**
  - Atretic bronchus; mucocele develops distal to point of atresia
  - CT is imaging modality of choice
    - Mucocele (focal bronchiectasis with inspissated mucus): Nodular or branching opacity
    - Surrounding hyperlucent lung

Helpful Clues for Rare Diagnoses

- **Mounier-Kuhn Syndrome**
  - Thinning of airway wall elastic fibers, cartilage, smooth muscle
  - Bronchiectasis involving trachea and 1st- to 4th-generation bronchi
- **Williams-Campbell Syndrome**
  - Cartilage deficiency involving mid order (4th-6th generation) bronchi
  - Bronchiectasis that spares trachea and mainstem bronchi

SELECTED REFERENCES

1. Aksamit TR et al: Adult patients with bronchiectasis: a first look at the US Bronchiectasis Research Registry. Chest. 151(5):982-92, 2017
2. Milliron B et al: Bronchiectasis: mechanisms and imaging clues of associated common and uncommon diseases. Radiographics. 35(4):1011-30, 2015
3. Cantin L et al: Bronchiectasis. AJR Am J Roentgenol. 193(3):W158-71, 2009

Sarcoidosis

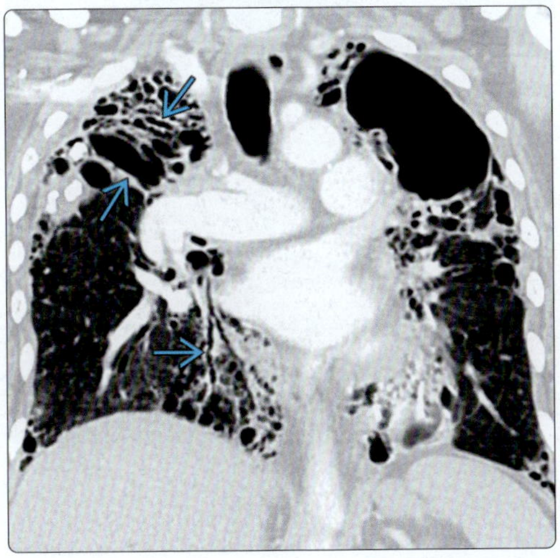

Cystic Fibrosis

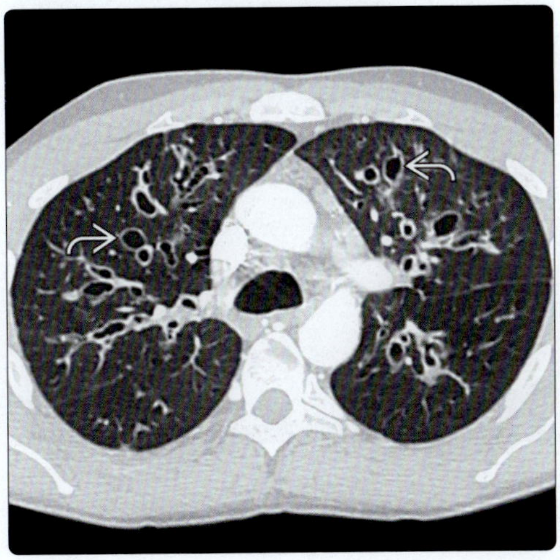

(Left) *Coronal CECT of a patient with a longstanding history of sarcoidosis shows upper lobe predominant cylindrical and cystic bronchiectasis ➔ amid peribronchovascular fibrosis. The upper lobe predominant cystic spaces may become colonized by aspergillus, and affected patients are at risk of developing life-threatening hemoptysis.* **(Right)** *Axial CECT of a young patient with cystic fibrosis shows diffuse bilateral multifocal saccular bronchiectasis ➔ and bronchial wall thickening with upper lobe predominance.*

(Left) *Coronal CECT of a patient with tuberculosis shows left upper lobe cicatricial atelectasis characterized by volume loss and architectural distortion with intrinsic cylindrical bronchiectasis →.* **(Right)** *Coronal NECT of a patient with nontuberculous mycobacterial infection shows left lung cavitation →, volume loss, and bronchiectasis →. Note scattered centrilobular micronodules → from associated cellular bronchiolitis. The findings are indistinguishable from those of cavitary tuberculosis.*

Tuberculosis

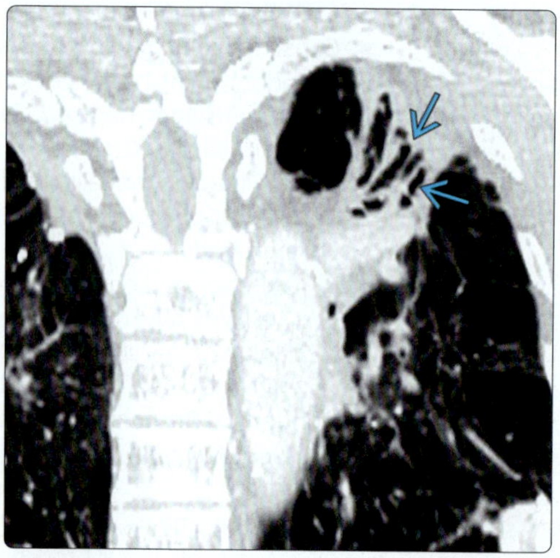

Nontuberculous Mycobacterial Infection (Cavitary)

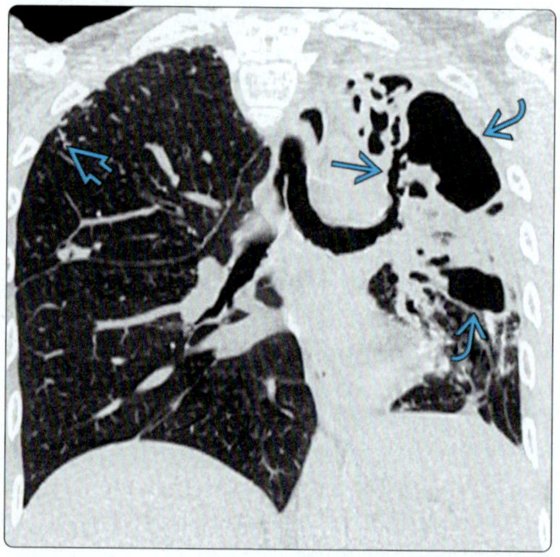

(Left) *Axial HRCT of a patient with idiopathic pulmonary fibrosis shows extensive lower lobe predominant subpleural honeycombing with multifocal areas of traction bronchiectasis →.* **(Right)** *Sagittal HRCT of the same patient demonstrates to better advantage the apicobasilar gradient of disease distribution and helps differentiate areas of honeycombing from bronchiectasis →, which may be challenging on axial imaging alone.*

Idiopathic Diffuse Fibrosing Lung Disease

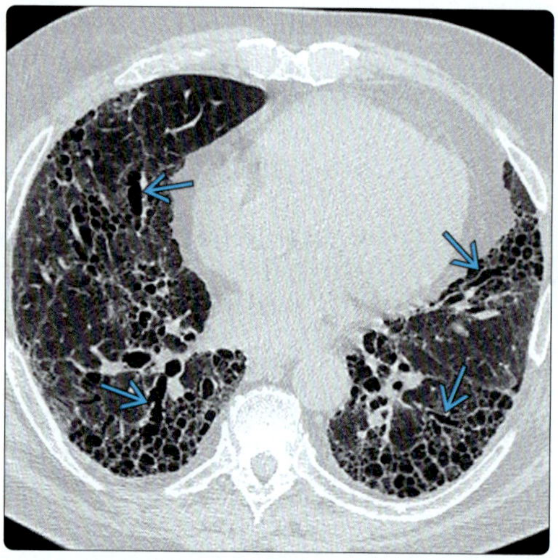

Idiopathic Diffuse Fibrosing Lung Disease

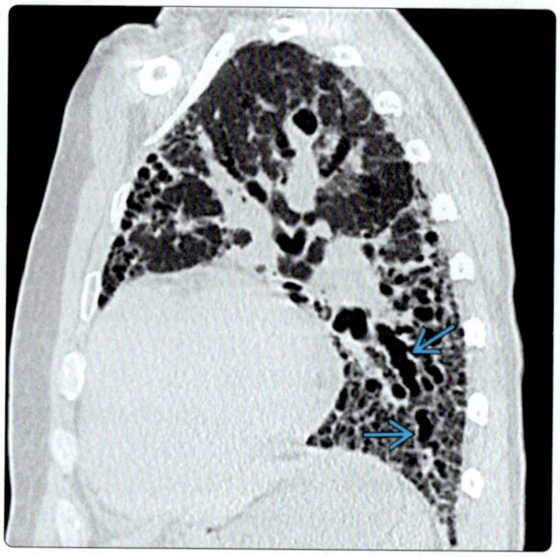

(Left) *Axial HRCT of a patient with connective tissue disease-related interstitial lung disease due to scleroderma shows bilateral ground-glass opacities and mild reticulation but no honeycombing. Note "out of proportion" varicoid traction bronchiectasis →, a finding frequently identified in patients with fibrosis due to progressive systemic sclerosis.* **(Right)** *Sagittal HRCT of the same patient shows marked basilar traction bronchiectasis →. Multiplanar imaging allows differentiation of bronchiectasis from honeycombing.*

Connective Tissue Disease-Related Interstitial Lung Disease

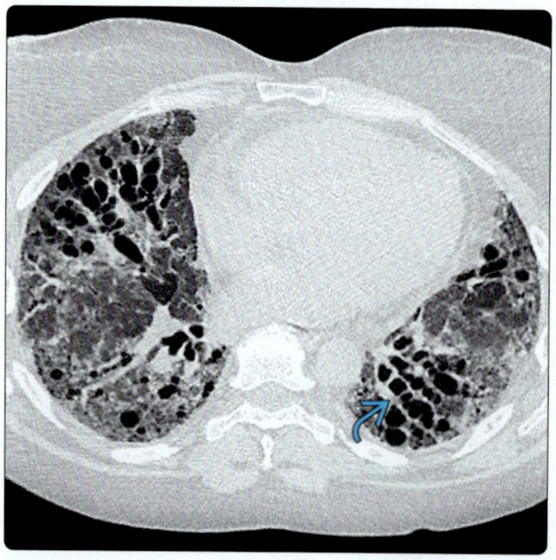

Connective Tissue Disease-Related Interstitial Lung Disease

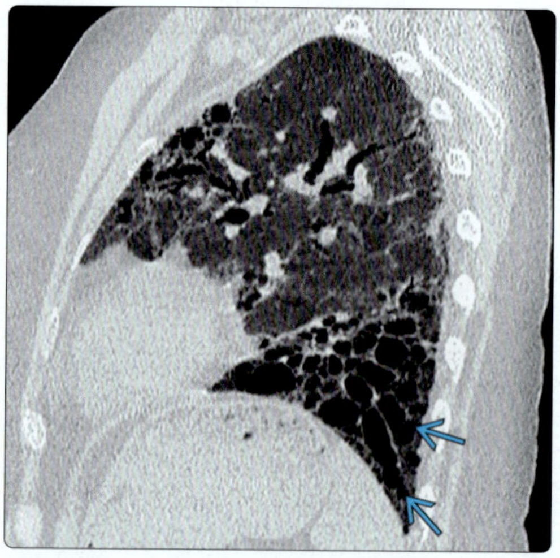

Aspiration Bronchiolitis

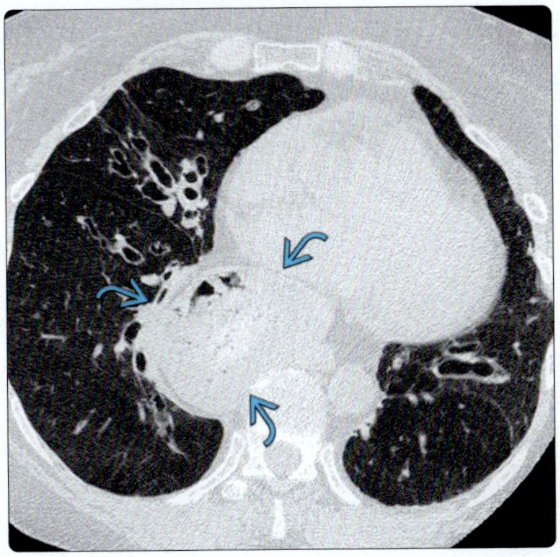

Nontuberculous Mycobacterial Infection (Bronchiectatic)

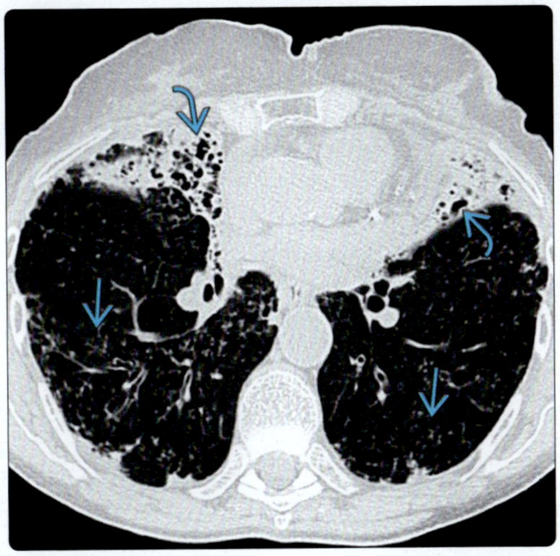

(Left) *Axial HRCT of a patient with diffuse aspiration bronchiolitis shows multifocal basilar predominant cylindrical bronchiectasis and bronchial wall thickening. Note the presence of large hiatus hernia* ↷*, which is a common predisposing factor for aspiration bronchiolitis.* **(Right)** *Axial HRCT of a patient with bronchiectatic nontuberculous mycobacterial infection shows multifocal bilateral cellular bronchiolitis* → *and middle lobe and lingular volume loss with intrinsic bronchiectasis* ↷.

Endobronchial Neoplasm

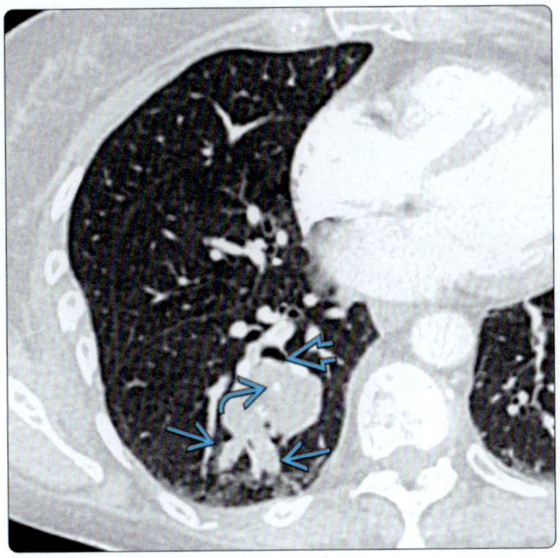

Post Radiation

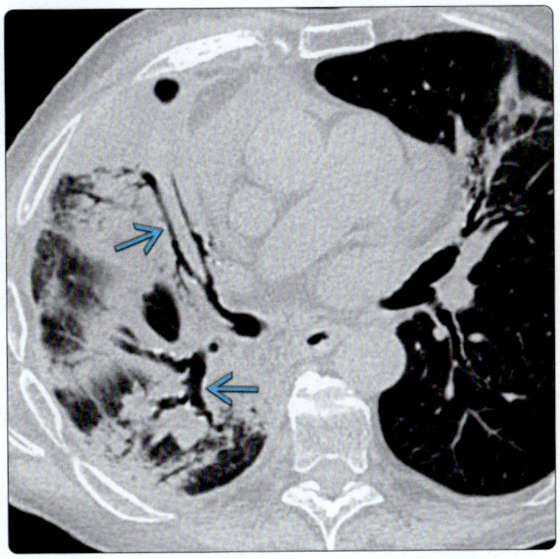

(Left) *Axial CECT of a patient with a right lower lobe bronchial carcinoid tumor shows a polylobular mass with an endobronchial component* ⇨*, intrinsic calcifications* ↷*, and distal bronchiectasis with inspissated mucus* →*. Carcinoid tumors are commonly endobronchial and may produce postobstructive abnormalities.* **(Right)** *Axial CECT of a patient with a history of lung cancer treated with radiation shows band-like consolidations with volume loss and intrinsic traction bronchiectasis* → *limited to the radiation field.*

Allergic Bronchopulmonary Aspergillosis

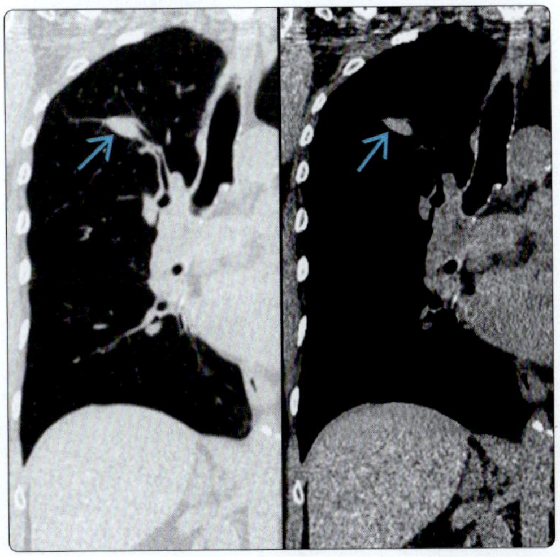

Hypersensitivity Pneumonitis

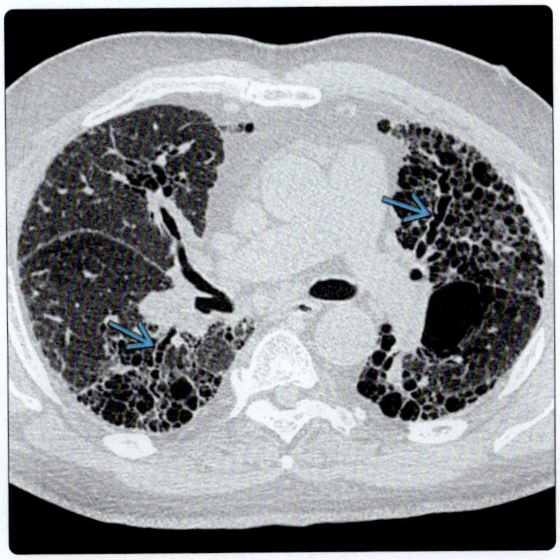

(Left) *Composite image with coronal NECT in lung (left) and soft tissue (right) window of a patient with allergic bronchopulmonary aspergillosis shows right upper lobe bronchiectasis with high-attenuation inspissated mucus* →*.* **(Right)** *Axial HRCT of a patient with hypersensitivity pneumonitis shows peribronchovascular and subpleural reticulation, honeycombing, and scattered traction bronchiectasis* → *that may be indistinguishable from usual interstitial pneumonia or nonspecific interstitial pneumonia.*

(Left) *Axial NECT of a patient with human immunodeficiency virus (HIV) infection shows lower lobe predominant cylindrical bronchiectasis* ➔. *Bronchiectasis is a common pulmonary manifestation of congenital and acquired immunodeficiencies.* **(Right)** *Axial HRCT of a patient with Kartagener syndrome shows extensive mid and lower lung zone predominant bronchial wall thickening and bronchiectasis* ➔. *Dextrocardia, left middle lobe atelectasis* ↪*, and bronchiectasis are features of Kartagener syndrome.*

Immunodeficiency

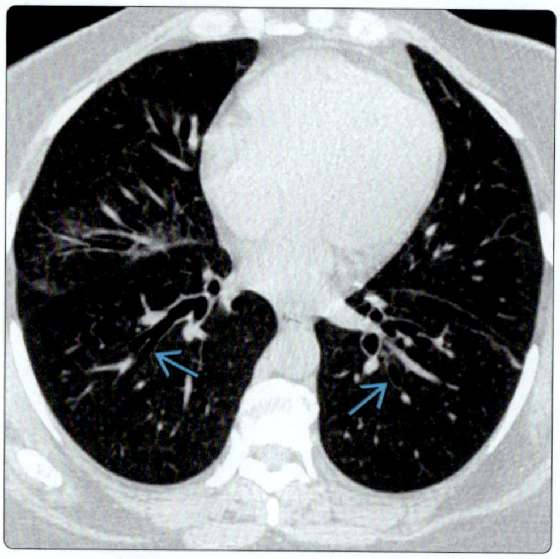

Primary Ciliary Dyskinesia

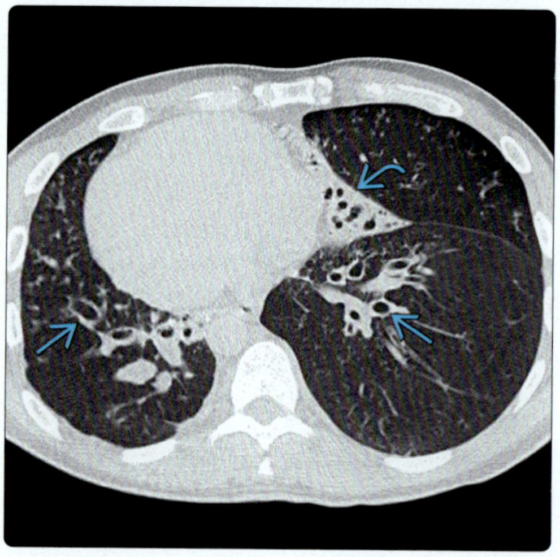

(Left) *Axial CECT of a patient with prior acute respiratory distress syndrome shows nondependent reticulation and honeycombing amid areas of traction bronchiectasis* ➔. **(Right)** *Coronal NECT of a patient status post bilateral lung transplantation with longstanding bronchiolitis obliterans syndrome shows extensive bilateral lower lobe predominant cylindrical and cystic bronchiectasis* ↪*. Constrictive bronchiolitis is a manifestation of chronic rejection as a complication of organ and bone marrow transplantation.*

Acute Respiratory Distress Syndrome

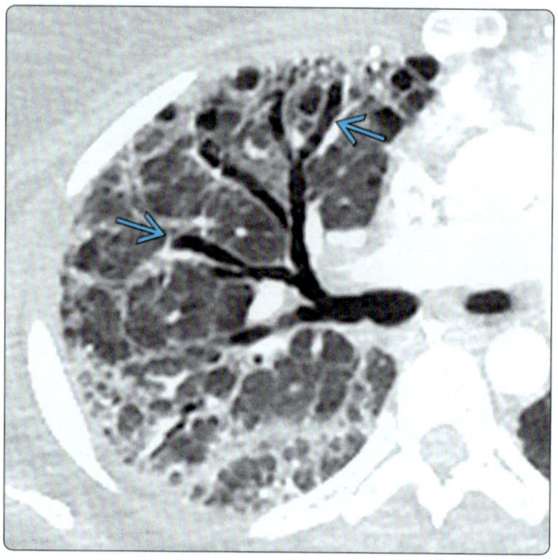

Constrictive Bronchiolitis

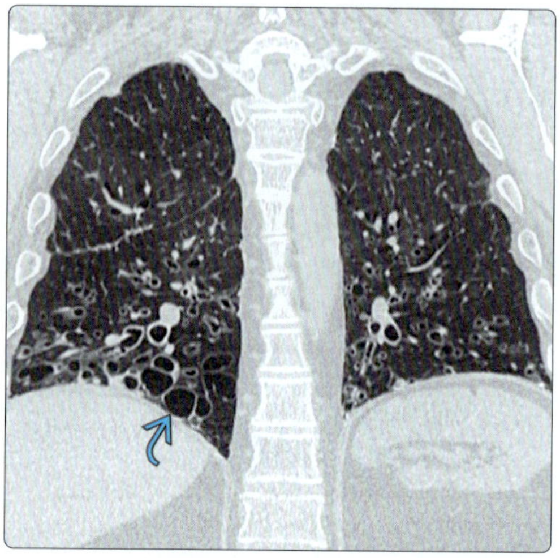

(Left) *Coronal NECT of a patient with Swyer-James syndrome shows extensive mosaic attenuation with associated bronchial wall thickening and bronchiectasis* ➔*. The syndrome is characteristically related to childhood infection, typically Adenovirus.* **(Right)** *Composite image with axial CECT of a patient with broncholithiasis shows a calcified nodule* ➔ *in the lumen of the distal left mainstem bronchus with extensive postobstructive pneumonia with intrinsic bronchiectasis* ↪*.*

Constrictive Bronchiolitis

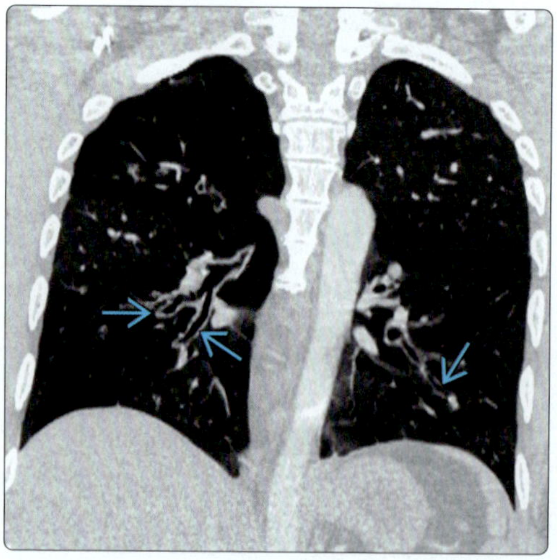

Broncholithiasis

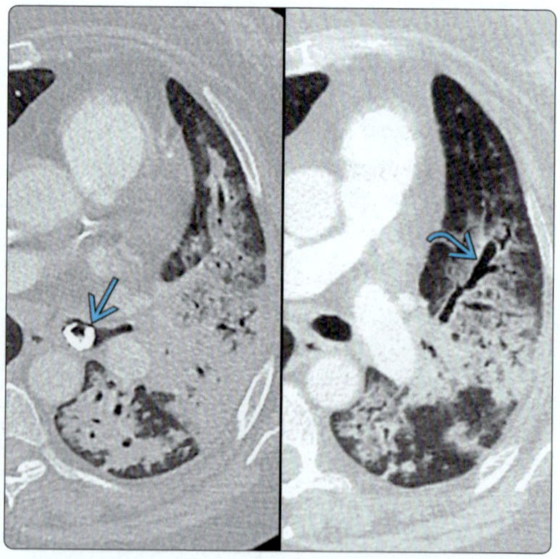

Foreign Body

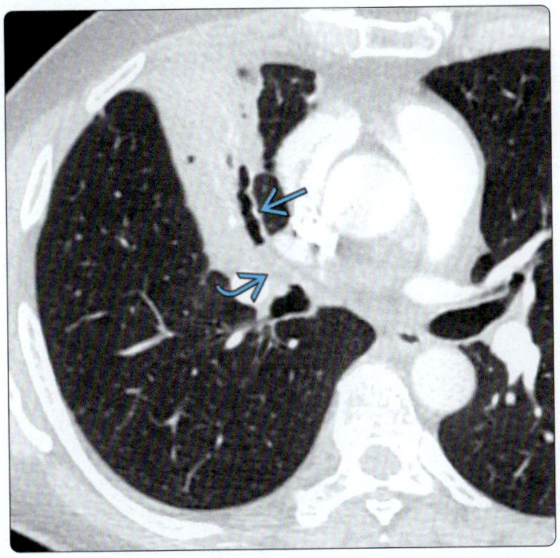

Congenital Bronchial Atresia

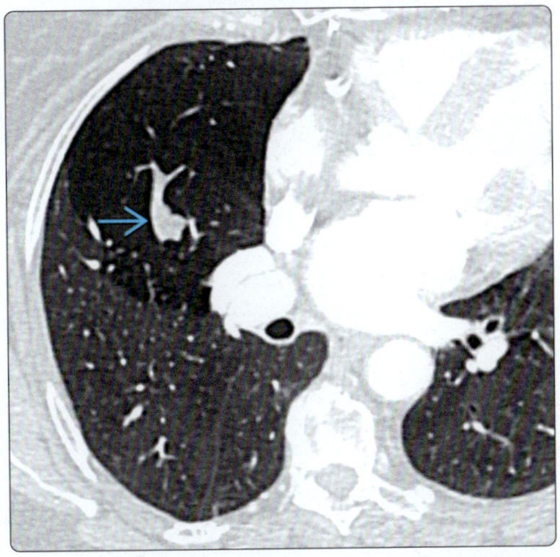

(Left) *Axial CECT of a patient with an aspirated foreign body that lodged in the lumen of the proximal middle lobe bronchus shows proximal luminal obstruction and postobstructive pneumonitis, atelectasis, and bronchiectasis.* **(Right)** *Axial CECT of a patient with congenital bronchial atresia shows a branching mucocele (i.e., inspissated mucus within a dilated bronchus distal to the point of atresia) surrounded by hyperlucent lung. These findings are considered diagnostic of congenital bronchial atresia.*

Mounier-Kuhn Syndrome

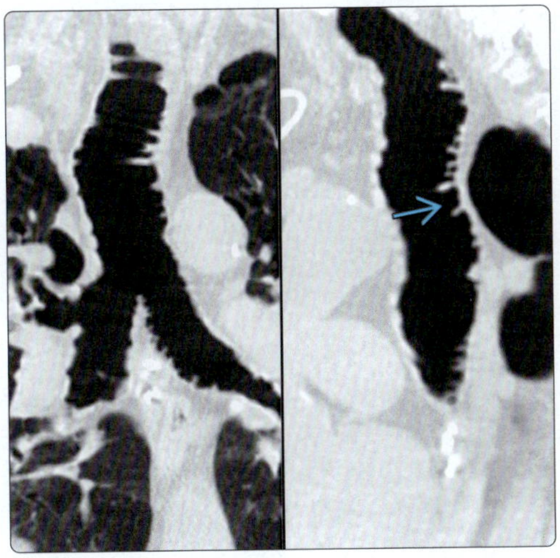

Mounier-Kuhn Syndrome

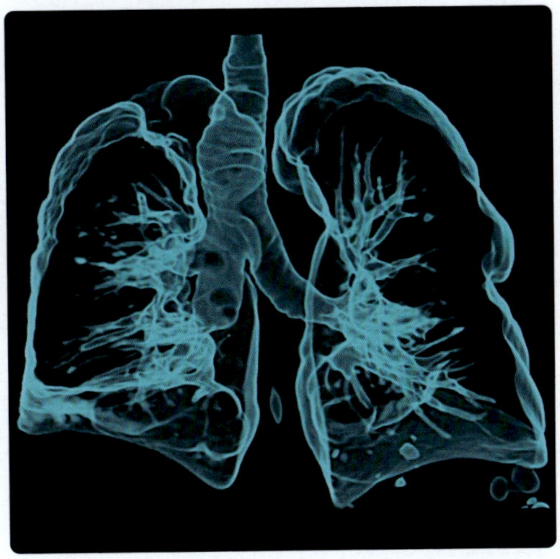

(Left) *Composite image with coronal (left) and sagittal (right) NECT of a patient with Mounier-Kuhn syndrome shows dilatation of the trachea and mainstem bronchi. Note small sacculations along the airway walls characteristic of this disorder.* **(Right)** *3D surface-rendered display of the same patient shows tracheobronchial dilatation that spares the distal bronchi. Mounier-Kuhn syndrome, or tracheobronchomegaly, may manifest with recurrent cough and respiratory tract infections.*

Williams-Campbell Syndrome

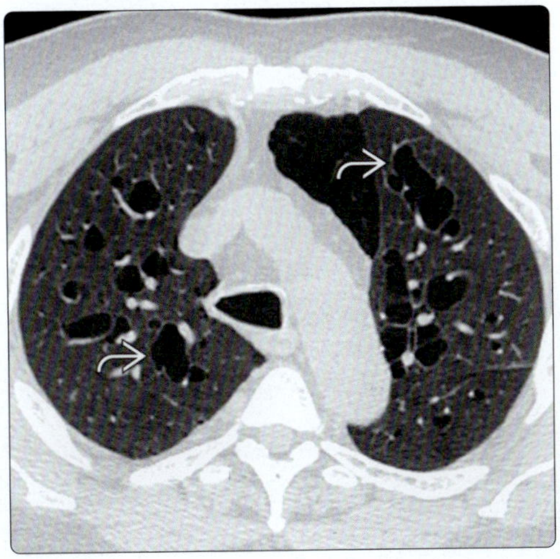

Williams-Campbell Syndrome

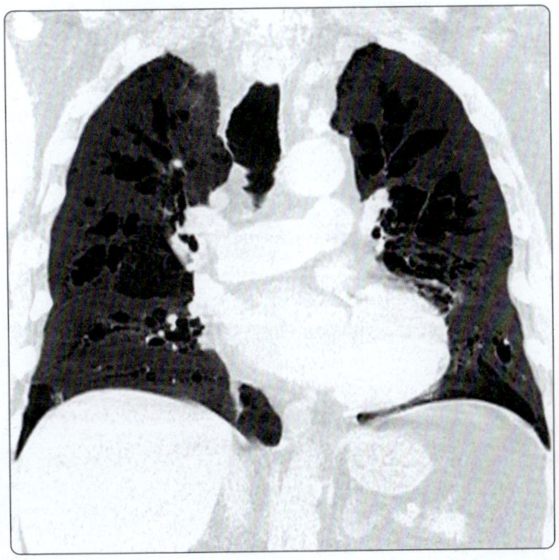

(Left) *Axial NECT of a patient with Williams-Campbell syndrome shows extensive bronchiectasis involving mid-order bronchi. Note sparing of the trachea.* **(Right)** *Coronal NECT (minIP reformatted image) of the same patient shows bronchiectasis involving mid-order bronchi. Williams-Campbell syndrome is thought to be related to deficient cartilage in the subsegmental bronchi with resultant bronchiectasis and is often associated with recurrent infection.*

SECTION 5

Mediastinum and Hila

Approach to Mediastinum and Hila

General Imaging Patterns

Modality-Specific Imaging Findings: Radiography

Modality-Specific Imaging Findings: Computed Tomography

Modality-Specific Imaging Findings: Magnetic Resonance Imaging

Mediastinum

General Concepts

The mediastinum is the zone between the lungs and pleural spaces that extends from the thoracic inlet to the diaphragm and is bound anteriorly by the sternum and posteriorly by the vertebral bodies. It contains a number of vital structures, including the heart and pericardium, the pulmonary trunk and central pulmonary veins, the thoracic aorta and branch vessels, the esophagus, the trachea and carina, and the thoracic duct. The mediastinum also contains fat, lymph nodes, and nerves. Abnormalities may arise from any of these structures and may produce mediastinal contour abnormalities or masses. Radiographic identification of such abnormalities relies on knowledge of the normal imaging anatomy of the mediastinum and its lines, stripes, and interfaces. Mediastinal abnormalities are optimally assessed with cross-sectional imaging with CT or MR for accurate localization, characterization, identification of mass effect on or invasion of adjacent structures, and associated findings, such as lymphadenopathy.

Mediastinal Abnormalities

Radiography

Mediastinal abnormalities are often detected on radiography based on identification of an abnormal mediastinal contour. Approximately 10% of mediastinal contour abnormalities are vascular and include anomalous vessels and aneurysms. Mediastinal masses may be focal and unilateral or diffuse and bilateral. Diffuse mediastinal enlargement suggests lymphadenopathy, while focal enlargement is typical of primary neoplasms. Once a mediastinal abnormality is identified on frontal chest radiography, it is localized within a mediastinal compartment (anterior, middle, or posterior) based on lateral chest radiography. The radiographic features are then correlated with the patient's age, sex, and clinical presentation in order to provide a focused differential diagnosis and suggest the next most appropriate imaging study or management step. For example, a unilateral anterior mediastinal mass in a patient over the age of 40 years is often a thymoma. The next imaging study should be a contrast-enhanced chest CT. On the other hand, a focal posterior mediastinal mass with benign pressure erosion on the adjacent skeleton in an asymptomatic adult is most likely a neurogenic neoplasm, and the most appropriate next imaging study is MR to exclude intraspinal extension, which occurs in approximately 10% of cases.

CT and MR

CT and MR allow further characterization of mediastinal abnormalities. Vascular lesions may be contiguous with other vascular structures and are optimally evaluated with intravenous contrast. Focal lesions can be analyzed for the presence or absence of cystic change, calcification, fat, or necrosis. Adjacent structures can be assessed for identification of mass effect or local invasion. Diffuse mediastinal enlargement often represents lymphadenopathy, which can be identified based on involvement of one or several intrathoracic lymph node stations. Lymphadenopathy may manifest as discrete enlarged lymph nodes or as a diffuse locally invasive soft tissue mass (nodal coalescence). Mediastinal masses can be localized to one or more mediastinal compartments, which include prevascular, visceral, and paravertebral compartments, for the formulation of a differential diagnosis.

Hilum

General Concepts

The pulmonary hilum is the point of connection between the lung and mediastinum and provides a passage through which airways and vessels course from the mediastinum into the lungs. The hila also contain fat, lymph nodes, nerves, and lymphatics.

Hilar Abnormalities

Radiography

The hila are readily assessed on radiography, and the pulmonary arteries form most of the normal hilar opacity. In the majority of cases, the left hilum is higher than the right, and in 3% of cases, the right and left hila are at the same level. The normal right hilum is never higher than the left. Alteration of the hilar relationships may be due to lobar collapse or volume loss. On lateral radiography, the right hilar vascular opacity is located anterior to the central airways and the left hilum (comprised by the left pulmonary artery) is located posteriorly. Recognition of the normal hilar anatomy is crucial for the identification of hilar masses, lymphadenopathy, and central vascular enlargement.

Hilar enlargement may be secondary to a mass, lymphadenopathy, or enlargement of the pulmonary arteries. Unilateral hilar masses are often due to lymphadenopathy, and primary lung cancer and lymphoma are important diagnostic considerations. A hilar mass may produce lobar collapse due to central bronchial obstruction. Hilar lymphadenopathy may be unilateral or bilateral and may occur in cases of lymphoma, fungal infection, and lymph node metastases. Bilateral hilar lymphadenopathy is a typical finding of sarcoidosis.

Hilar enlargement may also be secondary to pulmonary artery enlargement from pulmonary hypertension (often with associated enlargement of the pulmonary trunk) or pulmonic stenosis (characterized by unilateral left pulmonary artery enlargement). The hilum convergence sign allows identification of a vascular etiology for the hilar enlargement, as enlarged pulmonary arteries converge on the enlarged hilum. The hilum overlay sign indicates that a mass is not in the hilum and is typically described in anterior mediastinal masses through which there is radiographic visualization of the hilum.

CT and MR

Cross-sectional imaging with CT and MR is helpful in evaluating the abnormal hilum and allows characterization of hilar masses. Enlarged lymph nodes manifest as soft tissue lesions located within anatomic lymph node stations and characteristically exhibit a short axis diameter > 1 cm. Nodal coalescence obliterates individual enlarged lymph nodes and manifests as a conglomerate soft tissue mass. CT allows identification of lymph node calcification, which is commonly seen in remote granulomatous infection secondary to histoplasmosis. Contrast-enhanced CT is preferred for the assessment of hilar lymphadenopathy, as it allows differentiation between lymph nodes and adjacent blood vessels.

Radiographic identification of mediastinal and hilar abnormalities allows the formulation of a focused differential diagnosis. Cross-sectional imaging allows further characterization of the abnormalities and enables the suggestion of a specific diagnosis &/or management recommendations.

Diffuse Mediastinal Enlargement

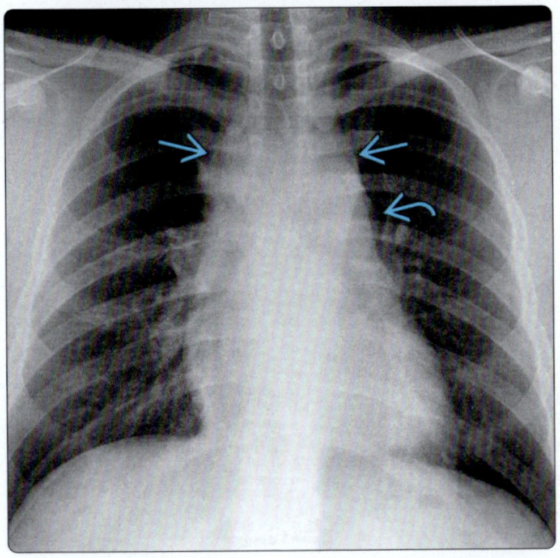

Diffuse Mediastinal Enlargement

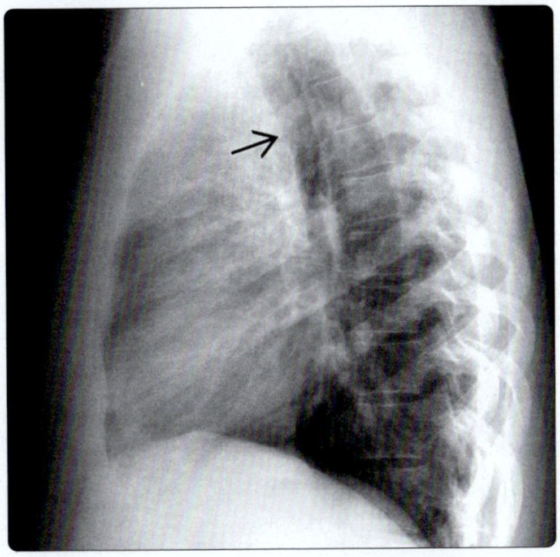

(Left) *PA chest radiograph of a 30-year-old man with chest pain and weight loss shows diffuse mediastinal enlargement manifesting as abnormal upper mediastinal contours ➔ involving both sides of midline. Note abnormal opacity in the AP window ➔.* **(Right)** *Lateral chest radiograph of the same patient shows that the mass is located in the anterior mediastinum and produces mass effect on the anterior tracheal wall ➔. Based on the findings and the patient's demographic, the most likely diagnosis is lymphoma.*

Prevascular Mass: Lymphadenopathy

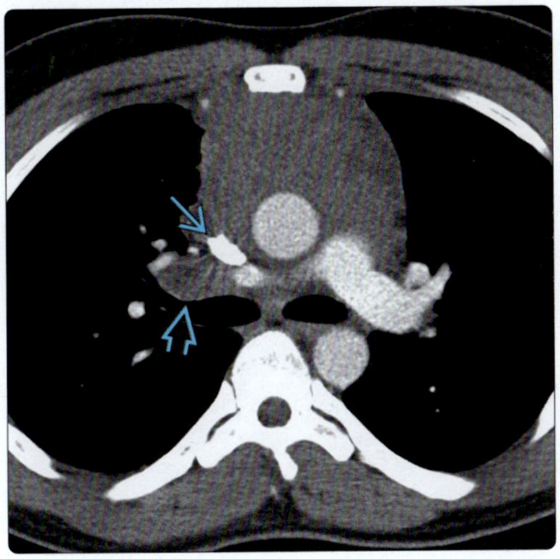

Prevascular Mass: Lymphadenopathy

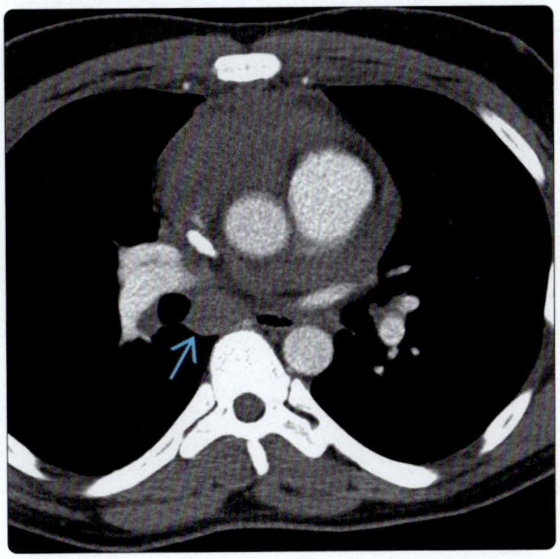

(Left) *CECT of the same patient shows nodal coalescence that manifests as a prevascular soft tissue mass that encases vascular structures, obliterates the brachiocephalic veins, and narrows the superior vena cava ➔. Note associated right hilar soft tissue ➔, which helps suggest lymphadenopathy.* **(Right)** *Axial CECT of the same patient shows coalescent prevascular and right paraesophageal ➔ lymphadenopathy in this patient with Hodgkin lymphoma.*

Posterior Mediastinal Mass

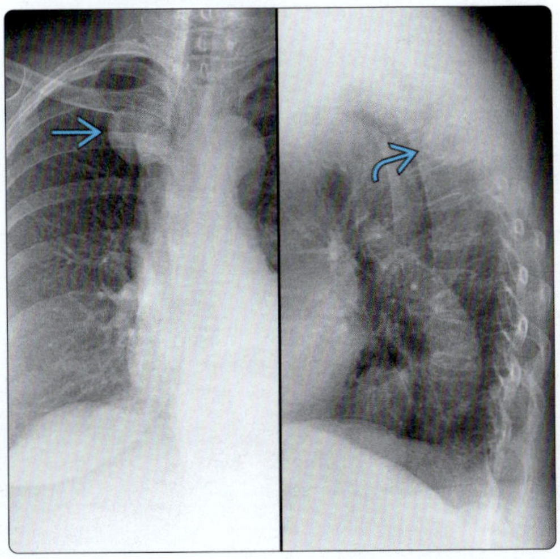

Paravertebral Mediastinal Mass

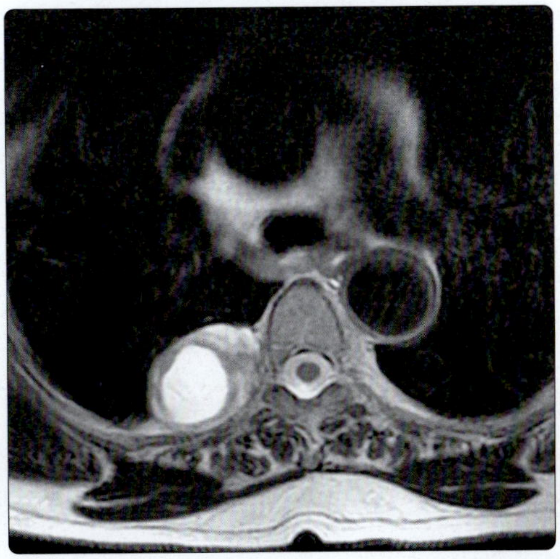

(Left) *Composite image with PA (left) and lateral (right) chest radiographs of an asymptomatic woman shows a focal right upper mediastinal mass ➔, which is localized to the posterior mediastinum ➔ on the lateral radiograph. The most likely diagnosis is neurogenic neoplasm.* **(Right)** *Axial T2W MR of the same patient shows a cystic right paravertebral schwannoma. MR is the imaging modality of choice for assessment of paravertebral masses, as it allows identification of intraspinal &/or neuroforaminal involvement.*

(Left) *PA chest radiograph of a 31-year-old man with dysphagia shows a large retrocardiac mediastinal mass with well-defined borders, which extends to both sides of midline. The upper mediastinum is normal, and there is no evidence of hilar enlargement as would be seen with lymphadenopathy.* **(Right)** *Lateral chest radiograph of the same patient shows the large mediastinal mass located behind the heart in the middle mediastinum. Foregut cyst is a common etiology for these imaging findings.*

Middle Mediastinal Mass

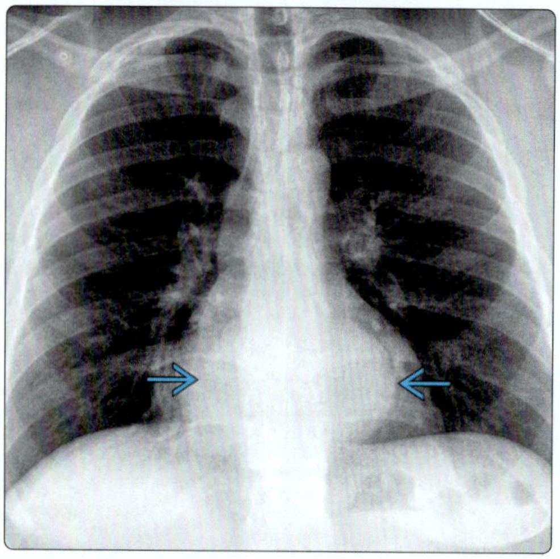

Middle Mediastinal Mass

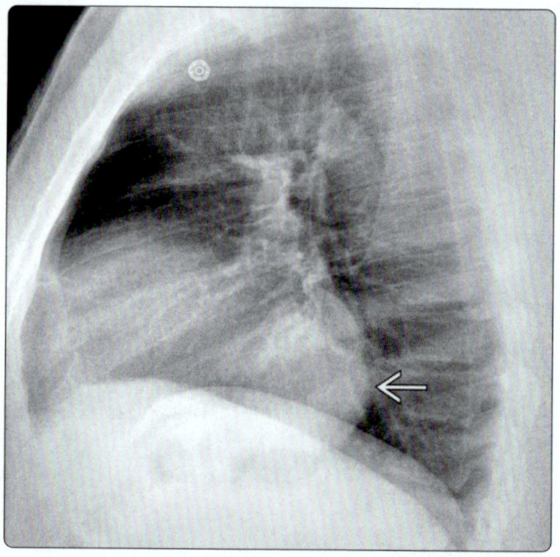

(Left) *Lateral esophagram of the same patient shows that the lesion produces smooth mass effect on and posterior displacement of the mid to lower esophagus. The visualized esophageal mucosa is normal.* **(Right)** *Axial CECT of the same patient shows the mass in the visceral mediastinum. The lesion exhibits intrinsic water attenuation and a thin enhancing wall. Note small bilateral pleural effusions. The imaging features are characteristic of congenital foregut cyst, in this case, a bronchogenic cyst.*

Middle Mediastinal Mass

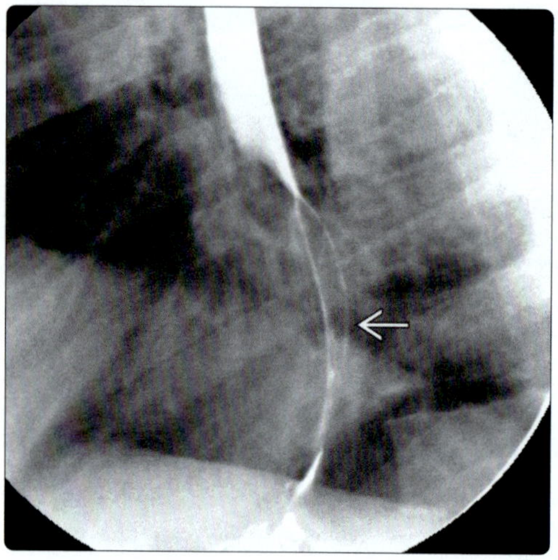

Visceral Mediastinal Mass

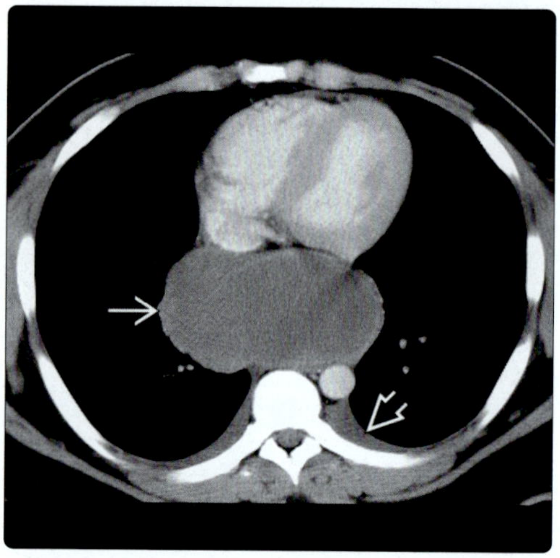

(Left) *PA chest radiograph of an asymptomatic elderly patient shows an abnormal mediastinal contour due to a right aortic arch, which descends on the right and exhibits a right para-aortic interface. Approximately 10% of mediastinal contour abnormalities are of a vascular etiology, as in this case.* **(Right)** *Lateral chest radiograph of the same patient shows that the right aortic arch has non-mirror image branching as evidenced by mass effect on the posterior trachea secondary to an aberrant left subclavian artery.*

Mediastinal Contour Abnormality

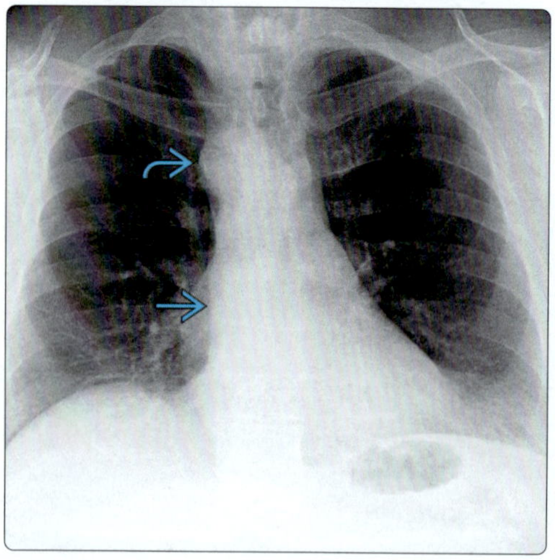

Mediastinal Contour Abnormality

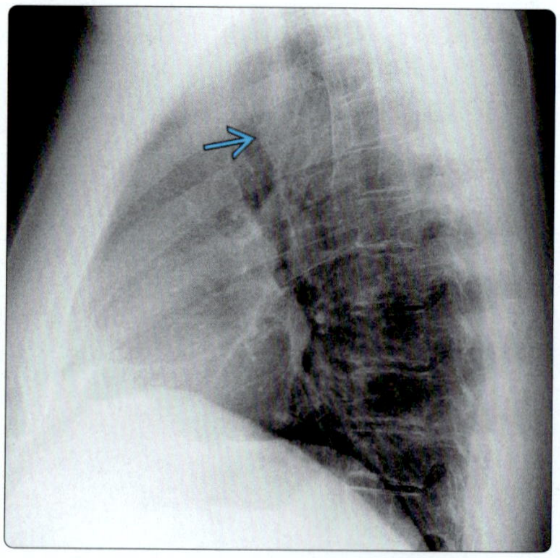

Unilateral Hilar Enlargement: Lymphadenopathy

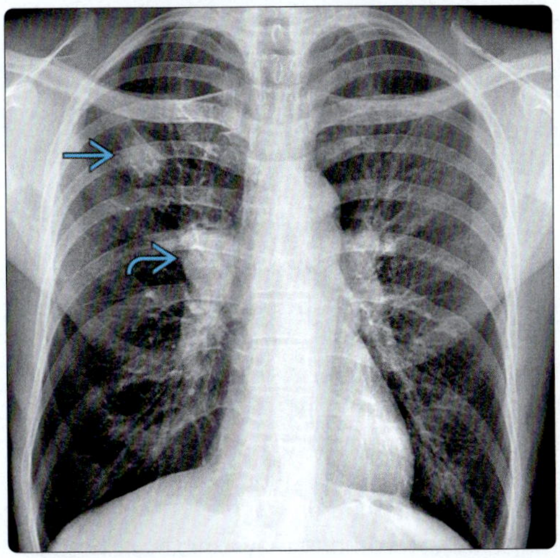

Unilateral Hilar Enlargement: Lymphadenopathy

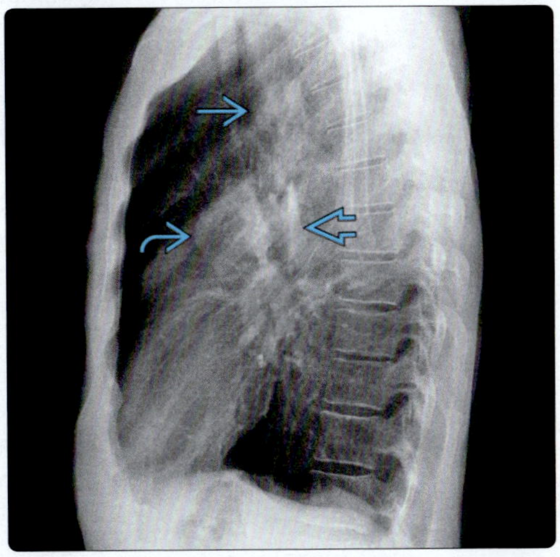

(Left) *PA chest radiograph of a 54-year-old man with primary lung cancer shows a right upper lobe mass and ipsilateral right hilar enlargement, consistent with right hilar lymphadenopathy.* **(Right)** *Lateral chest radiograph of the same patient shows the right upper lobe mass, right hilar enlargement, and a thick intermediate stem line, consistent with metastatic hilar lymphadenopathy. Unilateral hilar enlargement may be due to hilar lymphadenopathy or hilar mass.*

Bilateral Hilar Enlargement: Lymphadenopathy

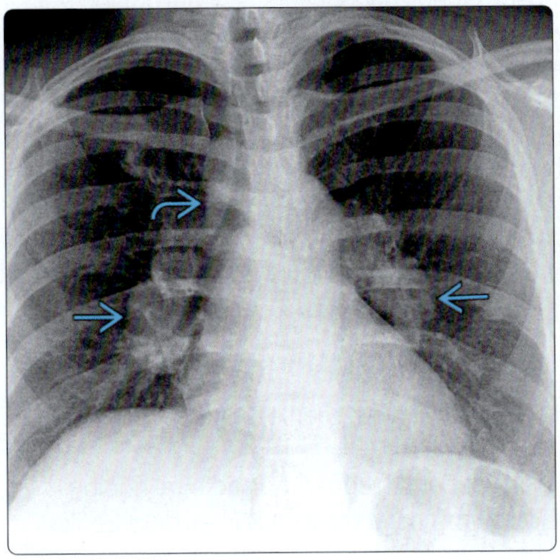

Bilateral Hilar Enlargement: Lymphadenopathy

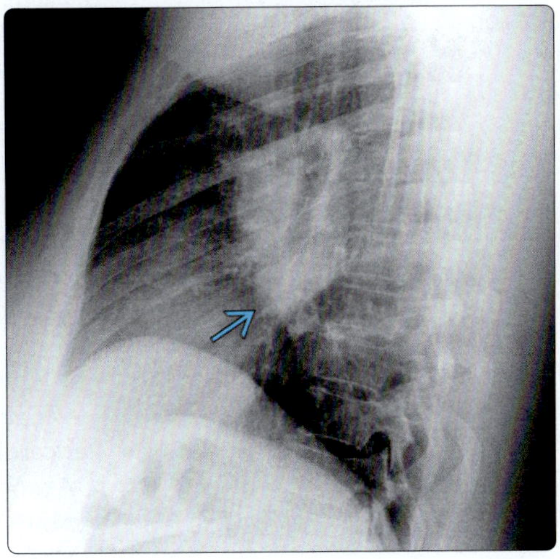

(Left) *PA chest radiograph of a 32-year-old man with sarcoidosis shows bilateral hilar lymphadenopathy manifesting as bilateral hilar enlargement with lobular contours. Note the thick right paratracheal stripe, also consistent with lymphadenopathy.* **(Right)** *Lateral chest radiograph of the same patient shows bilateral hilar lymphadenopathy producing the so-called doughnut sign. Note abnormal soft tissue in the inferior hilar window indicative of subcarinal lymphadenopathy.*

Bilateral Hilar Enlargement: Pulmonary Hypertension

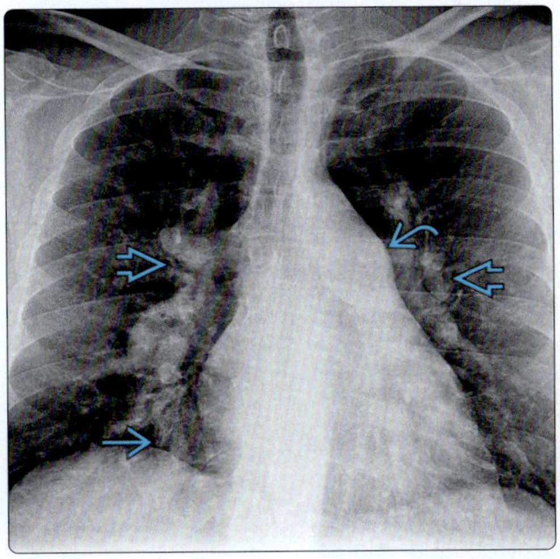

Bilateral Hilar Enlargement: Pulmonary Hypertension

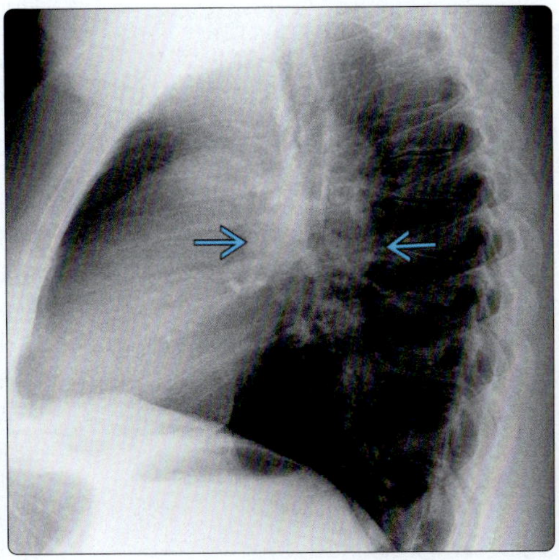

(Left) *PA chest radiograph of a patient with pulmonary hypertension shows bilateral enlarged hila and the hilum convergence sign as enlarged peripheral pulmonary arteries course to or converge with the abnormal hila, characteristic of a vascular etiology of the hilar enlargement. Note pulmonary trunk enlargement.* **(Right)** *Lateral chest radiograph of the same patient shows bilateral hilar enlargement from pulmonary hypertension. Note the normal inferior hilar window and the normal intermediate stem line.*

DIFFERENTIAL DIAGNOSIS

Common

- Lymphadenopathy
- Aneurysm
- Thyroid Goiter
- Pericardial Cyst

Less Common

- Foregut Cyst
- Thymic Cyst
- Thymic Malignancy
- Neurogenic Neoplasm

Rare but Important

- Mature Teratoma
- Extramedullary Hematopoiesis
- Lateral Thoracic Meningocele

ESSENTIAL INFORMATION

Key Differential Diagnosis Issues

- Typically primary mediastinal lesion
  - Benign primary neoplasm
  - Malignant primary neoplasm
  - Congenital or acquired cyst
  - Glandular enlargement
  - Vascular lesion
    - Typically saccular aortic aneurysm
  - Lymphadenopathy
    - Typically manifests with diffuse bilateral mediastinal enlargement
    - Focal lymphadenopathy may also occur
- Imaging assessment
  - Identification of focal mediastinal mass or contour abnormality on PA chest radiography
  - Localization to mediastinal compartment on lateral chest radiography
    - Anterior
    - Middle
    - Posterior
  - Formulation of focused differential diagnosis based on demographic (age, sex) and clinical (presenting complaints) information
  - Cross-sectional imaging with contrast-enhanced CT
    - Localization to mediastinal compartment
      - Prevascular
      - Visceral
      - Paravertebral
    - Identification of relationship to mediastinal organs/structures
    - Characterization of focal mediastinal lesion
      - Attenuation
      - Presence or absence of calcification, fat, necrosis
      - Assessment of mass effect &/or invasion of adjacent structures
    - Formulation of focused differential diagnosis &/or most likely diagnosis
    - Recommendation for further imaging &/or management

Helpful Clues for Common Diagnoses

- **Lymphadenopathy**
  - May manifest as focal mediastinal mass
  - May affect any mediastinal compartment
  - Etiologies
    - Infectious/inflammatory
    - Lymphatic malignancy
    - Metastatic malignancy
- **Aneurysm**
  - Asymptomatic patient with incidental imaging abnormality versus symptomatic patient with chest pain
  - Saccular aneurysm more likely to manifest with focal mediastinal enlargement than fusiform aneurysm
  - Frequent peripheral curvilinear calcification
  - Continuity with vascular structures
    - Contrast enhancement contiguous with and similar to that of adjacent vessel lumen
  - ± endoluminal mural thrombus, may exhibit calcification
  - Mediastinal hemorrhage in cases of rupture
- **Thyroid Goiter**
  - Asymptomatic elderly patient versus symptomatic patient with airway compression
  - Mediastinal extension in 35% of cervical goiters versus ectopic thyroid goiter
  - May affect any mediastinal compartment
  - Cervicothoracic sign, frequent focal tracheal deviation &/or tracheal stenosis
  - High attenuation on unenhanced CT
  - Intense and sustained contrast enhancement
  - Heterogeneous soft tissue mass
    - Low-attenuation areas
    - Cystic change
    - Calcification: Curvilinear, coarse, punctate
- **Pericardial Cyst**
  - Asymptomatic patient, frequently incidental finding
  - Abuts pericardium; characteristically in cardiophrenic angle, R > L
  - Well-defined lesion
    - Imperceptible wall
    - Fluid attenuation/signal content
    - No mural nodules; very rarely soft tissue septa

Helpful Clues for Less Common Diagnoses

- **Foregut Cyst**
  - Symptomatic or asymptomatic patient; wide age range
  - Bronchogenic
    - Middle/visceral mediastinum
    - Frequent subcarinal location; abuts trachea and mainstem bronchi
    - Unilocular spherical or ovoid; ± mural calcification
    - Variable attenuation/signal ranging from fluid to soft tissue; may contain milk of calcium
  - Esophageal duplication or enteric
    - Middle/visceral mediastinum
    - Abuts esophagus ± mass effect
    - Variable attenuation/signal
  - Neuroenteric
    - Posterior/paravertebral mediastinum
    - Associated with congenital spinal anomaly
    - Fluid attenuation/signal

- **Thymic Cyst**
  - Congenital (unilocular) or acquired (internal septa)
  - Anterior/prevascular mediastinum, in anatomic location of thymus gland
  - May exhibit mural &/or septal calcification
  - Water attenuation/signal
  - Hemorrhage and infection may produce increased attenuation or increased signal on T1W MR
- **Thymic Malignancy**
  - Thymoma, thymic carcinoma, thymic carcinoid
  - Adult patient > 40 years
    - Asymptomatic
    - Signs/symptoms of mass effect, local invasion, or metastatic disease
    - Parathymic syndrome
  - Focal unilateral anterior/prevascular mediastinal mass
    - Cystic change, necrosis, and calcification
    - May exhibit heterogeneous attenuation/signal
    - May produce mass effect &/or local invasion
    - May produce drop pleural metastases, typically ipsilateral to lesion
- **Neurogenic Neoplasm**
  - Well-defined posterior/paravertebral mediastinal mass
    - Benign pressure erosion of adjacent skeleton
    - Intraspinal extension in 10% of cases
    - Multifocal lesions in patients with neurofibromatosis 1
  - Nerve sheath origin: Schwannoma, neurofibroma, malignant peripheral nerve sheath tumor
    - Typically asymptomatic adult
    - Spherical morphology
    - May exhibit heterogeneous attenuation and cystic change
  - Sympathetic ganglia origin: Ganglioneuroma, ganglioneuroblastoma, neuroblastoma
    - Young adults and children
    - Elongate morphology
    - Spans several vertebral bodies
    - May exhibit heterogeneous attenuation, including calcification

Helpful Clues for Rare Diagnoses

- **Mature Teratoma**
  - Benign anterior/prevascular mediastinal germ cell neoplasm
  - Children and young adults < 40 years
  - Asymptomatic patient versus symptoms related to mass effect
  - Spherical heterogeneous prevascular mediastinal mass
    - Frequent cystic changes with fluid attenuation/signal
    - Fat attenuation elements in 75% of lesions
    - Soft tissue elements &/or tissue septa
    - Frequent calcification
  - May produce mass effect on adjacent structures
  - No lymphadenopathy
  - No local invasion or metastatic disease
  - May rarely rupture
    - Mediastinal fat stranding, fluid
    - Pleural or pericardial effusion
- **Extramedullary Hematopoiesis**
  - Asymptomatic patient, typically incidental imaging abnormality
    - Hemoglobinopathy or hemolytic anemia
    - Myeloproliferative disorder
  - Posterior/paravertebral mediastinal soft tissue mass or masses
    - Typically involvement of lower posterior/paravertebral mediastinum
    - ± expansion or trabecular conspicuity of adjacent ribs
    - ± fat attenuation
- **Lateral Thoracic Meningocele**
  - Asymptomatic patient, incidental imaging abnormality
    - Typically patients with neurofibromatosis 1
    - Isolated lateral thoracic meningocele also occurs
  - Posterior/paravertebral mass
    - Water attenuation/signal
    - Continuity with adjacent thecal sac
    - ± benign pressure erosion of adjacent ribs, vertebral bodies, neuroforaminal enlargement

Lymphadenopathy

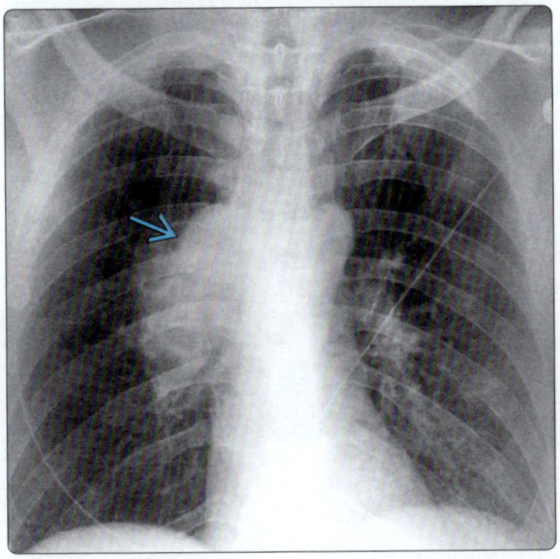

Lymphadenopathy

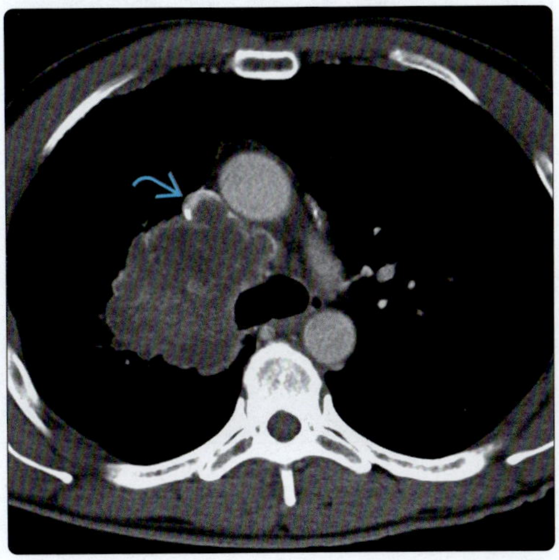

(Left) *AP chest radiograph of a 67-year-old man who presented for evaluation of a brain mass suspected to represent a metastasis shows a polylobular right mediastinal mass ➡ that produces mass effect on the right tracheobronchial tree.* **(Right)** *CECT of the same patient demonstrates a polylobular heterogeneously enhancing mediastinal mass that encases the right tracheobronchial tree and invades the superior vena cava ↗, consistent with metastatic lymphadenopathy from advanced primary lung cancer.*

(Left) *AP chest radiograph of a 94-year-old man who presented with signs and symptoms of pneumonia shows a large left upper mediastinal thoracic aortic saccular aneurysm that produces mass effect on the adjacent trachea.* **(Right)** *NECT of the same patient demonstrates a large left upper mediastinal saccular aneurysm. Note characteristic features, including peripheral curvilinear calcification and heterogeneous attenuation from endoluminal thrombus. Vascular lesions are optimally evaluated with CECT or MR.*

Aneurysm

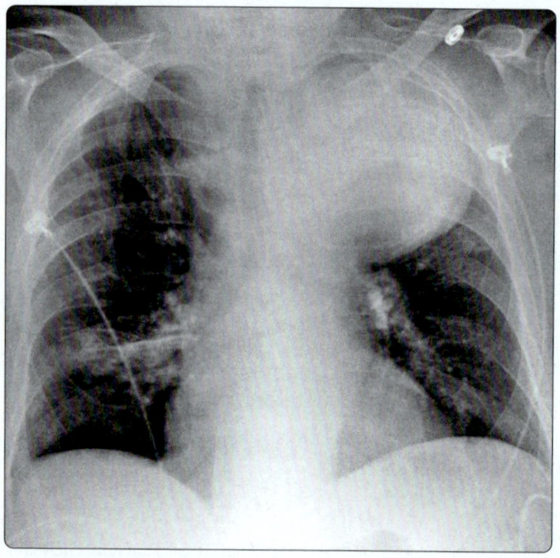

Aneurysm

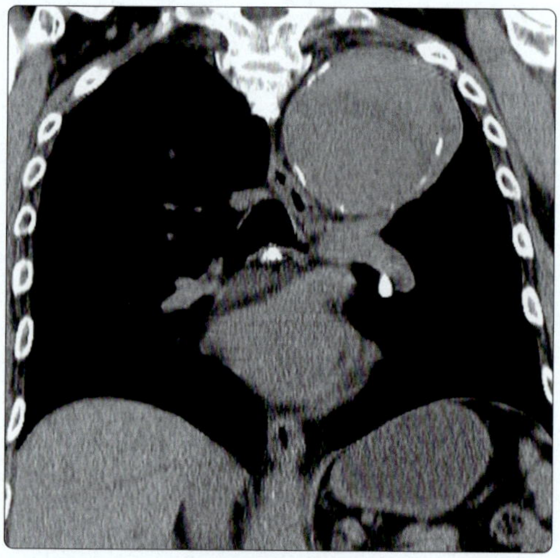

(Left) *Coronal CECT of an asymptomatic 54-year-old man shows an incidentally diagnosed ectopic thyroid goiter in the visceral mediastinum that exhibits heterogeneous intense contrast enhancement. Note the tissue plane ➡ between the mass and the cervical thyroid.* **(Right)** *Composite image with axial (left) and coronal (right) CECT of an asymptomatic 24-year-old man shows a well-defined water attenuation pericardial cyst with an imperceptible cyst wall located in the right cardiophrenic angle.*

Thyroid Goiter

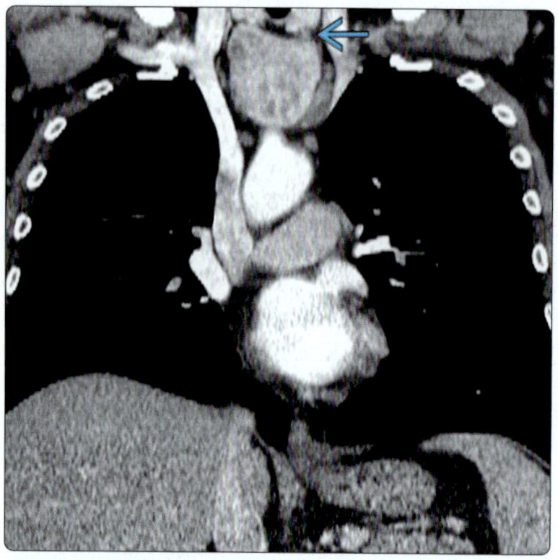

Pericardial Cyst

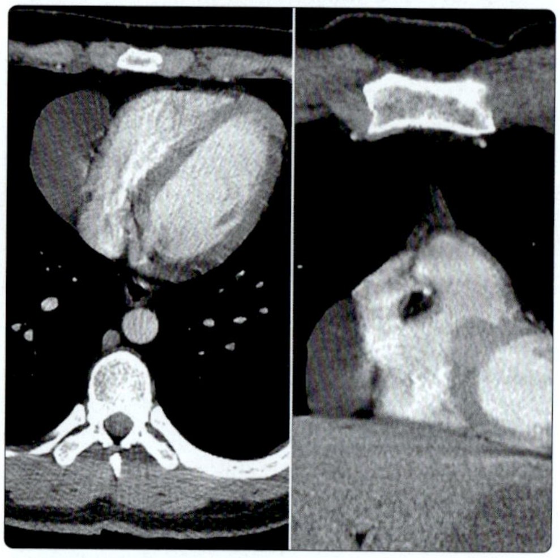

(Left) *Axial CECT of an asymptomatic 46-year-old man with an incidentally discovered radiographic abnormality shows a water attenuation bronchogenic cyst located in the right visceral mediastinum. The lesion abuts the trachea and the esophagus.* **(Right)** *Axial CECT of an asymptomatic 30-year-old man shows a thymic cyst that manifests as a water attenuation lesion ➡ in the prevascular mediastinum. MR imaging of this lesion (not shown) demonstrated absence of mural nodules or intrinsic soft tissue septa.*

Foregut Cyst

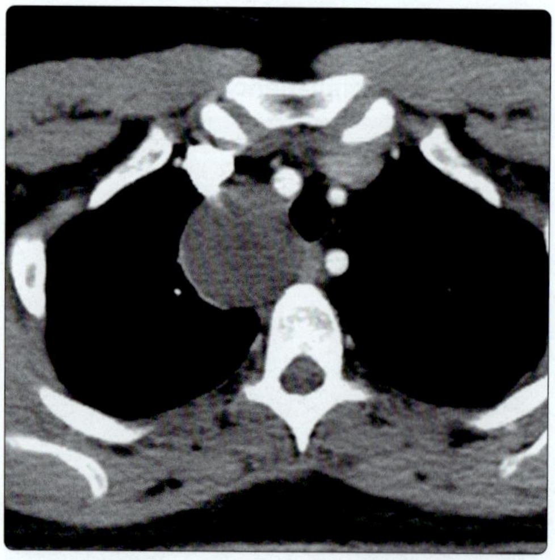

Thymic Cyst

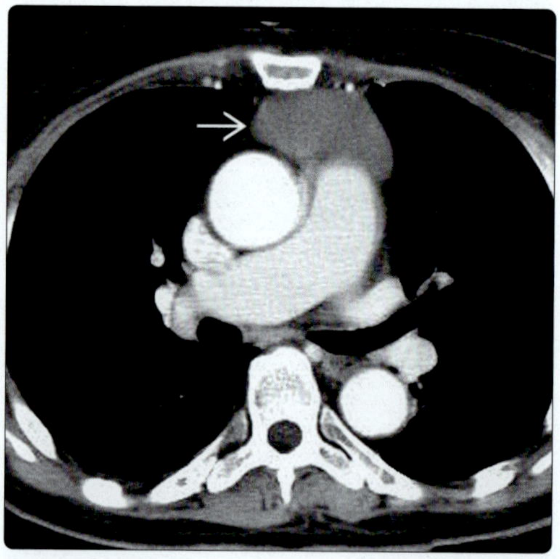

Thymic Malignancy

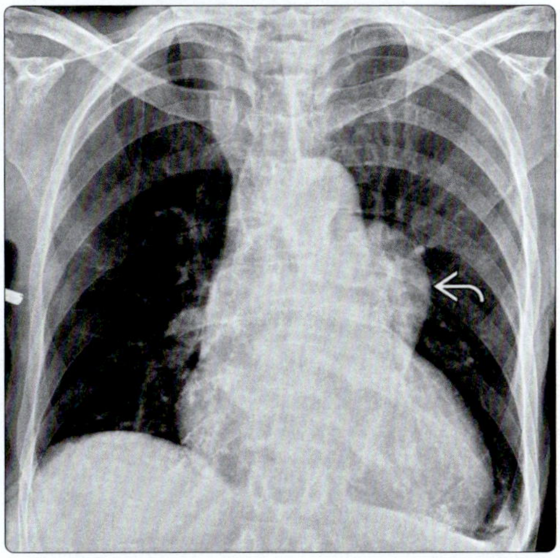

Thymic Malignancy

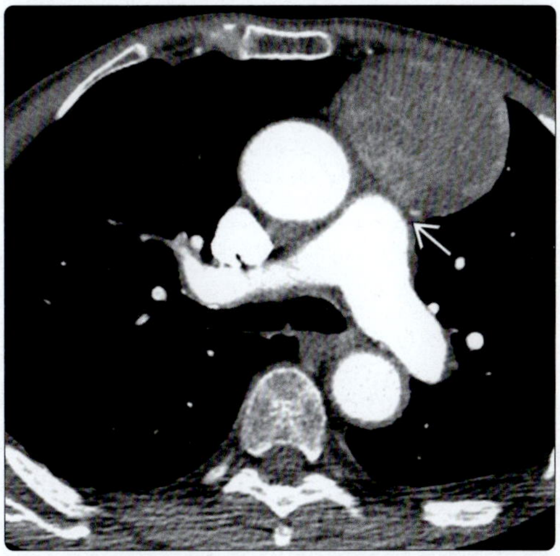

(Left) *AP chest radiograph of a 77-year-old woman who presented with chest discomfort shows a well-defined focal soft tissue mass → located in the left anterior mediastinum on lateral chest radiography (not shown). Note the small left pleural effusion.* **(Right)** *Axial CECT of the same patient shows a spherical left prevascular heterogeneously enhancing mediastinal soft tissue mass with a preserved tissue plane → between the lesion and the adjacent vascular structures. An encapsulated thymoma was diagnosed at surgery.*

Neurogenic Neoplasm

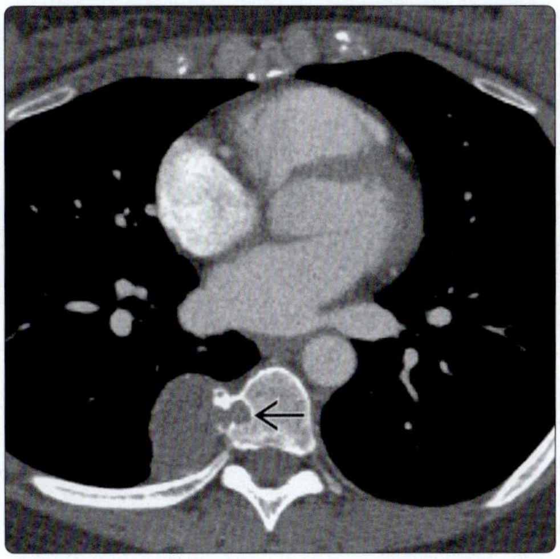

Mature Teratoma

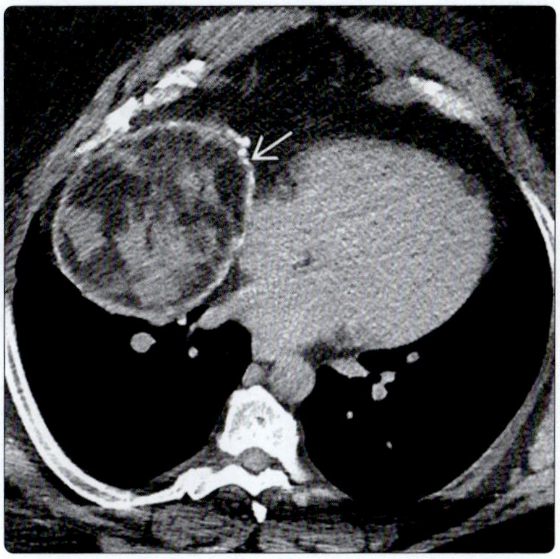

(Left) *Axial CECT of a 29-year-old woman with neurofibromatosis 1 shows a well-defined right paravertebral soft tissue mass that produces pressure erosion of the adjacent vertebral body → but no intraspinal extension. Biopsy demonstrated a schwannoma.* **(Right)** *Axial NECT of a 40-year-old man with abdominal pain shows a right cardiophrenic angle mature teratoma with typical imaging features that include a partially calcified soft tissue tumor capsule → and intrinsic fat and fluid attenuation.*

Extramedullary Hematopoiesis

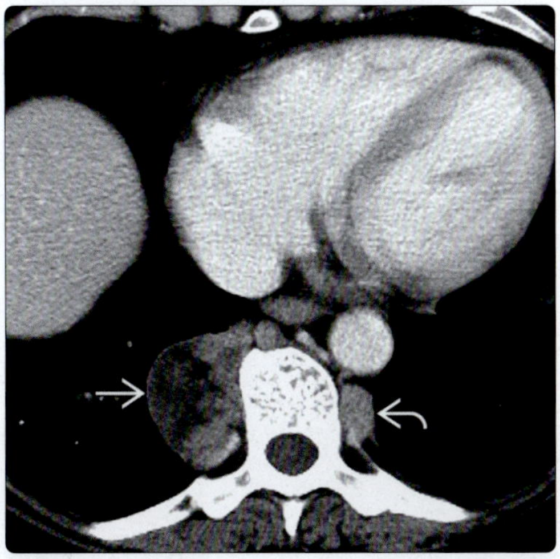

Lateral Thoracic Meningocele

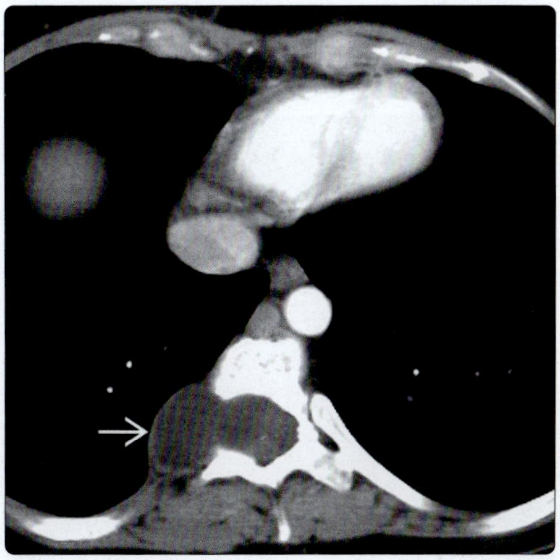

(Left) *Axial CECT of a 42-year-old man with hemolytic anemia and extramedullary hematopoiesis shows a dominant right paravertebral mass → with internal fat attenuation and a small left paravertebral soft tissue nodule →.* **(Right)** *Axial CECT of a 28-year-old woman with neurofibromatosis 1 shows an incidentally discovered right lateral thoracic meningocele that manifests as a right paravertebral fluid attenuation mass → that connects with the adjacent thecal sac via an enlarged right neuroforamen.*

DIFFERENTIAL DIAGNOSIS

Common

- Lung Cancer
- Lymphoma
- Metastatic Lymphadenopathy
- Lipomatosis

Rare but Important

- Malignant Germ Cell Neoplasm
- Lymphangioma
- Thymolipoma
- Castleman Disease
- Sarcoma

ESSENTIAL INFORMATION

Key Differential Diagnosis Issues

- Imaging assessment of diffuse mediastinal enlargement
  - Chest radiography
    - Diffuse mediastinal enlargement involving both sides of midline on PA radiography
    - Localization to mediastinal compartment(s) on lateral radiography: Anterior, middle, posterior
    - Formulation of focused differential diagnosis
  - Contrast-enhanced CT or MR
    - Lesion characterization: Morphology, density, cystic change, enhancement pattern, calcification
    - Identification of affected mediastinal compartment
      - Prevascular, visceral, paravertebral
    - Identification of affected mediastinal organs/structures for mass effect &/or invasion
    - Presence or absence of lymphadenopathy
    - Refinement of differential diagnosis

Helpful Clues for Common Diagnoses

- **Lung Cancer**
  - Typically small cell lung cancer
  - Mediastinal mass; lung lesion may not be evident
  - Mediastinal &/or hilar lymphadenopathy
  - Encasement &/or invasion of mediastinal structures
- **Lymphoma**
  - Primary mediastinal lymphoma: Hodgkin, non-Hodgkin
  - Typically anterior/prevascular mediastinum
  - Enlarged lymph nodes, nodal coalescence, local invasion
- **Metastatic Lymphadenopathy**
  - Typically intrathoracic malignancies: Lung cancer, esophageal cancer, malignant mesothelioma
  - Extrathoracic malignancies: Genitourinary, head/neck, and breast cancers and melanoma
  - Enlarged lymph nodes, nodal coalescence, local invasion
- **Lipomatosis**
  - Excessive non-encapsulated mediastinal fat
  - Smooth mediastinal widening, no mass effect
  - Cardiophrenic angle and subpleural fat deposition
  - Fat attenuation or signal, no dominant soft tissue

Helpful Clues for Rare Diagnoses

- **Malignant Germ Cell Neoplasm**
  - Seminoma, non-seminomatous malignant germ cell neoplasm
  - Men; 20-40 years
  - Prevascular mediastinal soft tissue mass; may exhibit heterogeneous enhancement and central low attenuation from necrosis
- **Lymphangioma**
  - Cystic mass ± soft tissue septa
  - Displacement/encasement of adjacent structures; no obstruction
- **Thymolipoma**
  - Lower prevascular mediastinum; connection to thymus
  - Admixture of fat and soft tissue attenuation/signal
- **Castleman Disease**
  - Multicentric type; mediastinal/hilar lymphadenopathy
  - Enhancing lymphadenopathy; Ca++ in up to 10%
- **Sarcoma**
  - Liposarcoma: Fat attenuation, soft tissue septa, &/or dominant soft tissue nodules
  - Synovial sarcoma: Heterogeneous attenuation from hemorrhage or necrosis
  - Encasement &/or invasion of adjacent structures

Lung Cancer

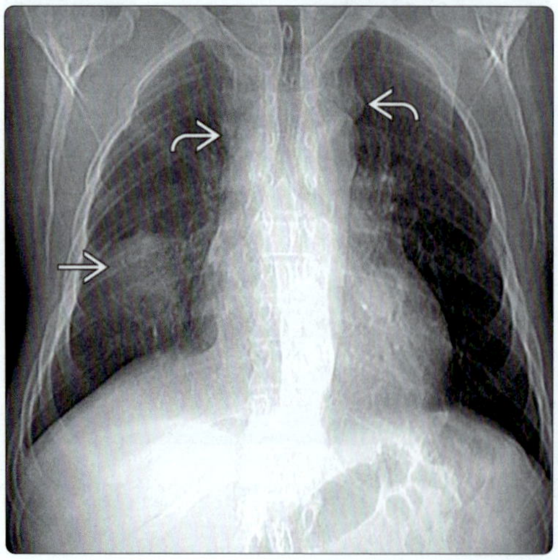

Lung Cancer

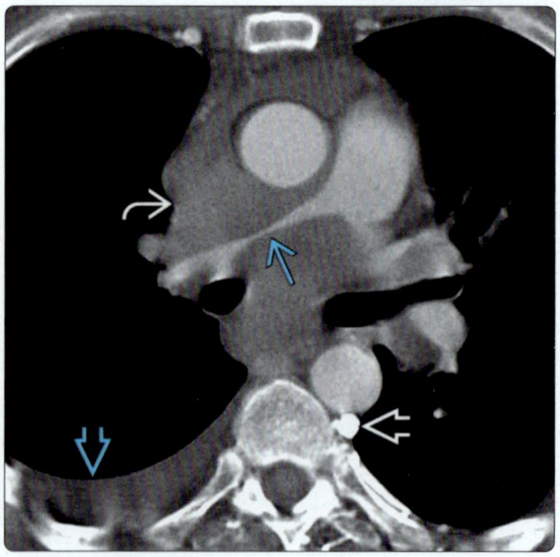

(Left) *PA chest radiograph of a 54-year-old man with small cell lung cancer shows a right mid lung zone mass and diffuse bilateral mediastinal enlargement with lobular contours concerning for diffuse lymphadenopathy.* **(Right)** *Axial CECT of the same patient shows locally invasive coalescent lymphadenopathy that obliterates the superior vena cava and encases and narrows the right pulmonary artery. Note mediastinal vascular collaterals from superior vena cava obstruction and a small right pleural effusion.*

Lung Cancer

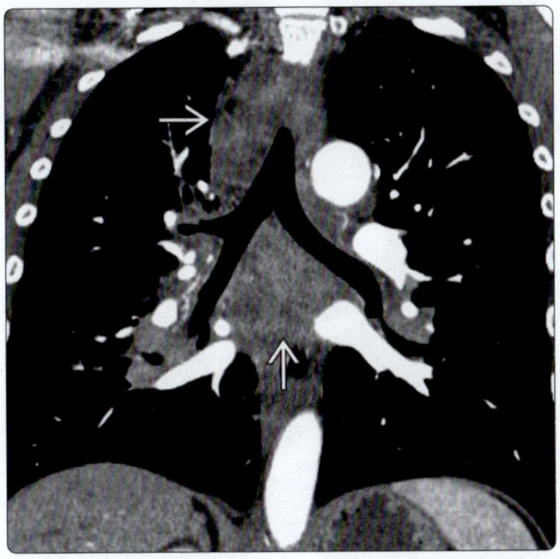

Lung Cancer

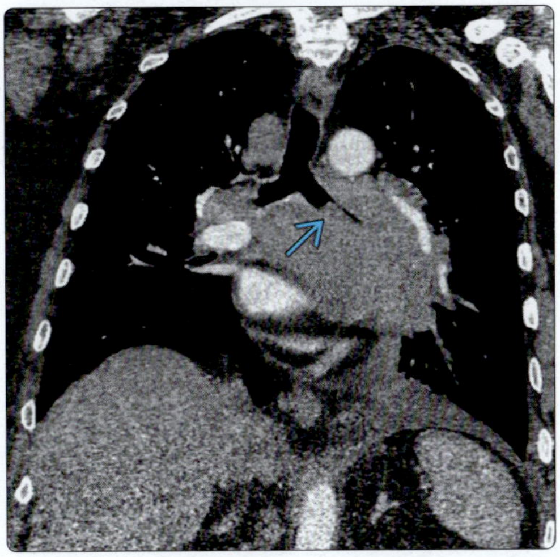

(Left) *Coronal CECT of a 44-year-old man with small cell lung cancer shows diffuse locally invasive mediastinal soft tissue →, consistent with coalescent lymphadenopathy. Small cell carcinoma may initially manifest with lymphadenopathy.* **(Right)** *Coronal CECT of a 79-year-old man with small cell lung cancer shows a diffuse locally invasive soft tissue mass that represents coalescent lymphadenopathy. The left mainstem bronchus endobronchial lesion → may represent the primary lung cancer.*

Lung Cancer

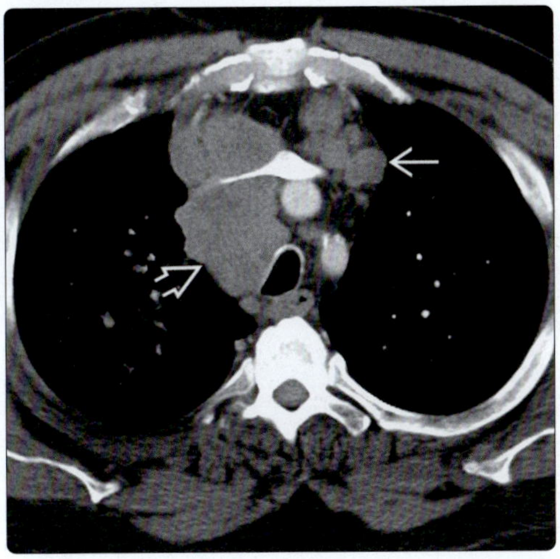

Lung Cancer

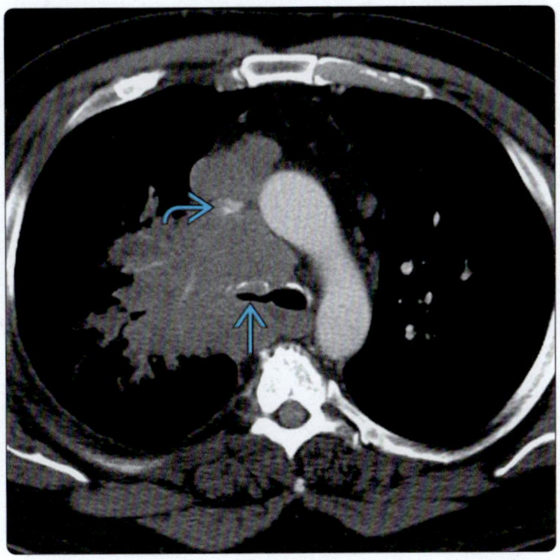

(Left) *Axial CECT of a 58-year-old man with small cell lung cancer and diffuse mediastinal enlargement from lymphadenopathy shows discrete enlarged prevascular mediastinal lymph nodes → and coalescent visceral mediastinal lymphadenopathy →.* **(Right)** *Axial CECT of a 58-year-old man shows small cell lung cancer manifesting as a large right hilar mass and mediastinal lymphadenopathy that encases and obliterates the right mainstem bronchus → and obstructs the superior vena cava →.*

Lymphoma

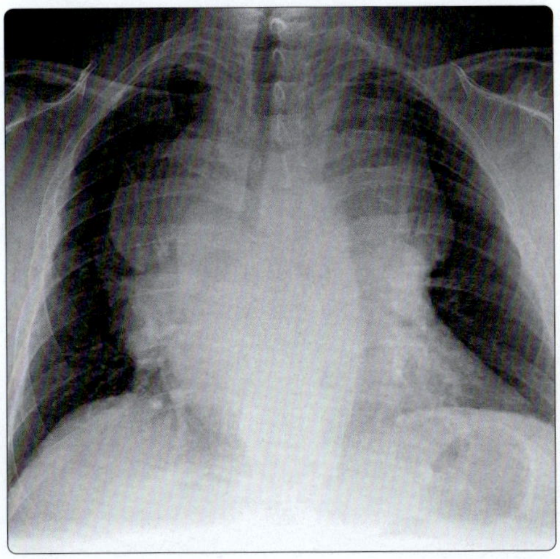

Lymphoma

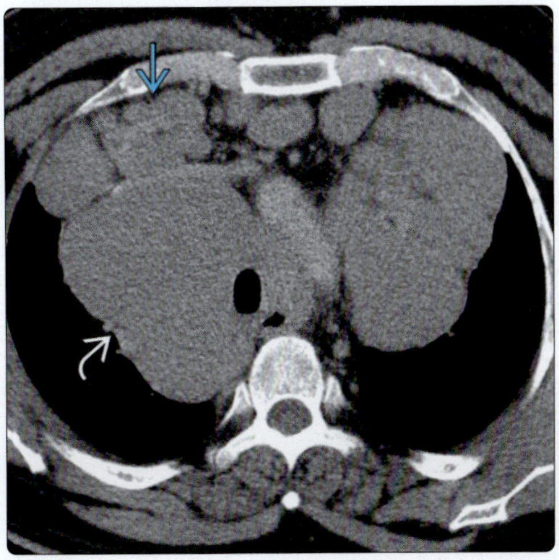

(Left) *PA chest radiograph of a 56-year-old man who presented with chest pain and dyspnea shows marked diffuse bilateral mediastinal enlargement with polylobular borders that produces mass effect on the trachea. Note obliteration of nearly all normal mediastinal interfaces.* **(Right)** *Axial CECT of the same patient shows bulky mediastinal lymphadenopathy in the prevascular → and visceral → mediastinal compartments, which encases the trachea and great vessels. Biopsy revealed non-Hodgkin lymphoma.*

Lymphoma

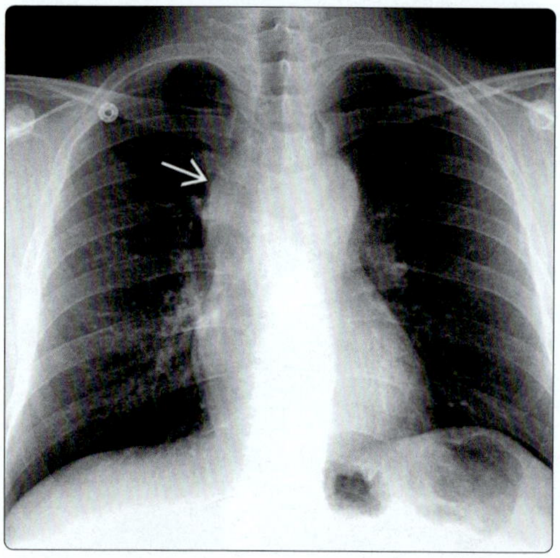

Lymphoma

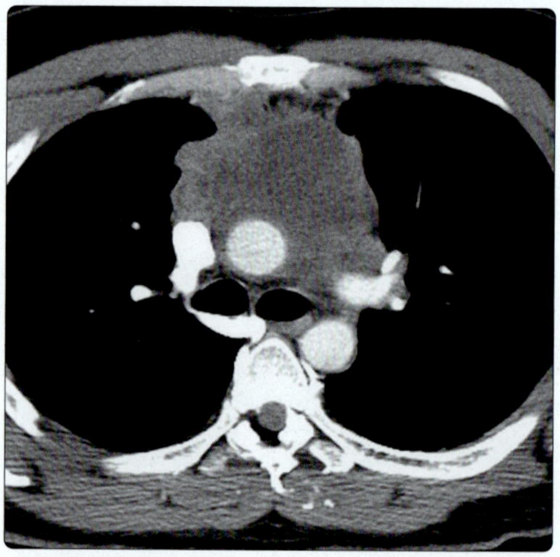

(Left) *PA chest radiograph of a 52-year-old man with Hodgkin lymphoma shows diffuse enlargement of the upper mediastinum that manifests with abnormal bilateral mediastinal contours and a thick right paratracheal stripe* ➡. **(Right)** *Axial CECT of the same patient shows a locally invasive heterogeneously enhancing mediastinal mass with internal low attenuation related to tumor necrosis that involves both sides of the midline and encases the ascending aorta and left pulmonary artery.*

Metastatic Lymphadenopathy

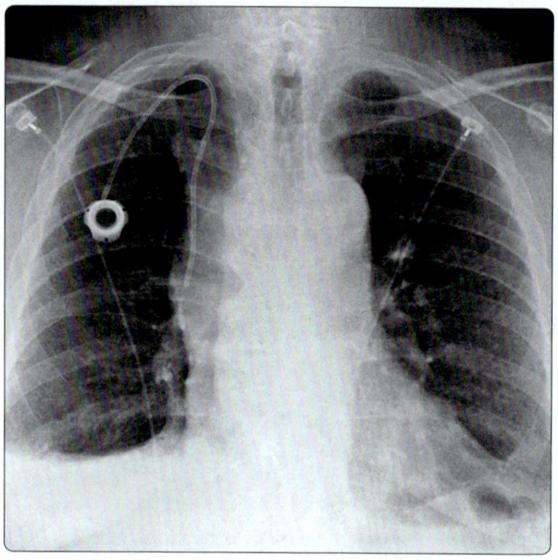

Metastatic Lymphadenopathy

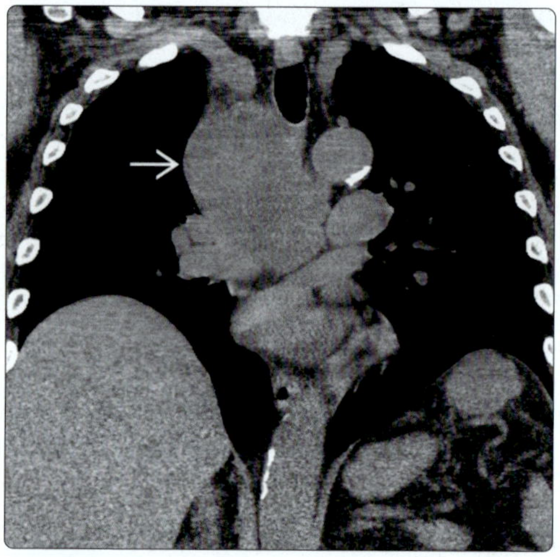

(Left) *PA chest radiograph of a 72-year-old man who presented with weight loss and chest pain shows a large mediastinal mass and a small right pleural effusion. Note lateral displacement of the distal aspect of the port catheter, which indicates mass effect on the superior vena cava by the lesion.* **(Right)** *Coronal NECT of the same patient shows a large soft tissue mass* ➡ *that invades adjacent mediastinal structures. Biopsy demonstrated metastatic carcinoma of unknown primary source.*

Lipomatosis

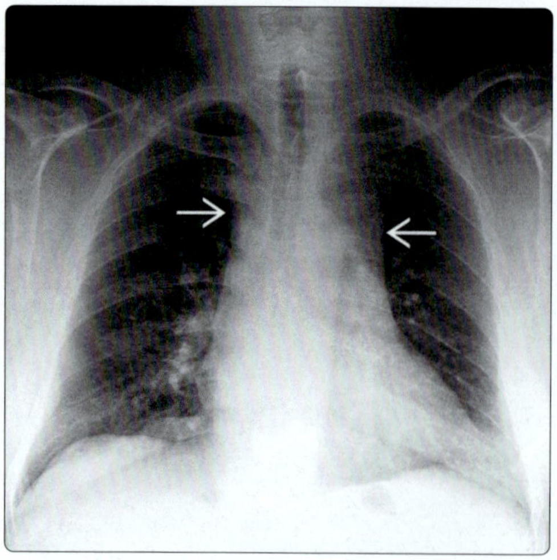

Lipomatosis

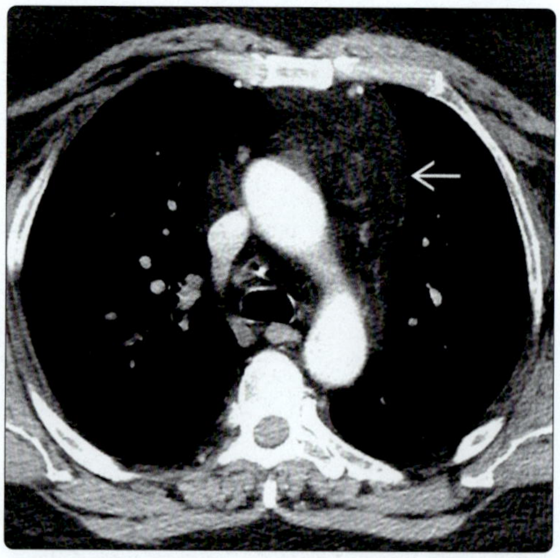

(Left) *PA chest radiograph of an asymptomatic 65-year-old man shows an abnormal featureless diffusely enlarged upper mediastinum* ➡. *Note that many of the normal mediastinal interfaces are still visible through the lesion.* **(Right)** *Axial CECT of the same patient shows that the radiographic abnormality corresponds to diffuse mediastinal fat attenuation* ➡, *consistent with mediastinal lipomatosis. Although the mediastinal fat encases adjacent normal structures, it does not narrow or obstruct them.*

Malignant Germ Cell Neoplasm

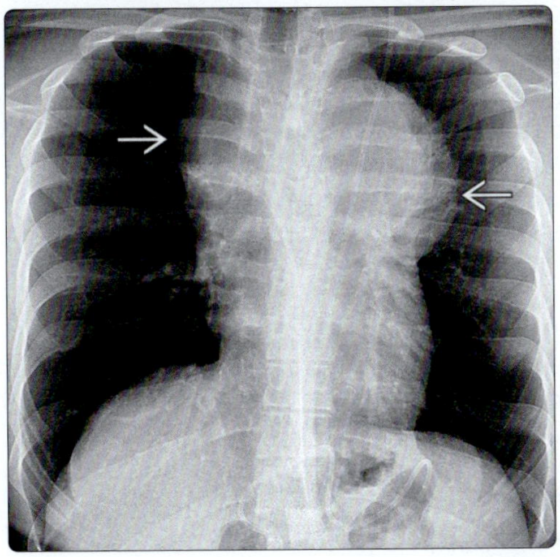

Malignant Germ Cell Neoplasm

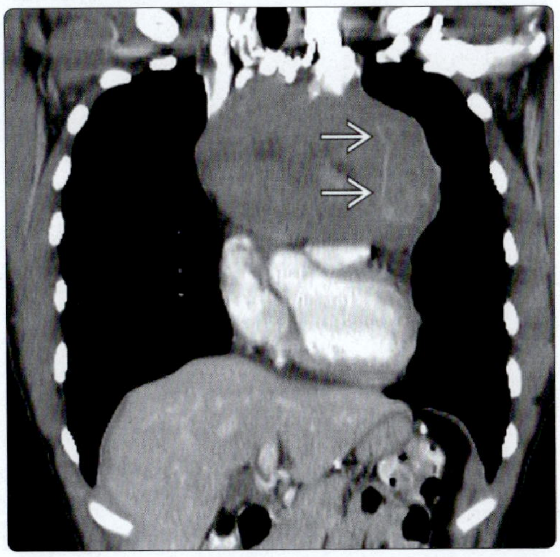

(Left) *PA chest radiograph of a 29-year-old man shows diffuse bilateral polylobular enlargement of the upper mediastinum. The differential diagnosis includes both lymphoma and malignant germ cell tumor given patient demographics.* **(Right)** *Coronal CECT of the same patient shows a large heterogeneous prevascular mediastinal mass that produces mass effect on adjacent vascular structures. Note partial encasement of the left internal mammary artery by the tumor. Biopsy confirmed mixed malignant germ cell neoplasm.*

Lymphangioma

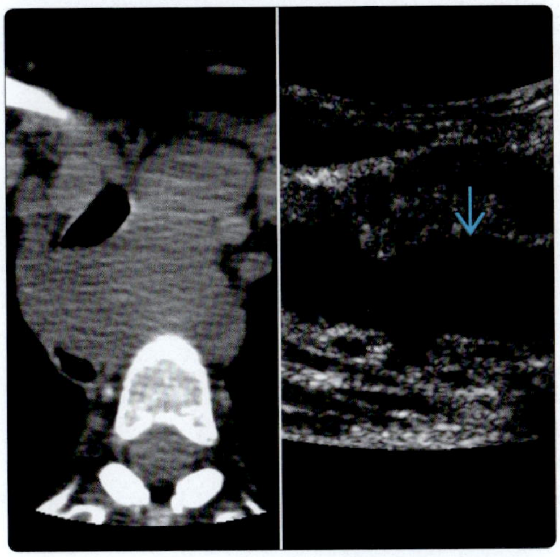

Thymolipoma

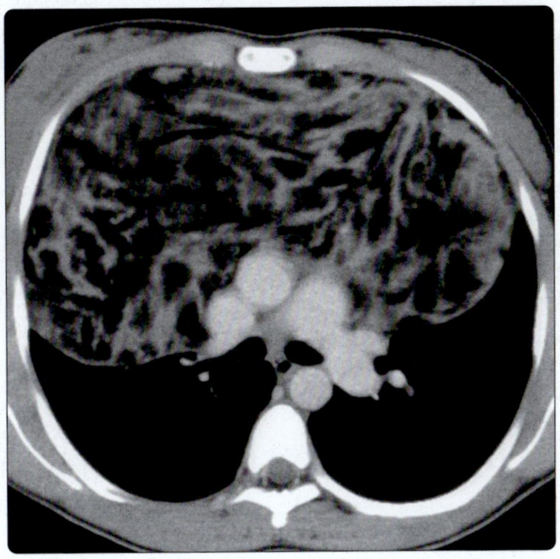

(Left) *Composite image with axial NECT (left) and longitudinal ultrasound (right) of a 33-year-old man shows a homogeneous infiltrative low-attenuation visceral mediastinal mass that exhibits intrinsic cystic change. The findings are consistent with mediastinal lymphangioma.* **(Right)** *Axial CECT shows a large prevascular mediastinal thymolipoma with typical imaging features that include an anatomic connection to the thymus and an admixture of soft tissue and fat attenuation elements. (Courtesy E. Marom, MD.)*

Castleman Disease

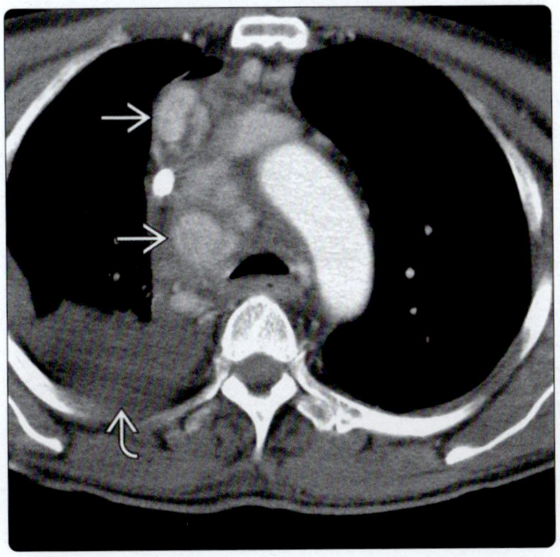

Sarcoma

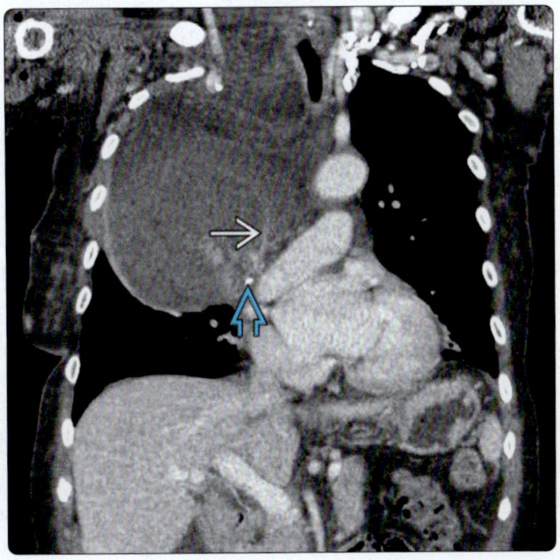

(Left) *Axial CECT of a 56-year-old man with multicentric Castleman disease, plasma cell variant, shows multifocal enhancing lymphadenopathy in the prevascular and visceral mediastinum and a large right pleural effusion.* **(Right)** *Coronal CECT of a 77-year-old woman shows a large cervicothoracic fat attenuation mass that produces mass effect on adjacent structures, narrows the trachea, and exhibits internal soft tissue septa and calcifications. Biopsy showed a well-differentiated liposarcoma.*

DIFFERENTIAL DIAGNOSIS

Common

- Thymoma
- Lymphoma
- Mature Teratoma
- Thyroid Goiter
- Thymic Hyperplasia
- Metastatic Disease

Less Common

- Thymic Carcinoma
- Thymic Cyst
- Seminoma
- Lipomatosis

Rare but Important

- Nonseminomatous Germ Cell Neoplasm
- Lipoma
- Liposarcoma
- Thymic Carcinoid
- Thymolipoma
- Ectopic Parathyroid Adenoma
- Lymphangioma

ESSENTIAL INFORMATION

Key Differential Diagnosis Issues

- Anterior compartment
  - Felson approach based on lateral radiography
    - Vertical line drawn from anterior tracheal wall to posterior inferior vena cava separates anterior mediastinum from middle mediastinum
  - Boundaries
    - Superior: Thoracic inlet
    - Inferior: Diaphragm
    - Anterior: Sternum
    - Posterior: Pericardium, aorta, and brachiocephalic vessels
  - Contents
    - Nonvascular: Thymus, pericardium, lymph nodes, adipose tissue
    - Vascular: Ascending aorta, great vessels, part of main pulmonary artery, heart
  - Anterior mediastinal lesion may disrupt normal lines, stripes, and interfaces
- Prevascular compartment
  - Defined by International Thymic Malignancy Interest Group (ITMIG) classification based on cross-sectional imaging
  - Boundaries
    - Superior: Thoracic inlet
    - Inferior: Diaphragm
    - Anterior: Sternum
    - Posterior: Anterior aspect of pericardium as it wraps around heart in curvilinear fashion
  - Contents
    - Nonvascular: Thymus, fat, lymph nodes
    - Vascular: Left brachiocephalic vein

Helpful Clues for Common Diagnoses

- **Thymoma**
  - Most common in 6th decade
  - Associations
    - Myasthenia gravis
    - Other paraneoplastic syndromes: Pure red cell aplasia/Diamond-Blackfan syndrome, hypogammaglobulinemia, aplastic anemia
  - Radiography: Round or lobulated and usually homogeneous
  - CT
    - Solid, homogeneous or slightly heterogeneous mass
    - Areas of necrosis, hemorrhage, calcification, and cyst formation may be present
    - Pleural or pericardial dissemination may be present in advanced disease
    - Lymphadenopathy is typically absent
- **Lymphoma**
  - Hodgkin lymphoma (HL) more common than non-Hodgkin lymphoma (NHL) in anterior/prevascular compartment
  - "B" symptoms (fever, weight loss, and night sweats) may be present
  - CT
    - HL commonly involves several contiguous lymph node groups
    - Involvement of single lymph node group is more common with NHL
    - Enlarged lymph nodes or mass, usually displaying homogeneous soft tissue attenuation
    - Infiltrative nature of some types enables differentiation from other neoplasms
      - Lesions may encase or encircle vascular structures without invading them
- **Mature Teratoma**
  - 25% of prevascular lesions in patients 10-19 years of age
  - Most common benign germ cell neoplasm
  - CT
    - Combination of fat, fluid, calcification, and soft tissue
      - Intralesional fat in 50% of cases
      - Fat-fluid levels are specific but much less common
      - Bone and tooth-like elements are rare
- **Thyroid Goiter**
  - Accounts for 10% of mediastinal masses
  - Mediastinal extension of thyroid goiter or ectopic goiter
  - CT
    - High attenuation on noncontrast CT is due to iodine content
    - Direct connection to thyroid is usually evident on CT
    - Cystic regions, calcifications may be present
- **Thymic Hyperplasia**
  - True thymic hyperplasia: Chemotherapy, radiation therapy, corticosteroids, burns, injuries
  - Thymic lymphoid (follicular) hyperplasia: Immunologic diseases (myasthenia gravis, hyperthyroidism, collagen vascular diseases) or human immunodeficiency virus (HIV) infection
  - CT
    - True thymic hyperplasia: Thymic enlargement or focal soft tissue mass

- Thymic lymphoid hyperplasia: Normal thymus, thymic enlargement, or focal soft tissue mass
- Regions of low density due to deposition of fat between hyperplastic thymic tissue

- **Metastatic Disease**
  - Lung and breast cancers are common
  - May involve thymus or mediastinal lymph nodes

Helpful Clues for Less Common Diagnoses

- **Thymic Carcinoma**
  - Large mass that can have areas of necrosis
  - Associated with aggressive features
    - Increased heterogeneity, local invasion, lymphadenopathy, &/or distant metastasis
  - Metastases often involve lungs, skeleton, liver, and brain
- **Thymic Cyst**
  - Fluid attenuation, unilocular or multilocular
    - High attenuation due to hemorrhage or infection, proteinaceous components
  - Thin or imperceptible wall
- **Seminoma**
  - Young men usually affected
  - 10% with elevated serum levels of β-human chorionic gonadotropin (β-HCG); α-fetoprotein (AFP) level is usually normal
  - Homogeneous or slightly heterogeneous soft tissue mass
  - Pleural effusions are rare; pulmonary metastases are relatively common
- **Lipomatosis**
  - Excessive unencapsulated fat in mediastinum associated with Cushing syndrome, steroids, obesity
  - Radiography: Smooth, symmetric mediastinal widening
  - CT: Homogeneous increased amount of mediastinal fat with smooth margins

Helpful Clues for Rare Diagnoses

- **Nonseminomatous Germ Cell Neoplasm**
  - Young men usually affected
  - Aggressive neoplasms with poor prognoses
  - 90% of patients present with markedly elevated serum levels of AFP or β-HCG
  - Infiltrative and heterogeneous with areas of hemorrhage and necrosis
  - Pulmonary metastases may be present
- **Lipoma**
  - Encapsulated lesions composed predominantly of fat
  - Small amount of soft tissue and blood vessels
- **Liposarcoma**
  - Comprised predominantly of fat but with more soft tissue than lipoma
  - Aggressive features compared to benign lesions
    - Greater proportion of soft tissue components; local invasion; intrathoracic lymphadenopathy; metastatic disease
- **Thymic Carcinoid**
  - Commonly secretes ACTH, which results in Cushing syndrome
  - Appears similar to thymic carcinoma on imaging
- **Thymolipoma**
  - Typically located in cardiophrenic angle
  - Encapsulated mass comprised of 50-85% fat (up to 95% fat has been reported)
  - Tend be very large at presentation; average reported size of 20 cm
  - Direct connection with thymus may be identified
- **Ectopic Parathyroid Adenoma**
  - Mediastinum is most common ectopic location
  - 4D CT: Intense contrast enhancement in arterial phase, washout of contrast material in delayed phase, and low attenuation on unenhanced imaging
- **Lymphangioma**
  - Usually congenital and often presents in childhood
  - Well circumscribed with homogeneous water attenuation
  - May wrap around mediastinal structures, such as great vessels

Thymoma

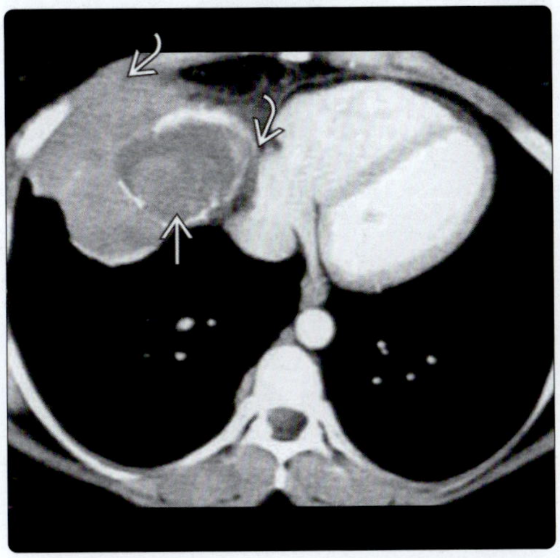

Thymoma

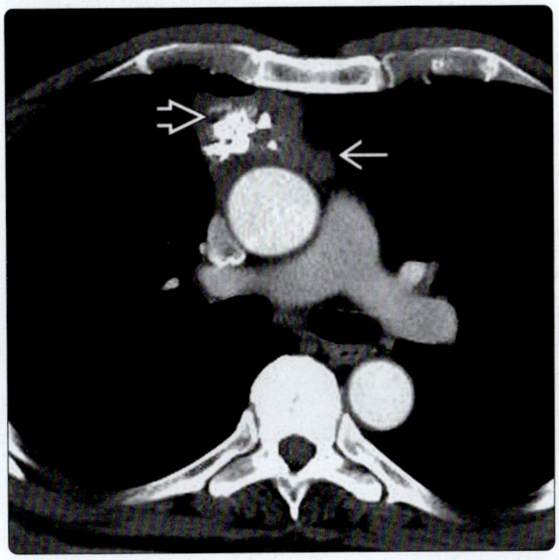

(Left) *Axial CECT shows a prevascular mediastinal soft tissue mass with rim calcifications →. The mass infiltrates the adjacent heart and chest wall →. Biopsy revealed thymoma.* **(Right)** *Axial CECT shows a heterogeneous prevascular mediastinal mass → with regions of soft tissue and coarse internal calcifications →. Calcifications are occasionally present within a thymoma and can be coarse, punctate, or peripheral.*

(Left) *Axial CECT shows a homogeneous soft tissue mass in the left prevascular mediastinal compartment. This lesion was radiographically occult and subsequent biopsy revealed non-Hodgkin lymphoma.* **(Right)** *Axial CECT demonstrates a heterogeneous soft tissue mass arising from the right prevascular mediastinum that compresses the superior vena cava and right pulmonary artery. Regions of low attenuation represent necrosis. A right pleural effusion is also present.*

Lymphoma

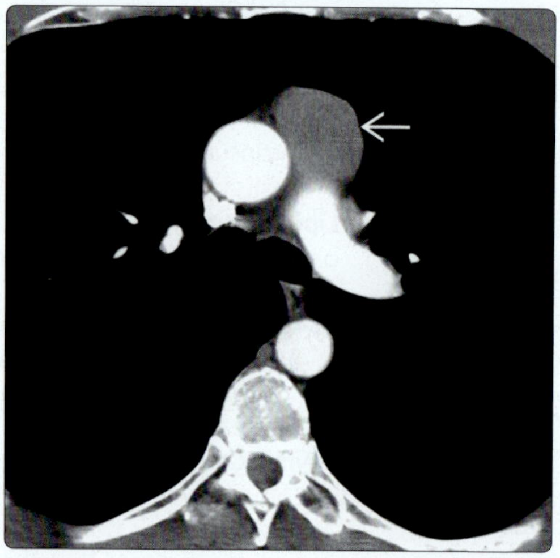

Lymphoma

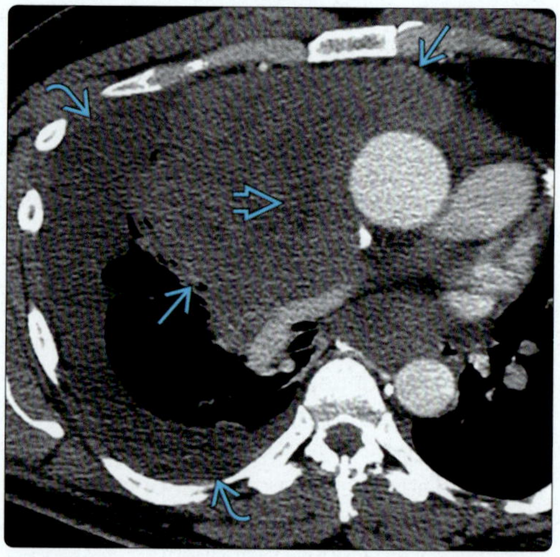

(Left) *Axial CECT demonstrates a fluid attenuation mass with peripheral soft tissue in the left prevascular mediastinum. Due to presenting symptoms of chest pain and shortness of breath, surgical resection was performed and revealed mature teratoma.* **(Right)** *Axial CECT shows a heterogeneous mass in the left prevascular mediastinum that is predominantly composed of soft tissue with a smaller amount of fluid. Surgical resection revealed mature teratoma.*

Mature Teratoma

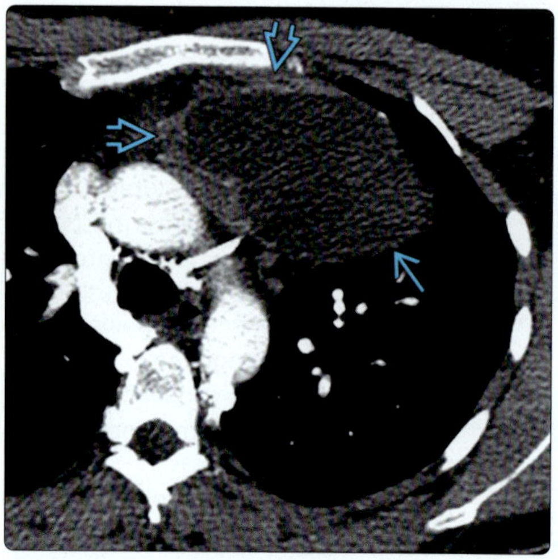

Mature Teratoma

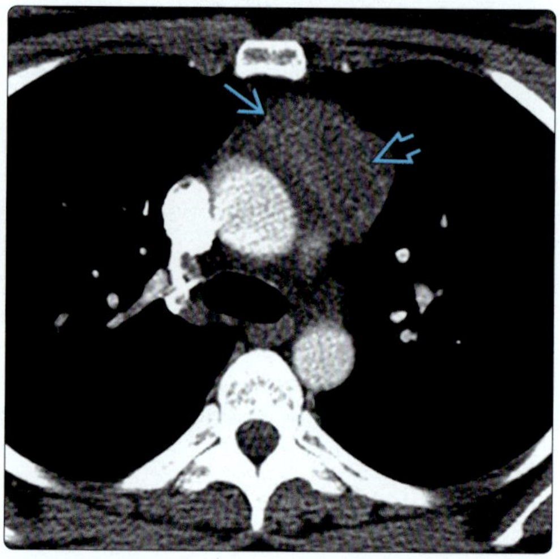

(Left) *Axial CECT shows a large mediastinal mass with displacement of the trachea and great vessels and no evidence of invasion. Other images showed communication with the thyroid in this patient with a large substernal goiter.* **(Right)** *Axial CECT shows an enlarged substernal thyroid with numerous nodules. Notice compression of the trachea. Also notice the increased attenuation of the lesion due to internal iodine content.*

Thyroid Goiter

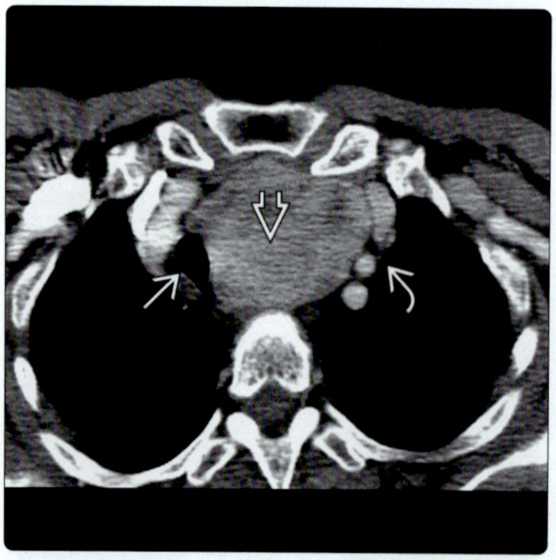

Thyroid Goiter

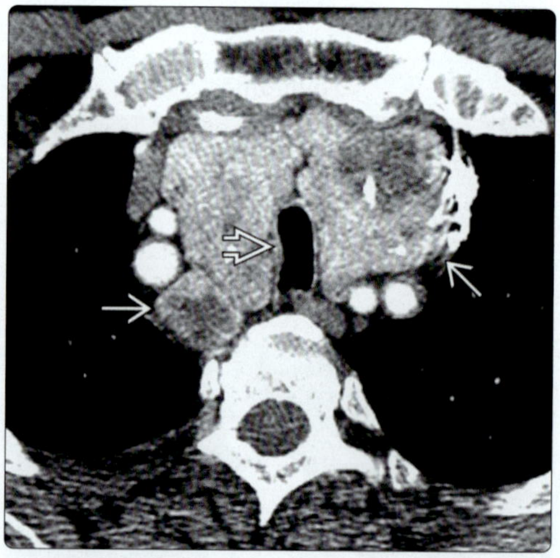

Thymic Hyperplasia

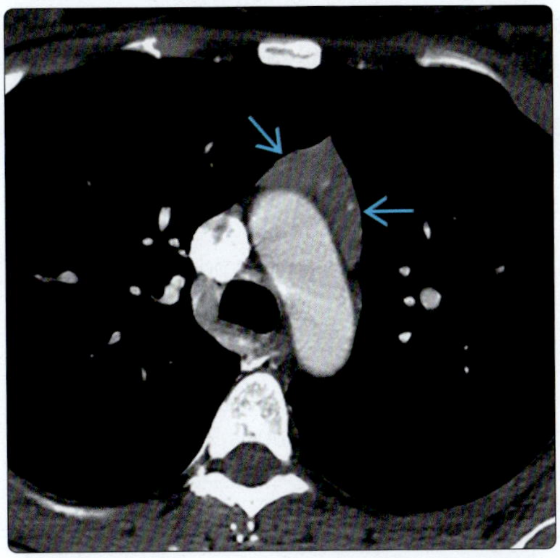

Thymic Hyperplasia

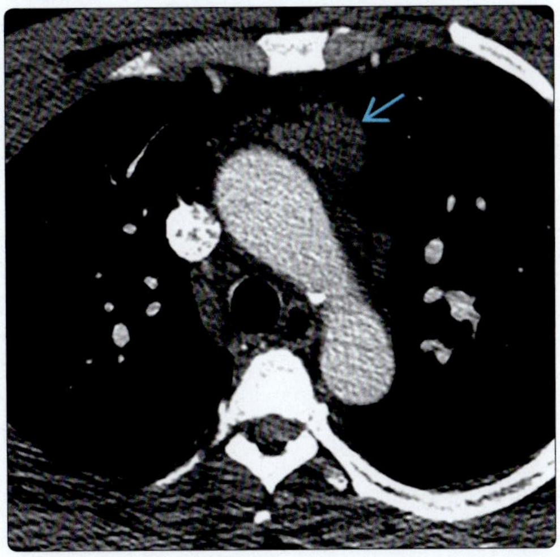

(Left) *Axial CECT of a patient treated with chemotherapy for non-Hodgkin lymphoma shows diffuse enlargement of the thymus consistent with thymic hyperplasia →.* **(Right)** *Axial CECT of a patient with hyperthyroidism shows a focal soft tissue mass in the left prevascular mediastinum that resolved over time and represented thymic hyperplasia →. Based on the etiology, thymic hyperplasia may manifest as diffuse thymic enlargement, a focal nodule or mass, or a normal appearance of the thymus.*

Seminoma

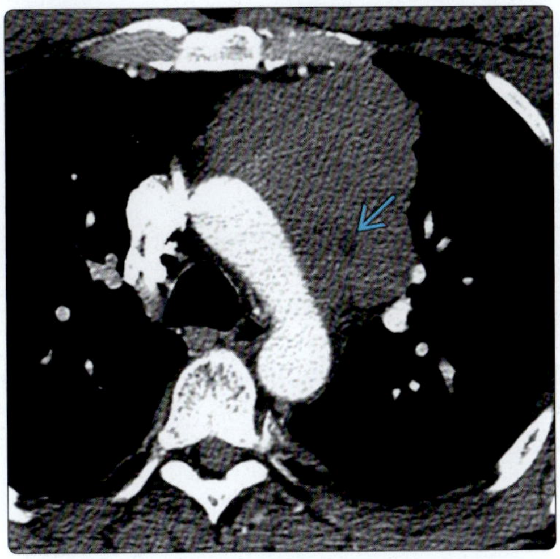

Lipomatosis

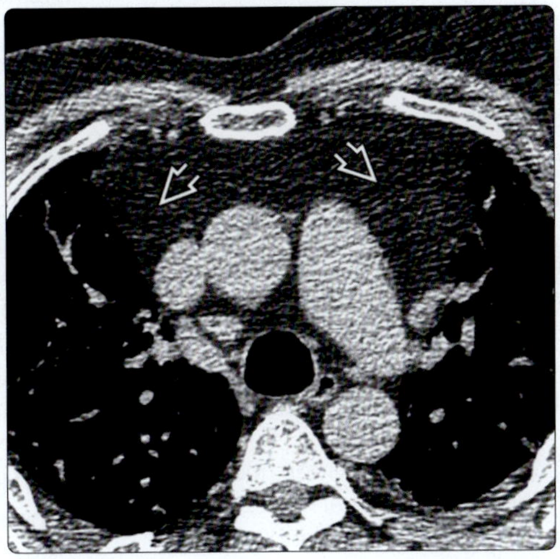

(Left) *Axial CECT of a young man presenting with chest pain and elevated serum β-HCG demonstrates a predominantly homogeneous soft tissue mass in the left prevascular mediastinum. Biopsy revealed seminoma, which typically affects young men. A small focus of necrosis is present →.* **(Right)** *Axial HRCT shows symmetric expansion of the mediastinal fat ➡ without associated mass effect in this patient on steroid therapy for pulmonary fibrosis. This is typical of mediastinal lipomatosis.*

Nonseminomatous Germ Cell Neoplasm

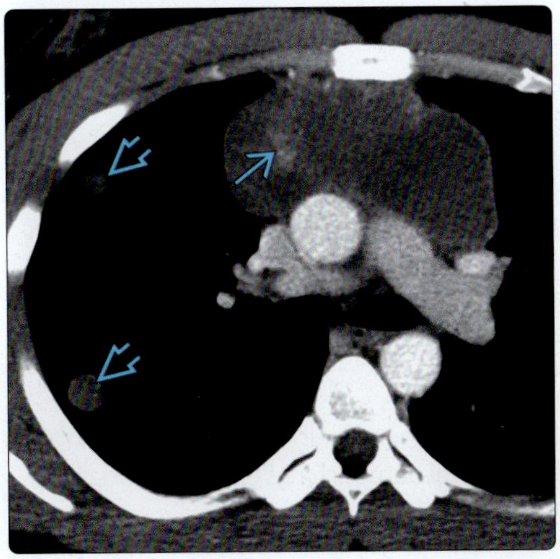

Nonseminomatous Germ Cell Neoplasm

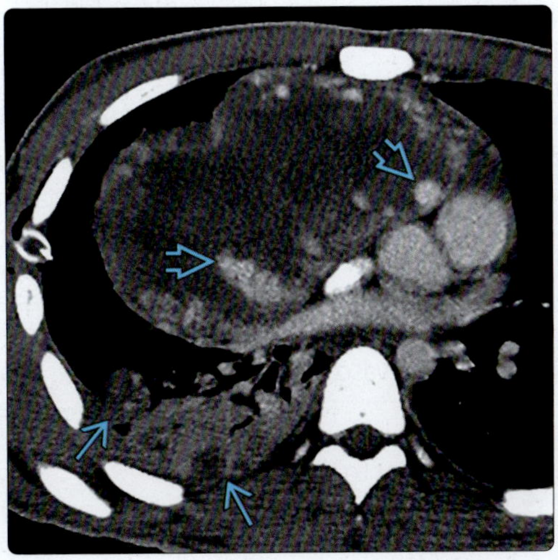

(Left) *Axial CECT of a patient with a nonseminomatous germ cell neoplasm shows a heterogeneous low-density mass in the prevascular mediastinum. Note the regions of internal enhancement → and the metastases in the right lung ⇒.* **(Right)** *Axial CECT of a patient with nonseminomatous germ cell neoplasm demonstrates a large heterogeneous mass in the prevascular mediastinum with regions of internal enhancement ⇒. Pulmonary and pleural metastases are present in the lower right hemithorax →.*

DIFFERENTIAL DIAGNOSIS

Common

- Lymphadenopathy
  - Infection
  - Metastatic Disease
  - Lymphoma
  - Sarcoidosis
- Foregut Duplication Cysts
- Hiatus Hernia

Less Common

- Aortic Aneurysm
- Lipomatosis
- Thyroid Goiter
- Esophageal Neoplasms
- Esophageal Varices

Rare but Important

- Mediastinitis
- Mediastinal Hemorrhage
- Tracheal Neoplasms

ESSENTIAL INFORMATION

Key Differential Diagnosis Issues

- Middle compartment
  - Defined on lateral chest radiograph
  - Boundaries
    - Anterior: Vertical line extending from diaphragm to thoracic inlet along back of heart and anterior to trachea
    - Posterior: Vertical line that connects points 1 cm behind anterior margins of vertebral bodies
  - Contents
    - Nonvascular: Trachea and main bronchi; lymph nodes; phrenic, vagus, and left recurrent laryngeal nerves
    - Vascular: Heart and pericardium; ascending and transverse aorta; superior vena cava; inferior vena cava; brachiocephalic vessels; pulmonary vessels
  - Middle mediastinal lesion may disrupt normal lines, stripes, and interfaces, such as
    - Right paratracheal stripe ≤ 4 mm
    - Concave interface in aortopulmonary window
    - Reverse S contour of azygoesophageal recess
    - Posterior tracheal stripe ≤ 6 mm on lateral radiograph
- Visceral compartment
  - Defined in ITMIG cross-sectional classification
  - Boundaries
    - Superior: Thoracic inlet
    - Inferior: Diaphragm
    - Anterior: Posterior boundaries of prevascular compartment
    - Posterior: Vertical line connecting point on each thoracic vertebral body 1 cm posterior to its anterior margin
  - Contents
    - Nonvascular: Trachea, carina, esophagus, lymph nodes
    - Vascular: Heart, ascending thoracic aorta, aortic arch, descending thoracic aorta, superior vena cava, intrapericardial pulmonary arteries, thoracic duct

Helpful Clues for Common Diagnoses

- **Lymphadenopathy**
  - Radiography
    - Right paratracheal stripe thickening: Right paratracheal lymphadenopathy
    - Convexity in superior azygoesophageal recess: Subcarinal lymphadenopathy
  - CT
    - Calcified nodes
      - Dense calcification usually from prior granulomatous infection
      - Rim calcification, "eggshell" appearance with sarcoidosis, silicosis, and treated lymphoma
    - Necrotic or low-density lymph nodes
      - Tuberculosis and histoplasmosis
      - Lymphoma, thymoma, metastases, and lung carcinoma
    - Enhancing lymphadenopathy
      - Vascular metastases (renal, thyroid, and melanoma)
      - Tuberculosis
      - Castleman disease
- **Foregut Duplication Cysts**
  - Radiography
    - Soft tissue density rounded structure
  - CT
    - Typically water or fluid attenuation
    - Round and well circumscribed
    - High density in setting of hemorrhage, infection, or proteinaceous contents
    - Bronchogenic cysts most commonly subcarinal or right paratracheal in location
      - Less commonly peripheral, hilar
    - Esophageal duplication cyst location
      - Paraesophageal or within esophageal wall
- **Hiatus Hernia**
  - Superior herniation of stomach through esophageal hiatus
  - Radiography
    - Convexity of lower azygoesophageal recess
  - CT
    - Easily diagnosed by protrusion of stomach through esophageal hiatus

Helpful Clues for Less Common Diagnoses

- **Aortic Aneurysm**
  - May involve aortic arch or descending aorta
  - True aneurysm: Most commonly due to atherosclerotic disease
  - False aneurysm: Most commonly due to trauma
  - Other definitions
    - Dilated ≥ 4 cm
    - Aneurysmal ≥ 5 cm
    - High risk of rupture ≥ 6 cm
    - Saccular are focal outpouchings and are associated with trauma or infection
    - Fusiform is circumferential
    - Annuloaortic ectasia is dilated aortic root and associated with Marfan syndrome
- **Lipomatosis**
  - Etiologies

- Obesity, long-term steroid therapy, Cushing disease
- Radiography
  - Smooth mediastinal widening without compression of trachea
- CT
  - Homogeneous fat causing bulging of mediastinal contours

- **Thyroid Goiter**
  - Radiography: Upper mediastinal mass with deviation of trachea
  - CT
    - Heterogeneous lesions with soft tissue, calcification, and cystic regions
    - Connection to thyroid gland
      - Coronal images very helpful
    - Enhance avidly with contrast and are high in density on pre-contrast exams
- **Esophageal Neoplasms**
  - Carcinoma
    - Thickening of esophageal wall, may be eccentric
    - Focal soft tissue mass
    - Smooth margins
    - Luminal narrowing
    - Invasion of adjacent structures
  - Mesenchymal neoplasm
    - Leiomyoma is most common histology
    - Often asymptomatic
    - Margins are smooth
- **Esophageal Varices**
  - Result of liver disease with chronic portal hypertension
  - Radiography
    - Abnormal convexity of lower azygoesophageal recess or paravertebral widening
  - CT
    - Vascular serpiginous masses
    - Connect with azygos system to bypass portal drainage

Helpful Clues for Rare Diagnoses

- **Mediastinitis**
  - Associated with sternotomy, esophageal perforation, or spread of infection
  - Radiography
    - Widening of mediastinal contours
  - CT
    - Diffuse fat stranding replacing normal mediastinal fat
    - Pneumomediastinum
    - Fluid collections
  - Difficult to differentiate normal postoperative appearance from mediastinitis
    - Resolution of expected fluid collections occurs within 2-3 weeks after surgery
- **Mediastinal Hemorrhage**
  - Etiologies
    - Acute aortic injury or venous bleeding secondary to severe blunt or penetrating trauma
    - Aneurysm or dissection rupture
  - Radiography
    - Nonspecific mediastinal widening
  - CT
    - High-attenuation fluid within mediastinum
    - Hematoma not adjacent to aorta is secondary to venous bleeding
- **Tracheal Neoplasms**
  - Squamous cell carcinoma or adenoid cystic carcinoma are most common primary malignancies
  - Uncommonly single or multiple metastases
    - Melanoma, breast carcinoma, colon carcinoma, or adjacent tumor extension
  - CT
    - Polypoid, sessile, or circumferential lesion
    - Adenoid cystic carcinoma usually originates from posterolateral wall
    - Important to define extraluminal extent of disease for surgical planning

Infection

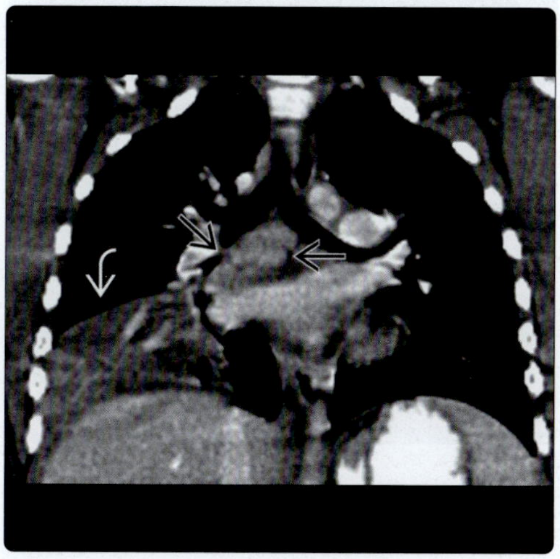

Metastatic Disease

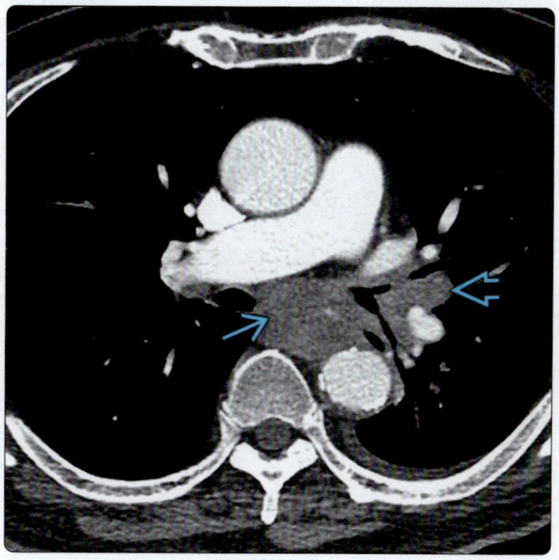

(Left) *Coronal CECT shows subcarinal lymphadenopathy ➞ and right lower lung consolidation ➞ in this patient with bacterial pneumonia.* **(Right)** *Axial CECT of a patient with lung cancer (not shown) demonstrates subcarinal ➞ and left hilar lymphadenopathy ➞, compatible with metastatic disease. Lymphadenopathy involving the visceral compartment may be caused by infection, metastatic disease, sarcoidosis, or lymphoma.*

Sarcoidosis

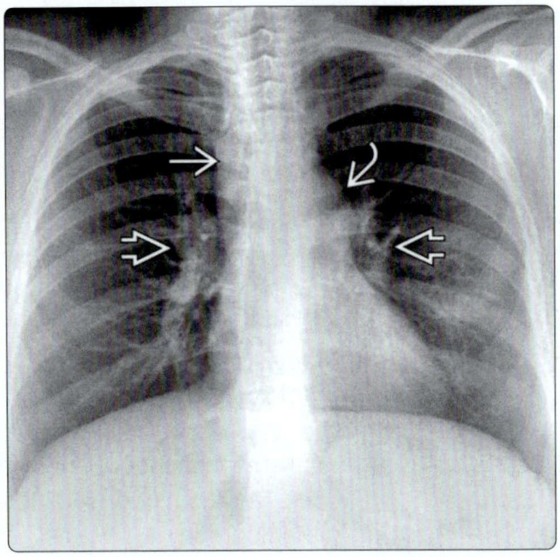

Sarcoidosis

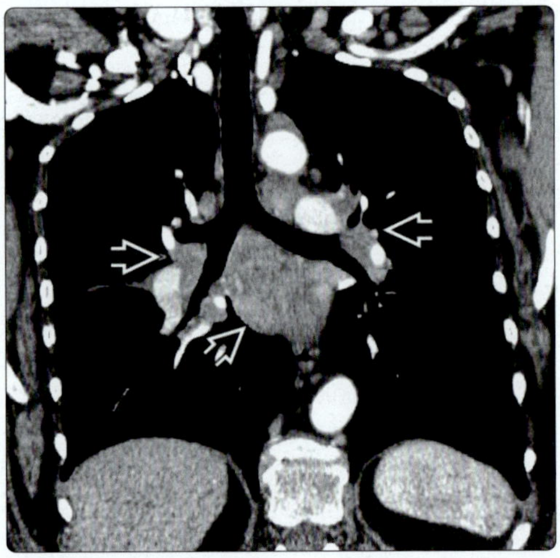

(Left) *Frontal chest radiograph shows enlarged bilateral hilar ➡, right paratracheal ➡, and left aortopulmonary lymph nodes ➡. This is a common finding in sarcoidosis. The presence of right paratracheal and bilateral hilar lymphadenopathy constitutes Garland's triad.* **(Right)** *Coronal CECT shows typical CT features of lymphadenopathy in sarcoidosis. Note the diffuse hilar and mediastinal lymphadenopathy ➡.*

Foregut Duplication Cysts

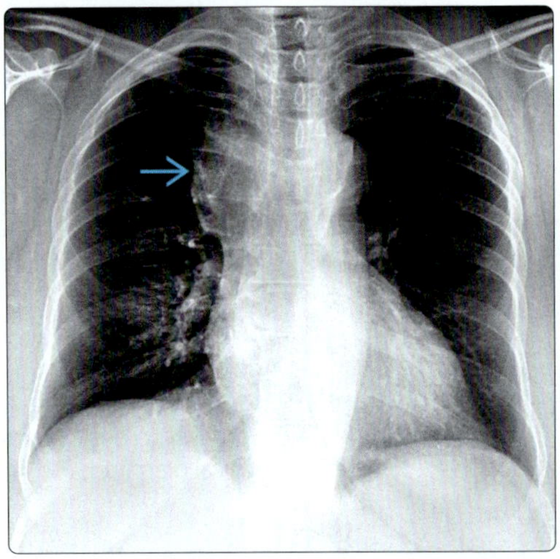

Foregut Duplication Cysts

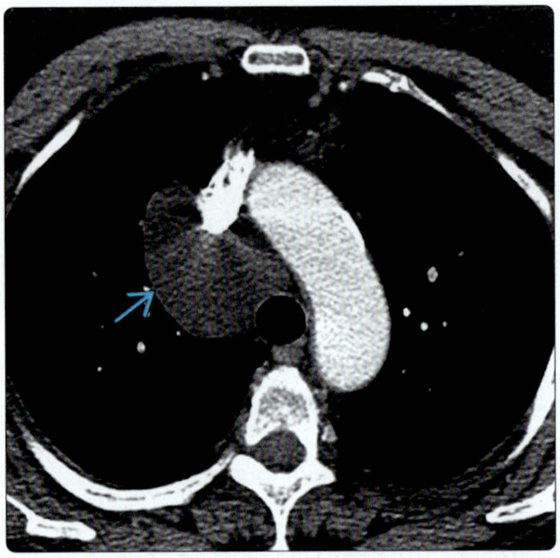

(Left) *PA chest radiograph demonstrates a lobulated contour of the right paratracheal region concerning for a mass ➡.* **(Right)** *Axial CECT of the same patient demonstrates a well-defined lesion of water attenuation in the right paratracheal region, compatible with a bronchogenic cyst ➡. Bronchogenic cysts are typically seen in the subcarinal and right paratracheal regions as rounded water or fluid attenuation structures.*

Hiatus Hernia

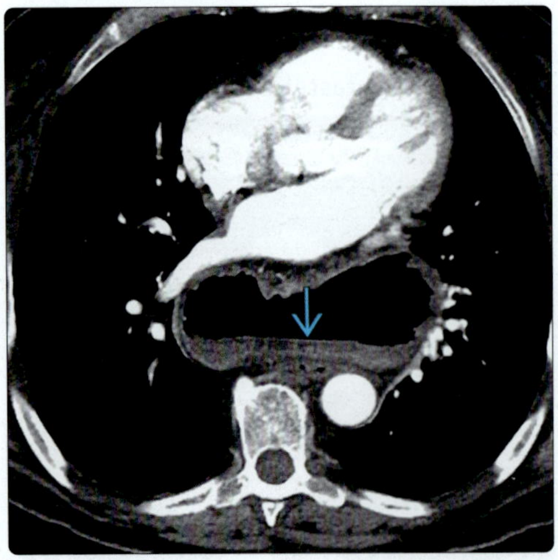

Aortic Aneurysm

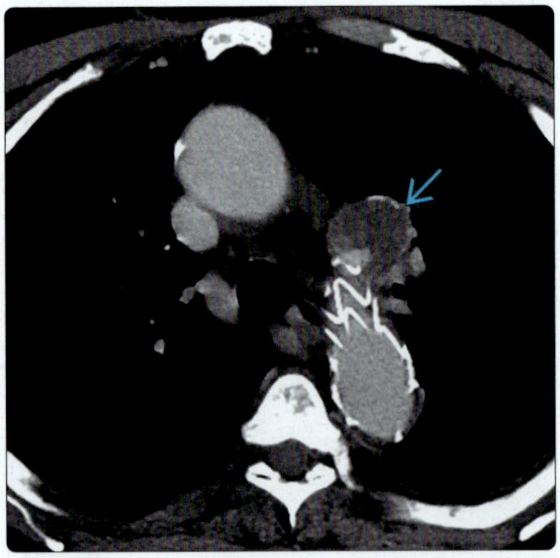

(Left) *Axial CECT shows a large hiatus hernia in the visceral compartment with an air-fluid level ➡. A hiatus hernia represents superior herniation of the stomach through the esophageal hiatus.* **(Right)** *Axial CECT of a patient with prior endograft stent placement in the descending thoracic aorta demonstrates focal outpouching of the aortic arch representing a saccular aneurysm ➡. Saccular aneurysms are focal outpouchings and are associated with trauma or infection.*

Lipomatosis

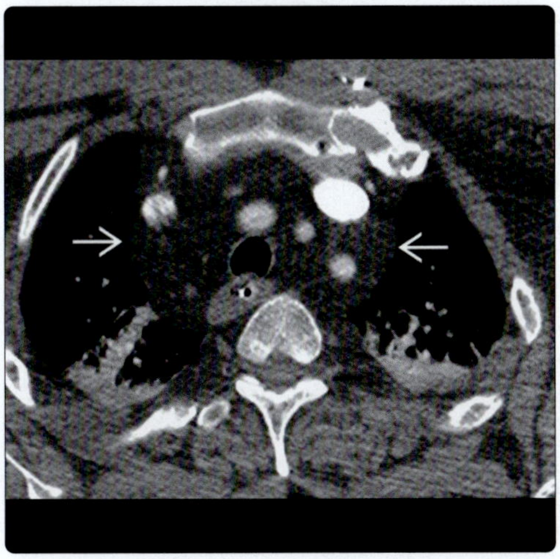

Esophageal Neoplasms

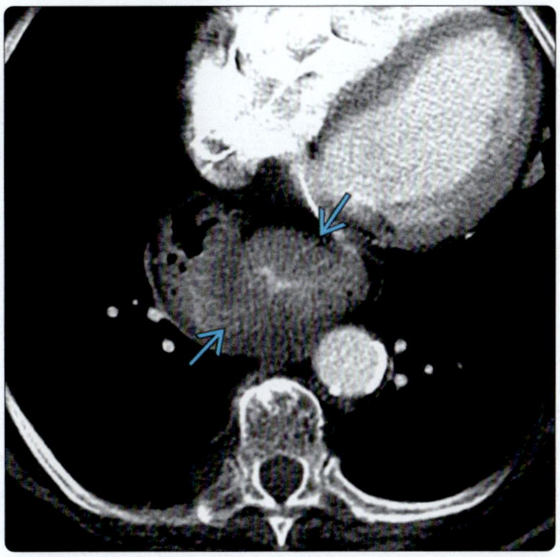

(Left) *Axial CECT shows typical CT features of mediastinal lipomatosis with diffuse smooth mediastinal widening from fat ➡. Etiologies of mediastinal lipomatosis include obesity, long-term steroid therapy, and Cushing disease.* **(Right)** *Axial CECT of a patient with esophageal cancer demonstrates a hiatus hernia and marked thickening of the esophageal wall representing the primary malignancy ⇨.*

Esophageal Neoplasms

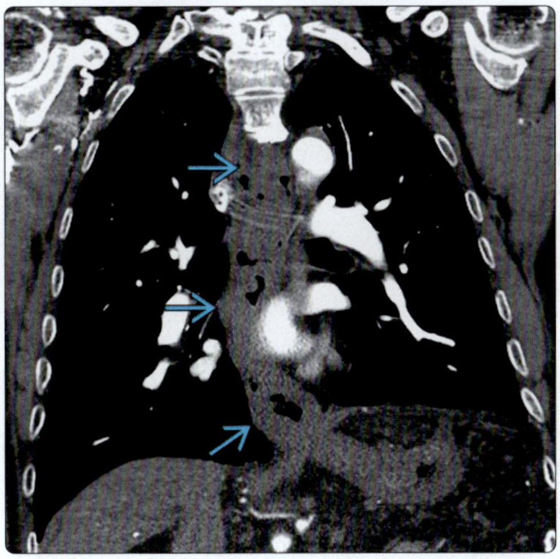

Esophageal Varices

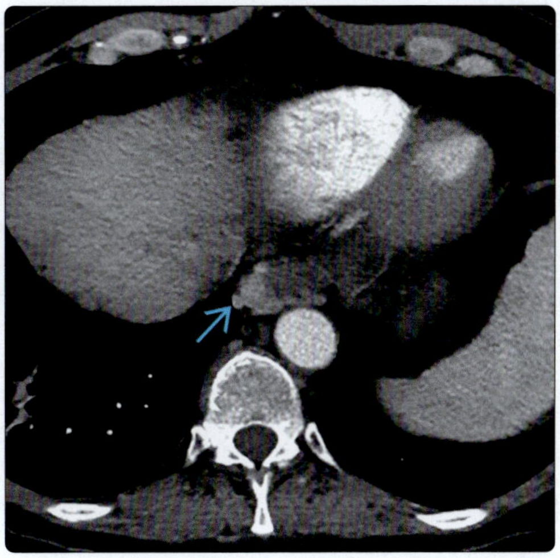

(Left) *Coronal CECT of a patient with esophageal cancer shows extensive irregular thickening of most of the esophageal wall representing a combination of malignancy and esophagitis related to therapy ⇨. Esophageal cancer may manifest as wall thickening &/or a focal mass.* **(Right)** *Axial CECT of a patient with chronic portal hypertension shows numerous enhancing serpiginous vessels adjacent to the distal thoracic esophagus representing varices ⇨.*

Mediastinitis

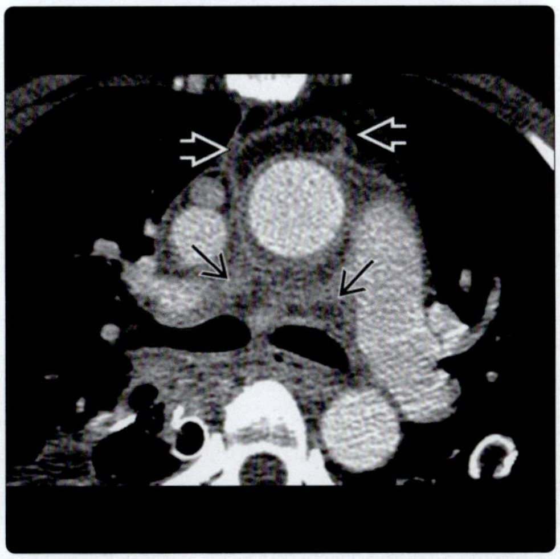

Mediastinitis

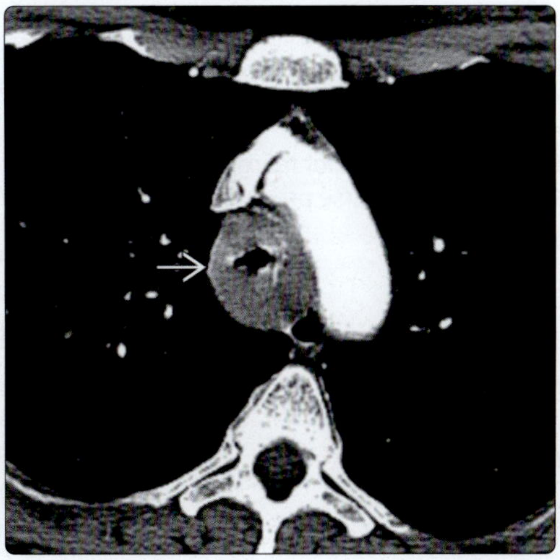

(Left) *Axial CECT shows thickening and abnormal fluid collections within prevascular mediastinum ➡ and visceral mediastinum ⇨ in this patient with mediastinitis secondary to a spreading pharyngeal infection. Presence of infectious symptoms is an important factor in diagnosing this condition.* **(Right)** *Axial CECT shows diffuse circumferential tracheal wall thickening from adenoid cystic carcinoma ➡. Squamous cell carcinoma and adenoid cystic carcinoma are the most common primary tracheal malignancies.*

DIFFERENTIAL DIAGNOSIS

Common

- Neurogenic Neoplasms
  - Peripheral Nerve Sheath Tumor
  - Sympathetic Ganglion Tumor
- Lymphoma

Less Common

- Metastatic Disease
- Foregut Duplication Cyst
- Infection

Rare but Important

- Lateral Thoracic Meningocele
- Extramedullary Hematopoiesis
- Hemangioma
- Lymphangioma
- Mediastinal Abscess
- Pancreatic Pseudocyst

ESSENTIAL INFORMATION

Key Differential Diagnosis Issues

- Posterior compartment
  - Felson approach based on lateral radiography
    - Line that connects points 1 cm behind anterior margins of vertebral bodies separates middle and posterior mediastinal compartments
  - Normal contents
    - Vertebral bodies
    - Descending thoracic aorta
    - Azygos vein
    - Esophagus
    - Lymph nodes
    - Adipose tissue
- Paravertebral compartment
  - Defined by International Thymic Malignancy Interest Group (ITMIG) classification based on cross-sectional imaging
  - Boundaries
    - Superior: Thoracic inlet
    - Inferior: Diaphragm
    - Anterior: Posterior boundaries of visceral compartment
    - Posterolateral: Vertical line against posterior margin of chest wall at lateral margin of transverse process of thoracic spine
  - Normal contents
    - Thoracic spine
    - Paravertebral soft tissues

Helpful Clues for Common Diagnoses

- Neurogenic Neoplasms
  - **Peripheral Nerve Sheath Tumor**
    - More common in adults than children
    - Schwannoma, neurofibroma, plexiform neurofibroma
    - Imaging
      - Smooth, round or oval, often less dense than muscle
      - Enlargement of adjacent neural foramina with occasional extension into spinal canal
      - Often have internal foci of decreased attenuation due to lipid or cyst formation
      - Increased signal on T2 MR and heterogeneous enhancement
  - **Sympathetic Ganglion Tumor**
    - More common in children and young adults
    - Ganglioneuroma
      - Benign neoplasm of ganglion cells and Schwann cells
      - Most common in 2nd and 3rd decades
      - Calcification in 20%
      - May have 'whorled' appearance on MR
    - Ganglioneuroblastoma
      - Intermediate histology between ganglioneuroma and neuroblastoma
      - Most common in older children
      - Imaging resembles neuroblastoma
    - Neuroblastoma
      - Malignant neoplasm associated with systemic symptoms
      - Most common in children < 5 years old
      - Curvilinear and speckled calcification in 40%
      - May invade adjacent structures
- **Lymphoma**
  - Non-Hodgkin lymphoma (NHL) is more common than Hodgkin lymphoma (HL)
  - "B" symptoms (fever, weight loss, and night sweats) may be present
  - Imaging
    - HL commonly involves several contiguous lymph node groups
    - Involvement of single lymph node group is more common with NHL
    - Enlarged lymph nodes or mass, usually displaying homogeneous soft tissue attenuation
    - Necrosis is occasionally present, usually detected after contrast administration
    - Infiltrative nature of some types enables differentiation from other neoplasms
      - Lesions may encase or encircle structures without invading them
- **Metastatic Disease**
  - Often involves lymph nodes
  - Involvement of posterior/paravertebral compartment lymph nodes is suggestive of primary malignancy within abdomen
  - Can involve osseous structures

Helpful Clues for Less Common Diagnoses

- **Foregut Duplication Cyst**
  - Neurenteric cyst
    - Composed of neural and gastrointestinal components
    - Imaging
      - Water or fluid attenuation
      - Cyst contents may be proteinaceous with increased attenuation and increased signal on T1 MR
      - Round or oval with smooth borders
      - Thin wall with no enhancement; wall calcification is uncommon

- Connection to meninges through vertebral defect
- Associated with vertebral anomalies (scoliosis or hemivertebrae)

- **Infection**
  - Spondylitis, paraspinal abscess
  - Imaging
    - Evaluation for disc space and vertebral body destruction
    - If mass is present, determine if it appears to arise from bone or soft tissues

Helpful Clues for Rare Diagnoses

- **Lateral Thoracic Meningocele**
  - Anomalous herniation of leptomeninges through intervertebral foramen or vertebral body defect
  - Strong association with neurofibromatosis type 1
  - More common in adults than in children
  - Imaging
    - Water or fluid attenuation
    - Direct communication with subarachnoid space around spinal cord
    - Associated with vertebral anomalies, such as hemivertebrae, butterfly vertebra, or spina bifida
- **Extramedullary Hematopoiesis**
  - Associations
    - Thalassemia
    - Sickle cell anemia
    - Spherocytosis
  - Imaging
    - Multiple bilateral paraspinal masses
    - May contain fat in long-standing lesions
    - Sharp borders with homogeneous attenuation
    - May be associated with skeletal abnormalities
- **Hemangioma**
  - Soft tissue mass
  - Internal phleboliths
  - Appearance similar to soft tissue hemangiomas elsewhere in body
- **Lymphangioma**
  - Benign hyperplasia of lymphatic vessels
  - Imaging
    - Low-density mass that insinuates between adjacent structures
    - Unilocular or multilocular
    - ± thin septations ± soft tissue components
- **Mediastinal Abscess**
  - Recent clinical history important
    - Median sternotomy
    - Esophageal perforation
    - Head and neck infection
  - Imaging
    - Rim-enhancing lesion with central low density
    - May demonstrate internal foci of air
    - Communication may be seen with coexisting subphrenic abscesses or empyema
    - May be difficult to differentiate from postoperative hematoma/seroma
      - May require needle aspiration
      - Postoperative hematoma/seroma should resolve after several weeks
- **Pancreatic Pseudocyst**
  - Develops over short period of time in clinical setting of pancreatitis
  - Contain pancreatic secretions, blood, and necrotic material
  - Accesses mediastinum via esophageal or aortic hiatus
  - Thin-walled masses that may be low or high density
  - High density results from hemorrhage or infection
  - Lesion tracks from abdomen; separate intra-abdominal pseudocysts may or may not be present

SELECTED REFERENCES

1. Carter BW et al: ITMIG classification of mediastinal compartments and multidisciplinary approach to mediastinal masses. Radiographics. 37(2):413-36, 2017
2. Carter BW et al: A modern definition of mediastinal compartments. J Thorac Oncol. 9(9 Suppl 2):S97-101, 2014

Peripheral Nerve Sheath Tumor

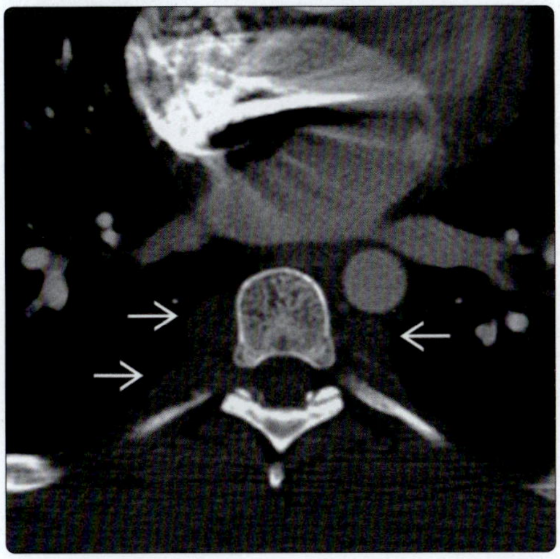

Peripheral Nerve Sheath Tumor

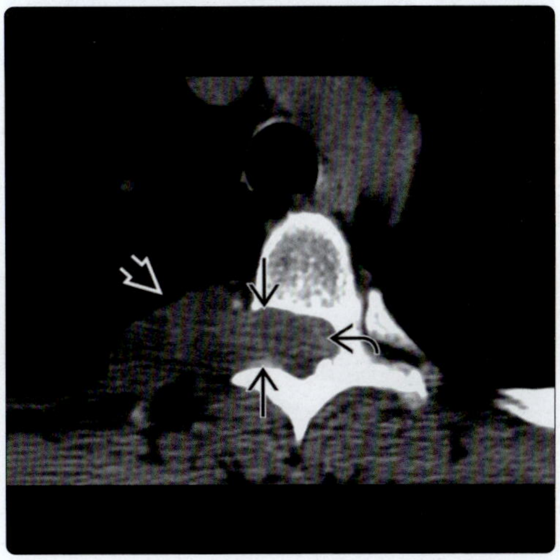

(Left) *Axial NECT demonstrates multiple round and oval nonenhancing soft tissue masses bilaterally within the paravertebral mediastinum ➡. This is a typical appearance of multiple neurofibromas in a patient with neurofibromatosis.* **(Right)** *Axial NECT shows a schwannoma within the paravertebral mediastinum ➡ that has expanded the right neural foramen ➡ and extends into the central canal ➡. Neurogenic neoplasms are the most common paravertebral masses.*

(Left) *Axial CECT of a 28-year-old man shows a nonenhancing lobulated paravertebral mediastinal mass . This was proven to represent a ganglioneuroma. Notice the lack of invasion into adjacent structures.* **(Right)** *Axial CECT shows a large mass in the left paravertebral mediastinum . There is invasion of the adjacent chest wall . Notice the internal calcifications. In a young child, this is highly suggestive of neuroblastoma.*

Sympathetic Ganglion Tumor

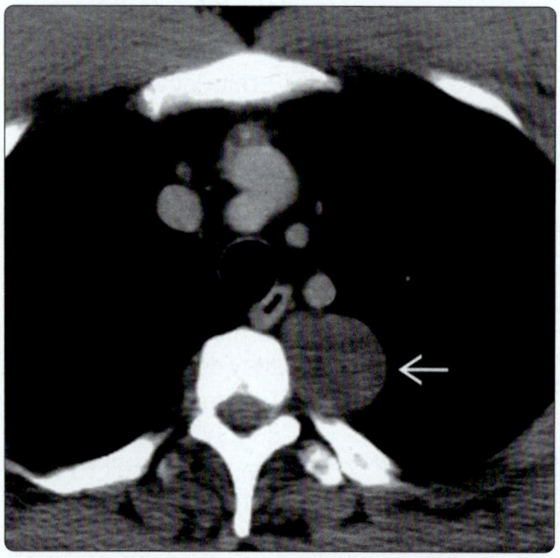

Sympathetic Ganglion Tumor

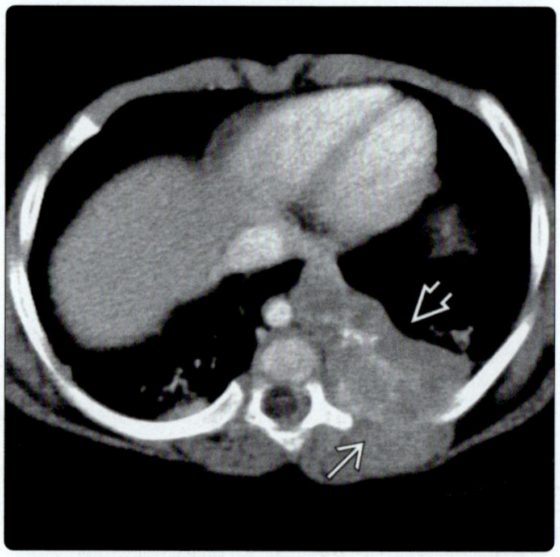

(Left) *Axial CECT of a patient with non-Hodgkin lymphoma demonstrates a homogeneous soft tissue mass in the paravertebral compartment that extends into the visceral compartment.* **(Right)** *Axial CECT of a patient with non-Hodgkin lymphoma demonstrates an infiltrative soft tissue mass in the paravertebral and visceral compartments . A small left pleural effusion is present . The infiltrative nature of some lymphomas enables differentiation from other neoplasms.*

Lymphoma

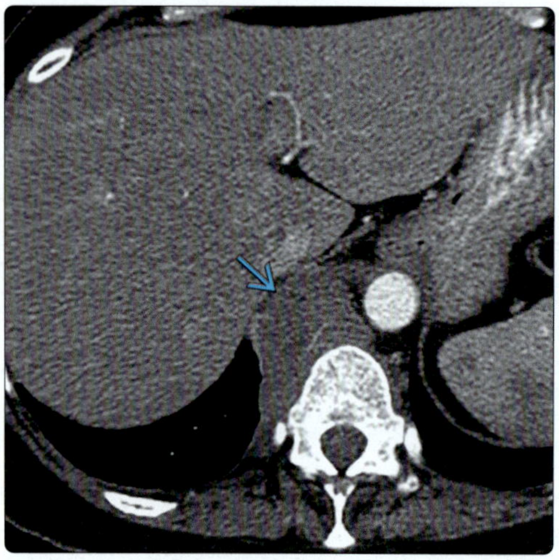

Lymphoma

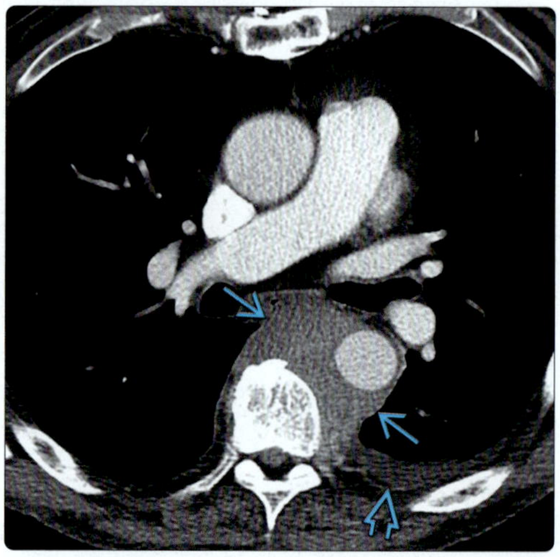

(Left) *Axial CECT of a patient with salivary gland malignancy demonstrates a lobular soft tissue lesion in the right paravertebral compartment representing a metastasis .* **(Right)** *Axial CECT shows a well-defined, water attenuation lesion in the left paravertebral mediastinum representing a neurenteric cyst . Neurenteric cysts connect with meninges through vertebral defects and are associated with vertebral anomalies, such as scoliosis or hemivertebrae.*

Metastatic Disease

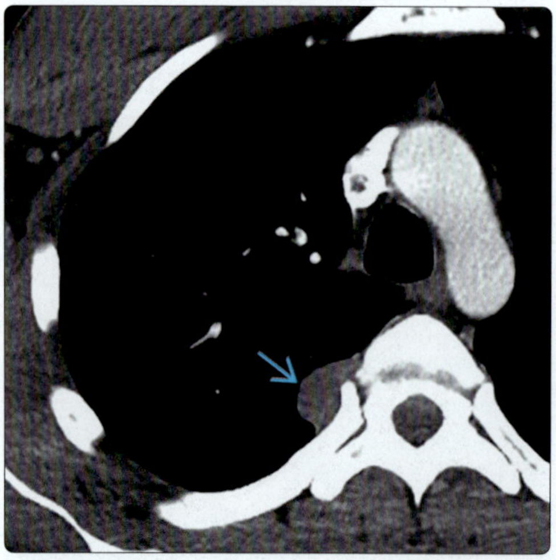

Foregut Duplication Cyst

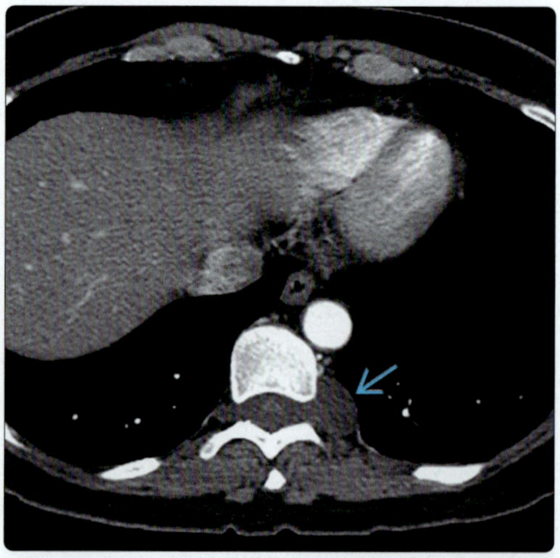

Infection

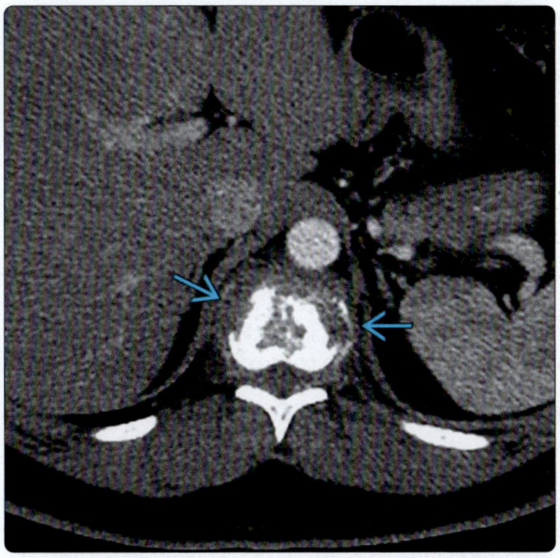

Infection

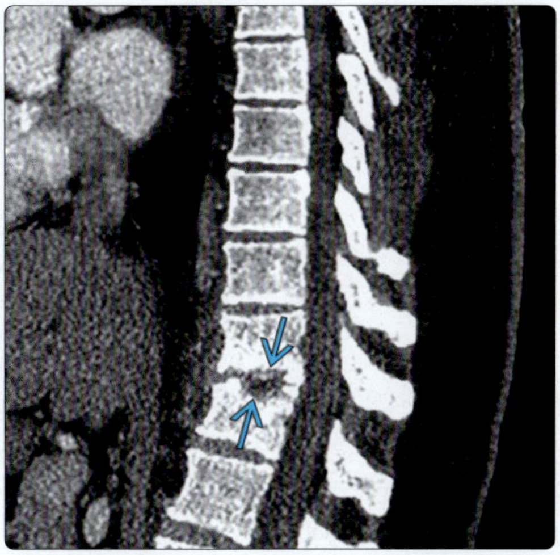

(Left) *Axial CECT of a patient presenting with low back pain demonstrates ill-defined soft tissue and inflammation in the paraspinal soft tissues adjacent to a lower thoracic vertebral body and osseous destruction* ➙. **(Right)** *Sagittal CECT of the same patient shows loss of the intervertebral disc space, osseous destruction, and paraspinal soft tissue, consistent with discitis and osteomyelitis* ➙. *In suspected cases of spinal infection, evaluation for disc space and osseous destruction is paramount.*

Lateral Thoracic Meningocele

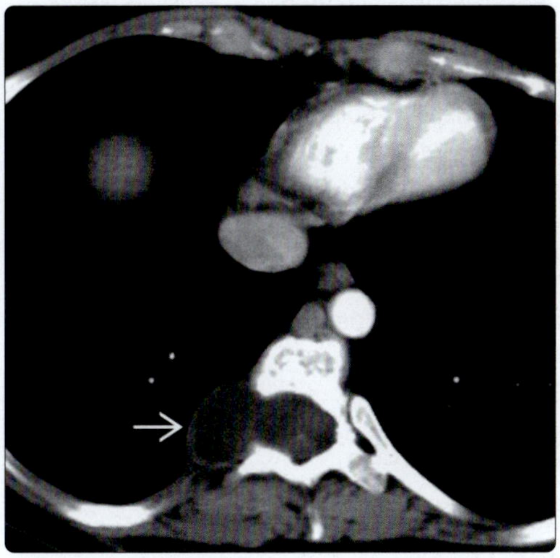

Lateral Thoracic Meningocele

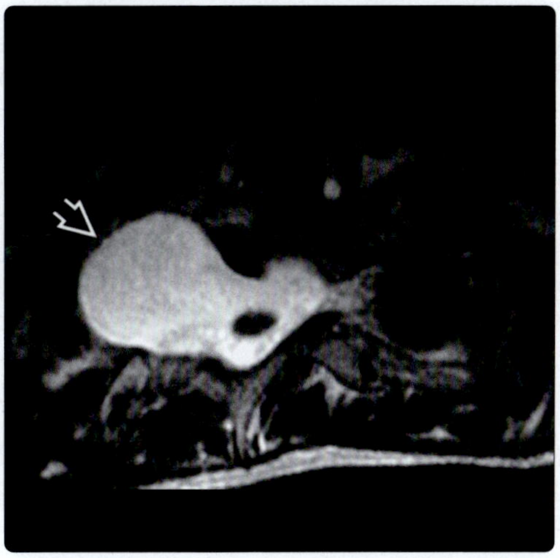

(Left) *Axial CECT shows a typical lateral meningocele* ➙ *in a patient with neurofibromatosis. Notice the low density, consistent with cerebrospinal fluid (CSF) and expansion of the neural foramen.* **(Right)** *Axial T2 MR shows a large lateral meningocele arising from the right neural foramen of an upper thoracic vertebra* ➙. *Notice the contiguity with the central canal and homogeneous increased T2 signal, consistent with CSF.*

Extramedullary Hematopoiesis

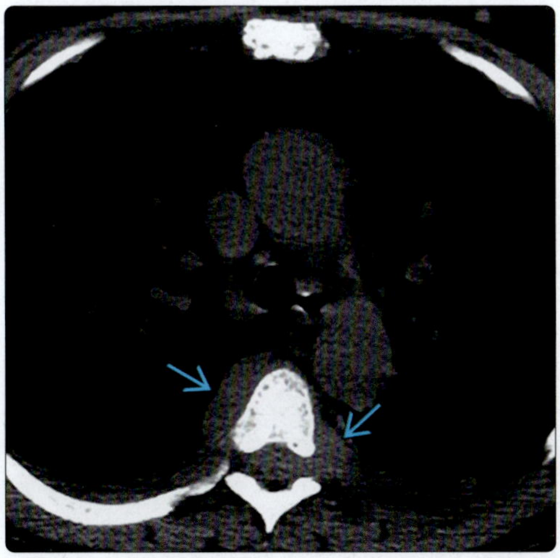

Lymphangioma

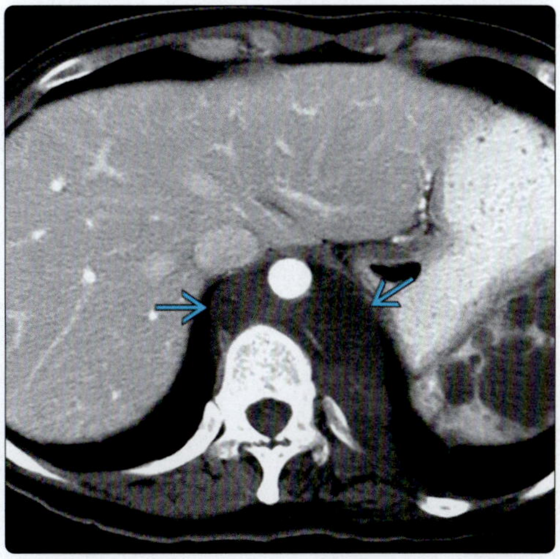

(Left) *Axial NECT of a patient with sickle cell anemia demonstrates lobular and infiltrative soft tissue lesions in the paravertebral space representing extramedullary hematopoiesis* ➙. *Extramedullary hematopoiesis is typically associated with thalassemia, sickle cell anemia, and spherocytosis.* **(Right)** *Axial CECT shows a low-attenuation mass in the paravertebral compartment that has insinuated itself between the descending thoracic aorta and the thoracic spine* ➙, *representing a lymphangioma.*

Cardiophrenic Angle Lesion

DIFFERENTIAL DIAGNOSIS

Common

- Pericardial Fat Pad
- Pericardial Cyst
- Morgagni Hernia
- Lymphadenopathy

Less Common

- Thymoma

Rare but Important

- Mediastinal Fat Necrosis

ESSENTIAL INFORMATION

Key Differential Diagnosis Issues

- Mnemonic for common diagnoses: **Fat PAD**
    - **Fat, P**ericardial cyst, **A**denopathy, **D**iaphragmatic hernia

Helpful Clues for Common Diagnoses

- **Pericardial Fat Pad**
    - Accumulation of fat between pericardium and parietal pleura; may be associated with obesity
    - Common normal finding; may mimic pneumonia, cardiomegaly, or mass on radiography
    - Cardiophrenic angle mass
        - Less opaque than heart, more opaque than lung
        - Homogeneous fat attenuation on CT
- **Pericardial Cyst**
    - Benign lesion thought to arise from defective pericardial development; may be secondary to previous surgery
    - 5-10% of all mediastinal masses
    - Right (78%) or left (22%) cardiophrenic angle
    - Size: 2-30 cm in diameter
    - Morphology: Spherical or ovoid, well-defined margins
        - Unilocular (80%) or multilocular (20%)
        - CT: Imperceptible wall, water attenuation, no contrast enhancement
        - MR: Low-to-intermediate signal on T1WI, high signal on T2WI
- **Morgagni Hernia**
    - 1-3% of diaphragmatic hernias, female predominance
    - Parasternal or retrosternal herniation through diaphragmatic sternocostal hiatus
    - Right (90%), bilateral (8%), left (2%)
    - Morphology
        - Sharply marginated, fat-attenuation lesion
        - Content: Fat > colon > stomach > small bowel
            - Omental vessels course from abdomen into hernia
- **Lymphadenopathy**
    - Lymphoma is most common etiology
    - Metastatic lymphadenopathy from thoracic neoplasms: Mesothelioma, breast and thymic malignancies

Helpful Clues for Less Common Diagnoses

- **Thymoma**
    - Homogeneous lobular, spherical, or ovoid soft tissue mass
    - CT: Ca++ in 1/3; usually thin and linear within capsule
        - Cystic change and necrosis in 1/3, typically in large tumors
        - May exhibit local invasion, drop pleural metastases
    - Paraneoplastic syndromes in 40% of cases
- **Mediastinal Fat Necrosis**
    - Also called pericardial or epipericardial fat necrosis
    - More common on left
    - Sudden, excruciating chest pain, typically pleuritic
    - CT: Increased mediastinal fat density/stranding, fat-attenuation lesion with peripheral soft tissue ring or "capsule"
        - Thickening of adjacent pericardium, small ipsilateral pleural effusion
        - May mimic liposarcoma

SELECTED REFERENCES

1. Tower-Rader A et al: Pericardial masses, cysts and diverticula: a comprehensive review using multimodality imaging. Prog Cardiovasc Dis. 59(4):389-97, 2017
2. Goldstein AJ et al: A tour of the thymus: a review of thymic lesions with radiologic and pathologic correlation. Can Assoc Radiol J. 66(1):5-15, 2015

Pericardial Fat Pad

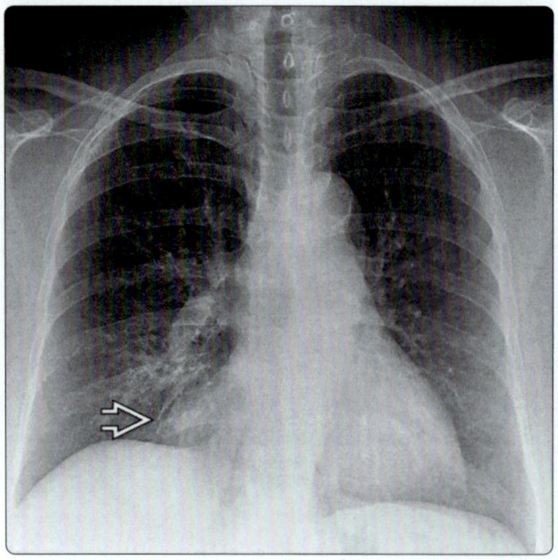

Pericardial Fat Pad

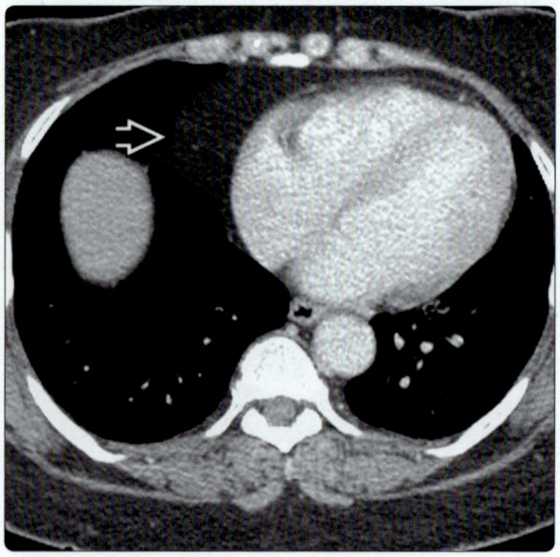

(Left) *PA chest radiograph of an asymptomatic woman shows mass-like opacity in the right cardiophrenic angle ➡. The lesion is denser than the adjacent lung but not as dense as the heart.* **(Right)** *Axial CECT of the same patient shows accumulation of mediastinal fat ➡ in the right cardiophrenic angle corresponding to the abnormal opacity identified on the PA chest radiograph. Pericardial fat pad may or may not be associated with obesity. Although termed "pericardial," the fat is located in the mediastinum.*

Pericardial Cyst

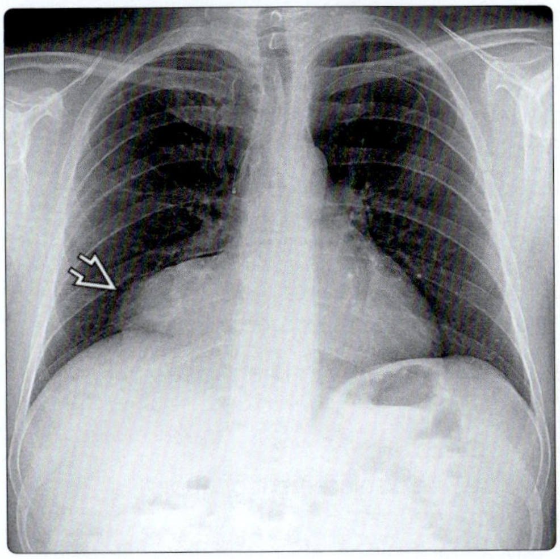

Pericardial Cyst

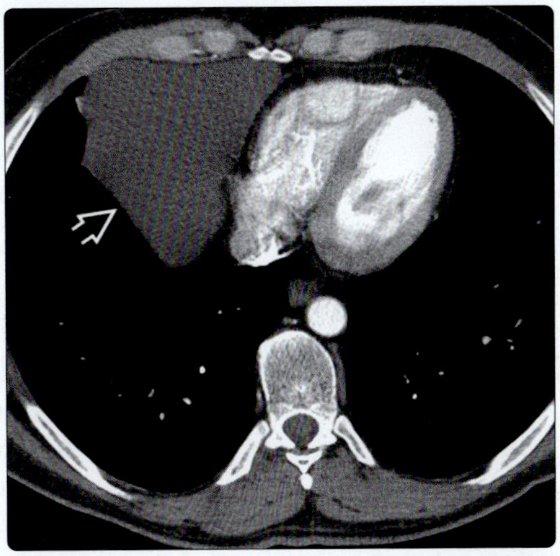

(Left) *PA chest radiograph of an asymptomatic young man shows a well-defined mass-like lesion in the right cardiophrenic angle, which alters the expected contour of the right heart border .* **(Right)** *Axial CECT of the same patient shows a sharply marginated water-attenuation mass with an imperceptible wall typical of a pericardial cyst. Pericardial cysts are located in the right cardiophrenic angle in ~ 78% of cases. These are usually unilocular cystic lesions.*

Morgagni Hernia

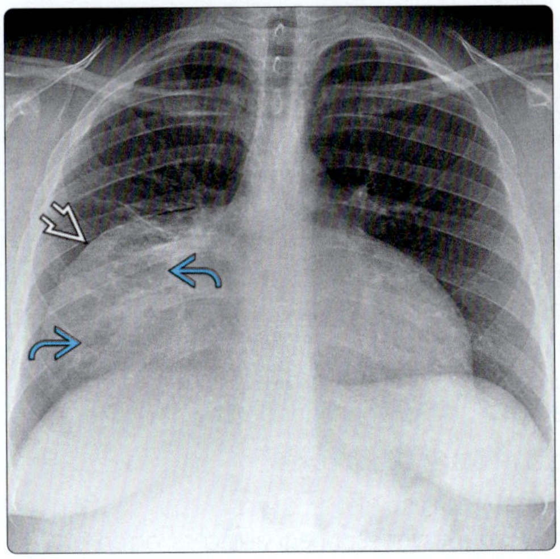

Morgagni Hernia

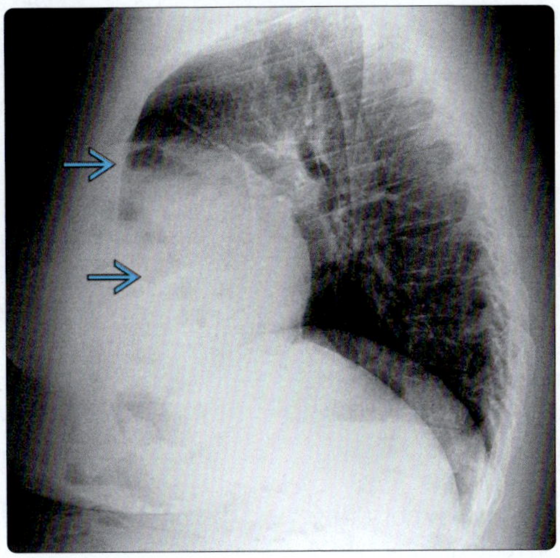

(Left) *PA chest radiograph of an asymptomatic man shows a large right cardiophrenic angle mass with well-defined borders. Note gas-containing structures within the lesion.* **(Right)** *Lateral chest radiograph of the same patient shows the anterior location of the lesion and multifocal intrinsic air and air-fluid levels , consistent with herniated bowel into the thorax secondary to a Morgagni hernia. Morgagni hernias result from a congenital defect in the anterior diaphragm.*

Lymphadenopathy

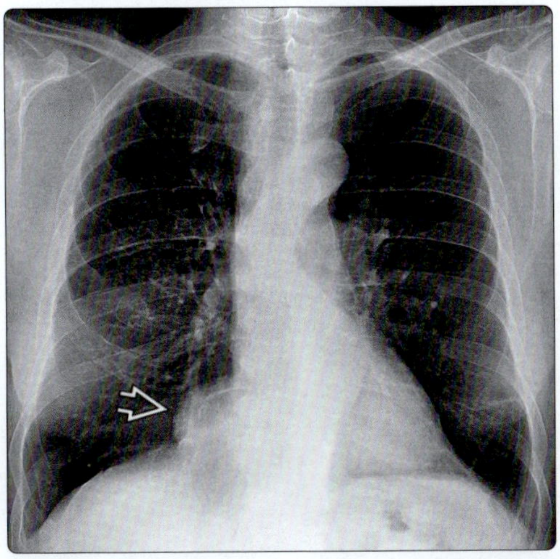

Lymphadenopathy

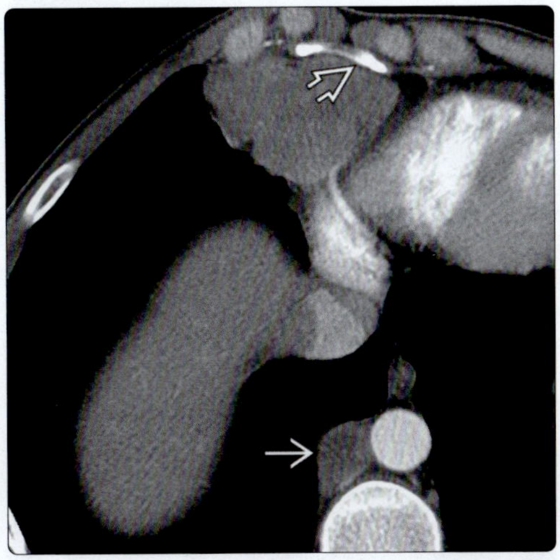

(Left) *PA chest radiograph of a 49-year-old man with previously treated lymphoma shows a right cardiophrenic angle mass , which should suggest lymphadenopathy from recurrent malignancy in this clinical scenario.* **(Right)** *Axial CECT of the same patient shows bulky right cardiophrenic angle and right retrocrural lymphadenopathy, consistent with recurrent lymphoma. Lymphadenopathy secondary to lymphoma is the most common cause of cardiophrenic angle lymph node enlargement.*

DIFFERENTIAL DIAGNOSIS

Common

- Lymphadenopathy
- Hiatus Hernia
- Esophageal Carcinoma

Less Common

- Congenital Foregut Cyst

Rare but Important

- Paraesophageal Varices

ESSENTIAL INFORMATION

Key Differential Diagnosis Issues

- Azygoesophageal recess formed by contact of aerated right lower lobe with mediastinum adjacent to esophagus (anteriorly) and azygos vein (posteriorly)
- Azygoesophageal recess: Interface between lung and adjacent mediastinum on frontal chest radiography
  - From azygos arch superiorly to diaphragm inferiorly
  - Mild leftward convexity in upper third
  - Straight or mild leftward convexity in middle third
  - Straight or mild leftward convexity in lower third
- Rightward convexity of upper or lower azygoesophageal recess is abnormal
- Obscuration of azygoesophageal recess interface may reflect abnormality of adjacent right lower lobe

Helpful Clues for Common Diagnoses

- **Lymphadenopathy**
  - Most common abnormality (rightward displacement) of upper azygoesophageal recess
    - Neoplastic: Lymphoma, lymph node metastases
    - Nonneoplastic: Sarcoidosis, histoplasmosis, tuberculosis
  - Enlarged lymph nodes < 15 mm may not alter azygoesophageal recess on radiography
  - Radiography: Subcarinal opacity, inferior hilar window fullness/mass, thick or mass-like intermediate stem line
  - CT: Soft tissue attenuation, low-attenuation areas may denote necrosis, variable contrast enhancement, ± Ca++
- **Hiatus Hernia**
  - Most common abnormality (rightward displacement) of lower azygoesophageal recess
    - Sliding versus paraesophageal morphologic types
    - May contain stomach, bowel, and other organs
  - Elderly subjects, obesity
  - Visualization of intrinsic air-fluid level allows confident diagnosis on radiography
  - CT imaging allows assessment of morphologic type and identification of herniated structures

Helpful Clues for Less Common Diagnoses

- **Congenital Foregut Cyst**
  - **Bronchogenic Cyst**
    - Typically rightward displacement of upper azygoesophageal recess
    - Classic subcarinal location, abuts trachea/mainstem bronchi
    - Unilocular, thin-wall ± Ca++, fluid or soft tissue attenuation
    - MR helpful for diagnosis of bronchogenic cyst with high-attenuation content on CT
  - **Esophageal Duplication Cyst**
    - May be indistinguishable from bronchogenic cyst
    - Abuts adjacent esophagus, ± mass effect on esophageal lumen
- **Esophageal Carcinoma**
  - Large tumors may show displacement or interruption of azygoesophageal recess
  - Dysphagia is common clinical manifestation
  - CT allows characterization and identification of associated metastatic lymphadenopathy

Helpful Clues for Rare Diagnoses

- **Paraesophageal Varices**
  - Abnormal inferior azygoesophageal recess; often imperceptible on radiography
  - Serpiginous enhancing paraesophageal structures
  - Signs of portal venous hypertension, including ascites

Lymphadenopathy

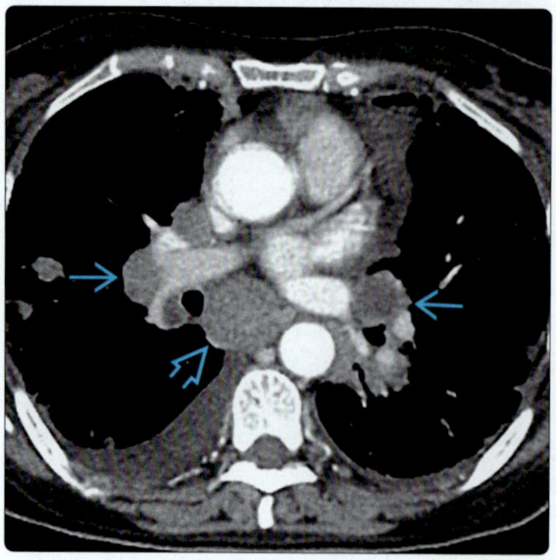

Lymphadenopathy

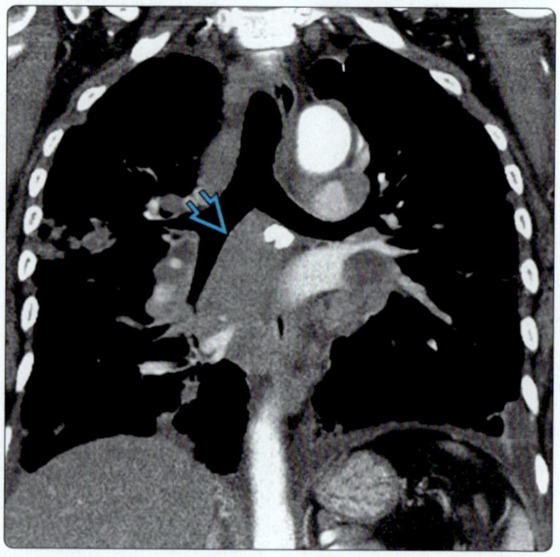

(Left) *Axial CECT of a 53-year-old man with lymphoma shows extensive mediastinal and hilar → lymphadenopathy. A large right paraesophageal lymph node → produces an abnormal convexity of the azygoesophageal recess. Note small bilateral pleural effusions and multiple pulmonary nodules.* **(Right)** *Coronal CECT of the same patient shows marked coalescent mediastinal lymphadenopathy involving subcarinal and paraesophageal lymph nodes →.*

Hiatus Hernia

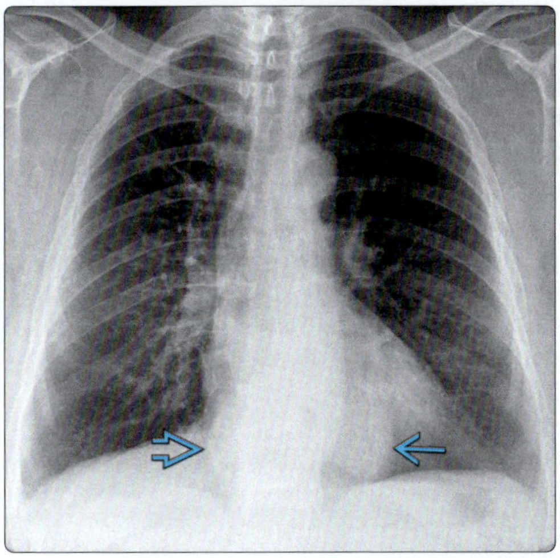

Hiatus Hernia

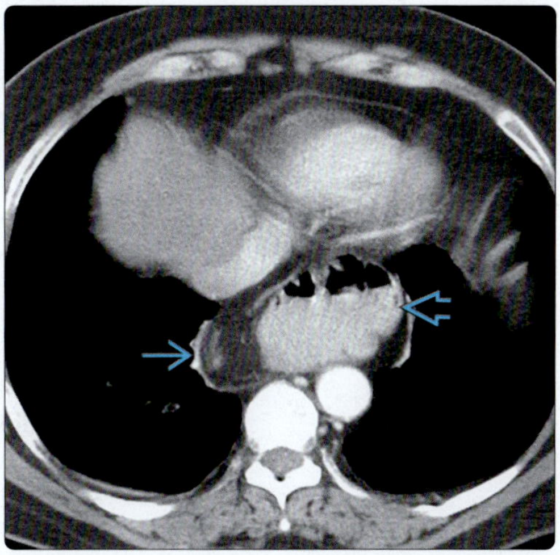

(Left) *PA chest radiograph of an asymptomatic 49-year-old man with a large hiatus hernia shows abnormal convexity and lateral displacement of the lower third of the azygoesophageal recess and a left retrocardiac opacity. Gas within the lesion is consistent with a hiatus hernia.* **(Right)** *Axial CECT of the same patient confirms the presence of a paraesophageal hiatus hernia, which contains a portion of the stomach. Note lateral displacement of the inferior aspect of the azygoesophageal recess.*

Esophageal Carcinoma

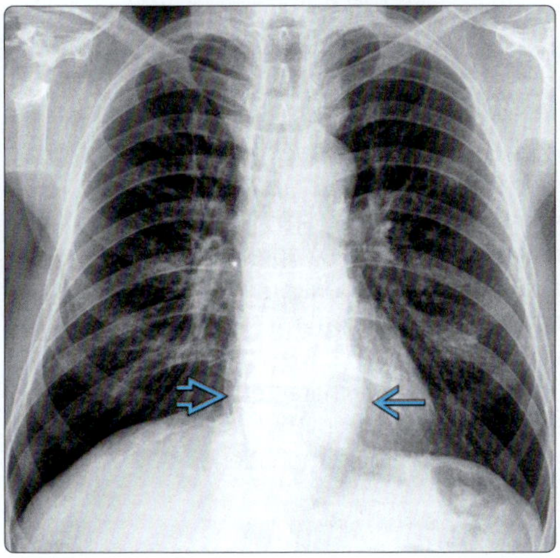

Esophageal Carcinoma

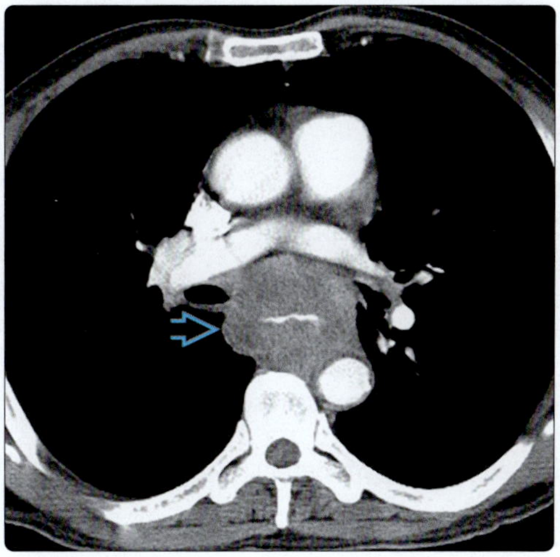

(Left) *PA chest radiograph of a 63-year-old man who presented with severe dysphagia shows abnormal convexity of the lower third of the azygoesophageal recess and a left retrocardiac mass-like opacity.* **(Right)** *Axial CECT of the same patient shows that the radiographic abnormality corresponds to marked circumferential mural thickening of the lower esophagus, which produces an abnormal convexity of the azygoesophageal recess. Biopsy confirmed esophageal carcinoma.*

Congenital Foregut Cyst

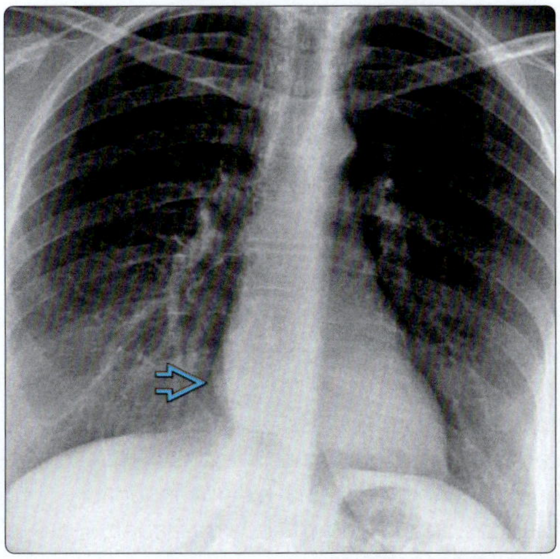

Congenital Foregut Cyst

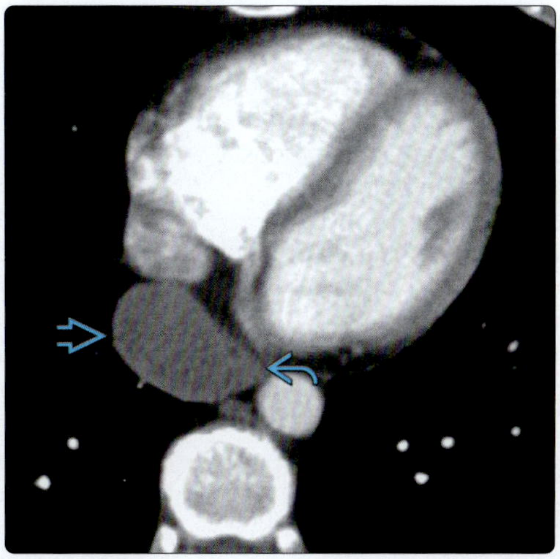

(Left) *PA chest radiograph of a 63-year-old man with an esophageal duplication cyst shows subtle abnormal convexity of the lower third of the azygoesophageal recess.* **(Right)** *Axial CECT of the same patient shows an ovoid water attenuation mass in the visceral mediastinum, which abuts the esophagus and is consistent with a congenital foregut cyst. In this case, an esophageal duplication cyst was diagnosed, which may be indistinguishable from bronchogenic cyst on imaging.*

DIFFERENTIAL DIAGNOSIS

Common

- Lung Cancer
- Lymphoma
  - Non-Hodgkin Lymphoma
  - Hodgkin Lymphoma
- Metastases
- Tuberculosis
- Fungal Infection
- Sarcoidosis
- Heart Failure

Less Common

- Viral Infection
- Nontuberculous Mycobacterial Infection
- Berylliosis
- Silicosis
- Amyloidosis
- Castleman Disease

Rare but Important

- Drug-Induced Lymphadenopathy
- Interstitial Lung Disease

ESSENTIAL INFORMATION

Key Differential Diagnosis Issues

- Increased hilar density: Most common radiographic manifestation of hilar mass
- Lymphadenopathy: Common cause of unilateral or bilateral hilar enlargement
  - Considerable overlap in differential diagnosis
  - Unilateral hilar enlargement: Lung cancer, metastases, lymphoma, infection
  - Bilateral hilar enlargement: Sarcoidosis (symmetric), metastases, lymphoma, infection
- Enlarged pulmonary artery may mimic hilar mass or lymphadenopathy
- CECT is modality of choice for evaluation of hilar lymphadenopathy
  - Low-attenuation/minimal enhancement lymphadenopathy: Tuberculosis, nontuberculous mycobacterial infection, metastases (testicular tumors), Hodgkin lymphoma
  - Calcified lymphadenopathy: Remote granulomatous disease, sarcoidosis, silicosis, metastases (colon adenocarcinoma, osteosarcoma, papillary thyroid carcinoma, lung cancer), amyloidosis, radiated lymphoma
  - Size criteria for mediastinal/hilar lymph node enlargement: > 10 mm in short axis diameter
  - Pericardial recesses may mimic lymphadenopathy

Helpful Clues for Common Diagnoses

- **Lung Cancer**
  - Pulmonary nodule or mass
    - ± locally invasive, spiculated, large, hilar/mediastinal lymphadenopathy
    - Frequent associated with emphysema
  - Lymphadenopathy
    - Ipsilateral lymphadenopathy
      - Soft tissue attenuation, no cavitation, no avid contrast enhancement
      - Rare calcification
    - Associated mediastinal &/or contralateral lymphadenopathy
- **Lymphoma**
  - **Non-Hodgkin Lymphoma**
    - Bilateral, typically asymmetric, mediastinal/hilar lymphadenopathy
      - May exhibit nodal coalescence
    - Involvement of multiple noncontiguous lymph node stations; distant lymph node and extranodal involvement
    - Mild to moderate uniform enhancement
  - **Hodgkin Lymphoma**
    - Frequent intrathoracic involvement and mediastinal lymphadenopathy
    - Homogeneous lobulated anterior/prevascular mediastinal mass ± discrete lymphadenopathy
    - Low attenuation with necrosis, hemorrhage, or cystic change
    - Lymph nodes may calcify following radiation therapy
- **Metastases**
  - Lung cancer
    - Hilar lymphadenopathy (30%)
    - Mediastinal involvement depends on location of primary malignancy
  - Extrapulmonary malignancy: Hilar metastases without mediastinal metastases are exceptional
    - Head and neck cancers, genitourinary cancers, breast cancer, malignant melanoma
- **Tuberculosis**
  - Primary pattern of disease characterized by consolidation ± lymphadenopathy
  - Unilateral hilar/mediastinal lymphadenopathy (80-90% of cases)
  - CECT
    - Lymph nodes with low-attenuation centers and peripheral enhancement
    - Enlarged calcified hilar or mediastinal lymph nodes suggestive of healing
- **Fungal Infection**
  - Histoplasmosis
    - Lymph node involvement by histoplasmosis
    - CECT: Enlarged lymph nodes with central low attenuation from caseous necrosis; frequent calcification with healing
  - Coccidioidomycosis
    - Bronchopneumonia with hilar lymphadenopathy (20%)
    - Rarely bilateral hilar lymphadenopathy without pulmonary involvement
  - Paracoccidioidomycosis (*P. brasiliensis*)
    - More common in Latin America
    - Frequent hilar and mediastinal lymphadenopathy
    - Complications: Suppuration, fistula formation, scarring, pulmonary fibrosis
- **Sarcoidosis**
  - Most common cause of bilateral symmetric hilar lymphadenopathy

- Radiographic 1-2-3 sign or Garland triad: Lymphadenopathy affecting right paratracheal, right hilar, and left hilar lymph nodes
- Lymph nodes may exhibit calcification
  - Amorphous
  - Punctate
  - Eggshell
- Associated perilymphatic micronodules

- **Heart Failure**
  - Frequent mediastinal lymph node enlargement; possibly related to mediastinal edema
  - Enlargement of several mediastinal nodes; less likely to affect hilar lymph nodes or isolated lymph node stations
  - Small size, < 2 cm in short axis
  - Strongly associated with acute volume overload and pleural effusion

Helpful Clues for Less Common Diagnoses

- **Viral Infection**
  - Epstein-Barr virus
    - Generalized lymphadenopathy, including hilar and mediastinal involvement
    - Splenomegaly in 50% of cases
  - Rubeola (measles)
    - Hilar lymphadenopathy (74%) early in course of disease
    - Pulmonary involvement (55%)
- **Nontuberculous Mycobacterial Infection**
  - Extensive hilar (unilateral or bilateral) and paratracheal lymphadenopathy
  - ± parenchymal disease
  - Lymph nodes may exhibit extensive necrosis
- **Berylliosis**
  - Mimics appearance of sarcoidosis
    - Diagnosis supported by documentation of beryllium exposure
  - Hilar or mediastinal lymphadenopathy (40%)
    - Lymph nodes may exhibit diffuse or eggshell calcification
  - Lymphadenopathy always associated with lung involvement
- **Silicosis**
  - Silicosis and coal workers' pneumoconiosis are similar on imaging
    - Lung disease usually less severe in coal workers pneumoconiosis
  - Frequent hilar and mediastinal lymphadenopathy
    - Eggshell calcification (5%)
- **Amyloidosis**
  - Rarely isolated lymphadenopathy, associated with nodular parenchymal and airway involvement
  - Mediastinal and hilar lymphadenopathy may be massive
    - Stippled, diffuse, or eggshell calcification
- **Castleman Disease**
  - Hyaline-vascular type (> 90%): Children and young adults; focal mass; asymptomatic
  - Plasma cell type: 40-50 years of age; lymphadenopathy; systemic illness
  - CECT
    - Lobular contours and well-defined borders
    - Avid contrast enhancement (both forms)
    - Less common: Non- or poorly enhancing areas secondary to focal fibrosis, edema, &/or necrosis

Helpful Clues for Rare Diagnoses

- **Drug-Induced Lymphadenopathy**
  - Phenytoin, bleomycin, carbamazepine, indomethacin, minocycline, interferon-β, penicillin
- **Interstitial Lung Disease**
  - Nonneoplastic lymph node enlargement reported in affected patients

SELECTED REFERENCES

1. Nin CS et al: Thoracic lymphadenopathy in benign diseases: a state of the art review. Respir Med. 112:10-7, 2016
2. Shweihat YR et al: Congestive adenopathy: a mediastinal sequela of volume overload. J Bronchology Interv Pulmonol. 23(4):298-302, 2016
3. Kahraman H et al: Cryptogenic organising pneumonia presenting with bilateral hilar and mediastinal lymphadenopathy. BMJ Case Rep. 2013, 2013

Lung Cancer

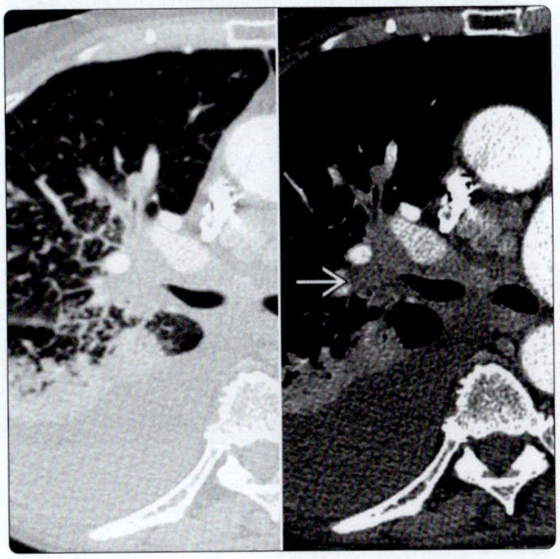

Hodgkin Lymphoma

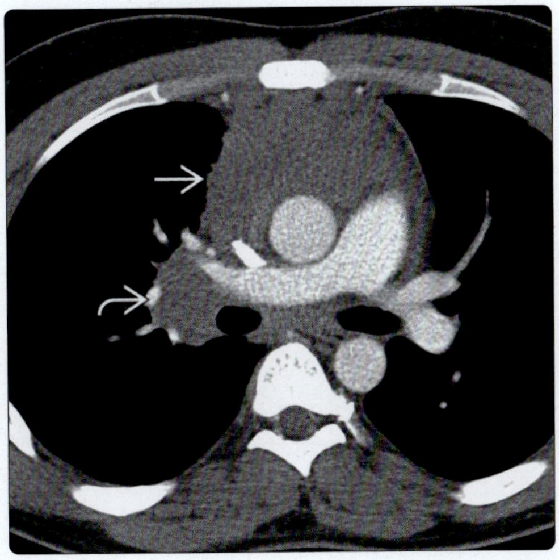

(Left) *Composite image with axial CECT in lung (left) and soft tissue (right) window of a patient with advanced lung cancer shows right hilar lymphadenopathy ➔, a moderate right pleural effusion, and right lung lymphangitic carcinomatosis (left).* **(Right)** *Axial CECT of a 23-year-old man with Hodgkin lymphoma shows coalescent prevascular mediastinal ➔ and right hilar lymphadenopathy ➔. Unilateral hilar lymphadenopathy should raise concern for malignancy.*

(Left) *Axial CECT of a patient with metastatic intrathoracic lymphadenopathy shows multifocal enlarged lymph nodes involving the right paratracheal* ➔*, subcarinal* ➔*, and bilateral hilar* ➔ *lymph node stations. Low-attenuation areas are consistent with necrosis.* **(Right)** *Coronal CECT of a patient with the post primary pattern of tuberculosis shows multiple calcified mediastinal and hilar lymph nodes* ➔ *and a chronic right upper lobe cavitary lesion with an intrinsic mycetoma* ➔*.*

Metastases

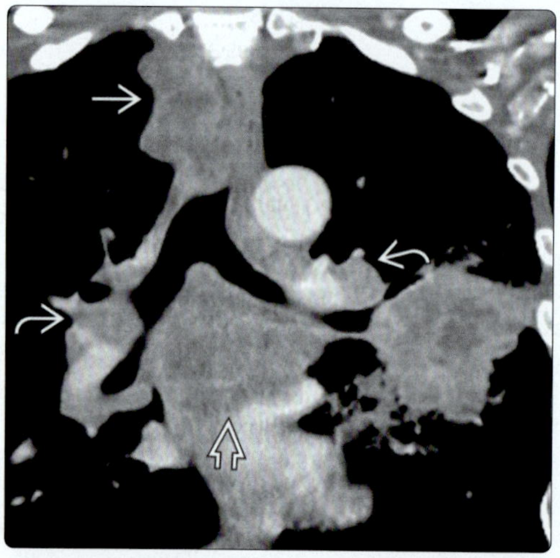

Tuberculosis

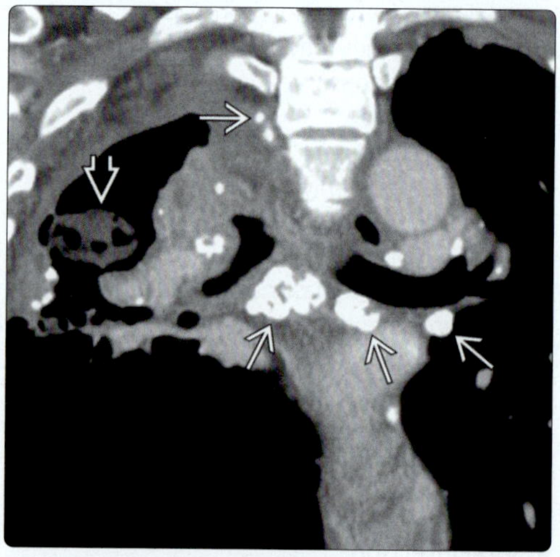

(Left) *Axial CECT of an immunocompromised patient with the primary pattern of tuberculosis shows bilateral lower paratracheal lymphadenopathy* ➔ *with central low attenuation and peripheral enhancement.* **(Right)** *Axial CECT of a patient with acute histoplasmosis shows heterogeneously enhancing right hilar lymphadenopathy* ➔ *with intrinsic low-attenuation foci. A primary pulmonary site of infection is not always identified in these cases. Such necrotic lymph nodes often heal with calcification.*

Tuberculosis

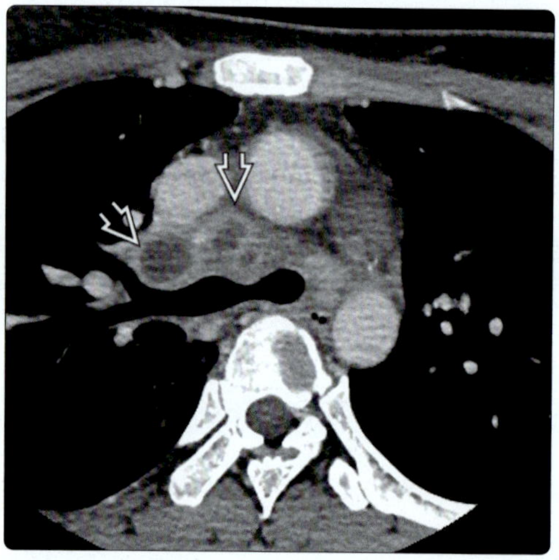

Fungal Infection

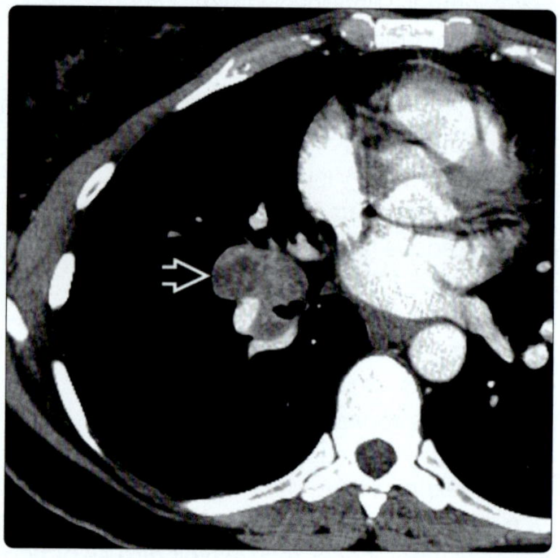

(Left) *PA chest radiograph of a patient with sarcoidosis shows bilateral hilar* ➔ *and right paratracheal* ➔ *lymphadenopathy and the 1-2-3 sign or Garland triad. Note AP window* ➔ *and subcarinal lymphadenopathy.* **(Right)** *Composite image with axial CECT in lung (left) and soft tissue (right) window of a patient with pulmonary edema shows interlobular septal thickening, bilateral pleural effusions, and lymphadenopathy* ➔*. Nonneoplastic lymph node enlargement is described in pulmonary edema.*

Sarcoidosis

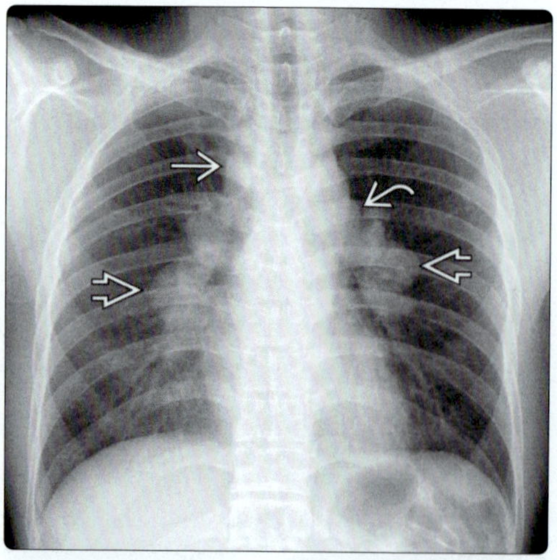

Heart Failure

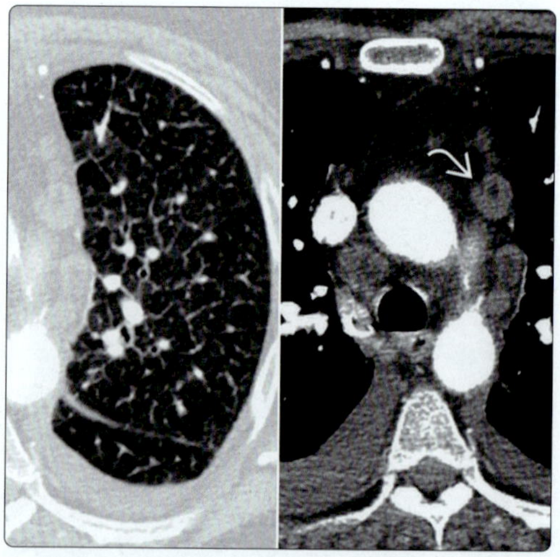

- Benign pressure erosion of adjacent ribs, neuroforamen, vertebrae
- Neurofibromatosis: Multifocal neurogenic tumors

- **Thymic Cyst**
  - Congenital: Unilocular, thymopharyngeal duct remnant
  - Acquired: Multilocular
  - Uncommon: 1% of mediastinal masses
  - CT
    - Prevascular well-circumscribed thymic lesion
      - Spherical, ovoid, elongate
      - Homogeneous water attenuation
      - High-attenuation content: Hemorrhage, proteinaceous fluid
  - MR
    - Distinction between cystic and solid lesions, identification/characterization of solid components
      - Unilocular cyst versus internal septations
      - Mural nodules should suggest cystic neoplasm

Helpful Clues for Rare Diagnoses

- **Thymolipoma**
  - Rare, benign primary encapsulated thymic neoplasm
    - Admixture of thymic and adipose tissue
    - Variable size; average reported size of 20 cm
  - Typically asymptomatic patient
    - May be associated with myasthenia gravis or immune disorders
  - CT/MR
    - Inferior aspect of prevascular mediastinum
    - Anatomic connection to thymus
    - Admixture of fat and soft tissue attenuation/signal
- **Liposarcoma**
  - Mediastinal liposarcoma: < 1% of mediastinal tumors
  - Symptoms: Dyspnea, wheezing, chest pain, superior vena cava compresssion/syndrome
  - CT
    - Manifestations depend on degree of differentiation
    - Greater amount of soft tissue typically denotes higher grade liposarcoma
      - Well differentiated: Fatty mass with soft tissue septa; at least 75% adipose tissue
      - Intermediate grade: < 25% adipose tissue
      - High grade: No fat attenuation, 20% of cases
    - Local invasion, intrathoracic lymphadenopathy, metastatic disease
- **Extramedullary Hematopoiesis**
  - May be asymptomatic; symptoms usually relate to mass effect
  - Compensatory mechanism of red cell production outside of bone marrow
    - Common etiologies
      - Myelofibrosis
      - Thalassemia: Hemosiderosis or hemochromatosis (multiple transfusions)
      - Chronic hemolysis
      - Sickle cell disease
      - Diffuse osseous metastases, leukemia, bone marrow irradiation
    - Fat-containing paravertebral soft tissue mass(es)
    - Expansion of adjacent ribs/osseous structures
  - CT
    - Paravertebral soft tissue mass(es)
      - Typically bilateral
      - May exhibit intrinsic fat
      - Differential diagnosis: Neurogenic neoplasm, lymphoma, Castleman disease

SELECTED REFERENCES

1. Rosti G et al: Primary mediastinal germ cell tumors. Semin Oncol. 46(2):107-11, 2019
2. Roberts AS et al: Extramedullary haematopoiesis: radiological imaging features. Clin Radiol. 71(9):807-14, 2016
3. Occhipinti M et al: Imaging the posterior mediastinum: a multimodality approach. Diagn Interv Radiol. 21(4):293-306, 2015
4. Carter BW et al: Approaching the patient with an anterior mediastinal mass: a guide for radiologists. J Thorac Oncol. 9(9 Suppl 2):S110-8, 2014
5. Juanpere S et al: A diagnostic approach to the mediastinal masses. Insights Imaging. 4(1):29-52, 2013
6. Hahn HP et al: Primary mediastinal liposarcoma: clinicopathologic analysis of 24 cases. Am J Surg Pathol. 31(12):1868-74, 2007

Thymoma

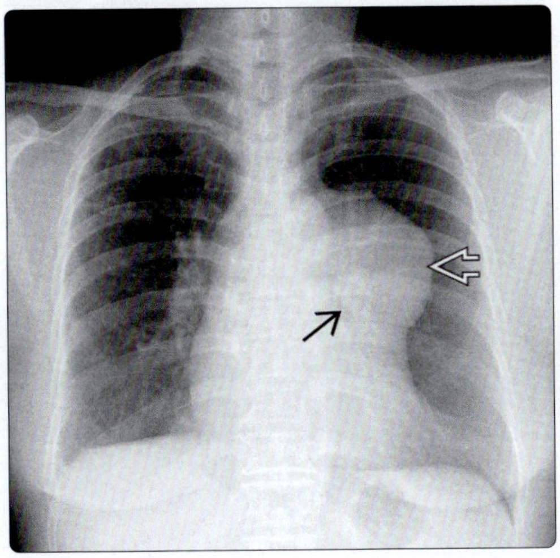

Thymoma

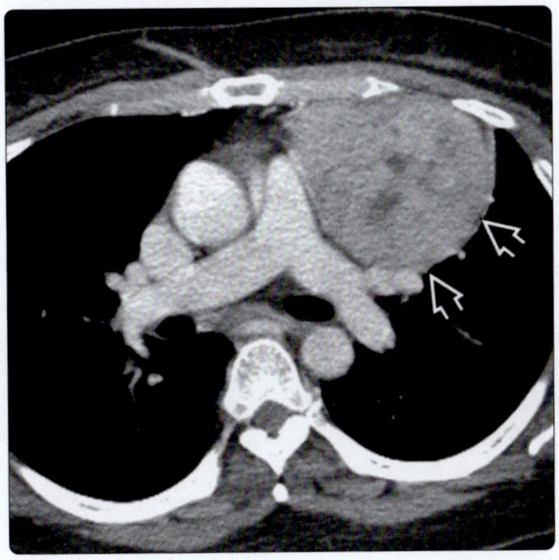

(Left) *PA chest radiograph of an asymptomatic woman shows an incidentally discovered left anterior mediastinal mass ➡. The left pulmonary artery ⇨ is visible through the lesion, consistent with the hilum overlay sign.* **(Right)** *Axial CECT of the same patient confirms the left prevascular heterogeneously enhancing mediastinal soft tissue mass ➡. The lesion is sharply marginated, and there is a visible tissue plane between it and the adjacent pulmonary artery. An encapsulated thymoma was diagnosed at surgery.*

(Left) *PA chest radiograph of an asymptomatic 34-year-old woman shows a left anterior mediastinal mass that demonstrates the hilum overlay sign with visualization of the left pulmonary artery through the lesion.* **(Right)** *Axial CECT of the same patient shows a left prevascular mediastinal mass of heterogeneous attenuation. The lesion exhibits soft tissue, fluid, and fat attenuation, virtually diagnostic of a mature teratoma. Note mass effect on the left pulmonary artery.*

Germ Cell Neoplasm

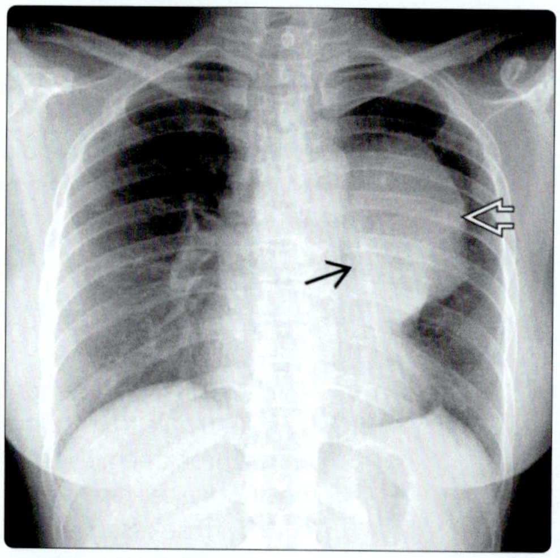

Germ Cell Neoplasm

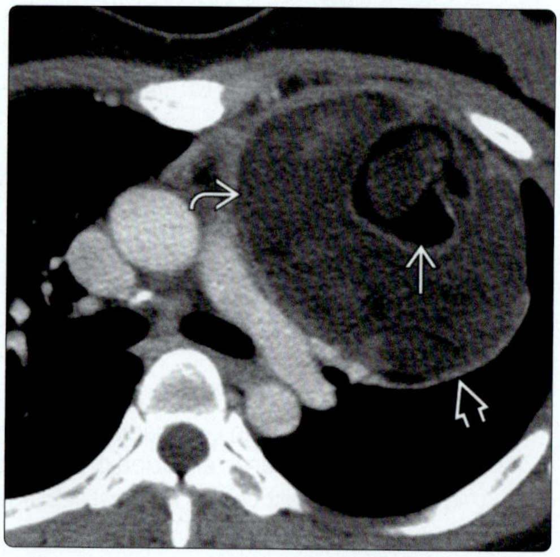

(Left) *PA chest radiograph of a patient with night sweats and weight loss shows a well-defined left anterior mediastinal mass that exhibits the hilum overlay sign with visualization of the left pulmonary artery through the lesion.* **(Right)** *Axial CECT of the same patient shows a heterogeneously enhancing soft tissue mass in the prevascular mediastinum involving both sides of midline. Note absence of a tissue plane between the lesion and the pulmonary trunk. Biopsy confirmed the diagnosis of Hodgkin lymphoma.*

Lymphoma

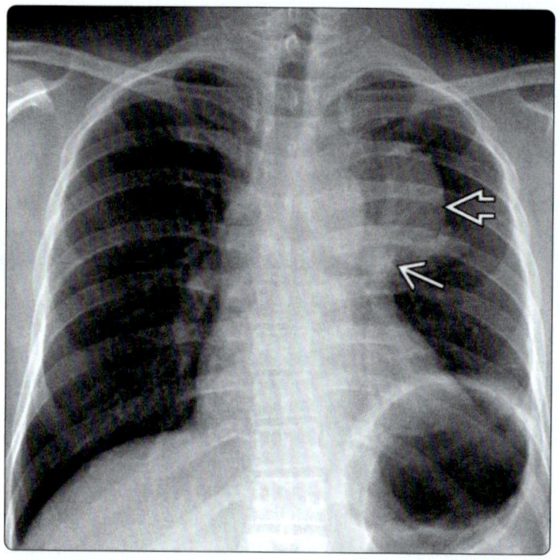

Lymphoma

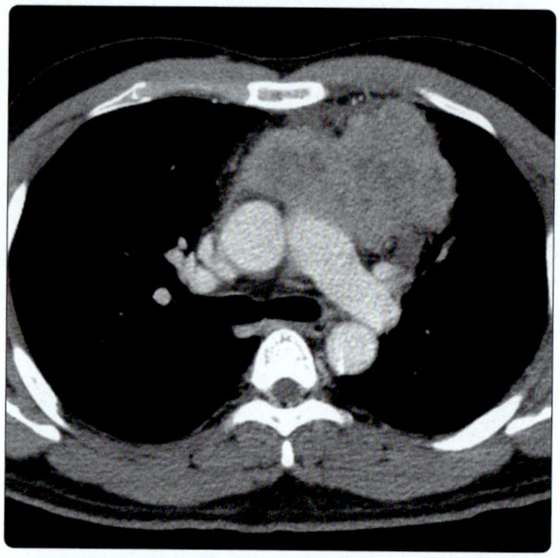

(Left) *PA chest radiograph of an asymptomatic older woman shows a large left anterior mediastinal mass. Note the normal left hilum visible through the lesion. A portion of the mass extends superiorly into the neck and produces mass effect on the left trachea.* **(Right)** *Coronal CECT of the same patient shows a large mass continuous with a thyroid goiter and an exophytic mediastinal component. The lesions exhibit Ca^{++} and cystic changes. The findings are consistent with a thyroid goiter.*

Thyroid Goiter

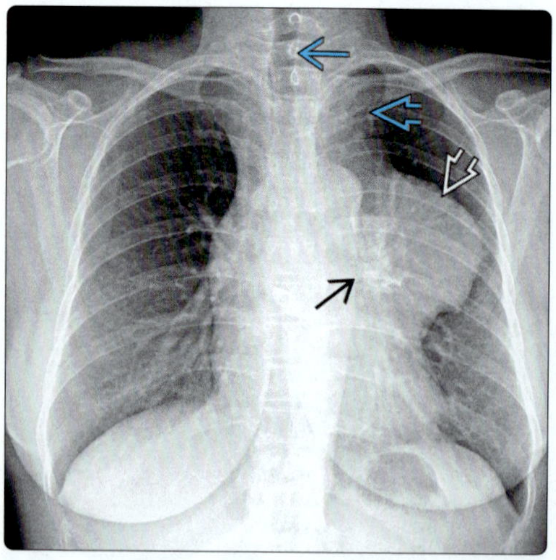

Thyroid Goiter

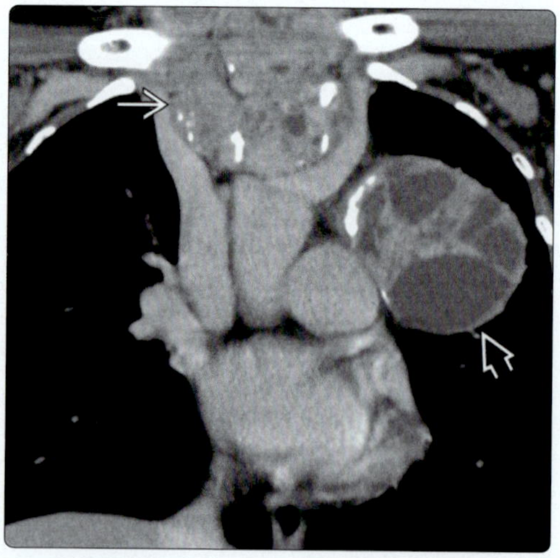

Schwannoma

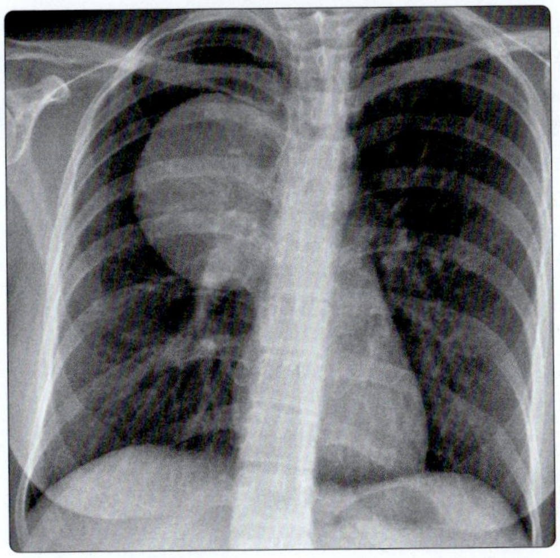

Schwannoma

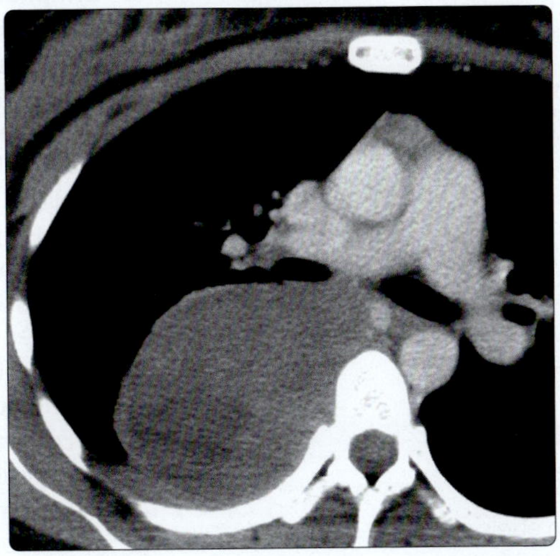

(Left) *PA chest radiograph of an asymptomatic 34-year-old woman shows a large mediastinal mass that projects over the right hilum and exhibits the hilum overlay sign. Thus, the lesion is located either anterior or posterior to the hilum.* **(Right)** *Axial CECT of the same patient demonstrates a heterogeneously enhancing right paravertebral mediastinal mass. A mediastinal schwannoma was diagnosed on surgical excision. Imaging evaluation should always include MR to exclude intraspinal involvement.*

Ganglioneuroma

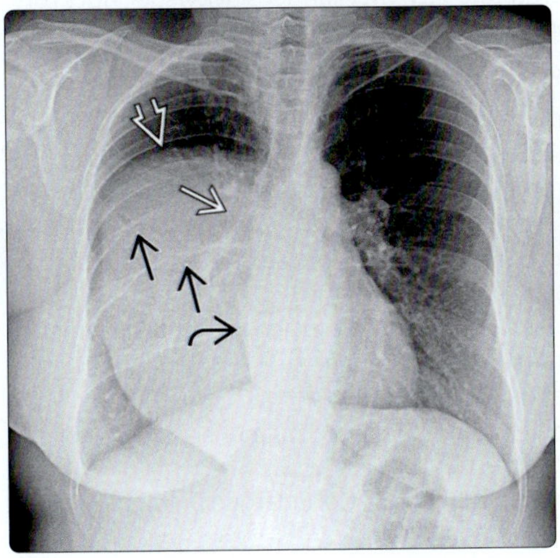

Ganglioneuroma

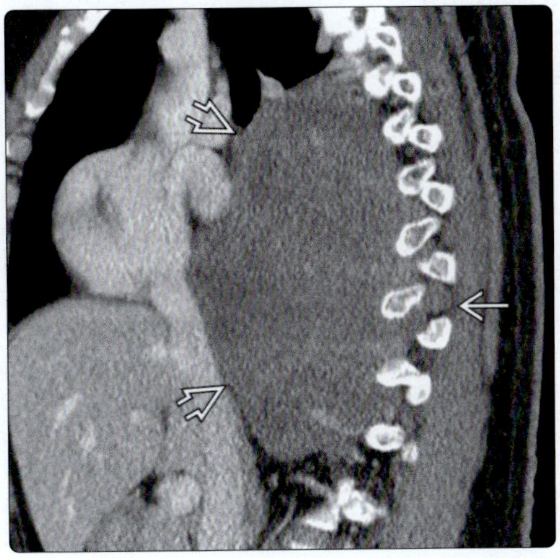

(Left) *PA chest radiograph of an adolescent girl shows a well-demarcated right mediastinal mass ➡ through which the right hilum ➡ and the right heart border ➡ are visible. Note benign pressure erosion of the adjacent right posterior ribs ➡, suggestive of neurogenic neoplasm.* **(Right)** *Sagittal CECT shows a heterogeneously enhancing right paravertebral mass ➡ with associated neuroforaminal involvement ➡. The elongate morphology of the lesion is consistent with a ganglioneuroma.*

Extramedullary Hematopoiesis

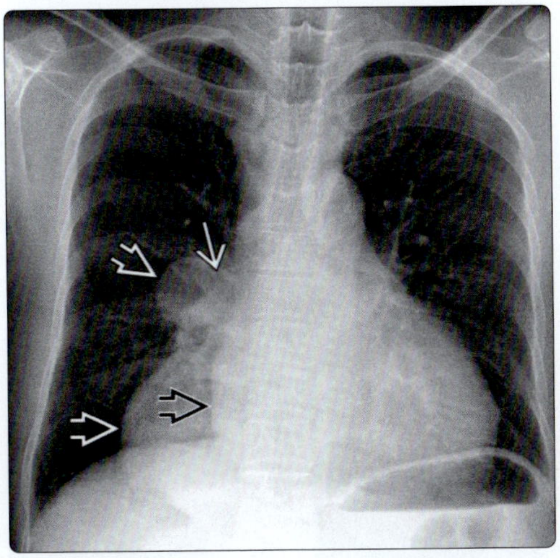

Extramedullary Hematopoiesis

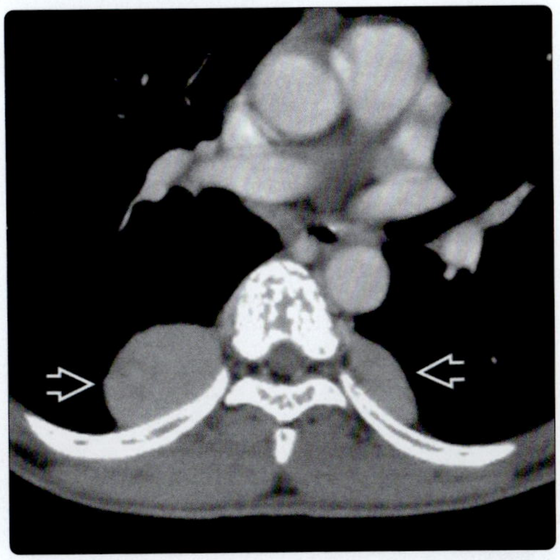

(Left) *PA chest radiograph of an adult patient with hemolytic anemia shows a polylobular right mediastinal mass ➡. The right hilum ➡ and right cardiac border ➡ are visible through the lesion, indicating that while the mass overlies the hilum it does not involve it.* **(Right)** *Axial CECT of the same patient shows bilateral paravertebral mediastinal soft tissue masses ➡. Associated abnormal vertebral mineralization is consistent with suspected extramedullary hematopoiesis.*

DIFFERENTIAL DIAGNOSIS

Common

- Lung Cancer
- Reactive Lymphadenopathy

Less Common

- Lymphoma
- Metastatic Disease
- Carcinoid Tumor

Rare but Important

- Castleman Disease
- Pulmonary Artery Enlargement

ESSENTIAL INFORMATION

Key Differential Diagnosis Issues

- Malignancy is most common etiology
  - Risk factors for lung cancer &/or known malignancy
- Reactive lymphadenopathy may occur with some infections

Helpful Clues for Common Diagnoses

- **Lung Cancer**
  - Squamous cell carcinoma
    - Central location, ± bronchial obstruction, postobstructive atelectasis/pneumonia
    - ± hilar/mediastinal lymphadenopathy
  - Small cell carcinoma
    - Typically central mass, rapid growth
    - Frequent lymphadenopathy
    - Encasement/invasion of adjacent structures
    - 60-70% of patients have metastases at diagnosis
    - Osseous metastases or direct osseous invasion
    - Associated paraneoplastic syndromes
- **Reactive Lymphadenopathy**
  - Typically related to pulmonary infection
    - Fungi, tuberculosis, bacteria, mononucleosis
  - Ipsilateral consolidation, nodules, bronchiolitis
  - Tuberculosis: Central low attenuation, peripheral enhancement

Helpful Clues for Less Common Diagnoses

- **Lymphoma**
  - Mediastinal ± hilar lymphadenopathy
  - Typically Hodgkin lymphoma
    - Frequent hilar and extramediastinal lymphadenopathy; may be asymmetric
- **Metastatic Disease**
  - History of malignancy
    - Head and neck cancer, breast cancer, melanoma, genitourinary malignancy
  - Enhancing lymph nodes: Renal cell and thyroid cancers, melanoma
  - Necrotic lymph nodes: Breast, testicular, renal cancers
- **Carcinoid Tumor**
  - Low-grade neuroendocrine malignancy
  - Typically central location
  - Frequent bronchial relationship: Endobronchial, partially endobronchial, abutting bronchus
    - ± postobstructive atelectasis/pneumonia
  - May exhibit contrast enhancement &/or calcification
  - Gallium-Dotatate PET/CT: High sensitivity/specificity for detection of carcinoid tumors

Helpful Clues for Rare Diagnoses

- **Castleman Disease**
  - Unicentric Castleman disease
  - Typically asymptomatic
  - 70% of cases involve thorax
    - Solitary or multiple tracheobronchial, hilar, mediastinal lymph nodes
  - May exhibit calcification, intense contrast enhancement
- **Pulmonary Artery Enlargement**
  - Various etiologies
    - Pulmonic stenosis: Enlarged pulmonary trunk and left pulmonary artery
    - Absence of pulmonic valve: Enlarged pulmonary trunk and left pulmonary artery
    - Pulmonary artery aneurysm or pseudoaneurysm
    - Intravascular tumor: Primary pulmonary artery sarcoma, endovascular metastasis

Lung Cancer

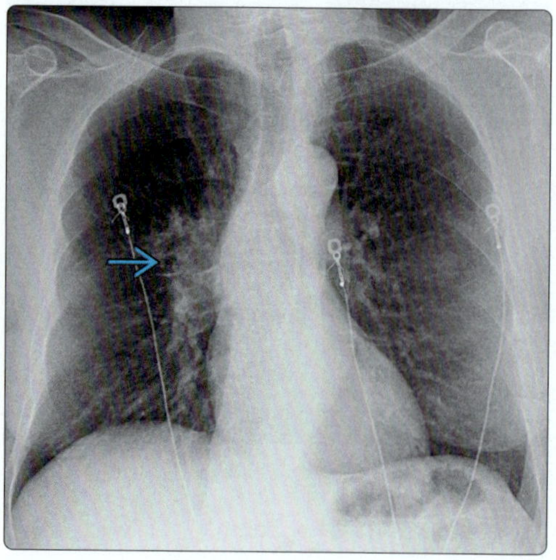

Lung Cancer

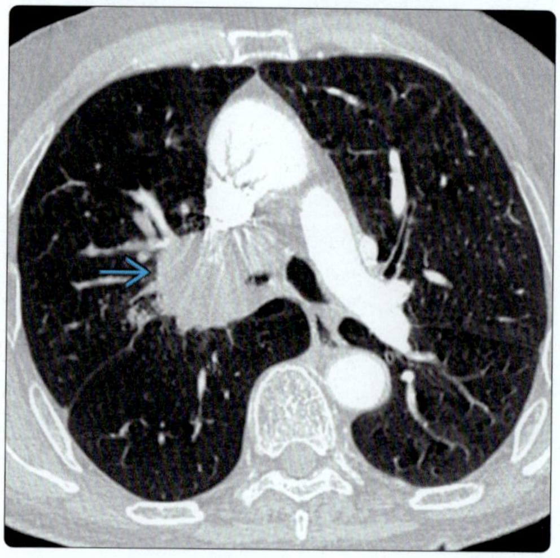

(Left) *PA chest radiograph of a 62-year-old man who presented with cough and chest pain shows asymmetric enlargement and abnormal convexity of the right hilum* ➔ *secondary to a large centrally obstructing primary lung cancer.* **(Right)** *Axial CECT of the same patient shows a large right hilar mass* ➔ *that encases and nearly obliterates the right mainstem bronchus and its branches and the right pulmonary arteries and veins, which accounts for the radiographic abnormality. Biopsy demonstrated squamous cell carcinoma.*

Lung Cancer

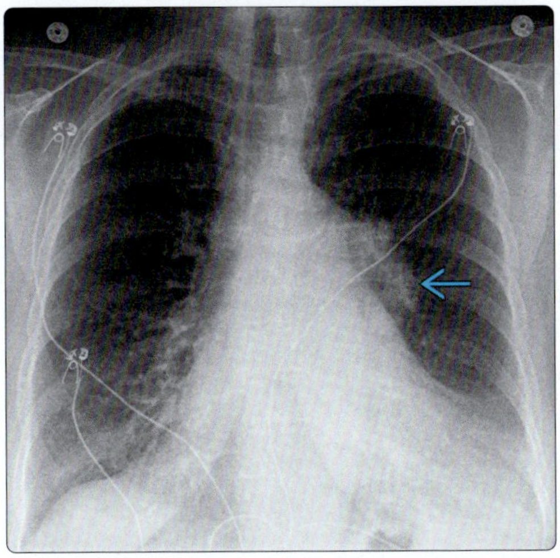

Lung Cancer

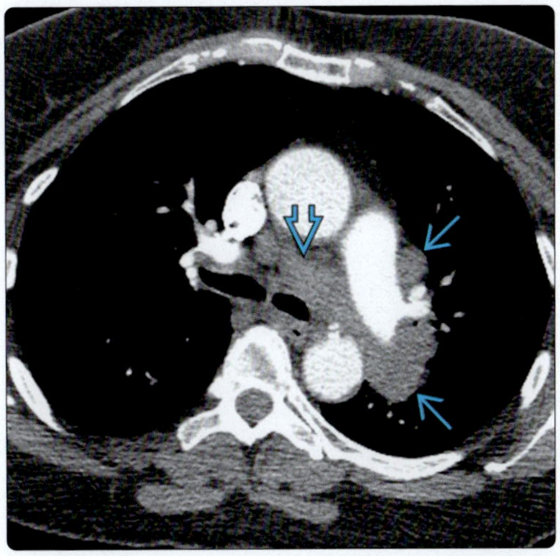

(Left) *PA chest radiograph of a 60-year-old woman who presented with dyspnea and chest pain shows asymmetric enlargement of the left hilum secondary to a left hilar mass. The findings are highly concerning for primary lung cancer.* **(Right)** *Axial CECT of the same patient shows extensive left hilar lymphadenopathy that encases the left pulmonary artery as well as mediastinal lymphadenopathy. A pulmonary mass was not visualized. Biopsy revealed small cell lung cancer.*

Reactive Lymphadenopathy

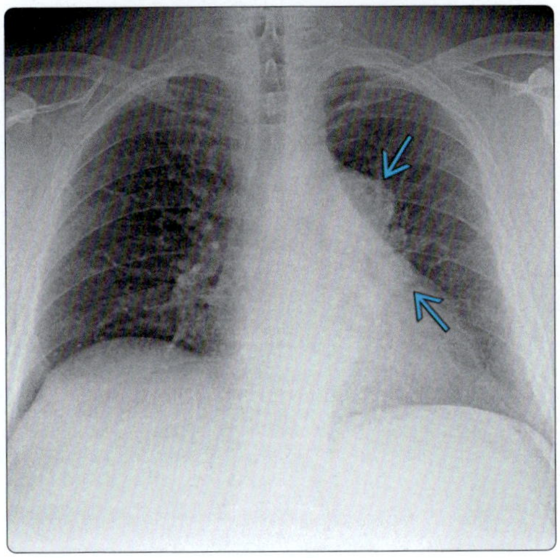

Reactive Lymphadenopathy

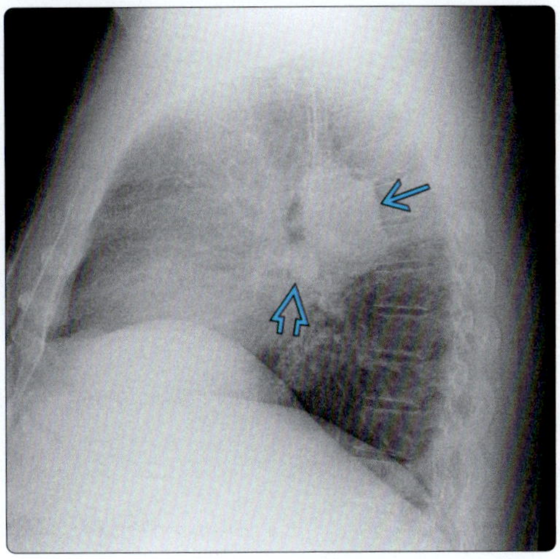

(Left) *PA chest radiograph of a 45-year-old man shows asymmetric left hilar masses that exhibit intrinsic calcification and are most consistent with residual calcified hilar lymph nodes from remote histoplasmosis infection.* **(Right)** *Lateral chest radiograph of the same patient confirms enlargement of the left hilum secondary to enlarged calcified lymph nodes. Note calcified soft tissue in the infrahilar window, consistent with subcarinal lymph node involvement.*

Reactive Lymphadenopathy

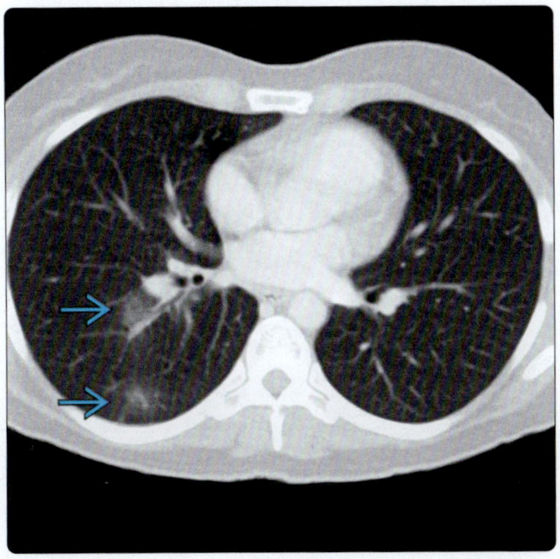

Reactive Lymphadenopathy

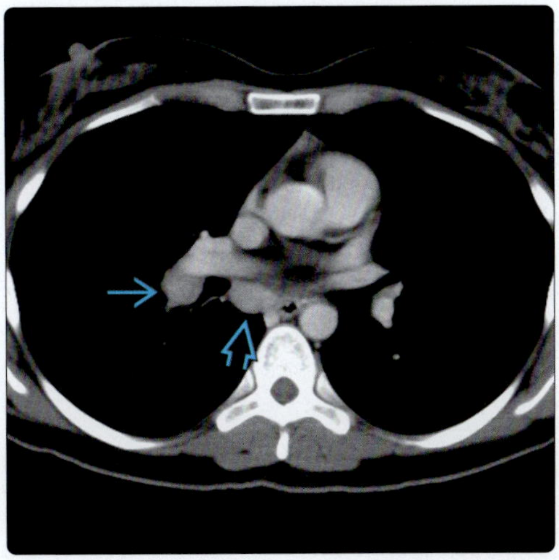

(Left) *Axial CECT (lung window) of a 29-year-old man who presented with cough and fever shows multifocal right lower lobe ground-glass opacity nodules.* **(Right)** *Axial CECT (soft tissue window) of the same patient shows asymmetric right hilar and paraesophageal lymphadenopathy. Reactive unilateral lymphadenopathy may occur in patients with acute fungal infection. Bacterial and mycobacterial pulmonary infections may also produce reactive lymphadenopathy.*

(Left) *PA chest radiograph of a 34-year-old woman who presented with malaise and fatigue shows right hilar lymphadenopathy and polylobular enlargement of the upper mediastinum, consistent with multifocal intrathoracic lymphadenopathy. In this patient demographic, the most likely diagnosis is lymphoma. Hodgkin lymphoma was confirmed on biopsy.* **(Right)** *Axial CECT of the same patient shows right hilar and subcarinal lymphadenopathy.*

Lymphoma

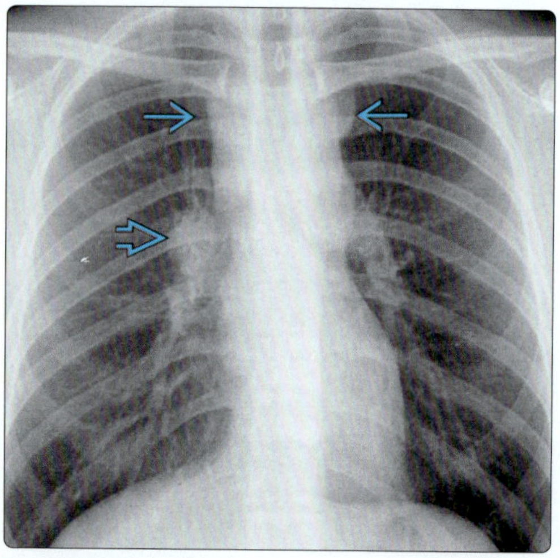

Lymphoma

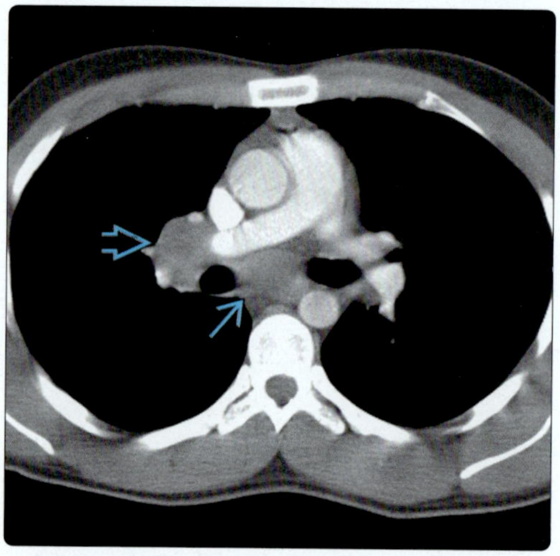

(Left) *PA chest radiograph of a 59-year-old man with metastatic renal cell carcinoma shows right hilar and mediastinal lymphadenopathy. Mass effect on the medial aspect of the bronchus intermedius is consistent with subcarinal lymphadenopathy.* **(Right)** *Axial CECT of the same patient shows right hilar and subcarinal lymphadenopathy. Lymphadenopathy is a characteristic manifestation of intrathoracic metastatic renal cell carcinoma.*

Metastatic Disease

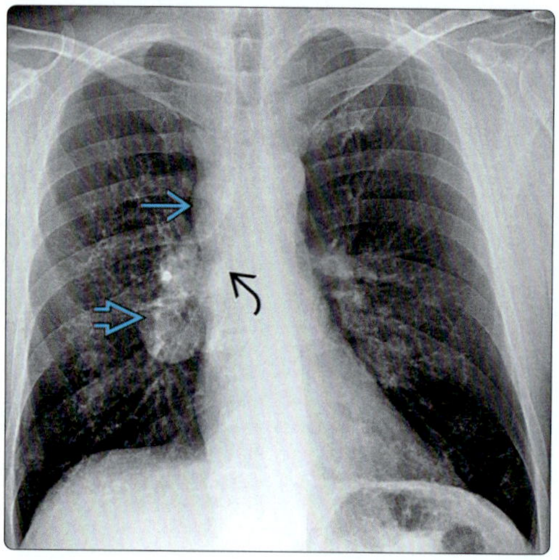

Metastatic Disease

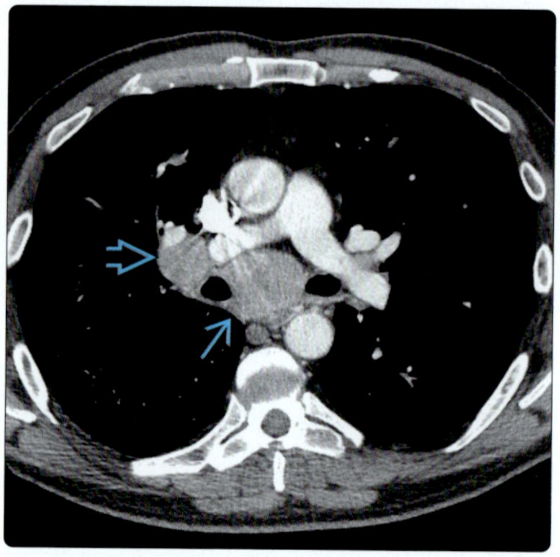

(Left) *Axial CECT (lung window) of a 58-year-old woman with metastatic adrenal cortical carcinoma shows left hilar lymphadenopathy and an enlarged left lower lobe perifissural intrapulmonary lymph node.* **(Right)** *Axial CECT (soft tissue window) of the same patient shows heterogeneously enhancing left hilar lymphadenopathy with low attenuation areas, consistent with necrosis. Metastatic genitourinary malignancies often involve hilar and mediastinal lymph nodes.*

Metastatic Disease

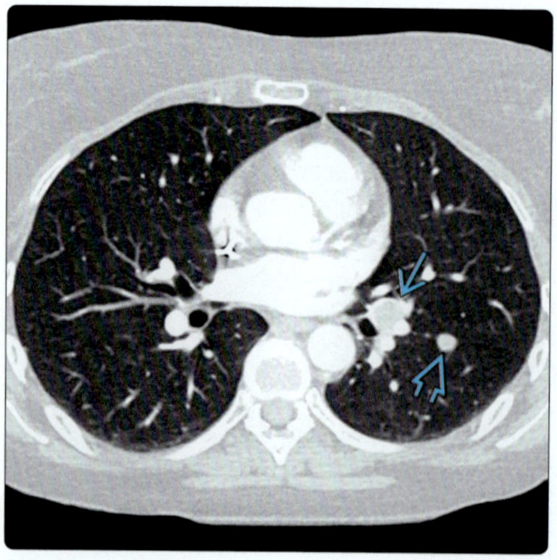

Metastatic Disease

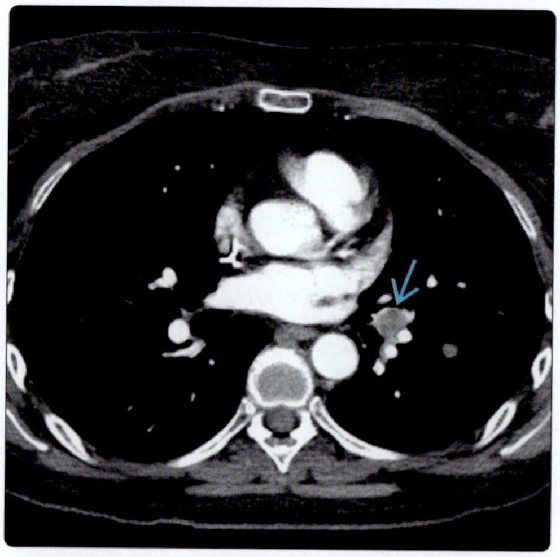

Lymphoma

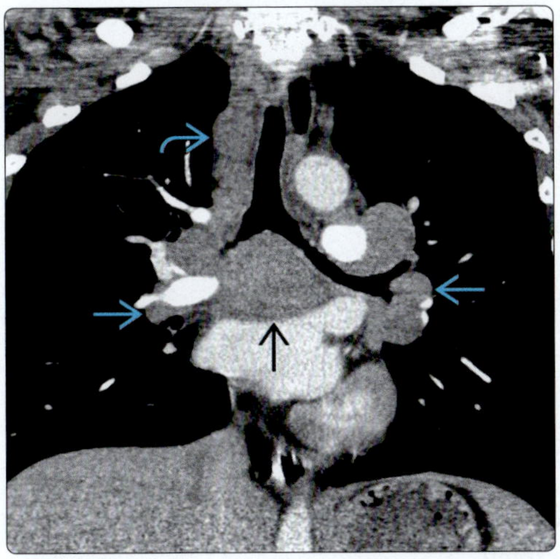

Metastatic Lymphadenopathy

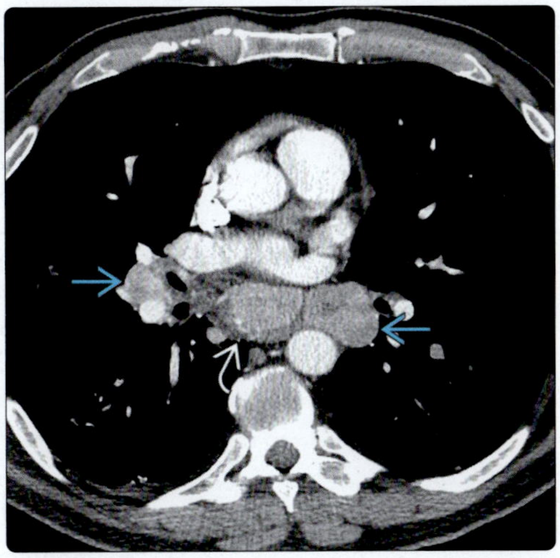

(Left) *Coronal CECT of a 34-year-old man with Hodgkin lymphoma shows multifocal intrathoracic lymphadenopathy that affects the bilateral hila* → *as well as the subcarinal* → *and right paratracheal* → *regions.* **(Right)** *Axial CECT of a 55-year-old man with renal cell carcinoma shows enhancing metastatic lymphadenopathy involving the bilateral hila* → *and the subcarinal* → *regions. Neoplastic lymphadenopathy may mimic reactive lymphadenopathy and sarcoidosis.*

Silicosis/Coal Workers' Pneumoconiosis

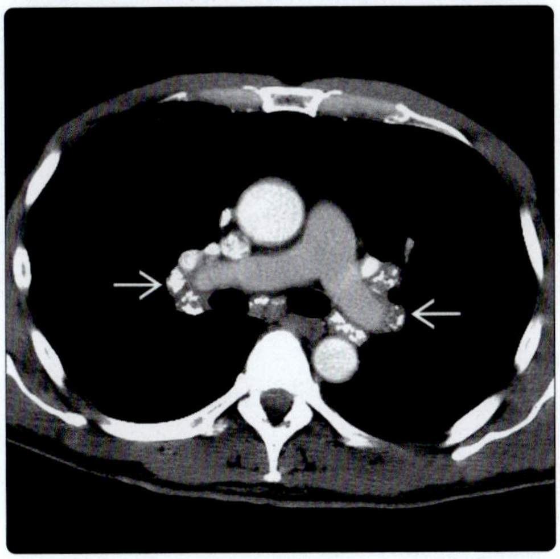

Silicosis/Coal Workers' Pneumoconiosis

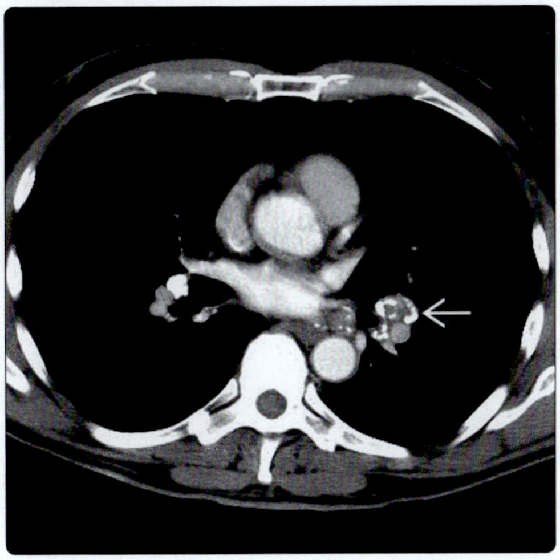

(Left) *Axial CECT of a 70-year-old man with silicosis shows multifocal bilateral enlarged and nonenlarged mediastinal and hilar* → *lymph nodes that exhibit complete and clustered punctate calcifications. Associated upper lung zone-predominant small nodules &/or upper lobe mass-like fibrosis and a history of exposure help support the diagnosis.* **(Right)** *Axial CECT of the same patient shows asymmetric bilateral calcified hilar and interlobar lymph nodes. Note eggshell pattern of lymph node calcification* →.

Amyloidosis

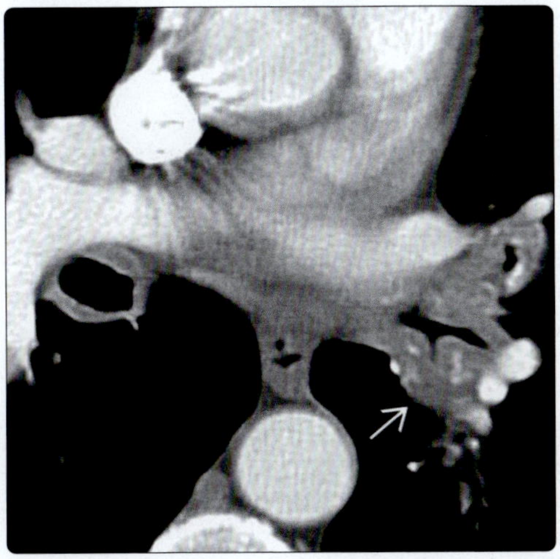

Multicentric Castleman Disease

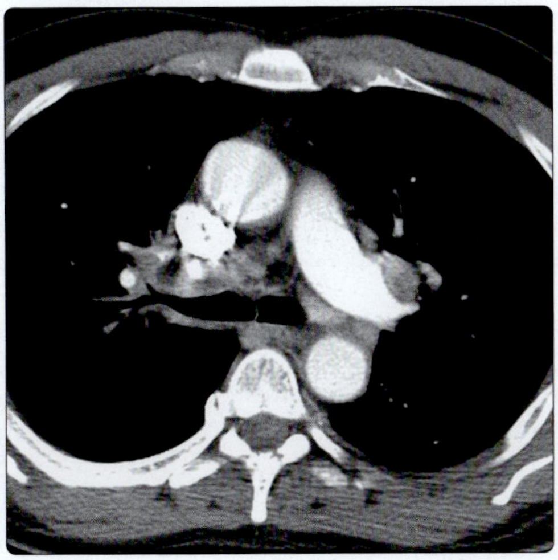

(Left) *Axial CECT of a patient with proven tracheobronchial amyloidosis shows bilateral nodular central bronchial wall thickening with intrinsic punctate calcifications that produces hilar enlargement* → *and mimics lymphadenopathy.* **(Right)** *Axial CECT of a 60-year-old man with multicentric Castleman disease shows bilateral hilar and mediastinal lymphadenopathy. Affected lymph nodes exhibit heterogeneous contrast enhancement, a characteristic imaging feature.*

DIFFERENTIAL DIAGNOSIS

Common

- Pleural Effusion
- Atelectasis
- Pneumothorax

Less Common

- Pneumonectomy
- Radiation Fibrosis
- Tuberculosis

Rare but Important

- Hemothorax
- Fibrothorax
- Malignancy
- Chylothorax
- Diaphragmatic Hernia
- Scimitar Syndrome

ESSENTIAL INFORMATION

Key Differential Diagnosis Issues

- Direction of mediastinal shift
  - Ipsilateral shift
    - Loss of volume in affected hemithorax
    - Atelectasis, pneumonectomy, fibrothorax
  - Contralateral mediastinal shift
    - Increased volume in affected hemithorax
    - Pleural effusion, pneumothorax, hemothorax, diaphragmatic hernia

Helpful Clues for Common Diagnoses

- **Pleural Effusion**
  - Opaque hemithorax
  - Etiology of large pleural effusion
    - Empyema, malignant pleural effusion, chylothorax, hemothorax
  - CT
    - Malignancy: Circumferential nodular pleural thickening > 1 cm
    - Smooth pleural thickening and parietal pleural enhancement seen in exudative pleural effusion
- **Atelectasis**
  - Diminished expansion of all or part of lung with corresponding diminution in lung volume
    - Collapse: Term reserved for complete atelectasis
    - Acute: Aspirated foreign material, mucus plug
    - Chronic: Endobronchial neoplasm, compression by adjacent mass
  - Direct signs: Fissural displacement toward collapsed lobe, ipsilateral mediastinal shift
  - Indirect signs: Pulmonary opacification, shift of other structures to compensate for volume loss
  - Patterns of mediastinal shift
    - Lobar collapse
      - Triangular shape, homogeneous opacity
      - Anterior and middle mediastinal compartments more mobile
    - Total lung collapse
      - Opaque affected hemithorax
      - Mediastinal and hilar shift toward affected side
      - Elevation of ipsilateral hemidiaphragm
      - Hyperinflation of contralateral lung (enlarged retrosternal air space)
- **Pneumothorax**
  - Convex thin pleural line paralleling chest wall
  - Air density without intrinsic vascular markings adjacent to pleural line
  - Tension pneumothorax
    - Clinical diagnosis: Chest pain, hypoxia, circulatory collapse
    - Imaging
      - Contralateral mediastinal shift
      - Diaphragmatic flattening
      - Widened rib interspaces
      - Complete lung collapse

Helpful Clues for Less Common Diagnoses

- **Pneumonectomy**
  - Ipsilateral mediastinal shift
  - Small hemithorax + ipsilateral surgical changes
  - Opaque hemithorax secondary to fluid in pneumonectomy space
- **Radiation Fibrosis**
  - Important threshold doses
    - Seldom visible with ≤ 30 Gy
    - Nearly always visible with ≥ 40 Gy
  - Incidence increases with 2nd course of therapy
  - Occurs 6-12 months after radiotherapy
  - No progression 2 years after radiotherapy
  - Imaging
    - Ipsilateral mediastinal shift
    - Volume loss, traction bronchiectasis, pleural thickening
    - Fibrosis does not conform to lobar or segmental boundaries
    - Sharp straight demarcation corresponding to radiation portals
- **Tuberculosis**
  - Cicatrization atelectasis and lung destruction from severe or untreated infection
  - Activity difficult to determine in destroyed lung without comparison radiographs
  - Common locations
    - Upper lobes, lower lobe superior segments
  - Imaging
    - Parenchyma
      - Upper lobe atelectasis, ipsilateral mediastinal shift
      - Fibrosis, traction bronchiectasis, hilar retraction, adjacent emphysema
      - Cavities
    - Airways: Tracheobronchial stenosis with long segment luminal narrowing and mural thickening
    - CT features of active disease
      - Tree-in-bud opacities indicating endobronchial spread of infection
      - Cavitation
      - Consolidation
      - Rim-enhancing lymphadenopathy

Helpful Clues for Rare Diagnoses

- **Hemothorax**
  - Most common cause: Penetrating or blunt trauma
  - Less common associations
    - Aortic dissection, ruptured aneurysm, coagulopathy
  - Radiography
    - Rapidly increased pleural effusion
    - Contralateral mediastinal shift
  - CT
    - High-attenuation pleural fluid (≥ 30 HU)
    - May see fluid-fluid levels; hematocrit effect
- **Fibrothorax**
  - Marked unilateral pleural thickening ± calcification
  - Ipsilateral mediastinal shift
  - Severe pleural inflammation
    - Hemothorax
    - Empyema, tuberculosis
    - Therapeutic pleurodesis
- **Malignancy**
  - Airways: Endobronchial lesion or extraluminal airway compression with resultant atelectasis
  - Mediastinum: Germ cell neoplasm, thymoma, thymic carcinoma
  - Pleura: Malignant mesothelioma, pleural metastases with large malignant pleural effusion
- **Chylothorax**
  - Obstruction by tumor, complication of surgery or trauma, infection (tuberculosis), idiopathic
  - CT
    - Variable attenuation or near water density
    - Indistinguishable from transudative pleural effusion
  - MR
    - Signal intensity similar to that of subcutaneous fat
- **Diaphragmatic Hernia**
  - Diaphragmatic rupture with intrathoracic herniation of abdominal organs
    - High-energy blunt or penetrating trauma
    - Associated injuries: Pneumo-/hemothorax, rib fractures, pulmonary contusion/laceration
    - Radiography: Intrathoracic herniation of hollow viscus (stomach, colon, small bowel) ± focal constriction of viscus at site of diaphragmatic tear (collar sign)
    - CT: Diaphragmatic discontinuity, intrathoracic herniation of abdominal organ(s), focal constriction of viscus at site of diaphragmatic tear (collar sign)
  - Bochdalek hernia
    - Location: Posterior, L > R
    - Majority are small, contain fat, and are incidental findings
    - May be large and contain bowel or kidney; contralateral mediastinal shift
  - Morgagni hernia
    - Anterior and right-sided
    - Contains omental fat with small omental vessels
    - Most common herniated viscera is colon
  - Congenital diaphragmatic hernia
    - Developmental agenesis of portion of diaphragm
    - May be diagnosed prenatally with fetal ultrasound or MR
- **Scimitar Syndrome**
  - Right lung hypoplasia with ipsilateral mediastinal shift
  - Anomalous pulmonary venous return of portion of or all of affected lung
    - Vein (scimitar vein) parallels right heart border (scimitar sign)
  - Decreased size of right pulmonary artery
  - Systemic collaterals to portions of right lung
  - Associated congenital heart disease in 25%

SELECTED REFERENCES

1. Alhassan S et al: Extensive calcified fibrothorax. Am J Respir Crit Care Med. 195(4):e25-6, 2017
2. Iochum S et al: Imaging of diaphragmatic injury: a diagnostic challenge? Radiographics. 22 Spec No:S103-16; discussion S116-8, 2002
3. Proto AV: Lobar collapse: basic concepts. Eur J Radiol. 23(1):9-22, 1996
4. Woodring JH et al: Radiographic manifestations of lobar atelectasis. J Thorac Imaging. 11(2):109-44, 1996
5. Wiegel BJ et al: General case of the day. Idiopathic chylothorax. Radiographics. 13(6):1403-6, 1993

Pleural Effusion

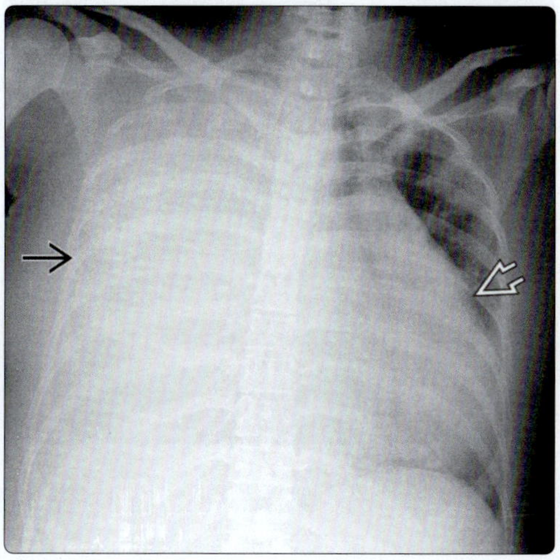

Atelectasis

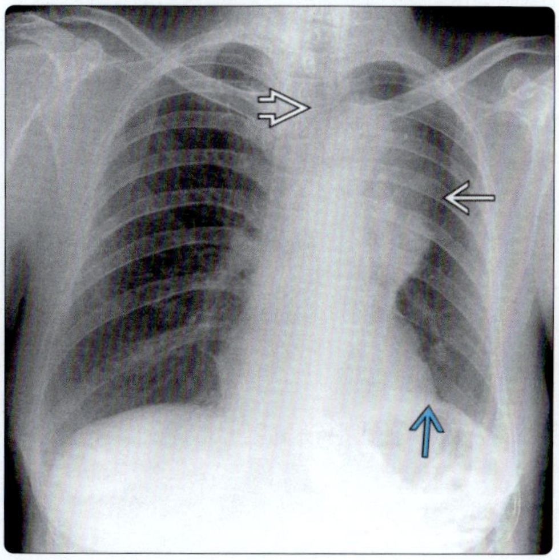

(Left) *PA chest radiograph of a patient who presented with progressive dyspnea shows an opaque right hemithorax ➔ secondary to a massive right pleural effusion. Note contralateral shift of the mediastinum ➔ secondary to mass effect from the large pleural effusion.* **(Right)** *PA chest radiograph shows complete left upper lobe atelectasis manifesting with an ill-defined left upper lung zone opacity ➔. Note associated ipsilateral shift of the trachea ➔ and mediastinum, and elevation of the left hemidiaphragm ➔.*

(**Left**) *Axial CECT of a patient with acute hypoxia shows complete left lung atelectasis → secondary to a centrally obstructive mucus plug → that fills the lumen of the left mainstem bronchus. Note mediastinal shift to the left and a small left pleural effusion →.* (**Right**) *AP chest radiograph of a patient who presented with acute chest pain and dyspnea shows a large left tension pneumothorax → with contralateral mediastinal shift due to mass effect and complete left lung atelectasis →.*

Atelectasis

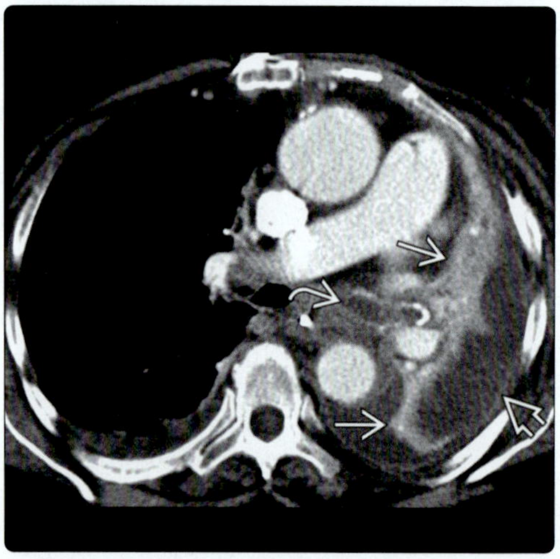

Pneumothorax

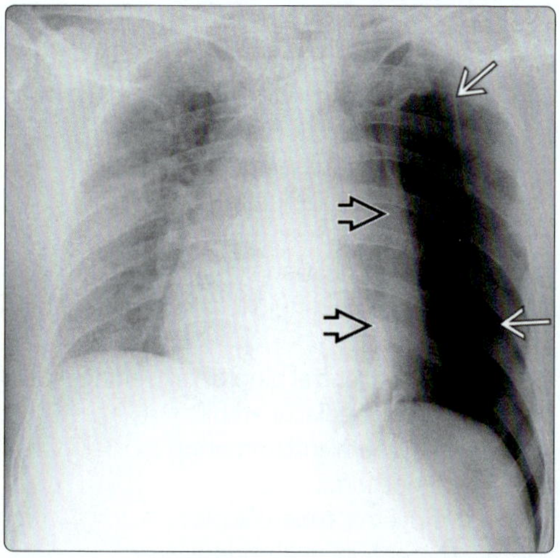

(**Left**) *PA chest radiograph of a patient who underwent a left pneumonectomy shows an opaque left hemithorax → with ipsilateral shift of the mediastinum →. Note the presence of multiple surgical clips → overlying the region of the left hilum.* (**Right**) *Axial NECT shows typical features of post-pneumonectomy syndrome, a complication of left pneumonectomy in this case. Note marked mediastinal shift → to the left and narrowing of the right mainstem bronchus → as it courses and drapes over the thoracic spine.*

Pneumonectomy

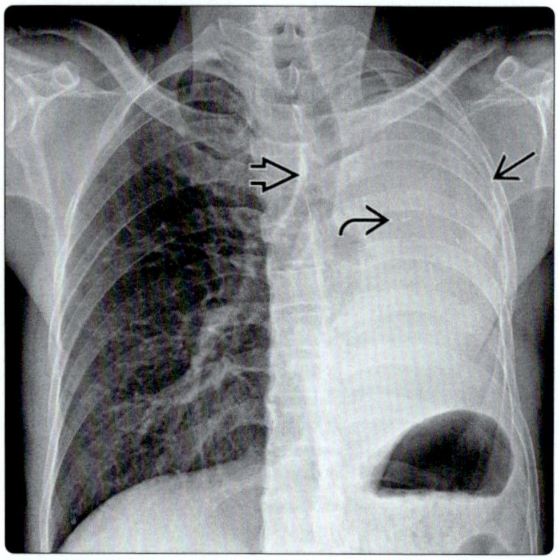

Pneumonectomy

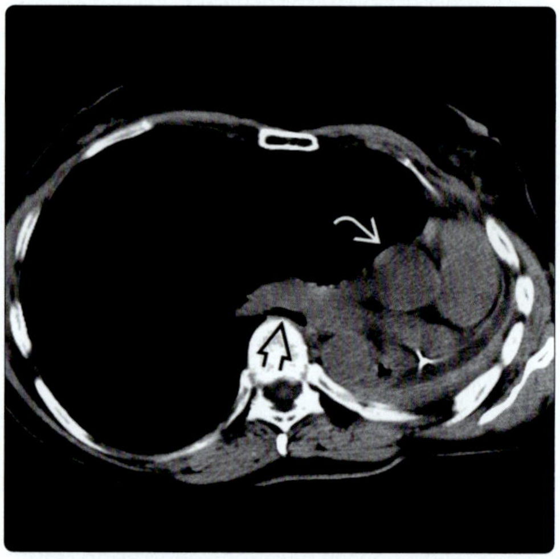

(**Left**) *PA chest radiograph of an 85-year-old man status post right lung irradiation for primary lung cancer shows right perihilar architectural distortion and volume loss with mild ipsilateral mediastinal shift.* (**Right**) *Axial CECT of a patient with chronic cavitary tuberculosis shows marked right lung volume loss and right upper lobe cavitary disease → with an intrinsic mycetoma in the dependent aspect of the cavity. Note marked mediastinal shift to the right manifesting with rightward displacement of the anterior junction line →.*

Radiation Fibrosis

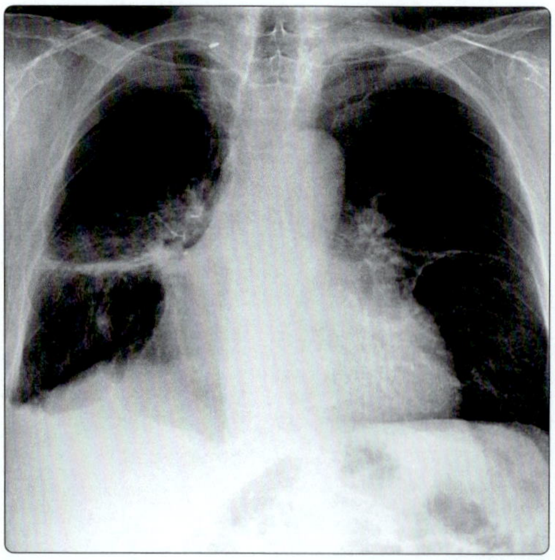

Tuberculosis

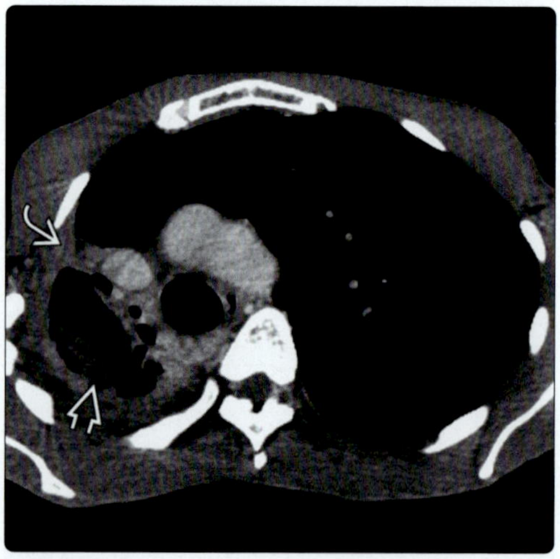

Hemothorax

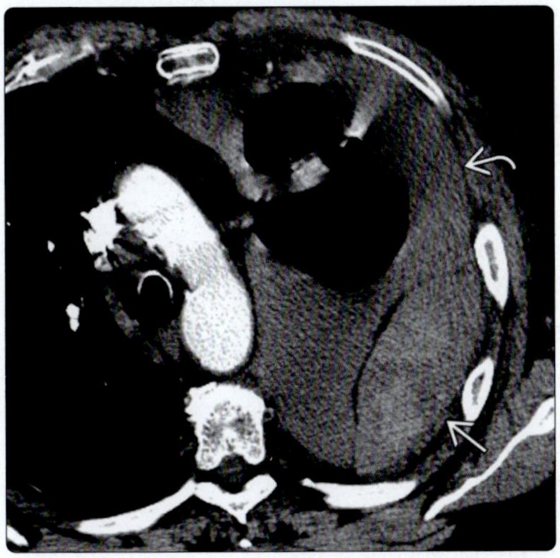

Fibrothorax

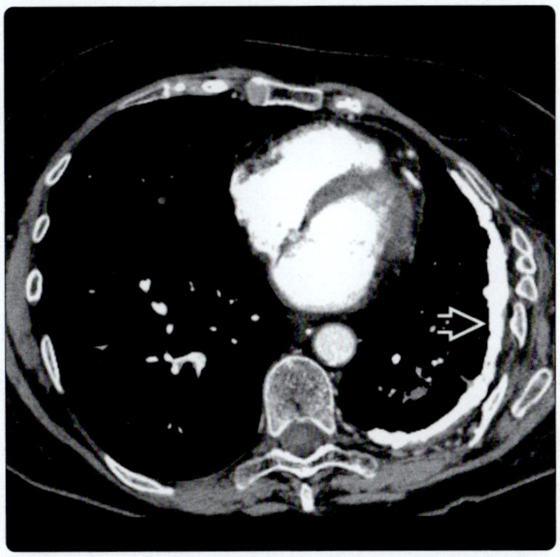

(Left) *Axial CECT of a patient who sustained blunt chest trauma with multiple left rib fractures (not shown) shows a large free left pleural effusion secondary to a hemothorax and a loculated extrapleural hematoma that displaces the extrapleural fat. Note associated shift of the mediastinum to the right.* **(Right)** *Axial CECT shows calcified left pleural thickening and left lung volume loss secondary to fibrothorax from remote tuberculous empyema. Note ipsilateral shift of the mediastinum to the left.*

Malignancy

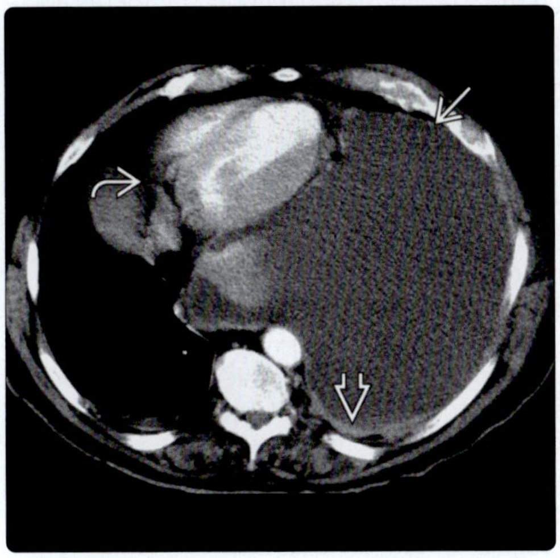

Chylothorax

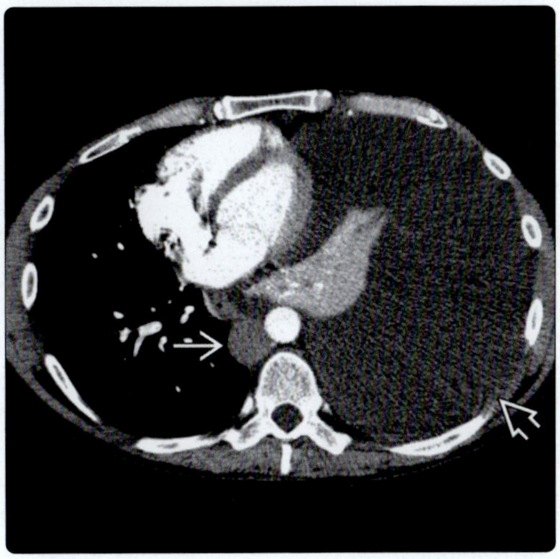

(Left) *Axial CECT of a patient with malignant pleural mesothelioma shows a massive malignant left pleural effusion and nodular pleural thickening that produce rightward shift of the mediastinum.* **(Right)** *Axial CECT of a patient with malignancy and secondary obstruction of the thoracic duct shows a massive left pleural effusion with associated complete left lung atelectasis due to a large chylothorax. Note contralateral mediastinal shift and lymphadenopathy.*

Diaphragmatic Hernia

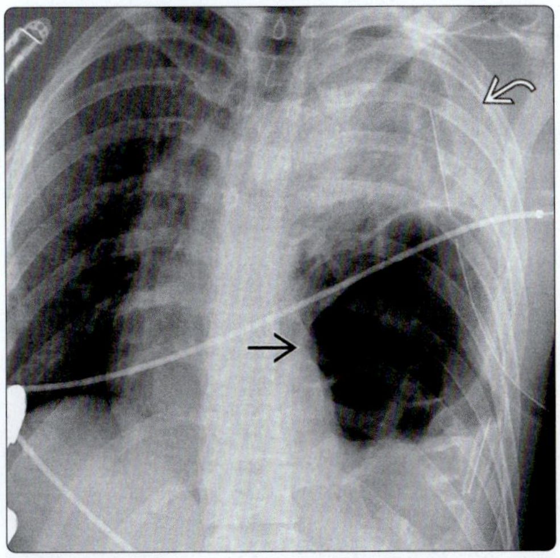

Scimitar Syndrome

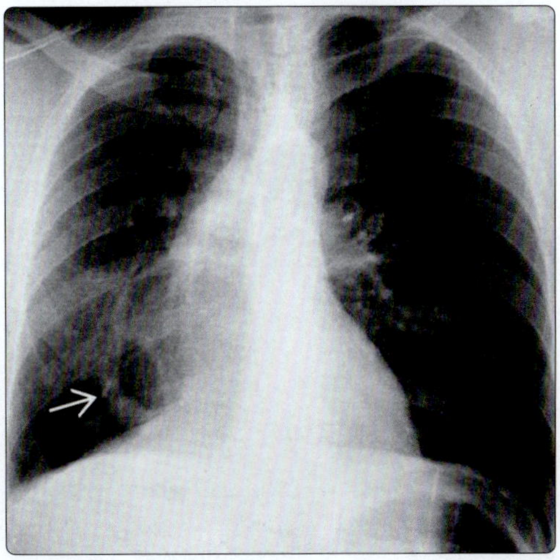

(Left) *AP chest radiograph of a patient who sustained blunt chest trauma shows typical features of acute diaphragmatic tear with resultant intrathoracic bowel herniation. Note shift of the mediastinum to the right. Associated left pleural effusion suggests bowel strangulation.* **(Right)** *PA chest radiograph of an asymptomatic patient with scimitar syndrome shows a small right lung volume, a characteristic scimitar vein draining into the inferior vena cava, and ipsilateral shift of the mediastinum.*

DIFFERENTIAL DIAGNOSIS

Common

- Mature Teratoma

Less Common

- Thymolipoma
- Thymic Hyperplasia

Rare but Important

- Lipoma
- Liposarcoma
- Malignant Teratoma
- Extramedullary Hematopoiesis

ESSENTIAL INFORMATION

Key Differential Diagnosis Issues

- Intralesional fat on CT; -40 to -120 Hounsfield units
- Chemical shift MR useful for indeterminate lesions

Helpful Clues for Common Diagnoses

- **Mature Teratoma**
  - 25% of prevascular lesions in patients 10-19 years of age
  - Combination of fat, fluid, calcification, and soft tissue
    - Intralesional fat in 50% of cases
    - Fat-fluid levels are specific but much less common
    - Bone and tooth-like elements are rare

Helpful Clues for Less Common Diagnoses

- **Thymolipoma**
  - Accounts for < 5% of prevascular mediastinal masses
  - 50-85% fat; scattered soft tissue and septa
  - Most common in cardiophrenic angle; large (average size: 20 cm)
  - Direct connection with thymus may be present
- **Thymic Hyperplasia**
  - True thymic hyperplasia: Chemotherapy, radiation therapy, corticosteroids, burns, injuries
  - Thymic lymphoid (follicular) hyperplasia: Immunologic diseases (myasthenia gravis, hyperthyroidism, collagen vascular diseases) or human immunodeficiency virus (HIV) infection
  - Imaging
    - True thymic hyperplasia: Thymic enlargement or focal soft tissue mass
    - Thymic lymphoid hyperplasia: Normal thymus, thymic enlargement, or focal soft tissue mass
    - Regions of low density due to deposition of fat between hyperplastic thymic tissue

Helpful Clues for Rare Diagnoses

- **Lipoma**
  - 2% of all primary mediastinal neoplasms
  - Encapsulated lesions composed predominantly of fat
  - Small amount of soft tissue and blood vessels
- **Liposarcoma**
  - Comprised predominantly of fat
  - Aggressive features compared to benign lesions
    - Greater proportion of soft tissue components; local invasion; intrathoracic lymphadenopathy; metastatic disease
- **Malignant Teratoma**
  - Also known as teratocarcinoma
  - More nodular or poorly defined than benign teratomas; mold to and compress surrounding structures
  - Demonstrate fat less often than benign teratomas (40% vs. 90%); more likely to appear solid
  - Thick enhancing capsule may be present on CECT
- **Extramedullary Hematopoiesis**
  - Hematologic disorders resulting in bone marrow replacement (myelofibrosis or chronic myelogenous leukemia) or hemolytic anemia (thalassemia, sickle cell anemia, or hereditary spherocytosis)
  - Large or small and unilateral or bilateral; typically enhance on post-contrast CT due to high vascularity
  - Fat infiltration in longstanding lesions

Mature Teratoma

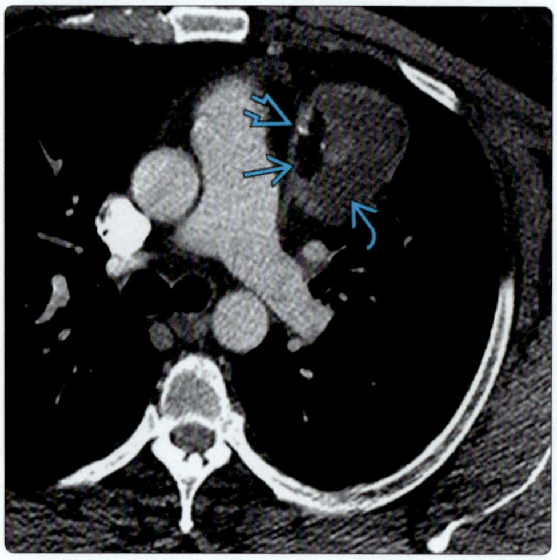

Thymolipoma

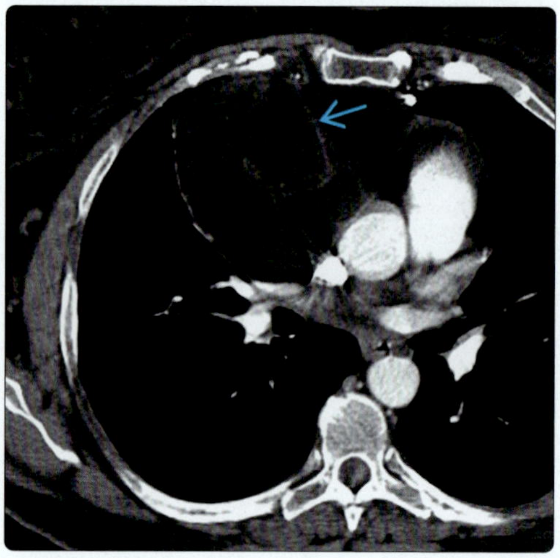

(Left) *Axial CECT of a patient with mature teratoma demonstrates a heterogeneous mass in the left prevascular mediastinum composed of fat ➡, fluid ➡, and calcification ➡. Although fat-fluid levels are highly specific for mature teratoma, this feature is only rarely seen.* **(Right)** *Axial CECT of a patient with thymolipoma shows a predominantly fat-containing mass in the right prevascular mediastinum with thin fibrous septa ➡.*

Thymic Hyperplasia

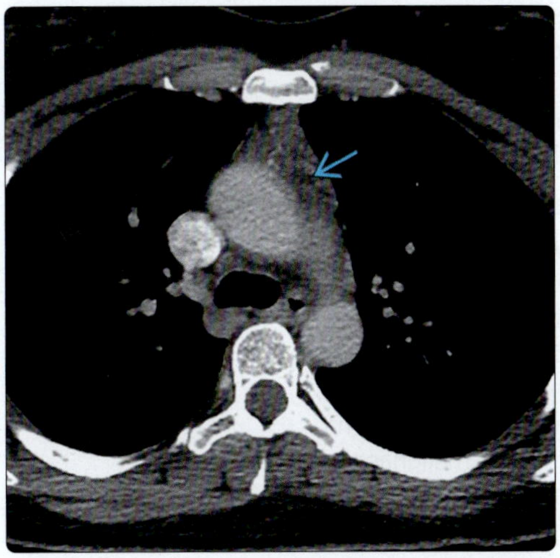

Thymic Hyperplasia

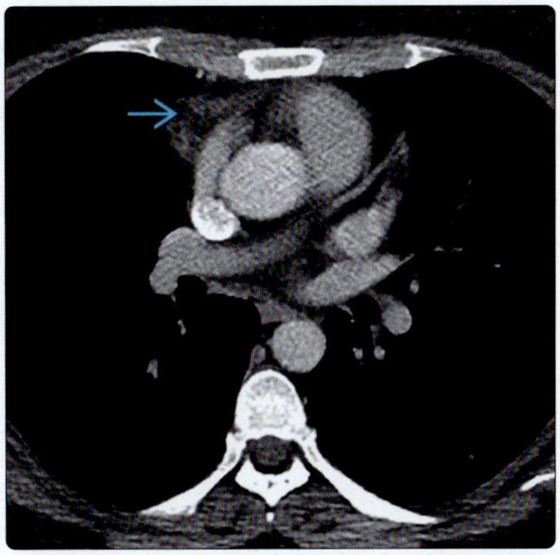

(Left) *Axial CECT of a patient with Hodgkin lymphoma following treatment demonstrates soft tissue in the prevascular mediastinum with interspersed regions of fat attenuation* →. **(Right)** *Axial CECT of a patient with myasthenia gravis shows focal soft tissue with interspersed fat attenuation* → *in the right prevascular mediastinum. Although thymic hyperplasia typically appears as increased soft tissue or a focal mass, regions of low density due to deposition of fat between hyperplastic thymic tissue may be seen.*

Lipoma

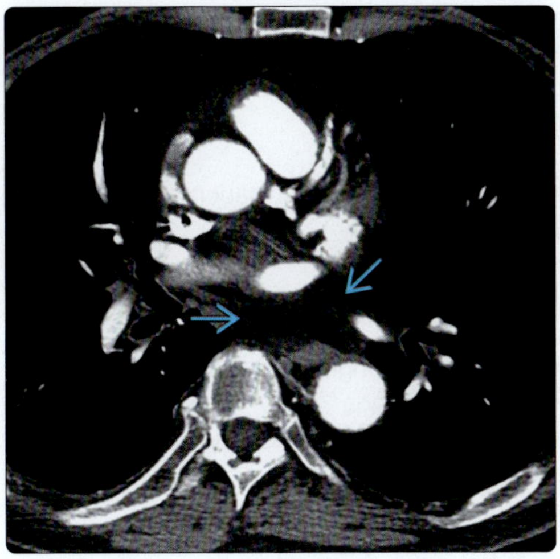

Liposarcoma

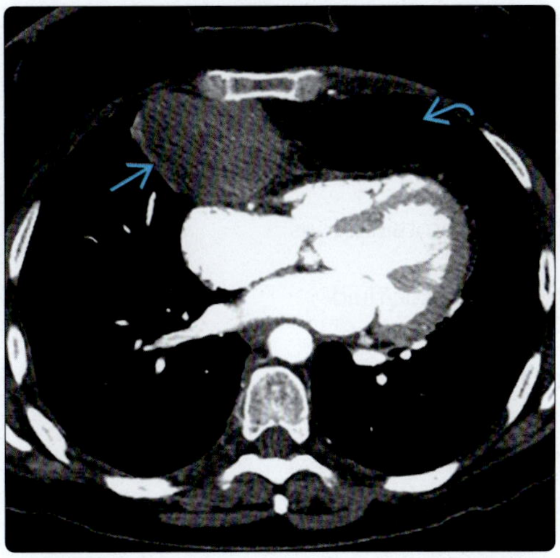

(Left) *Axial CECT of a patient with mediastinal lipoma shows an ill-defined mass* → *in the visceral mediastinum containing only fat and no soft tissue or fibrous septa.* **(Right)** *Axial CECT of a patient with mediastinal liposarcoma demonstrates a heterogeneous mass in the prevascular mediastinum containing prominent regions of enhancing soft tissue* → *and fat* →. *Liposarcomas show features such as a greater proportion of soft tissue, local invasion, or spread.*

Malignant Teratoma

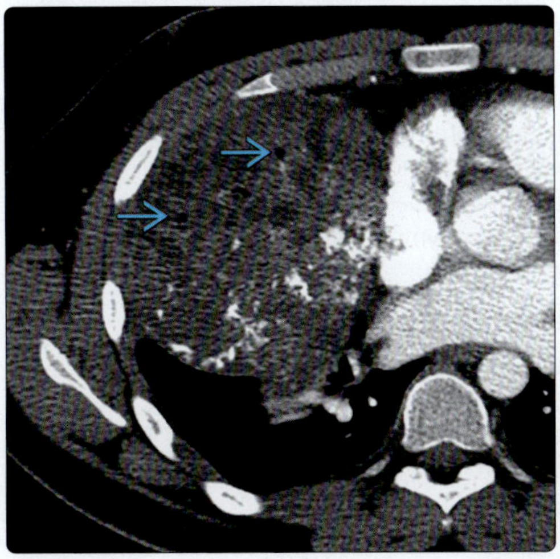

Extramedullary Hematopoiesis

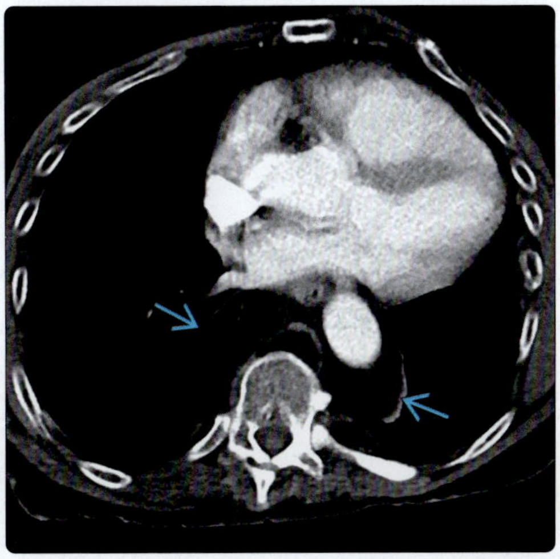

(Left) *Axial CECT of a patient with malignant teratoma demonstrates a large mass composed primarily of soft tissue and calcification but with a small amount of fat* →. *Compared to benign teratomas, malignant lesions are more nodular or poorly defined than benign teratomas and contain less fat.* **(Right)** *Axial CECT of a patient with myelofibrosis and longstanding extramedullary hematopoiesis shows predominantly fat-containing masses in the visceral and paravertebral compartments* →.

DIFFERENTIAL DIAGNOSIS

Common

- Bronchogenic Cyst
- Thyroid Goiter
- Pericardial Cyst

Less Common

- Necrotic Lymph Nodes
- Necrotic or Cystic Neoplasm

Rare but Important

- Thymic Cyst
- Other Foregut Duplication Cysts
- Lymphangioma
- Lateral Thoracic Meningocele
- Mediastinal Abscess
- Pseudocyst

ESSENTIAL INFORMATION

Key Differential Diagnosis Issues

- 10% of mediastinal masses in adults and children are cysts
- Most mediastinal cysts are congenital in origin
- Differential diagnosis primarily depends on location
- Hallmark on CT is mediastinal lesion measuring water or fluid attenuation with HU between 0 and 20
- MR useful for indeterminate lesions
  - T1WI: High signal intensity due to proteinaceous components
  - T2WI: High signal intensity due to cystic/fluid components

Helpful Clues for Common Diagnoses

- **Bronchogenic Cyst**
  - Most common foregut duplication cyst
  - Location
    - Typically occur in visceral and paravertebral compartments
    - Paratracheal or subcarinal regions
  - Imaging
    - Round and smooth in contour
    - Thin or imperceptible wall
    - Water or fluid attenuation
    - Hemorrhage or infection may result in abrupt increase in size &/or density
    - No enhancement on CECT
- **Thyroid Goiter**
  - Accounts for 10% of mediastinal masses
  - Location
    - May be identified in prevascular or visceral compartment
  - Imaging
    - Cystic regions in otherwise high-density or heterogeneous lesion
    - Demonstrates connection to thyroid gland
  - Factors that suggest thyroid neoplasm
    - Invasion of adjacent structures
    - Lymphadenopathy
    - Metastatic disease
- **Pericardial Cyst**
  - Composed of single layer of mesothelial cells
  - Location
    - Prevascular compartment
    - Most occur in cardiophrenic angles, right > left
  - Imaging
    - Homogeneous water or fluid attenuation
    - No enhancement on CECT

Helpful Clues for Less Common Diagnoses

- **Necrotic Lymph Nodes**
  - Etiologies
    - Infection
      - Tuberculosis, histoplasmosis
    - Intrathoracic malignancies
      - Lung cancer, lymphoma
    - Extrathoracic malignancies
      - Head and neck and gastric cancers, seminoma
  - Location
    - Prevascular, visceral, or paravertebral compartment
  - Imaging
    - Heterogeneous appearance of lymph nodes
      - Central low density secondary to necrosis
      - Peripheral (rim) enhancement
- **Necrotic or Cystic Neoplasms**
  - Germ cell neoplasms
    - Mature teratoma
      - 25% of prevascular lesions in patients 10-19 years of age
      - Prevascular in location
      - Well-defined cystic lesion ± fat, calcification
    - Seminoma
      - Typically affects younger men
      - Prevascular in location
      - Homogeneous lesion ± cystic regions
    - Nonseminomatous neoplasms
      - Prevascular in location
      - Heterogeneous lesion, which may have cystic regions
  - Thymic epithelial neoplasms
    - Thymoma and thymic carcinoma are most common
    - Located in prevascular mediastinum
    - May have cystic or necrotic centers
      - More common with larger neoplasms
    - Thymic carcinoma demonstrates more aggressive behavior than thymoma
      - Invasion of mediastinal structures
      - Intrathoracic lymphadenopathy
      - Metastatic disease

Helpful Clues for Rare Diagnoses

- **Thymic Cyst**
  - Etiologies
    - Congenital
    - Acquired
      - Most arise due to inflammation
      - Iatrogenic: Surgery, radiation therapy, chemotherapy
      - Associated with malignant neoplasms
  - Location
    - Prevascular compartment

- Imaging
  - Usually incidental finding
  - Unilocular or multilocular
  - Thin or imperceptible wall
  - Water or fluid attenuation on CT
    - High attenuation due to hemorrhage or infection, proteinaceous components
- **Other Foregut Duplication Cysts**
  - Esophageal duplication cyst
    - Lesion lined by gastrointestinal mucosa
    - Location
      - Visceral compartment
    - Imaging
      - Features are similar to those of bronchogenic cyst
      - Arises from esophageal wall/contacts esophagus
  - Neurenteric cyst
    - Composed of neural and gastrointestinal components
    - Location
      - Paravertebral compartment
    - Imaging
      - Imaging appearance is similar to that of other duplication cysts
      - Connection to meninges through vertebral defect
      - Associated with vertebral anomalies (scoliosis or hemivertebrae)
- **Lymphangioma**
  - Location
    - Prevascular, visceral, or paravertebral compartment
    - Extends into neck, axilla, or chest wall
  - Imaging
    - Unilocular or multilocular
    - ± thin septations ± soft tissue components
- **Lateral Thoracic Meningocele**
  - Anomalous herniation of leptomeninges through intervertebral foramen or vertebral body defect
  - Strong association with neurofibromatosis type 1
  - More common in adults than in children
  - Location
    - Paravertebral compartment
  - Imaging
    - Water or fluid attenuation
    - Associated with vertebral anomalies, such as hemivertebrae, butterfly vertebra, or spina bifida
- **Mediastinal Abscess**
  - Recent clinical history important
    - Median sternotomy, esophageal perforation, or head and neck infection
  - Location
    - Paravertebral compartment most common
  - Imaging
    - Rim-enhancing lesion with central low density
    - May demonstrate internal foci of air
    - Communication may be seen with coexisting subphrenic abscesses or empyema
    - May be difficult to differentiate from postoperative hematoma/seroma
      - May require needle aspiration
      - Postoperative hematoma/seroma should resolve after several weeks
- **Pseudocyst**
  - Develops over short period of time in clinical setting of pancreatitis
  - Contain pancreatic secretions, blood, and necrotic material
  - Location
    - Paravertebral compartment most common
    - Accesses mediastinum via esophageal or aortic hiatus
  - Imaging
    - Thin-walled masses that may be low or high density
      - High density results from hemorrhage or infection
    - Lesion tracks from abdomen; separate intra-abdominal pseudocysts may or may not be present

SELECTED REFERENCES

1. Madan R et al: Cystic mediastinal masses and the role of MRI. Clin Imaging. 50:68-77, 2018
2. Carter BW et al: ITMIG classification of mediastinal compartments and multidisciplinary approach to mediastinal masses. Radiographics. 37(2):413-36, 2017

Bronchogenic Cyst

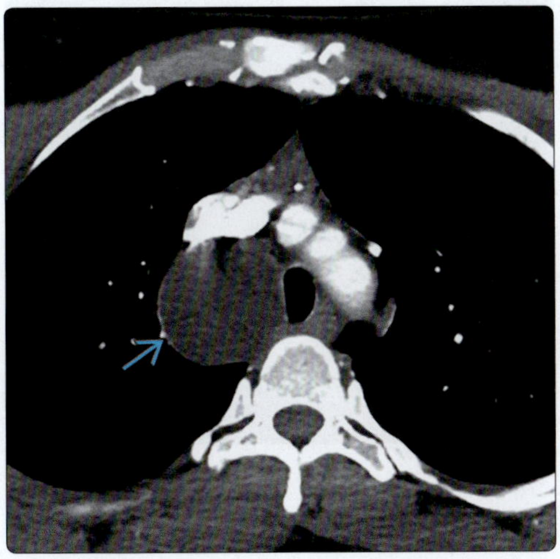

Bronchogenic Cyst

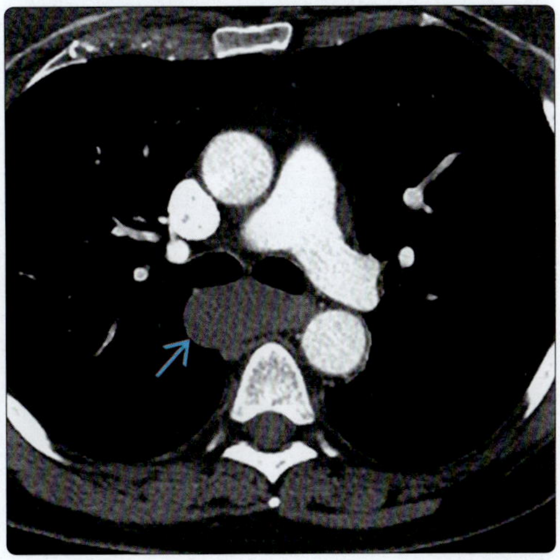

(Left) *Axial CECT demonstrates a well-circumscribed, water attenuation mass in the right paratracheal region ➔ representing a bronchogenic cyst.* **(Right)** *Axial CECT of a 41-year-old woman shows a bronchogenic cyst in the subcarinal region ➔. Bronchogenic cysts typically demonstrate water or fluid attenuation but may be hyperdense on CT due to hemorrhage or infection.*

(Left) *Axial NECT shows an enlarged, somewhat necrotic/cystic-appearing thyroid goiter → descending into the right paratracheal space. Leftward deviation of the trachea → and esophagus → are noted. Cystic regions may be seen in thyroid goiters with otherwise high density or heterogeneous soft tissue.* **(Right)** *Axial CECT demonstrates a well-defined water attenuation lesion in the right prevascular mediastinum, compatible with a pericardial cyst →.*

Thyroid Goiter

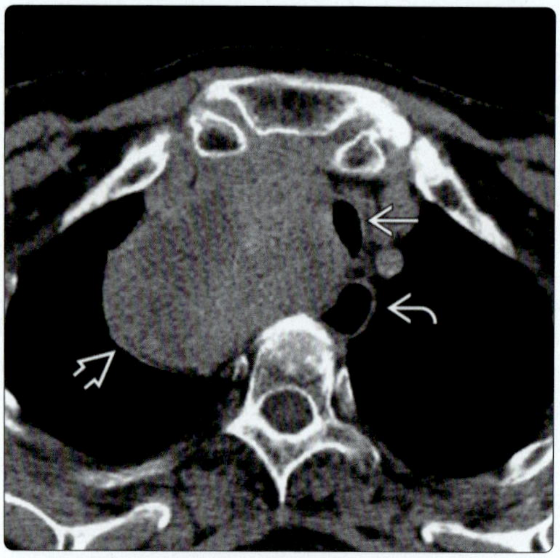

Pericardial Cyst

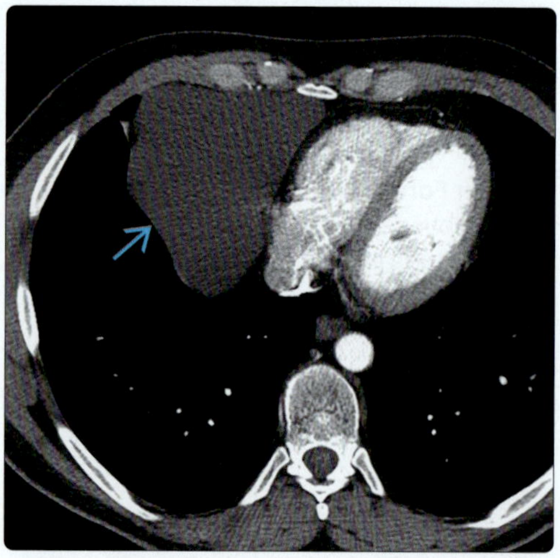

(Left) *Axial CECT shows right upper lobe lobulated consolidation → and multiple coalescent lymph nodes in the right paratracheal region with low-density centers → in this patient with tuberculosis.* **(Right)** *Axial CECT of a patient with metastatic head and neck cancer shows an enlarged lymph node in the prevascular mediastinum with central low density and peripheral (rim) enhancement →. Necrotic lymph nodes may be seen in the spread of intrathoracic and extrathoracic malignancies.*

Necrotic Lymph Nodes

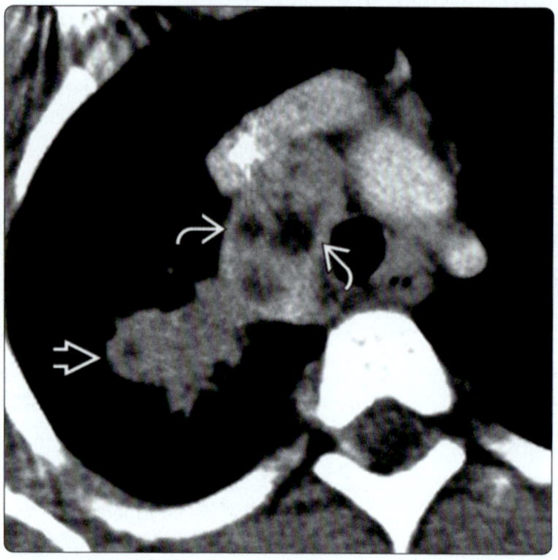

Necrotic Lymph Nodes

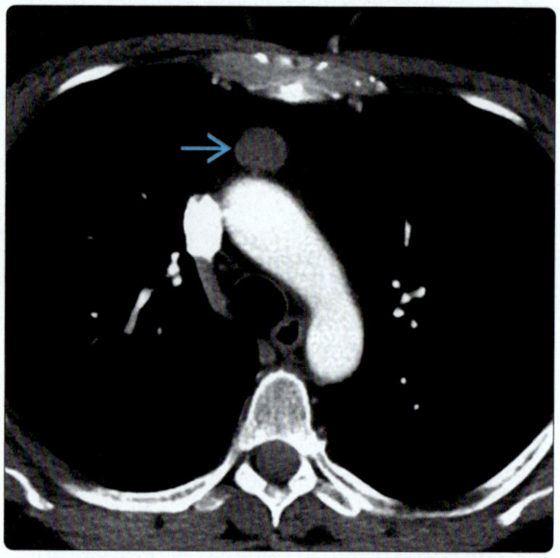

(Left) *Axial CECT of a patient with myasthenia gravis demonstrates a large low-density mass in the prevascular mediastinum →. Biopsy revealed a cystic thymoma.* **(Right)** *Axial CECT shows a heterogeneous prevascular mediastinal cystic, calcified →, and solid lesion →. There is thrombosis and expansion of the superior vena cava secondary to tumor invasion →. Note the hematogenous lung metastasis → in this patient with thymic carcinoma.*

Necrotic or Cystic Neoplasm

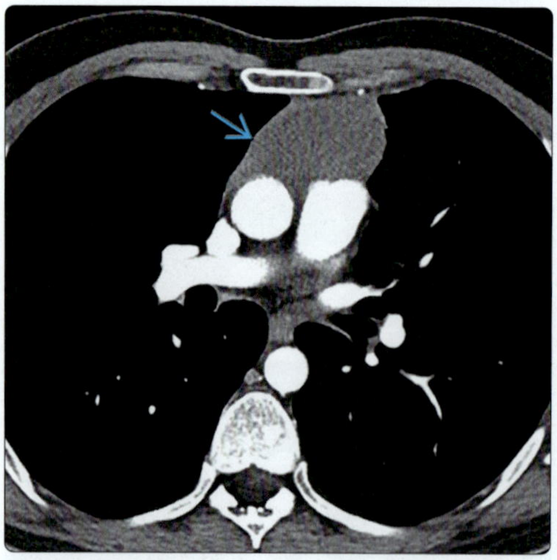

Necrotic or Cystic Neoplasm

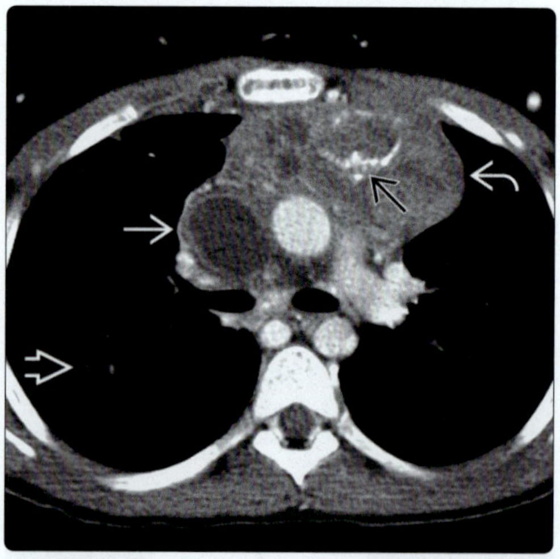

Thymic Cyst

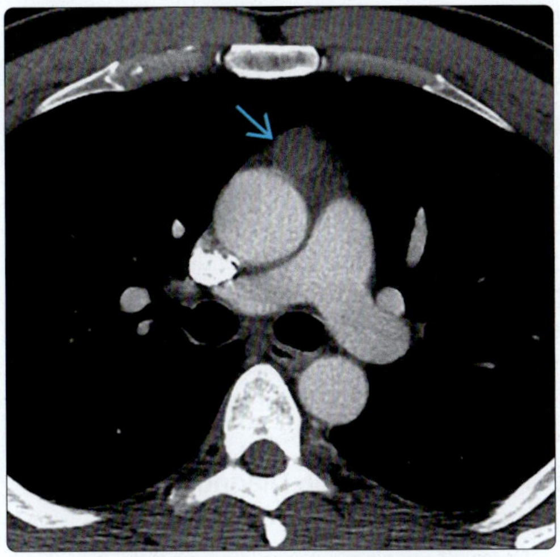

Thymic Cyst

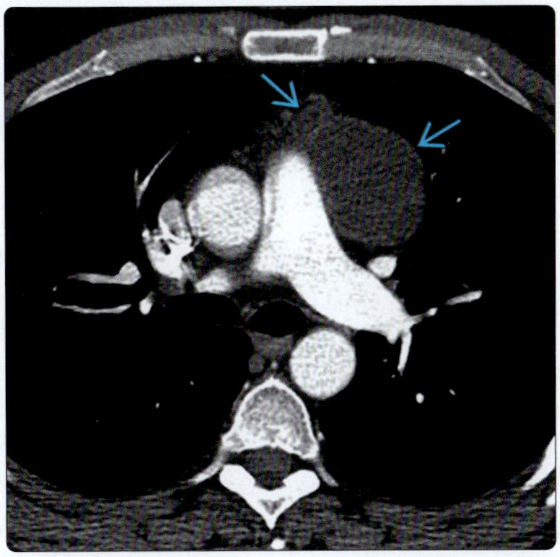

(Left) *Axial CECT demonstrates a focal low-density nodule in the prevascular mediastinum that measures fluid attenuation, consistent with a unilocular thymic cyst* →. **(Right)** *Axial CECT of a patient with a history of radiation to the mediastinum for lymphoma shows a complex low-density mass in the left prevascular mediastinum with multiple components, compatible with a multilocular thymic cyst* →. *Acquired thymic cysts are associated with radiation therapy, chemotherapy, surgery, and neoplasms.*

Lymphangioma

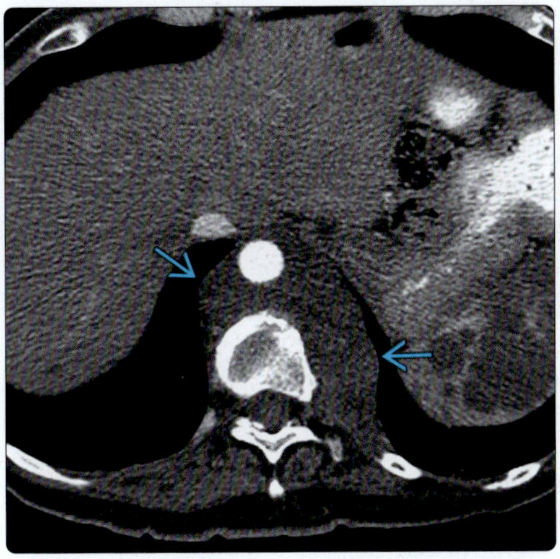

Lateral Thoracic Meningocele

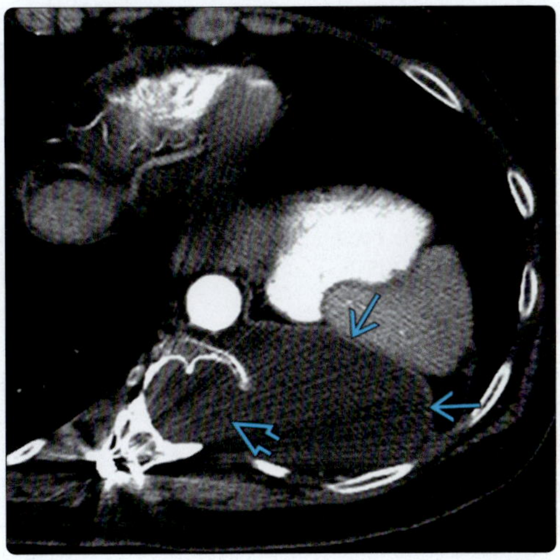

(Left) *Axial CECT shows a heterogeneous mass in the visceral and paravertebral compartments with both fluid attenuation and soft tissue components* →. *Biopsy revealed lymphangioma.* **(Right)** *Axial CECT of a patient with neurofibromatosis type 1 demonstrates a water attenuation lesion arising from the spinal canal and extending into the posterior left hemithorax* →. *Note widening of the left neural foramen and communication with the spinal canal* ⇨.

Mediastinal Abscess

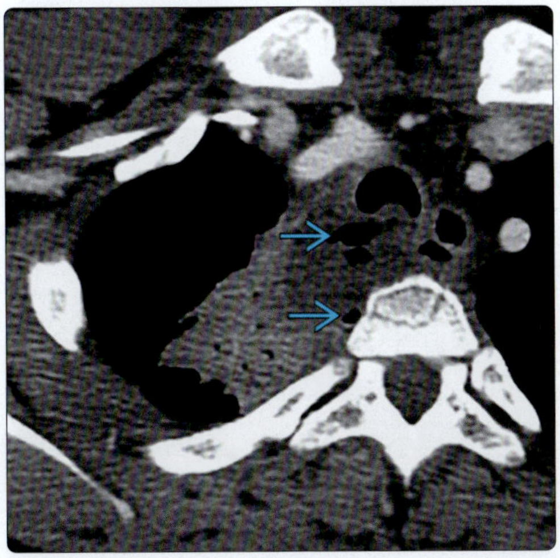

Pseudocyst

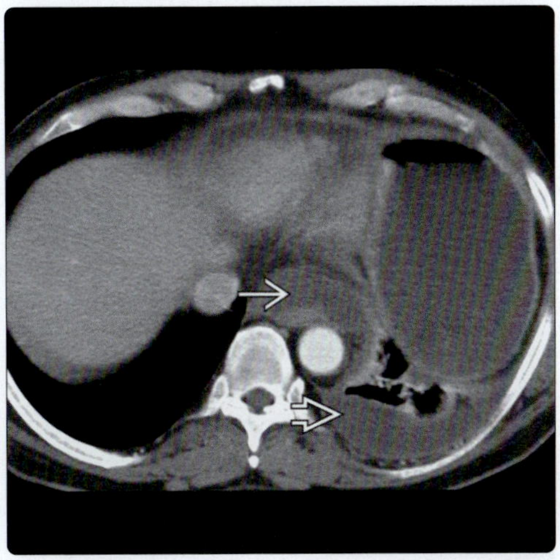

(Left) *Axial CECT of a patient with recent history of esophagitis and a perforated esophagus demonstrates an ill-defined low-density lesion in the right mediastinum containing foci of air* →. *These findings represent mediastinal abscess.* **(Right)** *Axial CECT demonstrates fluid surrounding the aorta* ➡. *Note left pleural effusion* ➡. *Lower sections revealed a peripancreatic cyst, and the patient had a remote history of severe pancreatitis. The pseudocyst resolved on follow-up imaging.*

DIFFERENTIAL DIAGNOSIS

Common

- Lymphadenopathy
- Thyroid Goiter
- Mediastinal Fibrosis
- Thymic Hyperplasia

Less Common

- Thymic Malignancy
- Neurogenic Neoplasm

Rare but Important

- Malignant Germ Cell Neoplasm
- Extramedullary Hematopoiesis

ESSENTIAL INFORMATION

Key Differential Diagnosis Issues

- Primary neoplasms
  - Thymic neoplasms
  - Primary mediastinal lymphoma
  - Malignant germ cell neoplasms
  - Neurogenic neoplasms
  - Rare miscellaneous primary malignancies
- Secondary neoplasms
  - Lymphadenopathy from lymphoproliferative disorders
  - Metastatic lymphadenopathy from thoracic or extrathoracic primary malignancies
- Glandular enlargement of thyroid or thymus
- Imaging manifestations
  - Focal mass: Well circumscribed &/or encapsulated
  - Locally invasive mass ± lymphadenopathy
  - Coalescent lymphadenopathy; may be locally invasive; may mimic primary neoplasia

Helpful Clues for Common Diagnoses

- **Lymphadenopathy**
  - Focal or multifocal involvement of mediastinal lymph node stations
  - Nodal coalescence; may be locally invasive
- **Thyroid Goiter**
  - Mediastinal extension of thyroid goiter or ectopic goiter
  - Cervicothoracic sign; mass effect on trachea
  - Heterogeneous, high attenuation, intense enhancement
  - Substernal versus retrotracheal/retroesophageal
- **Mediastinal Fibrosis**
  - Granulomatous versus nongranulomatous
  - Locally invasive mediastinal soft tissue with frequent calcification
  - Vascular, airway or esophageal obstruction
- **Thymic Hyperplasia**
  - Types: Rebound, lymphoid follicular
  - Diffuse or focal thymic enlargement
  - Chemical shift MR for diagnosis and exclusion of thymic neoplasia

Helpful Clues for Less Common Diagnoses

- **Thymic Malignancy**
  - Thymoma, thymic carcinoma, thymic carcinoid
  - Anterior/prevascular mediastinal mass ± local invasion &/or drop pleural metastases
- **Neurogenic Neoplasm**
  - Paravertebral mediastinal mass
  - Peripheral nerve sheath neoplasms, sympathetic ganglia neoplasms, paragangliomas
  - MR assessment for exclusion of neuroforaminal/intraspinal growth

Helpful Clues for Rare Diagnoses

- **Malignant Germ Cell Neoplasm**
  - Seminoma, nonseminomatous germ cell neoplasm
    - Symptomatic male patient; 20-40 years of age
  - Anterior/prevascular mediastinal mass: Homogeneous or heterogeneous, local invasion, ± mediastinal lymphadenopathy
- **Extramedullary Hematopoiesis**
  - Asymptomatic patient with hemoglobinopathy or myeloproliferative disorder
  - Lower posterior mediastinal/paravertebral soft tissue mass(es), often bilateral

Lymphadenopathy

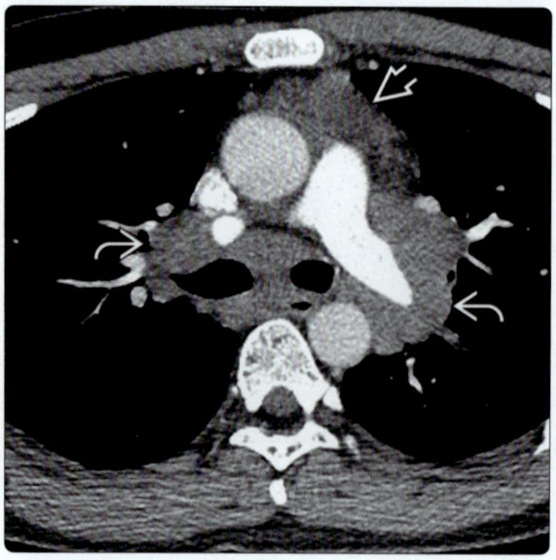

Lymphadenopathy

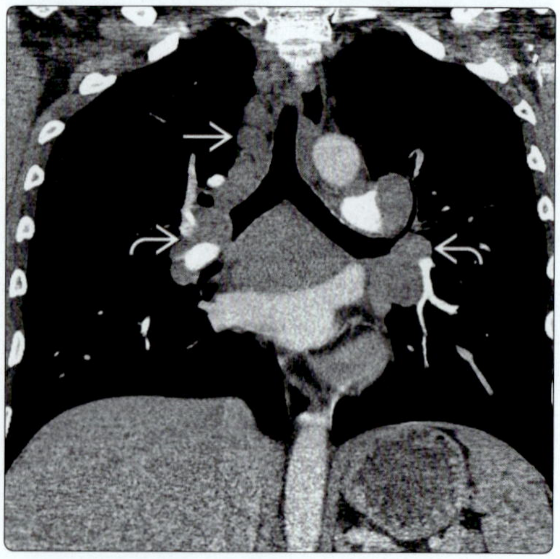

(Left) *Axial CECT of a 34-year-old man shows bilateral hilar, subcarinal, and coalescent prevascular lymphadenopathy.* **(Right)** *Coronal CECT of the same patient shows bilateral symmetric hilar, paratracheal, and coalescent subcarinal lymphadenopathy. Given the demographic features and the distribution of enlarged lymph nodes, sarcoidosis should be considered in the differential diagnosis, but is a diagnosis of exclusion. Biopsy demonstrated Hodgkin lymphoma.*

Lymphadenopathy

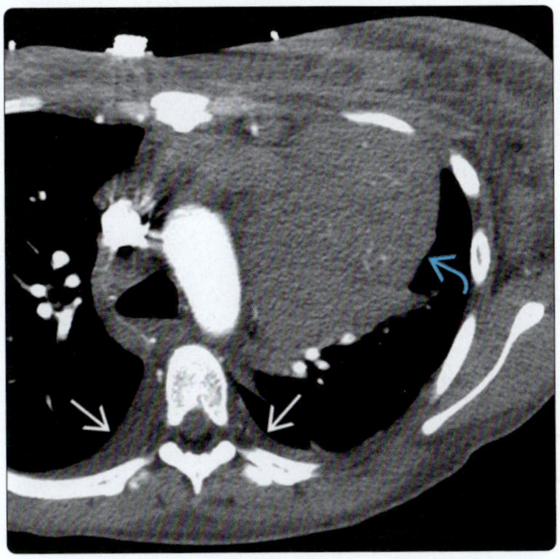

Lymphadenopathy

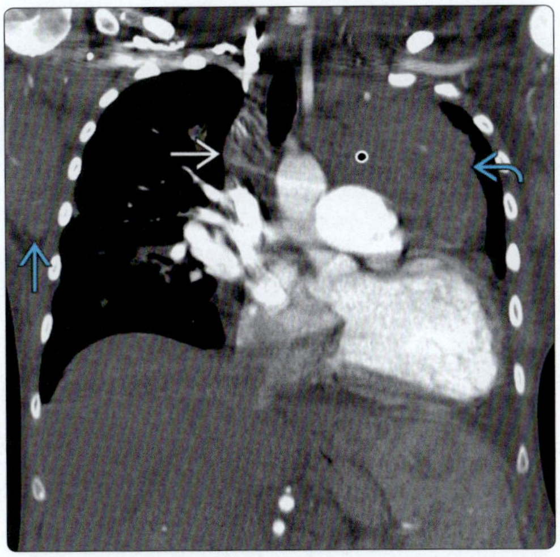

(Left) *Axial CECT of a 31-year-old woman with Hodgkin lymphoma shows coalescent left prevascular lymphadenopathy that mimics a primary mediastinal malignancy. Note small bilateral pleural effusions.* **(Right)** *Coronal CECT of the same patient shows coalescent left mediastinal lymphadenopathy, right paratracheal, and right axillary lymphadenopathy. Mediastinal lymphadenopathy may manifest as discrete soft tissue lesions in 1 or more lymph node stations &/or as a coalescent soft tissue mass.*

Thyroid Goiter

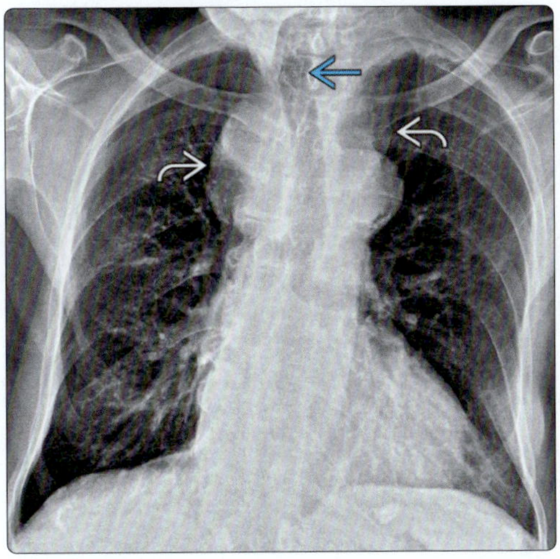

Thyroid Goiter

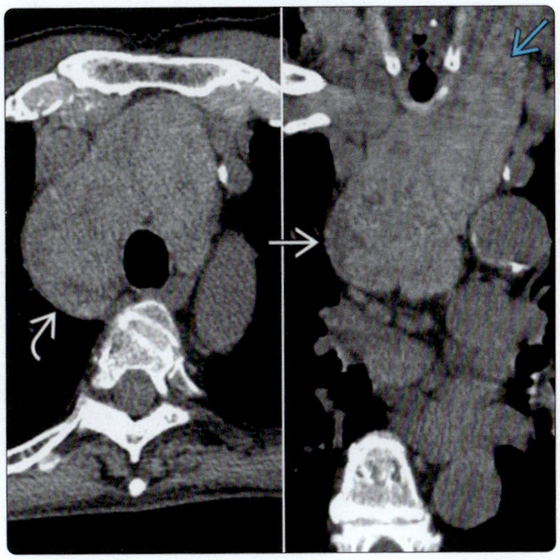

(Left) *PA chest radiograph of a 90-year-old man with thyroid goiter shows bilateral polylobular upper mediastinal enlargement with mass effect on the left suprasternal trachea and the cervicothoracic sign, consistent with a thyroid lesion.* **(Right)** *Composite image with axial (left) and coronal (right) NECT of the same patient shows a heterogeneous soft tissue mass with high attenuation. Note continuity between the mediastinal mass and the cervical component of the goiter.*

Mediastinal Fibrosis

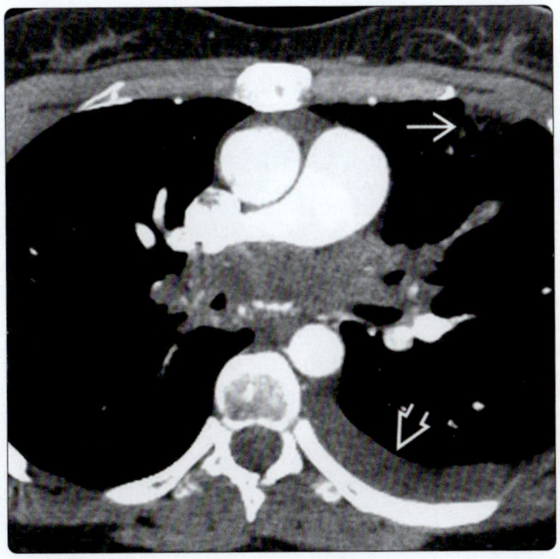

Mediastinal Fibrosis

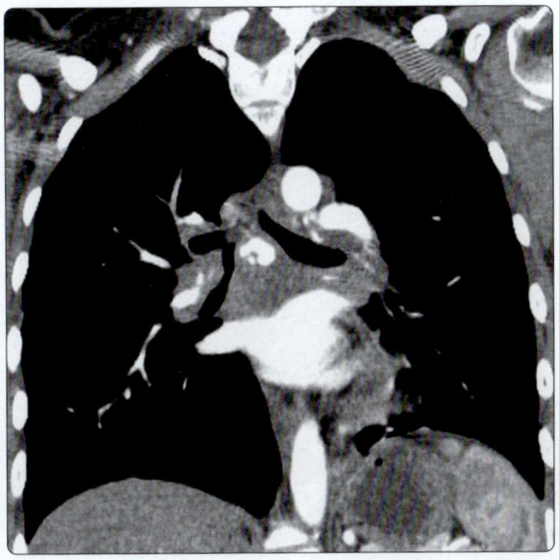

(Left) *Axial CECT of a 34-year-old woman with chronic dyspnea secondary to mediastinal fibrosis shows a coalescent soft tissue mass with intrinsic calcifications in the visceral mediastinum that produces mass effect on the right pulmonary artery and obliterates the bilateral superior pulmonary veins. Note left upper lobe venous infarct and left pleural effusion.* **(Right)** *Coronal NECT of the same patient shows the infiltrative mediastinal soft tissue mass with intrinsic calcifications, typical of mediastinal fibrosis.*

(Left) *Composite image with axial CECT obtained at baseline (left) and 5 years later (right) of an asymptomatic 26-year-old woman shows interval development of a prevascular mediastinal soft tissue mass .* **(Right)** *Composite image with axial in-phase (left) and out-of-phase (right) chemical shift MR of the same patient shows that the prevascular soft tissue mass exhibits signal drop on out-of-phase imaging. These findings are most consistent with thymic hyperplasia and help exclude thymic neoplasia.*

Thymic Hyperplasia

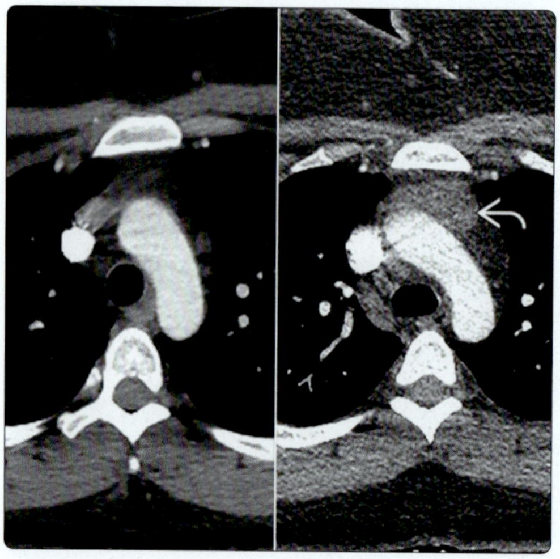

Thymic Hyperplasia

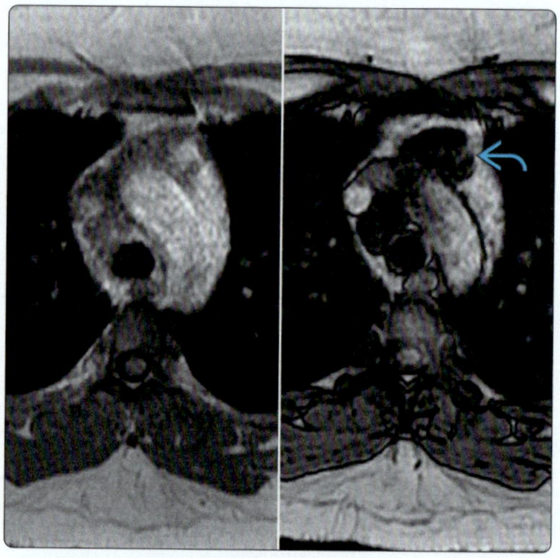

(Left) *AP chest radiograph of a 75-year-old woman who presented with chest pain shows a focal left mediastinal soft tissue mass located in the anterior mediastinum, a finding confirmed on lateral chest radiography (not shown).* **(Right)** *Axial CECT of the same patient shows a discrete heterogeneous soft tissue mass in the left prevascular mediastinum with an intact tissue plane between the lesion and the adjacent mediastinal great vessels. A type AB encapsulated thymoma was diagnosed at surgery.*

Thymic Malignancy

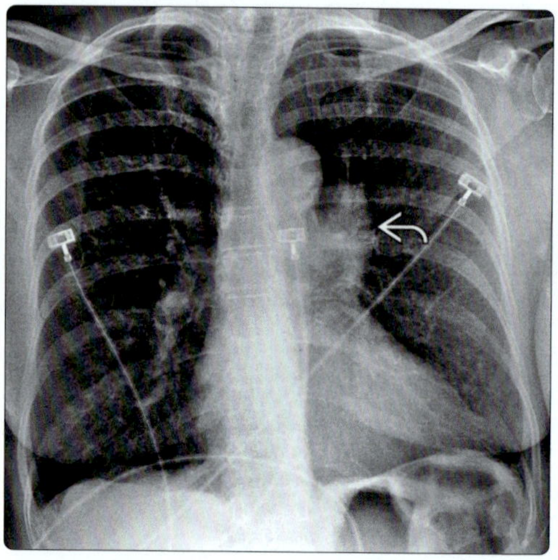

Thymic Malignancy

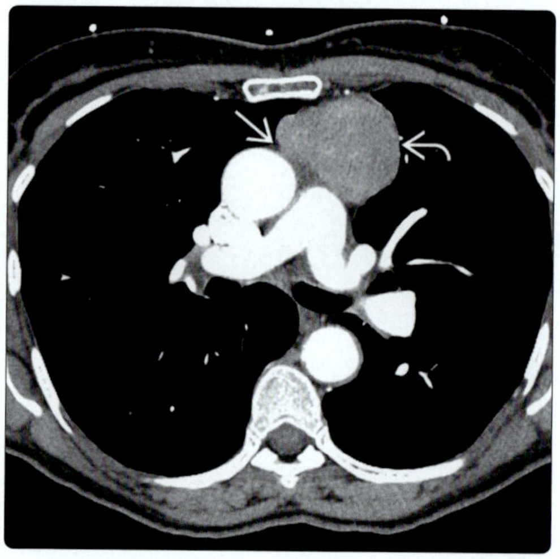

(Left) *Axial CECT of a 69-year-old woman who presented with chest pain shows a heterogeneously enhancing prevascular mediastinal mass that partially encases the ascending aorta and invades the superior vena cava . Thymic carcinoma was diagnosed at surgery.* **(Right)** *Axial CECT of a 50-year-old man with multiple endocrine neoplasia 1 shows a locally invasive left mediastinal mass that involves the prevascular and visceral compartments and encases mediastinal great vessels. Biopsy demonstrated thymic carcinoid.*

Thymic Malignancy

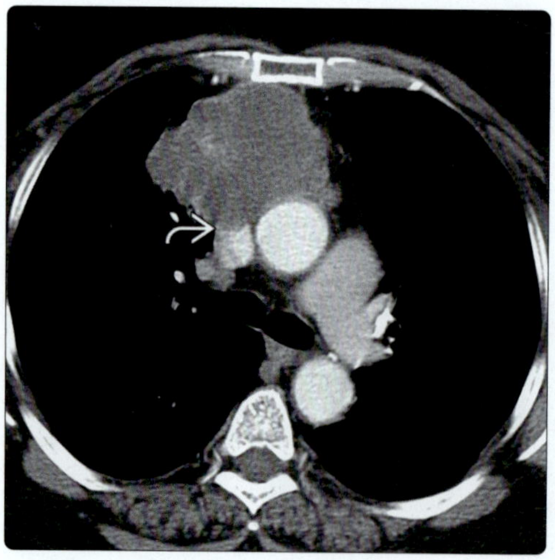

Thymic Malignancy

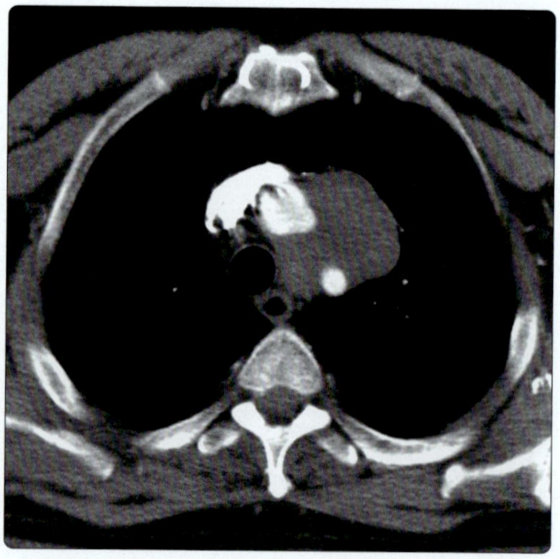

Neurogenic Neoplasm

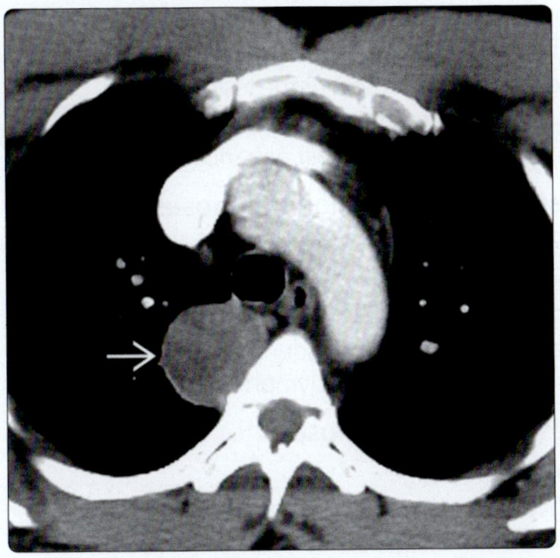

Neurogenic Neoplasm

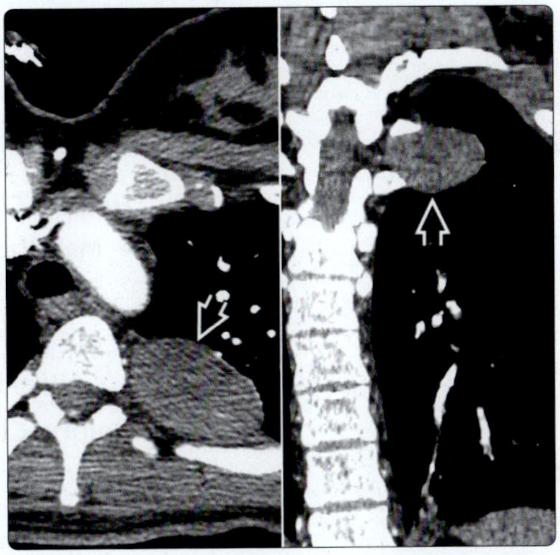

(Left) *Axial CECT of an asymptomatic 58-year-old man shows a spherical right paravertebral soft tissue mass* ➡*. Mediastinal schwannoma was diagnosed at surgery. Schwannoma is the most common mediastinal peripheral nerve sheath tumor.* **(Right)** *Composite image with axial (left) and coronal (right) CECT of a 26-year-old woman with neurofibromatosis 1 shows a left paravertebral neurofibroma* ➡ *that extends toward an adjacent neuroforamen. Note mild upper thoracic dextroscoliosis.*

Neurogenic Neoplasm

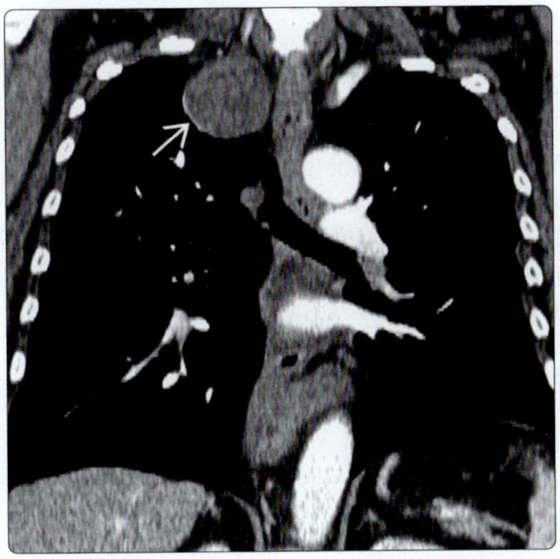

Neurogenic Neoplasm

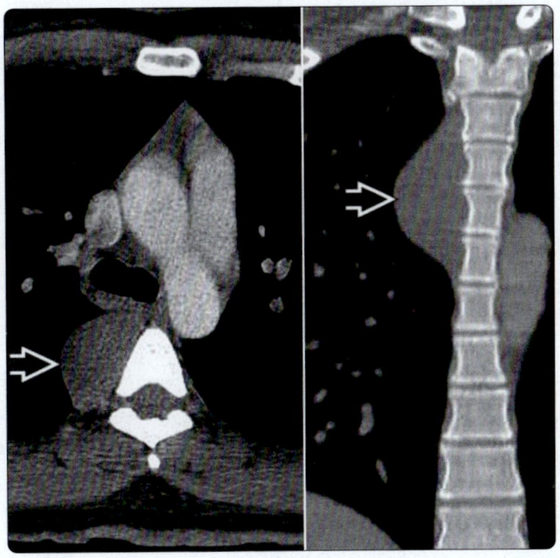

(Left) *Coronal CECT of an asymptomatic 28-year-old woman shows a spherical right paravertebral neurofibroma* ➡*. Neurofibroma is the 2nd most common mediastinal peripheral nerve sheath tumor.* **(Right)** *Composite image with axial (left) and coronal (right) CECT of an asymptomatic 21-year-old woman shows a right paravertebral ganglioneuroma* ➡ *that exhibits an elongate morphology and spans 4 vertebral bodies. Note that the mass produces pressure erosion of adjacent vertebral bodies.*

Malignant Germ Cell Neoplasm

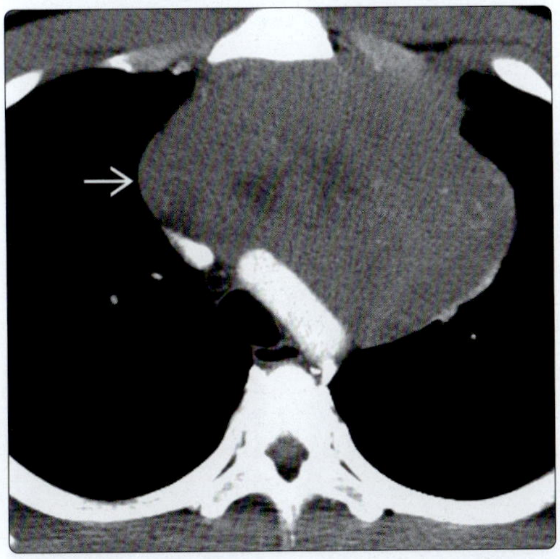

Extramedullary Hematopoiesis

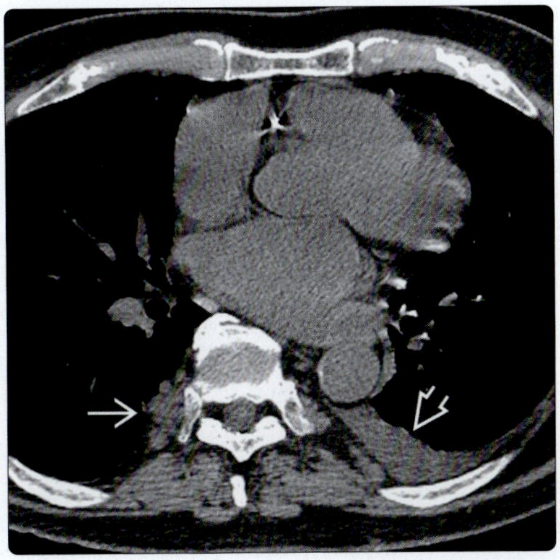

(Left) *Axial CECT of a 29-year-old man with chest pain shows a heterogeneously enhancing prevascular mediastinal soft tissue mass* ➡ *that produces mass effect on the aorta and superior vena cava and obliterates the bilateral brachiocephalic veins. Biopsy showed mixed malignant germ cell neoplasm.* **(Right)** *Axial NECT of a 90-year-old man with hemolytic anemia shows a polylobular right paravertebral soft tissue mass* ➡ *and a small left pleural effusion* ➡*. Extramedullary hematopoiesis was confirmed on CT-guided biopsy.*

DIFFERENTIAL DIAGNOSIS

Common

- Aneurysm
- Thyroid Goiter
- Varices

Less Common

- Metastases

Rare but Important

- Parathyroid Adenoma
- Castleman Disease
- Hemangioma
- Paraganglioma

ESSENTIAL INFORMATION

Key Differential Diagnosis Issues

- Hypervascular soft tissue tumors and neoplasms
- Vascular lesions: 10% of mediastinal contour abnormalities

Helpful Clues for Common Diagnoses

- **Aneurysm**
  - Typically aortic aneurysm or pseudoaneurysm; also aneurysms of other arteries and venous aneurysms
  - Enhancement of vascular lumen, similar to that of adjacent normal arteries
  - ± endoluminal mural thrombus &/or calcification
- **Thyroid Goiter**
  - Intramediastinal extension or ectopic thyroid tissue
  - Radiographic cervicothoracic sign; mass effect on suprasternal trachea
  - Well-defined soft tissue nodule or mass
    - Anterior/prevascular mediastinum or retroesophageal/visceral mediastinum
    - Heterogeneous attenuation: Cystic change, low-attenuation areas, calcification
    - High attenuation on unenhanced CT due to iodine content
    - Intense and sustained contrast enhancement
- **Varices**
  - Uphill varices: Portal hypertension, lower visceral (paraesophageal) mediastinum
  - Downhill varices: Superior vena cava obstruction
  - Serpiginous mediastinal soft tissue lesions
    - May be unopacified on arterial-phase imaging
    - May exhibit delayed contrast enhancement

Helpful Clues for Less Common Diagnoses

- **Metastases**
  - Hypervascular malignancies: Renal and thyroid cancers, melanoma, sarcoma
  - Metastatic mediastinal lymphadenopathy; may involve other intra- and extrathoracic lymph nodes

Helpful Clues for Rare Diagnoses

- **Parathyroid Adenoma**
  - Primary hyperparathyroidism: ↑ serum Ca^{++} and parathyroid hormone levels
  - Ectopic mediastinal parathyroid adenoma
  - Technetium-99m sestamibi (99mTc MIBI) SPECT/CT, parathyroid 4D CT
  - Intense enhancement on arterial-phase CT
- **Castleman Disease**
  - Localized Castleman disease: Hyaline vascular and plasma cell histologic types
  - Mediastinal/hilar lymph node(s) or soft tissue mass(es)
    - Intense enhancement; Ca^{++} in up to 10%
    - Axillary and cervical lymph nodes may be affected
- **Hemangioma**
  - Well-defined soft tissue mass; often in anterior or prevascular mediastinum
  - Central, peripheral or heterogeneous enhancement
  - Intrinsic small punctate calcifications: Phleboliths
- **Paraganglioma**
  - Neoplasm of paraganglion cells; affected patients may present with hypertension from catecholamine production
  - Paravertebral, aortopulmonary, juxtacardiac
  - Intense contrast enhancement

(Left) *PA chest radiograph of an asymptomatic 64-year-old woman shows a well-defined right retrocardiac soft tissue mass ➙.* **(Right)** *Coronal CECT of the same patient shows that the radiographic abnormality corresponds to a saccular aneurysm ➙ arising from the right side of the lower descending thoracic aorta, which exhibits partial enhancement of the vascular lumen and extensive endoluminal mural thrombus. Note diffuse aortic atherosclerosis and left renal atrophy ➙.*

Aneurysm

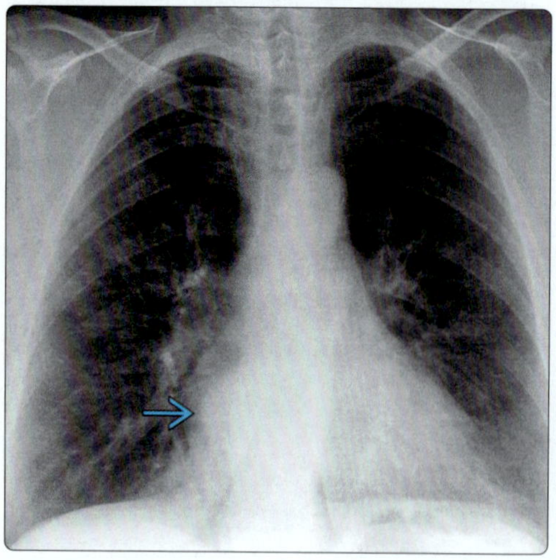

Aneurysm

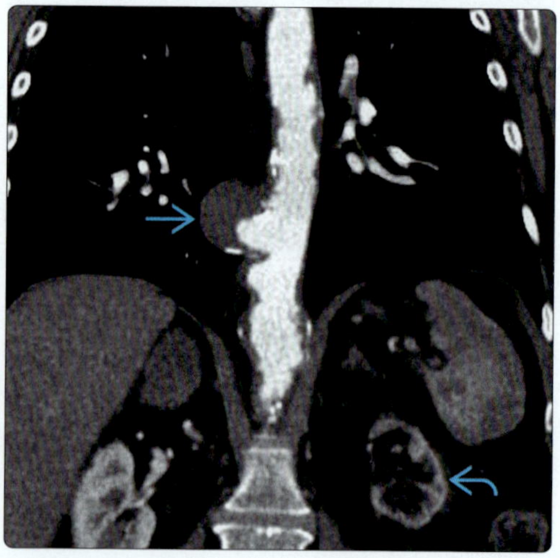

Aneurysm

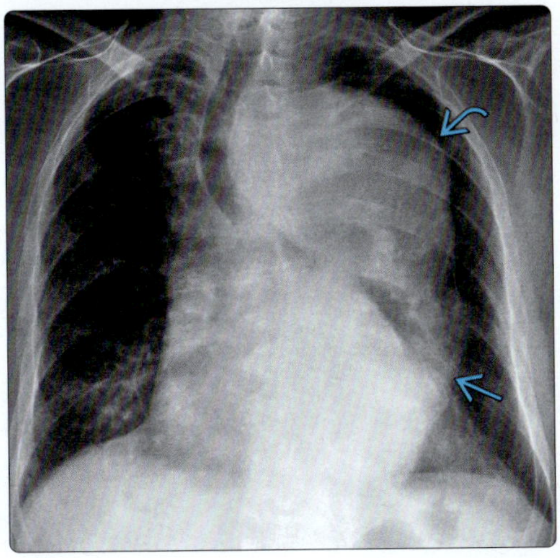

Aneurysm

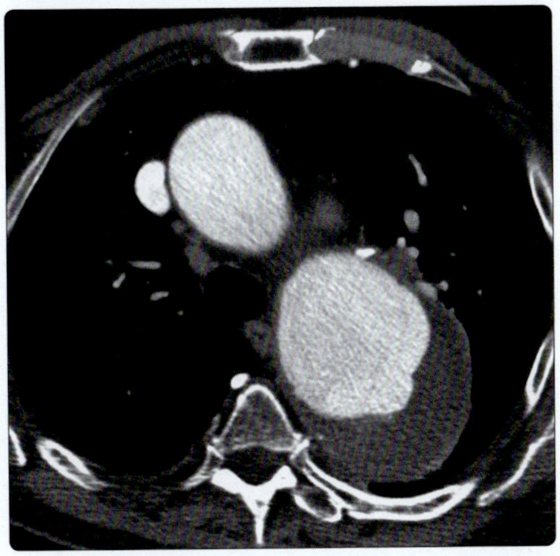

(Left) *PA chest radiograph of a 75-year-old man who presented with chest pain shows a large soft tissue mass of the left upper mediastinum with contours that are contiguous with the tortuous descending thoracic aorta. Note mass effect on the left lower trachea in the anatomic location of the aortic arch.* **(Right)** *Axial CECT of the same patient shows a large aneurysm of the proximal descending thoracic aorta with enhancement of the vascular lumen and peripheral crescentic low-attenuation mural thrombus.*

Aneurysm

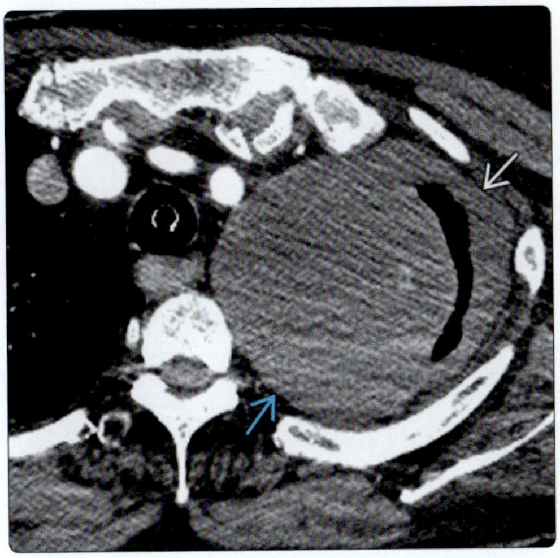

Aneurysm

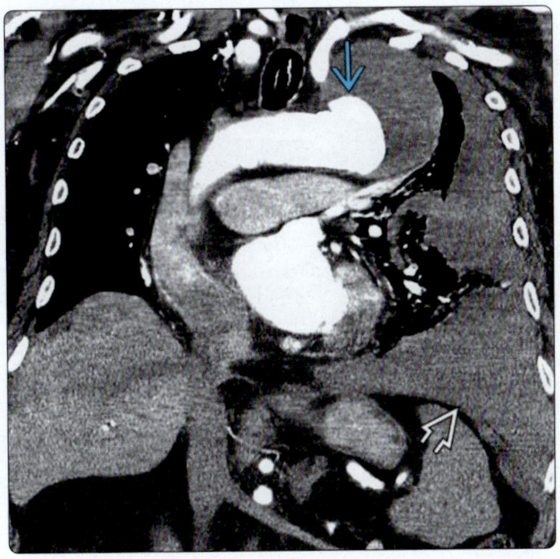

(Left) *Axial CECT of an 88-year-old man with acute chest pain shows a large left apical soft tissue mass and adjacent left apical pleural fluid.* **(Right)** *Coronal CECT of the same patient shows that the left apical soft tissue mass corresponds to the upper aspect of a large aneurysm of the aortic arch with contrast opacification of a small portion of its lumen. Note the large ipsilateral high-attenuation left pleural effusion. The findings were concerning for ruptured aortic aneurysm, confirmed at surgery.*

Thyroid Goiter

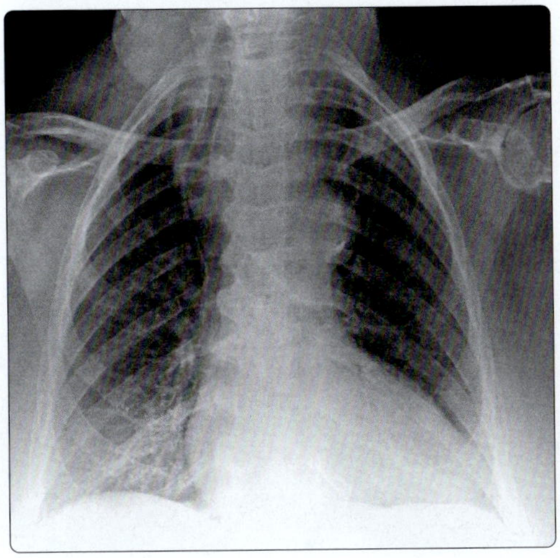

Thyroid Goiter

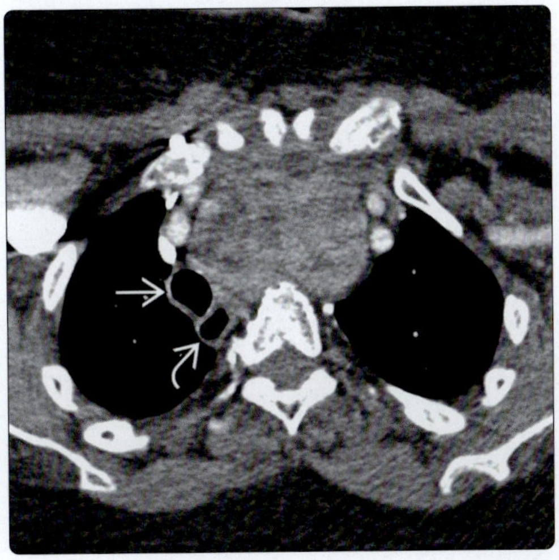

(Left) *PA chest radiograph of a 67-year-old woman shows suprasternal and mediastinal soft tissue that produces marked mass effect on the left trachea and exhibits the radiographic cervicothoracic sign indicating that the mass is both in the neck and the mediastinum.* **(Right)** *Axial CECT of the same patient shows a large intramediastinal soft tissue mass with heterogeneous contrast enhancement, which produces marked mass effect on the trachea, esophagus, and adjacent vessels, consistent with thyroid goiter.*

Varices

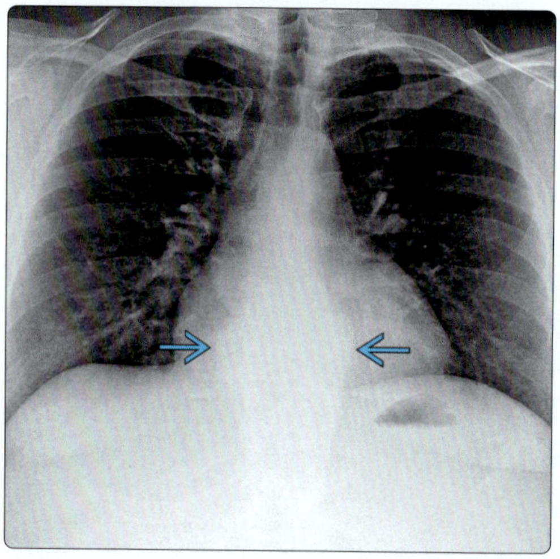

Varices

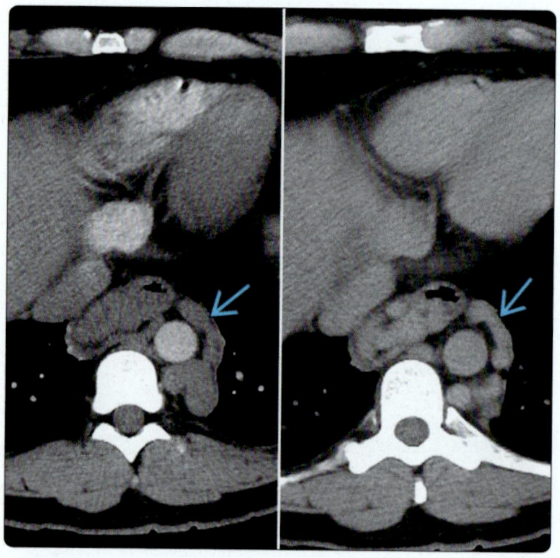

(Left) *PA chest radiograph of a 39-year-old man with end-stage liver disease shows bilateral polylobular lower paravertebral soft tissue masses.* **(Right)** *Composite image with axial CECT in arterial (left) and venous (right) phases shows that the mediastinal masses correspond to serpiginous soft tissue lesions that enhance on delayed venous-phase imaging, consistent with paraesophageal varices. Varices may not exhibit contrast enhancement on arterial-phase imaging.*

Metastases

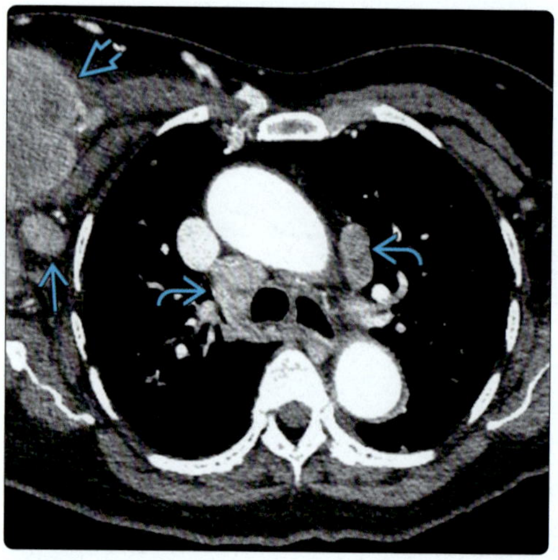

Metastases

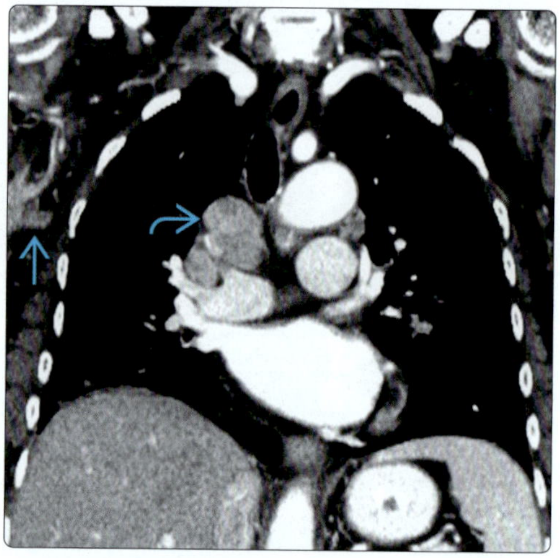

(Left) *Axial CECT of an 85-year-old woman with a palpable right breast mass shows enhancing right axillary and bilateral mediastinal lymphadenopathy concerning for lymph node metastases. Note the partially imaged heterogeneously enhancing right breast mass.* **(Right)** *Coronal CECT of the same patient shows enhancing enlarged mediastinal lymph nodes that represented lymph node metastases from primary breast cancer. Note partially imaged right axillary lymphadenopathy.*

Parathyroid Adenoma

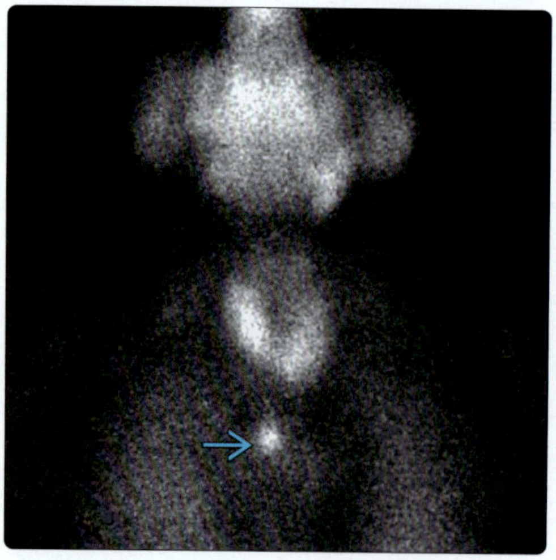

Parathyroid Adenoma

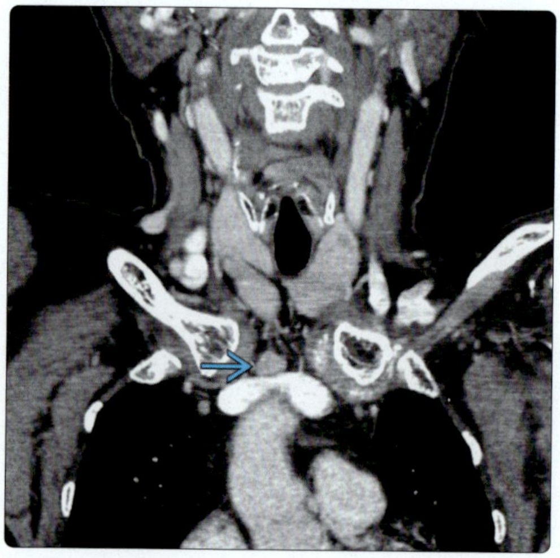

(Left) *Anterior Tc-99m sestamibi parathyroid scintigraphy of a 73-year-old woman with primary hyperparathyroidism and elevated serum calcium and parathormone levels shows abnormal uptake in the upper mediastinum, consistent with an ectopic parathyroid adenoma.* **(Right)** *Coronal 4D CECT of the same patient shows an enhancing nodule in the upper mediastinum that corresponds to the abnormal radiotracer uptake on scintigraphy and represents an ectopic parathyroid adenoma.*

Castleman Disease

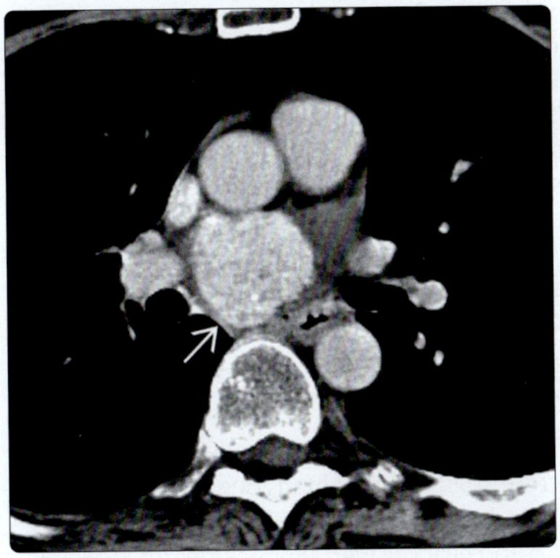

Castleman Disease

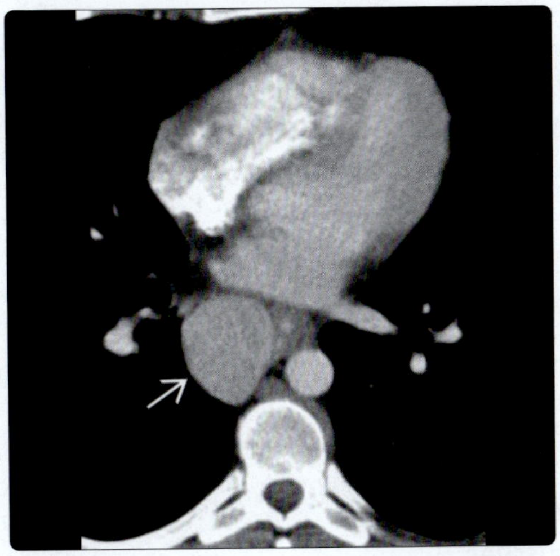

(Left) *Axial CECT of a 44-year-old man with localized Castleman disease shows an intensely enhancing soft tissue mass* ➡ *in the subcarinal visceral mediastinum, which exhibits a small punctate calcification.* **(Right)** *Axial CECT of a 32-year-old man with localized Castleman disease shows an enhancing soft tissue mass* ➡ *in the right visceral mediastinum. Castleman disease may manifest with localized or multicentric disease and may demonstrate focal or multifocal enhancing nodules, masses, &/or lymph nodes.*

Hemangioma

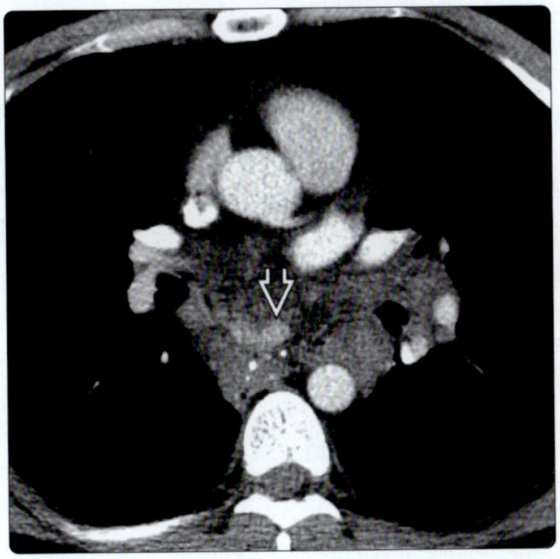

Hemangioma

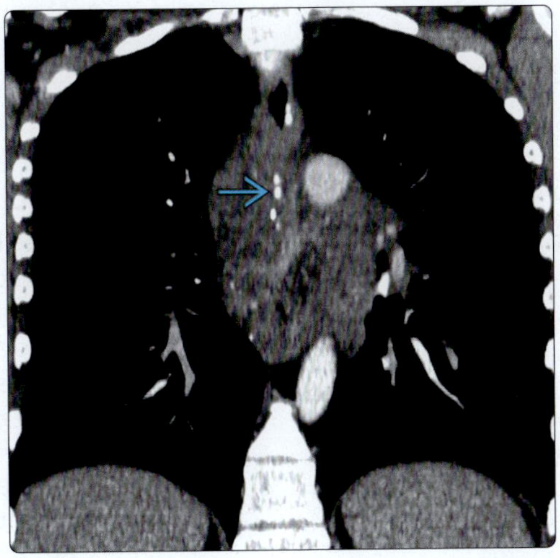

(Left) *Axial CECT of an asymptomatic 38-year-old man with mediastinal hemangioma shows an infiltrative soft tissue mass in the visceral mediastinum that exhibits heterogeneous attenuation, foci of contrast enhancement* ➡*, and multifocal punctate calcifications that likely represent phleboliths.* **(Right)** *Coronal CECT of the same patient shows the infiltrative soft tissue mass in the visceral mediastinum. Note multifocal punctate calcifications* ⇨*, consistent with phleboliths.*

Paraganglioma

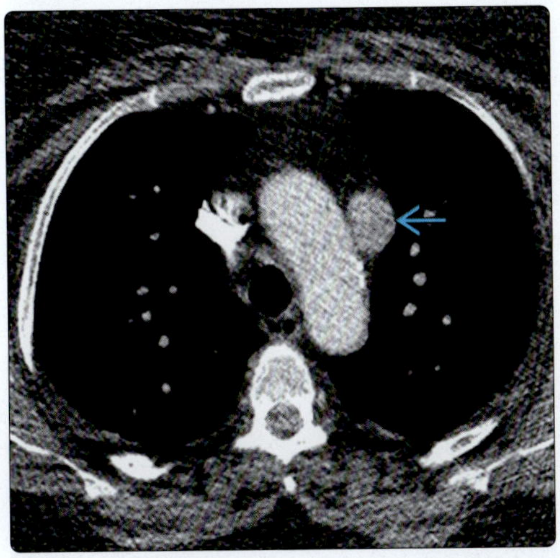

Paraganglioma

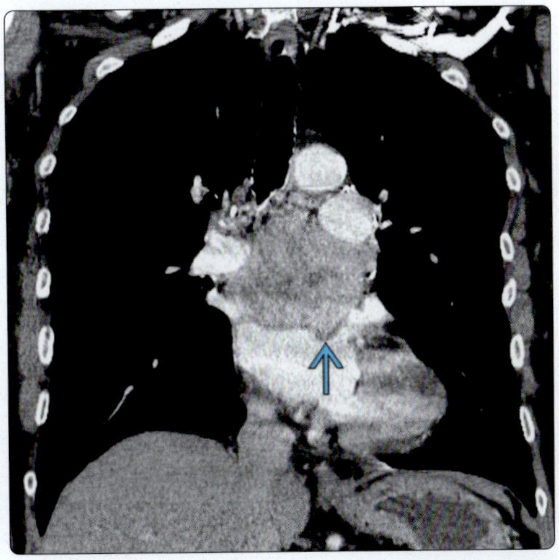

(Left) *Axial CECT of a 60-year-old woman with hypertension shows a well-defined left prevascular soft tissue lesion* ⇨ *that demonstrates contrast enhancement. Mediastinal paraganglioma was diagnosed on surgical excision.* **(Right)** *Coronal CECT of an 85-year-old woman with chest pain shows a large subcarinal heterogeneously enhancing mass in the visceral mediastinum, which was diagnosed as a paraganglioma on biopsy. Note local invasion of the upper aspect of the left atrium* ⇨*.*

DIFFERENTIAL DIAGNOSIS

Common

- Histoplasmosis
- Cardiovascular Calcification
- Mediastinal Goiter
- Sarcoidosis

Less Common

- Silicosis
- Mediastinal Fibrosis

Rare but Important

- Treated Lymphoma
- Metastases
- Congenital Cyst

ESSENTIAL INFORMATION

Key Differential Diagnosis Issues

- Lymph nodes
  - Remote granulomatous disease: Infectious, noninfectious
  - Pneumoconiosis
  - Metastases: Bone-forming and treated malignancies
- Cardiovascular: Vessel walls, myocardium, pericardium
- Congenital cysts
- Abnormal protein deposition in tissue

Helpful Clues for Common Diagnoses

- **Histoplasmosis**
  - Infection with fungus *Histoplasma capsulatum*
  - Remote granulomatous infection: Calcified mediastinal/hilar lymph nodes, may be large and coalescent; calcified pulmonary granulomas
- **Cardiovascular Calcification**
  - Atherosclerosis; intimal calcification, ± endoluminal mural thrombus, ulcerated plaque
  - Mural calcification in aneurysms
  - Constrictive pericarditis; pericardial Ca++ and mass effect on cardiac chambers
- **Mediastinal Goiter**
  - Continuity with cervical goiter; cervicothoracic sign; mass effect on trachea and adjacent structures
  - Heterogeneous: High attenuation on unenhanced CT, intense/sustained contrast enhancement, cystic change
  - Calcification: Amorphous, coarse, punctate, ring-like
- **Sarcoidosis**
  - Chronic systemic granulomatous disease; unknown etiology; non-caseating granulomas
  - Bilateral hilar and mediastinal lymphadenopathy
  - Chronic sarcoidosis: Lymph node calcification in 3-20%
  - Amorphous, cloud-like, punctate, or eggshell calcification

Helpful Clues for Less Common Diagnoses

- **Silicosis**
  - Occupational inhalation of silica; decades of exposure
  - Small discrete 2-5 mm upper lung zone nodules ± Ca++
  - Nodules may coalesce as progressive massive fibrosis
  - Mediastinal and hilar calcified lymph nodes; may exhibit eggshell (peripheral) calcification
- **Mediastinal Fibrosis**
  - Abnormal mediastinal widening
  - Mediastinal soft tissue nodule or mass
    - May exhibit calcification
    - May be localized or infiltrative
    - May obstruct vessels, airways, &/or esophagus

Helpful Clues for Rare Diagnoses

- **Treated Lymphoma**
  - Calcification in small percentage of cases
    - Typically 1 year after treatment
  - Punctate or dense and coalescent Ca++
- **Metastases**
  - Calcified metastatic lymphadenopathy
    - Thyroid cancer, mucinous adenocarcinoma, osteosarcoma
- **Congenital Cyst**
  - Bronchogenic, esophageal duplication
  - Mural calcification
  - Milk of calcium: Diffuse Ca++, milk of Ca++-fluid level

Histoplasmosis

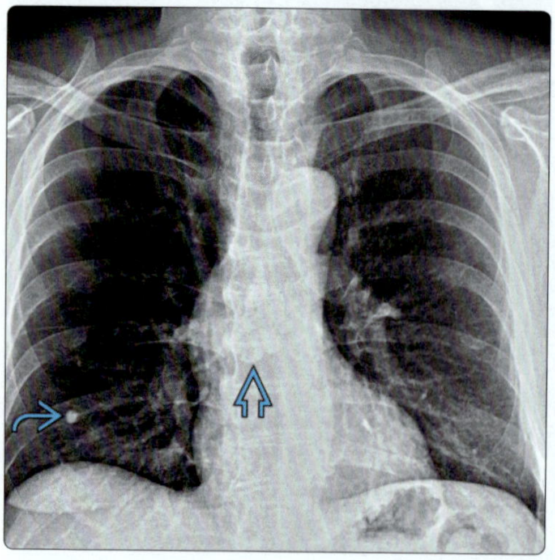

Histoplasmosis

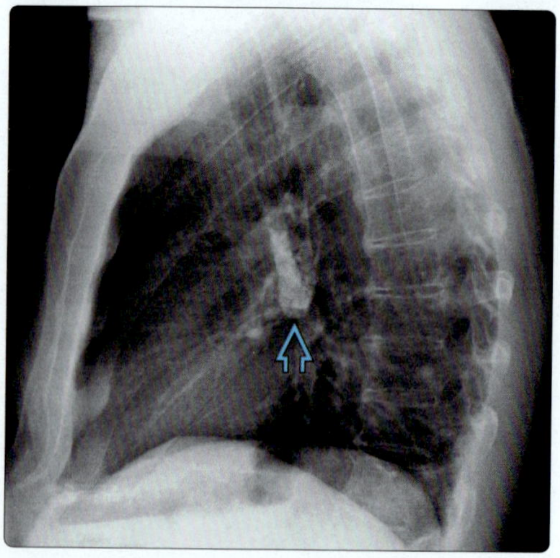

(Left) *PA chest radiograph of an asymptomatic 64-year-old man shows a right lower lobe calcified pulmonary granuloma and a large polylobular calcification projecting over the subcarinal region.* **(Right)** *Lateral chest radiograph of the same patient shows the large subcarinal calcification that likely corresponds to clustered or coalescent calcified mediastinal lymph nodes. The findings are consistent with remote granulomatous infection, a typical imaging feature of prior histoplasmosis.*

Histoplasmosis

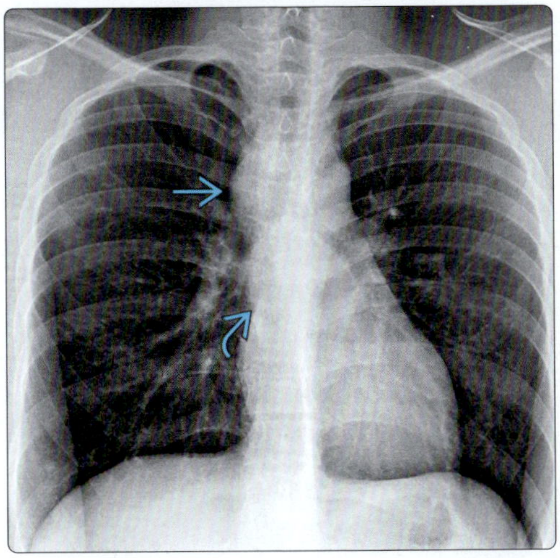

Histoplasmosis

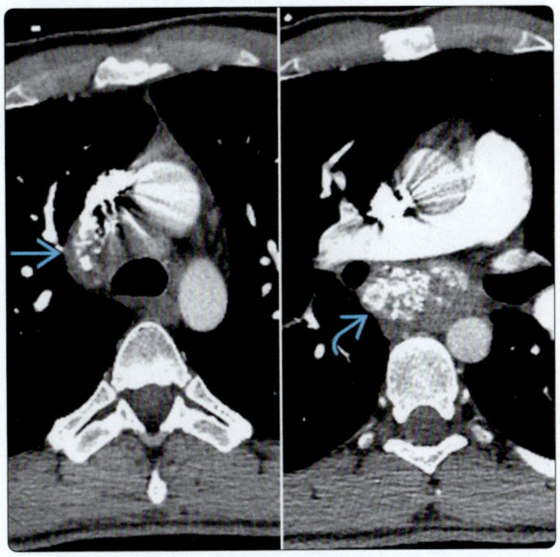

(Left) *PA chest radiograph of an asymptomatic 20-year-old man shows right paratracheal* *and subcarinal* *soft tissue masses, consistent with lymphadenopathy.* **(Right)** *Composite image with axial CECT of the same patient shows multifocal clustered punctate and coalescent calcifications within right lower paratracheal* *and subcarinal* *enlarged lymph nodes, consistent with sequela of remote granulomatous disease, a typical imaging finding of remote histoplasmosis.*

Cardiovascular Calcification

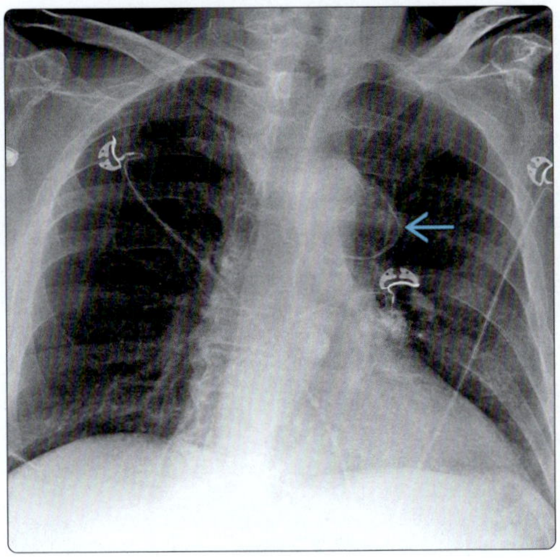

Cardiovascular Calcification

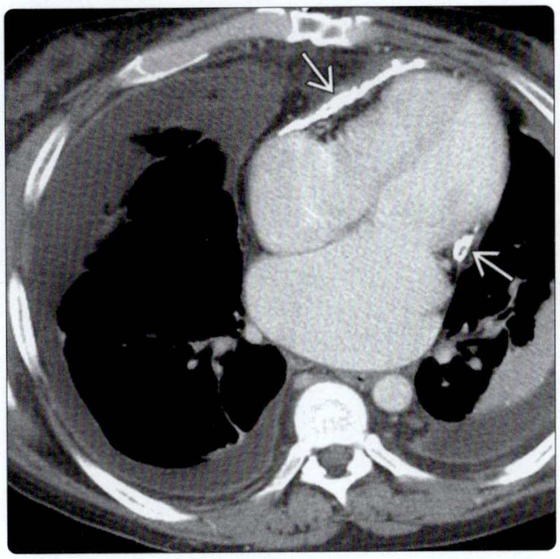

(Left) *AP portable chest radiograph of an 88-year-old man with chest pain shows a soft tissue mass in the aortopulmonary window with peripheral curvilinear calcification, consistent with a saccular aortic aneurysm, which was confirmed on chest CT (not shown).* **(Right)** *Axial CECT of a 44-year-old man with chest pain and peripheral edema shows pericardial calcification* *that produces mass effect on the right and left ventricles, consistent with suspected constrictive pericarditis. Note bilateral pleural effusions.*

Cardiovascular Calcification

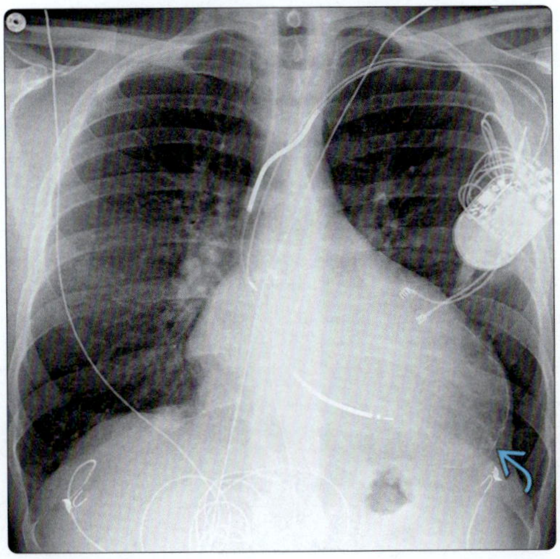

Cardiovascular Calcification

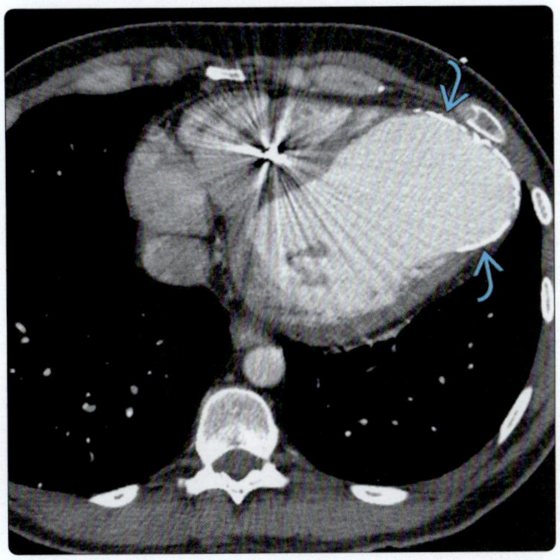

(Left) *PA chest radiograph of a 46-year-old man with a history of remote myocardial infarction shows curvilinear calcification projecting over the left ventricular apex, consistent with a postinfarction left ventricular aneurysm.* **(Right)** *Axial CECT of the same patient shows a large left ventricular true aneurysm characterized by thinning and calcification* *and the left apical ventricular myocardium. Cardiovascular calcifications may affect the vessel walls, the myocardium, or the pericardium.*

(Left) *Axial NECT of an 89-year-old woman shows a mediastinal goiter that involves the right prevascular and visceral compartments and exhibits intrinsic high attenuation and coarse calcifications. Note mass effect on the right trachea and upper mediastinal vessels.* **(Right)** *Coronal oblique NECT of the same patient shows continuity between the cervical and mediastinal portions of the goiter, which exhibits heterogeneous high attenuation, coarse calcifications, and mass effect on adjacent structures.*

Mediastinal Goiter

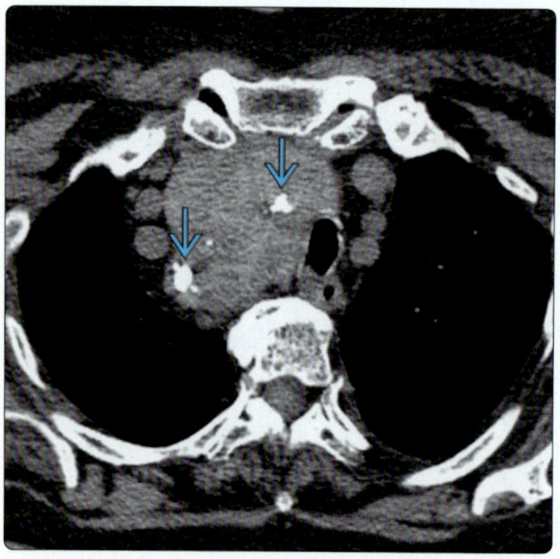

Mediastinal Goiter

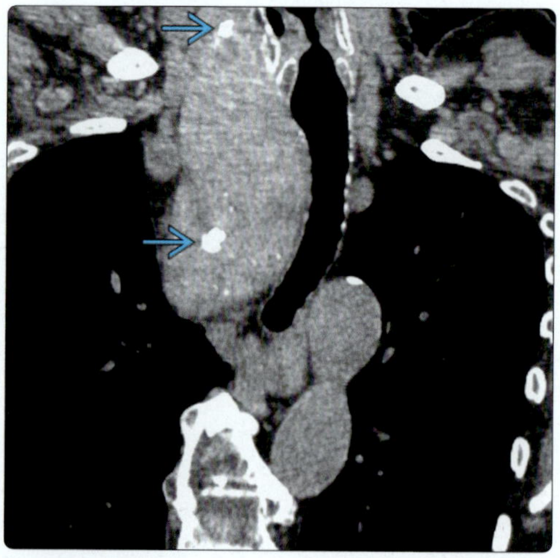

(Left) *PA chest radiograph of a 76-year-old woman with chronic dyspnea and end-stage sarcoidosis shows bilateral architectural distortion and bilateral hilar and mediastinal lymphadenopathy with intrinsic calcifications.* **(Right)** *Axial CECT of the same patient shows enlarged right lower paratracheal and left mediastinal lymph nodes with intrinsic dense calcifications. Calcification is seen in up to 20% of intrathoracic lymph nodes in the setting of chronic sarcoidosis.*

Sarcoidosis

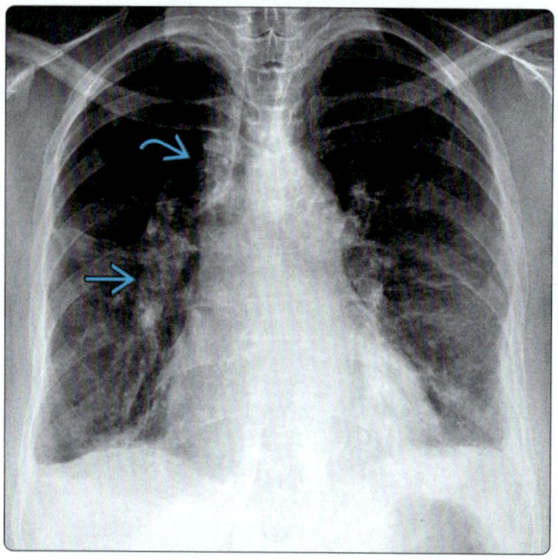

Sarcoidosis

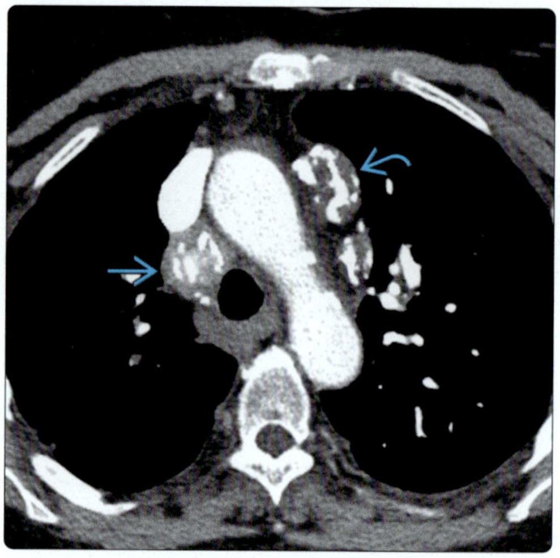

(Left) *Axial NECT of a 75-year-old male sandblaster with complicated silicosis shows multifocal partially calcified nonenlarged mediastinal lymph nodes. Note peripheral curvilinear calcification of a nonenlarged paraaortic lymph node, consistent with eggshell calcification, characteristic of silicosis.* **(Right)** *Coronal NECT of the same patient shows bilateral hilar and aortopulmonary lymph node calcifications and multifocal calcifications in an enlarged subcarinal lymph node. Note calcified pulmonary nodules.*

Silicosis

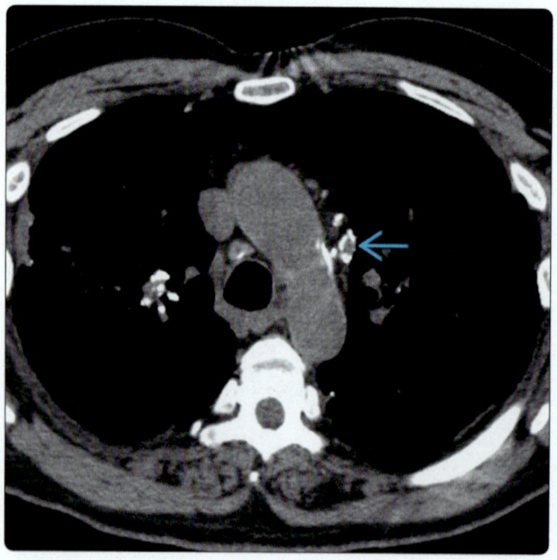

Silicosis

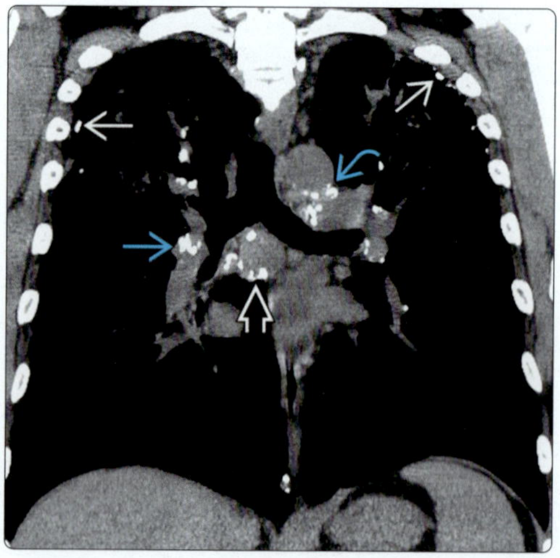

Mediastinal Fibrosis

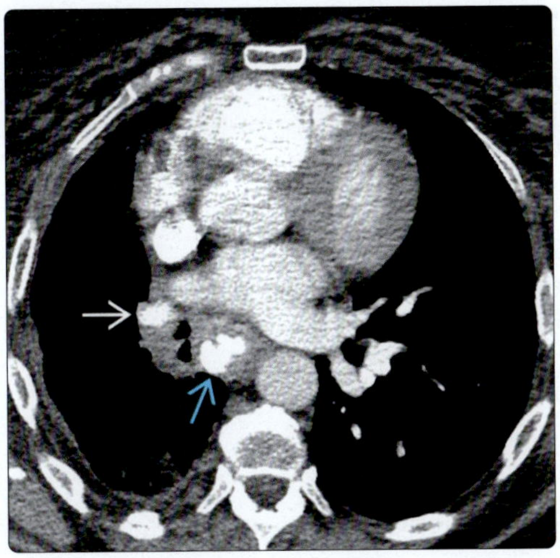

Mediastinal Fibrosis

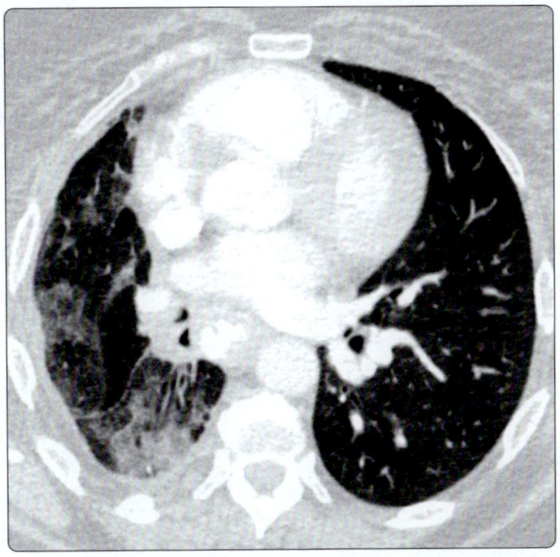

(Left) *Axial CECT of a 56-year-old woman with mediastinal fibrosis and chronic dyspnea shows densely calcified right hilar ➔ and mediastinal ⇨ soft tissue masses, which obliterate the right inferior pulmonary vein and branches of the right pulmonary artery, and diffuse right pleural thickening.* **(Right)** *Axial CECT of the same patient shows a small right lung volume and multifocal right lung ground-glass and linear opacities and consolidations thought to represent sequela of chronic right-sided arterial and venous obstruction.*

Treated Lymphoma

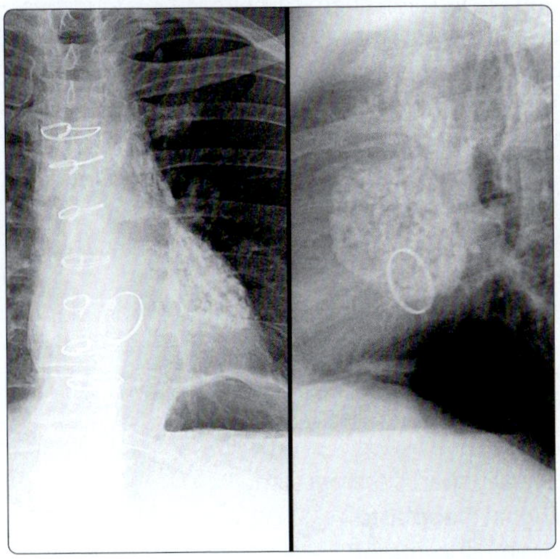

Metastases

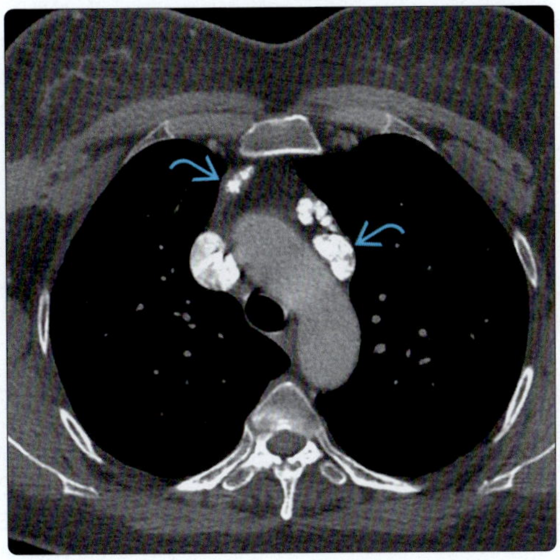

(Left) *Composite image with coned-down PA (left) and lateral (right) chest radiographs of an asymptomatic 50-year-old man with remote Hodgkin lymphoma treated with radiation shows dense left anterior mediastinal calcifications in the anatomic locations of previous neoplastic involvement.* **(Right)** *Axial CECT of a 58-year-old woman with metastatic breast cancer shows calcified prevascular mediastinal lymph nodes ⇨ representing calcified lymph node metastases.*

Congenital Cyst

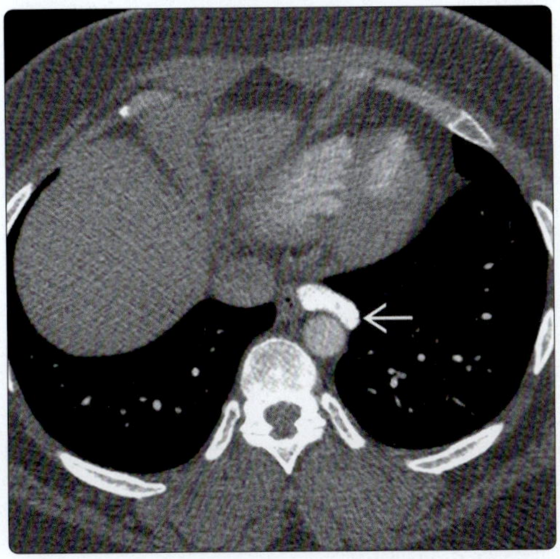

Congenital Cyst

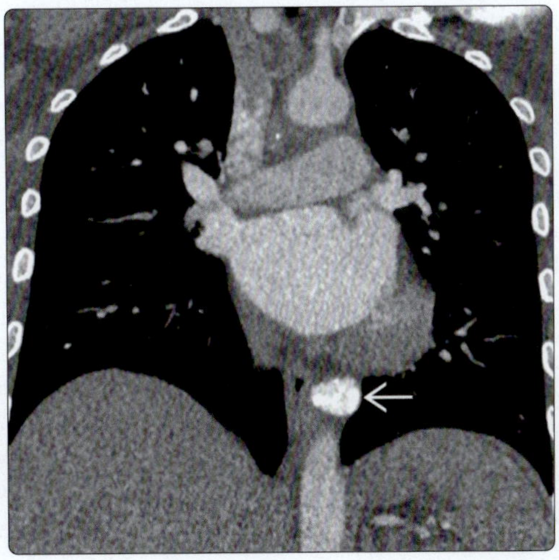

(Left) *Axial CECT of a 37-year-old woman demonstrates a densely calcified elongate left paraesophageal lesion ➔ in the visceral mediastinum representing a foregut cyst with intrinsic milk of calcium.* **(Right)** *Coronal CECT of the same patient shows the dense ovoid densely calcified cyst ➔ in the left visceral mediastinum adjacent to the esophagus. Bronchogenic cysts may exhibit high-attenuation fluid, mural calcification, and milk of calcium. The latter may be diffuse or may manifest as a fluid-milk of calcium level.*

DIFFERENTIAL DIAGNOSIS

Common

- Thymic Hyperplasia
- Thymic Epithelial Neoplasm
- Lymphoma
- Neurogenic Neoplasm

Less Common

- Thymic Cyst
- Foregut Duplication Cyst

Rare but Important

- Hemangioma
- Fibrosing Mediastinitis

ESSENTIAL INFORMATION

Key Differential Diagnosis Issues

- CT is imaging modality of choice for most mediastinal abnormalities
  - Some lesions may be indeterminate
- Advantages of MR
  - Higher soft tissue contrast compared to CT
  - MR is superior to CT for
    - Distinguishing cystic from solid lesions (e.g., thymic cysts from solid tumors)
    - Identifying cystic &/or necrotic components within solid masses
    - Identifying septations &/or soft tissue within cystic lesions
    - Distinguishing thymic hyperplasia and normal thymus from solid tumors
- Added value of MR in evaluation of mediastinal masses
  - Alter patient management
  - Reduce or eliminate need for subsequent follow-up
  - Reduce surgical intervention rate for mediastinal lesions
- MR protocol for assessment of mediastinal masses
  - T1WI
  - T2WI
  - In-phase and out-of-phase gradient echo (GRE)
  - Pre- and post dynamic contrast-enhanced FS T1WI
  - Other sequences as needed
    - Fat saturation techniques to detect macroscopic fat
    - Diffusion weighted imaging (DWI)
    - Short tau inversion recovery (STIR): Most sensitive pulse sequence for bone marrow edema
- Chemical shift GRE
  - Includes in-phase and out-of-phase sequences
  - Employed for detection of microscopic fat
  - Distinguish benign lesion from malignant tumors
    - Normal thymus and thymic hyperplasia demonstrate loss of signal on out-of-phase sequences
      - Due to suppression of microscopic fat interspersed between nonneoplastic thymic tissue
      - Malignant lesions, such as thymic epithelial neoplasms, lymphoma, and metastases do not suppress
  - Chemical shift ratio (CSR)
    - Tool used to calculate signal loss
    - Definition
      - CSR = (thymus SI OP/paraspinal muscle SI OP)/(thymus SI IP/paraspinal muscle SI IP)
      - Normal thymus and thymic hyperplasia: CSR of 0.5-0.6
      - Thymic epithelial neoplasms, lymphoma, and other lesions: CSR 0.9-1.0
  - Signal intensity index (SII)
    - Definition
      - SII = (thymus SI IP - thymus SI OP)/(thymus SI IP) x 100%
      - Normal thymus and thymic hyperplasia: > 9%
- Dynamic contrast enhancement (DCE)
  - Measure of tissue vascularity
  - Facilitates differentiation of lesions by enhancement pattern
  - Enables postprocessed subtraction
- DWI
  - Detect presence and extent of restricted diffusion

Helpful Clues for Common Diagnoses

- **Thymic Hyperplasia**
  - Suppression of signal on chemical shift MR is suggestive of thymic hyperplasia
  - Qualitative assessment of suppression is not as sensitive as quantitative evaluation
  - Quantitative assessment
    - CSR ≤ 0.7 and SII > 9% suggest either normal thymus or thymic hyperplasia
  - Few cases of nonsuppressing normal thymus and thymic hyperplasia
    - If other MR features may suggest thymic hyperplasia rather than malignancy, consider follow-up
      - Obtain MR in 3-6 months
      - Confirm stability, regression, &/or changes in suppression
      - Potentially spares thymectomy
- **Thymic Epithelial Neoplasm**
  - Thymoma is most common
    - T1WI: Low to intermediate signal intensity
      - Cystic regions and necrosis will show high signal intensity
    - T2WI: High signal intensity
  - Thymic carcinoma and thymic carcinoid
    - T1WI: Hyperintense to muscle
    - T2WI: Hyperintense to muscle
    - Heterogeneous signal: Cystic changes, necrosis, hemorrhage
    - Carcinoid tumors may show hyperenhancement on T1+C
  - Chemical shift MR
    - No or little suppression of tissue on out-of-phase MR imaging
  - DCE pattern
    - Low-risk thymomas vs. high-risk thymomas and other lesions
      - More rapid mean time-to-peak enhancement: 1.3 minutes vs. 2.5 minutes
  - DWI
    - Low-risk thymomas vs. high-risk thymomas and thymic carcinoma

  - High-risk thymomas may have lower apparent diffusion coefficient (ADC) than low-risk thymomas
  - Proposed ADC cutoff value: 1.56 x 10-3 mm²/second
- **Lymphoma**
  - MR appearance depends on several factors
    - Type of lymphoma
    - Treatment
  - Most untreated lymphomas
    - T1WI: Homogeneous hypointensity
    - T2WI: Homogeneous hypointensity
    - T1+C: Homogeneous enhancement is typical; heterogeneity may be due to necrosis
  - During and following therapy
    - Decrease in water content
    - Increase in collagen or fibrotic content
    - T2WI: Lower signal
    - T1+C: Decrease in enhancement
- **Neurogenic Neoplasm**
  - Neurofibroma
    - T2WI: Hypointense centrally with peripheral hyperintensity ("target" appearance)
    - Limited enhancement; cystic components are rare
    - Findings suggestive of malignant transformation
      - Cystic changes
      - Rapid or intense enhancement
  - Schwannoma
    - T2WI: Hyperintense centrally
    - T1+C: Moderate enhancement of solid components

Helpful Clues for Less Common Diagnoses

- **Thymic Cyst**
  - Unilocular or multilocular
  - MR can identify complex cystic lesions
    - Mural nodules
    - Wall thickening
    - Septations
  - T1WI: Homogeneous but variable signal intensity
    - Depends on serous, proteinaceous, and hemorrhagic components
  - T2WI: Homogeneous high signal intensity
    - Isointense to cerebrospinal fluid
  - T1+C: No internal enhancement
    - Thin, smooth enhancement of wall may be seen
  - Follow-up and management
    - Simple thymic cyst
      - Initially at 6 months
      - Annually for 5 years
    - Complex cyst
      - Followed by imaging or surgically resected
      - Depends on level of clinical and imaging concern
- **Foregut Duplication Cyst**
  - Includes bronchogenic and esophageal cysts
  - T1WI: Homogeneous but variable
    - Due to proteinaceous, hemorrhagic, and mucoid content
  - T2WI: High signal intensity
  - T1+C: No enhancement
    - Thin, smooth wall enhancement may be seen

Helpful Clues for Rare Diagnoses

- **Hemangioma**
  - T1+C: Findings similar to liver hemangiomas
    - Peripheral nodular enhancement
    - Fill-in or partial fill-in over time
    - Not always present
- **Fibrosing Mediastinitis**
  - May be focal or infiltrative
    - Infiltrative lesions may encase and narrow vessels and structures
  - T2WI
    - Acute: High signal intensity
    - Chronic: Low signal intensity

SELECTED REFERENCES

1. Carter BW et al: ITMIG classification of mediastinal compartments and multidisciplinary approach to mediastinal masses. Radiographics. 37(2):413-36, 2017
2. Ackman JB: MR imaging of mediastinal masses. Magn Reson Imaging Clin N Am. 23(2):141-64, 2015

Thymic Hyperplasia

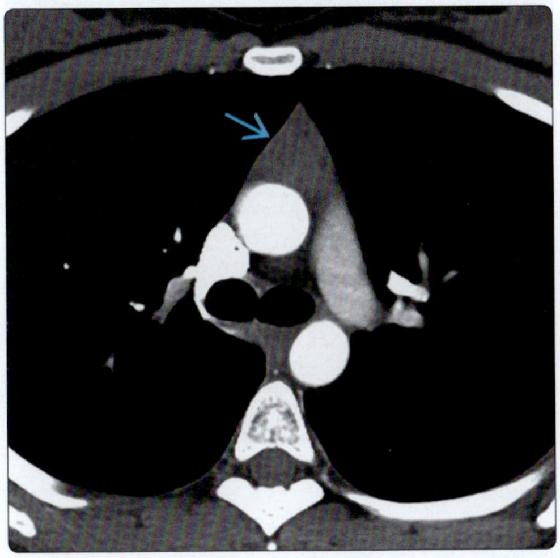

Thymic Hyperplasia

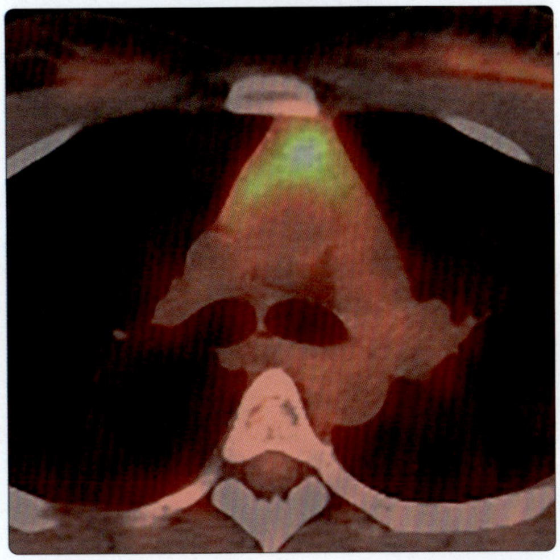

(Left) *Axial CECT of a patient with lymphoma treated with chemotherapy demonstrates triangular-shaped soft tissue in the prevascular mediastinum, representing thymic hyperplasia* ➡. **(Right)** *Fused axial FDG PET/CT of the same patient shows increased FDG uptake in the hyperplastic thymic tissue. Benign disease processes, such as thymic hyperplasia, can result in FDG-avid soft tissue in the prevascular mediastinum and potentially be misinterpreted as malignancy.*

Thymic Hyperplasia

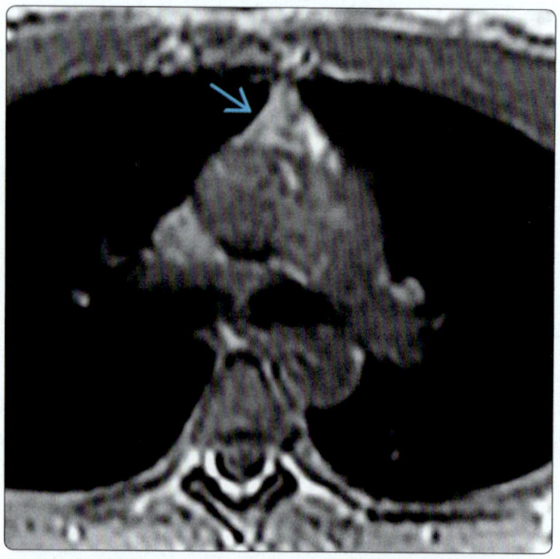

Thymic Hyperplasia

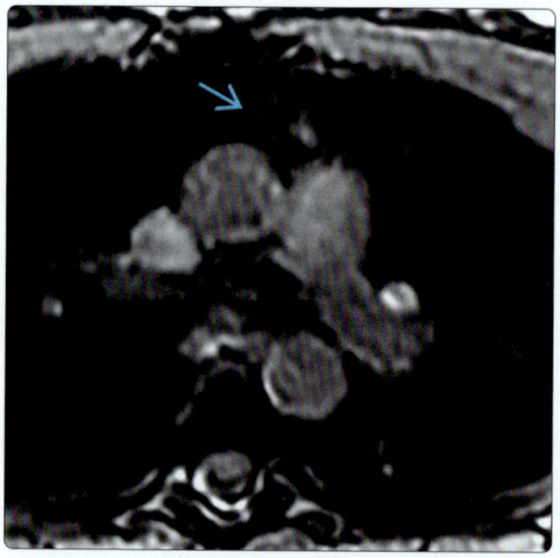

(Left) *Axial T1W in-phase MR of the same patient shows uniform high signal intensity in the region of thymic hyperplasia.* **(Right)** *Axial T1 out-of-phase MR demonstrates uniform loss of signal within the thymic tissue. On chemical shift MR, the loss of signal intensity on out-of-phase imaging indicates the presence of microscopic fat interspersed between hyperplastic thymic tissue. Other lesions, such as thymic epithelial neoplasms, lymphoma, and metastases, will not lose signal in this fashion.*

Thymic Epithelial Neoplasm

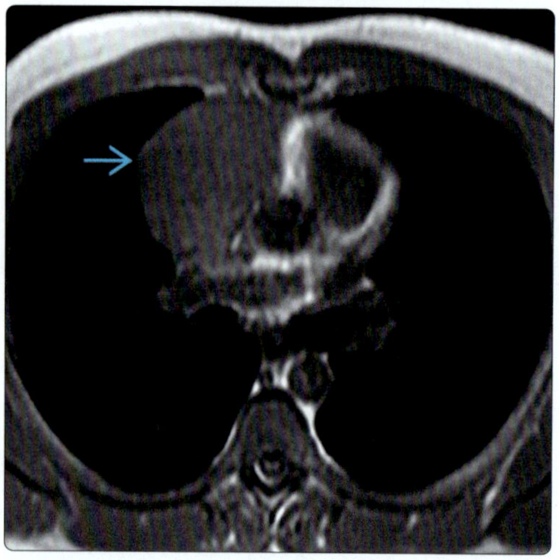

Thymic Epithelial Neoplasm

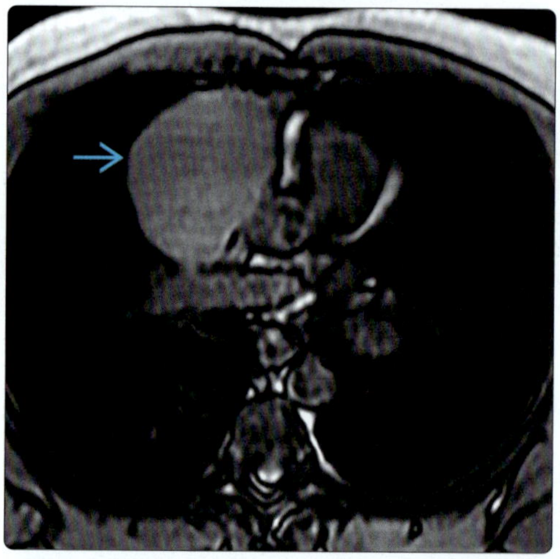

(Left) *Axial T1 in-phase MR demonstrates a right prevascular mediastinal mass that is of uniform signal intensity similar to that of the adjacent musculature of the chest wall.* **(Right)** *Axial T1 out-of-phase MR of the same patient shows no loss of signal intensity, indicating the presence of solid tissue. Biopsy revealed thymoma. In contrast to normal thymus and thymic hyperplasia, thymic epithelial neoplasms and other tumors will not demonstrate loss of signal intensity on chemical shift MR.*

Thymic Cyst

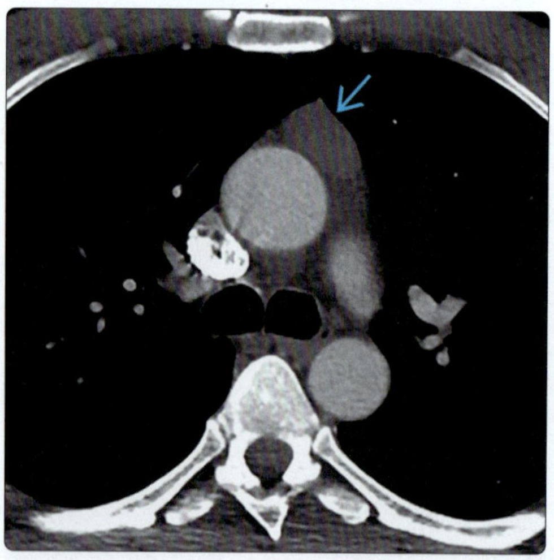

Thymic Cyst

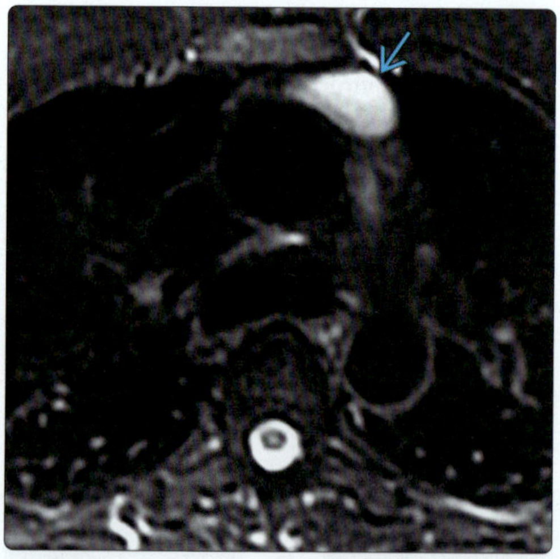

(Left) *Axial CECT of an asymptomatic patient shows a well-circumscribed low-attenuation lesion in the prevascular mediastinum. Although fluid attenuation was present in most of the lesion, regions of high (soft tissue) attenuation were present.* **(Right)** *Axial T2 FS MR of the same patient shows homogeneous high signal intensity within the lesion, reflecting its cystic nature. MR is superior to CT in differentiating cystic from solid lesions and revealing the presence of solid components in cystic lesions.*

Thymic Cyst

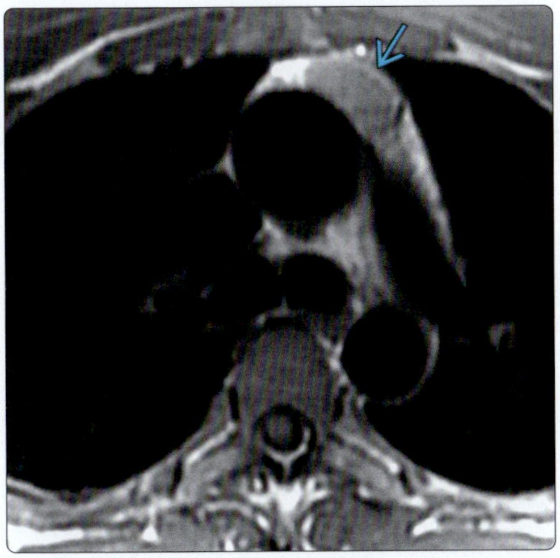

Thymic Cyst

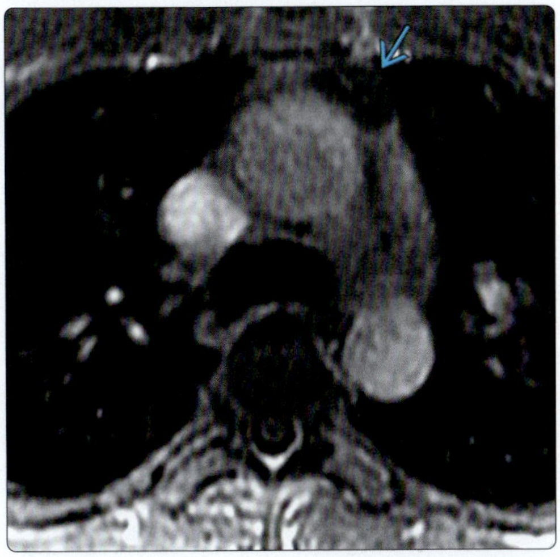

(Left) *Axial T1 MR of the same patient shows homogeneous signal intensity →.* **(Right)** *Axial T1 C+ FS MR of the same patient demonstrates normal enhancement in the mediastinal vessels but no regions of enhancement in the thymic cyst →. Following the administration of intravenous contrast, no enhancement should be identified within thymic cysts, although multilocular cysts complicated by infection or inflammation may show rim enhancement.*

Foregut Duplication Cyst

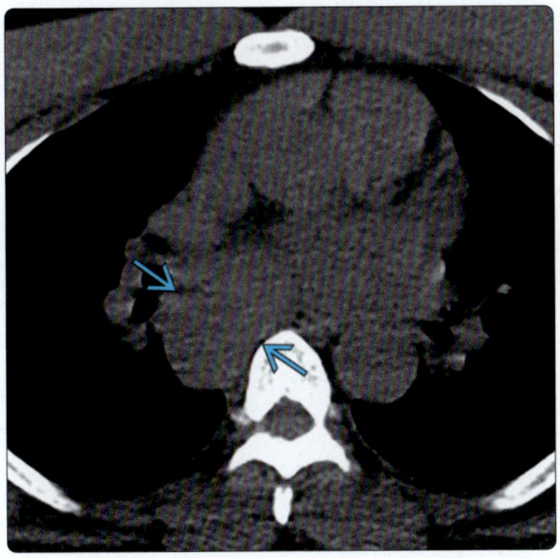

Foregut Duplication Cyst

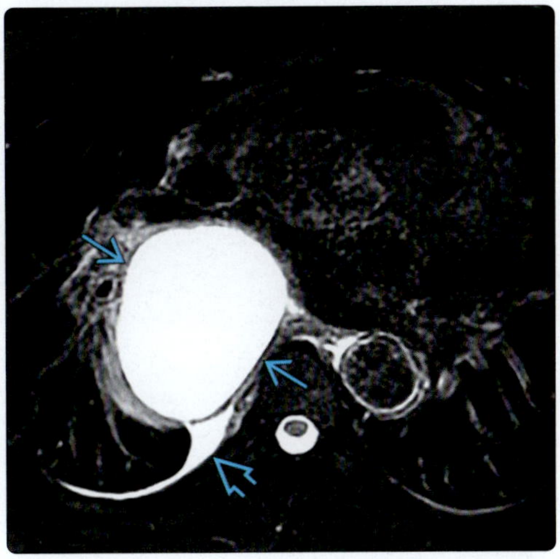

(Left) *Axial NECT of a patient presenting with dysphagia demonstrates a well-circumscribed lesion involving the visceral and paravertebral compartments that is isodense relative to other mediastinal structures →.* **(Right)** *Axial T2 FS MR of the same patient shows homogeneous high signal intensity within the lesion, representing a foregut duplication cyst, specifically a bronchogenic cyst →. The lesion was resected due to the presence of symptoms at the time of presentation. Note the small right pleural effusion ⇨.*

Foregut Duplication Cyst

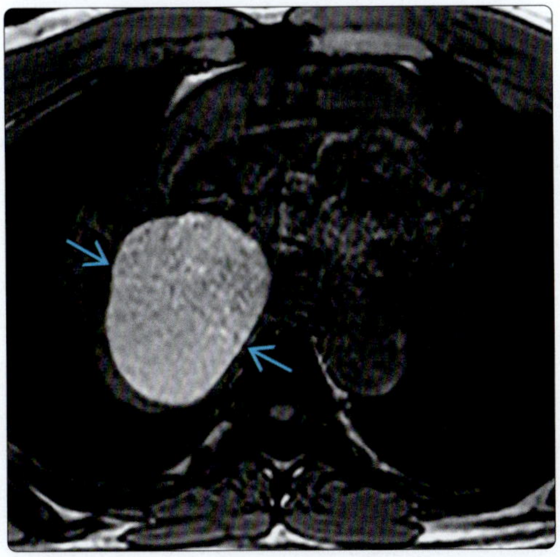

Foregut Duplication Cyst

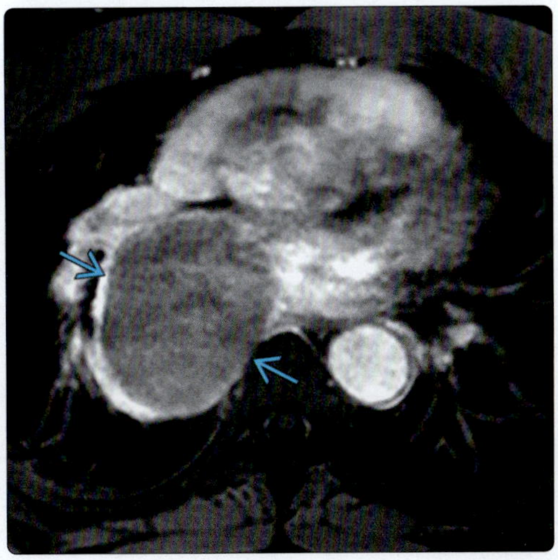

(Left) *Axial T1 MR of the same patient shows intrinsic high signal intensity in the cyst, representing the presence of hemorrhagic or proteinaceous components →.* **(Right)** *Axial T1 C+ MR of the same patient shows normal enhancement within the mediastinal blood pool but no contrast enhancement associated with the bronchogenic cyst →. Following the administration of intravenous contrast, no enhancement should be identified within bronchogenic cysts, although lesions complicated by infection may show rim enhancement.*

Pulmonary Artery Mass

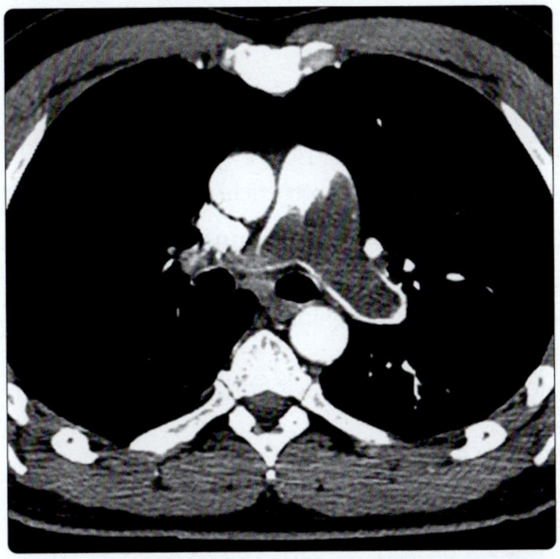

Pulmonary Artery Mass

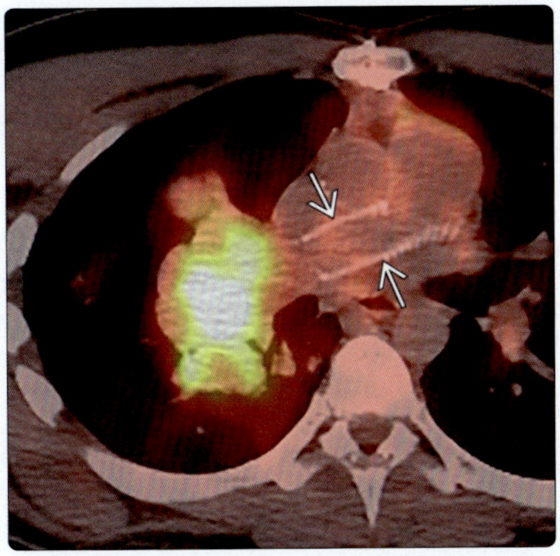

(Left) *Axial CECT of a patient presenting with chest pain shows a large mass in the pulmonary trunk extending into the proximal left and right pulmonary arteries. Biopsy revealed primary pulmonary artery sarcoma.* **(Right)** *Fused axial FDG PET/CT of a patient with prior resection of pulmonary artery sarcoma and reconstruction of the right pulmonary artery ➡ shows a large FDG-avid mass arising from the distal right pulmonary artery extending into the right lung, representing recurrent malignancy.*

Pulmonary Artery Mass

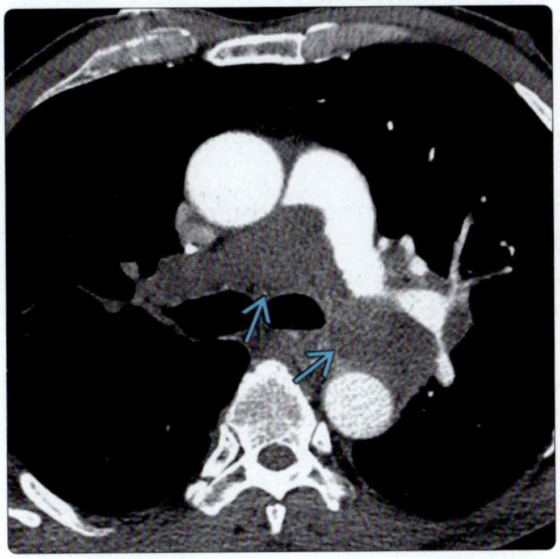

Pulmonary Artery Invasion

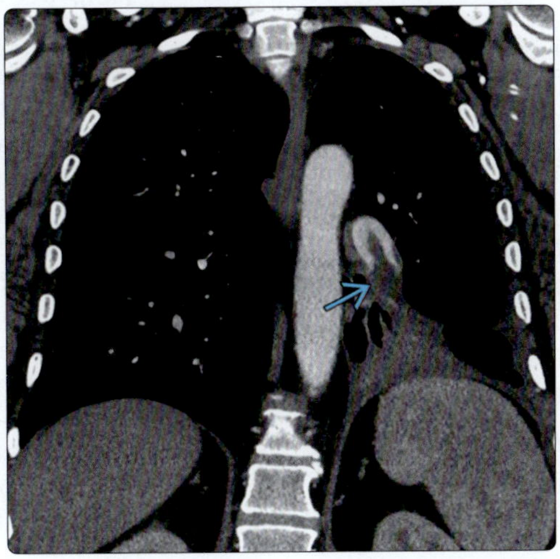

(Left) *Axial CECT of a patient with pulmonary artery sarcoma shows an ill-defined soft tissue mass arising from the pulmonary arteries and invading the adjacent mediastinum ➡. Pulmonary artery sarcoma is typically confined to the vessels but may invade adjacent structures in the mediastinum or lung.* **(Right)** *Coronal CECT of a patient with recurrent left lower lobe lung cancer demonstrates invasion of the left lower lobe pulmonary artery ➡.*

Pulmonary Artery Invasion

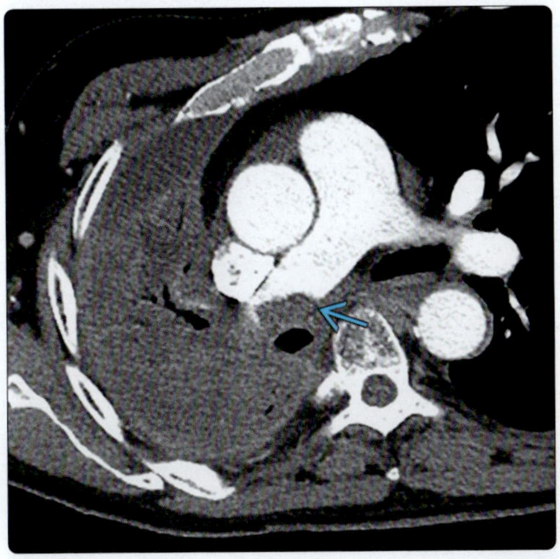

Pulmonary Artery Invasion

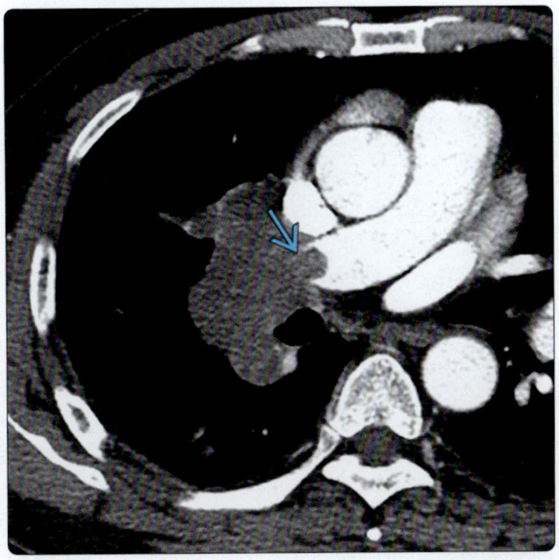

(Left) *Axial CECT of a patient with a history of malignant pleural mesothelioma who has received radiation therapy to the right hemithorax demonstrates recurrent tumor that invades the proximal right pulmonary artery ➡.* **(Right)** *Axial CECT of a patient with recurrent germ cell neoplasm of the right mediastinum shows invasion of the right pulmonary artery ➡. Pulmonary artery invasion is most commonly seen in lung cancer but may also occur in the setting of mediastinal, pleural, and chest wall neoplasms.*

DIFFERENTIAL DIAGNOSIS

Common

- Pulmonary Arterial Hypertension
- Pulmonic Valvular Stenosis
- Atrial Septal Defect

Less Common

- Takayasu Arteritis
- Pulmonary Artery Aneurysm

Rare but Important

- Mitral Stenosis or Regurgitation
- Pulmonary Venoocclusive Disease
- Pulmonary Capillary Hemangiomatosis

ESSENTIAL INFORMATION

Key Differential Diagnosis Issues

- Radiographic features of pulmonary arterial hypertension (PAH)
  - Disproportionate enlargement of central pulmonary arteries (PA)
  - Hilum convergence sign on radiography
    - Helps distinguish PA dilatation from hilar mass/enlarged hilar lymph node
    - Positive hilum convergence sign: If PA branches are visible through hilar opacity, then it is due to hilar mass/enlarged lymph node
    - Negative hilum convergence sign: If PA branches lead toward hilar opacity, then it is due to enlarged PA
- CT features of PAH
  - Pulmonary trunk > 3 cm in size
  - Main PA:ascending thoracic aortic ratio of ≥ 1

Helpful Clues for Common Diagnoses

- **Pulmonary Arterial Hypertension**
  - Resting mean PA pressure ≥ 25 mmHg at right heart catheterization
  - Variable causes or idiopathic
  - Enlargement of central PA and peripheral arterial pruning
- **Pulmonic Valvular Stenosis (Poststenotic Dilatation)**
  - Disproportionate enlargement of main and left PA
  - Right ventricle enlargement
- **Atrial Septal Defect (ASD)**
  - Increased pulmonary vascular flow
  - Cardiomegaly: Enlarged right ventricle and right atrium

Helpful Clues for Less Common Diagnoses

- **Takayasu Arteritis**
  - Pulmonary artery wall thickening (acute phase)
  - Aneurysmal dilatation
  - Common involvement of thoracic aorta and major branches
- **Pulmonary Artery Aneurysm**
  - Idiopathic: May be associated with PA valve insufficiency
    - Isolated dilatation of pulmonary trunk
  - Acquired: Behçet disease, mycotic aneurysms
    - Segmental and subsegmental branches

Helpful Clues for Rare Diagnoses

- **Mitral Stenosis or Regurgitation**
  - Cardiomegaly
  - Left atrial enlargement
- **Pulmonary Venoocclusive Disease (PVOD)**
  - Rare cause of PAH
  - Interlobular septal thickening and centrilobular ground-glass opacities
  - Signs of PA hypertension with normal pulmonary capillary wedge pressure
- **Pulmonary Capillary Hemangiomatosis**
  - Imaging findings may overlap with PVOD
  - Ground-glass opacities and reticular opacities represent capillary proliferation beyond resolution of imaging
  - Interlobular septal thickening and pleural effusions are unusual

Pulmonary Arterial Hypertension

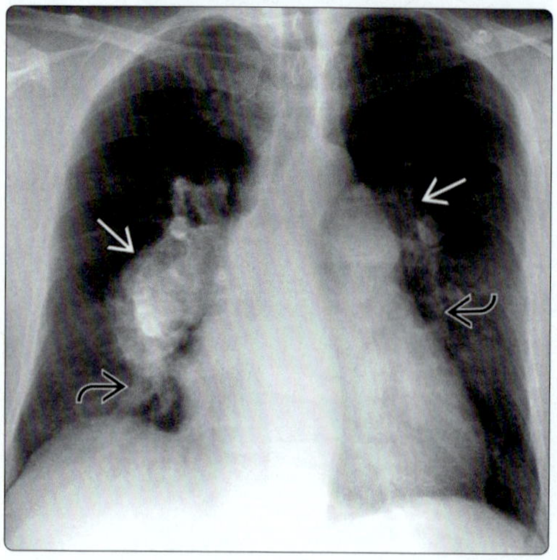

Pulmonic Valvular Stenosis

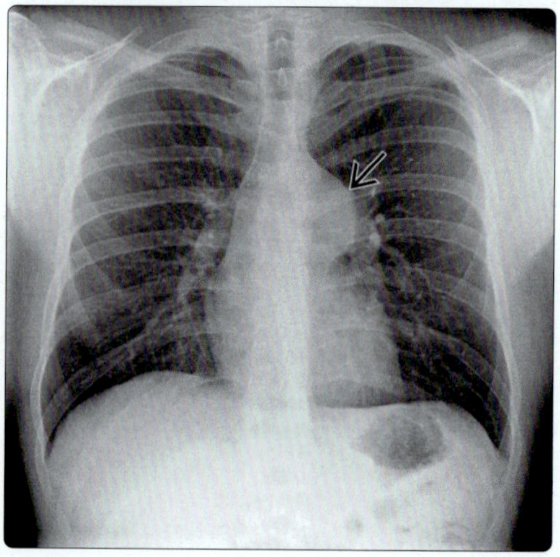

(Left) *Frontal chest radiograph shows massively enlarged main and bilateral pulmonary arteries ➡. Note rapid tapering of distal branches ⇨ and cardiomegaly.* **(Right)** *Frontal chest radiograph shows enlargement of the main and left pulmonary arteries ⇨ with a right pulmonary artery of normal caliber in this patient with pulmonary valve stenosis. The heart size and peripheral pulmonary markings are normal.*

Atrial Septal Defect

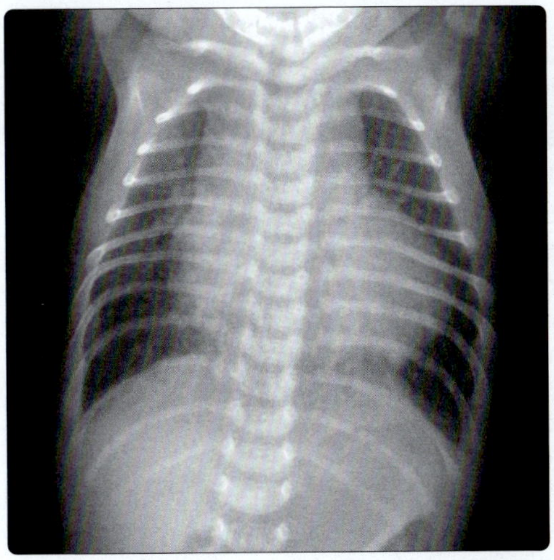

Takayasu Arteritis

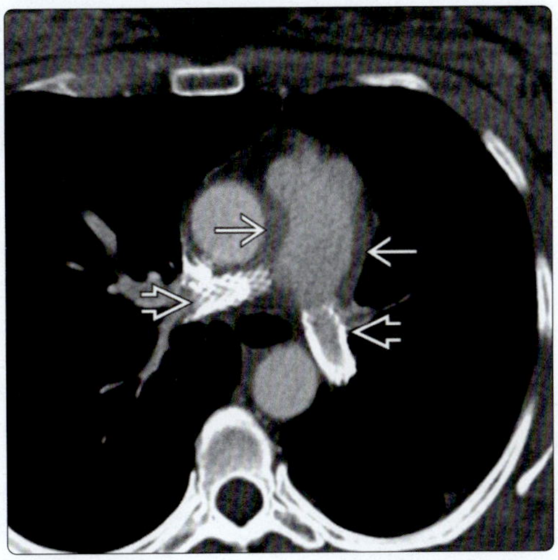

(Left) *AP chest radiograph of an infant demonstrates cardiomegaly and increased pulmonary vascular flow secondary to an underlying atrial septal defect. Mediastinal widening is due to normal thymic tissue in this patient.* **(Right)** *Axial CECT of a patient with Takayasu arteritis demonstrates dilatation and mural (wall) thickening → of the pulmonary trunk. Bilateral pulmonary artery stents were placed for vascular stenoses →, which is a common complication encountered in late-stage Takayasu arteritis.*

Pulmonary Artery Aneurysm

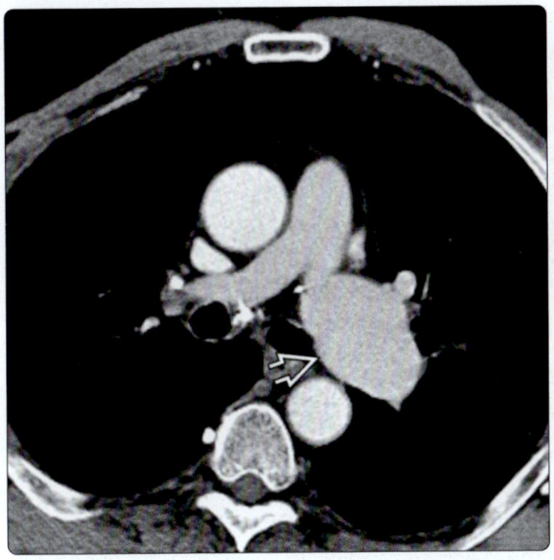

Mitral Stenosis or Regurgitation

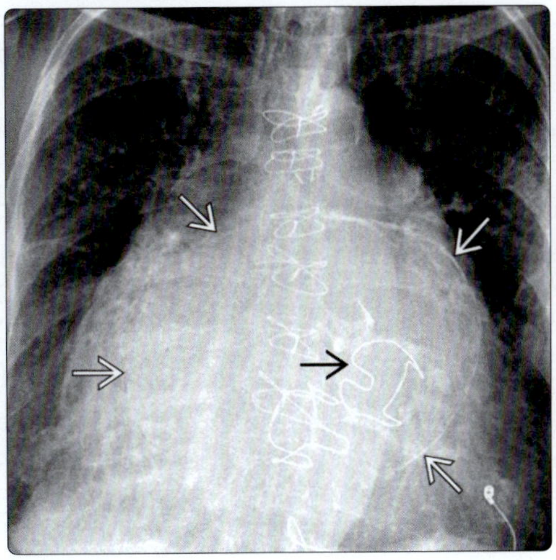

(Left) *Axial CECT of a patient with Hughes-Stovin syndrome demonstrates a left pulmonary artery aneurysm →. Hughes-Stovin syndrome is characterized by pulmonary artery and peripheral vein thrombosis and pulmonary artery aneurysms.* **(Right)** *Frontal chest radiograph of a patient with history of mitral regurgitation shows cardiomegaly with an enlarged left atrium, outlined by a peripheral rim of calcification →. The mitral valve has been replaced →.*

Pulmonary Venoocclusive Disease

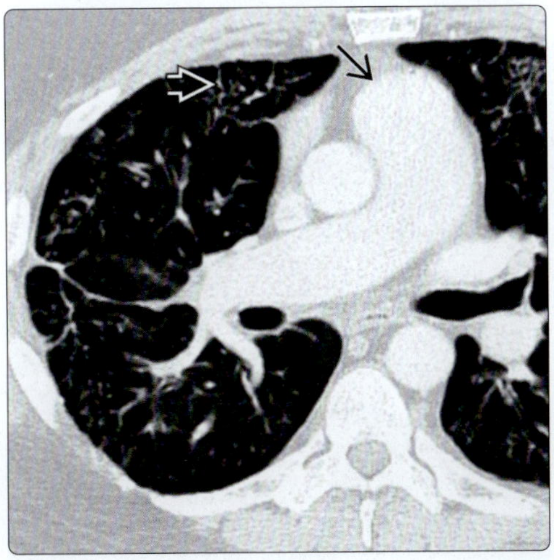

Pulmonary Capillary Hemangiomatosis

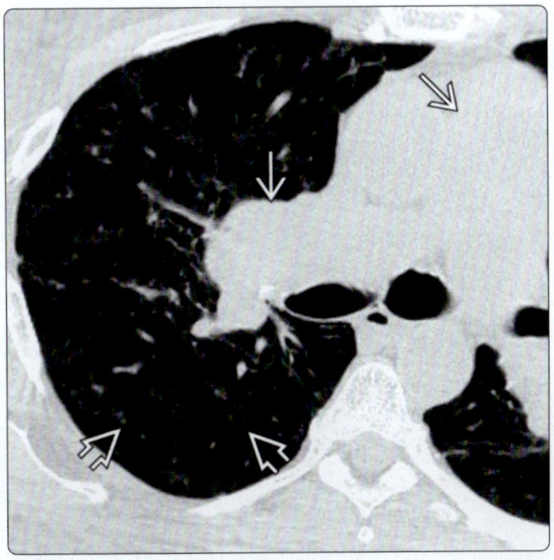

(Left) *Axial CECT of a patient with pulmonary arterial hypertension due to pulmonary venoocclusive disease shows interlobular septal thickening → and enlarged central pulmonary arteries →. Patchy ground-glass opacities are also present.* **(Right)** *Axial NECT of a patient with pulmonary capillary hemangiomatosis demonstrates enlarged central pulmonary arteries → and innumerable centrilobular ground-glass opacities → that represent capillary proliferation beyond the resolution of imaging.*

Pulmonary Artery Filling Defect

DIFFERENTIAL DIAGNOSIS

Common

- Pulmonary Embolism

Less Common

- Nonthrombotic Pulmonary Embolism
  - Tumor Embolism
  - Air Embolism
  - Polymethyl Methacrylate Embolism
  - Foreign Body Embolism

Rare but Important

- Pulmonary Artery Sarcoma

ESSENTIAL INFORMATION

Key Differential Diagnosis Issues

- Bland thrombus, tumor embolus, and pulmonary artery sarcoma can have similar imaging appearances
- Mimics
  - Suboptimal bolus timing: Too early or too late; contrast interruption artifact
  - Flow artifact from slow pulmonary arterial flow (e.g., heart failure, atelectasis)

Helpful Clues for Common Diagnoses

- **Pulmonary Embolism**
  - Acute pulmonary embolism
    - Low-attenuation filling defect
      - Partial ("rim", "railway-track", "tram-track" signs)
      - Occlusive (vessel "cut-off" sign)
    - ↑ diameter of occluded artery
    - Signs of right ventricular overload/strain
      - Right ventricular dilatation (i.e., RV:LV ratio > 1)
      - Interventricular septum shift
    - Pulmonary infarct: Peripheral consolidation &/or ground-glass opacity, often with intrinsic lucency or reversed halo sign
  - Chronic thromboembolic pulmonary hypertension
    - Peripheral filling defect
    - ↓ diameter of artery distal to obstruction
    - Signs of thrombus organization
    - Right ventricular hypertrophy
    - Bronchial artery dilatation
    - Mosaic attenuation pattern

Helpful Clues for Less Common Diagnoses

- **Nonthrombotic Pulmonary Embolism**
  - **Tumor Embolism**
    - Autopsy series incidence (2.5-26%)
    - Invasion of arterial wall
    - Occasional central pulmonary arterial filling defects
    - Alternating strictures and dilatation of vessel ("beading")
  - **Air Embolism**
    - Frequently iatrogenic
      - Insertion of central venous catheters
      - Barotrauma from positive-pressure ventilation
      - Administration of intravenous contrast
      - Transthoracic needle aspiration and biopsy
  - **Polymethyl Methacrylate Embolism**
    - Complication of percutaneous vertebroplasty and kyphoplasty
    - Leakage of cement into paraspinal veins
    - Tubular high-attenuation opacities within pulmonary arteries
  - **Foreign Body Embolism**
    - During insertion procedure or associated with spontaneous catheter breakage
      - Catheter fragment in abnormal location
    - Embolization of inferior vena cava filter strut(s)

Helpful Clues for Rare Diagnoses

- **Pulmonary Artery Sarcoma**
  - Central and unilateral filling defects
  - Acute angles with pulmonary artery wall
  - Extension outside of vessel lumen
  - Hemorrhage, necrosis, and ossification may be observed within mass
  - Enhancement on CT or MR or uptake on FDG PET/CT

Pulmonary Embolism

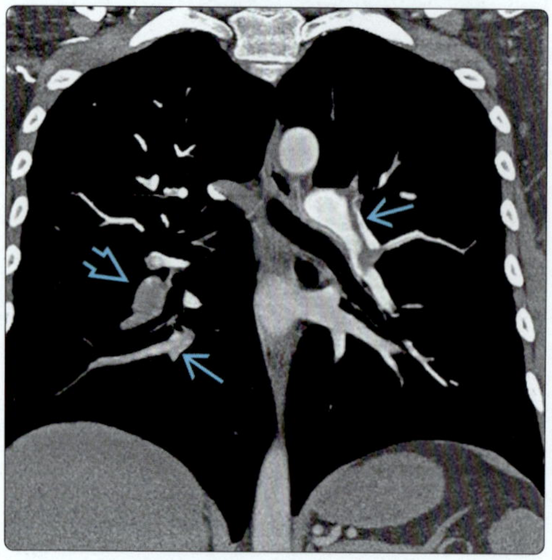

Pulmonary Embolism

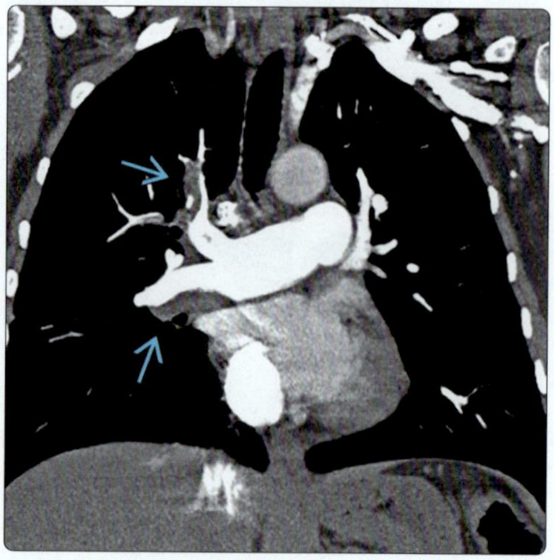

(Left) *Coronal CECT of a 53-year-old man with acute pulmonary embolism shows filling defects in the left pulmonary artery and segmental branches of the right lower lobe pulmonary artery ➔ and complete occlusion of the right interlobar artery ➔.* **(Right)** *Coronal CECT of a 72-year-old man with chronic thromboembolic pulmonary hypertension shows low-attenuation eccentric filling defects in branches of the right pulmonary artery ➔ and dilated pulmonary artery from pulmonary hypertension.*

Tumor Embolism

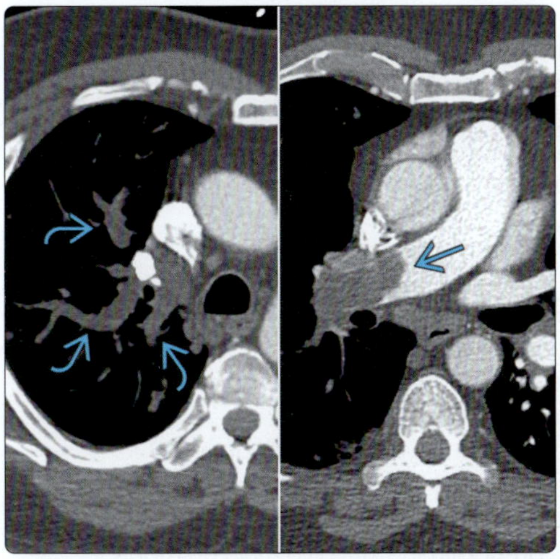

Air Embolism

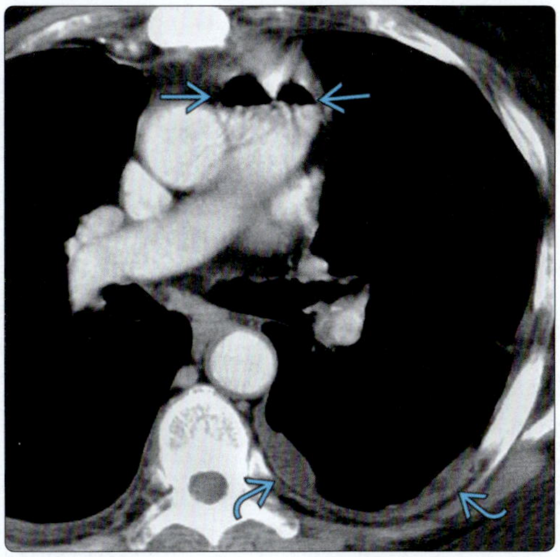

(Left) *Composite image with axial CECT (left and right) at different levels of a patient with pelvic chondrosarcoma and tumor embolism shows central arterial pulmonary filling defect, which propagates extensively into the right upper lobe.* **(Right)** *Axial CECT of a patient with history of cancer shows gas layering along the nondependent aspect of the pulmonary trunk. Often this is an incidental finding that poses no clinical consequences. Note the presence of left pleural metastases.*

Polymethyl Methacrylate Embolism

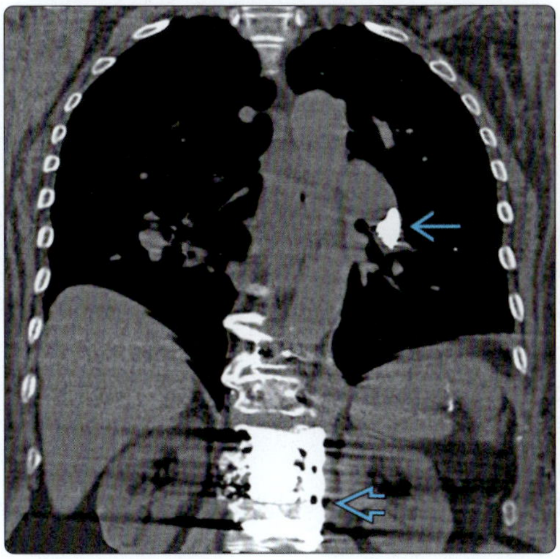

Foreign Body Embolism

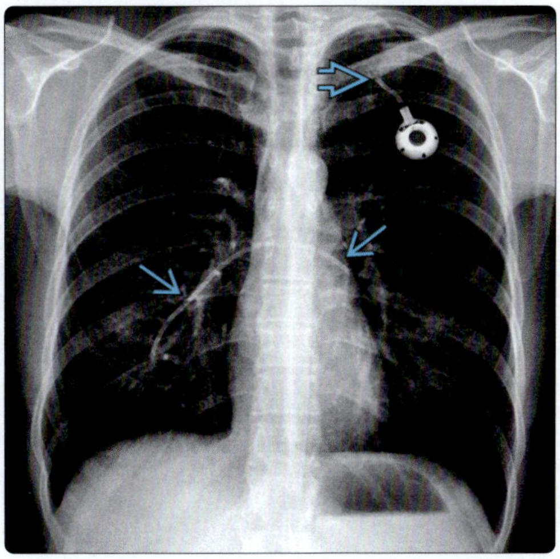

(Left) *Coronal NECT of a 76-year-old man with polymethyl methacrylate embolism secondary to vertebroplasty shows high-density material in the left pulmonary artery. Note cement along multiple thoracolumbar vertebral bodies.* **(Right)** *Chest radiograph of a patient with ruptured and embolized left subclavian central line shows a large catheter fragment within the central pulmonary arteries. Note the fracture site at the expected location of venous insertion of the tunneled catheter.*

Pulmonary Artery Sarcoma

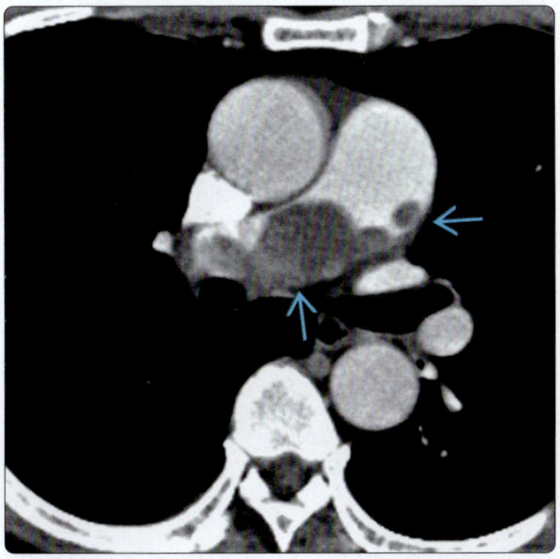

Pulmonary Artery Sarcoma

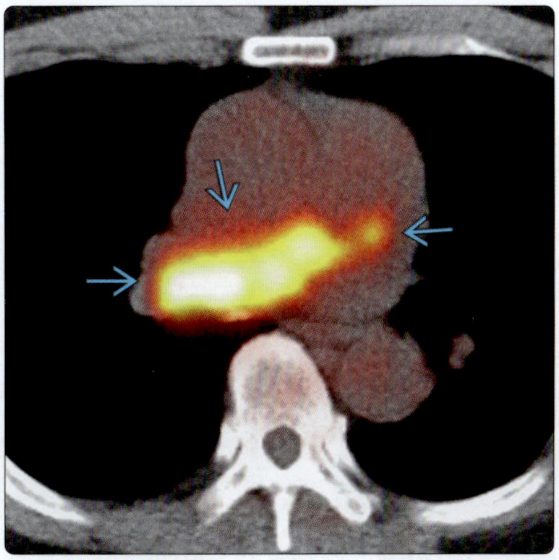

(Left) *Axial CECT of a patient with primary pulmonary artery pleomorphic sarcoma shows a large, nodular filling defect with heterogeneous enhancement in the pulmonary trunk extending into the right main pulmonary artery.* **(Right)** *Fused axial FDG PET/CT of the same patient shows markedly increased FDG uptake in the filling defect. Though uncommon, angiosarcoma is the most common primary malignancy involving the pulmonary arterial circulation and is associated with a dismal prognosis.*

DIFFERENTIAL DIAGNOSIS

Common

- Pulmonary Artery Invasion
- Tumor Embolism

Less Common

- Pulmonary Artery Sarcoma

Rare but Important

- Pulmonary Artery Myxoma

ESSENTIAL INFORMATION

Key Differential Diagnosis Issues

- Lung cancer is most common malignancy affecting the pulmonary arteries
- Sarcoma is most common primary malignant neoplasm of the pulmonary arteries
- Pulmonary artery sarcoma is frequently misdiagnosed as pulmonary embolism
  - Expansion of pulmonary artery, enhancement, and extramural extension of mass favors sarcoma
- Pulmonary artery sarcoma should be included in differential diagnosis if extensive filling defect remains after anticoagulant therapy

Helpful Clues for Common Diagnoses

- **Pulmonary Artery Invasion**
  - Lung cancer is most common malignancy that invades the pulmonary vessels
    - Centrally-located lung cancer can invade pulmonary artery and cause partial or complete pulmonary artery occlusion
      - Represents T4 in TNM staging system for lung cancer
  - CECT
    - Tumor infiltration of the mediastinum with concentric narrowing of pulmonary artery
    - Tumor occluding pulmonary artery
- **Tumor Embolism**
  - Most common associated malignancies: Hepatocellular carcinoma, breast cancer, and renal cancer
  - CECT
    - Low-density filling defect without expansion of pulmonary vessels, peripheral enhancement
    - In cases of renal cell carcinoma and hepatocellular carcinoma, tumor thrombus can be identified in inferior vena cava and right atrium
  - FDG PET/CT
    - Increased FDG uptake

Helpful Clues for Less Common Diagnoses

- **Pulmonary Artery Sarcoma**
  - Sarcomas are rare but the most common primary tumor of pulmonary arteries
  - Arises from mesenchymal cells of intima
    - Undifferentiated sarcoma and leiomyosarcomas are most common histopathological subtypes
  - Sarcomas predominantly involve main pulmonary arteries, pulmonary trunk (85%), right pulmonary artery (71%), and left pulmonary artery (65%)
  - CECT
    - Large, low-density mass/filling defect that expands and occupies lumen of main or proximal pulmonary arteries
      - Areas of enhancement within tumor
      - Extramural extension of mass
    - Direct tumor extension to mediastinal structures, pleura, and lung is more common than extrathoracic metastases
  - FDG PET/CT: Increased FDG uptake
  - T1WI C+ MR: Tumor enhances with contrast

Helpful Clues for Rare Diagnoses

- **Pulmonary Artery Myxoma**
  - Rare benign neoplasm
  - CT: Low-attenuation mass, no enhancement with contrast
    - Absence of lymph node and distant metastases

Pulmonary Artery Invasion

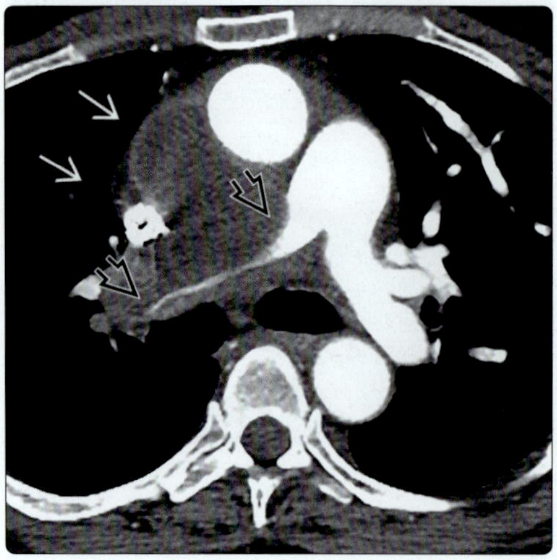

Pulmonary Artery Invasion

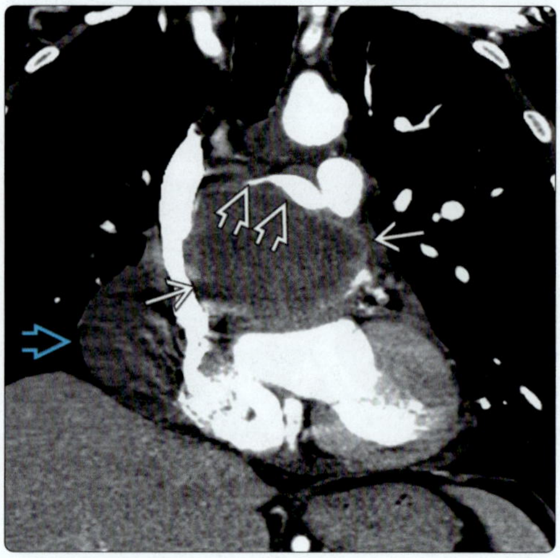

(Left) *Axial CECT of a 62-year-old man shows a right mediastinal mass representing small cell lung cancer ➡ that invades and markedly narrows the right main pulmonary artery ⇨.* **(Right)** *Coronal CECT of the same patient confirms invasion of the right pulmonary artery ➡ by the mass ➡. A pericardial effusion is also noted ⇨. Lung cancer is the malignancy that most commonly invades the pulmonary arteries, especially when the tumor is centrally located.*

Tumor Embolism

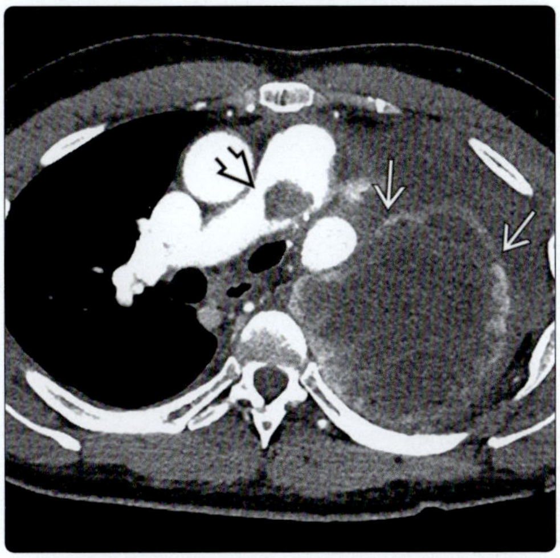

Tumor Embolism

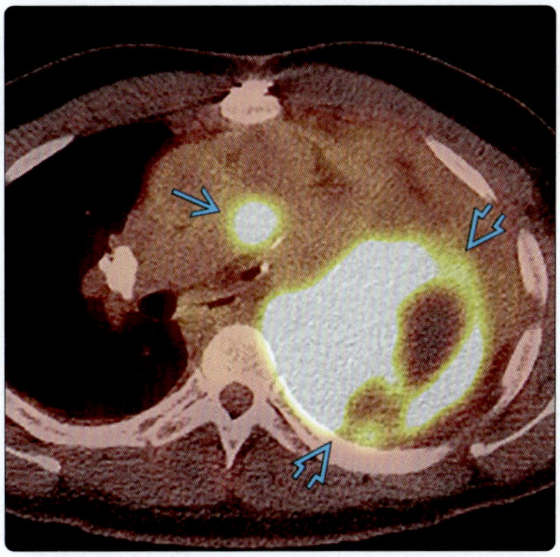

(Left) *Axial CECT of a 45-year-old man with spindle cell sarcoma of the pelvis shows a filling defect in the pulmonary trunk and extensive metastatic disease in the left lung.* **(Right)** *Fused axial FDG PET/CT of the same patient shows increased FDG uptake in the right pulmonary artery, consistent with tumor thrombus. Metastatic disease in the left lung is also FDG avid. Tumor emboli are most commonly reported in hepatocellular carcinoma and breast and renal cancers.*

Pulmonary Artery Sarcoma

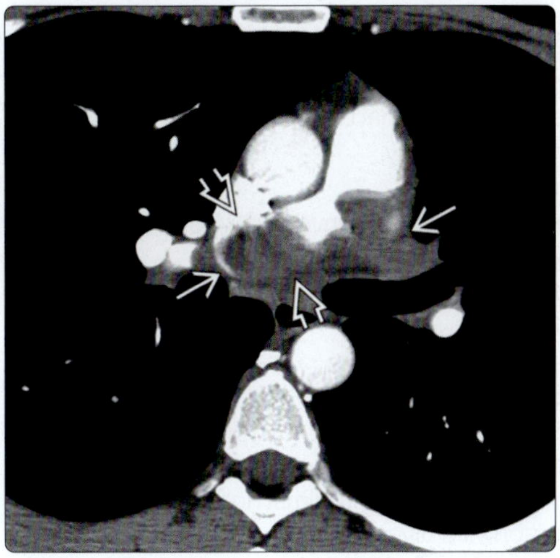

Pulmonary Artery Sarcoma

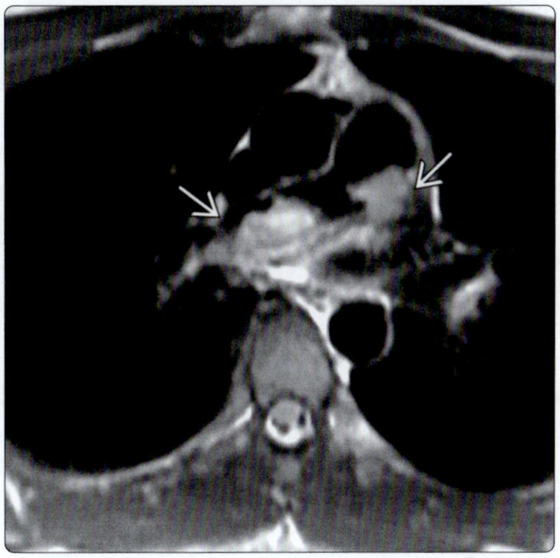

(Left) *Axial CECT of a 47-year-old man shows a large mass involving the right and left pulmonary arteries with expansion of the right main pulmonary artery, a finding which favors an intraluminal mass over bland thrombus.* **(Right)** *Axial T2 HASTE MR of the same patient shows an irregular, hyperintense mass in the right main pulmonary artery and proximal left pulmonary artery. Biopsy confirmed pulmonary artery sarcoma, specifically leiomyosarcoma.*

Pulmonary Artery Sarcoma

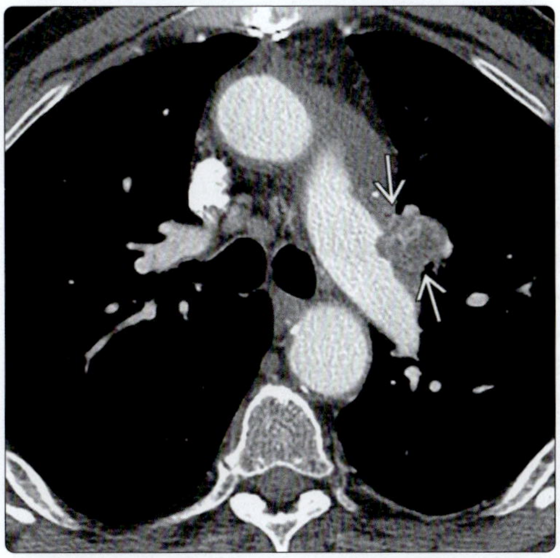

Pulmonary Artery Sarcoma

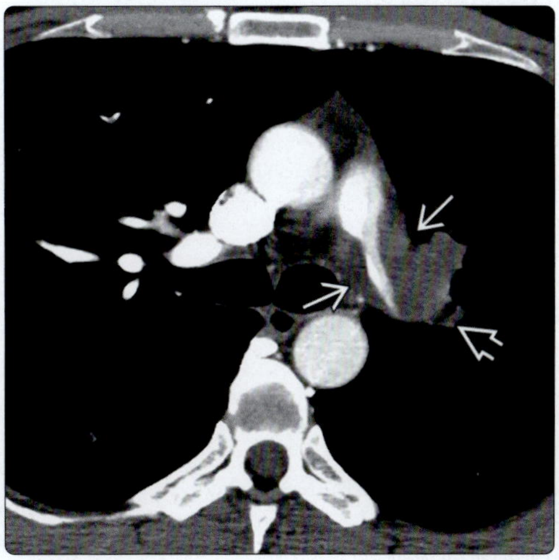

(Left) *Axial CECT of a 56-year-old man with undifferentiated sarcoma shows an enhancing mass expanding the left upper lobe pulmonary artery. Expansion of the vessel and enhancement are features that favor sarcoma over embolism.* **(Right)** *CECT of a 55-year-old woman with leiomyosarcoma shows circumferential narrowing of the left main pulmonary artery, consistent with tumor, that is also extending into the left upper lobe pulmonary artery. Pulmonary sarcoma tends to extend into the contiguous pulmonary vessels.*

DIFFERENTIAL DIAGNOSIS

Common

- Lung Cancer
- Metastasis

Less Common

- Pulmonary Artery Sarcoma
- Fibrosing Mediastinitis

Rare but Important

- Cardiac Sarcoma
- Tuberculosis

ESSENTIAL INFORMATION

Key Differential Diagnosis Issues

- Most common cause of pulmonary artery (PA) invasion is direct extension of primary lung cancer
- Surgeons, radiologists, and pathologists have different criteria for vascular invasion
- CT
  - CECT is imaging method of choice for diagnosis and follow-up
    - Arterial phase timed to optimize visualization of PA is best for assessment of vascular involvement
  - Vascular invasion
    - Primary lung cancer typically manifests as infiltrative central mass ± necrosis
    - Positive predictive value of CECT for detecting vascular invasion is low (< 35%)
    - 3 main findings that suggest vascular invasion
      - Obliteration of perivascular fat plane
      - Angle of tumor contact > 90°
      - Stenosis and deformation of vascular lumen
- FDG PET/CT
  - Assists in diagnosis of malignancy and response assessment
  - Limited role in initial diagnosis of fibrosing mediastinitis but can aid in treatment follow-up

Helpful Clues for Common Diagnoses

- **Lung Cancer**
  - Locally advanced lung cancer with invasion of mediastinal structures has significantly worse prognosis compared to earlier stage malignancies
  - Positive predictive value of CT in determining vascular invasion is low
  - Tumor (T) staging
    - Invasion of PA is considered T4 disease
      - T4 tumors have traditionally been considered unresectable
      - Limited invasion of proximal PA does not necessarily preclude surgical resection
  - Treatment
    - Surgical resection typically includes pneumonectomy
    - Procedures involving PA
      - Removal of portion of arterial wall
      - Circumferential resection with arterial reconstruction
    - Opportunity for complete cure diminishes when N1 or N2 disease is present
- **Metastasis**
  - Direct metastasis to PA as cause of vascular invasion is rare
    - Most cases are due to tumor embolism
  - Neoplasms associated with tumor embolism
    - Breast carcinoma
    - Renal cell carcinoma
    - Melanoma
    - Choriocarcinoma
    - Hepatocellular carcinoma
    - Gastric carcinoma
  - CT
    - Intravascular filing defect
      - Commonly involves segmental and subsegmental arterial branches
      - Enhancement of intravascular tissue may be seen if large enough
    - Alternating regions of vessel narrowing and dilatation
      - 'Beaded' appearance
    - Tree-in-bud opacities in lung periphery
  - May coexist with cardiac metastasis

Helpful Clues for Less Common Diagnoses

- **Pulmonary Artery Sarcoma**
  - Arises from mesenchymal cells of PA
  - Uncommon malignancy
  - Aggressive behavior
    - Occlusive growth within involved PA often seen
  - Poor prognosis
  - Difficult to differentiate from thromboembolic disease in early stages
  - Imaging
    - CT angiography
      - Intraluminal filling defect with soft tissue attenuation
      - Pulmonary trunk or proximal right or left PA most commonly involved
      - Enlargement of involved PA
      - Extraluminal tumor extension into adjacent mediastinal organs in advanced stages
    - MR
      - T1 C+: Tumor enhancement
      - Can be used to differentiate neoplasm from bland thrombus
    - FDG PET/CT
      - Typically demonstrate increased FDG uptake
      - Low-grade sarcomas may be mildly FDG avid and may be misdiagnosed as bland thrombus
- **Fibrosing Mediastinitis**
  - Nonmalignant condition
    - Deposition of fibrous tissue and collagen
  - Locally aggressive
  - May mimic malignancy
  - Etiologies
    - Idiopathic
    - Infection
      - Histoplasmosis
      - Tuberculosis
    - Radiation therapy
    - Exposure to drugs (methysergide)

- Young adults are typically affected
- Symptoms are typically related to central vascular occlusion
- 2 types
  - Focal (80%)
  - Diffuse (20%)
- Imaging
  - CT
    - Variable presentation according to extent of disease
    - Infiltrative soft tissue mass
    - Typically affects visceral mediastinal compartment &/or hilum
    - Encasement and narrowing/occlusion of PA, pulmonary veins, superior vena cava, &/or central airways
    - Enlarged bronchial collateral arteries are common
    - Coarse calcification of associated lymphadenopathy
    - Central venous occlusion may result in findings of edema: Interlobular septal thickening, ground-glass opacities, peribronchovascular thickening
    - Pulmonary infarction: Subpleural opacities that may be solid, ground-glass, or combination
  - FDG PET/CT
    - Variable FDG uptake
    - Controversial role in diagnosis as may be difficult to differentiate from malignancy
    - Role in follow-up after treatment: Lower metabolic activity may reflect decreased inflammatory reaction

Helpful Clues for Rare Diagnoses

- **Cardiac Sarcoma**
  - Angiosarcoma is most common histologic type
    - Uncommon malignant primary cardiac neoplasm
    - Most common sarcoma involving heart in adults
  - Involvement of right atrioventricular (AV) groove is common
  - Highly invasive locally
  - Transgression of pericardium is common
  - Large hemopericardium at presentation is common
    - Cardiac tamponade may develop
  - CT
    - Soft tissue mass
    - Involvement of right atrial wall and AV groove
    - Extension along pericardium, obliterates pericardial space
    - High propensity for necrosis and hemorrhage
    - Local invasion
      - Mediastinum
      - Right atrium
      - PA
      - Other adjacent mediastinal vessels
- **Tuberculosis**
  - Extrapulmonary tuberculosis
    - *Mycobacterium tuberculosis* involving organs other than lungs
  - More frequent form of disease in endemic areas of developing world
  - Vascular invasion is extremely rare form of presentation but has been described
  - Imaging
    - May be indistinguishable from malignancy
    - Associated with extensive lymphadenopathy
      - May be necrotic

SELECTED REFERENCES

1. Garrana SH et al: Multimodality imaging of focal and diffuse fibrosing mediastinitis. Radiographics. 39(3):651-67, 2019
2. Oka S et al: The major thoracic vascular invasion of lung cancer. Ann Med Surg (Lond). 20:13-8, 2017
3. Gleason JB et al: Pulmonary artery invasion caused by Mycobacterium tuberculosis. Chest. 150(4):e99-103, 2016
4. Carter BW et al: Acquired abnormalities of the pulmonary arteries. AJR Am J Roentgenol. 202(5):W415-21, 2014

Lung Cancer

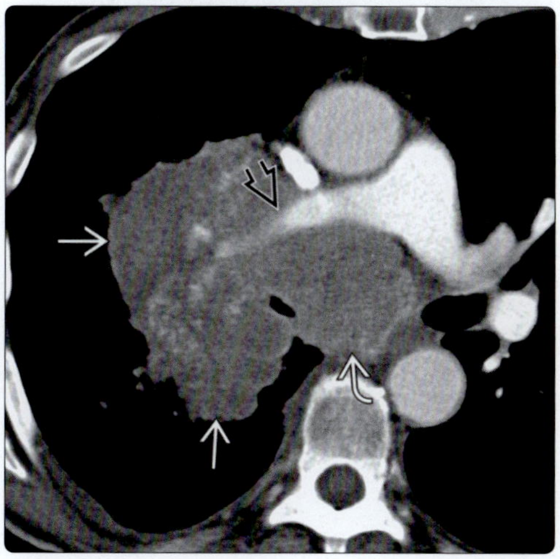

Lung Cancer

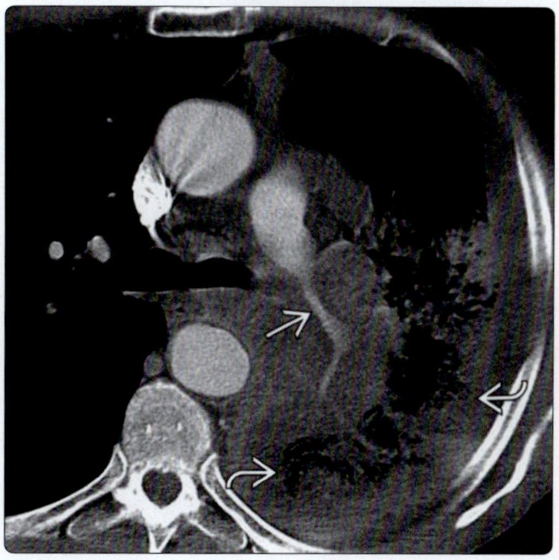

(Left) *Axial CECT of a patient with non-small cell lung cancer demonstrates a large right hilar mass* ➡ *encasing and severely compressing/narrowing the right pulmonary artery* ⇨ *and invading the mediastinum* ➡. **(Right)** *Axial CECT of a patient with small cell lung cancer shows severe narrowing of the left pulmonary artery* ➡. *Left lung consolidation* ➡ *represents postobstructive pneumonitis secondary to proximal bronchial occlusion by the mass.*

(Left) *Axial CECT of a patient with metastatic hepatocellular carcinoma demonstrates a solid, enhancing mass at the apex of the right ventricle, representing a cardiac metastasis.* **(Right)** *Axial CECT of the same patient shows a solid intraluminal mass in the proximal pulmonary trunk, representing a metastatic deposit. Direct metastasis to the pulmonary arteries as a cause of vascular invasion is rare, and most cases are due to tumor embolism.*

Metastasis

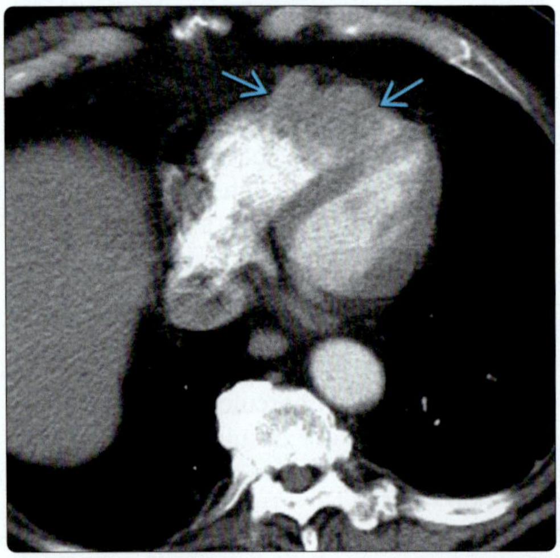

Metastasis

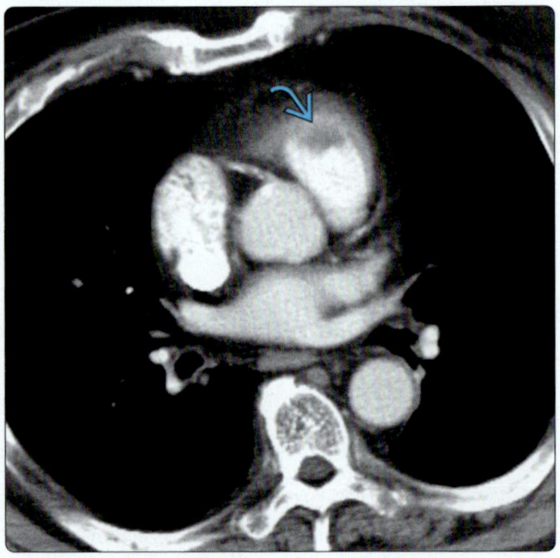

(Left) *Axial CECT of a patient with metastatic renal cell carcinoma shows a solid mass invading the inferior vena cava and extending into the right atrium. Transvenous extension of tumor thrombus is not uncommon in these patients.* **(Right)** *Axial CECT of the same patient shows filling defects in the left lower lobe pulmonary artery, representing tumor embolism. Tumor embolism may be initially indistinguishable from thromboembolic disease.*

Metastasis

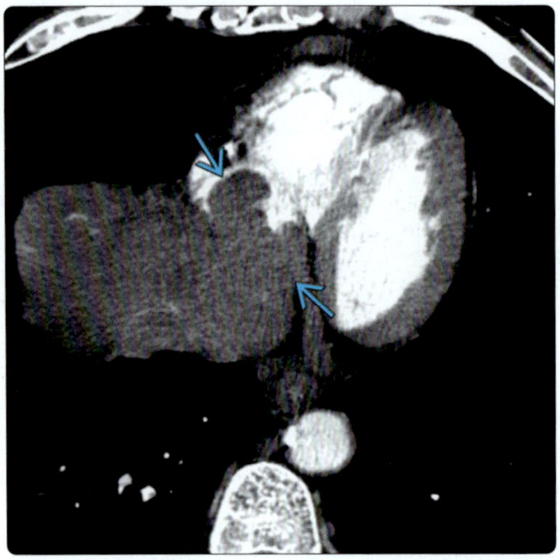

Metastasis

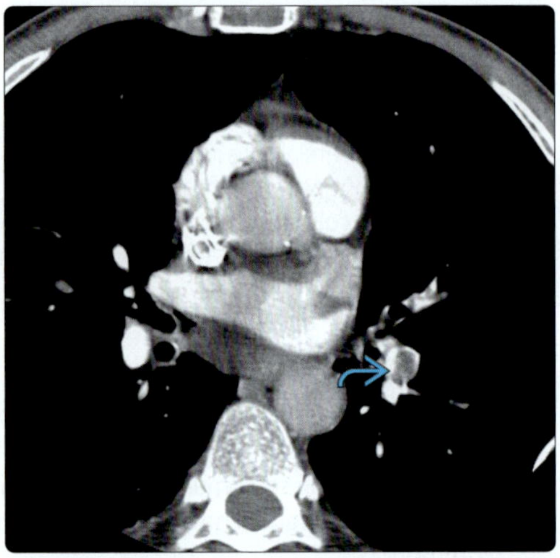

(Left) *Axial CECT of a patient with metastatic renal cell carcinoma shows focal enlargement of a segmental arterial branch in the right lung, a classic appearance of tumor embolism.* **(Right)** *Coronal reformatted image from CECT of a patient with a tumor embolism shows subsegmental artery branches in the left lower lobe with regions of narrowing and dilatation (or beading) due to tumor emboli. Other abnormalities such as tree-in-bud in the lung periphery may be identified on CT.*

Metastasis

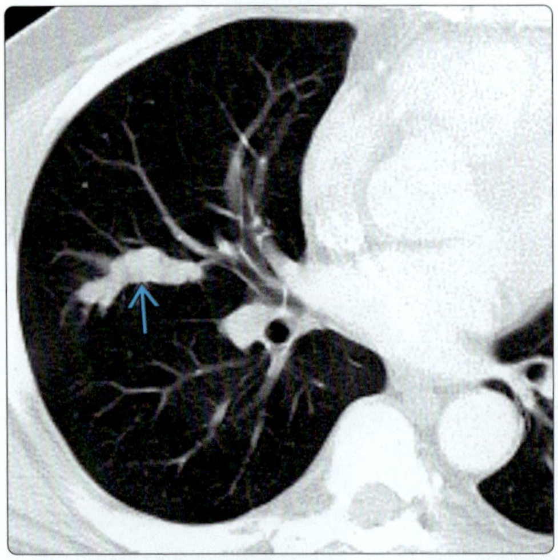

Metastasis

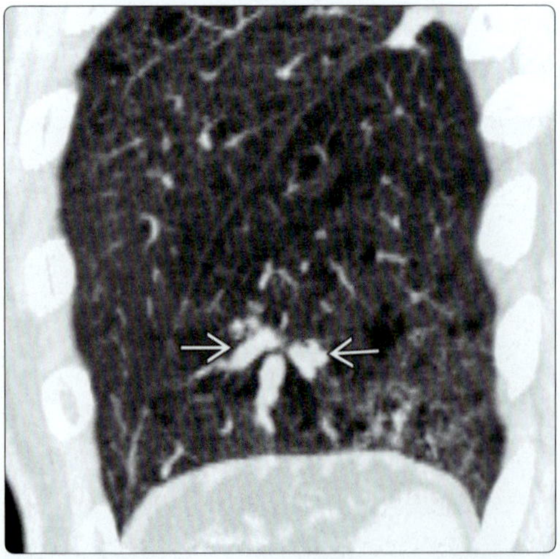

Fibrosing Mediastinitis

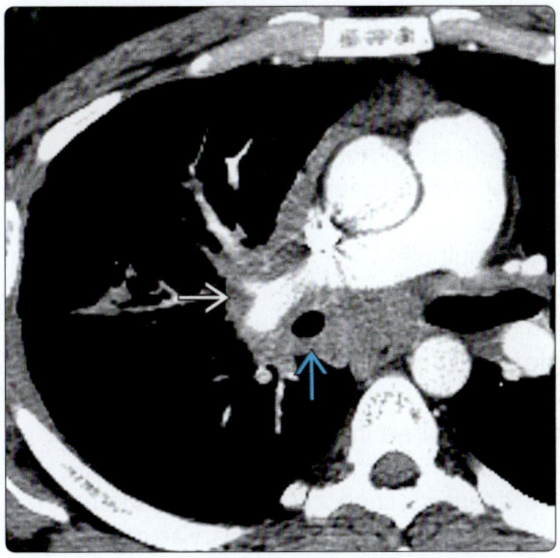

Fibrosing Mediastinitis

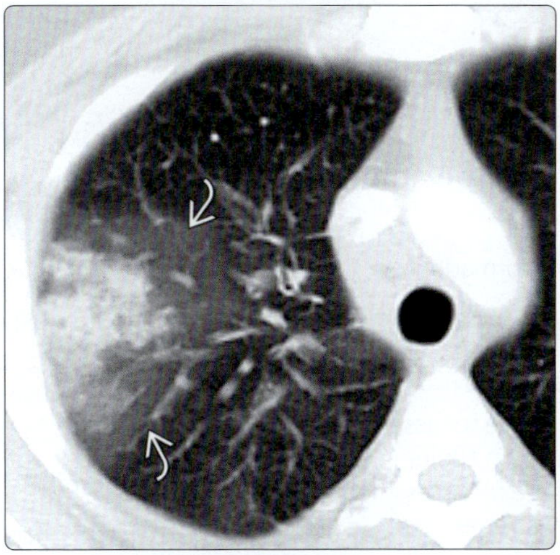

(Left) *Axial CECT of a patient with fibrosing mediastinitis demonstrates circumferential soft tissue encasing the right pulmonary artery, which is mildly narrowed. The bronchus intermedius is also encased by soft tissue resulting from inflammation.* **(Right)** *Axial CECT of the same patient shows focal consolidation with surrounding ground-glass opacities in the peripheral right upper lobe, representing pulmonary infarction due to focal occlusion of arterial and venous branches at the hilum.*

Fibrosing Mediastinitis

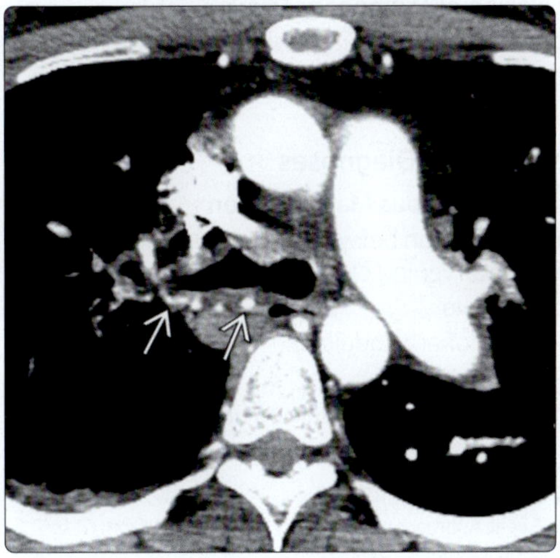

Fibrosing Mediastinitis

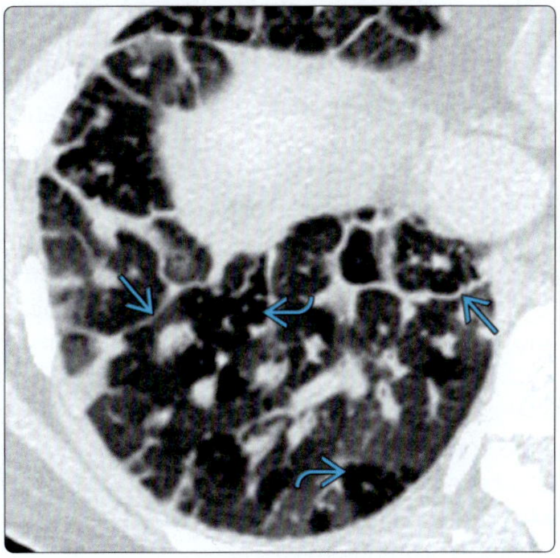

(Left) *Axial CECT of a patient with fibrosing mediastinitis due to histoplasmosis infection shows collateral circulation through enlarged bronchial arteries that developed as a result of complete occlusion of the right pulmonary artery.* **(Right)** *Axial CECT of the same patient shows bronchovascular and smooth interlobular septal thickening secondary to venous occlusion at the hilum (not shown). There is mosaic attenuation representing air-trapping.*

Cardiac Sarcoma

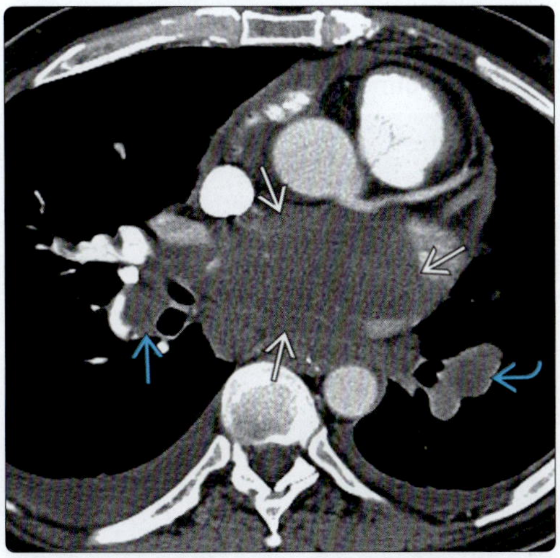

Cardiac Sarcoma

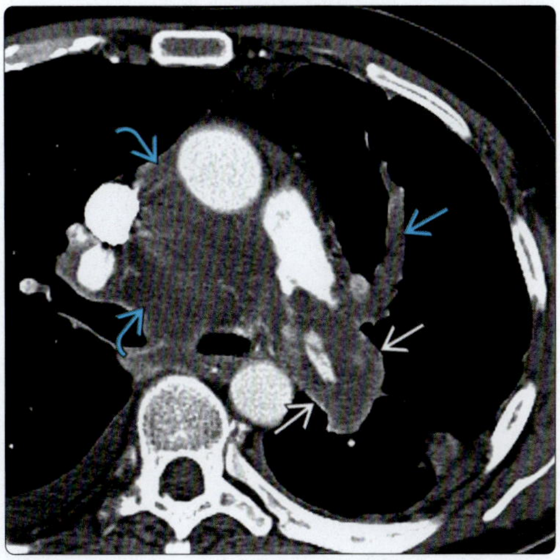

(Left) *Axial CECT of a patient with primary cardiac angiosarcoma shows extensive invasion of the left atrium by the soft tissue mass and invasion of the right interlobar pulmonary artery. There is also complete occlusion of the left lower lobe pulmonary arteries.* **(Right)** *Axial CECT of the same patient shows an infiltrative soft tissue mass with focal invasion and consequent occlusion of the left pulmonary artery and lobar branches in the left lung.*

Focal Pulmonary Artery Enlargement

DIFFERENTIAL DIAGNOSIS

Common

- Pulmonary Hypertension
- Pulmonary Artery Aneurysm/Pseudoaneurysm

Less Common

- Idiopathic Dilation of Pulmonary Trunk

Rare but Important

- Pulmonary Arteriovenous Malformation

ESSENTIAL INFORMATION

Key Differential Diagnosis Issues

- CECT is imaging method of choice for assessment of pulmonary artery abnormalities in adults
  - Timing of contrast optimized for assessment of central and peripheral pulmonary arteries
- MR is modality of choice for pulmonic valve assessment

Helpful Clues for Common Diagnoses

- **Pulmonary Hypertension (PH)**
  - Pulmonary pressure ≥ 25 mm Hg at rest
  - Secondary PH more common than idiopathic
  - Transthoracic 2-dimensional Doppler echocardiography is modality of choice
  - CT
    - Enlarged pulmonary artery > 29 mm: Measured on axial image at pulmonary trunk bifurcation
    - Increased segmental artery:bronchus ratio > 1:1 in ≥ 3 lobes
    - Peripheral pulmonary artery calcification in severe and late-stage PH
    - Pruning of distal pulmonary arteries
    - Eccentric filling defects in chronic thromboembolic PH
    - Hypertrophied bronchial arteries
    - Parenchymal findings: Mosaic attenuation, centrilobular nodules (cholesterol granulomas)
  - Cardiac MR: High accuracy for right ventricular size, morphology, and function
- **Pulmonary Artery Aneurysm/Pseudoaneurysm**
  - Focal dilation of vessel lumen
  - Saccular dilatation of segmental and subsegmental arteries
  - CTA is diagnostic modality of choice
  - Typically acquired
    - Vasculitis: Behçet syndrome
      - Recurrent oral and genital ulcerations, ocular anomalies
      - Single or multiple
      - Frequent in situ mural thrombosis
    - Infection (mycotic aneurysm/pseudoaneurysm)
      - Septic emboli, endocarditis
    - Neoplasm
      - Lung cancer: Direct invasion of pulmonary artery
      - Intravascular metastases: Renal, breast, gastric, and prostate cancers; choriocarcinoma; melanoma
    - Iatrogenic: Complication of pulmonary artery catheter placement

Helpful Clues for Less Common Diagnoses

- **Idiopathic Dilation of Pulmonary Trunk**
  - Rare congenital anomaly, diagnosis of exclusion
  - Right and left pulmonary arteries usually normal
  - Patients are asymptomatic

Helpful Clues for Rare Diagnoses

- **Pulmonary Arteriovenous Malformation**
  - Direct communication between pulmonary artery and vein without intervening capillary bed
  - Solitary or multiple
  - May mimic pulmonary nodule(s)
  - Right-to-left shunt
  - Most common in hereditary hemorrhagic telangiectasia

SELECTED REFERENCES

1. Aluja Jaramillo F et al: Approach to pulmonary hypertension: from CT to clinical diagnosis. Radiographics. 38(2):357-73, 2018
2. Carter BW et al: Acquired abnormalities of the pulmonary arteries. AJR Am J Roentgenol. 202(5):W415-21, 2014

Pulmonary Hypertension

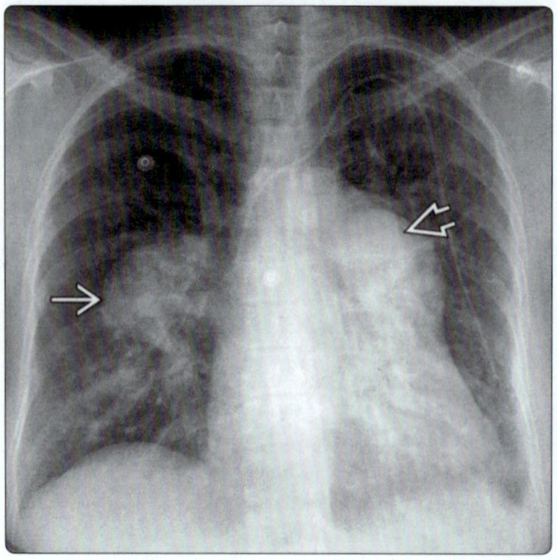

Pulmonary Hypertension

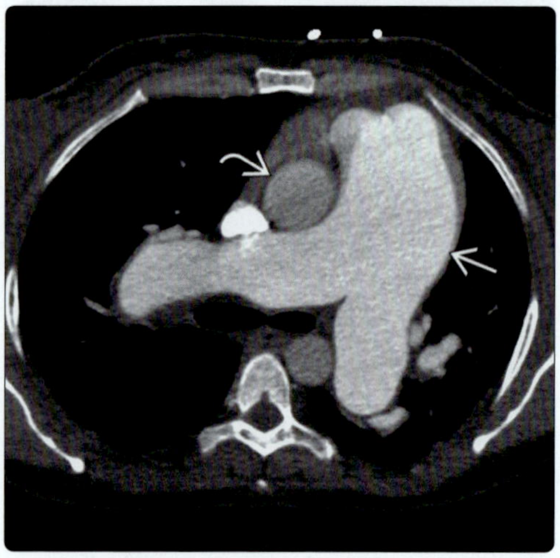

(Left) *PA chest radiograph of a patient with idiopathic pulmonary hypertension shows bilateral hilar enlargement from marked dilation of the right ➡ and left ➡ pulmonary arteries. The pulmonary trunk is also enlarged.* **(Right)** *Axial CECT of the same patient shows marked dilatation of the pulmonary trunk ➡ and central pulmonary arteries. The pulmonary trunk is measured on axial images at the level of the bifurcation. The pulmonary artery to ascending aorta ➡ ratio is > 1.*

Pulmonary Hypertension

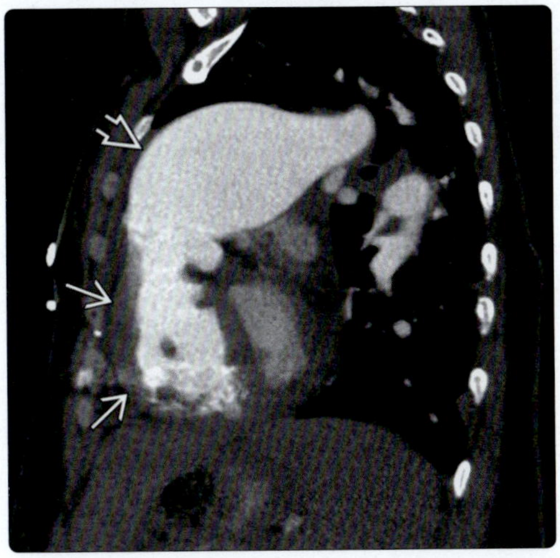

Pulmonary Hypertension

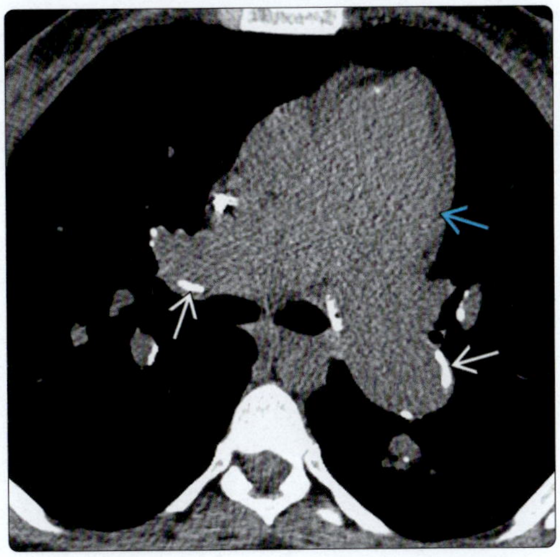

(Left) *Parasagittal CECT of the same patient shows a massively dilated pulmonary trunk ➡. The right ventricle is dilated and severely hypertrophic as manifested by thickening of the right ventricular myocardium ➡.* **(Right)** *Axial NECT of a patient with chronic pulmonary hypertension demonstrates an enlarged pulmonary trunk ➡ and peripherally located curvilinear calcifications ➡ in the pulmonary artery walls secondary to atherosclerosis from chronically elevated right heart pressures.*

Pulmonary Hypertension

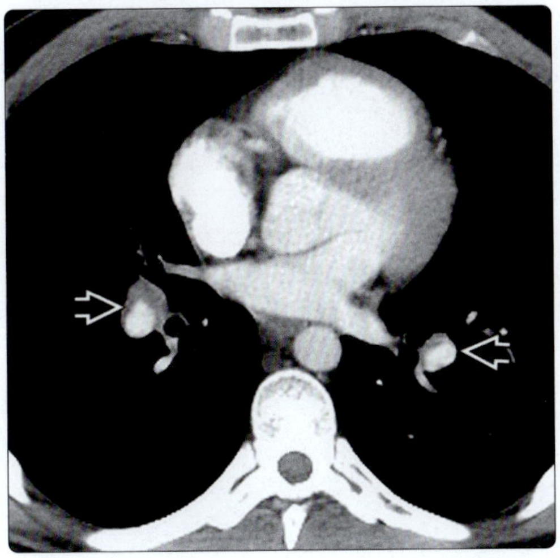

Pulmonary Hypertension

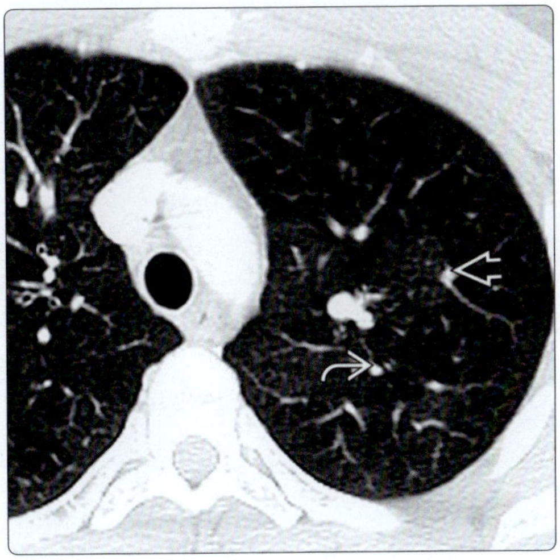

(Left) *Axial CECT (soft tissue window) of a patient with pulmonary hypertension secondary to chronic thromboembolic disease shows eccentric filling defects in the pulmonary arteries consistent with chronic PE ➡.* **(Right)** *Axial CECT (lung window) of the same patient shows alternating regions of high ➡ and low ➡ (mosaic) attenuation from variable pulmonary perfusion related to chronic pulmonary hypertension. Note attenuated caliber of the pulmonary arteries in the areas of low attenuation.*

Pulmonary Hypertension

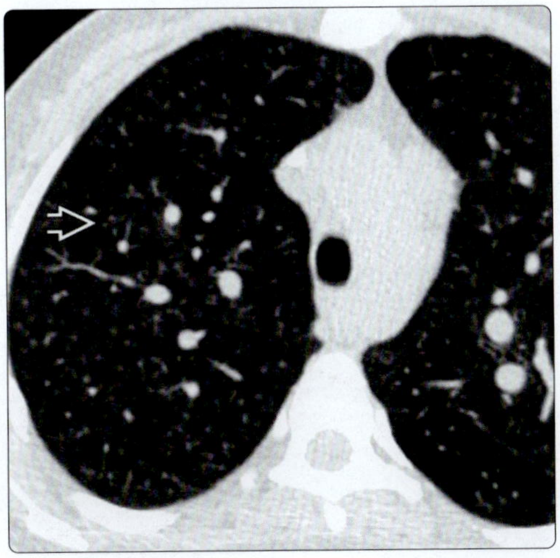

Pulmonary Hypertension

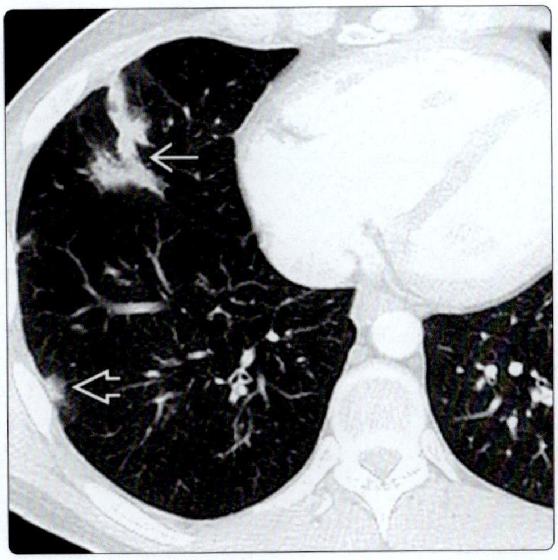

(Left) *Axial NECT of a patient with chronic pulmonary hypertension demonstrates numerous bilateral centrilobular ground-glass nodules ➡ representing cholesterol granulomas. These findings are seen in 25% of patients with severe pulmonary hypertension.* **(Right)** *Axial CECT of a patient with chronic thromboembolic pulmonary hypertension shows middle lobe irregular band-like opacities ➡ and right lower lobe subpleural nodules ➡ that represent the sequela of remote multifocal pulmonary infarcts.*

(Left) *Axial CECT of a patient with pulmonary hypertension secondary to pulmonic stenosis shows thickened and sclerotic pulmonary valve leaflets* ⇨. **(Right)** *Axial CECT of the same patient demonstrates the classic imaging findings of pulmonic stenosis characterized by an enlarged pulmonary trunk* ➡ *and asymmetric enlargement of the left pulmonary artery* ➡. *Note the normal caliber of the right pulmonary artery* ➡, *also a typical finding in this condition.*

Pulmonary Hypertension

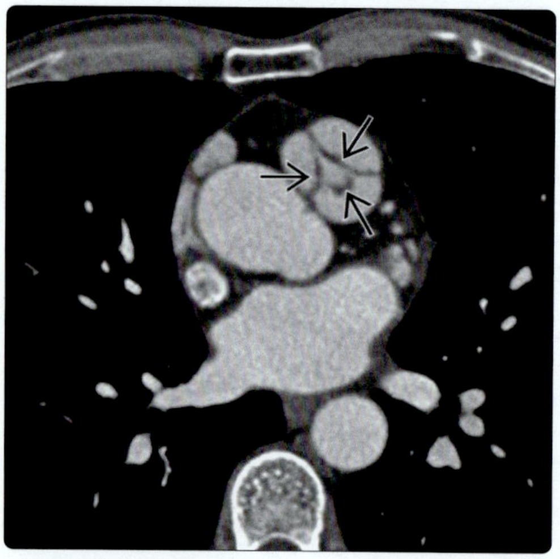

Pulmonary Hypertension

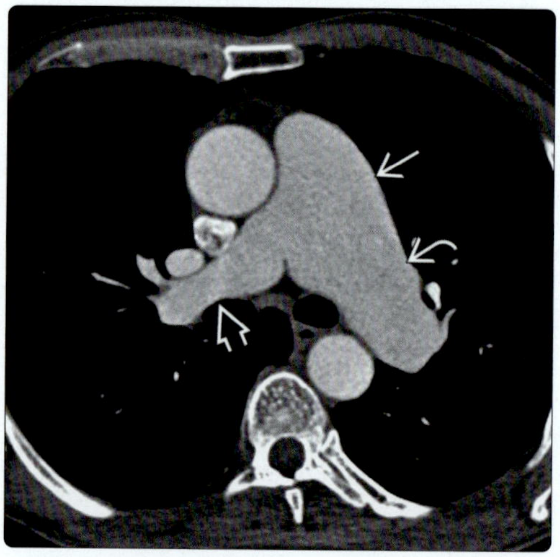

(Left) *PA chest radiograph of a patient with pulmonary hypertension and pulmonic valve stenosis demonstrates a dilated pulmonary trunk* ➡ *and an enlarged left pulmonary artery* ➡. *Note the normal appearance of the right pulmonary artery.* **(Right)** *Axial CECT of a patient with Hugh-Stovin syndrome, a rare variant of Behçet disease, demonstrates focal dilatation of the left pulmonary artery* ➡ *that represents a pulmonary artery aneurysm or pseudoaneurysm. Note the normal caliber of the pulmonary trunk.*

Pulmonary Hypertension

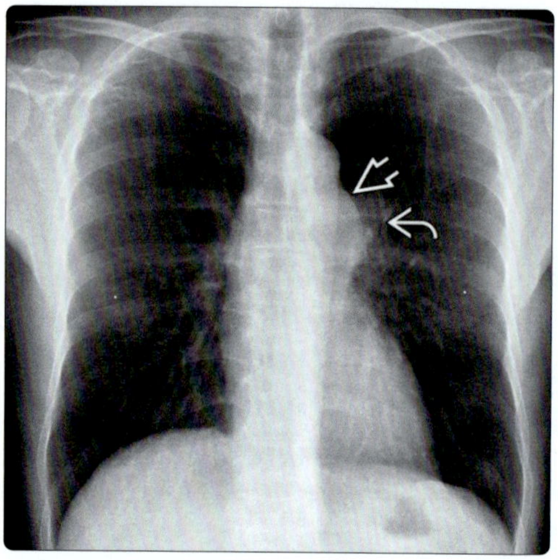

Pulmonary Artery Aneurysm/Pseudoaneurysm

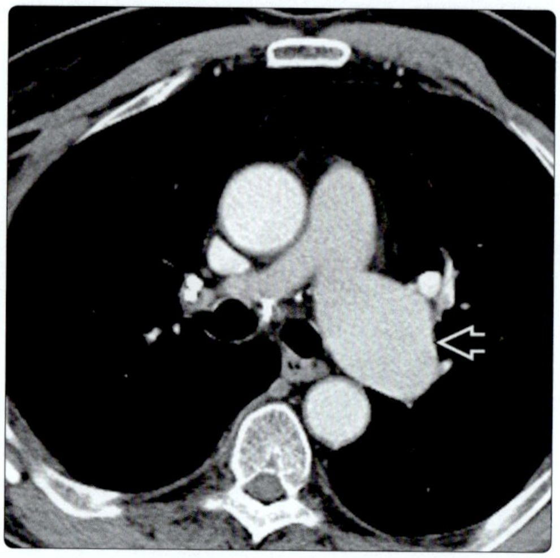

(Left) *AP chest radiograph coned down to the right lung base of a patient who previously underwent pulmonary artery catheterization shows a new 2 cm right basilar nodule* ➡ *concerning for pulmonary artery pseudoaneurysm, a known but rare complication of pulmonary artery catheterization.* **(Right)** *Coronal CECT of the same patient shows focal dilatation of a segmental branch of the right lower lobe pulmonary artery* ➡ *that confirms the suspected pseudoaneurysm.*

Pulmonary Artery Aneurysm/Pseudoaneurysm

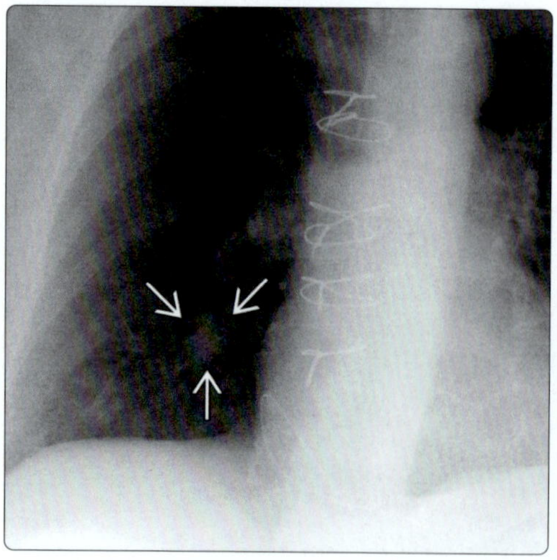

Pulmonary Artery Aneurysm/Pseudoaneurysm

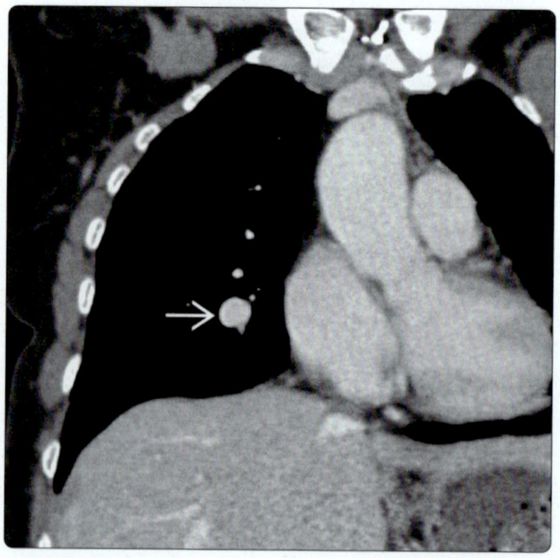

Pulmonary Artery Aneurysm/Pseudoaneurysm

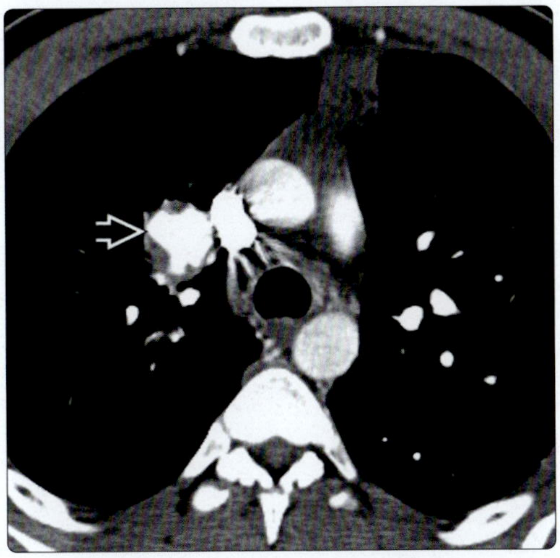

Pulmonary Artery Aneurysm/Pseudoaneurysm

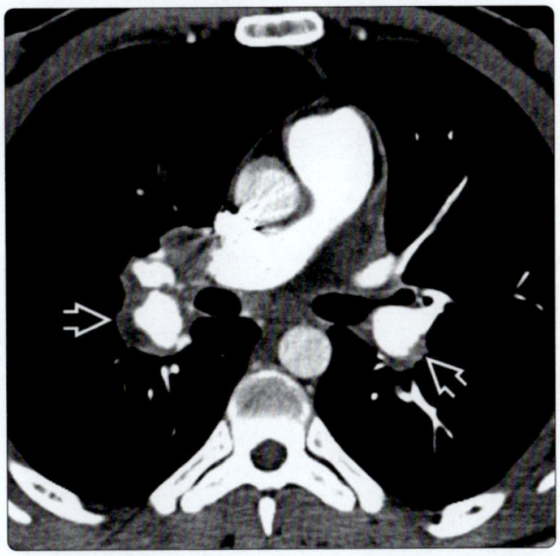

(Left) *Axial CECT of a patient with Behçet disease with multifocal pulmonary artery aneurysms/pseudoaneurysms demonstrates thick-walled dilatation of a right upper lobe segmental pulmonary artery ➡. Note associated mural thrombus.* **(Right)** *Axial CECT of the same patient shows bilateral partially thrombosed pulmonary artery aneurysms/pseudoaneurysms ➡ with peripheral mural thrombi. Although uncommon, Behçet disease is the most common etiology of pulmonary artery aneurysms or pseudoaneurysms.*

Idiopathic Dilation of Pulmonary Trunk

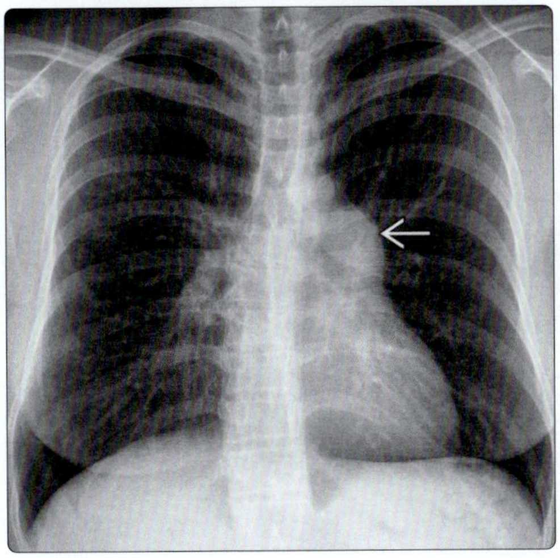

Idiopathic Dilation of Pulmonary Trunk

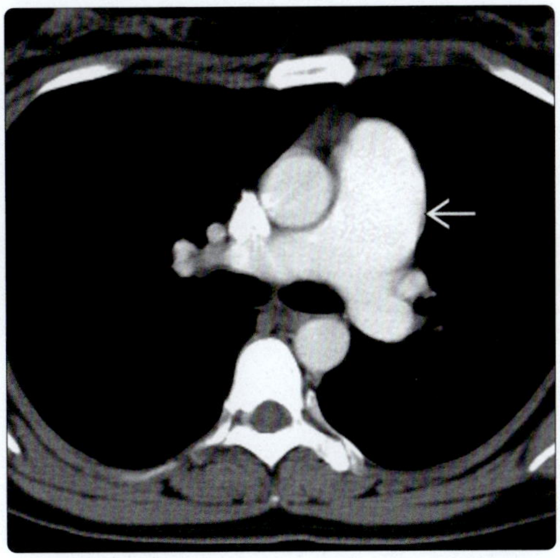

(Left) *PA chest radiograph of a patient with normal pulmonary artery pressures shows an enlarged pulmonary trunk ➡ secondary to idiopathic dilatation. Note the absence of pruning of the peripheral pulmonary artery branches.* **(Right)** *Axial CECT of the same patient shows marked isolated enlargement of the pulmonary trunk ➡ in the setting of normal pulmonary artery pressures. Note the normal caliber of the right and left pulmonary arteries consistent with idiopathic dilatation of the pulmonary trunk.*

Pulmonary Arteriovenous Malformation

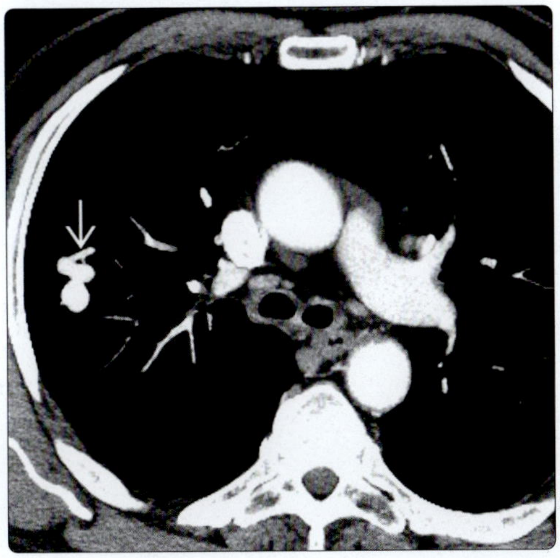

Pulmonary Arteriovenous Malformation

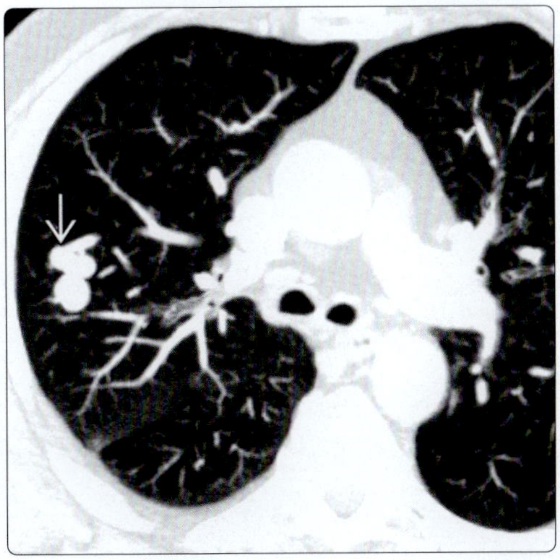

(Left) *Axial CECT (soft tissue window) of a patient with an incidentally discovered right pulmonary nodule demonstrates typical findings of pulmonary arteriovenous malformation ➡, which is an abnormal communication between a pulmonary artery and a pulmonary vein.* **(Right)** *Axial CECT (maximum intensity projection, lung window) of the same patient demonstrates the feeding pulmonary artery ➡. This lesion is amenable to management by catheter embolization.*

Traumatic Pseudoaneurysm

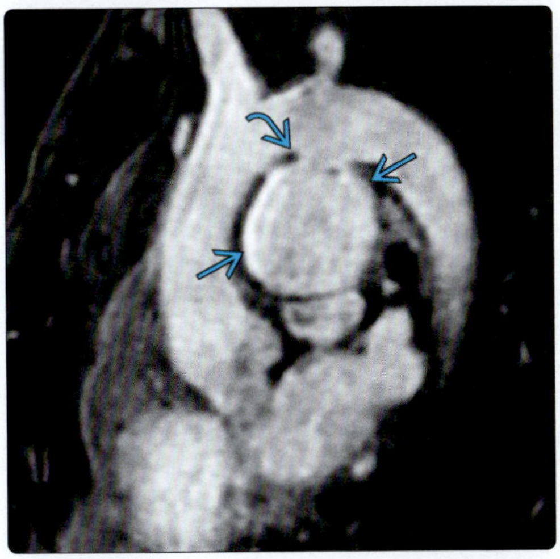

Traumatic Pseudoaneurysm

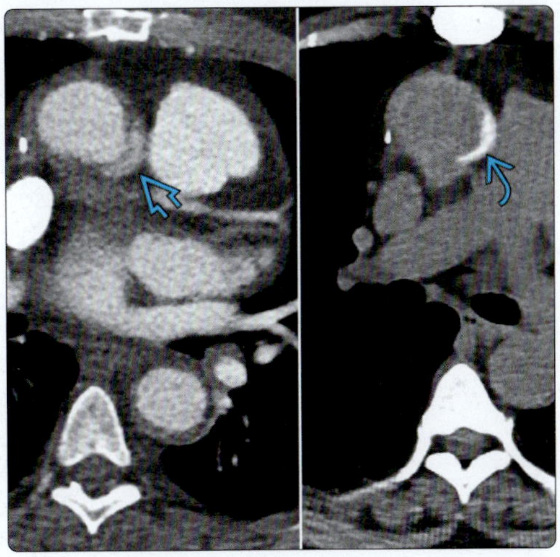

(Left) *Double oblique MRA of the thoracic aorta in a patient with a history of thoracic trauma shows a saccular aneurysm* → *of the aortic arch. Acute angles of the aneurysm* → *differentiate this pseudoaneurysm from a ductus diverticulum.* **(Right)** *Composite image with axial CECT (left) and NECT (right) shows focal dilation of the ascending aorta with high attenuation in the expected location of the medial aortic wall* → *representing postsurgical material* → *rather than aortic pathology.*

Postoperative Pseudoaneurysm

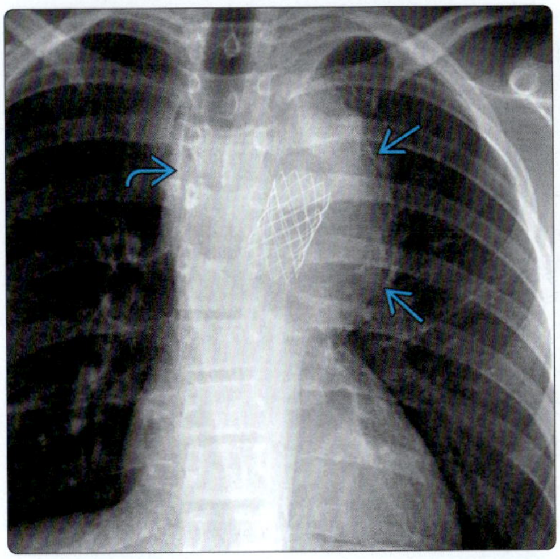

Postoperative Pseudoaneurysm

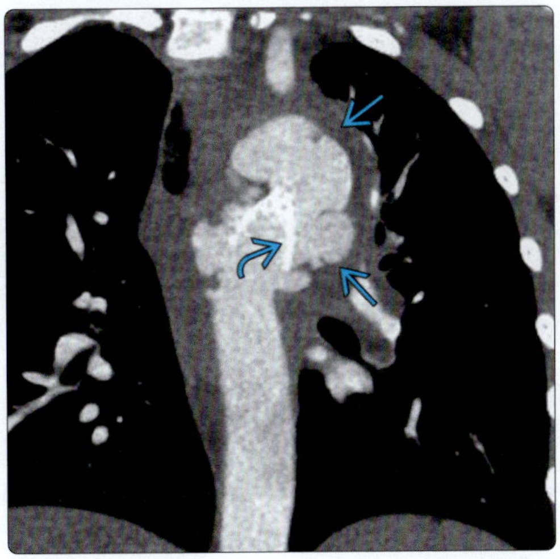

(Left) *PA chest radiograph of a patient with a history of bicuspid aortic valve and coarctation status post stent placement in the proximal descending thoracic aorta shows new dilation of the aortic arch and descending aorta* →*. The intrathoracic trachea is displaced to the right* →*.* **(Right)** *Coronal reformatted CECT of the same patient shows the descending thoracic aortic stent* → *complicated by large, complex contrast outpouchings* →*, consistent with postoperative pseudoaneurysms.*

Aortitis

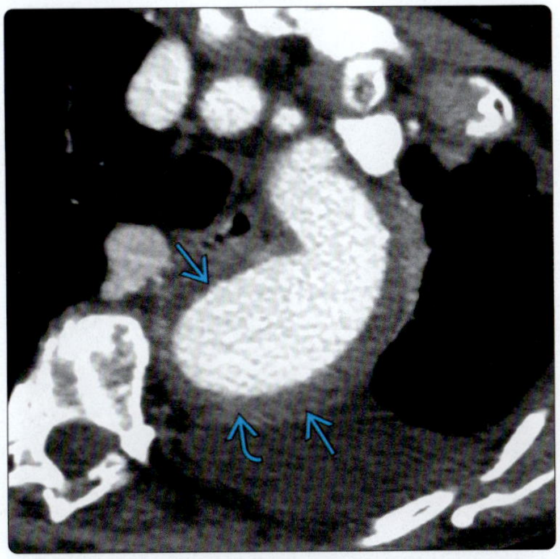

Aortitis

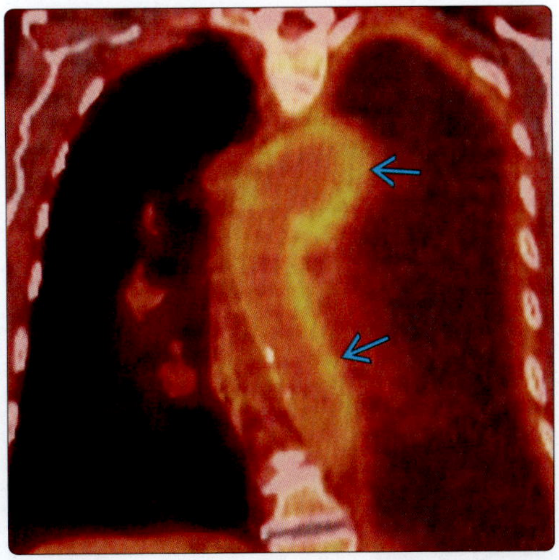

(Left) *Axial CECT of a patient with sepsis and chest pain shows aneurysmal dilation of the proximal descending thoracic aorta* → *with associated diffuse aortic wall thickening and enhancement* →*, consistent with infectious aortitis.* **(Right)** *Fused coronal reformatted FDG PET/CT of the same patient shows diffuse FDG avidity of the thickened, aneurysmal descending thoracic aorta* →*. A large left pleural effusion is also present. Staphylococcus and salmonella are frequent organisms causing infectious aortitis.*

Dilatation of Ascending Thoracic Aorta

DIFFERENTIAL DIAGNOSIS

Common

- Aging
- Hypertension
- Bicuspid Aortic Valve

Less Common

- Marfan Syndrome
- Turner Syndrome
- Aortitis
- Aortic Dissection

Rare but Important

- Loeys-Dietz Syndrome

ESSENTIAL INFORMATION

Helpful Clues for Common Diagnoses

- **Aging**
  - Growth rate of aorta is ~ 0.07-0.2 cm/year
  - Related to cystic medial degeneration (loss of muscle cells and fragmentation of elastic fibers)
  - Accelerated in setting of hypertension
- **Hypertension**
  - Elongated and tortuous thoracic aorta
  - Associated with left ventricular hypertrophy
- **Bicuspid Aortic Valve (BAV)**
  - Ascending aortic aneurysm considered combination of inherent aortopathy and abnormal hemodynamics in ascending aorta
  - Most common morphology is fusion of right and left cusps
  - Bicuspid morphology when evaluated *en face* on CT or MR, with or without raphe
  - Thickened aortic valve leaflets, early calcification (< 60 years)
  - BAV patients at higher risk of aortic dissection (5-10x)
  - Surgery recommended > 5.5 cm
    - Ascending aorta commonly replaced at > 4.5 cm if valve to be replaced

Helpful Clues for Less Common Diagnoses

- **Marfan Syndrome**
  - Autosomal dominant disease
  - Phenotype: Arachnodactyly, ectopia lentis, dural ectasia, scoliosis, pectus carinatum, or excavatum deformity
  - Aortic root dilatation resembles tulip bulb
  - Tubular portion of aorta may have normal diameter
  - Associated aortic insufficiency very common, leads to left ventricular enlargement and heart failure
  - Aortic dissection highly associated with caliber of ascending aorta
  - Surgery recommended > 5.0 cm; > 4.5 cm if considering pregnancy or if need for aortic valve replacement
- **Turner Syndrome**
  - Phenotype: Short stature, broad chest, neck hygroma, premature ovarian failure, cardiovascular defects
  - Ascending aortic aneurysm defined by aortic index of > 2.0 cm/m²
  - Ascending aortic aneurysm in 30-40% of patients
  - Other cardiovascular defects: Elongation of aortic arch, aortic coarctation, BAV, left superior vena cava, partial anomalous pulmonary venous return
  - Surgery recommended when aortic index > 2.5 cm/m²
- **Aortitis**
  - Large vessel vasculitis (Takayasu or giant cell arteritis): Thickened, edematous, enhancing aortic wall; periaortic stranding
    - Irregular aortic contours
    - Narrowed/occluded arch vessels (especially Takayasu)
- **Aortic Dissection**
  - Chronic type A dissection may lead to aortic dilation
  - Intimal flap in ascending aorta with or without thrombosis of false lumen

Helpful Clues for Rare Diagnoses

- **Loeys-Dietz Syndrome**
  - Autosomal dominant connective tissue disorder
  - Classic triad: Arterial tortuosity and aneurysms, hypertelorism, bifid uvula or cleft palate

(Left) *Axial CECT image of a patient with hypertension shows a large ascending aortic aneurysm. A descending aortic aneurysm is also present. Atherosclerosis and chronic hypertension are leading causes of ascending aortic enlargement. Short axis diameter ≥ 5.0 cm is considered aneurysmal.* **(Right)** *Double oblique noncontrast MRA of a patient with bicuspid aortic valve (BAV) shows enlargement of the ascending aorta. BAV patients have inherent aortopathy and flow dynamics in the ascending aorta.*

Hypertension

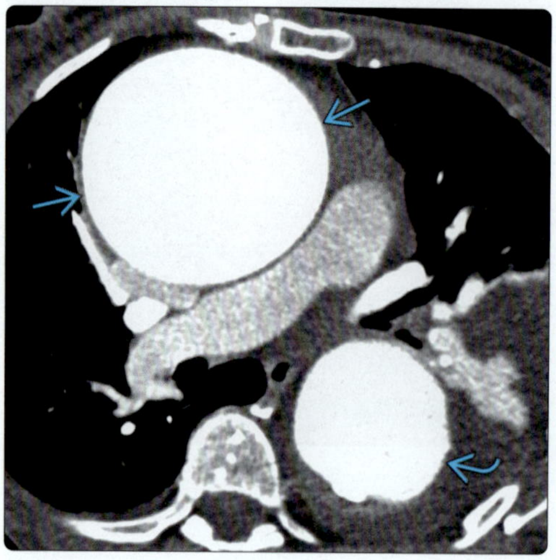

Bicuspid Aortic Valve

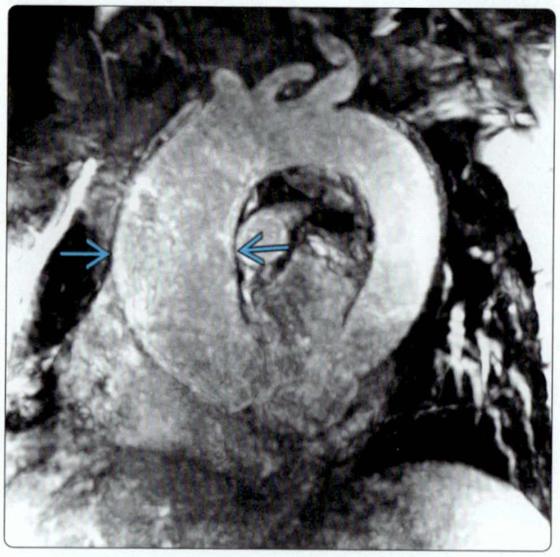

Marfan Syndrome

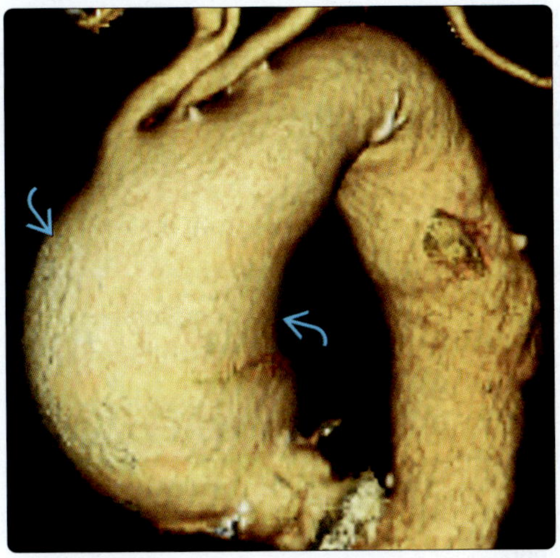

Marfan Syndrome

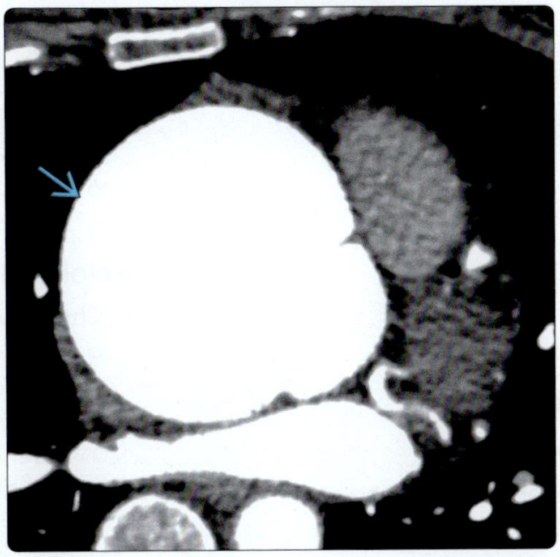

(Left) *Volume-rendered image from CECT of a patient with Marfan syndrome shows dilation of the ascending aorta. The degree of ascending aortic dilation is directly related to risk for ascending aortic dissection in patients with connective tissue disease-associated aortopathy.* **(Right)** *Axial CECT image of a patient with atypical chest pain shows large ascending aortic aneurysm also involving the aortic root. Patients with Marfan syndrome may have a normal tubular portion of the aorta ("tulip bulb").*

Aortitis

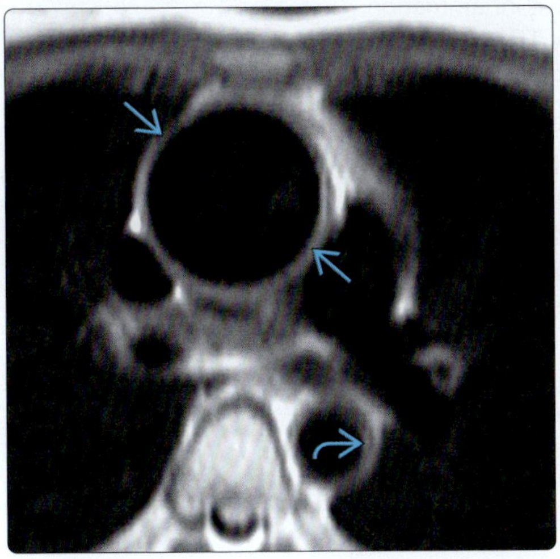

Aortitis

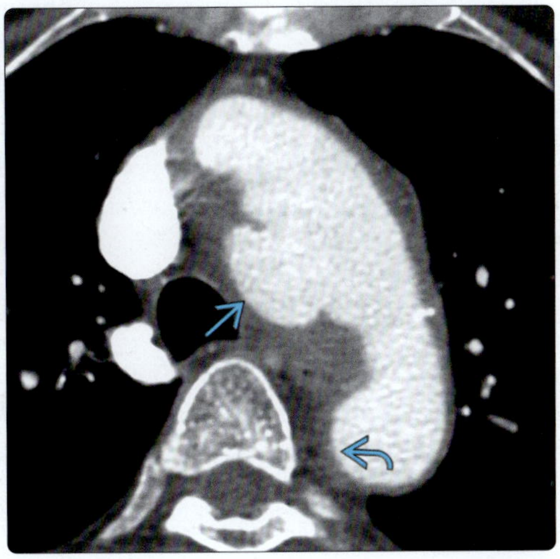

(Left) *Axial double inversion recovery MR of a patient with Takayasu arteritis shows an ascending aortic aneurysm. Aortic wall thickening and inflammatory changes are associated findings best depicted on MR in these patients. In the chronic setting, great arteries may be stenotic and calcify.* **(Right)** *Axial CECT image of a patient with giant cell arteritis shows saccular aneurysm of the ascending aorta and aortic arch. Note associated aortic wall thickening, a common finding in patients with aortitis.*

Aortic Dissection

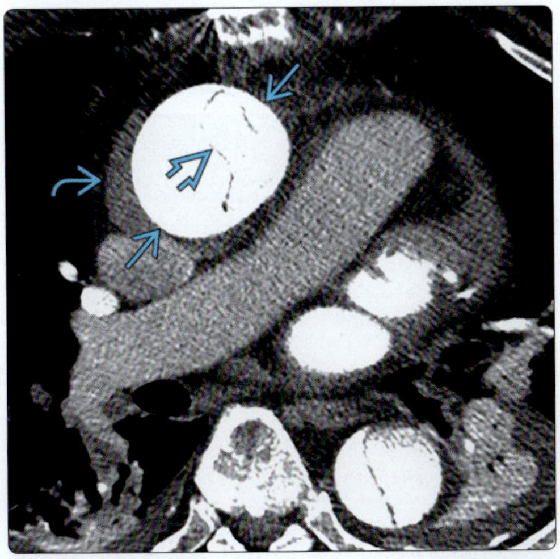

Aortic Dissection

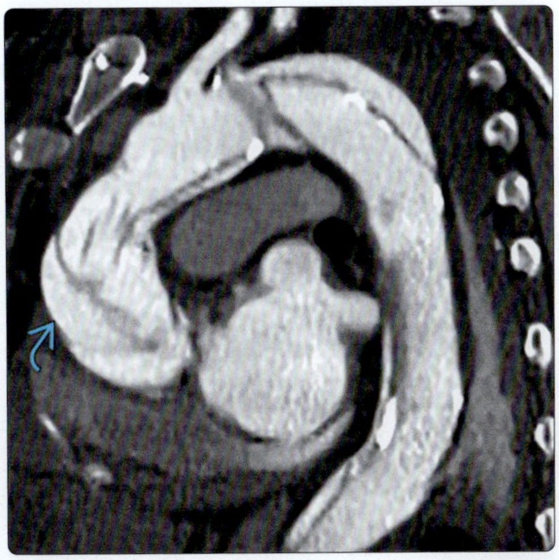

(Left) *Axial CECT image of a patient with acute chest pain shows dilation of the ascending aorta in the setting of ascending aortic dissection. Periaortic inflammatory stranding is also present.* **(Right)** *Double oblique sagittal reformatted CECT of a patient with aortic dissection shows irregularity and enlargement of the ascending aorta. Contrast enhanced CT or MR is necessary in cases of aortic enlargement to evaluate for dissection flaps and other aortic wall pathology.*

Aortic Calcification

DIFFERENTIAL DIAGNOSIS

Common

- Atherosclerotic Disease
- Calcified Mural Thrombus
- Chronic Kidney Disease/Diabetes Mellitus

Less Common

- Chronic Aortic Dissection/Intramural Hematoma
- Vasculitis

Rare but Important

- Post Radiation

ESSENTIAL INFORMATION

Key Differential Diagnosis Issues

- Frontal radiograph identifies arch/descending aortic calcification, ascending aorta identified on lateral radiograph
- Degree of atherosclerotic calcification advances with age
- Identification of heavy ascending aortic calcification may have surgical implications

Helpful Clues for Common Diagnoses

- **Atherosclerotic Disease**
  - More common in aortic arch and descending aorta than ascending aorta
  - Associated with noncalcified atherosclerotic plaque
  - Patchy distribution within atherosclerotic lesions and is most commonly amorphous without distinct architecture
    - At first, limited to intima
    - May progress to involve media
  - When circumferential in ascending aorta prevents surgical clamping and is termed porcelain aorta
  - Associated with increased cardiovascular morbidity and mortality
- **Calcified Mural Thrombus**
  - Atherosclerotic disease promotes formation of mural thrombus that may calcify
  - Low-attenuation nodular, sessile, or frond-like projections into aortic lumen
  - When chronic, these may calcify
  - Risk for distal embolization
  - Common in descending thoracic aorta
- **Chronic Kidney Disease/Diabetes Mellitus**
  - Calcification begins in medial smooth muscle
  - Diffuse calcification typically circumferential
  - Can be seen in addition to atherosclerotic disease

Helpful Clues for Less Common Diagnoses

- **Chronic Aortic Dissection/Intramural Hematoma**
  - False lumen may thrombose and subsequently calcify
  - Calcification occurs in false lumen, external to intima
  - Patients with higher flow through false lumen have lower risk of thrombosis
- **Vasculitis**
  - Takayasu arteritis in young patients; giant cell arteritis in older patients
  - Other vasculitides do not commonly involve aorta
  - Calcification within media but patchy as it follows areas of previous inflammation
  - Associated findings: Thickened aortic wall, aneurysmal foci, irregular aortic contours, aortic and branch stenosis

Helpful Clues for Rare Diagnoses

- **Post Radiation**
  - Calcification of medial smooth muscle, circumferential
  - Limited to radiation field with sharp margins
  - History of mediastinal or head and neck cancers
  - Associated findings: Paramediastinal fibrosis, calcified mediastinal mass or lymph nodes

SELECTED REFERENCES

1. Desai MY et al: Thoracic aortic calcification: diagnostic, prognostic, and management considerations. JACC Cardiovasc Imaging. 11(7):1012-26, 2018

Atherosclerotic Disease

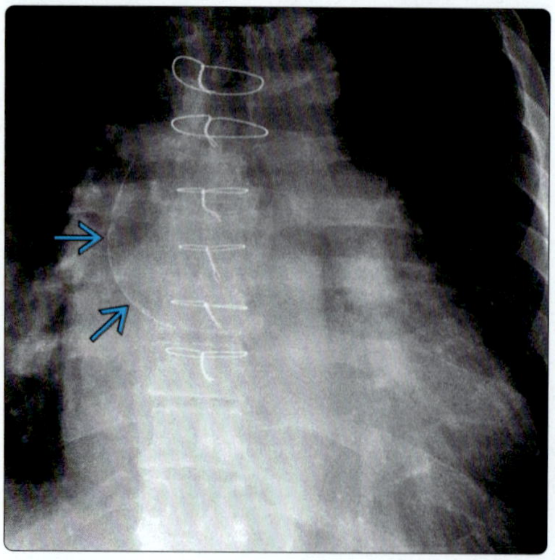

Atherosclerotic Disease

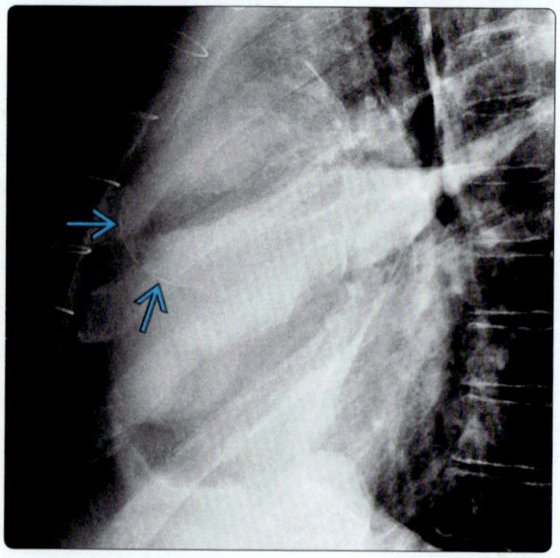

(Left) *PA chest radiograph of a patient status post median sternotomy shows curvilinear calcification ⇒ in the expected location of the ascending aorta.* **(Right)** *Lateral chest radiograph of the same patient shows opacity of the retrosternal clear space and curvilinear calcification ⇒ in the ascending aorta. Ascending aortic enlargement and calcification are often more visible on the lateral chest radiograph.*

Atherosclerotic Disease

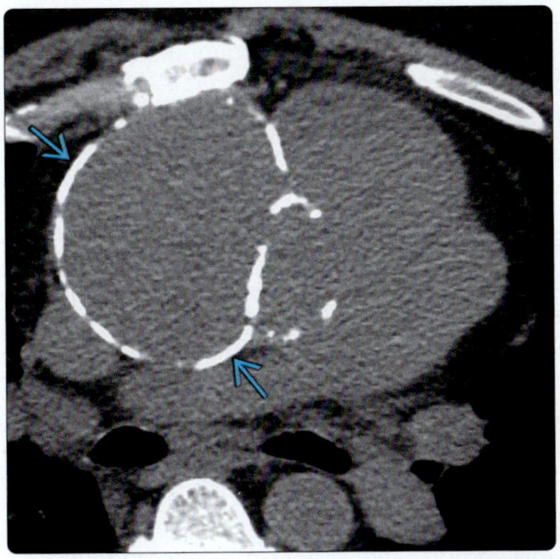

Atherosclerotic Disease

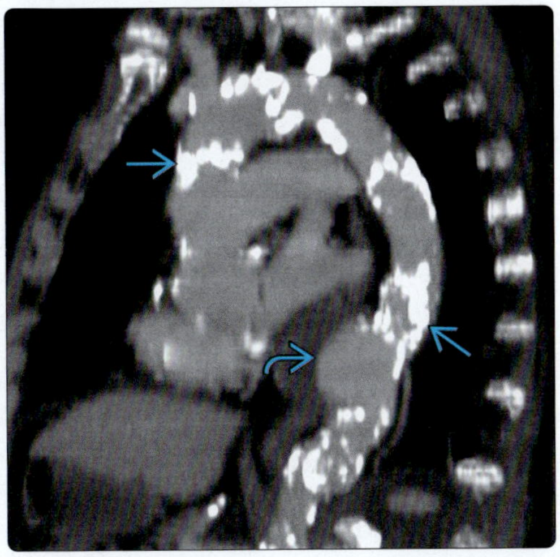

(Left) *Axial NECT of a patient status post median sternotomy shows aneurysmal dilation of the ascending aorta with aortic wall calcifications.* **(Right)** *Oblique sagittal CECT of a patient with focal aneurysm of the descending thoracic aorta shows diffuse, patchy calcification of the thoracic aorta, consistent with atherosclerosis. Atherosclerosis is the most common cause of aortic calcification. Circumferential and extensive ascending aortic calcification may complicate cardiac surgery.*

Atherosclerotic Disease

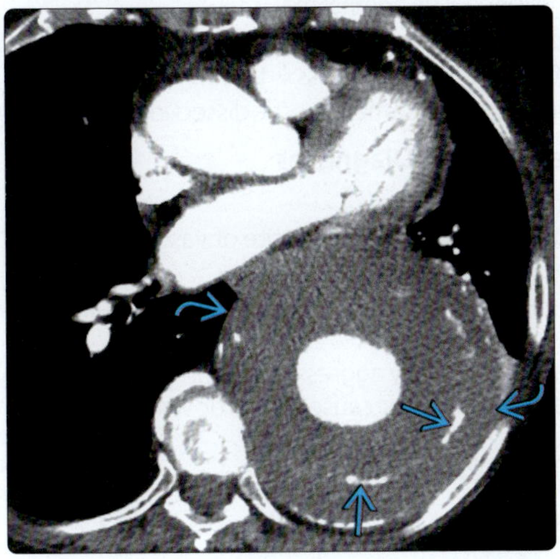

Atherosclerotic Disease

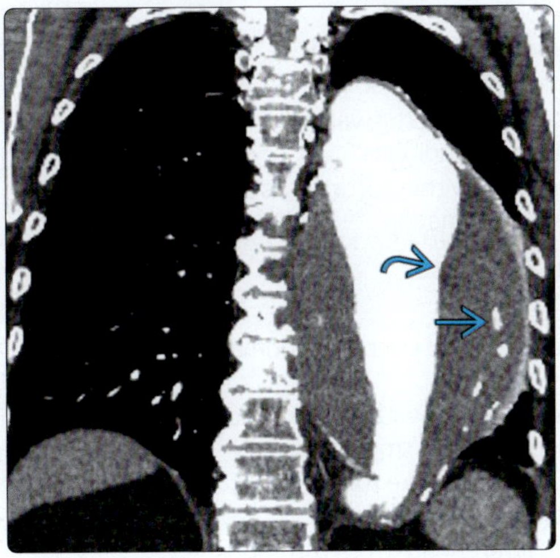

(Left) *Axial CECT of a patient with a descending thoracic aortic aneurysm shows circumferential thrombus within the aneurysm wall with internal curvilinear calcification.* **(Right)** *Coronal reformatted CECT of the same patient shows a long-segment fusiform aneurysm of the descending thoracic aorta with thrombus and internal calcification. Calcification of chronic thrombus is more common in the descending thoracic aorta and carries a risk for distal embolization.*

Chronic Aortic Dissection/Intramural Hematoma

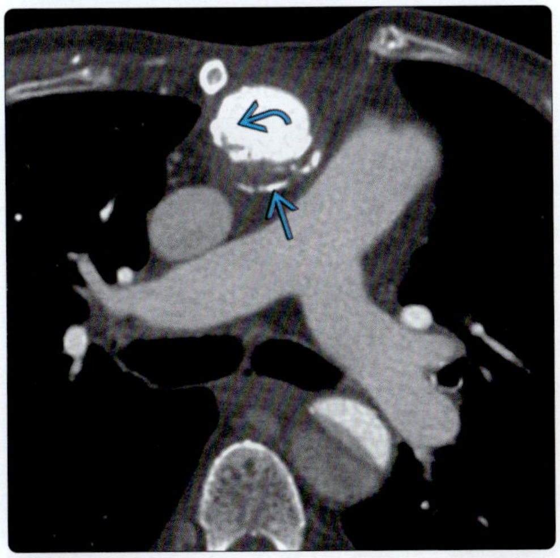

Vasculitis

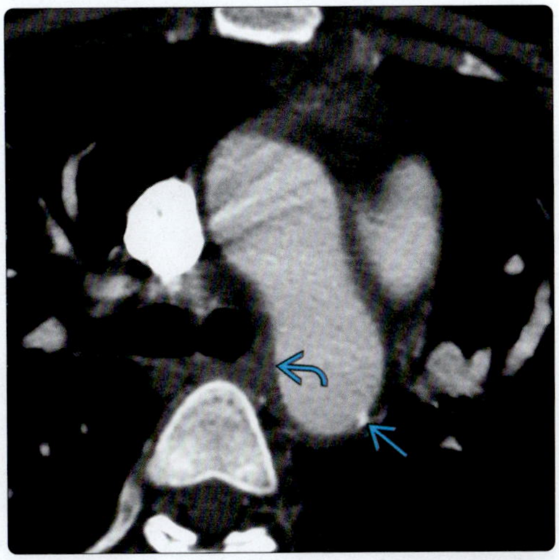

(Left) *Axial CECT of a patient status post remote median sternotomy shows aortic dissection of the ascending and descending thoracic aorta. Calcifications are present in both the intima and the thrombosed false lumen.* **(Right)** *Axial CECT of a 20-year-old woman with Takayasu arteritis shows diffuse thickening of the thoracic aorta and focal calcification in the descending thoracic aorta. Aortic calcification in vasculitis occurs in the media as a sequela of prior inflammation.*

DIFFERENTIAL DIAGNOSIS

Common

- Atherosclerosis
- Aortitis

Less Common

- Aortic Dissection
- Intramural Hematoma

Rare but Important

- Aortic Sarcoma

ESSENTIAL INFORMATION

Key Differential Diagnosis Issues

- Normal aortic wall thickness varies with sex and age, generally considered normal when ≤ 3 mm
- Aortic evaluation most frequently performed with CT, particularly in emergent setting
  - NECT is essential to problem solve aortic wall thickening
    - Postoperative material may be hyperattenuating and mimic aortic pathology post contrast
    - Blood in aortic wall easier to detect on NECT
  - CECT is used to evaluate integrity of aortic wall
    - May also show enhancement of aortic wall in infectious and inflammatory conditions
- MR allows characterization of flow within aorta and is more sensitive to subtle aortic wall inflammation

Helpful Clues for Common Diagnoses

- Atherosclerosis
  - Deposits of lipids, fibrous tissue, and calcium in intimal layer of aorta
  - Common imaging finding in patients with hypertension, hypercholesterolemia, diabetes, &/or smoking history
  - Characterized on imaging by plaque-like thickening of aortic wall and calcifications of intima
  - Plaque may be difficult to differentiate from thrombus, and these entities often coexist
  - Associated aneurysms from common etiologic factors
- Aortitis
  - Most common causes of inflammatory thoracic aortitis: Takayasu arteritis and giant cell arteritis
  - Wall thickening, irregular aortic contours, aneurysm formation, and narrowing/occlusion
  - Calcification may be present in chronic cases
  - Mycotic aortitis may cause aortic wall thickening
    - *Staphylococcus*, *Salmonella* spp. most common

Helpful Clues for Less Common Diagnoses

- Aortic Dissection
  - Intimal tear and subsequent blood propagation into subintimal layer of aortic wall, causing aortic wall thickening and intimomedial flap
  - Internally displaced intimal calcifications
  - May have associated mediastinal/pericardial hemorrhage
  - Ascending aortic dissection requires surgical repair
- Intramural Hematoma (IMH)
  - Aortic media hemorrhage, either from spontaneous rupture of vasa vasorum or small intimal tear
  - NECT findings include crescentic or eccentric wall thickening, periaortic hematoma
  - CECT shows no discernible intimal tear
  - Poor prognosis if IMH thickness > 10 mm
  - Treatment generally same as aortic dissection

Helpful Clues for Rare Diagnoses

- Aortic Sarcoma
  - Exceedingly rare, most common site of vascular sarcomas with pulmonary artery
  - May appear as intraluminal filling defect or irregular aortic wall thickening
  - Enhancement or locally aggressive features may differentiate from other causes of aortic wall thickening

SELECTED REFERENCES

1. Lichtenberger JP 3rd et al: MR imaging of thoracic aortic disease. Top Magn Reson Imaging. 27(2):95-102, 2018
2. Oyama-Manabe N et al: IgG4-related cardiovascular disease from the aorta to the coronary arteries: Multidetector CT and PET/CT. Radiographics. 38(7):1934-48, 2018

Atherosclerosis

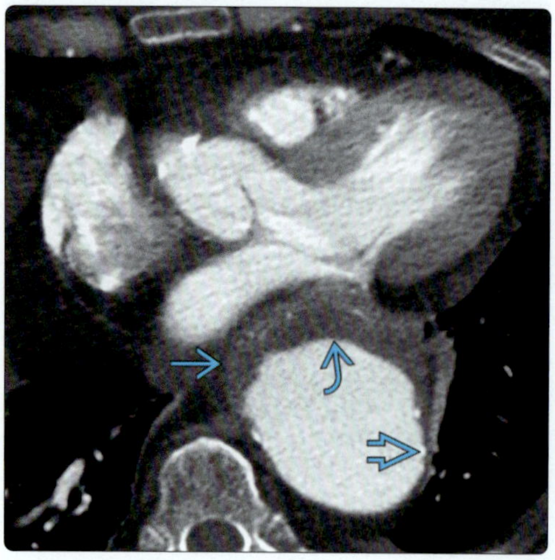

Aortitis

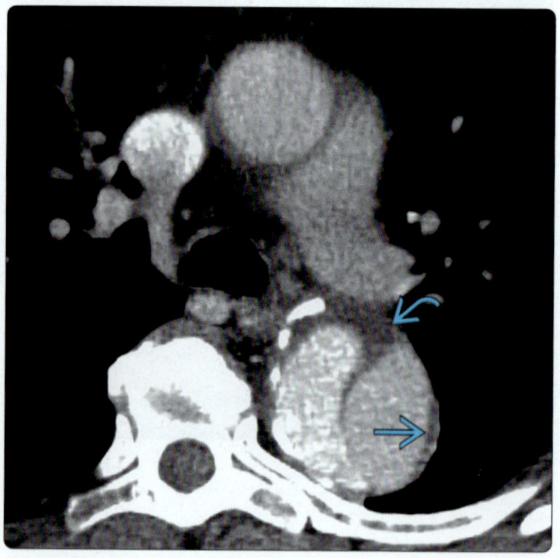

(Left) *Axial CECT of a patient with hypertension shows aortic wall thickening in the setting of atherosclerotic calcification and plaque within a descending thoracic aortic aneurysm. Atherosclerosis is a common cause of aortic wall thickening.* **(Right)** *Axial CECT of a patient with giant cell arteritis shows a descending thoracic aortic dissection with areas of aortic wall thickening and thrombus within the false lumen. Aortic dissection by definition results in thickening of the aortic wall.*

Aortitis

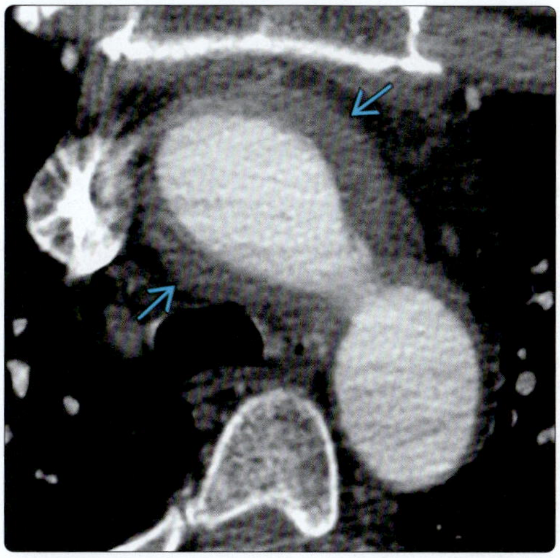

Aortitis

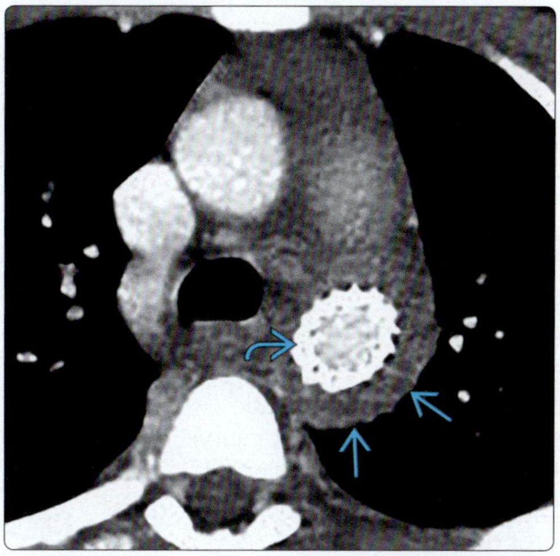

(Left) *Axial CECT of a patient with IgG4 aortitis shows thickening of the ascending aorta* → *extending toward the aortic arch. Inflammatory aortitis of the thoracic aorta is most commonly caused by Takayasu arteritis and giant cell arteritis.* **(Right)** *Axial CECT of a patient with a fever status post stent* ↪ *placement across a coarctation shows aortic wall thickening* →*, consistent with infectious aortitis. Infectious aortitis may be complicated by pseudoaneurysm and rupture.*

Aortic Dissection

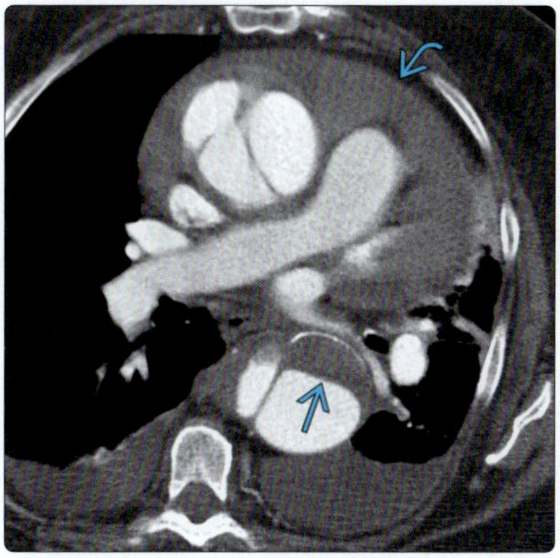

Intramural Hematoma

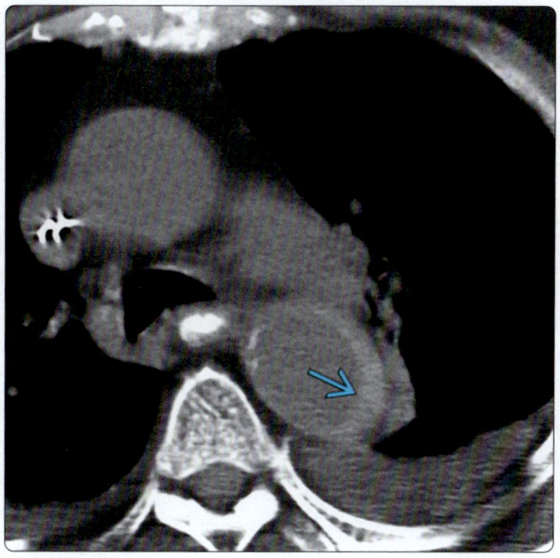

(Left) *Axial CECT of a patient with acute chest pain shows acute aortic dissection involving the ascending and descending thoracic aorta complicated by thrombus formation* → *in the descending aorta. Pericardial hemorrhage is also noted* ↪*.* **(Right)** *Axial NECT of a patient with chest pain shows high-attenuation wall thickening* →*, consistent with intramural hematoma. Note associated hemothorax in this patient with acute aortic syndrome. The aortic wall is considered normal when ≤ 3 mm.*

Aortic Sarcoma

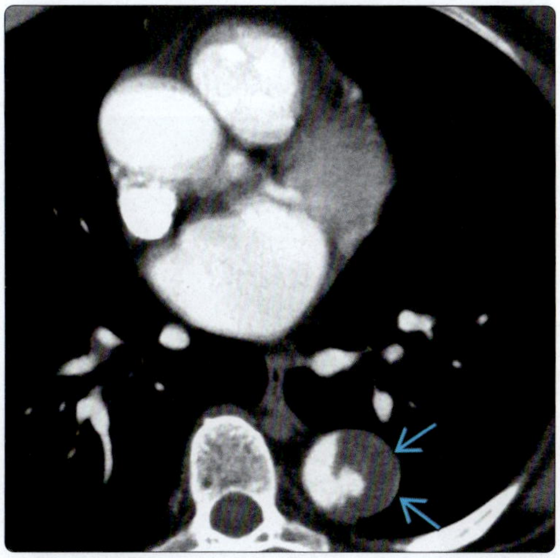

Aortic Sarcoma

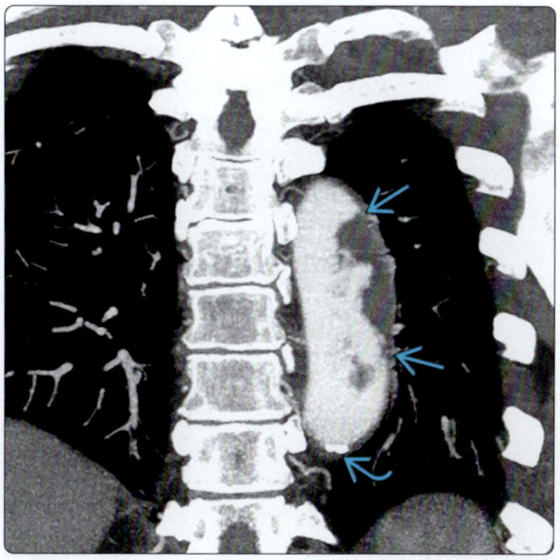

(Left) *Axial CECT of a patient with chest pain shows mass-like thickening* → *of the descending thoracic aorta. Biopsy subsequently revealed intimal sarcoma of the aorta.* **(Right)** *Coronal MIP reformation of a CECT of the same patient shows the craniocaudal extent of the mass-like aortic wall thickening* → *with minimal atherosclerotic calcification* ↪ *elsewhere. Although rare, aortic sarcoma is an important diagnosis to consider in young patients with mass-like thickening of the aorta.*

DIFFERENTIAL DIAGNOSIS

Common

- Aortic Dissection
- Intramural Hematoma

Less Common

- Penetrating Atherosclerotic Ulcer

ESSENTIAL INFORMATION

Key Differential Diagnosis Issues

- Understanding clinical presentation is important 1st step to appropriate discussion of aortic pathology
  - Acute aortic syndrome applies to acute nontraumatic clinical presentation (versus acute traumatic aortic injury)
    - Characteristically sudden tearing chest/back pain
  - Management decisions depend on accurate delineation and characterization of aortic disease
- NECT is important component of evaluation, allowing detection of intramural hematoma and problem-solving of hyperattenuation of aortic wall
- CECT is highly accurate and necessary for complete evaluation of aorta in acute setting
- MR has role in surveillance

Helpful Clues for Common Diagnoses

- Aortic Dissection
  - Intimal tear and subsequent blood propagation into subintimal layer of aortic wall
  - More common in men, peak age: 50-65 years
  - Most common signs/symptoms include sudden tearing chest pain, neck/jaw pain, or back pain
  - Classified based on location of proximal-most disease
    - Stanford A: Ascending aorta involved
    - Stanford B: Ascending aorta not involved
    - DeBakey I: Originates in ascending aorta and continues into arch or beyond
    - DeBakey II: Confined to ascending aorta
    - DeBakey IIIa: Confined to descending aorta; DeBakey IIIb: Extends below diaphragm
  - Intimomedial flap separates true and false lumen
    - False lumen often larger, may contain medial layer remnants, and delayed peak enhancement
    - False lumen may develop thrombus
    - Dissection may involve entire circumferential intima, leading to windsock appearance
  - Radiographic clues include aortic enlargement, mediastinal widening
  - NECT: Aortic dilation, mediastinal/pericardial hemorrhage, internally displaced intimal calcifications
  - CECT shows extent of intimal dissection, visceral malperfusion, and thrombus
  - Most acute ascending aortic dissections are surgically treated due to risk of aortic root and cardiac involvement
- Intramural Hematoma (IMH)
  - Aortic media hemorrhage, either from spontaneous rupture of vasa vasorum or small intimal tear
  - NECT: Crescentic or eccentric wall thickening, periaortic hematoma
  - CECT: No discernible intimal tear
    - May contain focal, small pool of contrast within intramural hematoma termed intramural blood pool
  - Poor prognosis if IMH thickness > 10 mm
  - Treatment generally same as aortic dissection

Helpful Clues for Less Common Diagnoses

- Penetrating Atherosclerotic Ulcer
  - Atherosclerotic lesion with disrupted internal elastic lamina of aortic wall and ulceration into media
  - More common in men; most prevalent in ages 60-70
  - 2-10% of all acute aortic syndrome cases
  - NECT may show associated IMH
  - CECT: Outpouching of contrast beyond aortic wall, irregular intima

SELECTED REFERENCES

1. Carroll BJ et al: Imaging for acute aortic syndromes. Heart. ePub, 2019
2. Gutschow SE et al: Emerging concepts in intramural hematoma imaging. Radiographics. 36(3):660-74, 2016

Aortic Dissection

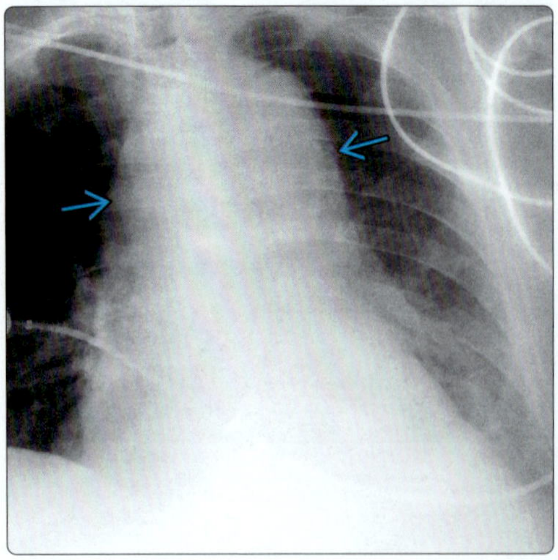

Aortic Dissection

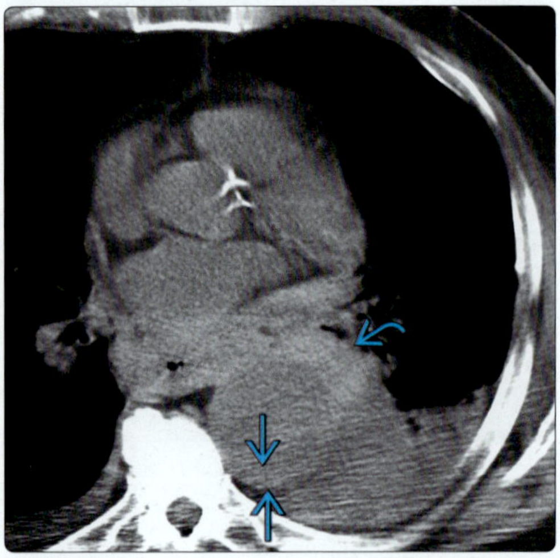

(Left) *Portable chest radiograph of a patient presenting with acute chest pain shows widening of the mediastinum ➔ and left pleural effusion. The normal features of the mediastinum are obscured, suggestive of mediastinal hemorrhage.* **(Right)** *Axial NECT of the same patient shows dilatation of the descending thoracic aorta and a thickened, hyperattenuating aortic wall, consistent with intramural hematoma ➔. Note the associated mediastinal hemorrhage ➔ and left hemothorax.*

Aortic Dissection

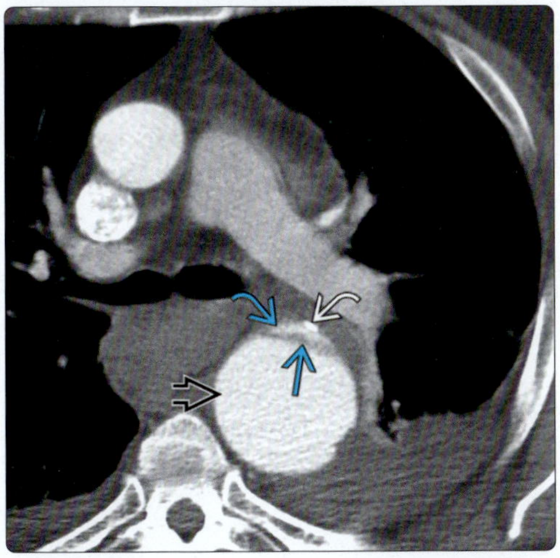

Aortic Dissection

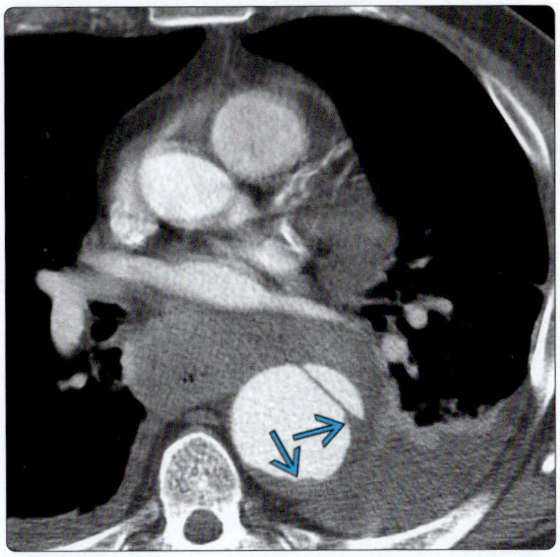

(Left) *Axial CECT of the same patient presenting with acute chest pain shows descending aortic dissection. An intimomedial flap* ➡ *is present with a compressed true lumen* ➡ *and a larger false lumen* ➡*. Atherosclerotic calcification* ➡ *is noted, an important marker for the intimal layer of the aortic wall.* **(Right)** *Axial CECT of the same patient shows irregularity of the wall of the false lumen and intimomedial flap* ➡*, evidence of the dissected medial layer of the aortic wall with associated hemorrhage.*

Aortic Dissection

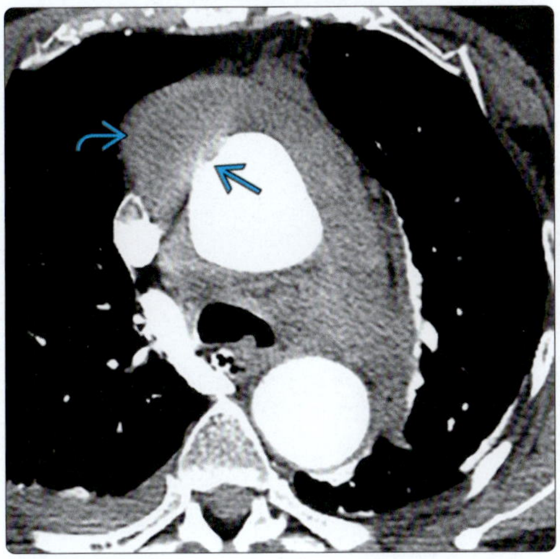

Aortic Dissection

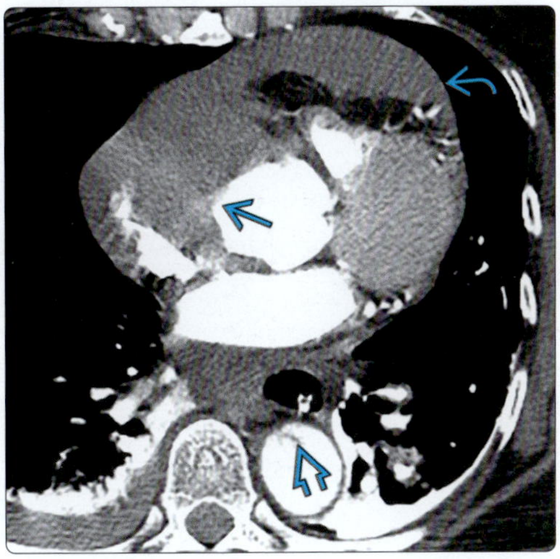

(Left) *Axial CECT of a patient with chest pain shows irregular morphology of the ascending aorta and focal irregularity of the anterolateral ascending aorta* ➡ *with mediastinal hemorrhage* ➡*, consistent with acute aortic dissection.* **(Right)** *Axial CECT of the same patient shows propagation of hemorrhage and dissection into the aortic root* ➡ *and pericardial space* ➡*. Dissection is also noted in the descending thoracic aorta* ➡*. Ascending aortic involvement of acute aortic syndrome is a surgical indication.*

Intramural Hematoma

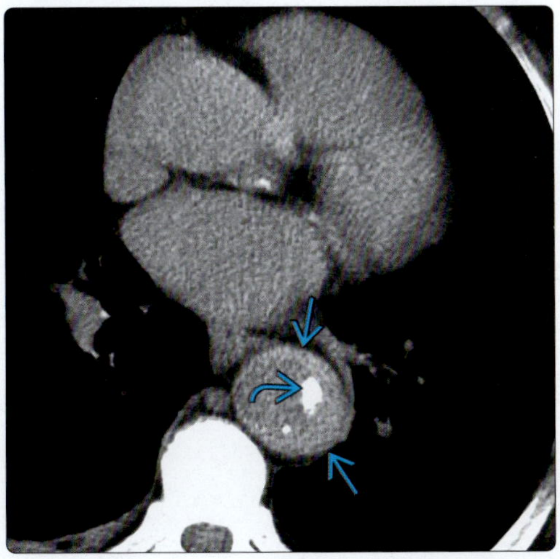

Intramural Hematoma

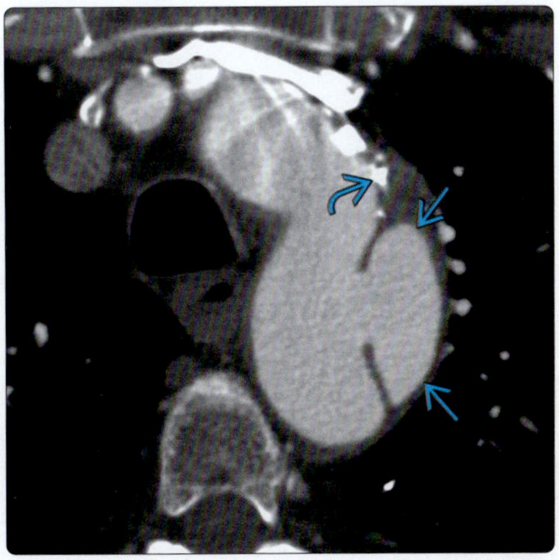

(Left) *Axial NECT of a patient with tearing back pain shows crescentic hyperattenuation in the descending thoracic aorta* ➡*, consistent with an intramural hematoma. Note the medial displacement of the intimal calcifications* ➡ *as hemorrhage expands the subintimal aorta.* **(Right)** *Axial CECT of a patient with chest pain shows focal protrusion of contrast* ➡ *beyond the wall of the aorta with associated intimal irregularity and atherosclerotic calcification* ➡*, consistent with a penetrating atherosclerotic ulcer.*

SECTION 8

Pleura

Approach to Pleura

General Imaging Patterns

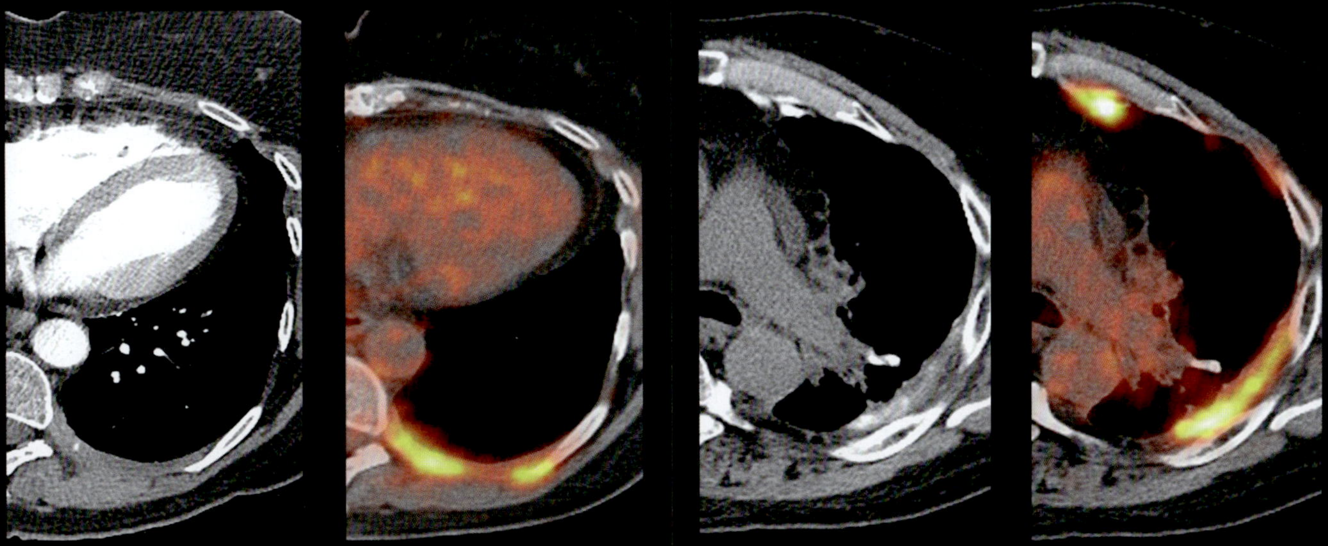

Anatomic Considerations

The pleural space is a potential space formed by 2 pleural surfaces: the visceral pleura lining the surface of the lungs that invaginates between the lobes to form the interlobar fissures and the parietal pleura covering the chest wall that extends onto the mediastinal and diaphragmatic surfaces. Each of the pleural membranes has several components. A thin sheet of mesothelial cells lines the surface of the pleura facing the pleural cavity, which are active in absorption and phagocytosis. Subjacent to the mesothelial lining are layers of connective tissue, including elastin and collagen fibers, which are thicker in the parietal pleura.

Under normal conditions, the pleural space helps to distribute and transmit the mechanical forces of breathing and reduces friction between the expanding and collapsing lung and the surrounding thoracic cage. There is a physiologic small amount of fluid in the pleural space, ~ 0.1-0.2 mL/kg, or less than 15 mL in the average individual. Turnover of this fluid is constant, with more than 1 L being cleared daily. Accumulation of pleural fluid is governed by Starling forces. Hydrostatic pressure within the capillary bed exceeds that of the pleural space, which has negative pressure, establishing a pressure gradient causing fluid movement into the pleural space, balanced by oncotic forces due to the much larger concentration of proteins and other molecules in plasma than in the pleural space.

Imaging of Normal Pleura

The normal parietal and visceral pleura are not visible on chest radiographs apart from the double layer of visceral pleura, which forms the interlobar fissures. The pleural layers are visualized on CT as part of the intercostal stripe. This thin line is seen extending between adjacent ribs, and is composed of the visceral pleura, a small amount of normal pleural fluid, the parietal pleura, the endothoracic fascia, and the innermost intercostal muscles. Most of the visible intercostal stripe is due to the intercostal muscles, which is why the stripe is not seen directly adjacent to the inner surface of the rib, where the intercostal muscles are naturally deficient.

Imaging of Abnormal Pleura

Pleural effusion occurs when fluid accumulation within the pleural space exceeds its clearance. Effusions may be either transudates or exudates depending on the etiology, which determines the fluid concentration of protein and lactate dehydrogenase. On upright radiographs, free-flowing pleural fluid will accumulate in the most dependent part of the chest, and smaller amounts of fluid will form a meniscus. 50-75 mL of fluid can be detected on lateral radiographs, whereas at least 175 mL must be present to create blunting of the lateral costophrenic angles on frontal radiographs. The lateral decubitus radiograph is most sensitive and can detect 5-10 mL of pleural fluid. On supine radiographs, pleural effusions become visible at 175 mL and may layer posteriorly creating an ill-defined opacity mimicking parenchymal disease. On CT, effusions appear posteriorly as a sickle-shaped opacity of fluid density. CT can also demonstrate higher density components, membranes, and septations in complex &/or loculated fluid.

Pleural thickening may be seen in both benign and malignant disease processes. For example, pleural thickening may be due to prior infection, asbestos exposure, hemothorax, or surgery. When pleural thickening is present alongside pleural nodules and masses, however, malignancy is much more likely.

Metastases are the most frequent cause of malignant pleural disease, whereas malignant pleural mesothelioma is the most common primary pleural malignancy. Circumferential pleural thickening and pleural nodules &/or masses are the most common findings on radiography. CT features that are highly suggestive of malignant pleural disease include circumferential pleural thickening, pleural nodularity, pleural thickening greater than 1 cm, and involvement of the mediastinal pleura. Metastases may demonstrate specific features of the primary malignancy, such as enhancement in thyroid and renal cancers, melanoma, and choriocarcinoma, and calcification or ossification in osteosarcoma, chondrosarcoma, and mucinous tumors of the gastrointestinal or genitourinary tract.

Pleural calcification is often visualized in the form of pleural plaques, which are a localized form of fibrosis involving only the parietal pleura that are histologically compatible with deposition of collagen fibers. They represent the most frequent manifestation of asbestos-related pleural disease, generally appearing up to 20-30 years following inhalational exposure to asbestos fibers. Plaques measure between 1-10 mm in thickness, extend up to 4 intercostal spaces, and may calcify over time, showing linear, punctate or "cake-like" patterns. They most often occur in the posterior and lateral lower thorax; the apices and costophrenic angles are usually not involved. Asbestos-related plaques are often bilateral, and diaphragmatic plaques are characteristic. Fibrothorax occurs when the visceral and parietal pleura fuse, leading to substantial compromise of the lung and thoracic cage. The process starts in the lower thorax and spreads cephalad. The fibrotic peel may be over 10 mm thick and will contract over time, causing rib crowding and volume loss in the ipsilateral hemithorax. Etiologies of fibrothorax include prior infection, hemothorax, and cardiac surgery, such as coronary artery bypass grafting.

Air in the pleural space may result from communication between alveolar spaces and the pleura, or connection between the outside atmosphere and the pleural space. Spontaneous pneumothorax is idiopathic and occurs primarily in tall, thin males who are smokers but have no apparent lung disease. Secondary pneumothorax is associated with multiple predisposing lung conditions, including cystic lung diseases, such as cystic fibrosis, Langerhans cell histiocytosis, and lymphangioleiomyomatosis; emphysema; alpha-1 antitrypsin deficiency; and infections, such as tuberculosis and *Pneumocystis jiroveci* pneumonia. Pneumothoraces may also be iatrogenic, from mechanical ventilation or line placement, or related to blunt or vehicular trauma. On radiographs, a pneumothorax is denoted by a very fine white line corresponding to the visceral pleural surface with absence of lung markings peripheral to it. CT is more sensitive for the detection of small pneumothoraces, especially in the trauma or ICU setting. Connection between the tracheobronchial tree and the pleural space constitutes a bronchopleural fistula (BPF), which is usually the result of previous surgery or radiation therapy. BPF may be suspected when there is persistent air with or without fluid on sequential chest radiographs. Following pneumonectomy, BPF is characterized by increasing air and decreasing fluid in the pneumonectomy space. Chest CT may demonstrate the bronchial connection with the air collection and is the most useful imaging modality for this entity.

Pleural Effusion

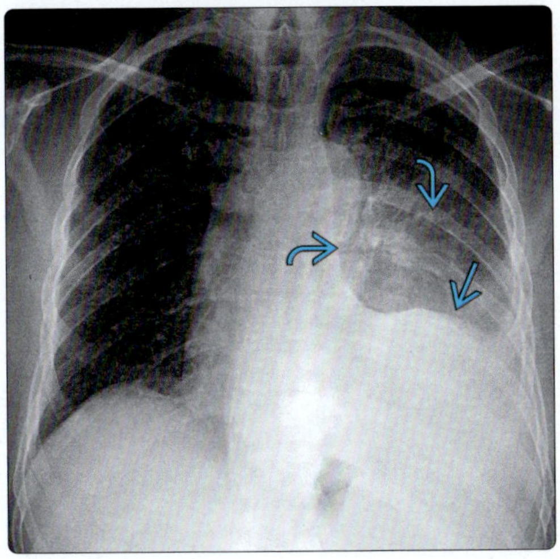

Pleural Effusion

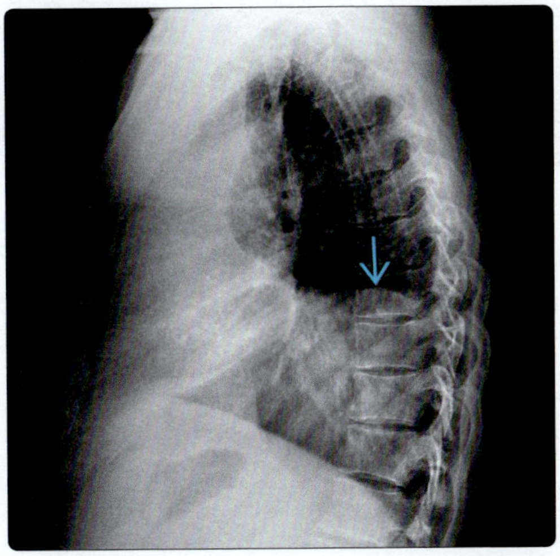

(Left) *PA chest radiograph of a patient with lung cancer demonstrates a left pleural effusion and vague opacity in the left hemithorax representing a combination of the malignancy and post-obstructive atelectasis.* **(Right)** *Lateral chest radiograph of the same patient better demonstrates the size of the left pleural effusion. On upright radiographs, free-flowing pleural fluid will accumulate in the most dependent part of the chest, and smaller amounts of fluid will form a meniscus.*

Pleural Effusion

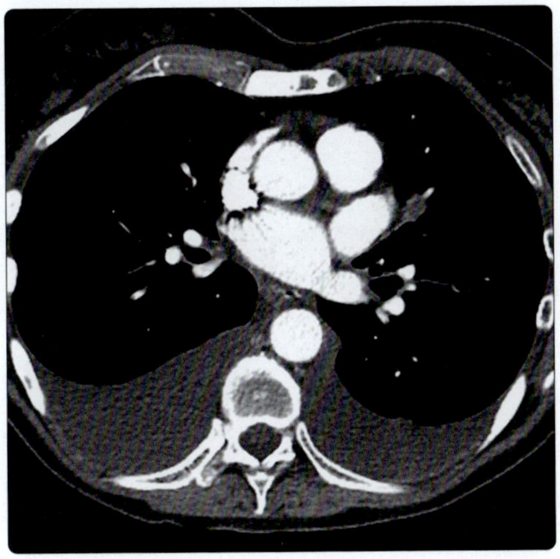

Pleural Effusion

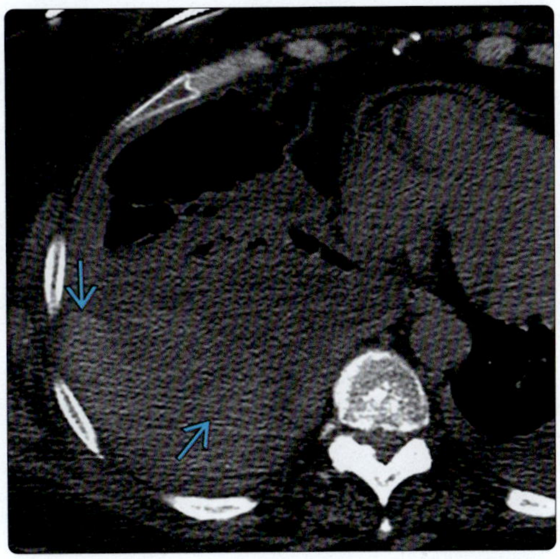

(Left) *Axial CECT of a patient with cirrhosis demonstrates small bilateral pleural effusions that measure fluid density.* **(Right)** *Axial NECT of a patient with metastatic lung cancer obtained after CT-guided biopsy of a right pleural metastasis shows regions of high attenuation in the right pleural space representing hemorrhage. CT can demonstrate higher density components, membranes, and septations in complex &/or loculated fluid.*

Pleural Effusion

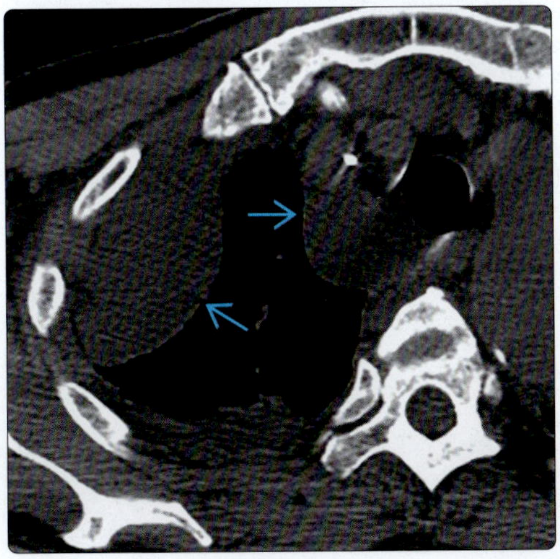

Pleural Effusion

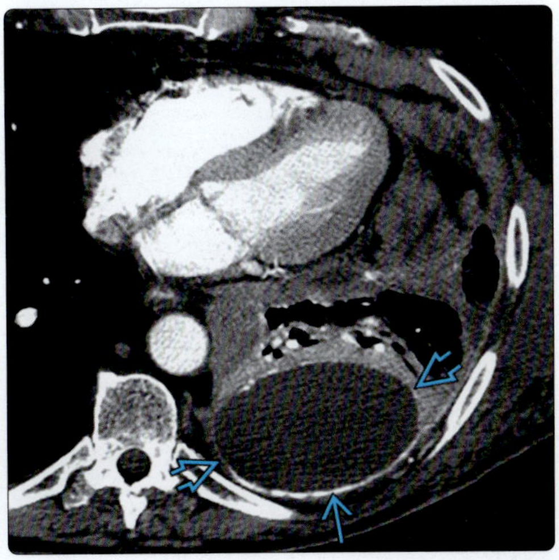

(Left) *Axial NECT of a patient with right lung cancer (not shown) demonstrates a multiloculated right pleural effusion following thoracentesis.* **(Right)** *Axial CECT of a patient with lung cancer shows a loculated left pleural effusion. Note high attenuation along the pleural surface representing the sequela of talc pleurodesis. Pleural fluid collections may become loculated following procedures such as thoracentesis or pleurodesis.*

(Left) *Axial CECT of a patient with right lung cancer demonstrates a large right pleural effusion and extensive pleural thickening in the right hemithorax representing pleural metastatic disease.* **(Right)** *Axial CECT of a patient with malignant pleural mesothelioma demonstrates pleural thickening and nodularity in the left hemithorax. Note the extension along the left interlobar fissure. A loculated left pleural effusion and a free right pleural effusion are present.*

Pleural Thickening

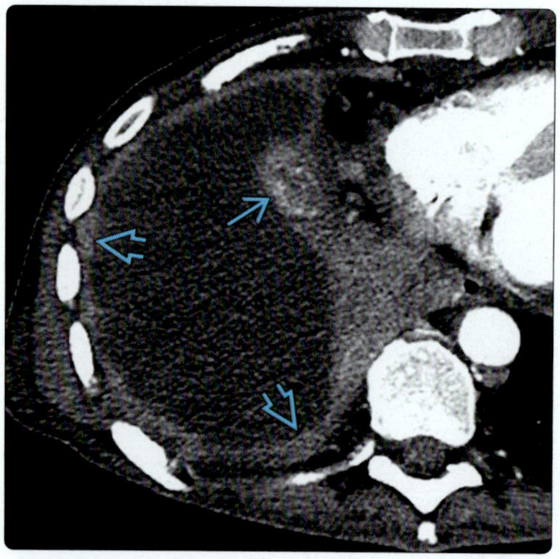

Pleural Thickening

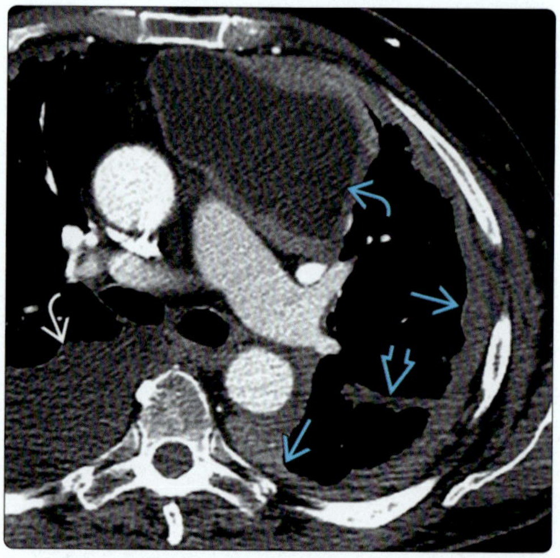

(Left) *Axial CECT of a patient with hemangiopericytoma demonstrates multiple solid pleural nodules and masses in the right hemithorax representing metastatic disease.* **(Right)** *Coronal CECT of a patient with thymoma shows pleural thickening and multiple pleural nodules and masses in the right hemithorax, consistent with metastatic disease. Metastases are the most frequent cause of malignant pleural disease.*

Pleural Nodules/Masses

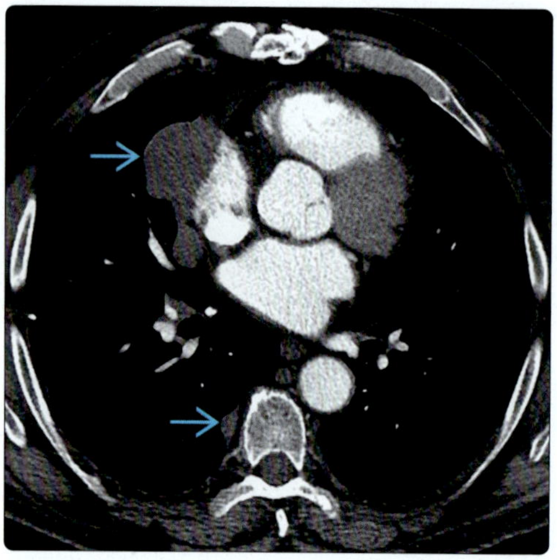

Pleural Nodules/Masses

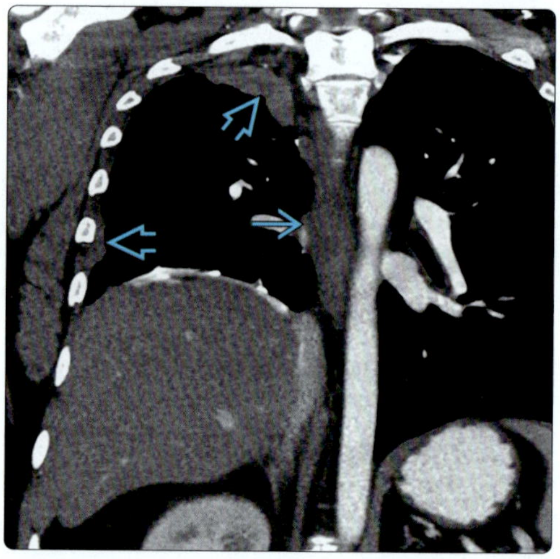

(Left) *Axial CECT of a patient with malignant pleural mesothelioma demonstrates extensive pleural thickening, nodules, and masses in the right hemithorax representing malignancy. Regions of high attenuation represent the sequela of prior talc pleurodesis.* **(Right)** *Axial fused FDG PET/CT of the same patient shows intense FDG uptake within these regions. When pleural thickening is present alongside pleural nodules and masses, malignancy is much more likely than benign disease processes.*

Pleural Nodules/Masses

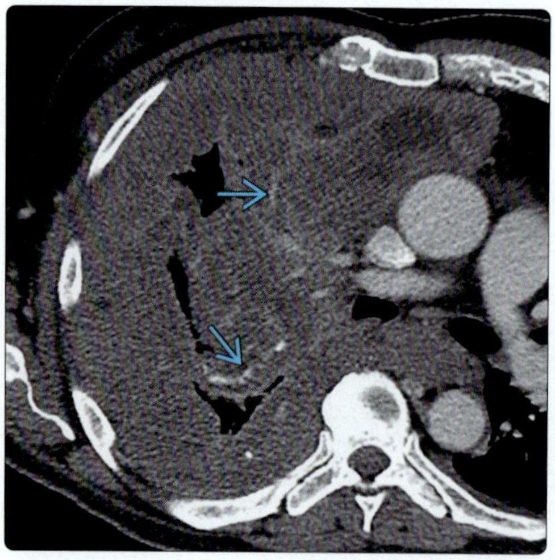

Pleural Nodules/Masses

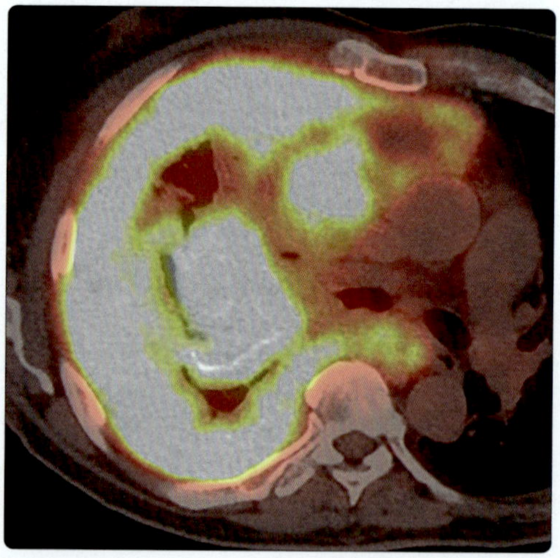

Pleural Calcification

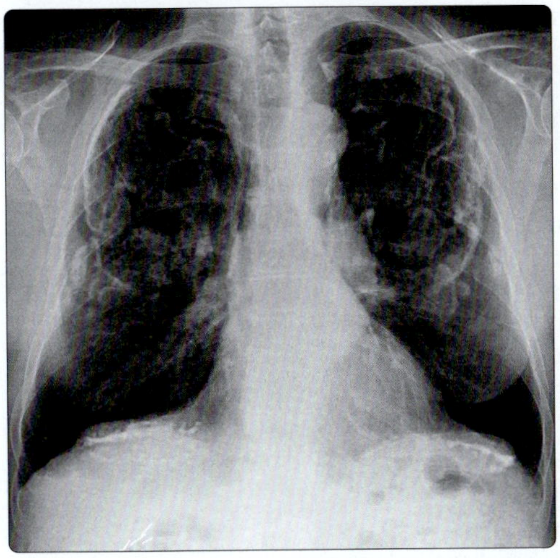

Pleural Calcification

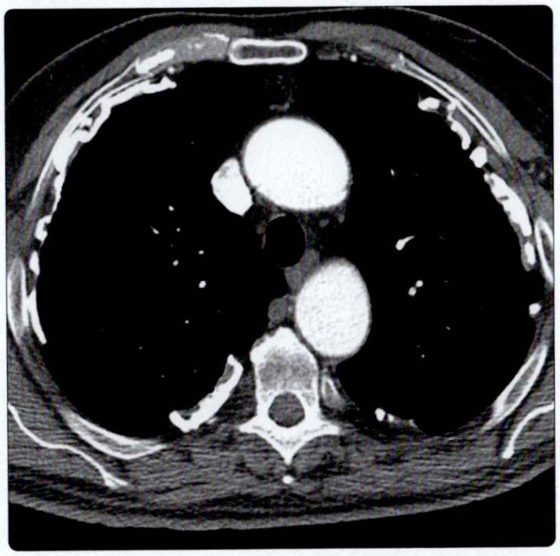

(Left) *PA chest radiograph of a patient employed for many years at a shipyard demonstrates extensive bilateral pleural plaques bilaterally representing asbestos-related pleural disease.* **(Right)** *Axial CECT of the same patient shows extensive calcified pleural plaques bilaterally. Pleural plaques are a localized form of fibrosis involving only the parietal pleura that are histologically compatible with deposition of collagen fibers in patients with prior asbestos exposure.*

Post Surgery

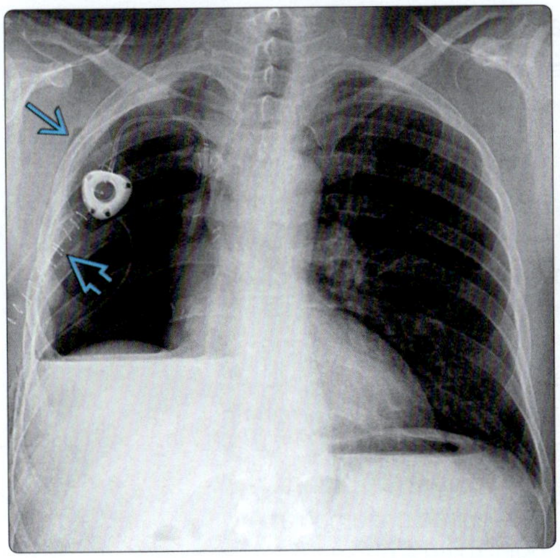

Post Surgery

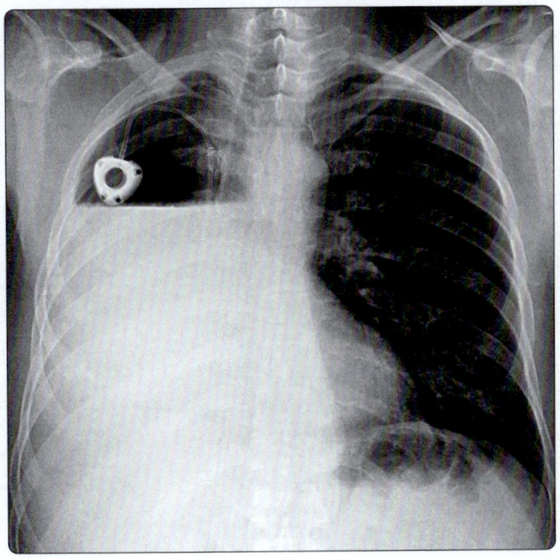

(Left) *PA chest radiograph of a patient following right pneumonectomy for lung cancer demonstrates air and fluid in the right pneumonectomy space. Note the surgical sutures* ➔ *and a small amount of subcutaneous air* ➔ *in the right chest wall.* **(Right)** *PA chest radiograph of the same patient 6 months later shows a decrease in the amount of air and an increase in the amount of fluid in the right pneumonectomy space. A gradual increase in the amount of fluid and decrease in the amount of air typically follows pneumonectomy.*

Bronchopleural Fistula

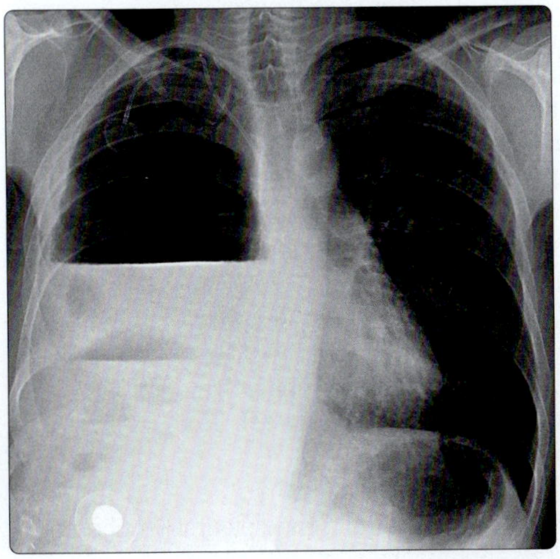

Bronchopleural Fistula

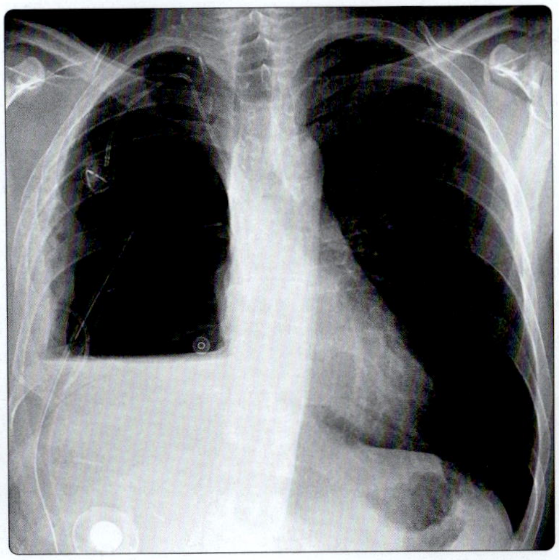

(Left) *PA chest radiograph of a patient following right pneumonectomy for lung cancer demonstrates air and fluid in the pneumonectomy space.* **(Right)** *PA chest radiograph of the same patient obtained 3 months later shows an increase in the amount of air and decrease in the amount of fluid in the pneumonectomy space suggestive of a bronchopleural fistula (BPF). BPF may be suspected when there is persistent air with or without fluid on sequential chest radiographs.*

DIFFERENTIAL DIAGNOSIS

Common

- Congestive Heart Failure
- Parapneumonic Pleural Effusion
- Malignant Pleural Effusion
- Hemothorax
- Pulmonary Embolism
- Connective Tissue Disease

Less Common

- Tuberculosis
- Hepatic Hydrothorax
- Chylothorax

Rare but Important

- Parasitic Infection
- Drug-Induced Pleuritis

ESSENTIAL INFORMATION

Key Differential Diagnosis Issues

- **Terminology**
  - Pleural effusion: Abnormal fluid accumulation within pleural space (dependent position)
  - Subpulmonic effusion: Fluid located between lung base and top of diaphragm
- **Pleural Effusions**
  - Transudative pleural effusion
    - Imbalance of hydrostatic and oncotic forces
      - Protein level < 30 g/L
      - Low specific gravity
    - Congestive heart failure, cirrhosis, hypoalbuminemia
  - Exudative pleural effusion
    - Increase in capillary permeability or decreased lymphatic drainage
      - Protein level > 30g/L
      - Pleural fluid protein level divided by serum protein level > 0.5
    - Infection(parapneumonic, empyema), malignancy, collagen vascular disease, drugs
- **Imaging**
  - Radiography
    - Chest radiography
      - 50 mL: Blunt costophrenic angle on lateral chest radiography
      - 200-300 mL: Blunt costophrenic angle on frontal radiography
      - > 1,000 mL: Contralateral mediastinal shift
      - Meniscus sign: Blunting of lateral costophrenic angles (concave upward slope)
      - Subpulmonic effusion: Lateral peaking of apparently raised hemidiaphragm; increased thickness between stomach gas bubble and lung base
    - Supine chest radiography
      - Decreased sensitivity for fluid
      - Homogeneous opacity in affected side with preservation of bronchovascular markings
      - Loss of sharp silhouette of hemidiaphragm
      - Blunting of costophrenic angle
      - Apical cap sign: Free fluid cap in lung apex
    - Lateral chest radiography
      - Best view to demonstrate small free-flowing pleural effusion
  - CT
    - Differentiation between transudate and exudate often not possible
    - Differentiation of ascites from pleural effusion
      - Diaphragm sign: Fluid between identifiable diaphragm and liver = ascites
      - Displaced-crus sign: Anterior and lateral displacement of crus away from spine = pleural effusion
      - Interface sign: Indistinct interface between pleural effusion and liver = pleural effusion
      - Bare-area sign: Pleural fluid behind liver at level of bare area
  - Ultrasonography
    - Detects small pleural effusions and guides thoracentesis
    - Fibrinous septations are better visualized than on CT

Helpful Clues for Common Diagnoses

- **Congestive Heart Failure**
  - Cardiomegaly, pleural effusions, and widened vascular pedicle
    - Abnormal accumulation of fluid in extravascular compartments
      - Perivascular and peribronchial cuffing
      - Bilateral perihilar opacities often exhibits bat-wing pattern
      - Interlobular septal thickening
    - Pleural effusion
      - Commonly bilateral, larger on right side
      - May be unilateral
- **Parapneumonic Pleural Effusion**
  - Community-acquired pneumonia
    - Develops in 20-60% of patients with acute bacterial pneumonia
    - Poses increased relative risk of mortality
      - Unilateral effusions (3.4x higher)
      - Bilateral effusions (7.0x higher)
    - < 10% progress to empyema
      - CT findings (e.g., loculation or air-fluid levels) may predict need for chest tube insertion
- **Malignant Pleural Effusion**
  - 10% of malignant pleural effusions are massive
    - 70% of massive pleural effusions are malignant
  - Pleural thickening/nodularity
    - Primary or secondary: Lung (36%), breast (25%), lymphoma (10%), ovary (5%)
    - Invasive thymoma may present with pleural metastases (i.e., drop metastases)
  - Diffuse pleural thickening
    - Malignant pleural mesothelioma
    - Metastatic adenocarcinoma and pleural lymphoma can mimic appearance of mesothelioma
  - CECT
    - Most sensitive modality
    - Contrast increases conspicuity of pleural thickening/nodularity

- **Hemothorax**
  - Diverse etiology (e.g., trauma, aortic rupture, iatrogenic, coagulopathy)
  - Fluid often hyperdense on CT (35-70 HU)
- **Pulmonary Embolism**
  - Pleural effusion in 30-50% of cases
    - Unilateral, small amount, exudative
    - More prevalent with lung infarct
- **Connective Tissue Disease**
  - **Systemic Lupus Erythematosus**
    - Commonly bilateral, small, exudative effusions; frequently associated with pericardial effusion
      - LE cells common in pleural fluid
      - Neutrophil with single reddish amorphous cytoplasmic inclusion representing damaged nucleus of another damaged leukocyte, which has been phagocytized
    - Primarily in reproductive-aged women
  - **Rheumatoid Arthritis**
    - Commonly unilateral and small associated with pericardial effusion and pleural thickening
    - Primarily in middle-aged men

Helpful Clues for Less Common Diagnoses

- **Tuberculosis**
  - Most common extrapulmonary manifestation of *Mycobacterium tuberculosis* infection
    - Adolescents and young adults
      - Delayed hypersensitivity
      - More common in immunocompromised and HIV-positive patients
    - Rare in absence of demonstrable pulmonary disease
      - ~ 80% of patients have concomitant pulmonary tuberculosis
      - Subpleural caseous focus: Rupture into pleural space
      - Ipsilateral pleural effusion
- **Hepatic Hydrothorax**
  - Recurrent moderate-to-large effusion in setting of cirrhosis and ascites, from direct diaphragmatic defects, in absence of other cause of pleural effusions; right > left
  - Fluid attenuation HU on CT
- **Chylothorax**
  - Diverse etiology (e.g., malignancy, iatrogenic, trauma, lymphangioleiomyomatosis)
  - Despite lipid content appears as fluid attenuation on CT
  - Diagnosis relies on pleural fluid sampling

Helpful Clues for Rare Diagnoses

- **Parasitic Infection**
  - Paragonimiasis
    - Associated with consumption of raw crawfish
    - Eosinophilia (peripheral and in pleural fluid)
    - Tracts from direct invasion across diaphragm into pleural space and lung parenchyma
- **Drug-Induced Pleuritis**
  - Small percentage of all pleural effusions
  - Parenchymal disease is typically absent
  - Lupus-like syndrome
    - Associated with many different drugs (e.g., hydralazine, procainamide, isoniazid, phenytoin, and chlorpromazine)

SELECTED REFERENCES

1. Porcel JM: Chest imaging for the diagnosis of complicated parapneumonic effusions. Curr Opin Pulm Med. 24(4):398-402, 2018
2. Hallifax RJ et al: State-of-the-art: radiological investigation of pleural disease. Respir Med. 124:88-99, 2017

Congestive Heart Failure

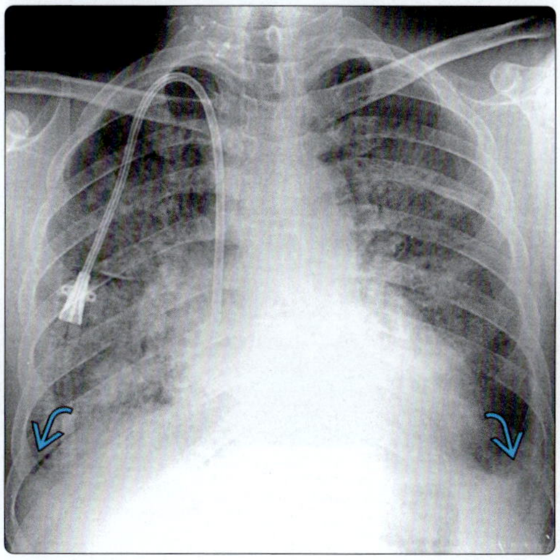

Parapneumonic Pleural Effusion

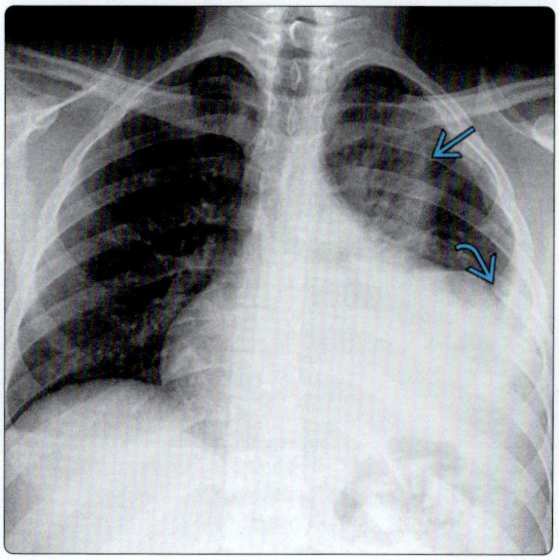

(Left) *PA chest radiograph of a patient with heart failure shows bilateral perihilar heterogeneous opacities, cardiomegaly, and blunting of the costophrenic angles bilaterally from small pleural effusions.* **(Right)** *PA chest radiograph of a patient with pneumonia and parapneumonic effusion shows left upper lobe consolidation and a moderate ipsilateral pleural effusion with blunting of the costophrenic angle and meniscus sign.*

(Left) *PA chest radiograph of a patient with lung cancer shows a spiculated left hilar mass with blunting of the ipsilateral costophrenic angle and meniscus sign, which indicates pleural effusion. Pleural effusions in the setting of cancer should always be surveilled for the possibility of malignant pleural effusion.* **(Right)** *PA chest radiograph of a patient with a large right malignant pleural effusion shows opacification of the right hemithorax secondary due to a large pleural effusion with leftward cardiomediastinal shift.*

Malignant Pleural Effusion

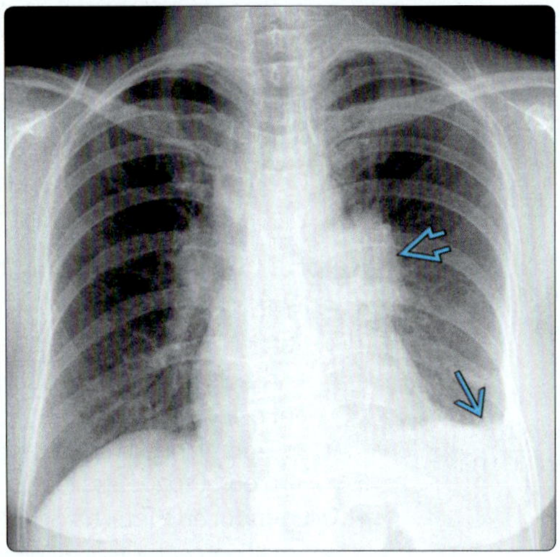

Malignant Pleural Effusion

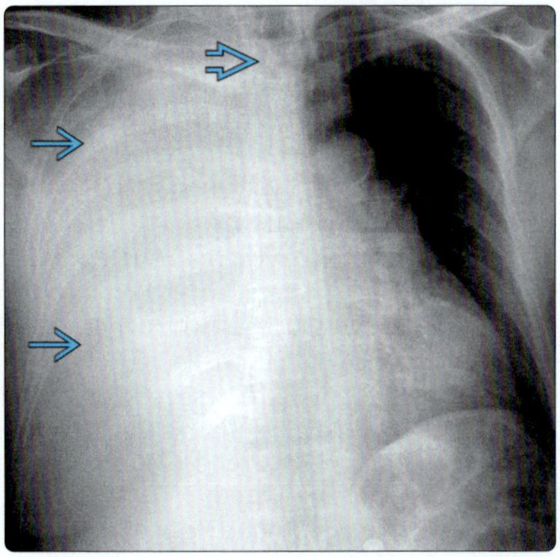

(Left) *AP chest radiograph of a patient with iatrogenic hemothorax from failed insertion of a left IJ port shows partial opacification of the left hemithorax. Note that on decubitus chest radiography, free-flowing effusion may not exhibit the classic meniscus sign as pleural fluid redistributes.* **(Right)** *Axial chest CECT of the same patient shows a large left pleural effusion, which exhibits heterogeneous density with higher dependent components related to clot.*

Hemothorax

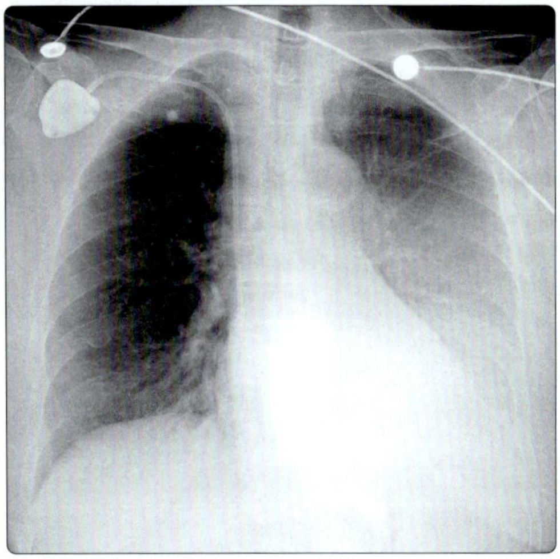

Hemothorax

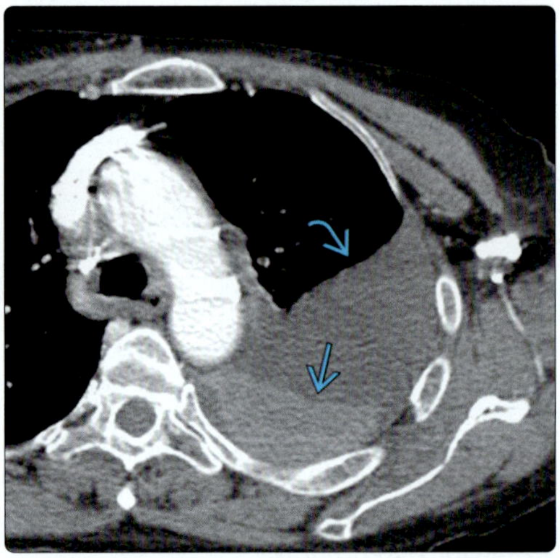

(Left) *PA chest radiograph of a patient with acute pulmonary thromboembolic disease shows scattered subsegmental atelectasis bilaterally. Note blunting of both costophrenic angles from associated pleural effusions.* **(Right)** *Axial chest CECT of the same patient shows multiple and bilateral pulmonary arterial filling defects with moderate dependent and free-flowing pleural effusions. While nonspecific, pleural effusions occur very commonly in the setting of acute thromboembolic disease.*

Pulmonary Embolism

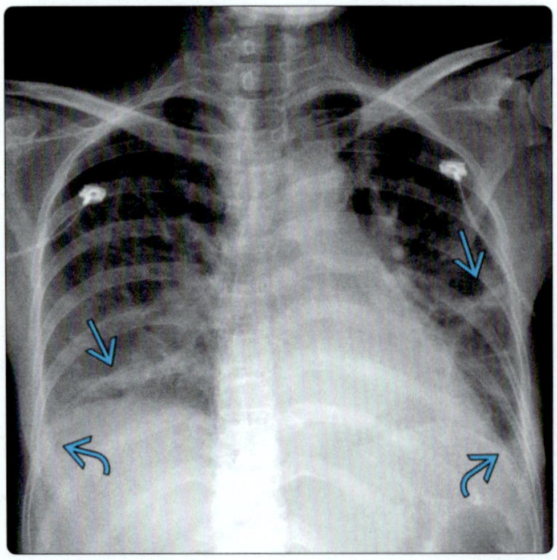

Pulmonary Embolism

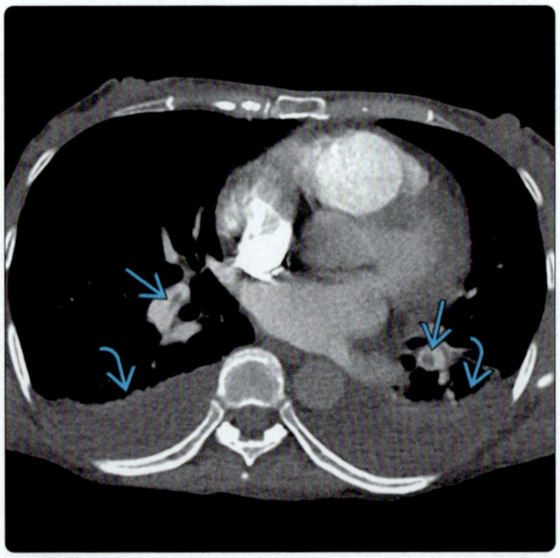

Connective Tissue Disease

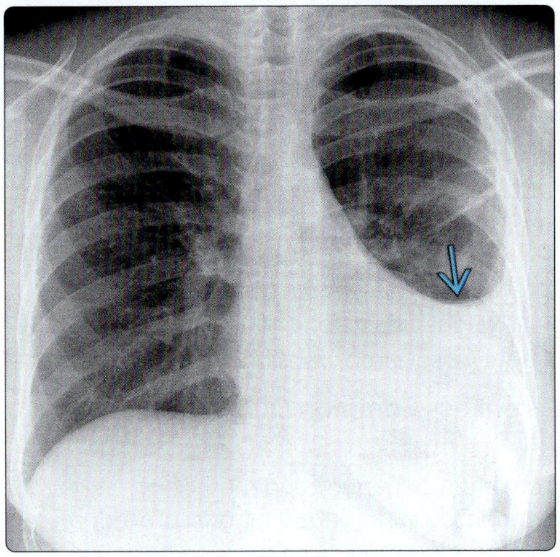

Connective Tissue Disease

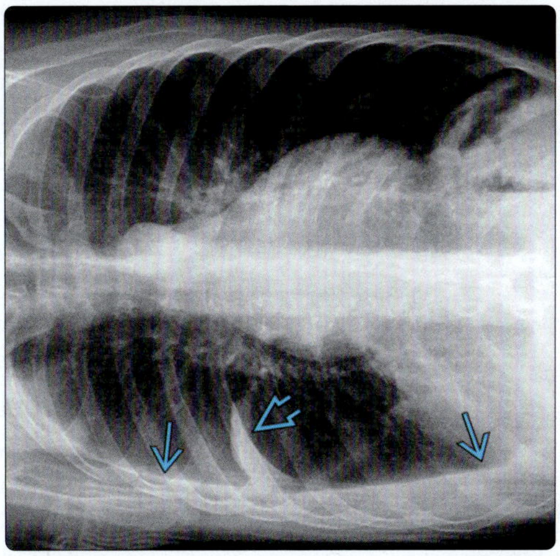

***(Left)** PA chest radiograph of a patient with systemic lupus erythematosus shows a well-defined meniscus sign ➡ from a left moderate pleural effusion. **(Right)** Right decubitus chest radiograph of a patient with connective tissue disease shows layering pleural fluid in the dependent hemithorax ➡ and along the minor fissure ➡. Decubitus radiographs are helpful to confirm small amounts of fluid when there is blunting of the costophrenic angle on erect views.*

Tuberculosis

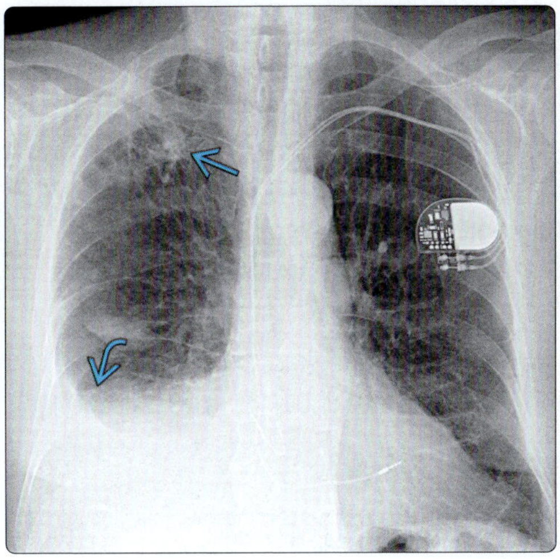

Tuberculosis

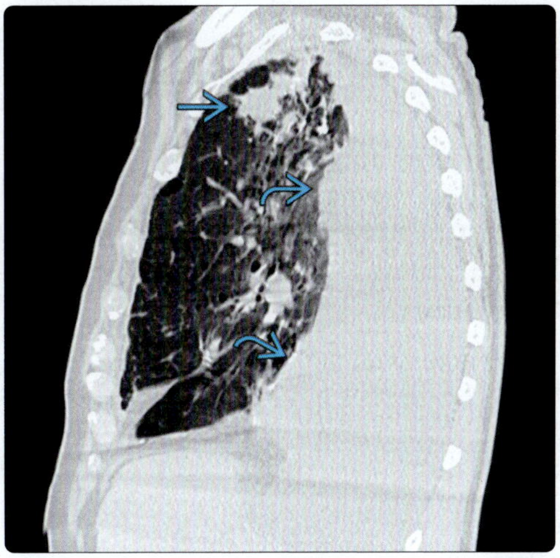

***(Left)** AP chest radiograph of a patient with pulmonary and pleural tuberculosis shows a moderate right pleural effusion ➡ and heterogeneous opacities in the right lung apex ➡. **(Right)** Sagittal NECT of the same patient shows a moderate-to-large pleural effusion ➡ with spiculated solid nodules in the right lung apex ➡. The nodules were not initially thought to represent tuberculosis, as no cavitation or tree-in-bud nodules were present. Diagnosis was achieved on pleural effusion sampling.*

Hepatic Hydrothorax

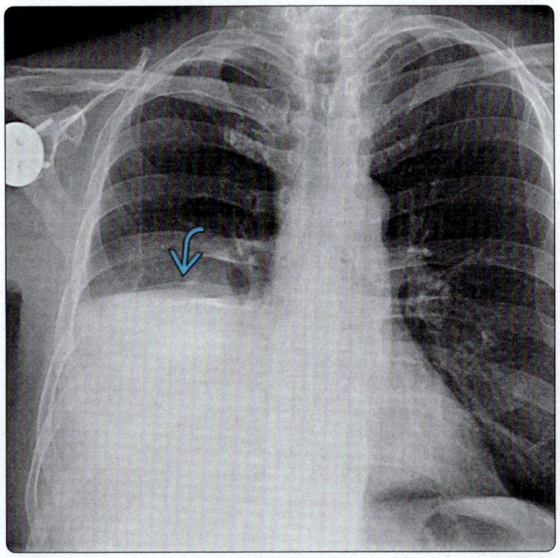

Hepatic Hydrothorax

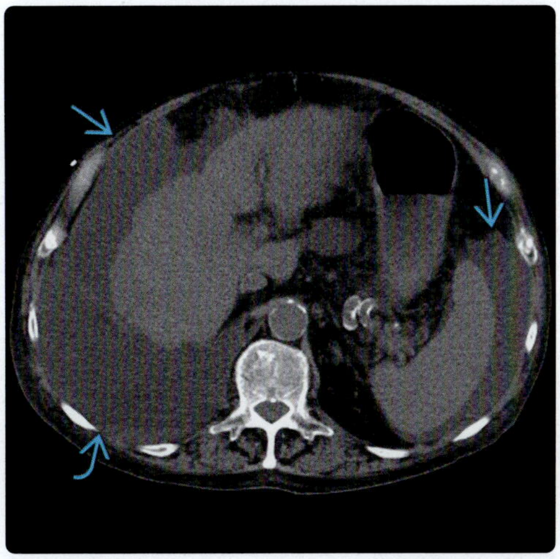

***(Left)** PA chest radiograph of a patient with cirrhosis and hepatic hydrothorax shows a moderate-to-large right pleural effusion ➡. **(Right)** Axial NECT of the same patient shows a small and nodular appearance of the liver, consistent with cirrhosis. Note abdominal ascites ➡ and large right pleural effusion ➡. Hepatic hydrothorax is often diagnosed after other causes of pleural effusion have been excluded in a patient with chronic liver disease and ascites.*

Loculated Pleural Effusion

DIFFERENTIAL DIAGNOSIS

Common

- Empyema
  - Tuberculous
  - Bacterial
- Malignant Pleural Effusion
- Pleural Pseudotumor

Less Common

- Hemothorax
- Postsurgical

Rare but Important

- Asbestos-Related Pleural Disease
- Pulmonary Embolism

ESSENTIAL INFORMATION

Key Differential Diagnosis Issues

- **Imaging**
  - Extrapulmonary disease
    - Lenticular shape with smooth margins, scalloped borders, and homogeneous attenuation
      - Obtuse angle with chest wall and tapered margin
      - Incomplete border sign
    - Split pleura sign: Fluid between enhancing thickened pleural layers
  - Ultrasonography: Good depiction of pleural septa and thickening

Helpful Clues for Common Diagnoses

- **Empyema**
  - Complication of ~ 10% of bacterial pneumonias
    - Fibrin strands within pleural exudate create loculations in nondependent location
  - Tuberculous
    - Rupture of postprimary tuberculosis into pleura
    - Empyema necessitatis: Rupture of tuberculous empyema through parietal pleura forms subcutaneous abscess
- **Malignant Pleural Effusion**
  - Primary or secondary cancer (e.g., lung cancer, breast cancer, and lymphoma)
    - Circumferential pleural thickening and mediastinal pleural involvement: Mesothelioma and metastatic adenocarcinoma
    - Associated with lung mass or nodule, liver metastasis, subdiaphragmatic tumor
- **Pleural Pseudotumor**
  - Also known as vanishing tumor or phantom tumor
  - Localized transudative interlobar fluid collection
  - Predominantly right-sided along minor fissure
  - Most commonly associated with congestive heart failure

Helpful Clues for Less Common Diagnoses

- **Hemothorax**
  - Sequela from blunt or penetrating thoracic or thoracoabdominal trauma, interventional procedures, bleeding diathesis, pulmonary infarct, and malignancy
  - May exhibit high attenuation on CT but can be fluid attenuation as it becomes chronic; can result in pleural calcification and fibrothorax
- **Postsurgical**
  - Can occur with any thoracic surgery violating pleura (common after coronary artery bypass grafting)
  - Commonly associated with rounded atelectasis

Helpful Clues for Rare Diagnoses

- **Asbestos-Related Pleural Disease**
  - Loculated pleural fluid; coexists with classic asbestos-related pleural plaques or rounded atelectasis
- **Pulmonary Embolism**
  - Late complication of pulmonary embolism
  - Pulmonary infarcts (often exhibiting intrinsic lucency)

SELECTED REFERENCES

1. Porcel JM: Chest imaging for the diagnosis of complicated parapneumonic effusions. Curr Opin Pulm Med. 24(4):398-402, 2018
2. Hallifax RJ et al: State-of-the-art: fadiological investigation of pleural disease. Respir Med. 124:88-99, 2017

Empyema

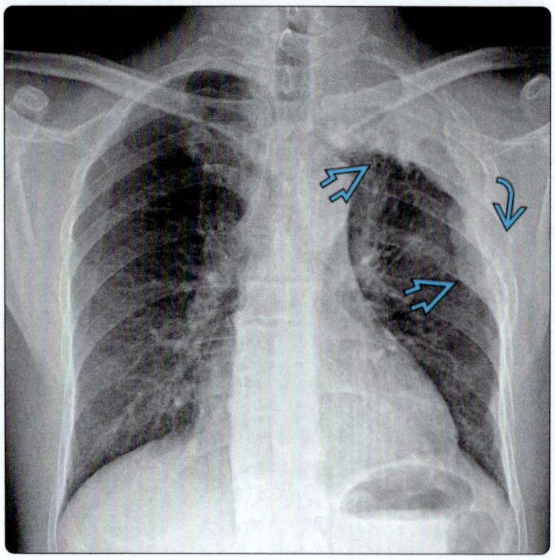

Empyema

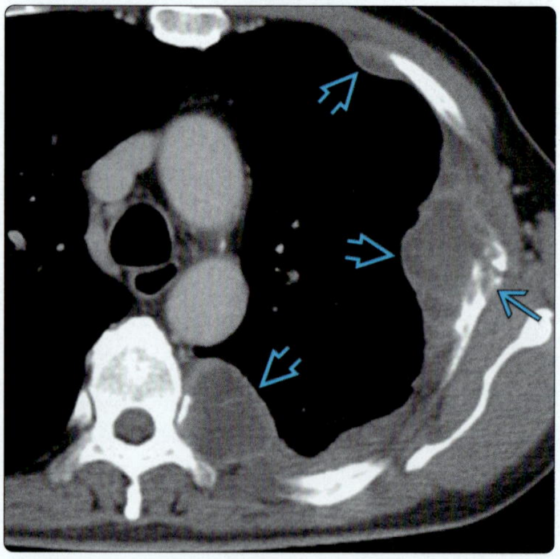

***(Left)** PA chest radiograph of a patient with tuberculous empyema shows a loculated pleural effusion ➡ in the upper left hemithorax. Note adjacent rib destruction ➡. **(Right)** Axial CECT of the same patient shows multiple rim-enhancing loculated pleural collections ➡ with adjacent rib destruction ➡, consistent with empyema necessitatis. Pleural tuberculosis is a common site of extrapulmonary tuberculous involvement. Pulmonary parenchymal and pleural tuberculosis often coexist.*

Connective Tissue Diseases

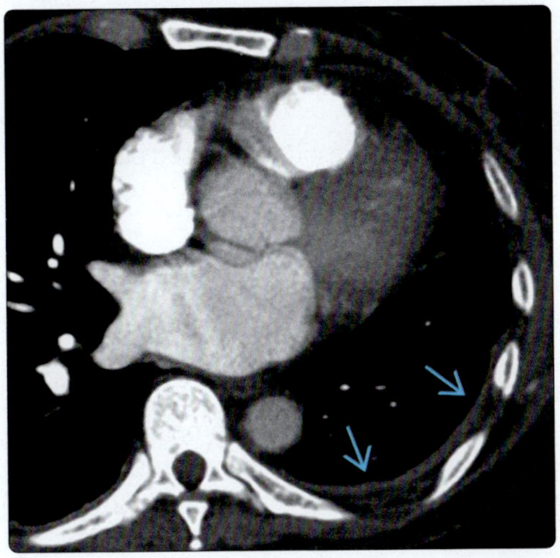

Connective Tissue Diseases

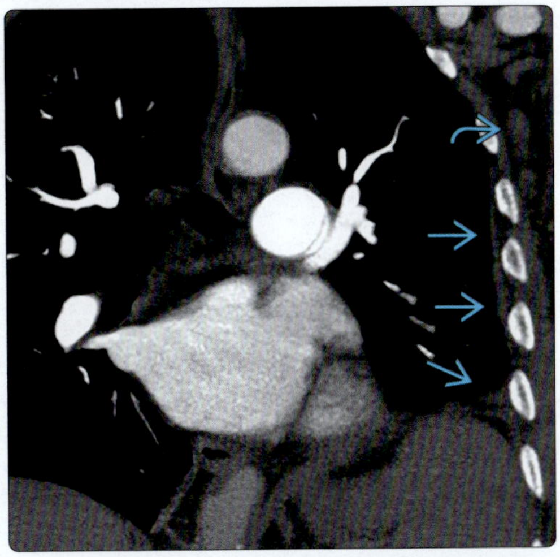

(Left) *Axial CECT of a patient with systemic lupus erythematosus and pleuritis shows smooth pleural thickening .* **(Right)** *Coronal CECT of the same patient shows left pleural thickening . Note left axillary lymphadenopathy . Pleural effusion and thickening are common manifestations of autoimmune diseases in the thorax and are often associated with reactive lymphadenopathy which may include mediastinal, hilar, axillary, and supraclavicular stations.*

Pleurodesis

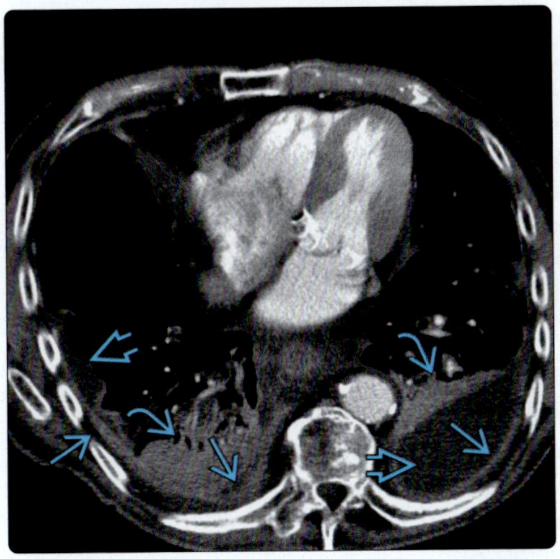

Malignant Pleural Mesothelioma

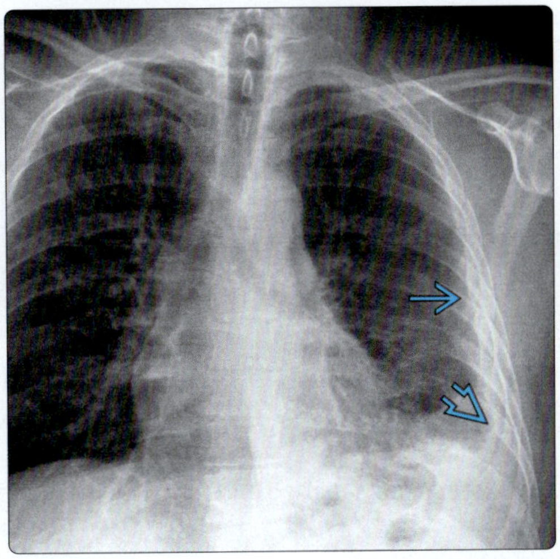

(Left) *Axial CECT of a patient who underwent talc pleurodesis for chronic pleural effusions from yellow nail syndrome shows bilateral pleural thickening and small effusions . Chronic lower lobe atelectasis is present bilaterally.* **(Right)** *Frontal chest radiograph of a 66-year-old man with history of exposure to asbestos and malignant pleural mesothelioma shows left pleural thickening with lung encroachment and pleural effusion .*

Malignant Pleural Mesothelioma

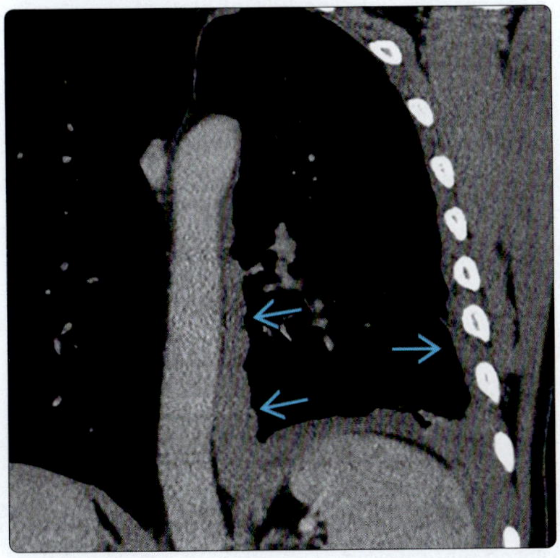

Drug Reaction

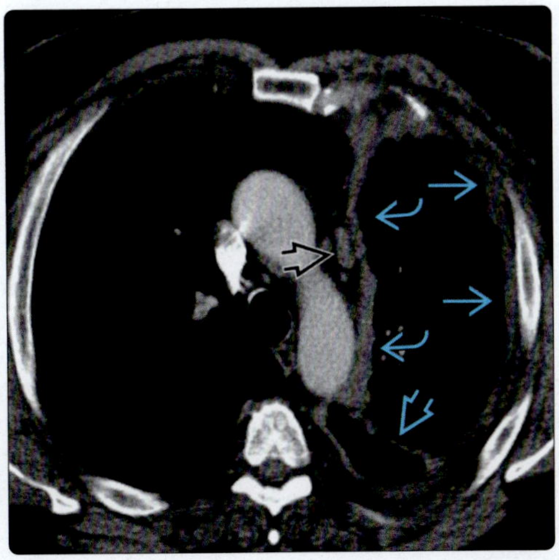

(Left) *Coronal CT of the same patient shows left pleural thickening . Mesothelioma is often related to asbestos, but an increasing number of cases not associated with asbestos exposure have been identified. Thus it is common to see coexisting calcified pleural plaques.* **(Right)** *Axial CECT of a patient with pleural drug reaction shows circumferential left pleural thickening and nodularity . Note involvement of mediastinal pleura and interlobar fissure . Mediastinal lymphadenopathy is also present .*

DIFFERENTIAL DIAGNOSIS

Common

- Pleural Pseudotumor
- Diffuse Pleural Thickening
- Empyema
- Rounded Atelectasis
- Pleural Plaque

Less Common

- Pleural Metastasis
- Pleurodesis

Rare but Important

- Malignant Pleural Mesothelioma
- Solitary Fibrous Tumor of Pleura
- Thoracic Splenosis
- Primary Lymphoma

ESSENTIAL INFORMATION

Key Differential Diagnosis Issues

- Split pleura sign: Fluid between thickened and enhancing visceral and pleural layers; often seen in empyema
- Findings suggestive of malignant pleural disease: Nodular and circumferential thickening
- Metastatic disease to pleura represents 90% of pleural malignancies

Helpful Clues for Common Diagnoses

- **Pleural Pseudotumor**
  - Loculated pleural fluid in interlobar fissure
  - History of congestive heart failure, hypoalbuminemia, cirrhosis, and renal insufficiency
  - Resolves after initiation of therapy
  - CT
    - Fluid with lenticular or biconvex shape; tapering ends along course of interlobar fissures
    - Associated with free pleural effusion
- **Diffuse Pleural Thickening**
  - Extensive inflammation of visceral pleura with secondary thickening of parietal pleura
  - Asbestos exposure, prior infection or inflammation, hemothorax, rheumatoid arthritis
    - Unilateral: Infection; bilateral: Asbestos exposure
  - CT
    - Affects posterolateral pleural cavity; obliteration of costophrenic sulci
    - Extends more than 8 cm in craniocaudal direction, more than 5 cm in cross section
    - Smooth thickening of pleura, foci of calcification in 15-20%
    - Increase in extrapleural fat thickness
    - Associated with parenchymal bands and rounded atelectasis
- **Empyema**
  - Pus in pleural space; most often from pneumonia/pulmonary abscess
  - CT
    - Loculated pleural effusion, lenticular or oblong shape
    - Nondependent location
    - Split pleura sign
    - Increase in attenuation of extrapleural fat
    - Displacement of adjacent lung and airways from pleura
- **Rounded Atelectasis**
  - Peripheral atelectatic lung adjacent to area of pleural thickening
  - Commonly associated with asbestos-related pleural disease
  - More common in men than women
  - 2.5-8 cm in size; usually located in lower lobes
  - CT
    - Round, lentiform, or irregular shape with air bronchograms
    - Subpleural location
    - Comet tail sign: Folded vessels and bronchi
    - Thickening of adjacent pleura; pleural effusion
- **Pleural Plaque**
  - Most common manifestation of asbestos exposure
    - Asbestos fibers migrate via lymphatic vessels to pleural space
  - Not associated with symptoms or impairment of lung function
  - CT
    - Focal parietal pleural thickening or nodularity ± calcification
    - Separate from extrapleural fat
    - Bilateral; may be symmetric
    - Posterolateral and diaphragmatic preponderance; sparing of apices and costophrenic angles
    - Associated lung abnormalities: Interstitial lines radiating from plaques (hairy plaques)

Helpful Clues for Less Common Diagnoses

- **Pleural Metastasis**
  - Represents 90% of malignant pleural disease
  - Affects both visceral and parietal pleura
  - Adenocarcinoma histology is most likely to produce pleural metastasis
    - Most common primary malignancies: Lung, breast, and ovarian carcinomas, and lymphoma
      - Lung cancer accounts for 40% of pleural metastases
  - Imaging
    - Most common finding is pleural effusion
    - CT
      - Irregular pleural thickening, nodules &/or masses ± enhancement
      - Rib destruction, chest wall invasion
- **Pleurodesis**
  - Iatrogenic fusion of visceral and parietal pleura; talc most often used
  - Treatment for recurrent pleural effusion (most often malignant etiology)
  - Imaging
    - CT: High attenuation in regions of treatment
      - Linear or nodular pleural thickening
      - Loculated pleural fluid
    - FDG PET/CT: Increased FDG uptake that can persist for years due to chronic inflammatory changes

Helpful Clues for Rare Diagnoses

- **Malignant Pleural Mesothelioma**
  - Strongly associated with prior asbestos exposure; risk increases with duration and intensity of exposure
  - Latency: 20-50 years
  - More common in men than in women, ratio of 4:1
  - Histologic types
    - Epithelioid: 55-65%
    - Sarcomatoid represents 10-15% and biphasic 20-35%
    - Biphasic: Includes epithelioid and sarcomatoid elements; 20-35%
  - Imaging
    - CT
      - Extensive circumferential thickening of pleura, including fissures
      - Encasement of lung: Rind-like appearance
      - Involvement of mediastinal pleura
      - Pleural thickening > 1 cm ± nodularity
      - Extension into chest wall, diaphragm, pericardium
      - Loculated or free pleural effusion
    - MR
      - Evaluation for invasion of endothoracic fascia and diaphragm
      - T1WI and T2WI: Iso- to moderately hyperintense
      - T1 C+: Enhancement
- **Solitary Fibrous Tumor of Pleura**
  - Occurs equally in men and women (60-70 years)
  - Arises from visceral pleural in 65-80%, from parietal pleura in 20-25%
    - Typically occurs in in middle or lower hemithorax
  - Benign or malignant
    - Differentiation primarily based on pathology findings
    - Rib erosion and extension into chest wall suggests malignant neoplasm
  - High incidence of local recurrence after resection
  - Symptoms
    - Symptomatic hypoglycemia in 5%; due to insulin-like growth factor
    - Hypertrophic osteoarthropathy in 3%
  - CT
    - Soft tissue mass
    - Obtuse or acute angles with chest wall depending on size and location
    - Enhancement varies with size
      - Small lesions: Homogeneous enhancement
      - Large lesions: Greater likelihood of heterogeneous enhancement due to necrosis, hemorrhage
- **Thoracic Splenosis**
  - Associated with diaphragmatic and splenic injury
  - Seeding of damage splenic tissue into pleural cavity
  - Males more frequently affected than females; 3-45 years of age
  - Consider if solitary or multiple pleural nodules + remote splenic trauma
  - Imaging
    - CT
      - Multiple pleural nodules up to 3 cm; density and enhancement similar to normal spleen
      - Absent spleen; splenules in left upper quadrant
    - Technetium 99m (99mTC)-sulfur colloid, indium 111-labeled platelets, or 99mTC-tagged heat-damaged red blood cells for confirmation
- **Primary Lymphoma**
  - Large B-cell lymphoma
  - Associated with human herpes virus 8 (HHV-8)/Kaposi sarcoma virus
  - Immunocompromised: HIV+, elderly, post transplant
  - Pyothorax-associated lymphoma (PAL)
    - Rare aggressive B-cell lymphoma presents in patients with history of chronic pyothorax
  - CT
    - Pleural nodule or mass
    - Unilateral large pleural effusion with pleural thickening
    - No lymphadenopathy, splenomegaly, or hepatomegaly
    - PAL: Pleural mass with invasion of chest wall, lung, &/or mediastinum

Pleural Pseudotumor

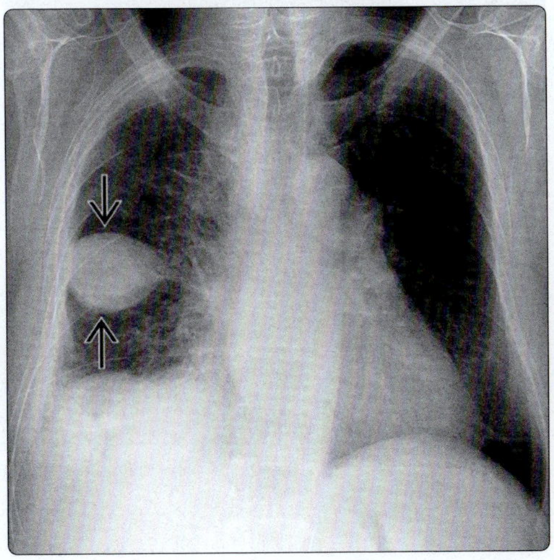

Pleural Pseudotumor

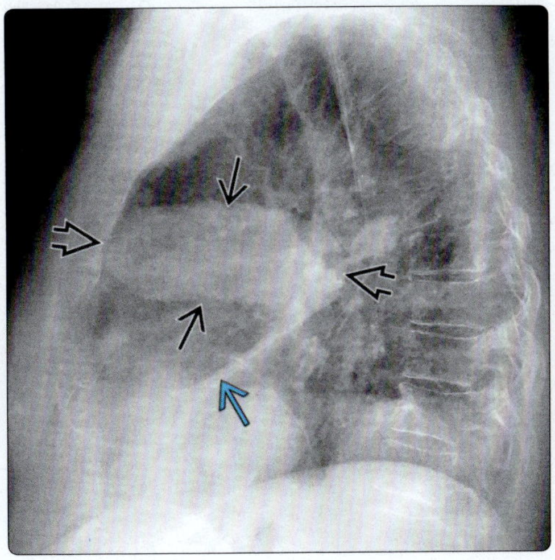

(Left) *PA chest radiograph of a 62-year-old woman with breast cancer and congestive heart failure shows an ovoid mass ➔ along the the minor fissure.* **(Right)** *Lateral radiograph of the same patient confirms that the mass is located within the minor fissure ➔ and has tapered anterior and posterior margins ➔ consistent with pleural pseudotumor, an entity associated with transudative effusion, especially congestive heart failure. Note also the presence of fluid along the major fissure ➔.*

(Left) *Axial CECT of a 51-year-old man with empyema shows a loculated pleural fluid collection. Both layers of the pleura show enhancement and come together at the margins of the collection, confirming the split pleura sign.* **(Right)** *Axial CECT of a 63-year-old woman shows an ovoid mass in the right lower lobe with broad-based attachment to calcified pleural thickening. Vessels and bronchi entering the mass are folded, representing the so-called "comet tail" sign characteristic of rounded atelectasis.*

Empyema

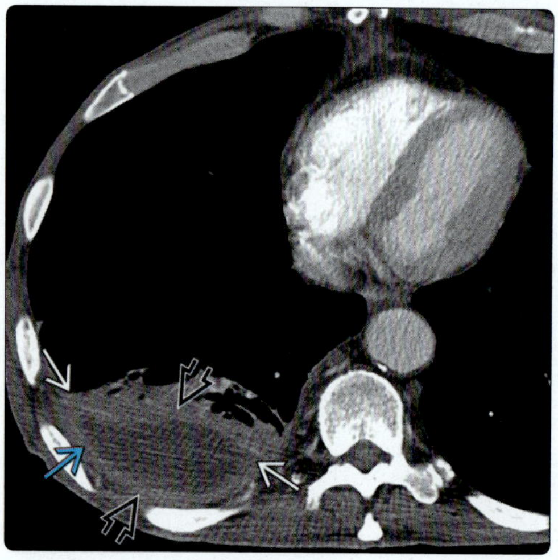

Rounded Atelectasis

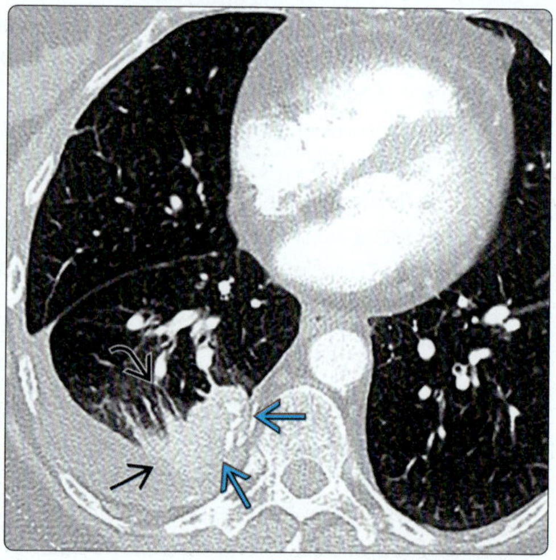

(Left) *Axial NECT of a 63-year-old man with history of asbestos exposure shows calcified and noncalcified pleural plaques in the inferior aspect of both hemithoraces. Note the presence of pleural plaques along the diaphragmatic pleura, a characteristic finding in asbestos-related pleural disease.* **(Right)** *Axial CECT of a 57-year-old woman with history of melanoma shows pleural nodules extending into the left major fissure consistent with metastases, the most common type of pleural malignancy.*

Pleural Plaque

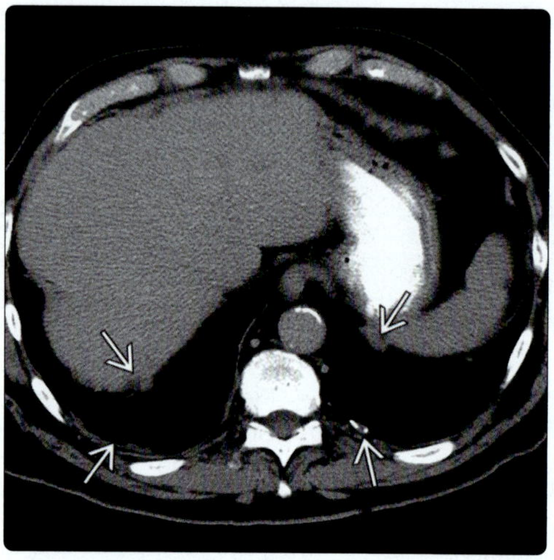

Pleural Metastasis

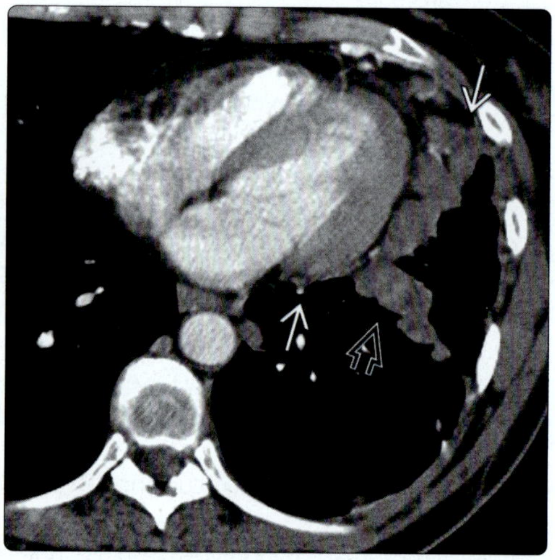

(Left) *Axial NECT of a 57-year-old woman treated with pleurodesis for recurrent right pleural effusion demonstrates high-attenuation material within the pleural space consistent with talc deposits.* **(Right)** *Fused axial FDG PET/CT of the same patient shows focal regions of increased FDG uptake corresponding to the talc deposits. Inflammatory response to talc can persist for years and result in misinterpretation on FDG PET/CT.*

Pleurodesis

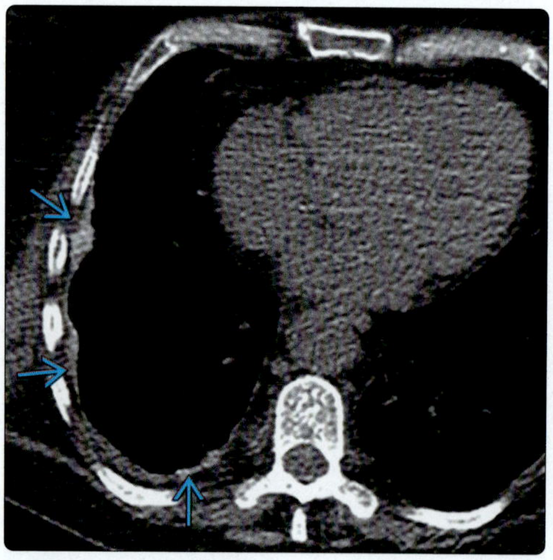

Pleurodesis

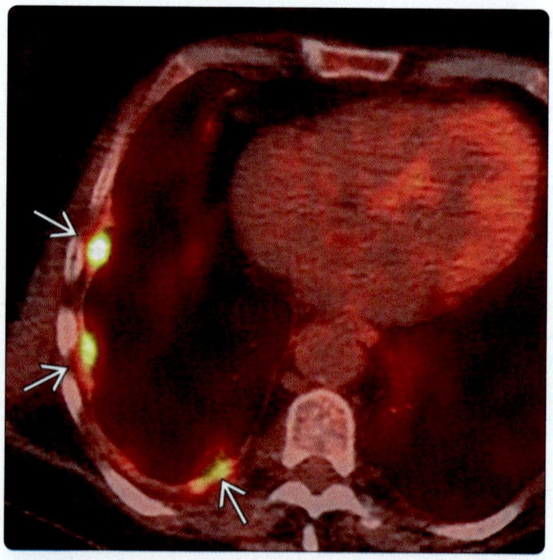

Malignant Pleural Mesothelioma

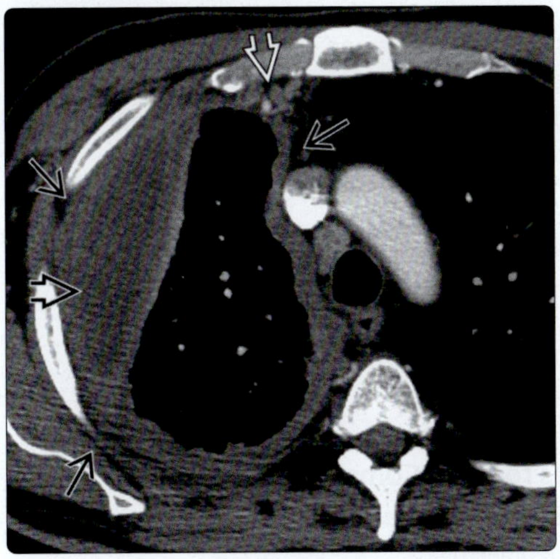

Malignant Pleural Mesothelioma

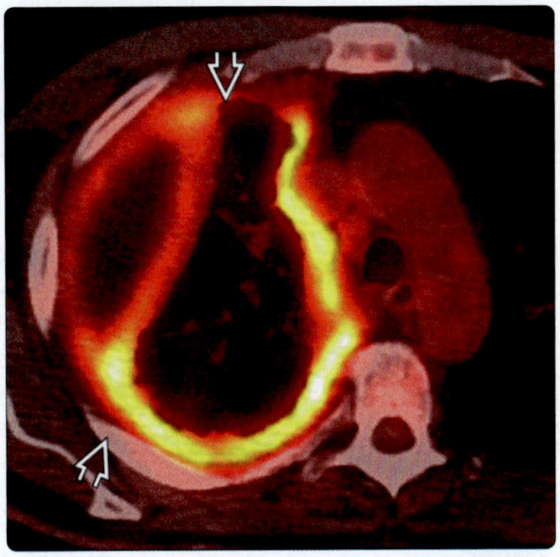

(Left) *Axial CECT of a 69-year-old man with malignant pleural mesothelioma shows a typical appearance of unilateral and circumferential pleural thickening* ⇨ *associated with effusion* ⇨ *and internal mammary lymphadenopathy* ➡*.* **(Right)** *Fused axial FDG PET/CT of the same patient shows increased FDG uptake within the tumor* ➡*. FDG PET/CT is useful in differentiating between benign and malignant causes of pleural thickening in patients with asbestos exposure.*

Solitary Fibrous Tumor of Pleura

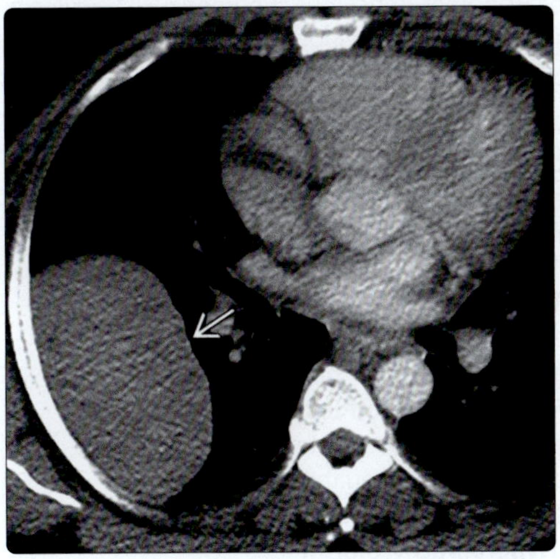

Thoracic Splenosis

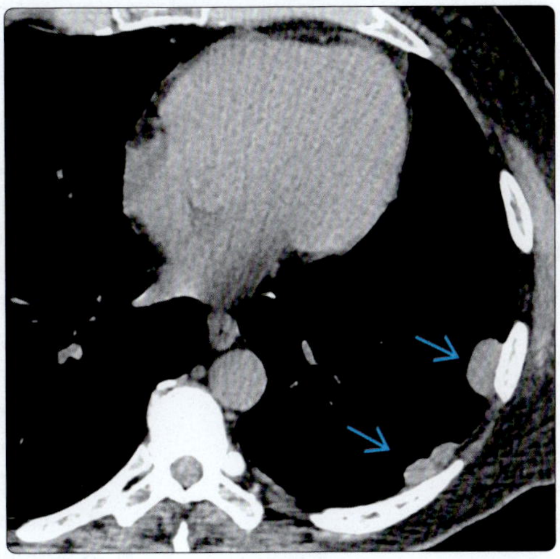

(Left) *Axial CECT of a 42-year-old woman with biopsy-proven solitary fibrous tumor of the pleura shows a homogenous oval mass* ➡*. The margins of the mass with the chest wall are obtuse, which is suggestive of pleural mass.* **(Right)** *Axial CECT of a 37-year-old patient demonstrates several enhancing pleural nodules* ⇨*. Biopsy showed splenic tissue. The patient had a history of splenic and diaphragmatic injury 5 years ago. The diagnosis of splenosis is difficult and requires a detailed clinical history.*

Primary Lymphoma

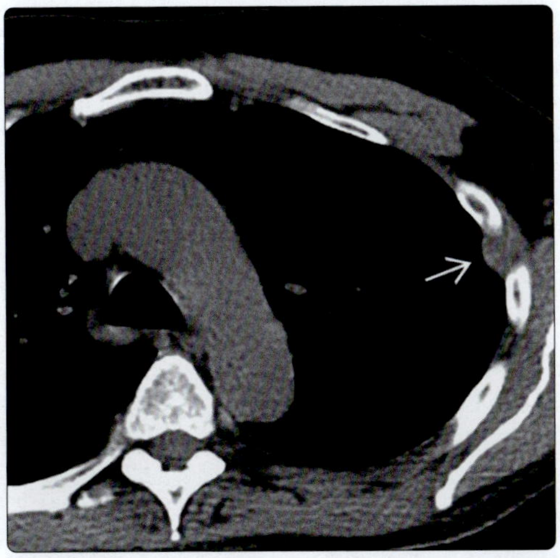

Primary Lymphoma

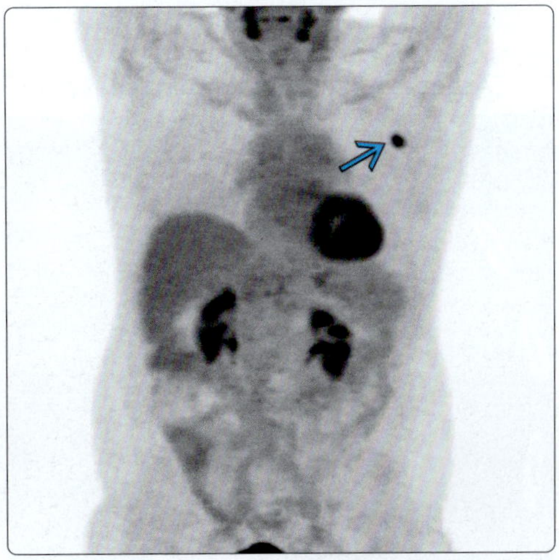

(Left) *Axial NECT of an 84-year-old man shows a small pleural nodule in the lateral aspect of the left hemithorax* ➡*. Biopsy demonstrated B-cell lymphoma.* **(Right)** *Coronal FDG PET of the same patient shows focal activity within the pleural nodule* ⇨*. There was no evidence of lymphadenopathy, splenomegaly, or hepatomegaly. Primary pleural lymphoma is uncommon and affects HIV(+), elderly, and posttransplant patients.*

DIFFERENTIAL DIAGNOSIS

Common

- Asbestos-Related Pleural Disease
- Pleural infection
- Hemothorax
- Pleurodesis

Less Common

- Pleural/Subpleural Metastasis

Rare but Important

- Osteoblastic Sarcomatoid Mesothelioma
- Calcifying Tumor of Pleura
- Localized Fibrous Tumor of Pleura
- Secondary Hyperparathyroidism

ESSENTIAL INFORMATION

Key Differential Diagnosis Issues

- Pleural thickening from any cause can calcify
- CT is more sensitive than radiography
- Unilateral
  - Pleural infection, hemothorax
- Bilateral
  - Asbestos-related pleural disease, pleural metastasis
- Pleural calcification suggests benign etiology in most cases

Helpful Clues for Common Diagnoses

- **Asbestos-Related Pleural Disease**
  - 20-30 years after exposure
  - Calcification occurs in ~ 15%, often bilateral
  - Typical location: Posterolateral chest wall, dome of diaphragm, mediastinal pleura
- **Pleural Infection**
  - Usually unilateral pleural calcifications
  - Bacterial infection
    - Results from prior pleural infection (i.e., empyema)
    - Associated pleural thickening
  - Tuberculosis
    - Rupture of subpleural pulmonary focus 6-12 weeks after primary infection
    - 50% of patients with tuberculous pleuritis have residual pleural thickening
- **Hemothorax**
  - Remote history of blunt, penetrating or iatrogenic trauma
  - Often unilateral and most extensive posterolaterally
  - Adjacent healed rib fractures
- **Pleurodesis**
  - Pleural inflammatory response (fibrosis and pleural thickening) induced by talc
  - Nodular or band-like foci of high-attenuation mimic pleural calcification
  - FDG avid on PET/CT

Helpful Clues for Less Common Diagnoses

- **Pleural/Subpleural Metastasis**
  - Primary neoplasm
    - Osteosarcoma
    - Chondrosarcoma
    - Adenocarcinomas (mucinous subtypes such as ovarian mucinous cystadenocarcinoma)
- Associated pleural effusion

Helpful Clues for Rare Diagnoses

- **Osteoblastic Sarcomatoid Mesothelioma**
  - Few cases reported
  - Pleural mass with irregular calcifications in thickened pleura
- **Calcifying Tumor of Pleura**
  - Few cases reported
  - Ovoid nodule or mass with intrinsic calcium
- **Localized Fibrous Tumor of Pleura**
  - 80% originate in the visceral pleura
  - Basal predominant extrapulmonary mass
  - Calcifications rare but may occur in large tumors
- **Secondary Hyperparathyroidism**
  - Chronic renal insufficiency
  - Pleural thickening with deposits of mineralization

Asbestos-Related Pleural Disease

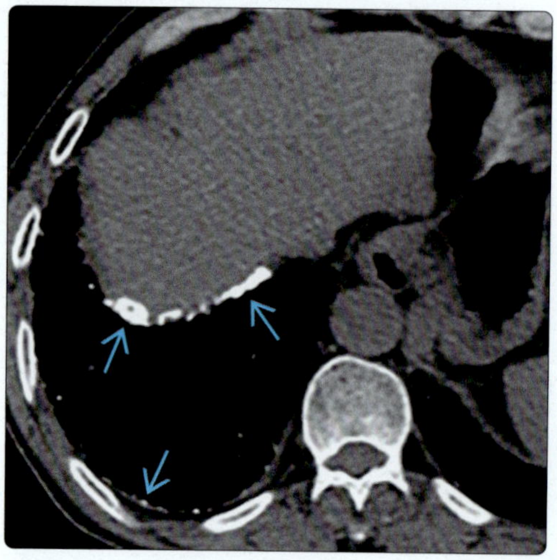

Asbestos-Related Pleural Disease

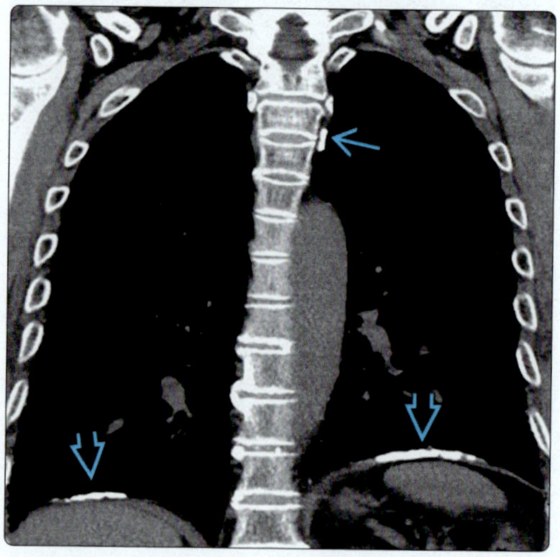

(Left) *Axial CT of a 57-year-old man with a history of exposure to asbestos shows discontinuous calcified plaques ➡ in the right hemithorax.* **(Right)** *Coronal NECT of the same patient shows bilateral discontinuous calcified plaques along the diaphragmatic surface of the pleura ⇨ and left paraspinal region ➡, which are in the classic distribution. The presence of bilateral pleural plaques is very suggestive of asbestos-related pleural disease.*

Pleural infection

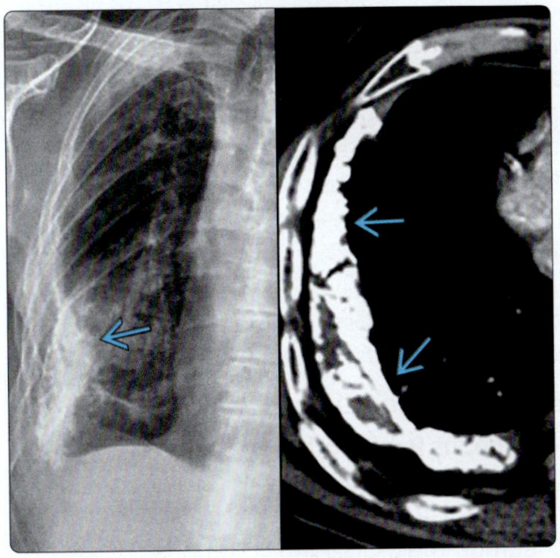

Hemothorax

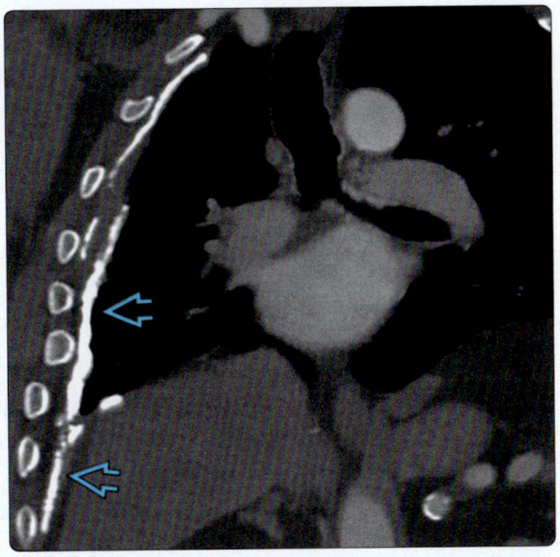

(Left) *Composite image with chest radiograph (left) and CECT (right) of a 76-year-old man with a history of tuberculosis shows calcified diffuse pleural thickening* → *with obliteration of the costophrenic angle.* **(Right)** *Coronal CT of a 42-year-old-man with a history of traumatic hemothorax shows calcified diffuse pleural thickening in the right hemithorax that extends to the costophrenic recess* →. *The abnormality occurs as non-drained hemothorax organizes and eventually calcifies.*

Pleurodesis

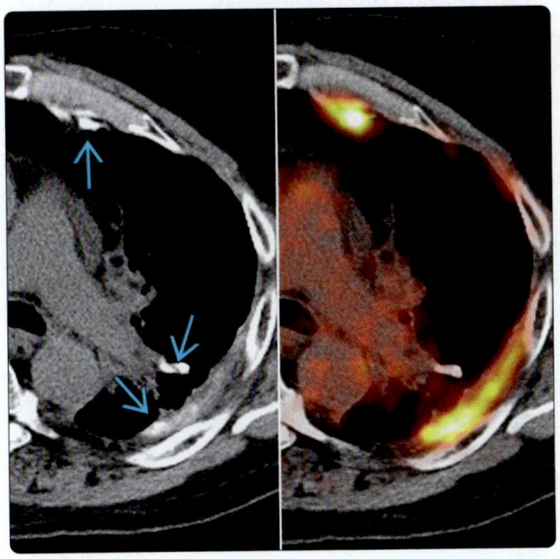

Pleural/Subpleural Metastasis

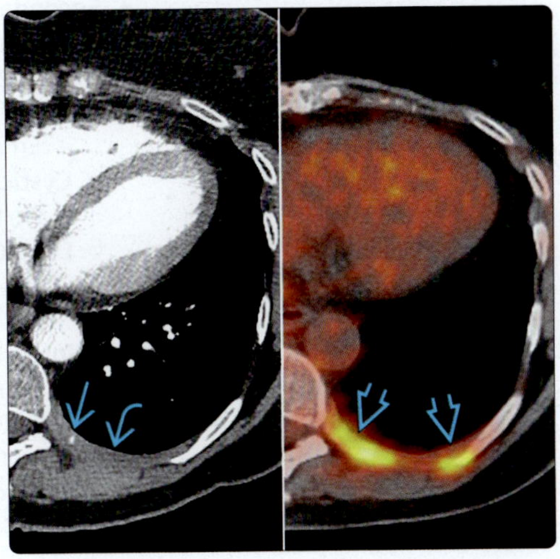

(Left) *Composite image with axial NECT (left) and axial fused FDG PET/CT (right) of a patient with lung adenocarcinoma who underwent talc pleurodesis shows high-attenuation regions of pleural thickening* →. *Note marked FDG avidity due to talc-induced granulomatous reaction.* **(Right)** *Composite image with axial CECT (left) and axial fused FDG PET/CT (right) of a patient with ovarian cancer and pleural metastases shows pleural thickening* → *with calcification* → *that is FDG avid* →.

Calcifying Tumor of Pleura

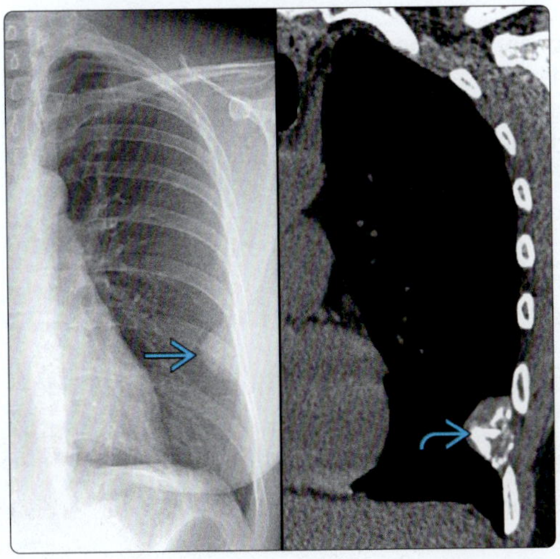

Localized Fibrous Tumor of Pleura

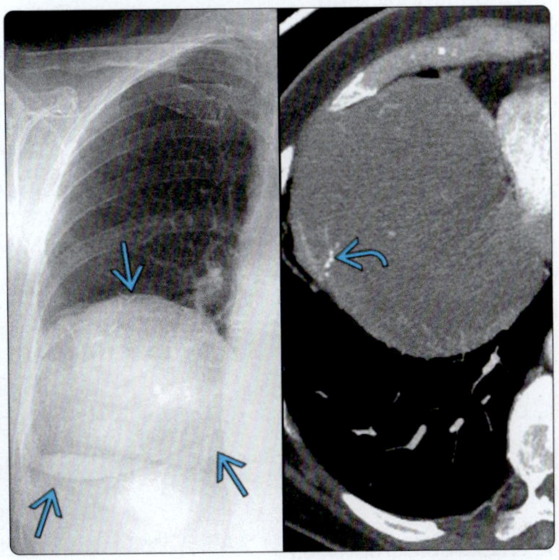

(Left) *Composite image with PA chest radiograph (left) and coronal NECT (right) of a patient with calcifying tumor of the pleura shows a homogenous well-defined extrapleural mass* →. *The mass exhibits marked intrinsic coarse calcifications* → *on CT.* **(Right)** *Composite image with PA chest radiograph (left) and axial CECT (right) of a patient with a large solitary fibrous tumor of the pleura shows a large mass occupying the inferior right hemithorax* →. *The mass is mostly soft tissue attenuation with a tiny amount of calcium* →.

DIFFERENTIAL DIAGNOSIS

Common

- Primary Spontaneous Pneumothorax
- Secondary Spontaneous Pneumothorax
  - COPD
  - Cystic Fibrosis
  - Lung Cancer
  - Interstitial Lung Disease
    - Pulmonary Fibrosis
    - Sarcoidosis
- Trauma
- Mimics

Less Common

- Secondary Spontaneous Pneumothorax
  - Infection
  - Cystic Lung Disease
    - Lymphangioleiomyomatosis
    - Langerhans Cell Histiocytosis
    - Birt-Hogg-Dubé Syndrome
    - Lymphoid Interstitial Pneumonia
  - Metastases
  - Pulmonary Infarct
  - Rheumatoid Nodules
  - Connective Tissue Disorders
  - Catamenial

Rare but Important

- Scuba Diving

ESSENTIAL INFORMATION

Key Differential Diagnosis Issues

- Most common symptoms: Sudden dyspnea and chest pain; may be asymptomatic
- Radiographic findings
  - Upright: Air in pleural space lateral to visceral pleura
    - Pleural line: Sharp thin radiopaque linear interface
    - Absence of lung marking beyond visceral pleural line
  - Supine: Air in anteromedial, subpulmonic, and posteromedial spaces
    - Anteromedial
      - Sharp delineation of mediastinal contour
      - Deep sulcus sign (lateral costophrenic angle deeper and more lucent)
    - Subpulmonic
      - Hyperlucent upper abdomen
      - Deep sulcus sign
    - Posteromedial: Lucent triangle with vertex at hilum, V-shaped base delineating costovertebral sulcus
      - Lucent triangle with vertex at hilum (V-shaped base) delineating costovertebral sulcus
  - Expiratory chest radiograph accentuates size of pneumothorax
- Sonographic diagnosis
  - More sensitive than supine chest radiography, as sensitive as CT to detect traumatic pneumothorax
  - Signs: Absence of lung sliding, absence of B lines, absence of lung pulse, presence of lung point
- Complications
  - Tension: Life-threatening complication and hemodynamic compromise
    - Radiography: Contralateral mediastinal displacement, diaphragmatic inversion, total or subtotal lung atelectasis
    - Commonly seen in trauma or mechanical ventilation
  - Reexpansion pulmonary edema
    - Lung reexpansion can cause capillary leak
    - Common after large primary pneumothorax in younger patients
  - Pneumomediastinum
    - Most common in neonates
    - Adults being mechanically ventilated

Helpful Clues for Common Diagnoses

- **Primary Spontaneous Pneumothorax**
  - Younger adults (age 10-30 years), tall individuals, and smokers
  - Familial pneumothorax: Occasionally reported
  - Rupture of either small subpleural bullae or blebs
  - May be treated conservatively with chest tube drainage
- **Secondary Spontaneous Pneumothorax**
  - Most common cause of spontaneous pneumothorax, related to underlying pulmonary pathology
  - **COPD**
    - Emphysema
  - **Cystic Fibrosis**
    - Up to 20% of affected patients older than 18 years
  - **Lung Cancer**
    - Pneumothorax in context of concerning pulmonary nodule or mass ± emphysema
  - **Interstitial Lung Disease**
    - **Pulmonary Fibrosis**
      - Pneumothorax or pneumomediastinum develops in 11% of cases
    - **Sarcoidosis**
      - Associated with upper lobe peribronchovascular fibrosis
      - Necrosis of subpleural granuloma
      - May be bilateral, recurrent
  - **Trauma**
    - Pulmonary lacerations in both blunt and penetrating trauma
    - Persistent pneumothorax due to air-leak or bronchopleural fistula
    - Fallen lung sign: Displaced lung to dependent side according to patient's position (i.e., inferior if patient erect, or posterior if patient in posterior decubitus)
    - Iatrogenic after procedure (i.e., drained pleural effusion, biopsy)
- **Mimics**
  - Skinfolds, chest tube tracks, giant bullae, scapular edge, and rib companion shadow

Helpful Clues for Less Common Diagnoses

- **Secondary Spontaneous Pneumothorax**
  - **Infection**
    - Bronchopleural fistula: May complicate necrotizing pneumonia (anaerobic, tuberculous, and pyogenic)
    - Postinfectious pneumatoceles resulting from *Pneumocystis jirovecii* or *Staphylococcus aureus*

- Angioinvasive aspergillosis: Hematogenous dissemination with invasion of small arteries, vascular occlusion, and often infarction
  - Particularly common in neutropenic stem cell transplant patients
- Immunocompromised HIV(+) patients
  - Bad prognosis and mortality 30-60%
  - Leading cause is *Pneumocystis jirovecii*

- **Cystic Lung Disease**
  - **Lymphangioleiomyomatosis**
    - Almost exclusively affects women of childbearing age
    - Pneumothorax develops in 80% of cases
    - CT: Normal or large lung volume and numerous, diffuse, thin-walled cysts without zonal predilection, normal intervening lung parenchyma
  - **Langerhans Cell Histiocytosis**
    - Tobacco-related disease in young adults, predominantly male
    - Pneumothorax develops in 25% of cases
    - CT: Irregular-shaped cyst, predominantly in upper and mid lung zones with sparing of costophrenic angles
  - **Birt-Hogg-Dubé Syndrome**
    - Dominantly inherited disease: Benign skin tumors, diverse types of renal cancer, pulmonary cysts (80%), and spontaneous pneumothorax
    - Lung cysts: Oval, round, lenticular, irregular, thin walled; bilateral with lower and medial lung predominance, and involve both costophrenic sulci
  - **Lymphoid Interstitial Pneumonia**
    - Occurs in context of Sjögren syndrome
- **Metastases**
  - Metastatic sarcomas: Osteosarcoma, synovial cell sarcoma, angiosarcoma, and leiomyosarcoma
    - Frequently after initiation of chemotherapy
- **Pulmonary Infarction**
  - May develop from septic embolism (from cavitary nodules)
    - Infective endocarditis in intravenous drug users
  - Rarely pulmonary infarcts in context of thromboembolic disease can cavitate and result in pneumothorax
- **Rheumatoid Nodules**
  - Subpleural necrobiotic nodules erode into pleural space; nodules are mostly well defined and can cavitate in up to 50% of cases
- **Connective Tissue Diseases**
  - Marfan syndrome
    - Pneumothoraces are reported 5-11%, commonly bilateral and recurrent
    - Apical blebs, bullae, abnormal connective tissue-related lung disease, or increased mechanical stresses in lung apices due to tall body habitus
  - Ehlers-Danlos syndromes
    - Pneumothorax is common in type IV Ehlers-Danlos syndrome; associated skeletal abnormalities are seen on chest radiograph
- **Catamenial**
  - Development of pneumothorax at time of menstruation from migrated endometrial tissue to pleura
  - 95% of cases occur on right side
  - CT: Pneumoperitoneum associated with right pneumothorax, diaphragmatic defect, diaphragmatic nodule/implant, and subpleural nodule/implant
  - < 1/3 associated with pelvic endometriosis

Helpful Clues for Rare Diagnoses

- **Scuba Diving**
  - Recent immersion history is critical

SELECTED REFERENCES

1. Onuki T et al: Primary and secondary spontaneous pneumothorax: prevalence, clinical features, and in-hospital mortality. Can Respir J. 2017:6014967, 2017
2. Rierson D et al: Pneumothorax in the supine patient: subtle radiographic signs. J Thorac Imaging. 31(4):W16-22, 2016
3. Bobbio A et al: Epidemiology of spontaneous pneumothorax: gender-related differences. Thorax. 70(7):653-8, 2015

Primary Spontaneous Pneumothorax

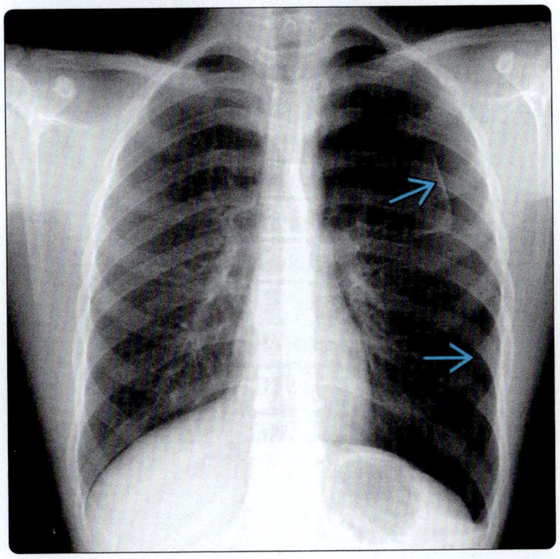

Primary Spontaneous Pneumothorax

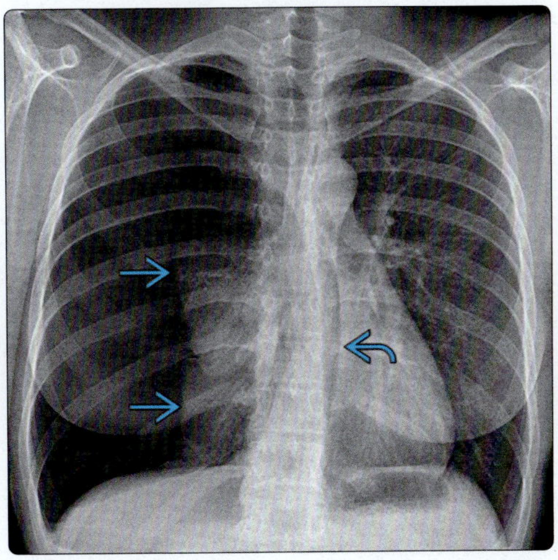

(Left) *PA chest radiograph of a patient with primary spontaneous pneumothorax shows a conspicuous pleural line* ➔ *along the periphery of the left hemithorax denoting the presence of a pneumothorax.* **(Right)** *PA chest radiograph of a young woman with a primary spontaneous pneumothorax with tension. Note marked atelectasis of the right lung* ➔ *with contralateral displacement of the cardiomediastinal silhouette and marked displacement of the anterior junction line* ↗.

(**Left**) *PA chest radiograph of a patient with COPD and secondary spontaneous pneumothorax shows a pleural line from a moderate to large pneumothorax and numerous bullae.* (**Right**) *Axial NECT of the same patient after insertion of a chest tube shows residual small anterior pneumothorax with extensive bullous disease bilaterally. Emphysema is a smoking-related disease and one of the most common causes of secondary spontaneous pneumothorax.*

COPD

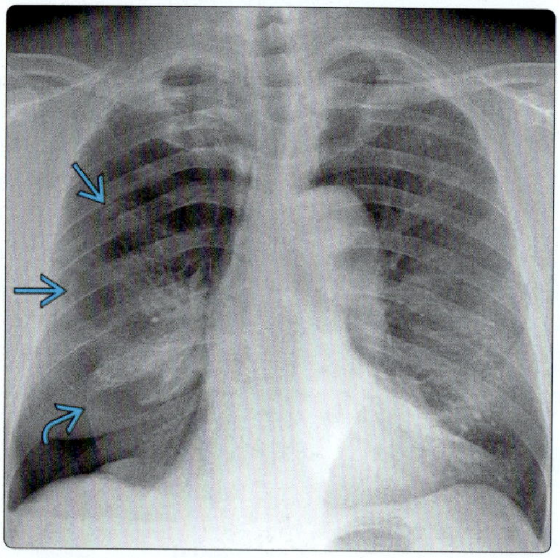

COPD

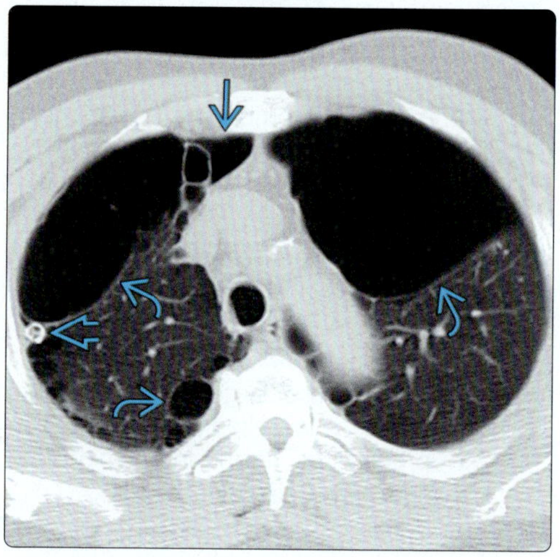

(**Left**) *Axial NECT of a patient with acute exacerbation of idiopathic pulmonary fibrosis (IPF) shows bilateral reticular and ground-glass opacities with traction bronchiectasis and a small anterior left pneumothorax.* (**Right**) *AP chest radiograph of a patient with blunt chest trauma shows multiple right rib fractures and a deep sulcus sign due to pneumothorax. This sign is extremely helpful, especially in the instances in which a definite pleural line to confirm pneumothorax is not identified.*

Pulmonary Fibrosis

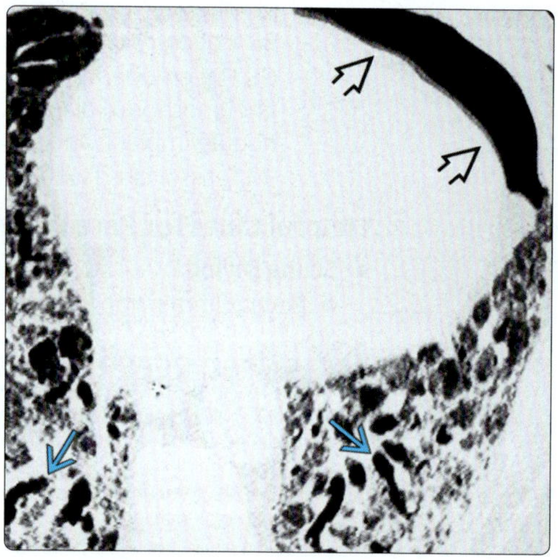

Trauma

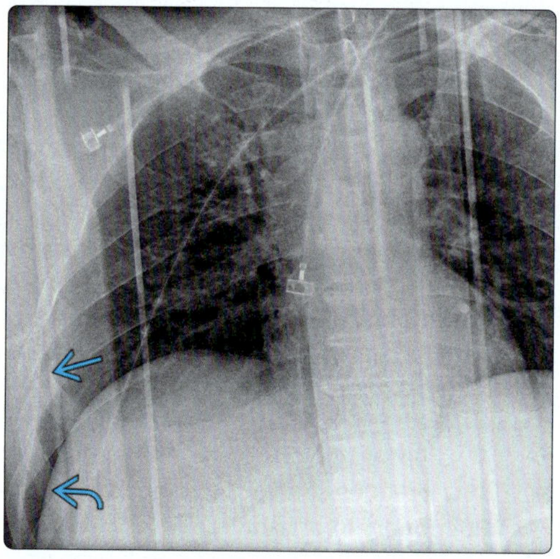

(**Left**) *AP chest radiograph with skinfold mimicking pneumothorax. Note the skinfold is an edge rather than a line and that pulmonary vessels are seen coursing beyond the skinfold.* (**Right**) *Composite image with PA chest radiograph (left) and coronal NECT (right) of a patient with bullous disease mimicking right basilar loculated pneumothorax is shown. Differentiation on radiography may be difficult or impossible, especially when apical in location, and chest tubes may be placed unnecessarily.*

Mimics

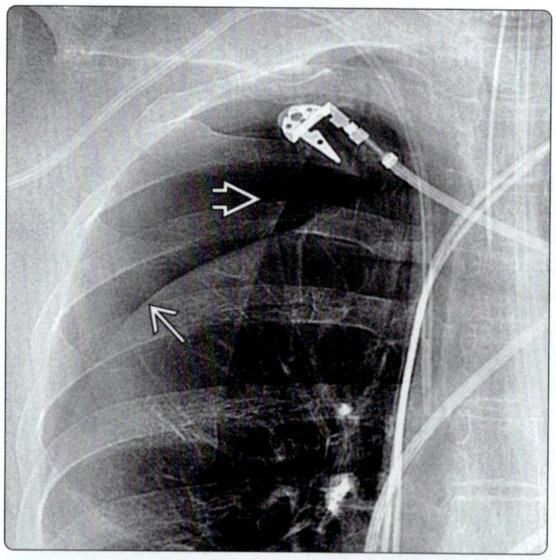

Mimics

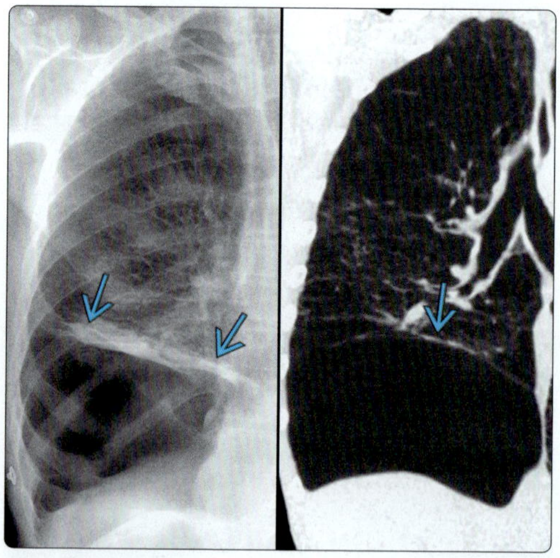

Lymphangioleiomyomatosis

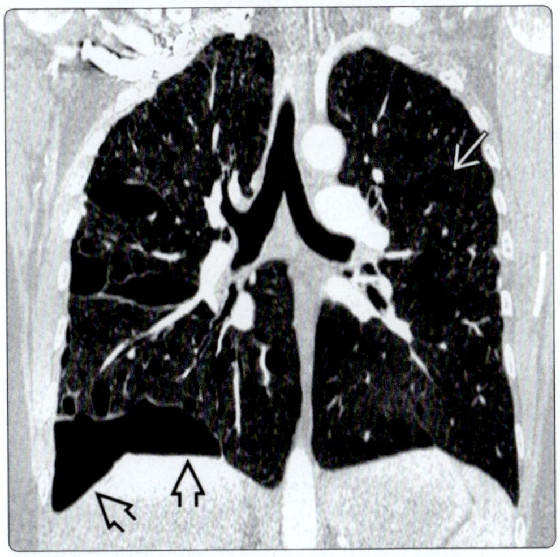

Langerhans Cell Histiocytosis

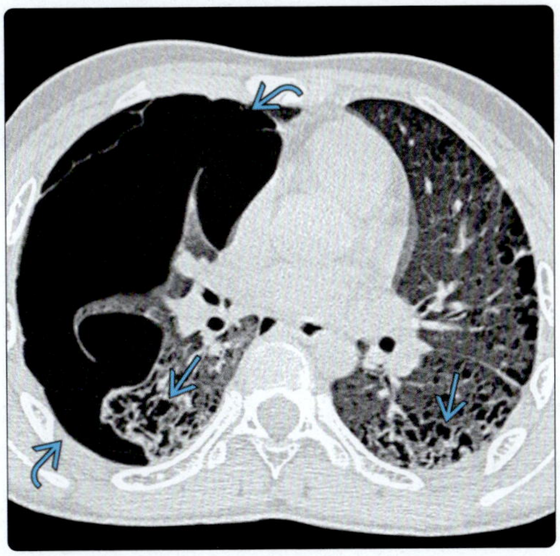

(Left) *Coronal NECT of a patient with lymphangioleiomyomatosis shows numerous thin-walled, round, and well-defined cysts scattered throughout both lungs* ➔ *and a loculated right basilar pneumothorax* ➔*. Secondary spontaneous pneumothorax is a common complication of lymphangioleiomyomatosis.* **(Right)** *Axial HRCT of a patient with Langerhans cell histiocytosis shows multiple irregular-shaped cysts* ➔ *bilaterally and a right pneumothorax* ➔*.*

Birt-Hogg-Dubé Syndrome

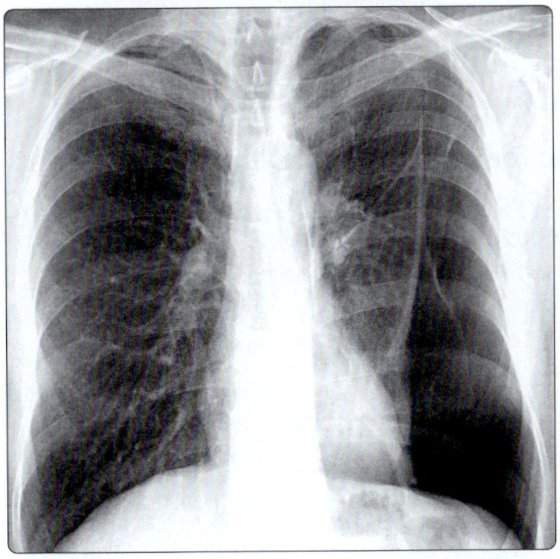

Birt-Hogg-Dubé Syndrome

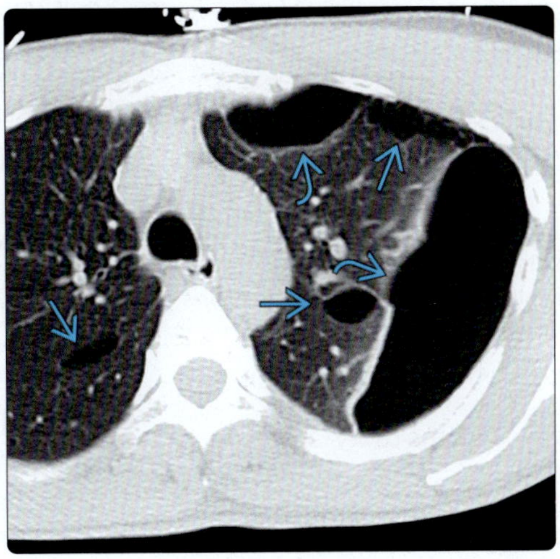

(Left) *PA chest radiograph of a patient with Birt-Hogg-Dubé syndrome shows a moderate left pneumothorax.* **(Right)** *Axial NECT of the same patient shows multiple subpleural round and lenticular cysts bilaterally* ➔ *with loculated left pneumothorax* ➔*. Secondary spontaneous pneumothorax is a common manifestation of Birt-Hogg-Dubé syndrome, a hereditary condition associated with multiple benign skin tumors, lung cysts, and increased risk of both benign and malignant kidney tumors.*

Rheumatoid Nodules

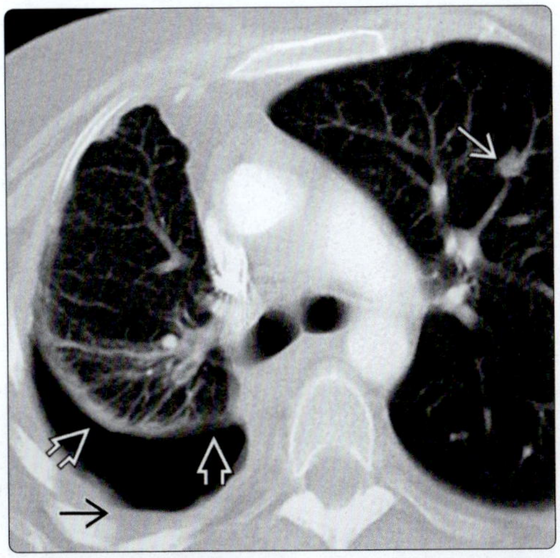

Catamenial

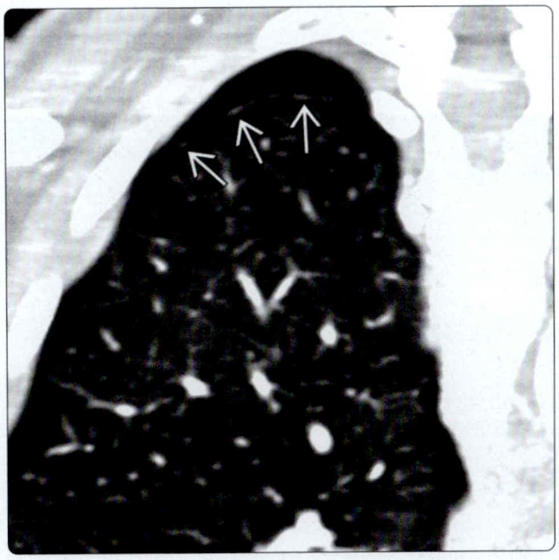

(Left) *Axial CECT of a 43-year-old woman with rheumatoid arthritis and necrobiotic nodules shows a small hydropneumothorax* ➔*. Note markedly thickened visceral pleura* ➔*, a common thoracic finding in rheumatoid arthritis, and a small rheumatoid nodule in the left lung* ➔*.* **(Right)** *Coronal CECT of a patient with catamenial pneumothorax shows subtle small visceral pleural nodules* ➔*, which represent endometrial tissue.*

DIFFERENTIAL DIAGNOSIS

Common

- Bronchopleural Fistula
  - Infection
  - Neoplasm
  - Thoracic Surgery
- Trauma
- Thoracentesis

Less Common

- Esophageal Rupture

Rare but Important

- Spontaneous Pneumothorax With Hemothorax

ESSENTIAL INFORMATION

Key Differential Diagnosis Issues

- Air-fluid level of pleural etiology
  - Elongated morphology (craniocaudal diameter > transverse and anteroposterior diameters)
  - Smooth/obtuse pleural angles
  - Displacement of adjacent lung ± atelectasis
- Mimics
  - Diaphragmatic hernia/rupture: History of trauma
  - Cavitary lung nodule/mass + air-fluid level
    - Lung abscess
    - Lung cancer: Smoker, upper lobe predominance
    - Infected bulla: Emphysema, upper lobe predominance
    - Pulmonary infarct: Complicates 1/3 of patients with pulmonary embolism, lower lobe predominance
    - Imaging features of pulmonary lesions
      - Spherical shape
      - Consolidated lung surrounds the cavity (abscess)
      - Acute pleural angles
  - Post pneumonectomy
    - Mediastinal shift to the opposite side of pneumonectomy
    - Air-fluid within pneumonectomy space simulates hydropneumothorax but anatomically not in pleural space
    - Progressively resolves after days-weeks

Helpful Clues for Common Diagnoses

- **Bronchopleural Fistula**
  - Secondary to infection, neoplasm, or thoracic surgery
  - Persistent air or air-fluid level in pleural space
  - Infection
    - Complicated parapneumonic effusion or empyema with bronchopleural fistula
      - Thickened enhancing parietal and visceral pleura separated by pleural fluid ("split pleura" sign)
      - Air-fluid level indicates bronchopleural fistula
    - Microorganisms: *S. pneumoniae, S. aureus,* aerobic gram (-), Anaerobes, and *M. tuberculosis*
  - Neoplasm
    - Cavitary lung cancer with pleural involvement/rupture
- **Trauma**
  - Blunt, penetrating or iatrogenic (i.e., postsurgical)
  - Injury of lung, pleura, diaphragm, or chest wall
  - Location of air-fluid level depends on patient position
- **Thoracentesis**
  - Air-fluid levels commonly follow this procedure

Helpful Clues for Less Common Diagnoses

- **Esophageal Rupture**
  - Spontaneous (Boerhaave syndrome)
    - Increased intraluminal esophageal pressure during vomiting
  - Secondary to trauma, foreign body perforation, or iatrogenic

Helpful Clues for Rare Diagnoses

- **Spontaneous Pneumothorax With Hemothorax**
  - Can be primary (without apparent lung pathology) or secondary (with intrinsic lung pathology; e.g., emphysema, cystic lung disease)
  - Pneumothorax may exhibit air-fluid levels from associated pleural effusion or hemothorax

Infection

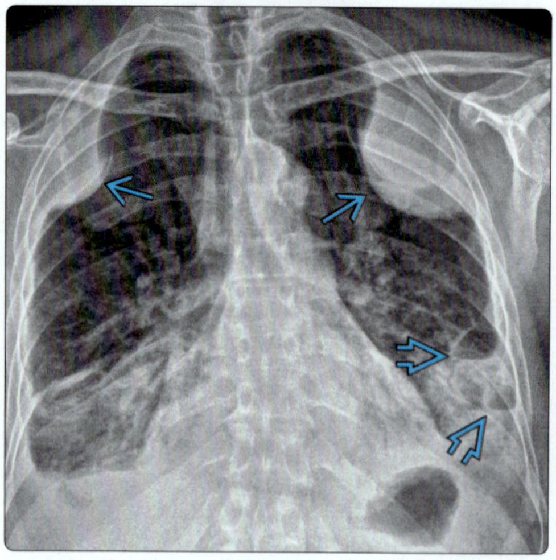

Infection

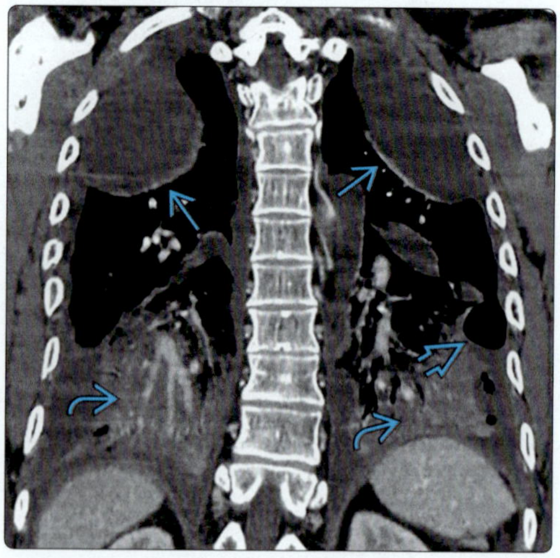

(Left) *Frontal chest radiograph of a 42-year-old-man with pneumonia due to Streptococcus pneumoniae complicated by empyema and bronchopleural fistula demonstrates loculated pleural effusions ➔ and a left basilar collection with an air-fluid level ➔.* **(Right)** *Coronal CECT of the same patient shows loculated pleural effusions ➔ with left basilar hydropneumothorax ➔ and multifocal lower lobe consolidations ➔ bilaterally. Bronchopleural fistula is an uncommon but well-known complication of pneumonia.*

Trauma

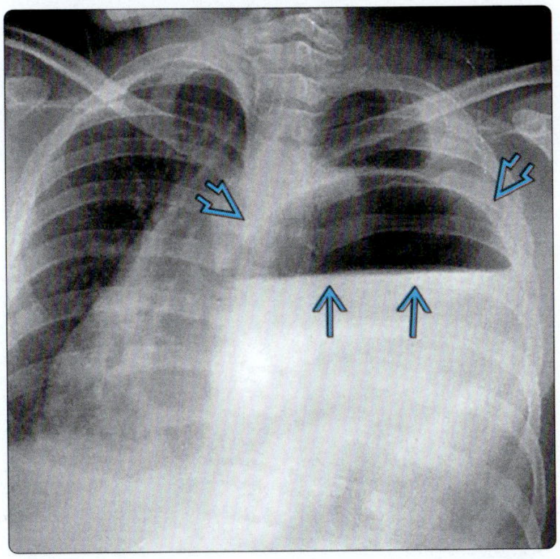

Trauma

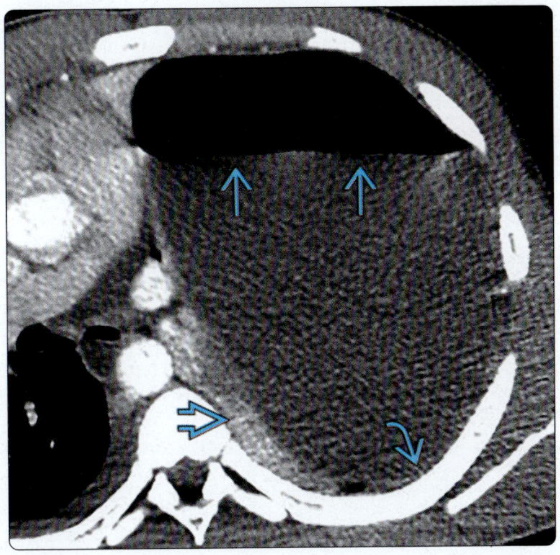

(Left) *Frontal chest radiograph of a 26-year-old man with traumatic diaphragmatic rupture shows a large air-fluid level in the left hemithorax, corresponding to an intrathoracic stomach.* ***(Right)*** *Axial CECT of the same patient shows an intrathoracic stomach with air-fluid level and marked compressive left lower lobe atelectasis. Note the so-called dependent viscera sign with the stomach contacting the posterior chest wall, commonly seen in diaphragmatic rupture.*

Esophageal Rupture

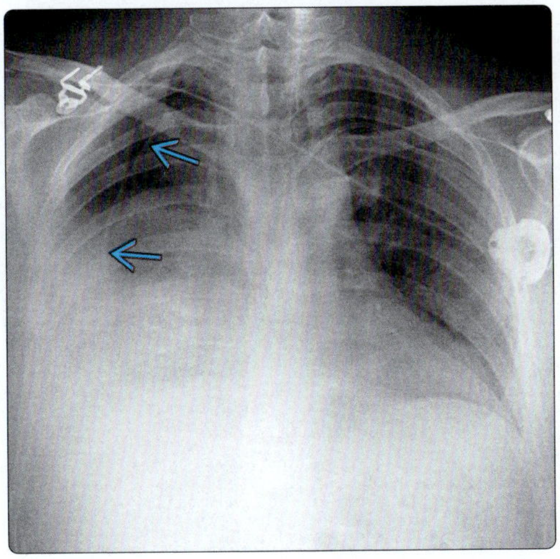

Esophageal Rupture

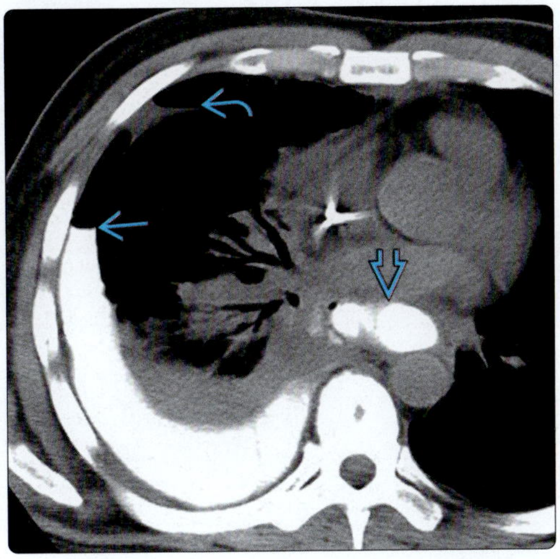

(Left) *Frontal chest radiograph of a patient with esophageal rupture from Boerhaave syndrome shows a moderate right hydropneumothorax. An air-fluid level is not apparent due to decubitus patient positioning.* ***(Right)*** *Axial NECT with oral contrast of the same patient shows extensive extravasation of oral contrast into the right pleural cavity with air-contrast and air space fluid levels. Note also the dilated and irregular esophagus. The presence of air-fluid levels is common in patients with esophageal rupture.*

Spontaneous Pneumothorax With Hemothorax

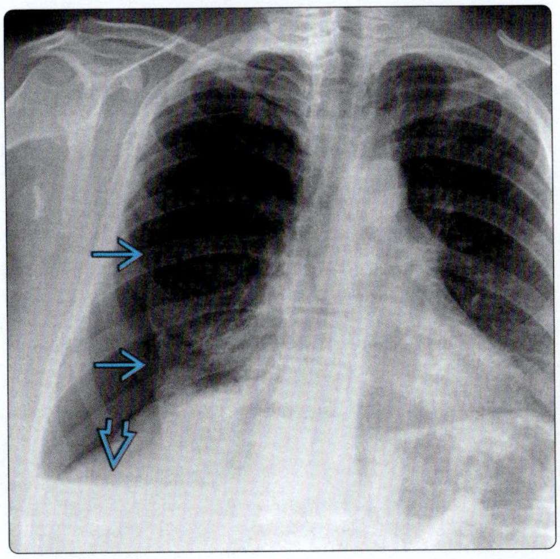

Spontaneous Pneumothorax With Hemothorax

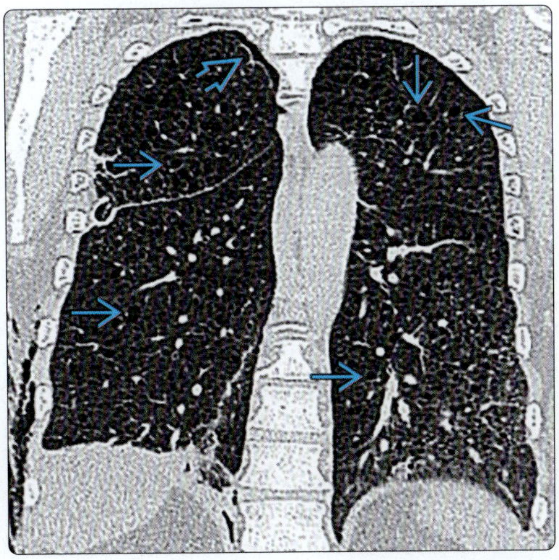

(Left) *Chest radiograph of a 35-year-old woman with lymphangioleiomyomatosis (LAM) and secondary spontaneous pneumothorax shows a right hydropneumothorax with an air-fluid level. In the context of LAM, pleural effusion may be secondary to associated hemothorax or chylous effusion.* ***(Right)*** *Coronal HRCT of the same patient shows numerous well-defined, thin-walled bilateral lung cysts and a right apical pneumothorax.*

SECTION 9

Chest Wall and Diaphragm

Approach to Chest Wall and Diaphragm

General Imaging Patterns

Modality-Specific Imaging Findings: Radiography

Modality-Specific Imaging Findings: Computed Tomography

Modality-Specific Imaging Findings: Magnetic Resonance Imaging

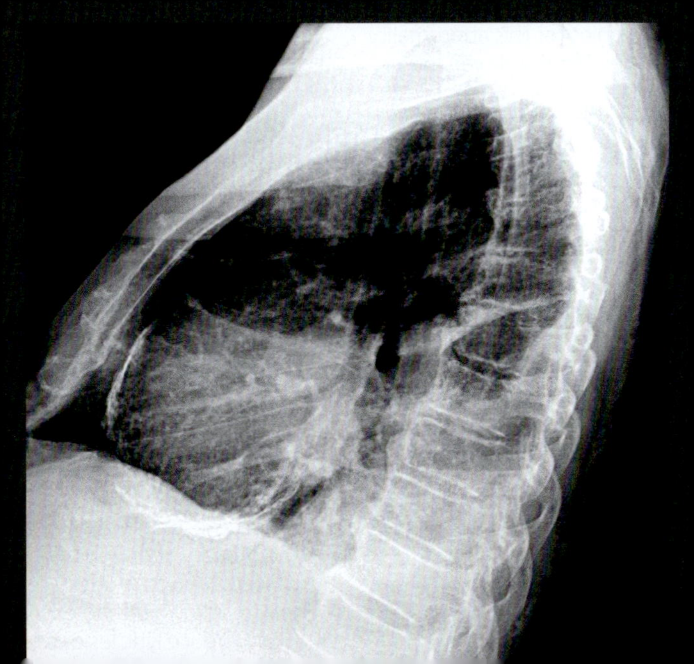

Introduction

The chest wall is a complex anatomical structure composed of many tissue types, presenting a challenge in both detection and diagnosis of disease. The spectrum of pathology involving the chest wall ranges from normal anatomical variants to benign and malignant diseases. Imaging plays a critical role in evaluating the chest wall, whether pathology is discovered incidentally or when imaging studies are performed for diagnosis of a specific clinical issue. Due to its widespread availability and use in clinical practice, chest radiography is often the first imaging modality to suggest the presence of a chest wall abnormality. However, cross-sectional imaging modalities, such as computed tomography (CT) and magnetic resonance (MR) imaging, are optimal for diagnosis and intervention planning. Other modalities, such as ultrasound and FDG positron emission tomography (PET)/CT, are not routinely used to evaluate patients with a chest wall abnormality but are useful in certain clinical scenarios. An understanding of the anatomy of the chest wall and knowledge of potential pitfalls are important to ensuring appropriate diagnosis and patient care and avoiding misdiagnosis.

Anatomic Considerations

The chest wall includes the tissue surrounding the lung and mediastinum, which is composed of mesenchymal elements, including bones and cartilage, muscles, vascular structures, and nerves. The intercostal neurovascular bundles are enveloped between the intercostal muscles and typically course beneath the rib. The endothoracic fascia is the deepest layer of the chest wall, serving as a surgical dissection plane for separating the underlying parietal pleura from the chest wall.

Imaging of Chest Wall and Diaphragm

Elevation of a hemidiaphragm is a frequent finding on chest radiography. A wide variety of etiologies for this abnormality have been described, including normal anatomic variant, phrenic nerve injury, eventration, iatrogenesis, and more sinister processes, such as neoplasm. One of the most important observations to make in the assessment of these cases is whether the elevation is focal or uniform. Important causes of focal elevation include eventration, prior lobectomy, diaphragmatic hernia, and diaphragmatic rupture, whereas key etiologies of uniform elevation include phrenic nerve paralysis, diaphragmatic weakness, and unilateral lung transplantation. CT is the imaging modality of choice for assessing these patients. Dynamic assessment of a hemidiaphragm with fluoroscopy or dynamic MR may be necessary when phrenic nerve function is uncertain.

Asymmetry of the chest wall may be encountered and has been described as either congenital or acquired. Congenital etiologies include pectus excavatum, pectus carinatum, and congenital rib deformities, whereas acquired abnormalities include deformities following trauma, infection, and surgery. Pectus excavatum is the most common chest wall deformity, occurring in ~ 1 in 1,000 live births with a strong male predominance (3-5:1), and is characterized by posterior bowing and rotation of the sternum and anterior ribs with decreased anteroposterior diameter of the chest. Findings on the lateral chest radiograph are diagnostic. Due to mass effect on the heart and medial aspect of the middle lobe, this abnormality may result in obscuration of the right heart border on the frontal chest radiograph and mimic middle lobe or pneumonia atelectasis. Other etiologies of chest wall asymmetry may not be readily identifiable on chest radiography and require assessment with CT or MR, the former of which is considered the imaging modality of choice, although the latter provides excellent visualization of soft tissue masses and most neoplasms.

Chest wall neoplasms may arise from the soft tissues or osseous structures and be malignant or benign. Approximately 20% of these lesions are visible on chest radiography, which can be helpful in demonstrating the location, size, and growth rate of neoplasms. In many cases, the "incomplete border" sign, which is characterized by both well-defined (when the x-ray beam hits the lesion tangentially) and ill-defined (when the x-ray beam hits the lesion en face) margins and indicates that a lesion is extrapulmonary in location, may be present; however, as the features identifiable on radiography are typically nonspecific, further evaluation with cross-sectional imaging is necessary, as CT and MR enable much more accurate identification and characterization of chest wall neoplasms. CT can demonstrate tumor site and tissue origin (bone and cartilage or soft tissues, such as muscle, fat, or skin), morphologic features, and internal components, such as fat and mineralization (calcification/ossification). MR provides superior soft tissue contrast compared with CT and is the optimal imaging modality for delineating extent of chest wall soft tissue involvement and enables the differentiation of malignancy from normal chest wall structures and nonneoplastic disease processes, such as infection and inflammation.

Greater than 50% of chest wall neoplasms are malignant and typically result from direct invasion by or metastasis from thoracic neoplasms; however, these lesions may also arise from the chest wall as primary lesions. The most frequent primary malignancies metastasizing to the chest wall are breast, lung, and prostate cancers and melanoma via direct extension or hematogeneous or lymphatic spread. The most common primary malignancies of bone and soft tissue origin include chondrosarcoma and undifferentiated pleomorphic sarcoma, respectively. Chondrosarcoma appears as a well-circumscribed mass of variable composition, usually soft tissue and mineralization, arising from the anterior chest wall with various configurations of calcification, such as rings, arcs, &/or a stippled pattern. On MR, the cartilage component is heterogeneous but frequently iso- to hypointense to muscle on T1WI and hyperintense to muscle on T2WI. The highly characteristic "rings and arcs" and other patterns of mineralization are hypointense to muscle on T1WI and T2WI. The imaging appearance of undifferentiated pleomorphic sarcoma is typically nonspecific, with the tumor manifesting as a heterogeneously enhancing mass centered on the deep fascial layers of the chest wall and commonly involving the adjacent rib. Metastatic lesions tend to manifest in ways that reflect the imaging characteristics of other metastases from the primary neoplasm. For example, prostate and breast cancers tend to produce sclerotic lesions, renal cell carcinoma may result in lytic and expansile lesions, and multiple myeloma may produce lytic lesions.

Chondrosarcoma

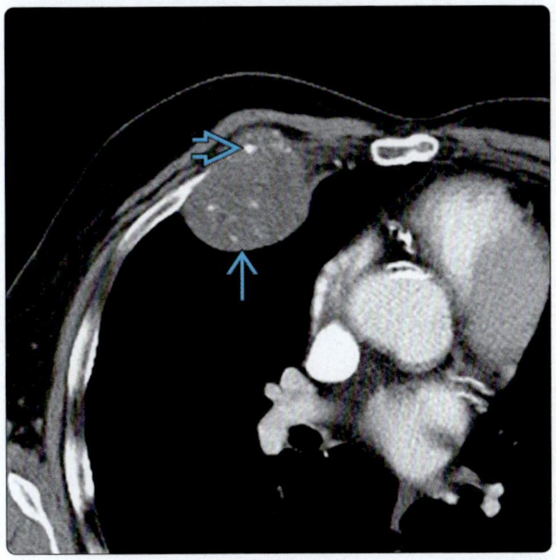

Osteosarcoma

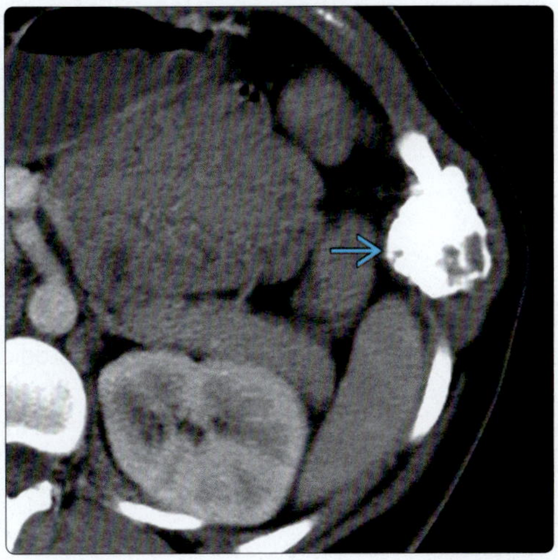

(Left) *Axial CECT of a patient presenting with right anterior chest wall pain shows a soft tissue mass with internal foci of mineralization. Biopsy revealed chondrosarcoma, which is the most common primary chest wall malignancy of osseous origin.* **(Right)** *Axial CECT of a patient presenting with left chest wall pain shows a soft tissue mass with extensive mineralization in the left anterolateral chest wall. Biopsy revealed osteosarcoma, which manifests as a soft tissue mass with variable mineralization.*

Lymphoma

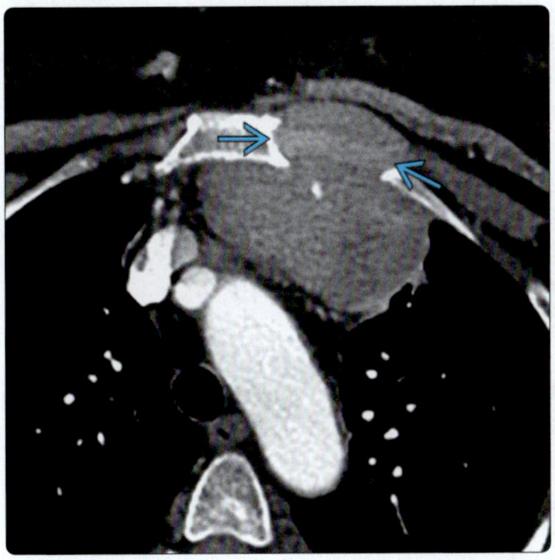

Osteochondroma

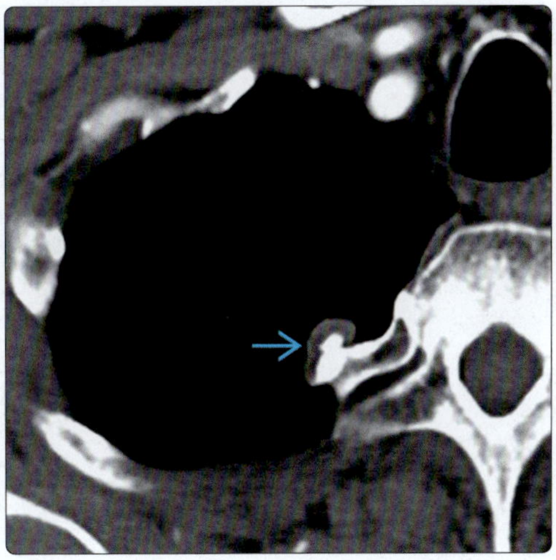

(Left) *Axial CECT of a patient presenting with fever, night sweats, and weight loss demonstrates a soft tissue mass arising from the left prevascular mediastinum and invading the left anterior chest wall. Biopsy revealed Hodgkin lymphoma.* **(Right)** *Axial CECT of an asymptomatic patient shows a soft tissue lesion with mineralization arising from the posterior aspect of an upper right rib that extends into the right hemithorax, representing a benign osteochondroma.*

Abscess

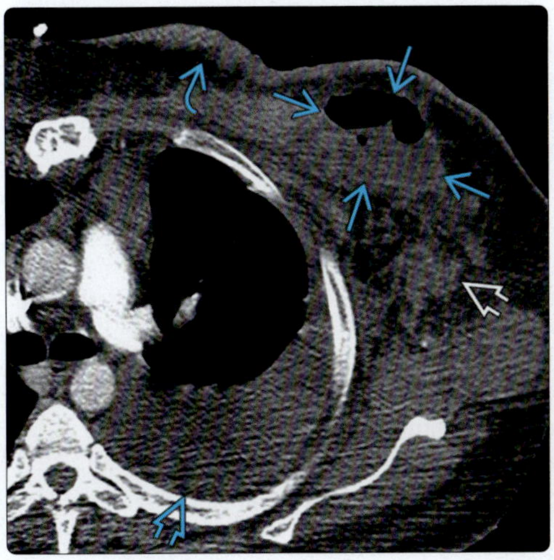

Abscess

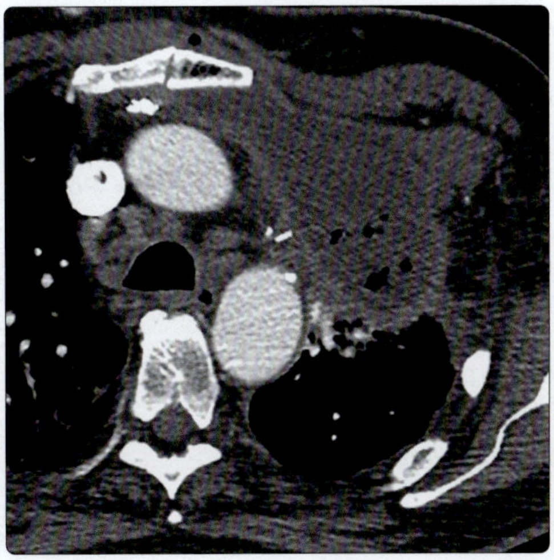

(Left) *Axial CECT of a patient status post surgical resection and radiation therapy for treatment of breast cancer demonstrates a fluid- and air-containing lesion in the left breast representing abscess. Note the adjacent skin thickening, inflammatory fat stranding, and left pleural effusion.* **(Right)** *Axial CECT of a patient status post partial resection of the left upper lobe for lung cancer demonstrates a fluid- and air-containing lesion compatible with abscess that extends into the left anterior chest wall.*

DIFFERENTIAL DIAGNOSIS

Common

- Normal Variant
- Phrenic Nerve Paralysis or Injury
- Eventration
- Diaphragmatic Weakness
- Postsurgical
- Lobar Atelectasis (Mimic)
- Bochdalek Hernia

Less Common

- Subpulmonic Pleural Effusion (Mimic)
- Hepatomegaly
- Unilateral Lung Transplantation
- Pleural, Diaphragmatic, Abdominal Tumor
- Ascites

Rare but Important

- Morgagni Hernia (Mimic)
- Diaphragmatic Tear (Mimic)

ESSENTIAL INFORMATION

Key Differential Diagnosis Issues

- Focal versus uniform elevation
    - Focal elevation
        - Eventration
        - Lobectomy
        - Diaphragmatic hernia
        - Diaphragmatic rupture
    - Uniform elevation
        - Phrenic nerve paralysis
        - Diaphragmatic weakness
        - Unilateral lung transplantation
- Imaging assessment of diaphragm
    - Diaphragm is very thin in elderly patients; difficult to visualize on cross-sectional imaging
    - CT: Imaging modality of choice for assessment of diaphragmatic defects and diaphragmatic hernia in adults
    - Ultrasound and MR: Very useful for assessment of diaphragmatic abnormalities in pediatric population
    - Dynamic assessment of diaphragm
        - Fluoroscopy
        - Dynamic MR
- Fluoroscopy
    - Differentiation of phrenic nerve paralysis from other causes of weakness or diaphragmatic eventration
    - Phrenic nerve paralysis: Paradoxical diaphragmatic motion on forced inspiration (sniff maneuver)
    - Diaphragmatic eventration: No paradoxical diaphragmatic motion on sniff maneuver

Helpful Clues for Common Diagnoses

- **Normal Variant**
    - Left hemidiaphragm is normally lower than right hemidiaphragm
    - Left hemidiaphragm may be slightly elevated or at same level as right hemidiaphragm in up to 10-15% of normal subjects
    - Dextrocardia or situs inversus: Left hemidiaphragm higher than right hemidiaphragm
- **Phrenic Nerve Paralysis or Injury**
    - Diaphragmatic dysfunction may be permanent or temporary, depending on etiology
    - Uniform, usually unilateral diaphragmatic elevation
        - Unilateral phrenic nerve paralysis: May be asymptomatic
        - Bilateral diaphragmatic dysfunction: Typically symptomatic, may be complicated by ventilatory failure
    - Abnormal nerve conduction at electromyography studies
    - Imaging
        - Fluoroscopy
            - Diaphragmatic paralysis: Absence of diaphragmatic excursion on quiet and deep breathing
            - Paradoxical motion on forced inspiration (sniff maneuver)
        - CT/MR
            - Phrenic nerve dysfunction may be 1st manifestation of locally invasive thoracic mass due to phrenic nerve invasion or compression by tumor
            - Diagnosis of phrenic nerve dysfunction should prompt further assessment with chest CT in high-risk patients
- **Eventration**
    - More common in elderly
    - Focal diaphragmatic bulge
        - Focal muscle weakness or thinning
        - Usually congenital
    - Typically affects anteromedial right hemidiaphragm
- **Diaphragmatic Weakness**
    - Indicates either neurogenic or muscular impairment
    - May be reversible
    - Etiologies
        - Recent surgery, typically cardiac surgery
        - Systemic lupus erythematosus: Vanishing lung syndrome from diaphragmatic myopathy
        - Guillain-Barré syndrome
        - Poliomyelitis
        - Polymyositis and dermatomyositis
    - Diaphragmatic weakness manifests with reduced or delayed excursion on deep breathing ± paradoxical motion on sniffing
- **Postsurgical**
    - History of lobectomy or pneumonectomy
    - Mediastinal shift to side of surgery
    - Signs of prior thoracotomy or lung resection are usually evident
    - Pneumonectomy may manifest with opaque hemithorax and crowding of ipsilateral ribs
- **Lobar Atelectasis (Mimic)**
    - Ipsilateral volume loss
    - Direct or indirect signs of lobar collapse
- **Bochdalek Hernia**
    - Focal diaphragmatic elevation
    - Posterior, more common on left
    - Often small incidental finding

Pectus Excavatum

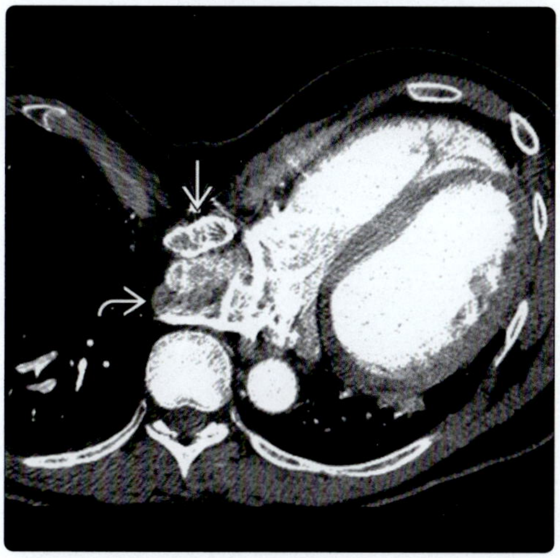

Pectus Excavatum

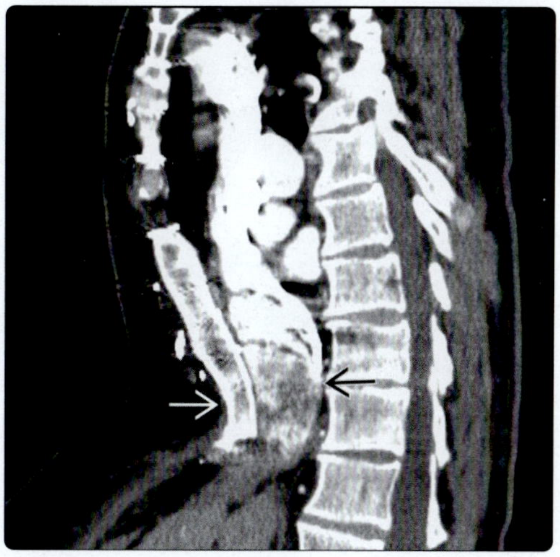

(Left) *Axial CECT of the same patient at the level of the heart shows severe concave deformity of the sternum with marked narrowing of the AP diameter of the thorax. Note displacement of the heart to the left, rotation of the heart, and severe compression of the right atrium.* **(Right)** *Sagittal CECT of the same patient shows severe pectus excavatum with marked posterior displacement of the lower sternum, narrow thoracic AP diameter, and loss of the retrosternal and retrocardiac spaces.*

Pectus Excavatum

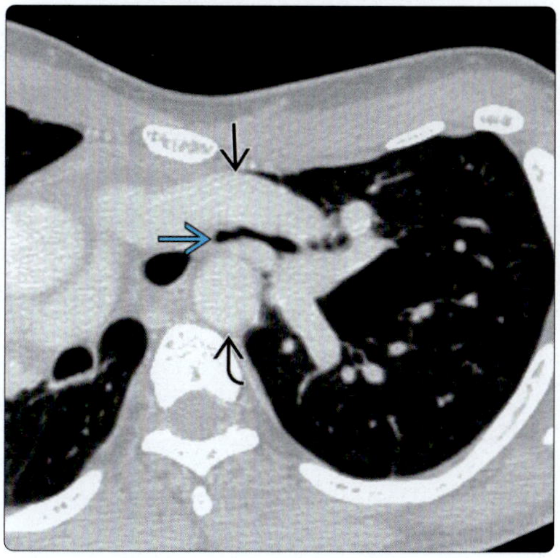

Pectus Excavatum

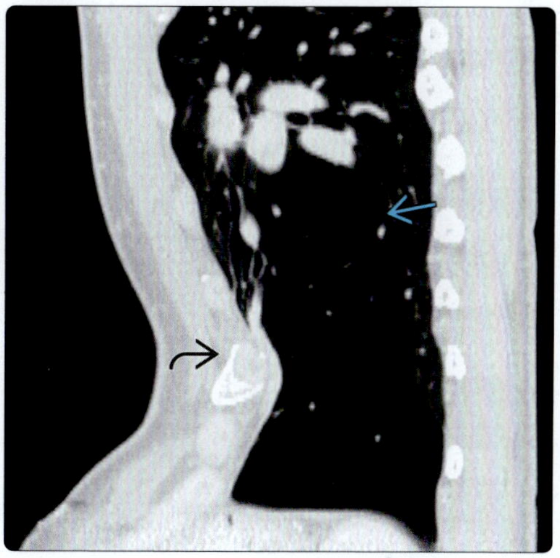

(Left) *Axial CECT of a patient with severe pectus excavatum deformity shows mediastinal shift to the right and severe compression of the left lower lobe bronchus between the left pulmonary artery anteriorly and the descending thoracic aorta posteriorly.* **(Right)** *Parasagittal CECT of the same patient shows severe left lower lobe hyperlucency, secondary to left lower lobe bronchus stenosis produced by the chest wall deformity. Note concavity of the lower anterior chest wall.*

Post Traumatic Deformity

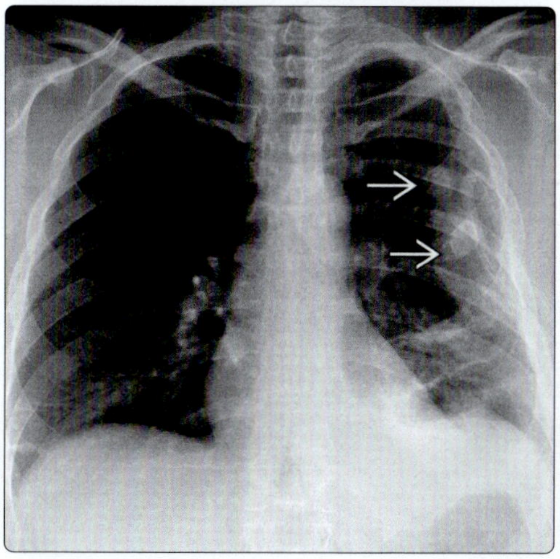

Post Traumatic Deformity

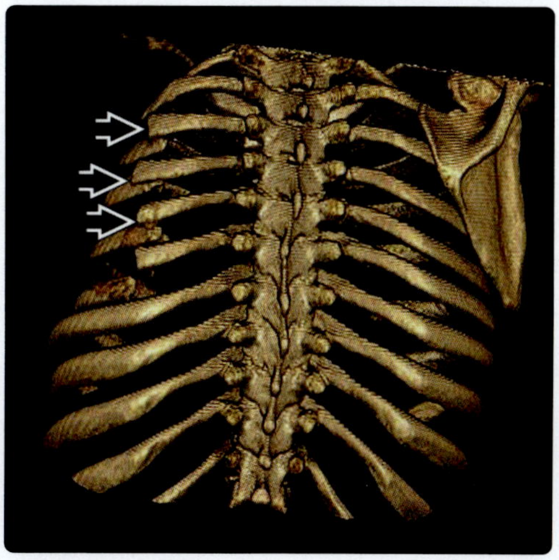

(Left) *PA chest radiograph of a patient with a remote history of blunt left chest trauma with multiple rib fractures and flail chest shows a low left lung volume secondary to left chest wall deformity from multiple healed contiguous rib fractures.* **(Right)** *NECT 3D reformatted image of the thoracic skeleton of the same patient shows deformity of the left rib cage secondary to multiple displaced acute left rib fractures.*

(Left) *Axial contrast-enhanced T1WI + FS MR of a patient with a left chest wall abscess that developed after coronary artery bypass surgery shows left anterolateral chest wall edema, abnormal enhancement of the soft tissues* ⇨*, and foci of susceptibility* ➔ *that suggest the presence of soft tissue gas.* **(Right)** *Axial NECT of the same patient obtained after chest wall debridement shows residual gas* ➔ *and fat stranding* ⇨ *at the surgical site, without evidence of organized fluid collections.*

Post Infectious Deformity

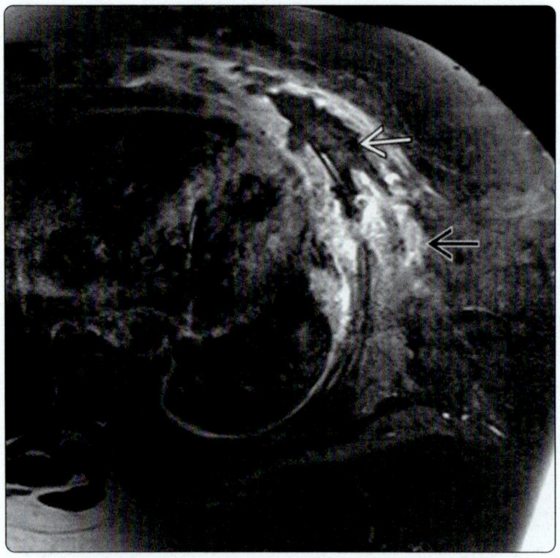

Post Infectious Deformity

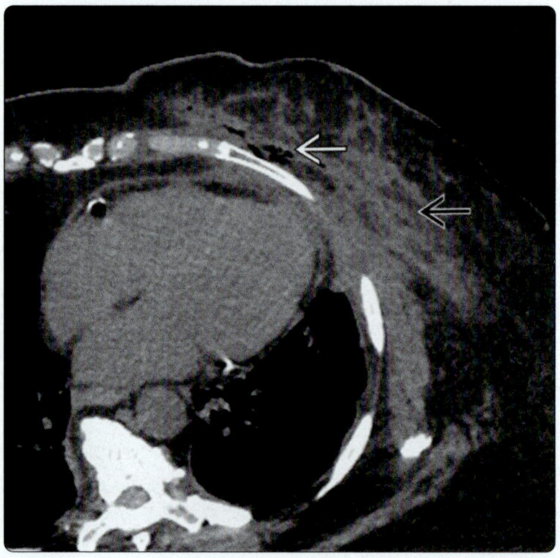

(Left) *PA chest radiograph of a patient with a history of recurrent right empyema treated surgically with an Eloesser flap shows deformity of the right lateral chest wall* ➔ *at the thoracostomy window.* **(Right)** *Axial CECT of the same patient shows a post surgical chest wall deformity due to open communication between the pleural space and the environment through a chest wall defect created surgically by the Eloesser flap thoracostomy* ➔*.*

Post Surgical Deformity

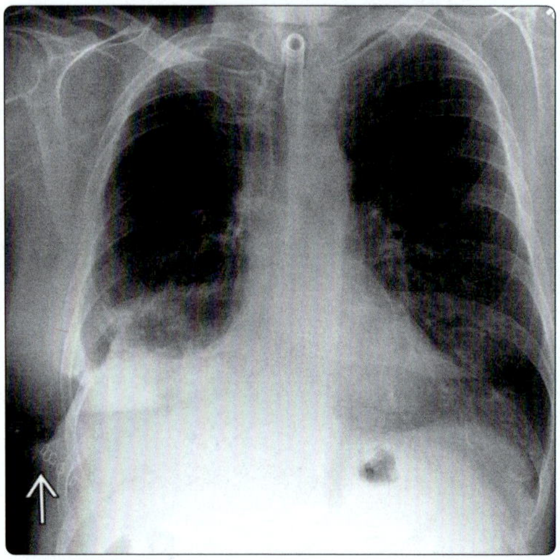

Post Surgical Deformity

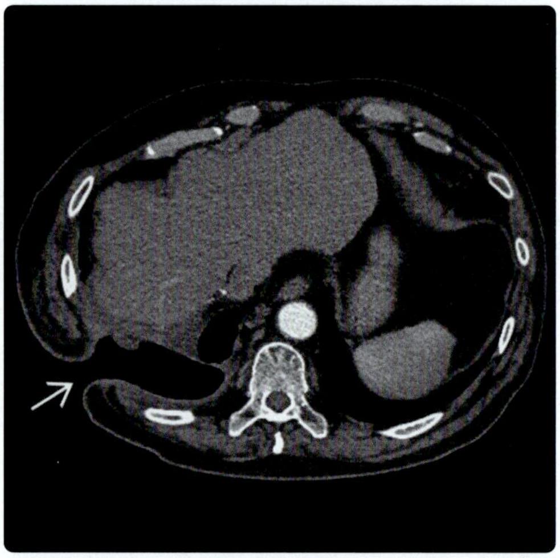

(Left) *Coned-down PA chest radiograph of a patient with a palpable right chest wall mass shows abnormal fat density* ↪ *within the thickened right chest wall soft tissues.* **(Right)** *Axial CECT of the same patient shows a well-circumscribed mass of homogeneous fat attenuation* ↪ *within the right serratus anterior muscle that represented a chest wall lipoma. Note absence of intrinsic soft tissue septa or nodules, which, if present, would raise suspicion for malignant degeneration.*

Chest Wall Tumor

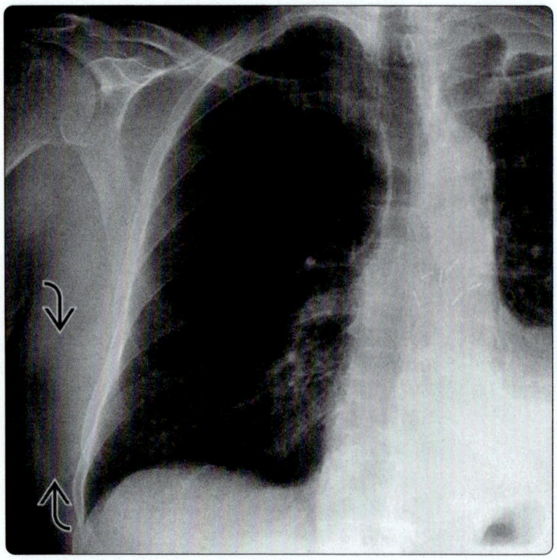

Chest Wall Tumor

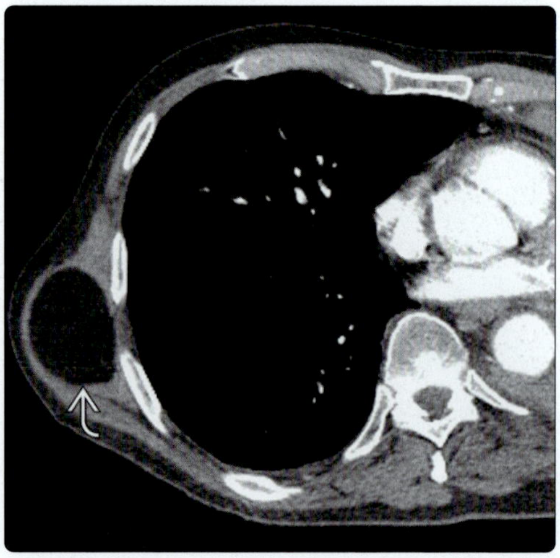

Chest Wall Tumor

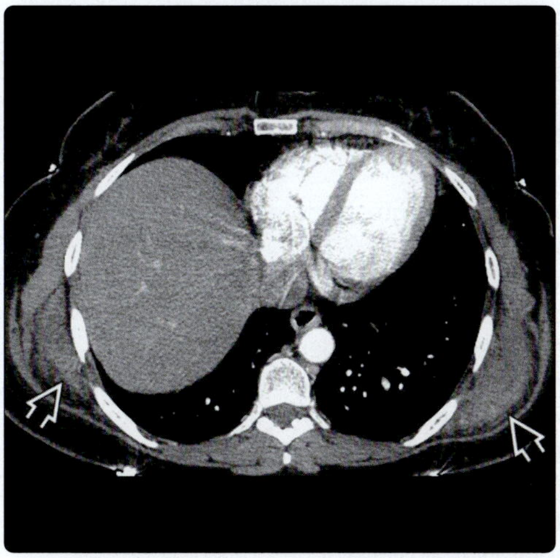

Chest Wall Tumor

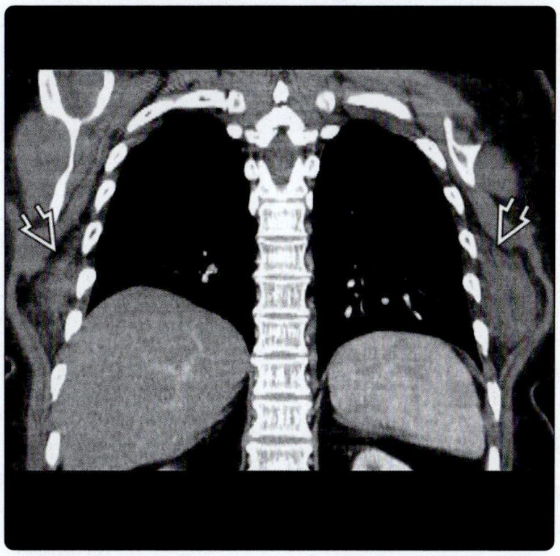

(Left) *Axial CECT of an asymptomatic patient shows relatively symmetric bilateral heterogeneous soft tissue masses in the subscapular spaces, characteristic of elastofibroma dorsi ➡.* **(Right)** *Coronal CECT of the same patient shows the typical subcapsular location and morphologic features of elastofibroma dorsi. These lesions typically manifest as soft tissue masses with areas of intrinsic fat attenuation ➡. Affected patients may present with pain &/or palpable chest wall mass(es).*

Chest Wall Tumor

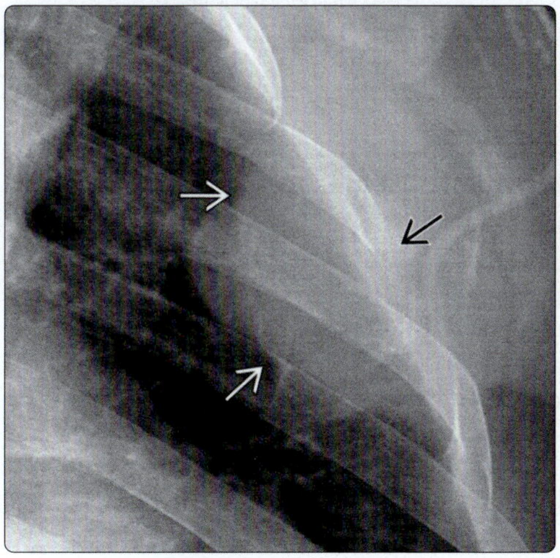

Chest Wall Tumor

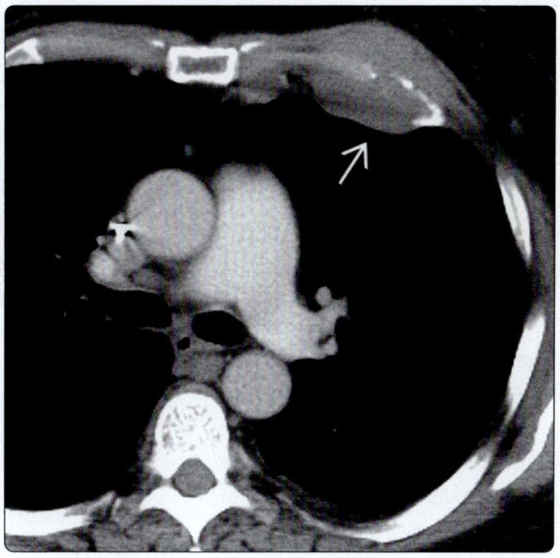

(Left) *Coned-down PA chest radiograph of a patient who presented with a palpable chest wall mass shows focal cortical disruption and fragmentation of a left rib ➡ secondary to an adjacent soft tissue mass ➡, which exhibits the incomplete border sign indicative of an extrapulmonary lesion.* **(Right)** *Axial CECT of the same patient shows an infiltrative soft tissue mass of the left anterior chest wall ➡ that produces local invasion of the intercostal muscles and rib destruction. Biopsy confirmed non-Hodgkin lymphoma.*

Poland Syndrome

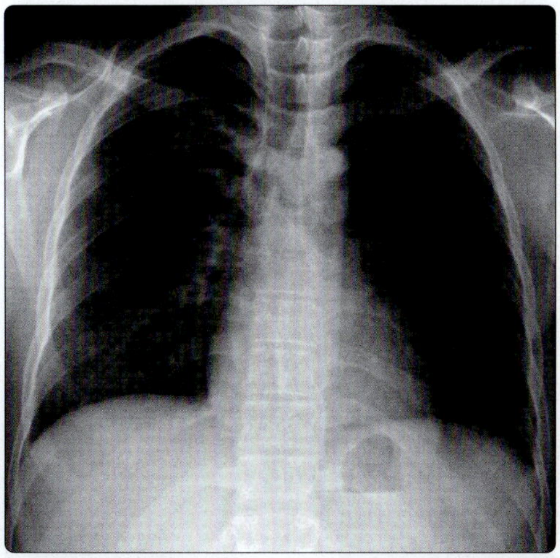

Poland Syndrome

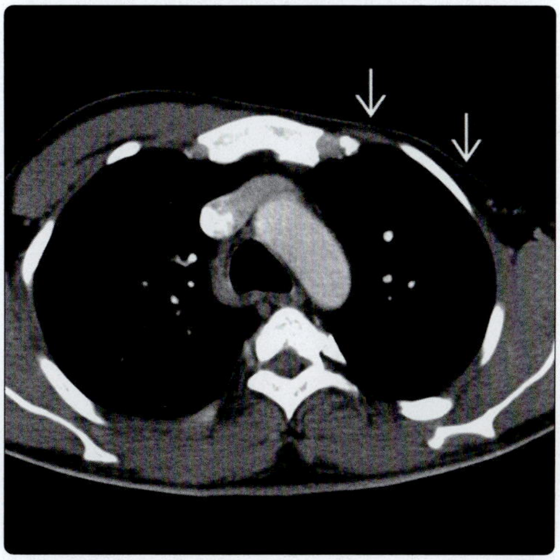

(Left) *PA chest radiograph of an asymptomatic patient with a chest wall deformity present since birth shows a hyperlucent left hemithorax due to congenital absence of the left pectoralis musculature.* **(Right)** *Axial CECT of the same patient shows complete absence of the left major and minor pectoralis muscles with resultant anterior chest wall asymmetry ➡ characteristic of Poland syndrome.*

DIFFERENTIAL DIAGNOSIS

Common

- Hiatal Hernia
- Bochdalek Hernia

Less Common

- Morgagni Hernia
- Traumatic Diaphragmatic Rupture

Rare but Important

- Lung Hernia
- Congenital Diaphragmatic Hernia
- Intrathoracic Fluid Collection (Mimic)

ESSENTIAL INFORMATION

Helpful Clues for Common Diagnoses

- **Hiatal Hernia**
  - Intramediastinal displacement of esophagus, stomach, &/or abdominal contents through esophageal hiatus
  - Sliding-type hiatal hernia: Most common
    - Gastroesophageal (GE) junction displaced superiorly; may contain entire stomach
  - Paraesophageal-type hiatal hernia
    - GE junction remains in peritoneal cavity; herniated stomach/abdominal contents through phrenoesophageal membrane defect alongside esophagus
  - Imaging
    - Radiography: Lateral displacement of azygoesophageal recess ± mediastinal air-fluid level
    - CT: Characterization of hernia type, identification of hernia contents, assessment of complications
    - Complications
      - □ *Volvulus*: At least 180° gastric rotation with gastric outlet obstruction; organoaxial > mesenteroaxial
      - □ *Incarceration*: Uncommon, may occur in large hernias that contain entire stomach
      - □ *Strangulation*: Uncommon, usually associated with volvulus, potential ischemia and perforation
- **Bochdalek Hernia**
  - 90% of developmental hernias; L > R
  - Herniation through remnant of pleuroperitoneal canal; posterior, posteromedial location
  - Retroperitoneal fat &/or portion of kidney

Helpful Clues for Less Common Diagnoses

- **Morgagni Hernia**
  - Anteromedial diaphragmatic defect between pars costalis and pars sternalis
  - R > L; incidental finding, mimics cardiophrenic angle mediastinal fat deposition
  - Multiplanar imaging allows identification of diaphragmatic defect and visualization of herniated abdominal contents
- **Traumatic Diaphragmatic Rupture**
  - Blunt trauma mechanism most commonly results in left diaphragmatic injury
  - Radiography: High position of nasogastric tube, intrathoracic gas-filled stomach/bowel loops
  - CT
    - Collar sign: Waist-like constriction of viscera at diaphragmatic defect
    - Dependent viscera sign: Intrathoracic abdominal organs which abut posterior ribs without intervening lung parenchyma

Helpful Clues for Rare Diagnoses

- **Lung Hernia**
  - May require surgical repair
  - Intercostal lung hernia: Postsurgical or posttraumatic; lung herniation into adjacent chest wall
  - Apical lung hernia: Defect in suprapleural membrane
    - Supraclavicular herniation
    - Increased intrathoracic pressure
    - Weight lifters, wind instrument players
- **Congenital Diaphragmatic Hernia**
  - Complete or partial diaphragmatic agenesis
  - L > R; identification of intrathoracic abdominal contents, mediastinal shift
  - May be associated with pulmonary hypoplasia

Hiatal Hernia

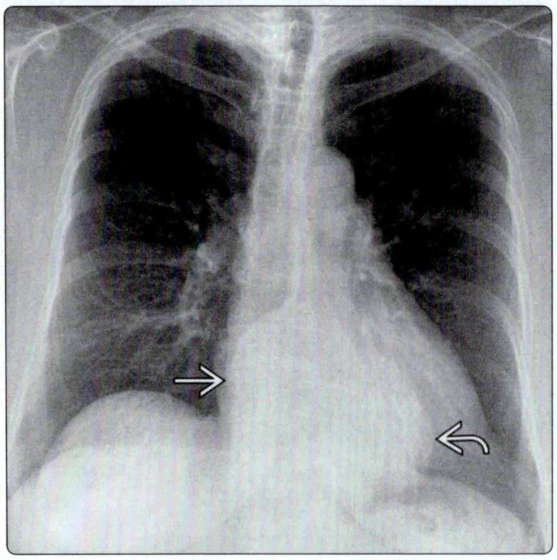

Hiatal Hernia

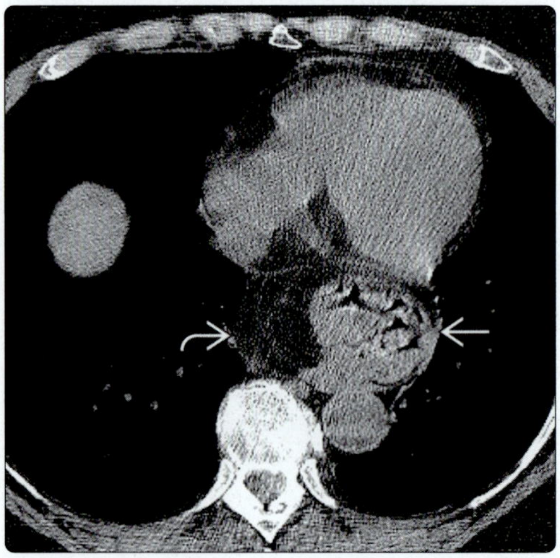

(Left) *PA chest radiograph of an asymptomatic woman shows a large hiatal hernia that manifests as a retrocardiac mass ➡ that produces lateral displacement of the inferior aspect of the azygoesophageal recess ➡. Identification of an intrinsic air-fluid level allows a confident radiographic diagnosis.* **(Right)** *Axial NECT of the same patient shows the retrocardiac hiatal hernia, which contains a portion of the stomach ➡ and omental fat ➡. Hiatal hernias are classified into sliding and paraesophageal types.*

Hiatal Hernia

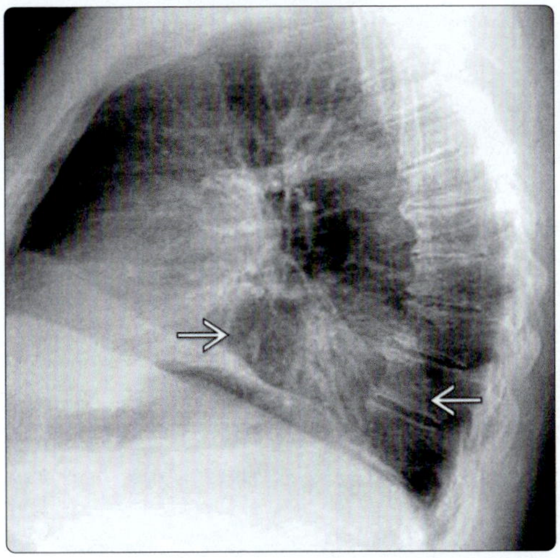

Hiatal Hernia

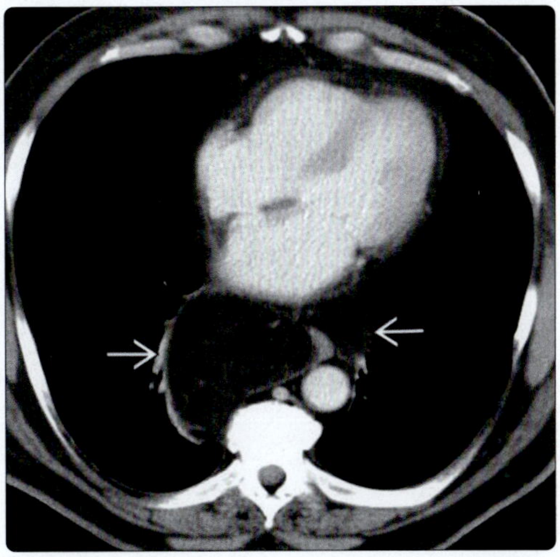

(Left) *Lateral chest radiograph shows a large retrocardiac mediastinal mass that represents a hiatal hernia. Note absence of an intrinsic air-fluid level, which makes the prospective radiographic diagnosis challenging.* **(Right)** *Axial CECT of the same patient shows the large hiatal hernia, which contains peritoneal fat . The stomach (not shown) remained in an intraabdominal location. Hiatal hernias characteristically contain portions of the stomach and fat but may also contain other abdominal organs.*

Hiatal Hernia

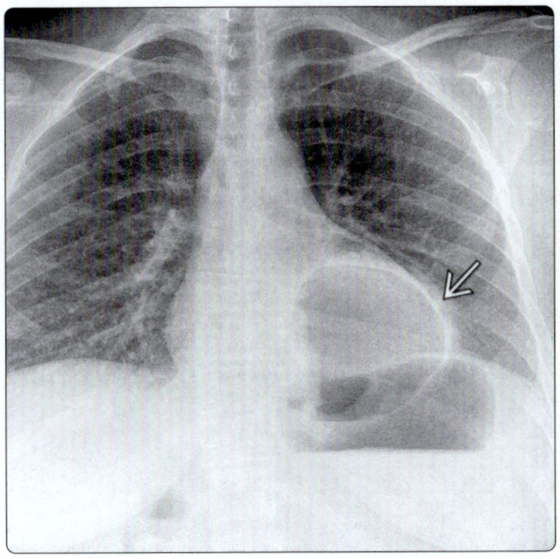

Hiatal Hernia

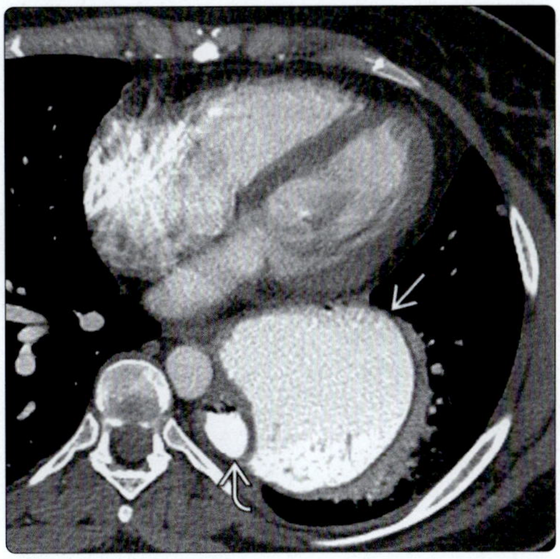

(Left) *PA chest radiograph of a patient with a large hiatal hernia shows a thin-walled, air-filled mass in the retrocardiac region that represents a herniated air-filled stomach .* **(Right)** *Axial CECT of the same patient shows oral contrast distending the herniated intrathoracic stomach . The esophagus is adjacent to the herniated stomach and the gastroesophageal junction (not shown) had an intraabdominal location, findings characteristic of the paraesophageal type of hiatal hernia.*

Hiatal Hernia

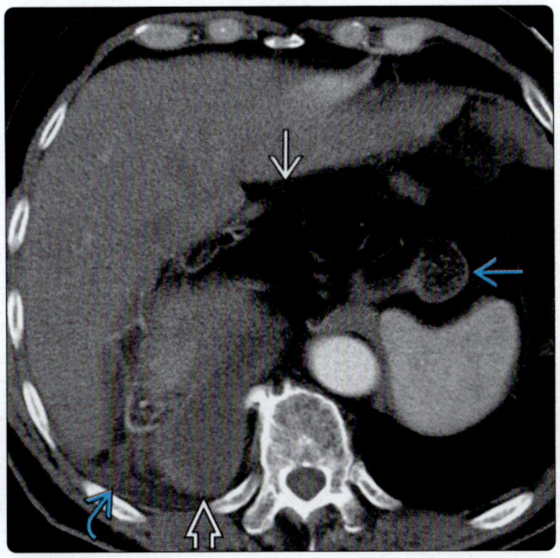

Hiatal Hernia

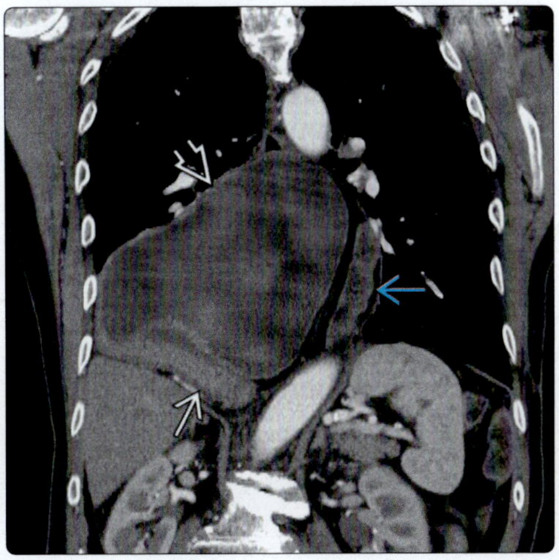

(Left) *Axial CECT of a patient with a large hiatal hernia complicated by strangulation shows the stomach , peritoneal fat , and transverse colon within the hernia sac. Perigastric fluid , mesenteric hyperemia, and fat stranding are signs of strangulation.* **(Right)** *Coronal CECT of the same patient shows a dilated fluid-filled gastric fundus , a collapsed distal stomach , and a portion of the transverse colon in the hernia. Strangulation is a known complication of hiatal hernia.*

Bochdalek Hernia

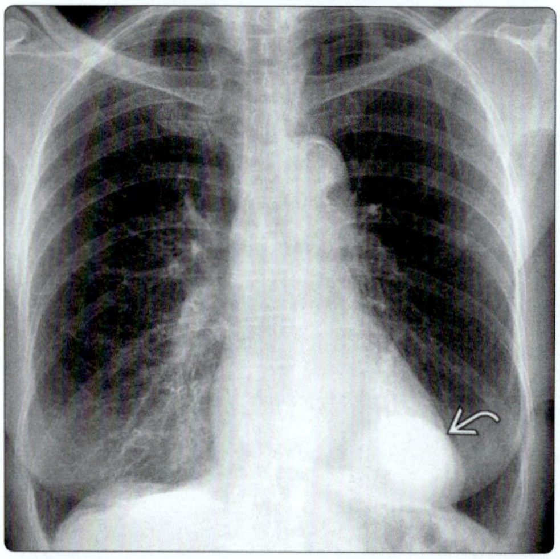

Bochdalek Hernia

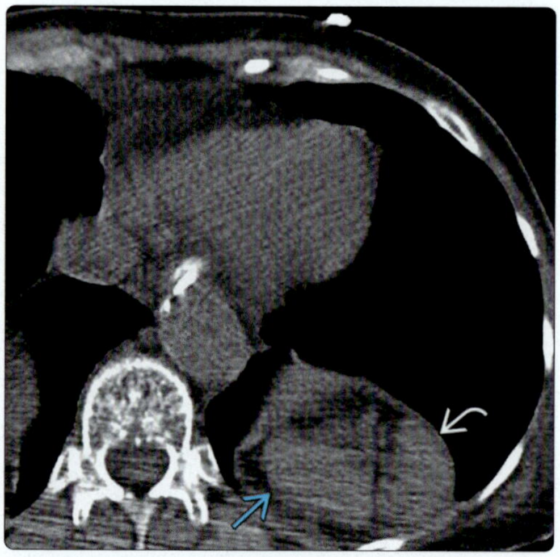

(Left) *PA chest radiograph of an asymptomatic 82-year-old woman shows a rounded left retrocardiac mass ➦ that obscures the adjacent hemidiaphragm and represents a Bochdalek hernia.* **(Right)** *Axial NECT of the same patient shows the left Bochdalek hernia, which contains fat, a portion of the upper pole of the left kidney ➡, and a portion of the spleen ➦. Bochdalek hernias result from intrathoracic herniation of abdominal contents through the embryologic remnant of the pleuroperitoneal canal.*

Morgagni Hernia

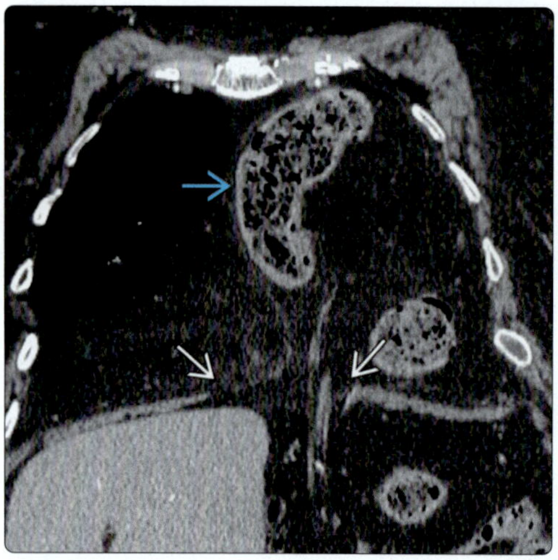

Morgagni Hernia

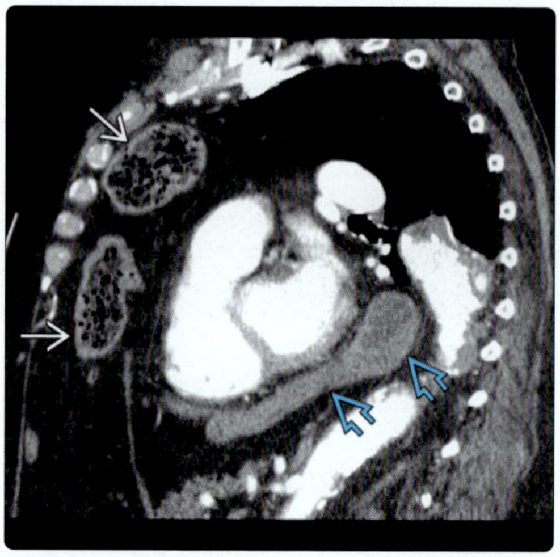

(Left) *Coronal CECT shows a large Morgagni hernia that contains mesenteric fat, mesenteric and omental vessels, and bowel ➡, which course into the thorax through an anterior diaphragmatic defect ➡.* **(Right)** *Sagittal CECT of the same patient shows the large anteriorly located Morgagni hernia, which contains bowel ➡ and mesenteric fat. There is also a moderate hiatus hernia that contains a portion of the stomach ➡ within the visceral mediastinum.*

Traumatic Diaphragmatic Rupture

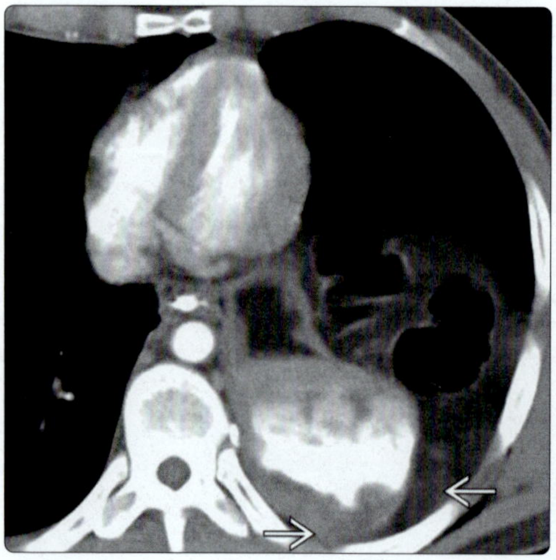

Traumatic Diaphragmatic Rupture

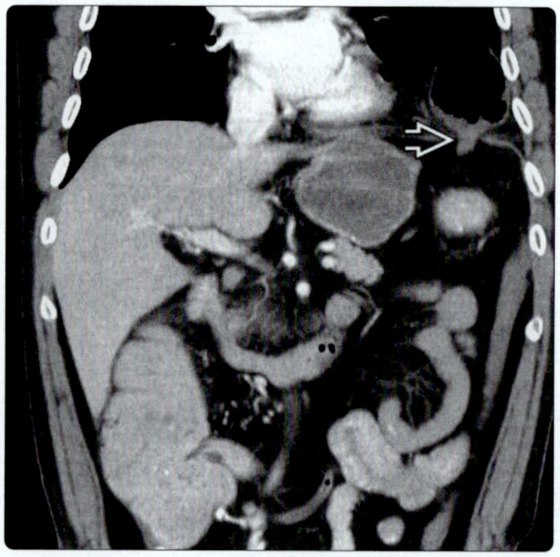

(Left) *Axial CECT of a patient with traumatic left diaphragmatic rupture shows an intrathoracic location of the stomach and bowel. The diagnosis is supported by the fact that abdominal organs abut the posterior ribs without intervening lung parenchyma, the so-called dependent visceral sign ➡.* **(Right)** *Coronal CECT of a patient with traumatic diaphragmatic rupture shows herniation of the gastric fundus through the left diaphragmatic defect ➡ and demonstrates the so-called collar sign.*

Traumatic Diaphragmatic Rupture

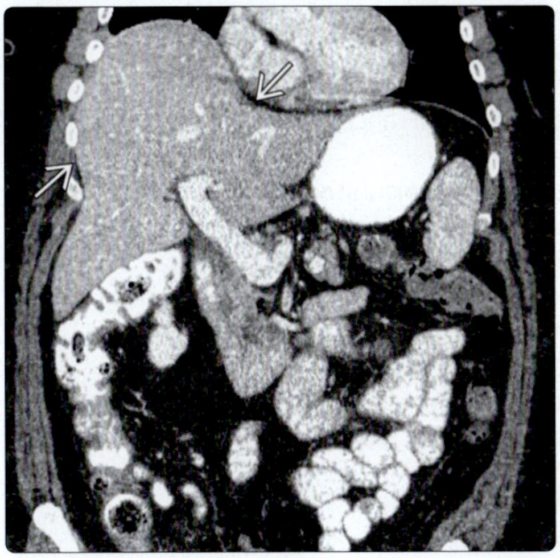

Lung Hernia

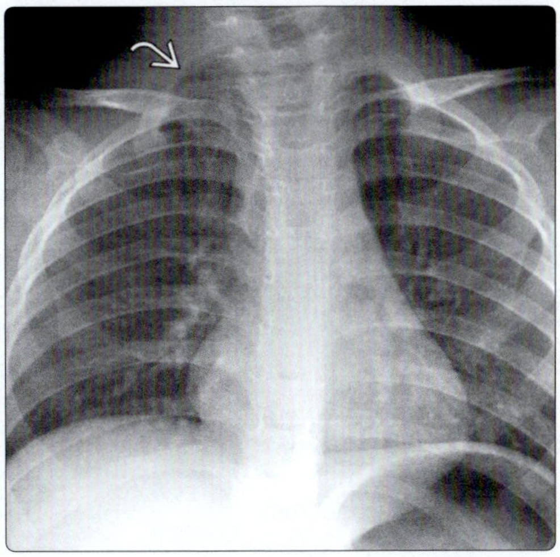

(Left) *Coronal CECT of a patient with chronic right hemidiaphragm rupture shows a mushroom-like morphology of the liver as it herniates through the right diaphragmatic defect.* **(Right)** *AP chest radiograph of a 3-year-old girl who presented with a palpable right supraclavicular mass shows a right apical lung hernia. These rare lung hernias are typically associated with repetitive maneuvers that increase intrathoracic pressures.*

Lung Hernia

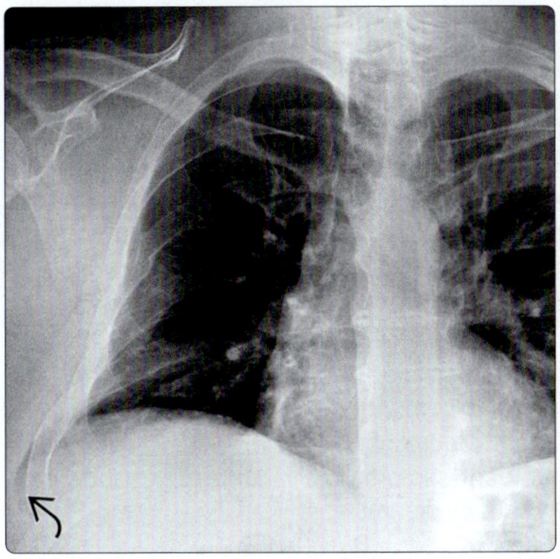

Lung Hernia

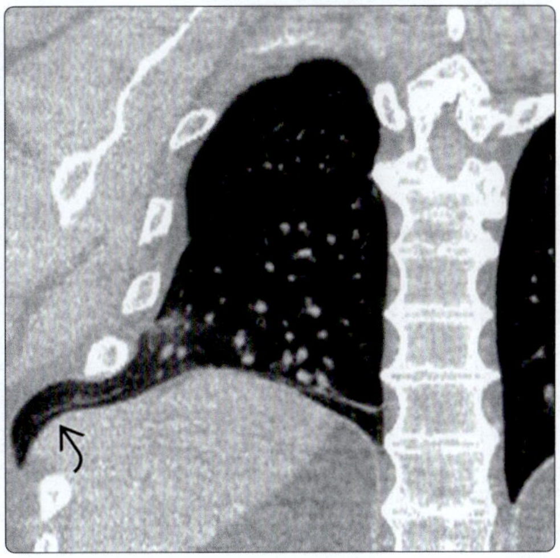

(Left) *PA chest radiograph of a 56-year-old man several years status post right diaphragmatic surgery shows lung herniation through the right lateral 6th intercostal space.* **(Right)** *Coronal NECT of the same patient shows a portion of the right lower lobe that herniates through the right lateral 6th intercostal space. Lung hernias are rare lesions and are typically complications of prior surgery or chest trauma.*

Congenital Diaphragmatic Hernia

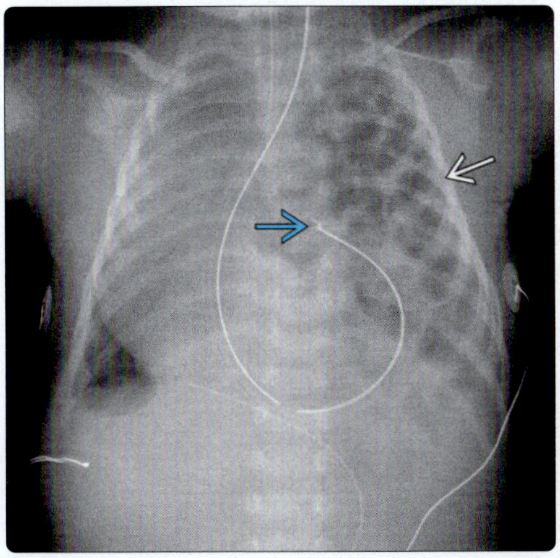

Congenital Diaphragmatic Hernia

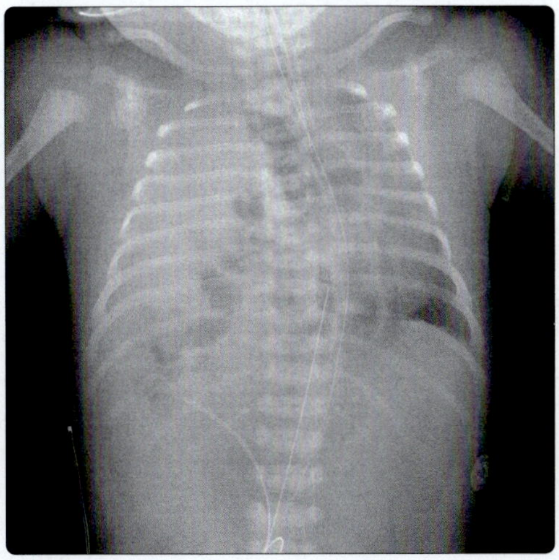

(Left) *AP chest radiograph of a neonate with respiratory distress shows multiple loops of bowel in the left hemithorax and shift of the mediastinum to the right. The nasogastric tube terminates in the herniated intrathoracic stomach.* **(Right)** *AP chest radiograph of an infant with respiratory distress shows a gasless abdomen, a nearly opaque right hemithorax, and a large right congenital diaphragmatic hernia with bowel and possibly liver in the right hemithorax as well as shift of the mediastinum to the left.*

DIFFERENTIAL DIAGNOSIS

Common

- Loculated Pleural Effusion
- Pleural Nodule/Mass
- Chest Wall Mass

Less Common

- Mediastinal Mass
- Pulmonary Mass

ESSENTIAL INFORMATION

Key Differential Diagnosis Issues

- Incomplete border sign
  - Characteristic of extrapulmonary lesions
  - Radiography
    - X-ray beam hits lesion tangentially: Well-defined portion of lesion border
    - X-ray beam hits lesion *en face*: Lesion border not discernible
    - Lesion may form obtuse angles with adjacent pleura/chest wall/mediastinum/diaphragm
  - Lung lesion: Surrounded by lung, visualization of entire lesion border
    - Pitfall: Peripheral lung lesion that abuts pleura, chest wall, mediastinum, diaphragm
      - May exhibit incomplete border sign on radiography
      - May form acute or obtuse angles with adjacent pleura/chest wall/mediastinum

Helpful Clues for Common Diagnoses

- **Loculated Pleural Effusion**
  - Empyema
    - Complex pleural fluid collection; typically multiloculated
    - Intrinsic gas, air-fluid level: Bronchopleural fistula
    - Associated smooth pleural thickening and pleural enhancement
    - Stranding of extrapleural fat
    - Predisposing conditions
      - Pneumonia and parapneumonic pleural effusion
      - Complication of surgical procedure
      - Complication of hemothorax
  - Loculated hemothorax
    - Density of pleural fluid varies with age of blood products
    - Acute: Low density (< 20 HU)
    - Subacute/chronic: High density (> 25 HU); frequent dependent clots if large volume
    - Pleural thickening and enhancement
    - Usually unilateral
    - Common causes: Trauma, surgery, complicated pneumonia
- **Pleural Nodule/Mass**
  - Pleural plaque
    - Asbestos-related pleural disease
      - Hallmark of occupational asbestos exposure
    - Multifocal discontinuous soft tissue pleural nodules ± complete or partial calcification
    - Normal pleura between pleural plaques
    - Typically spare costophrenic angles and apices
  - Pleural metastasis(es)
    - Most common cause of malignant pleural disease
      - Lung cancer
      - Breast cancer
      - Gastrointestinal cancer
      - Ovarian cancer
    - Single or multiple pleural nodules or masses; may
      - Produce circumferential nodular pleural thickening
      - Involve fissures and mediastinal pleura
      - Be associated with malignant pleural effusion
      - Mimic malignant pleural mesothelioma
  - Localized fibrous tumor of pleura
    - Most common benign primary pleural neoplasm
    - No reliable imaging features to distinguish benign from malignant lesions
      - 30% are malignant
    - Pleural lesion of variable size
    - Affected patients are often asymptomatic; patients with large lesions are often symptomatic
    - CT/MR
      - Pleural soft tissue nodule or mass
      - Vascular pedicle may allow lesion mobility within pleural space
      - Homogeneous or heterogeneous enhancement
      - Large lesions may exhibit necrosis &/or calcification
      - Areas of signal void in lesions with large internal vessels
  - Malignant pleural mesothelioma
    - Most common primary malignant pleural neoplasm
    - Imaging
      - Circumferential nodular pleural thickening with fissural involvement and lung encasement
      - Unilateral pleural effusion
      - Biphasic and sarcomatoid variants may manifest as bulky solitary pleural mass
- **Chest Wall Mass**
  - Abscess
    - May exhibit incomplete border sign with involvement of intercostal space &/or pleura
    - Predisposing conditions
      - Penetrating trauma
      - Surgery
      - Chest wall device placement or manipulation
  - Lipoma
    - Typically incidental finding in asymptomatic patient
    - CT/MR
      - Homogeneous fat attenuation/signal
      - No soft tissue components or thick septa
  - Metastasis
    - Hematogenous metastatic disease
    - Rib lesion with skeletal destruction ± soft tissue component
    - Soft tissue mass with variable cortical erosion/lysis of adjacent skeletal structures
  - Sarcoma
    - Painful palpable chest wall mass
    - Chondrosarcoma: Most common primary malignant chest wall neoplasm
      - Costosternal or costovertebral junction

- Variable imaging appearance according to size
- Frequent local invasion of adjacent structures
- Liposarcoma
  - 2nd most common primary malignant chest wall neoplasm
  - Usually in deep chest wall compartments: Axillary fossa, subscapular fossa, thoracic inlet
  - Variable appearance according to size
  - Fat attenuation mass with thick soft tissue septa &/or nodules
  - Locally invasive, imperceptible capsule
  - Lymphadenopathy is uncommon
  - Well-differentiated liposarcomas may be difficult to differentiate from benign atypical lipomas if there is paucity of soft tissue components
- Peripheral nerve sheath tumor
  - Origin from intercostal nerves, spinal nerve roots
  - Benign: Schwannoma, neurofibroma
    - Usually solitary, unless associated with neurofibromatosis (NF)
    - Schwannoma: Associated with NF type 2
    - Neurofibroma: Associated with NF type 1 (plexiform neurofibroma)
  - Malignant peripheral nerve sheath tumor

Helpful Clues for Less Common Diagnoses

- **Mediastinal Mass**
  - May exhibit incomplete border sign
  - Mediastinal contour abnormality on frontal radiography
  - Localization to mediastinal compartment on lateral radiography
    - Anterior
    - Posterior
    - Middle
  - CT/MR
    - Localization to mediastinal compartment
      - Prevascular
      - Visceral
      - Paravertebral
    - Characterization of tissue components
      - Soft tissue, fat, fluid, calcification
    - Evaluation of adjacent structures
      - Encasement, invasion
      - Lymphadenopathy
  - Differential diagnosis based on demographics, clinical presentation, mediastinal compartment, tissue characteristics, presence or absence of lymphadenopathy
- **Pulmonary Mass**
  - Etiologies
    - Lung cancer
    - Metastasis
  - Peripheral lung mass may exhibit incomplete border sign and mimic extrapulmonary lesion
    - Lung lesions that abut pleura, chest wall, mediastinum, diaphragm
    - Lung lesions that form acute angles with pleura, chest wall, mediastinum, or diaphragm may allow correct intrapulmonary localization
    - Lung lesions that invade chest wall or mediastinum
    - ± associated lymphadenopathy
  - Lung abscess
    - Usually in setting of complicated pneumonia
    - Radiography
      - Variable size, peripheral or central mass-like opacity, ± air-fluid level
      - ± lymphadenopathy
    - CT
      - Well-defined cavitary mass; may contain air &/or fluid
      - Variable wall thickness, usually > 3 mm
      - ± lymphadenopathy; may exhibit internal necrosis

SELECTED REFERENCES

1. Aluja Jaramillo F et al: Pleural tumours and tumour-like lesions. Clin Radiol. 73(12):1014-24, 2018
2. Hsu CC et al: The incomplete border sign. J Thorac Imaging. 29(4):W48, 2014
3. Walker CM et al: Tumorlike conditions of the pleura. Radiographics. 32(4):971-85, 2012

Loculated Pleural Effusion

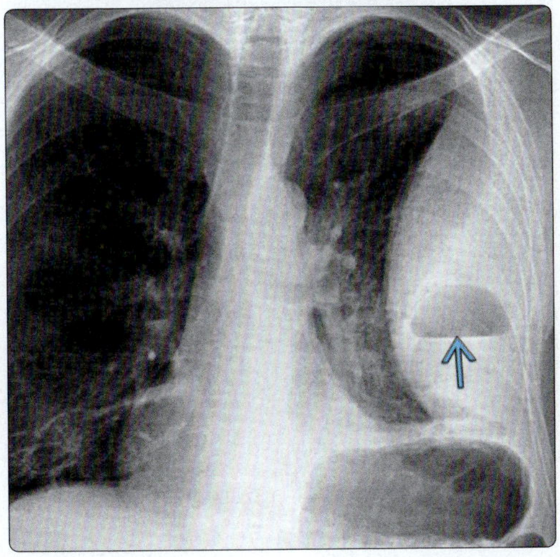

Loculated Pleural Effusion

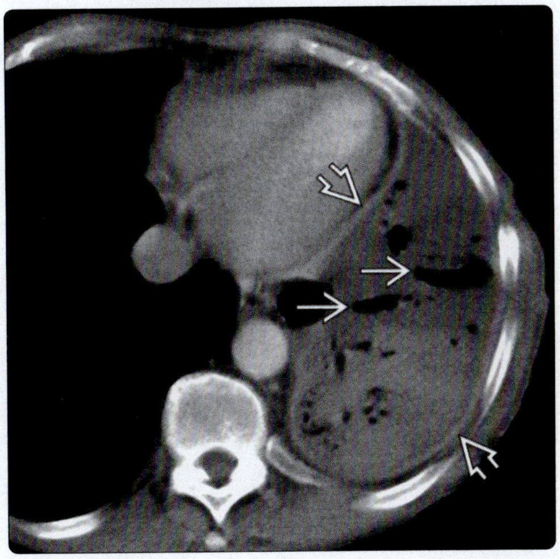

(Left) *AP chest radiograph of a patient who presented with fever, cough, and a history of prior complicated pneumonia shows a large loculated left pleural effusion with an intrinsic air-fluid level ➡, typical of empyema complicated by bronchopleural fistula.* **(Right)** *Axial CECT of a patient with a left empyema complicated by a bronchopleural fistula shows a complex loculated left pleural effusion that exhibits enhancement of the pleural surfaces ➡, heterogeneous pleural fluid, and multiloculated air pockets ➡.*

Incomplete Border Sign

Pleural Nodule/Mass

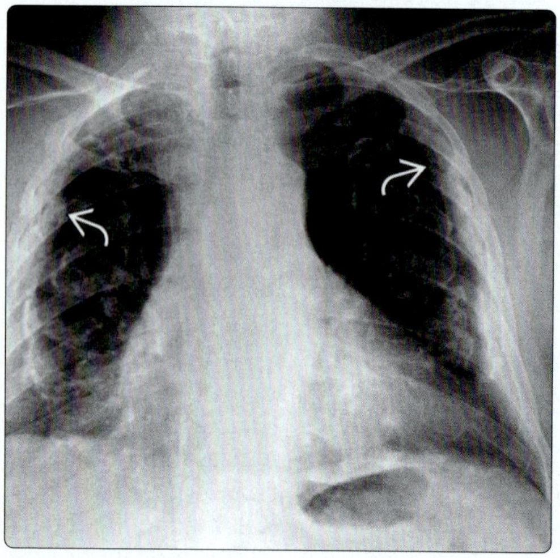

Pleural Nodule/Mass

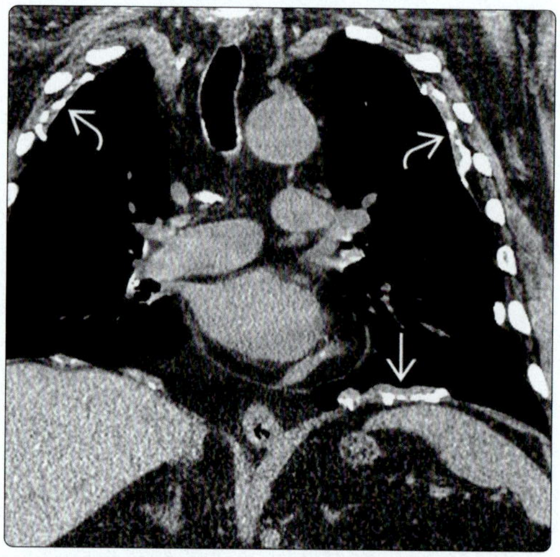

(Left) *PA chest radiograph of an 83-year-old man with prior occupational exposure to asbestos shows multifocal discontinuous nodular pleural thickening with calcification. Several lesions exhibit the incomplete border sign consistent with pleural plaques from asbestos-related pleural disease.* **(Right)** *Axial NECT of the same patient shows classic bilateral discontinuous calcified pleural plaques along the lateral pleural surfaces and the central tendinous portions of the hemidiaphragms with intervening normal pleura.*

Pleural Nodule/Mass

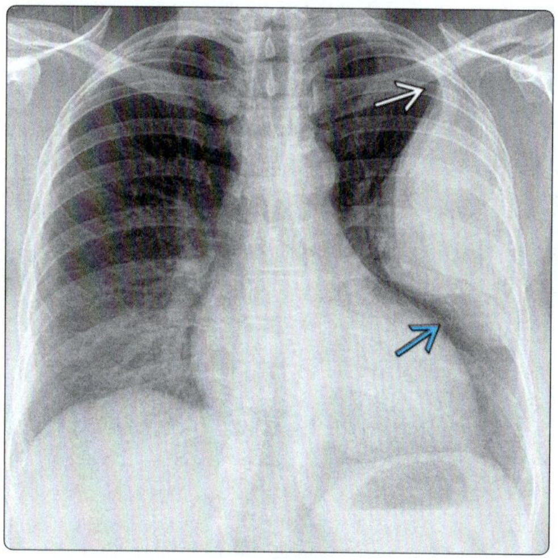

Pleural Nodule/Mass

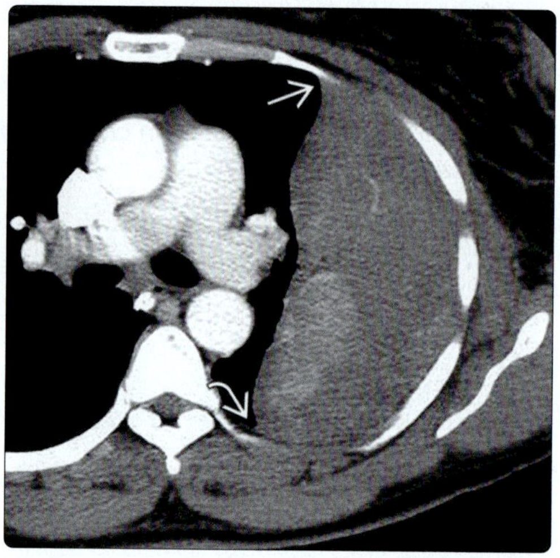

(Left) *PA chest radiograph of a patient with shortness of breath and chest pain shows a large soft tissue mass in the left hemithorax that exhibits the incomplete border sign and forms an obtuse angle with the adjacent pleura.* **(Right)** *Axial CECT of the same patient shows a large heterogeneously enhancing left pleural mass that forms both acute and obtuse angles with the adjacent pleura. Localized fibrous tumor of the pleura was diagnosed at surgical excision.*

Chest Wall Mass

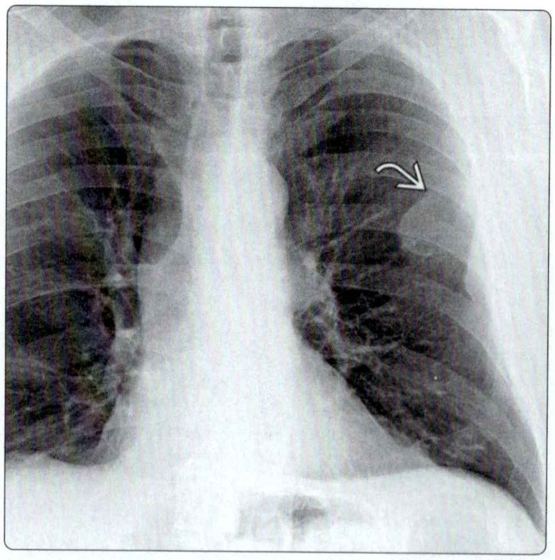

Chest Wall Mass

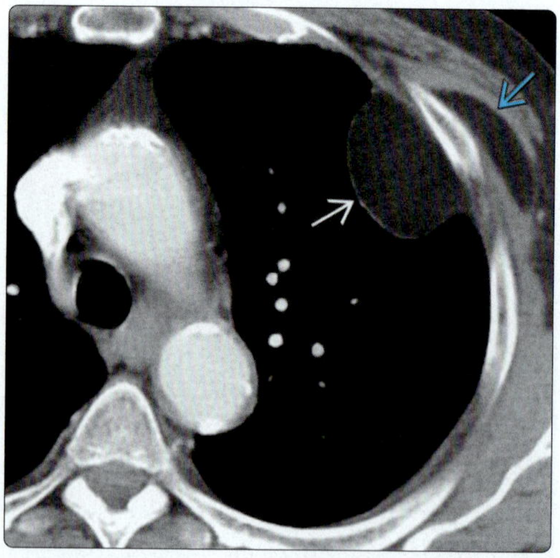

(Left) *PA chest radiograph of an asymptomatic patient with an incidentally discovered radiographic abnormality shows an ovoid mass in the left mid thorax that exhibits the incomplete border sign consistent with a pleural or chest wall lesion.* **(Right)** *Axial CECT of the same patient shows that the radiographic abnormality corresponds to a left chest wall lipoma. The lesion exhibits homogeneous fat attenuation as well as intrathoracic and intramuscular chest wall components.*

Chest Wall Mass

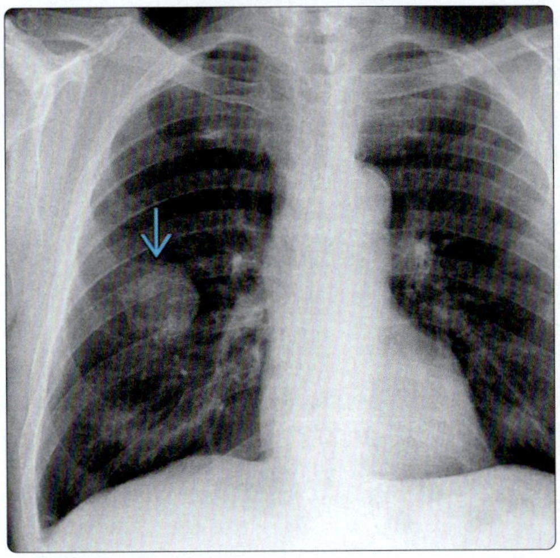

Chest Wall Mass

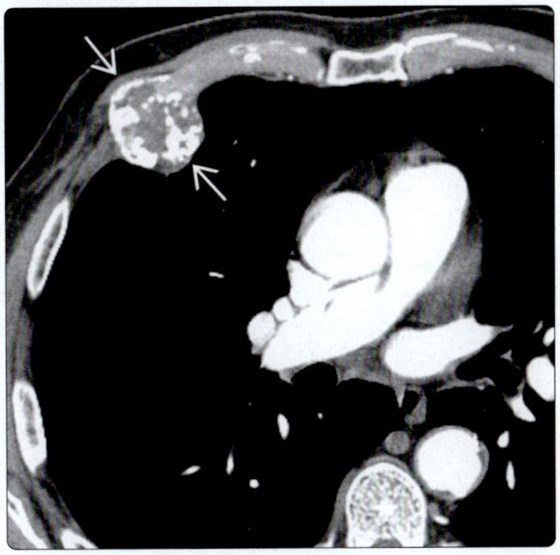

(Left) *Coned-down PA chest radiograph of a patient with right chest wall pain shows a focal heterogeneous mass* ⇨ *that exhibits the incomplete border sign and arises from the right anterior 4th rib. These findings are consistent with a chest wall lesion.* **(Right)** *Axial CECT of the same patient shows a heavily calcified mass* ➡ *arising from the cartilaginous portion of the right anterior 4th rib. The clinical presentation, chest wall location, and pattern of calcification are typical of chondrosarcoma.*

Chest Wall Mass

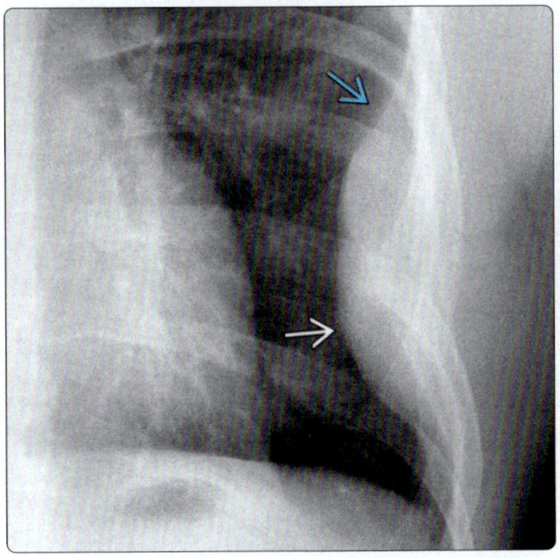

Chest Wall Mass

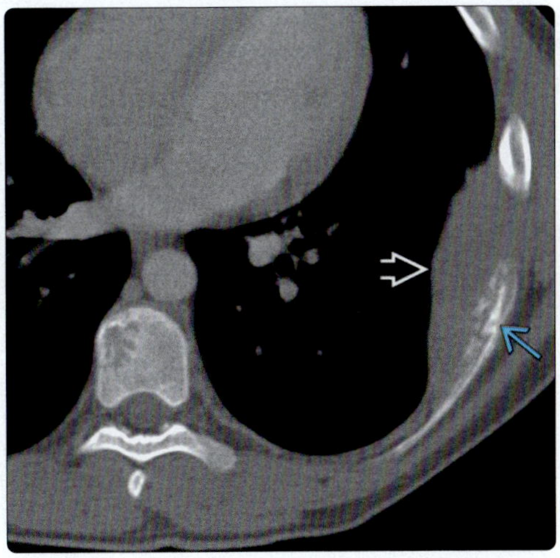

(Left) *Coned-down PA chest radiograph of a young patient with chest wall pain shows an elongate mass with a well-defined medial border* ➡ *and the incomplete border sign* ⇨ *along the superior aspect of the lesion. These findings together with the finding of erosion of an anterior rib are consistent with a chest wall location.* **(Right)** *Axial CECT of the same patient shows a left chest wall mass* ➡*, which produces cortical erosion and destruction of an adjacent rib* ⇨*. Biopsy confirmed the diagnosis of Askin tumor.*

Mediastinal Mass

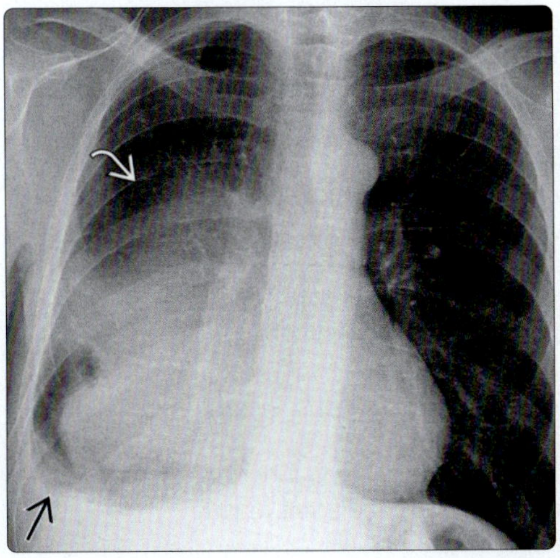

Mediastinal Mass

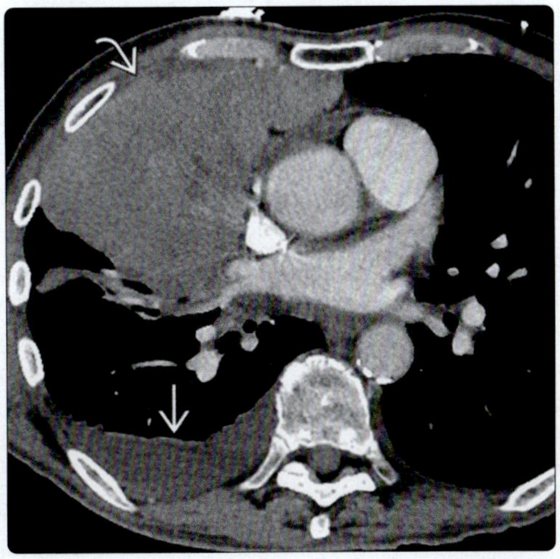

(Left) *PA chest radiograph of a 79-year-old man with a large anterior mediastinal thymoma shows a large opacity in the right hemithorax that exhibits the incomplete border sign manifesting as loss of the superolateral border of the lesion* ➡ *due to its extrapulmonary location. Note the small right pleural effusion* ⇨*.* **(Right)** *Axial CECT of the same patient shows a large right prevascular mediastinal soft tissue mass* ➡ *that corresponds to the radiographic abnormality and a small right pleural effusion* ➡*.*

DIFFERENTIAL DIAGNOSIS

Common

- Undifferentiated Pleomorphic Sarcoma
- Neurofibroma
- Schwannoma
- Hemangioma
- Lipoma
- Metastatic Disease

Less Common

- Secondary Invasion
- Elastofibroma Dorsi
- Fibromatosis

Rare but Important

- Lymphoma
- Liposarcoma
- Angiosarcoma
- Radiation-Associated Malignancy
- Malignant Peripheral Nerve Sheath Tumor

ESSENTIAL INFORMATION

Key Differential Diagnosis Issues

- Classification of primary soft tissue neoplasms of chest wall based on tissue type
  - Fibrohistiocytic
    - Undifferentiated pleomorphic sarcoma
  - Neurogenic
    - Benign peripheral nerve sheath: Neurofibroma, schwannoma
    - Malignant peripheral nerve sheath tumor
  - Adipocytic
    - Lipoma
    - Liposarcoma
  - Vascular
    - Hemangioma
    - Angiosarcoma
  - Fibroblastic-myofibroblastic
    - Elastofibroma dorsi
    - Fibromatosis

Helpful Clues for Common Diagnoses

- **Undifferentiated Pleomorphic Sarcoma**
  - Most common malignant soft tissue neoplasm of chest wall in adults
  - 3 histologic subtypes
    - High-grade pleomorphic sarcoma
    - Pleomorphic sarcoma with giant cells
    - Pleomorphic sarcoma with prominent inflammation
  - Imaging
    - Soft tissue mass that involves deep fascia or skeletal muscle
    - Enhances heterogeneously
    - Involvement of adjacent osseous structures is common
    - Internal mineralization often identified in periphery after treatment
- **Neurofibroma**
  - Benign neoplasm originating from nerve sheaths
  - Imaging
    - Low attenuation on CT
    - Heterogeneous enhancement
- **Schwannoma**
  - Benign neoplasm originating from nerve sheaths
  - Imaging
    - Smooth, rounded lesions that are isodense or hypodense to muscle
    - Variable enhancement
- **Hemangioma**
  - Vascular lesions that typically include nonvascular elements
  - Imaging
    - Soft tissue mass with poorly defined margins
    - Heterogeneous low attenuation on CT
    - Marked enhancement
    - Phleboliths may be present
- **Lipoma**
  - Most common benign soft tissue neoplasm
  - Imaging
    - Homogeneous fat attenuation is most common
    - Connective tissue septations or calcifications may be present
    - No enhancement is typical
      - Septations may demonstrate some enhancement
- **Metastatic Disease**
  - Typically seen only in setting of extensive metastatic disease elsewhere in body
  - Considered indicator of poor prognosis
  - Patterns of metastatic spread
    - Direct extension
    - Hematogenous
    - Lymphatic
  - Frequently demonstrate imaging characteristics specific to primary neoplasms from which they are derived

Helpful Clues for Less Common Diagnoses

- **Secondary Invasion**
  - Aggressive thoracic malignancies
    - Lung cancer
    - Breast cancer
    - Pleural neoplasms
    - Mediastinal neoplasms
  - CT considered inferior to MR due to differences in soft tissue contrast
- **Elastofibroma Dorsi**
  - Pseudotumor of soft tissues
  - Most occur in deep dorsal regions
    - Between chest wall and lower 1/3 of scapula
    - Beneath serratus anterior and latissimus dorsi muscles
  - Imaging
    - Poorly defined, lenticular-shaped, heterogeneous soft tissue mass
    - Linear regions of low attenuation secondary to fat
    - Similar attenuation as adjacent muscle
- **Fibromatosis**
  - a.k.a. desmoid tumor
  - Imaging
    - Soft tissue mass hypodense, isodense, or hyperdense to muscle

- Margins tend to be poorly defined

Helpful Clues for Rare Diagnoses

- **Lymphoma**
  - Typically results from direct invasion by Hodgkin lymphoma or large B-cell lymphoma arising from mediastinum, axilla, or bone
    - Direct invasion occurs in 6.4% of patients with Hodgkin lymphoma
  - Primary malignant lymphoma accounts for only 2.4% of primary chest wall tumors
  - Imaging
    - Infiltrative soft tissue masses in parasternal soft tissues
    - Direct extension of lymph nodes or masses in prevascular mediastinal compartment
    - Spread around bone and cartilage
- **Liposarcoma**
  - 2nd most common chest wall malignancy of soft tissue origin
  - Imaging appearance depends primarily on histologic features and internal composition
    - Well differentiated: 50-75% adipose tissue
      - Fat attenuation between -40 and -120 HU on CT
    - Imaging features differentiating liposarcoma from lipoma
      - > 10 cm in size
      - Internal septations thicker than 2 mm
      - Nodular regions of nonadipose tissue
      - Adipose tissue tissue accounting for < 75% of tumor's total content
- **Angiosarcoma**
  - Most common primary malignancy of vascular origin
  - Strongly associated with chronic lymphedema especially after mastectomy for breast cancer
  - Imaging features depend on lesion location
    - Superficial
      - Focal soft tissue mass with associated skin thickening and subcutaneous edema
    - Deep
      - Tend to manifest as focal mass without associated skin thickening and subcutaneous edema
    - Heterogeneous with internal regions of necrosis, hemorrhage, and vascularity
    - Enhancement of vascular tissue
- **Radiation-Associated Malignancy**
  - Most malignancies are histologically sarcomas
  - Aggressive lesions associated with high recurrence rate and distant metastatic spread
  - Most malignancies develop within or adjacent to radiation site
    - Correlating imaging findings with radiation treatment plan is helpful
  - Changes in appearance of previously irradiated bone, especially when associated soft tissue mass is present
  - Imaging
    - Osseous destruction and soft tissue mass are most common
      - Absence can help differentiate extensive benign osseous changes from tumor
    - Infiltration of adjacent structures
- **Malignant Peripheral Nerve Sheath Neoplasm**
  - Spindle cell sarcoma of nerve sheath origin that involves large and medium-sized nerves
  - Associated with neurofibromatosis type 1
    - Leading cause of cancer-related death in these patients
  - Imaging
    - Large soft tissue mass adjacent to 1 or more peripheral nerves
    - May invade adjacent osseous structures
    - Heterogeneity due to internal necrosis, hemorrhage, &/or cellularity
    - Malignant transformation
      - Sudden change in size of benign nerve sheath neoplasm
      - Heterogeneous attenuation on CT
      - Invasion of adjacent structures

Undifferentiated Pleomorphic Sarcoma

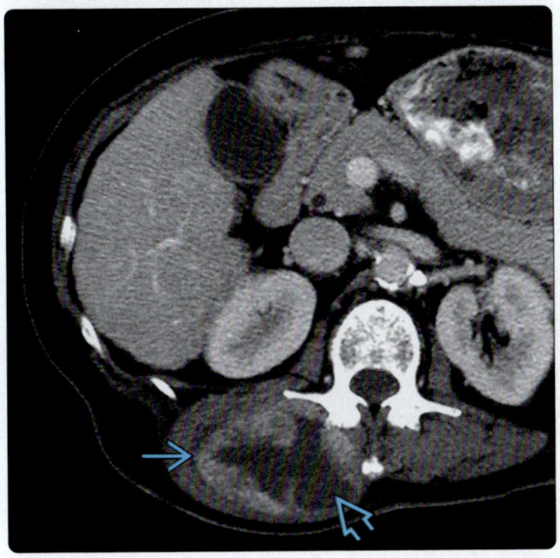

Undifferentiated Pleomorphic Sarcoma

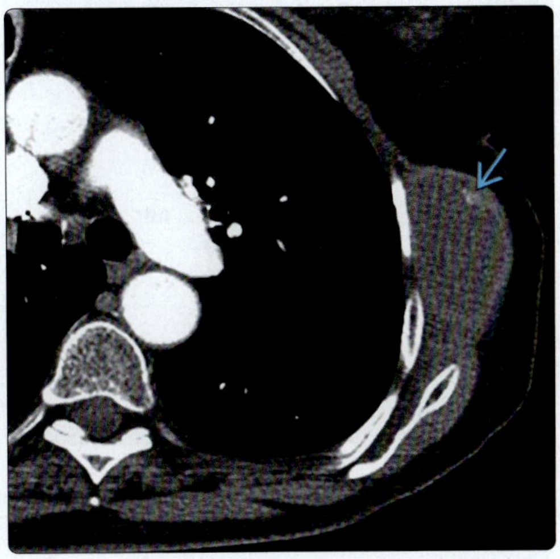

(Left) *Axial CECT of a patient with undifferentiated pleomorphic sarcoma (UPS) demonstrates a heterogeneous mass arising from the right posterior chest wall with regions of enhancing soft tissue and internal necrosis.* **(Right)** *Axial CECT shows a homogeneous soft tissue mass in the left chest wall with a small region of internal enhancement. UPS typically manifests as a soft tissue mass involving the deep fascia or skeletal muscle that enhances heterogeneously.*

(Left) *Axial CECT of a patient with neurofibromatosis type 1 demonstrates a predominantly low-attenuation mass in the right anterior chest wall consistent with a neurofibroma. This lesion typically manifests as a low-attenuation mass with heterogeneous enhancement.* **(Right)** *Axial CECT shows an ill-defined, heterogeneous lesion in the left chest wall composed of fat & soft tissue representing a hemangioma. Hemangiomas are vascular lesions that may contain nonvascular elements, such as fat.*

Neurofibroma

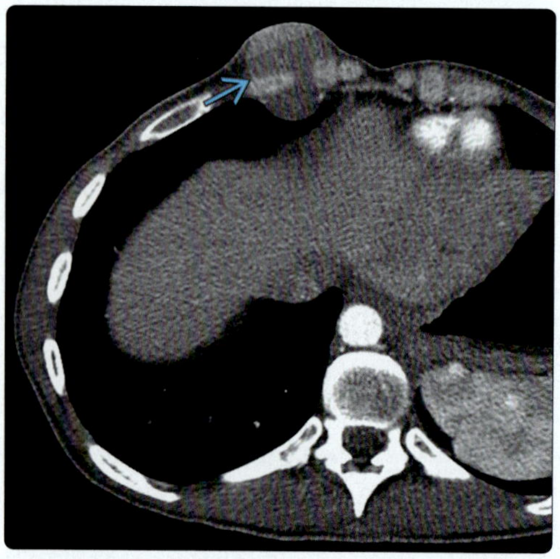

Hemangioma

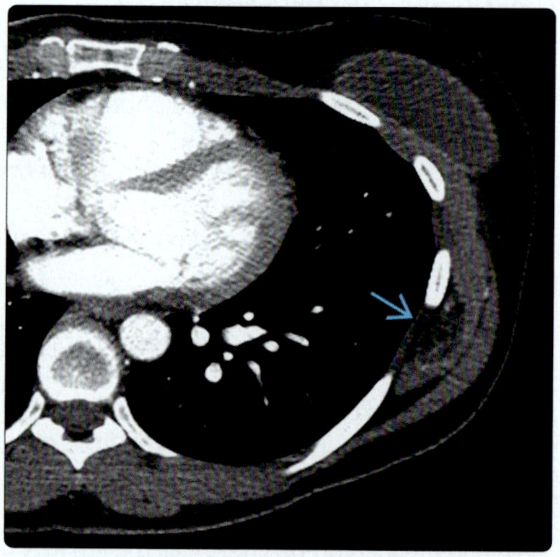

(Left) *Axial CECT demonstrates a well-defined lesion in the left chest wall consisting entirely of fat, consistent with a lipoma. Lipomas are predominantly fat-containing lesions, although thin septations or calcifications may be present.* **(Right)** *Axial CECT of a patient with non-Hodgkin lymphoma shows a soft tissue mass in the right prevascular mediastinum that results in multifocal chest wall invasion. A right pleural effusion is present.*

Lipoma

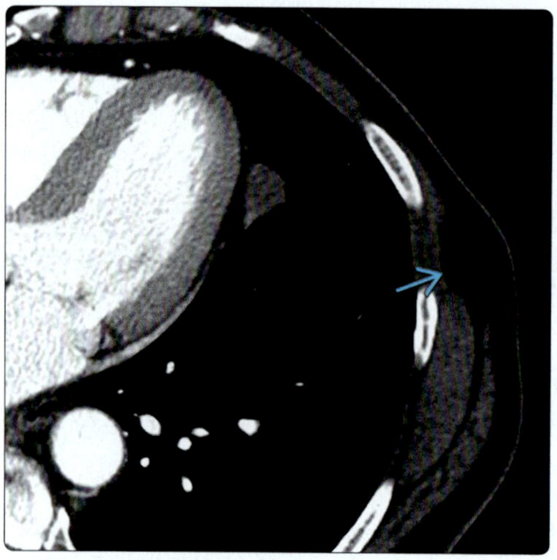

Secondary Invasion

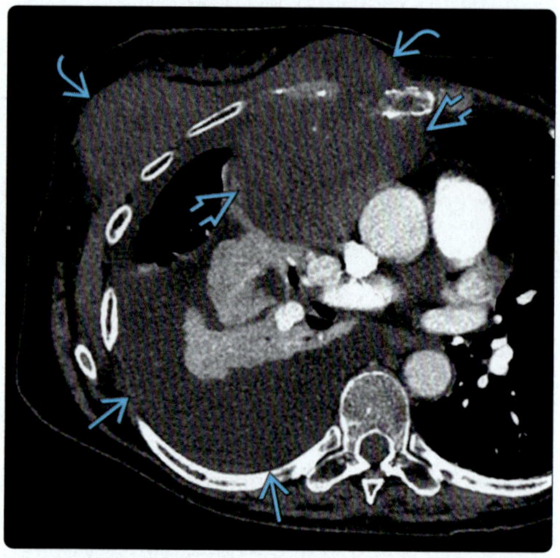

(Left) *Axial CECT of a patient with squamous cell carcinoma of the right lung demonstrates a large cavitary mass invading the right chest wall.* **(Right)** *Axial CECT of an asymptomatic patient demonstrates ill-defined lesions composed of soft tissue and fat located between the chest wall and scapula bilaterally characteristic of elastofibroma dorsi.*

Secondary Invasion

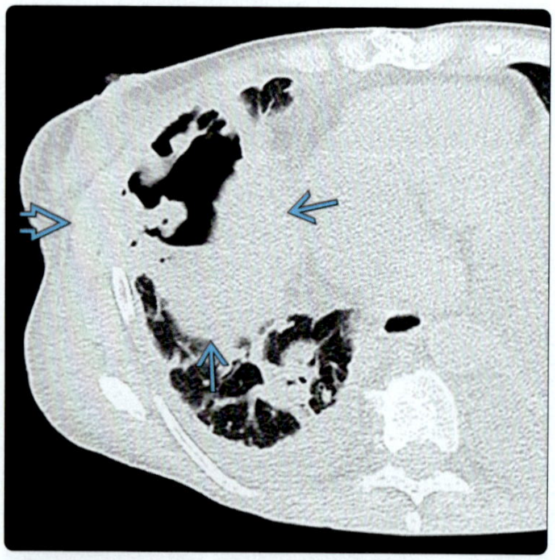

Elastofibroma Dorsi

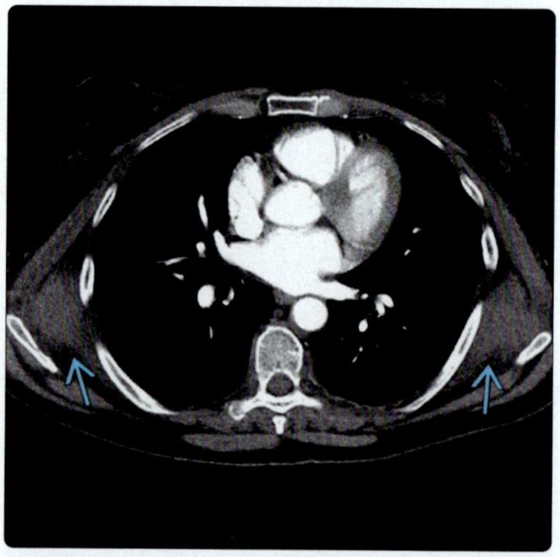

Fibromatosis

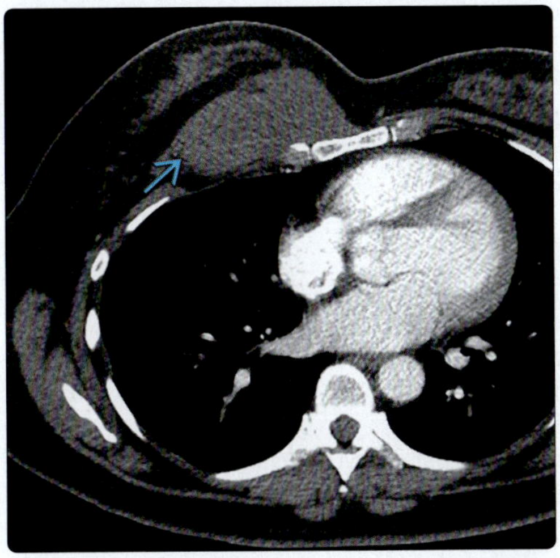

Liposarcoma

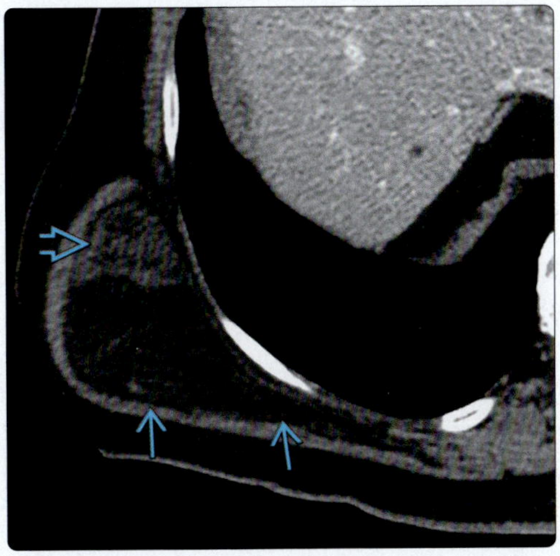

(Left) *Axial CECT of a patient presenting with a palpable mass in the right anterior chest wall shows a soft tissue mass isodense to muscle →. Biopsy revealed fibromatosis. This lesion may be hypodense, isodense, or hyperdense to muscle on CT.* **(Right)** *Axial CECT of an asymptomatic patient shows a right posterolateral chest wall mass that is composed primarily of fat → but also contains soft tissue elements →. Biopsy revealed liposarcoma.*

Liposarcoma

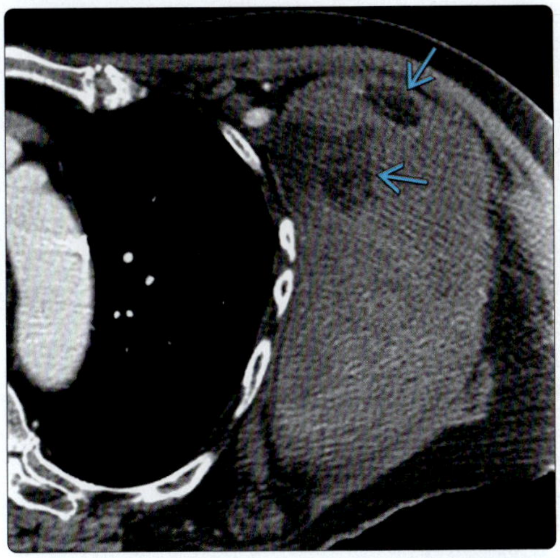

Angiosarcoma

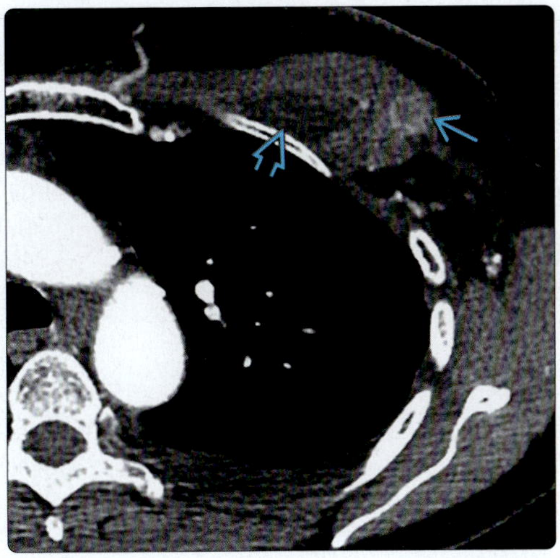

(Left) *Axial CECT of a patient with liposarcoma demonstrates a large heterogeneous mass in the left chest wall predominantly composed of soft tissue, although several foci of adipose tissue are present →.* **(Right)** *Axial CECT of a patient with prior breast cancer status post surgical resection shows an ill-defined mass in the left anterior chest wall composed of soft tissue, foci of enhancement →, & fluid →. Biopsy revealed angiosarcoma.*

Radiation-Associated Malignancy

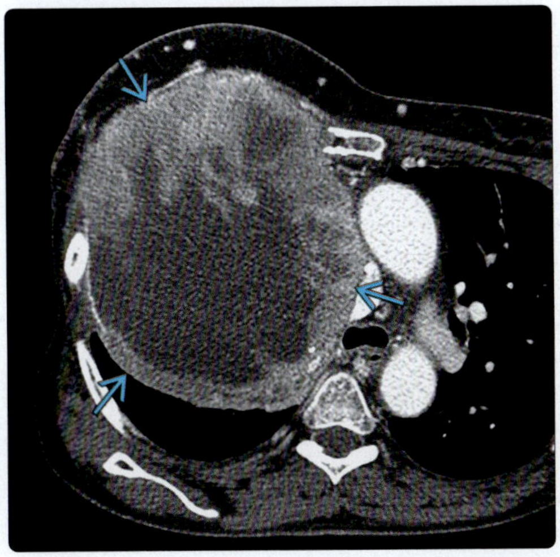

Malignant Peripheral Nerve Sheath Tumor

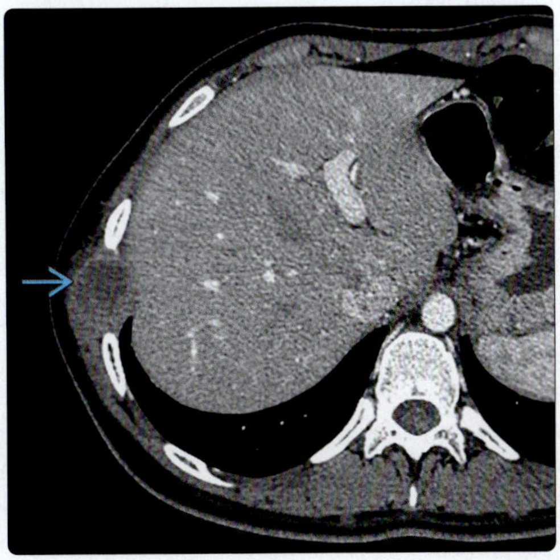

(Left) *Axial CECT of a patient with a history of right breast cancer treated with surgery and radiation therapy shows a large heterogeneous mass arising from the right anterior chest wall and extending into the right hemithorax →. Biopsy revealed a radiation-associated sarcoma.* **(Right)** *Axial CECT of a patient with neurofibromatosis type 1 shows a heterogeneous mass → arising from the right lateral chest wall at the site of a known neurofibroma. Biopsy confirmed malignant peripheral nerve sheath tumor.*

DIFFERENTIAL DIAGNOSIS

Common

- Malignant Neoplasms
  - Chondrosarcoma
  - Myeloma
  - Metastatic Disease
- Benign Neoplasms
  - Fibrous Dysplasia
  - Osteochondroma

Less Common

- Malignant Neoplasms
  - Osteosarcoma
  - Ewing Sarcoma
- Benign Neoplasms
  - Giant Cell Tumor
  - Aneurysmal Bone Cyst

Rare but Important

- Radiation-Associated Malignancies

ESSENTIAL INFORMATION

Key Differential Diagnosis Issues

- Differentiation between malignant and benign osseous neoplasms is critical
  - Malignancies frequently result in soft tissue mass formation
  - Benign neoplasms do not result in extraosseous soft tissue masses and typically exhibit nonaggressive imaging features
- CT helps determine
  - Location
  - Tissue origin (bone and cartilage)
  - Morphologic features
  - Internal components (fat, mineralization)
  - Tumor vascularity (via use of intravenous contrast)
- Limitations of CT
  - Reduced soft tissue contrast

Helpful Clues for Common Diagnoses

- **Chondrosarcoma**
  - Most common primary osseous malignancy of chest wall
    - 30% of all primary malignant osseous lesions
    - 33% of all primary rib neoplasms
  - Other etiologies
    - Malignant degeneration of benign chondromas
    - Trauma
    - Thoracic radiation therapy
  - Location
    - 10% occur in chest wall
      - Typically arise in anterior chest wall, from superior 5 ribs, adjacent to costochondral junctions, or in paravertebral regions
  - Imaging
    - Well-circumscribed mass of variable composition
    - Combination of soft tissue and mineralization
    - Patterns of calcification
      - Rings
      - Arcs
      - Stippled
    - Invasion and destruction of adjacent osseous structures are common
- **Myeloma**
  - Neoplasms composed of malignant plasmacytes
    - Multiple myeloma (MM)
      - Most common in patients 50-70 years of age
      - Affect bones with active hematopoiesis: Skull, thoracic skeleton, spine, pelvis, proximal humeri, and femora
    - Solitary plasmacytoma of bone (SBP)
      - Most common in patients ~ 50 years of age
      - Affect bones with active hematopoiesis: Skull, thoracic skeleton, spine, pelvis, proximal humeri, and femora
    - Extramedullary plasmacytoma (EP)
      - Most common in patients ~ 50 years of age
  - Imaging
    - MM: Multiple lytic lesions
    - SPB: Single expansile lytic bone lesion
    - EP: Focal soft tissue mass with attenuation characteristics similar to those of muscle
- **Metastatic Disease**
  - Osseous metastatic disease involving chest wall is usually seen in the setting of extensive disease elsewhere
  - May be encountered early in course of aggressive primary malignancies
  - Imaging
    - Metastases may demonstrate imaging characteristics of primary neoplasm
      - Prostate and breast cancers: Sclerotic lesions
      - Renal cell carcinoma: Lytic and expansile lesions
      - MM: Lytic lesions
- **FIbrous Dysplasia**
  - Developmental anomaly characterized by failure of osteoblasts to undergo normal morphologic differentiation and maturation
  - Commonly affects ribs
    - 6-20% of cases of monostotic fibrous dysplasia
    - 55% of cases of polyostotic fibrous dysplasia
  - Most common cause of osteolytic lesion by benign neoplasm or tumor-like lesion arising from osseous chest wall
  - Imaging
    - Expansile mass
    - Remodeling of protracted length of bone
    - Matrix may be completely osteolytic or show peripheral trabeculation or mineralization
    - Mineralization may be amorphous
    - Cartilage nodules may be present
- **Osteochondroma**
  - Hamartomatous, cartilage-capped osseous growth projecting from surface of affected bone
  - Imaging
    - Pedunculated osseous protuberance arising from surface of parent bone
    - Hallmark is continuity of marrow cavity between lesion and affected bone
      - Not always visualized for lesions involving ribs

- Complications: Fractures, deformity, vascular injury, neural compression, bursa formation, malignant transformation
- Findings suggesting malignant transformation
  - Pain at lesion site, bone erosion, irregular calcification, thickening of cartilage cap

Helpful Clues for Less Common Diagnoses

- **Osteosarcoma**
  - High-grade malignant mesenchymal neoplasm
  - Accounts for 10-15% of primary malignant chest wall neoplasms
  - 2 forms based on peak age
    - Osseous: Affects young adults
    - Extraosseous: Adults > 50 years of age
  - Imaging
    - Soft tissue mass with variable amounts of matrix mineralization
    - Matrix mineralization
      - Calcification or ossification
      - Dense, cloudy, or ivory-like
      - Greatest in central part, decreased in periphery
- **Ewing Sarcoma Family of Tumors**
  - Group of malignant neoplasms
    - Ewing sarcoma of bone
    - Extraosseous Ewing sarcoma
    - Askin tumor (peripheral primitive neuroectodermal tumor of chest wall)
  - Postulated to arise from embryonal neural crest cells
  - Highly aggressive lesions
  - Contain identical balanced, reciprocal translocation between chromosomes 11 and 22, t(11;22)
  - Imaging
    - Heterogeneous soft tissue masses
      - Regions of necrosis, hemorrhage, &/or cystic changes
    - Calcification is rarely seen
    - May invade adjacent structures, such as pleura, mediastinum, and lung
- **Giant Cell Tumor**
  - Comprised of vascular sinuses lined or filled with abundant giant cells and spindle cells
  - Imaging
    - Eccentric osteolytic lesions
    - Cortical thinning and expansion
    - CT shows extent and relationship to adjacent structures
- **Aneurysmal Bone Cyst**
  - Composed of network of multiple blood-filled cysts lined by fibroblasts and multinucleated giant cells of osteoclast type
  - Potential for rapid growth, bone destruction, and extension into adjacent soft tissue
  - Imaging
    - Expansile lesion with well-defined inner margin
    - CT helps delineate size and location of intraosseous and extraosseous components
    - Fluid-fluid levels may be seen on MR but are not specific for lesion

Helpful Clues for Rare Diagnoses

- **Radiation-Associated Malignancies**
  - Most malignancies are histologically sarcomas
  - Aggressive lesions associated with high recurrence rate and distant metastatic spread
  - Most malignancies develop within or adjacent to radiation site
    - Correlating imaging findings with radiation treatment plan used previously is helpful
  - Changes in appearance of previously irradiated bone, especially when associated soft tissue mass is present
  - Imaging
    - Osseous destruction and soft tissue mass are most common findings
      - Absence can help differentiate extensive benign osseous changes from radiation-associated sarcoma
    - Infiltration of adjacent structures

Chondrosarcoma

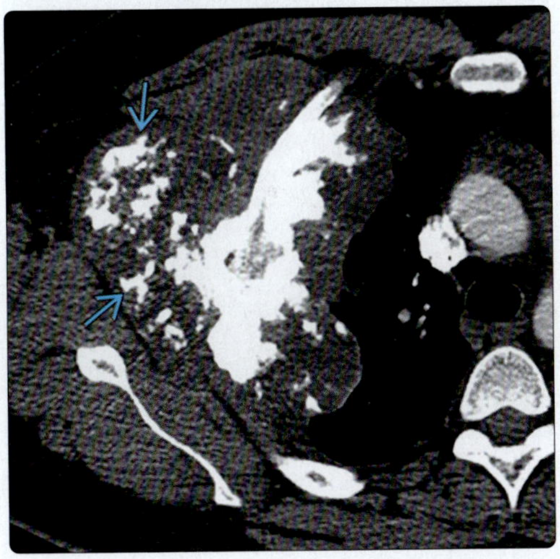

Chondrosarcoma

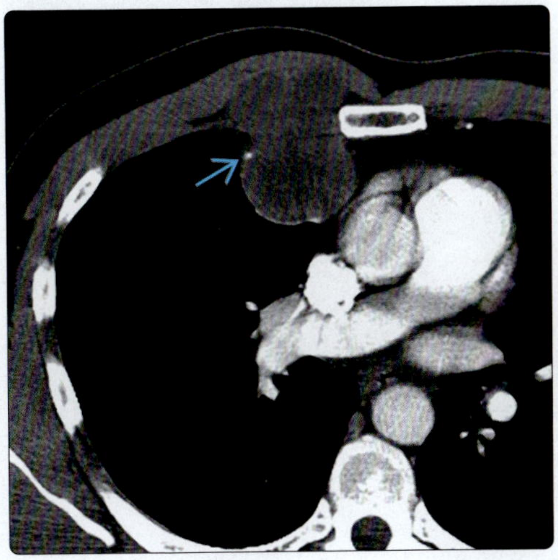

(Left) *Axial CECT of a patient with chondrosarcoma demonstrates a large destructive mass in the right chest wall with internal rings and arcs* →. **(Right)** *Axial CECT of a patient with chondrosarcoma shows a soft tissue mass involving the right anterior chest wall. Note that only a small amount of mineralization is present* →. *Chondrosarcoma is the most common primary osseous malignancy of the chest wall and demonstrates variable composition.*

(Left) *Axial CECT of a patient with multiple myeloma demonstrates numerous lytic lesions within the sternum and thoracic spine. Multiple myeloma classically results in multiple lytic lesions on CT.* **(Right)** *Axial CECT demonstrates a solitary plasmacytoma of bone appearing as a heterogeneous mass arising from the right posterior chest wall and invading the adjacent vertebral body.*

Myeloma

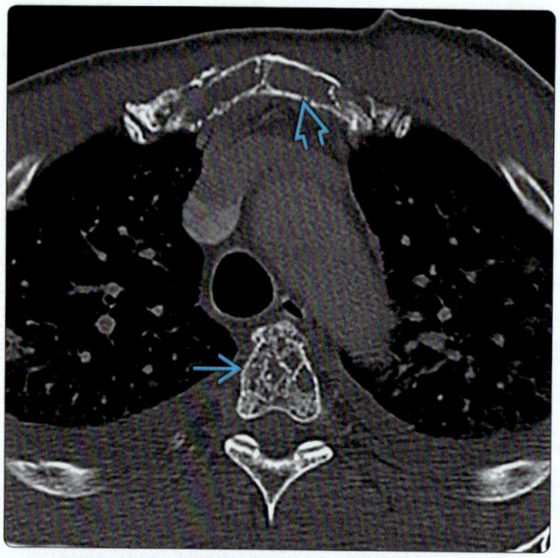

Myeloma

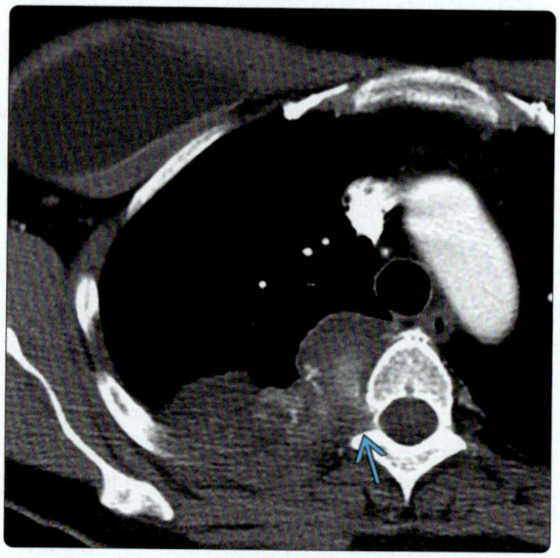

(Left) *Axial CECT of a patient with renal cell cancer demonstrates a soft tissue mass with peripheral enhancement in the right chest wall representing a metastasis.* **(Right)** *Axial CECT of a patient with osteosarcoma of the spine shows a calcified mass arising from the left posterior chest wall and extending into the left hemithorax. This metastasis demonstrates imaging features that are similar to those of the primary malignancy, including abundant mineralization.*

Metastatic Disease

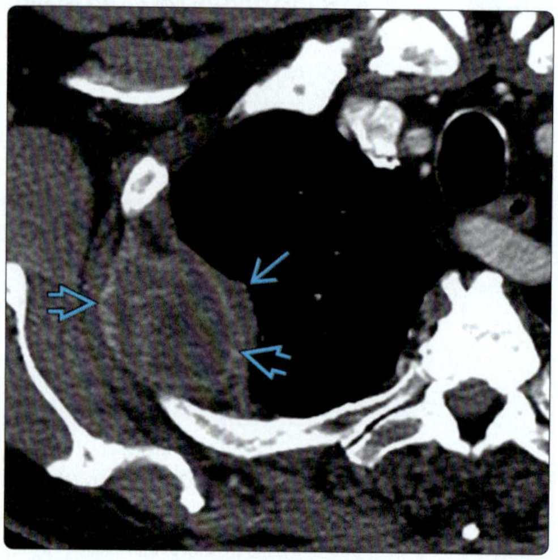

Metastatic Disease

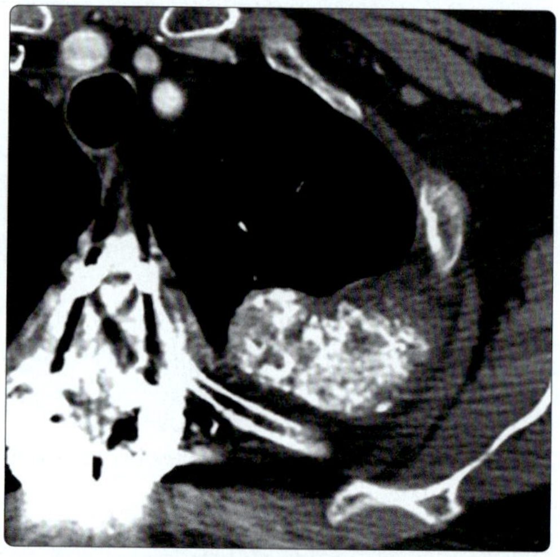

(Left) *Axial CECT of a patient with fibrous dysplasia shows a heterogeneous mass arising from the left chest wall with regions of mineralization, soft tissue, and fluid.* **(Right)** *Axial CECT of a patient with an osteochondroma demonstrates a mass-like protuberance arising from a rib with internal mineralization. Note the continuity of the marrow cavity between the lesion and the parent bone and extension of the lesion into the left lung.*

Fibrous Dysplasia

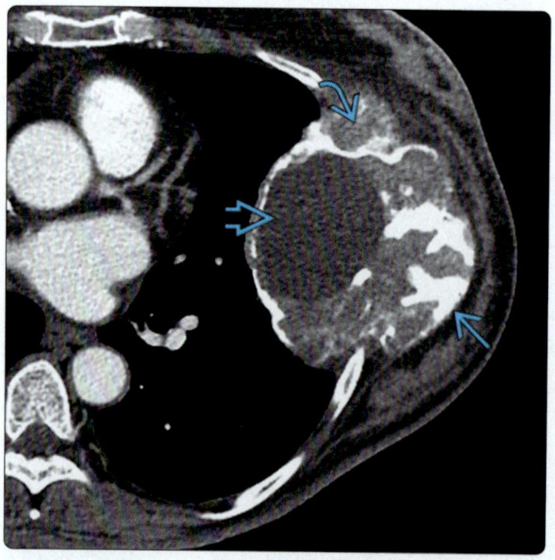

Osteochondroma

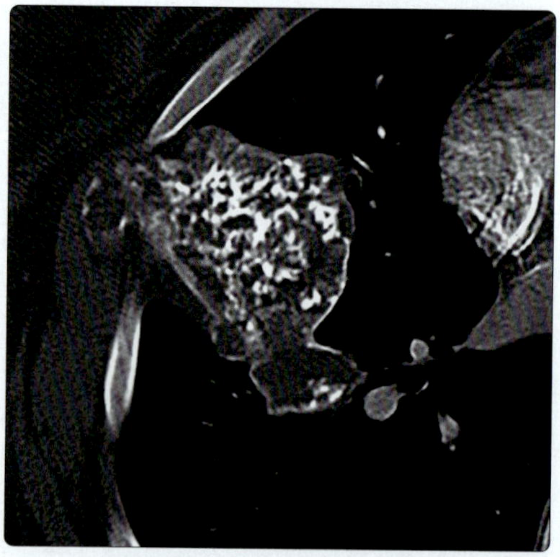

Osteosarcoma

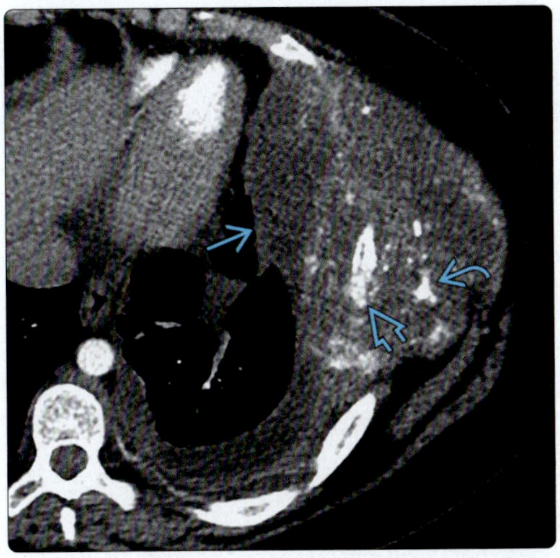

Ewing Sarcoma

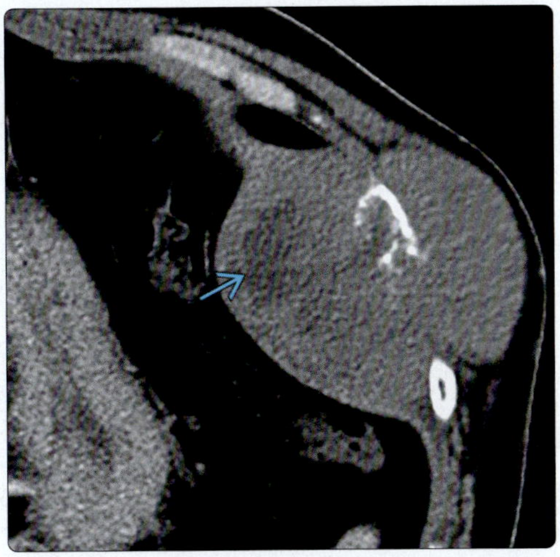

(Left) *Axial CECT of a patient with osteosarcoma shows a large soft tissue mass with internal foci of mineralization and destruction of an adjacent rib. The matrix of osteosarcoma is typically greatest in the central aspect of the lesion and decreased in the periphery.* **(Right)** *Axial CECT of a patient with Ewing sarcoma of bone demonstrates a heterogeneous soft tissue mass arising from the left chest wall with regions of low attenuation due to necrosis. Note destruction of an adjacent rib.*

Ewing Sarcoma

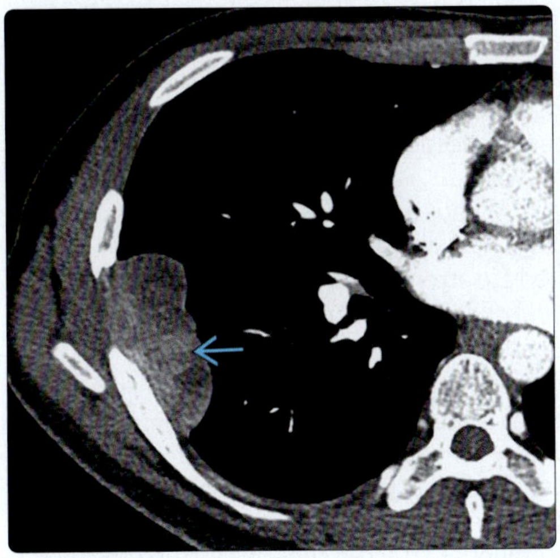

Giant Cell Tumor

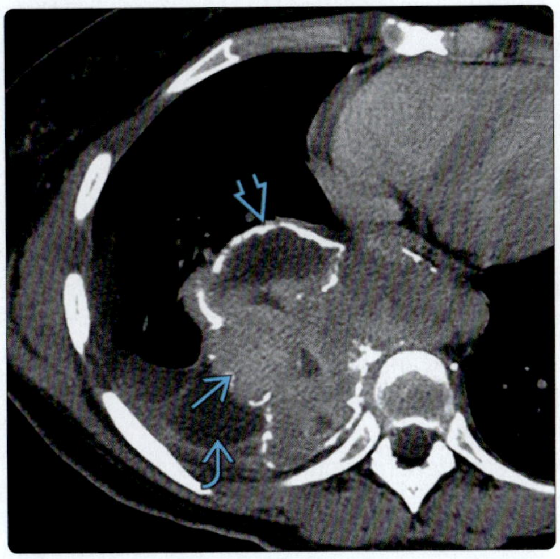

(Left) *Axial CECT of a patient with Ewing sarcoma of bone shows a heterogeneous mass arising from the right chest wall with regions of enhancement.* **(Right)** *Axial CECT demonstrates a heterogeneous mass arising from the right posterior chest wall containing soft tissue, fluid, and mineralization. Biopsy revealed giant cell tumor.*

Giant Cell Tumor

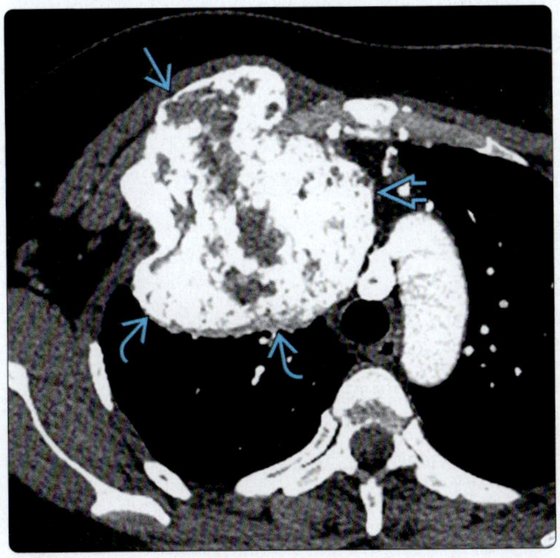

Aneurysmal Bone Cyst

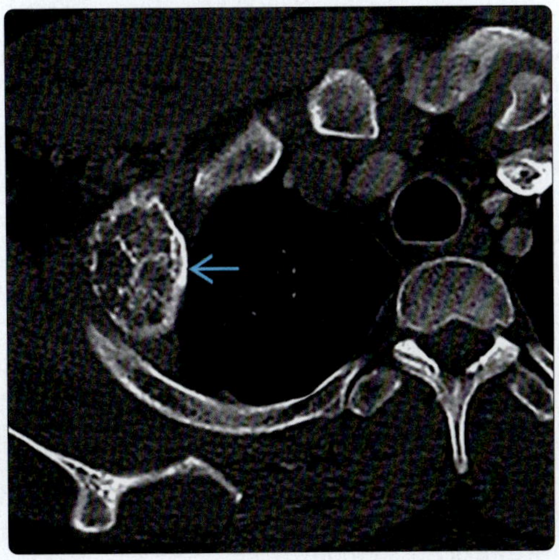

(Left) *Axial CECT of a patient with a giant cell tumor shows a large and extensively calcified mass arising from the right anterior chest wall with extension in the right hemithorax and mediastinum.* **(Right)** *Axial CECT of a patient with an aneurysmal bone cyst demonstrates an expansile lesion originating from a right-sided rib. Although there is thinning and disruption of the outer cortex, note the well-defined and intact inner margin, which is one of the features of aneurysmal bone cyst.*

Chest Wall Fluid Collection

DIFFERENTIAL DIAGNOSIS

Common

- Hematoma
- Abscess
- Postsurgical Seroma

Less Common

- Empyema Necessitans
- Chest Wall Neoplasm (Mimic)

Rare but Important

- Metastatic Disease (Mimic)
- Necrotizing Fasciitis

ESSENTIAL INFORMATION

Key Differential Diagnosis Issues

- Patients with chest wall fluid collections most commonly have history of recent surgery
- Chest wall trauma and surgery are common predisposing conditions for development of chest wall fluid collections
  - Hematoma
  - Infection
  - Seroma
- Spontaneous chest wall infections are rare but may occur in specific clinical settings
  - Diabetes mellitus
  - Immunosuppression
- Imaging
  - Ultrasound: Role in initial evaluation and diagnosis
    - Follow-up of noncomplicated fluid collections
    - Image guidance for fluid sampling and diagnosis
  - CT: Imaging method of choice for initial diagnosis and characterization of fluid collection
    - Determination of etiology and identification of complications
    - High sensitivity for detection of soft tissue gas and foreign bodies
  - MR: Mainstay in diagnosis and characterization of soft tissue infections and fluid collections
    - Excellent spatial and contrast resolution: Detailed assessment of chest wall bones and soft tissues
    - Contrast: Identification and assessment of complex collections, sinus tracts, devitalized soft tissue

Helpful Clues for Common Diagnoses

- **Hematoma**
  - Frequent history of trauma or recent surgery; minor trauma (accidental or iatrogenic) may inadvertently cause hematoma in anticoagulated patients
    - Gossypiboma: Foreign object (sponge) left inadvertently in body cavity; may predispose to abscess formation
  - Spontaneous chest wall hematoma is rare
  - Diagnostic clues
    - Bruising on physical exam
    - Associated displaced fracture of rib, sternum, spine
  - CT: Variable findings based on size and age of blood products
    - Hyperdense (> 20 HU) usually biconvex fluid collection
    - Heterogeneous attenuation ± fluid-fluid levels in large hematomas
    - Traumatic hematoma may exhibit contrast extravasation due to active bleeding from intercostal arteries
  - MR: Variable signal intensity according to age of blood products
    - Biconvex well-defined fluid collection
    - High-signal intensity on STIR images confirms fluid contents
    - Layering of intermediate-to-high-signal material
- **Abscess**
  - Typically caused by *Staphylococcus aureus*; less commonly *Actinomyces* and *Mycobacterium tuberculosis*
  - Most common after surgery and at sites of trauma or medical device insertion
    - May be associated with sternal osteomyelitis (as complication of sternotomy)
  - Spontaneous chest wall infection more common in diabetes, immunosuppression, and IV drug use
  - Clinical features: Pain, fever, redness, swelling
  - Ultrasound: Identification of fluid collection in area of inflammation
    - Modality of choice for image-guided drainage for diagnosis &/or treatment
    - Echogenic collection with enhanced through transmission
  - CT: Modality of choice for assessment of abscess and surrounding chest wall tissues
    - Intermediate attenuation, variable size/morphology
    - Stranding of adjacent subcutaneous fat
    - Identification of intrinsic gas
    - Peripheral enhancement
  - MR: Excellent spatial and contrast resolution; modality of choice for assessment of intercostal stripe
    - Complex fluid collection, variable signal intensity
    - Identification of surrounding soft tissue edema and enhancement of affected chest wall structures
- **Postsurgical Seroma**
  - History of sternotomy, thoracotomy, mastectomy, lymphadenectomy
  - Small seromas may resolve spontaneously; large seromas may require drainage
  - Imaging
    - Ultrasound
      - Simple fluid collection in surgical bed
      - Variable size
    - CT/MR
      - Variable size
      - Homogeneous fluid adjacent to surgical site
      - Hypodense/hyperintense on T2WI
      - No capsular/peripheral enhancement
  - Management
    - May resolve spontaneously or persist as chronic finding
    - No treatment necessary if small and uninfected

Helpful Clues for Less Common Diagnoses

- **Empyema Necessitans**
  - Pleural infection (empyema) complicated by extension of infection into adjacent chest wall

- Most commonly postsurgical; infection of surgical bed
- Spontaneous
  - Tuberculosis and *Actinomyces* are most common pathogens
- CT: Modality of choice for assessment of pleural empyema and involvement of adjacent chest wall
  - Complex multiloculated pleural fluid collection with pleural thickening and peripheral enhancement
  - Stranding and thickening of adjacent intercostal stripe and chest wall soft tissues
  - Variable size of chest wall fluid collection
- Treatment
  - Surgical evacuation
  - May require extensive debridement and open-window thoracotomy (Eloesser flap)

- **Chest Wall Neoplasm (Mimic)**
  - Primary chest wall neoplasms are uncommon
  - Chest wall neoplasms with intrinsic cystic change, hemorrhage or necrosis may mimic fluid chest wall fluid collections
    - Lipoma
      - Common
      - Homogeneous, fat attenuation, encapsulated mass
      - Involves subcutaneous chest wall fat, chest wall muscles, or extrapleural fat
    - Hemangioma, lymphangioma, hemangiolymphangioma
      - Uncommon
      - Variable size
      - CT/MR: Tortuous vessels/lymphatics, interspersed fat, heterogeneous enhancement, phleboliths
    - Lymphoma
      - Chest wall involvement by Hodgkin and non-Hodgkin lymphoma ± intrathoracic lymphadenopathy
      - Infiltrative soft tissue mass, invades multiple chest wall compartments, may extend to pleura
    - Soft tissue sarcoma
      - CT/MR: Soft tissue mass ± necrosis, hemorrhage, calcification, enhancement

Helpful Clues for Rare Diagnoses

- **Metastatic Disease (Mimic)**
  - Most common neoplasms
    - Melanoma
    - Renal cell carcinoma
    - Breast cancer
    - Lung cancer
    - Mesothelioma
  - Local chest wall invasion from intrathoracic malignancy versus hematogenous metastasis
  - CT: Variable findings according to size, presence of hemorrhage, &/or necrosis
- **Necrotizing Fasciitis**
  - Rapidly progressive infection of deep soft tissues with high mortality rate
  - Usually polymicrobial infection
  - Risk factors: IV drug use, diabetes mellitus, immunosuppression, obesity, peripheral vascular disease
  - Diagnostic dilemma: Differentiation of superficial from deep soft tissue infection; latter requires emergent debridement
  - CT
    - Focal subcutaneous fat stranding and asymmetric fascial thickening
    - ± soft tissue gas, highly specific in appropriate clinical setting
    - Variable amount of fluid
  - MR: High T2 signal intensity along deep fascia (mainly deep intermuscular fascia)

SELECTED REFERENCES

1. Hayeri MR et al: Soft-tissue infections and their imaging mimics: from cellulitis to necrotizing fasciitis. Radiographics. 36(6):1888-910, 2016
2. Jeung MY et al: Imaging of chest wall disorders. Radiographics. 19(3): 617-37, 1999

Hematoma

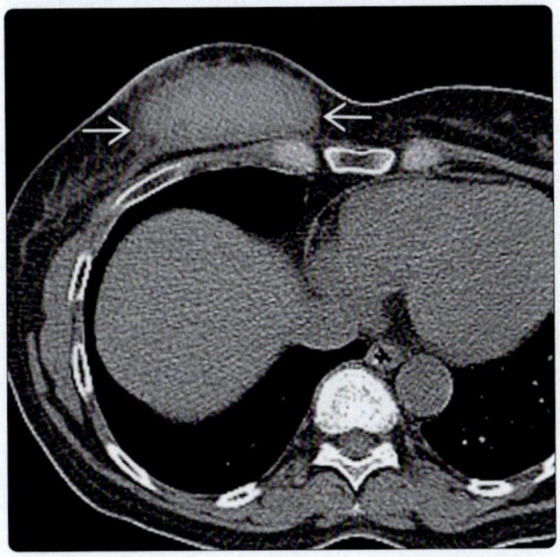

Abscess

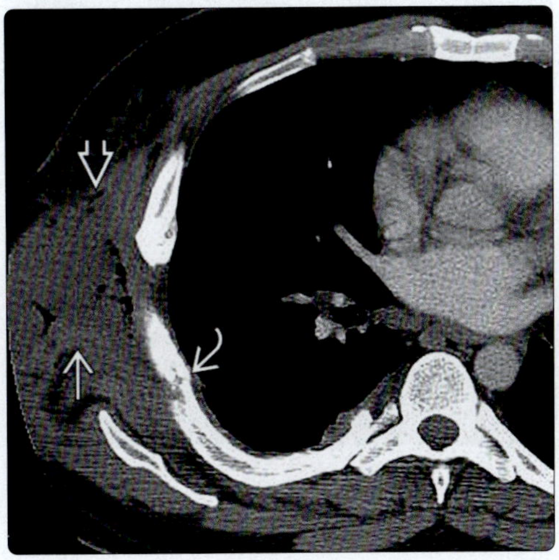

(Left) *Axial NECT of a patient with chest wall pain and swelling after right breast biopsy shows a large hyperdense right breast hematoma ➡. Hematoma attenuation varies with the age of the blood products.* **(Right)** *Axial CECT of a patient with a chest wall abscess shows a large complex fluid collection ➡ in the right chest wall with intrinsic gas ➡. Note cortical disruption and periosteal reaction of adjacent right ribs ➡ secondary to osteomyelitis. Chest wall abscess may be associated with adjacent osteomyelitis.*

(Left) *Axial CECT of a patient who presented with a painful anterior chest wall mass following a recent sternotomy shows a multiloculated subxyphoid fluid collection with enhancing borders → consistent with a chest wall abscess.* **(Right)** *Axial CECT of the same patient shows the complex anterior chest wall abscess → and surrounding fat stranding in the presternal space. In this case, CT allows identification of a sinus tract → that connected the abscess with the cardiac surgical bed.*

Abscess

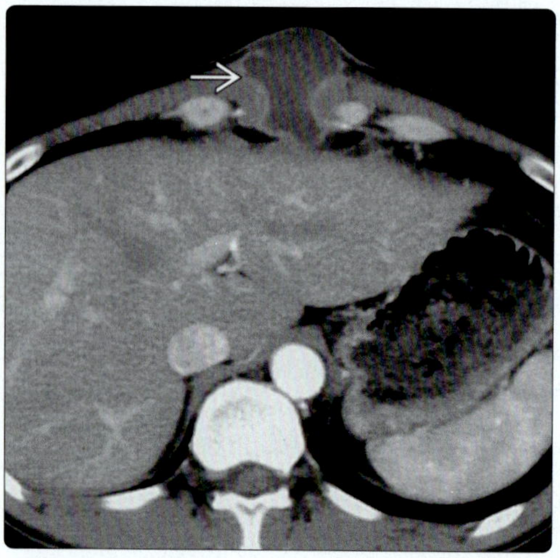

Abscess

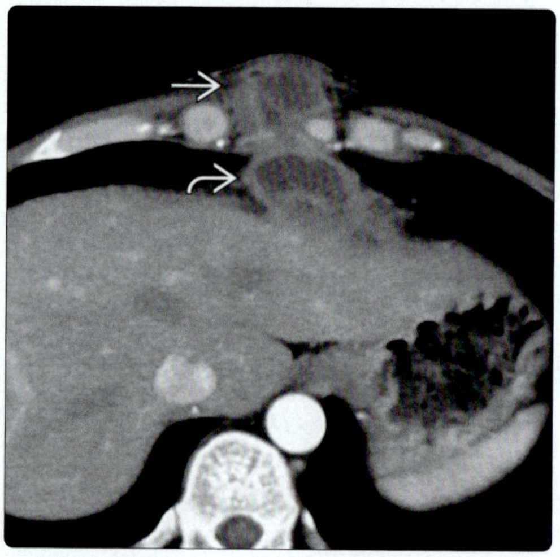

(Left) *Axial CECT of the same patient shows a complex loculated fluid collection or abscess → in the left posterior pericardial space surrounding a high-density serpiginous foreign body → that represented retained surgical material. This gossypiboma was the etiology of the chest wall abscess.* **(Right)** *Axial CECT of an asymptomatic patient status post left mastectomy shows a small elongate fluid collection in the surgical bed consistent with a postsurgical seroma →. Note absence of fat stranding or intrinsic gas.*

Abscess

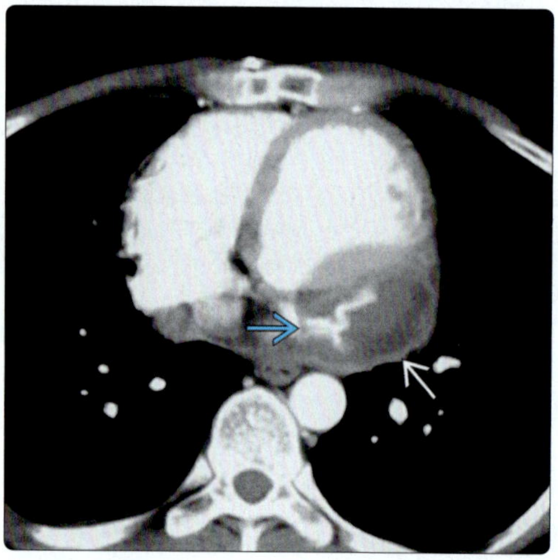

Postsurgical Seroma

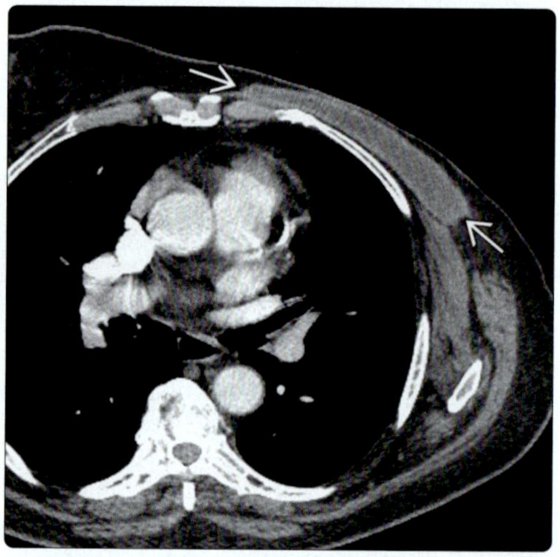

(Left) *Axial CECT of a patient who presented with fever, leukocytosis, and a right chest wall mass shows a large multiloculated empyema with multiple gas pockets and pleural enhancement →. Gas and fluid extend through the ribs into the right chest wall. Note peripheral enhancement of the chest wall abscess →.* **(Right)** *Axial NECT of a patient with empyema necessitans secondary to actinomycosis shows a moderate right pleural effusion → draining into a large right chest wall fluid collection with high-attenuation borders →.*

Empyema Necessitans

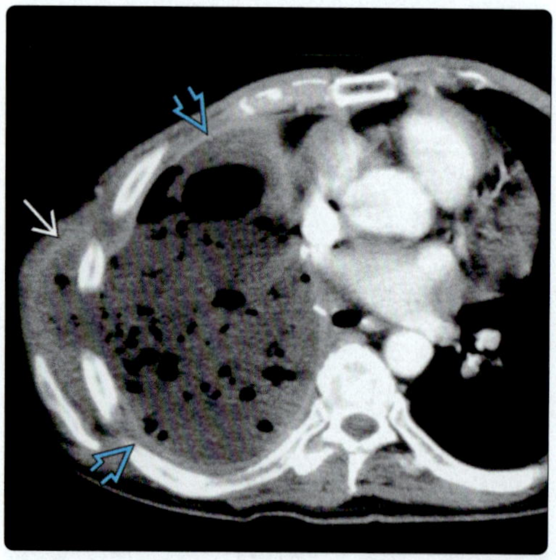

Empyema Necessitans

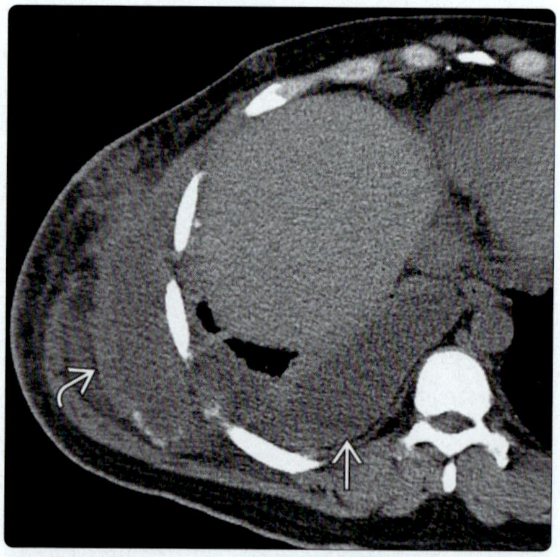

Chest Wall Neoplasm (Mimic)

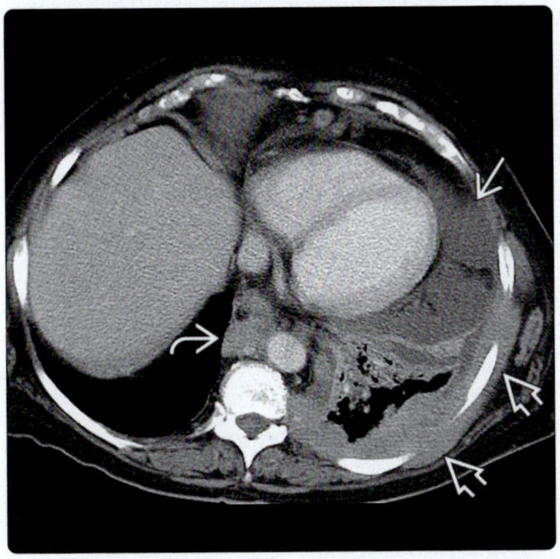

Chest Wall Neoplasm (Mimic)

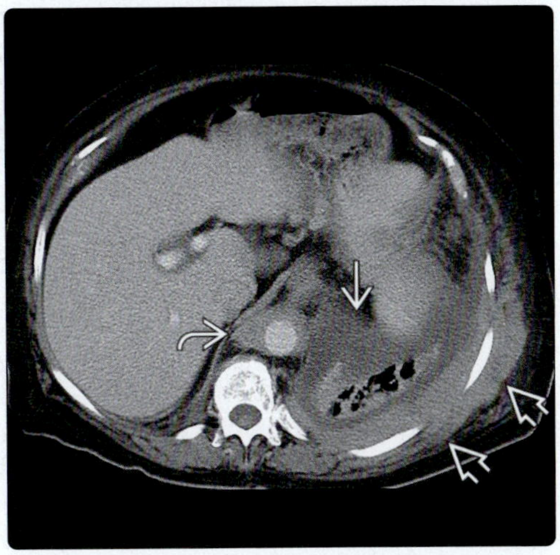

(Left) *Axial CECT of a patient with chest wall lymphoma shows a loculated left pleural effusion and an infiltrative chest wall soft tissue mass that encases the left ribs without skeletal destruction. Note mediastinal lymphadenopathy.* **(Right)** *Axial CECT of the same patient shows a left chest wall soft tissue mass that encases the left ribs, an adjacent left pleural effusion, and mediastinal lymphadenopathy. Chest wall neoplasms may mimic an empyema necessitans, as in this case.*

Chest Wall Neoplasm (Mimic)

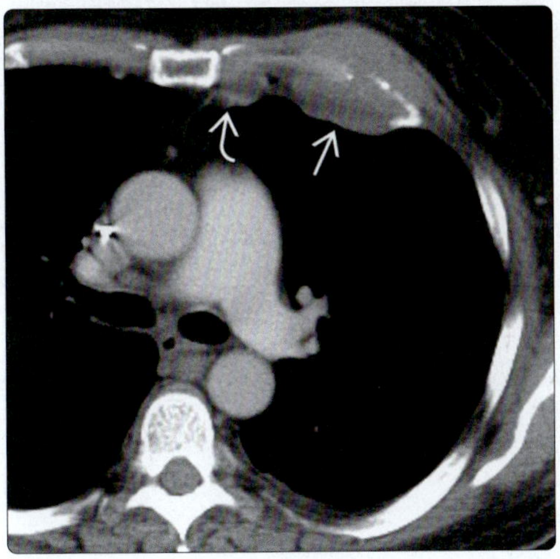

Chest Wall Neoplasm (Mimic)

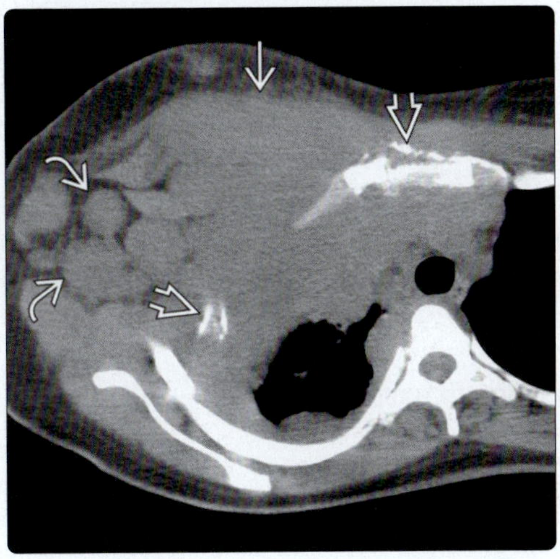

(Left) *Axial CECT of a patient with chest wall lymphoma shows a fusiform left anterior chest wall soft tissue mass that encases and destroys a left anterior rib and left internal mammary lymphadenopathy.* **(Right)** *Axial NECT of a patient with lymphoma shows a large soft tissue mass that involves the right pleura and chest wall, extensive right axillary lymphadenopathy, and skeletal destruction. A locally invasive chest wall neoplasm may mimic a chest wall abscess adjacent to osteomyelitis.*

Chest Wall Neoplasm (Mimic)

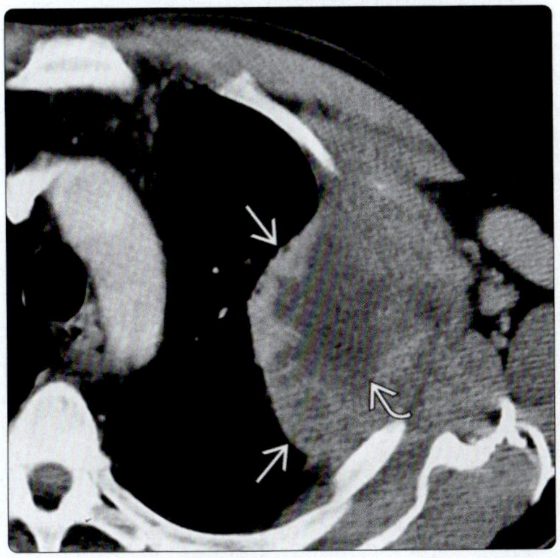

Chest Wall Neoplasm (Mimic)

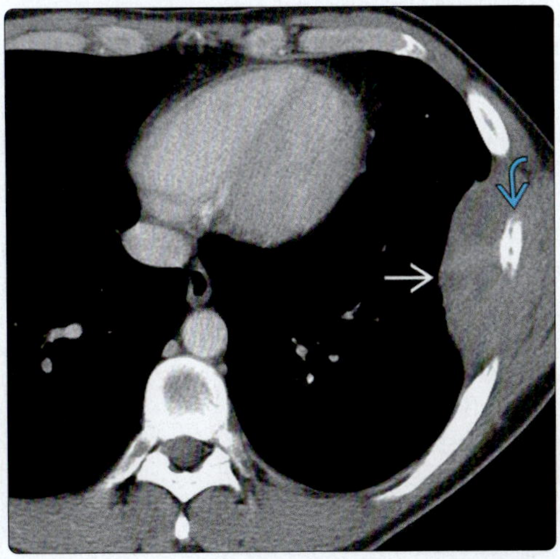

(Left) *Axial CECT of a patient with non-Hodgkin lymphoma shows a large infiltrative left chest wall mass with intrinsic low attenuation secondary to necrosis. Necrotic neoplasms may mimic chest wall fluid collections.* **(Right)** *Axial CECT of a patient with an Askin tumor shows an infiltrative heterogeneous left chest wall soft tissue mass that encases a left rib and produces skeletal destruction. Chest wall neoplasms may mimic chest wall fluid collections. Ultrasound allows identification &/or exclusion of intrinsic fluid components.*

DIFFERENTIAL DIAGNOSIS

Common

- Soft Tissue
  - Undifferentiated Pleomorphic Sarcoma
  - Neurofibroma
  - Schwannoma
  - Hemangioma
  - Lipoma
- Osseous
  - Chondrosarcoma
  - Myeloma
  - Fibrous Dysplasia
  - Osteochondroma
- Metastatic Disease

Less Common

- Soft Tissue
  - Elastofibroma Dorsi
  - Fibromatosis
- Osseous
  - Osteosarcoma
  - Ewing Sarcoma
  - Giant Cell Tumor
  - Aneurysmal Bone Cyst
- Secondary Invasion

Rare but Important

- Soft Tissue
  - Lymphoma
  - Liposarcoma
  - Angiosarcoma
  - Malignant Peripheral Nerve Sheath Tumor
- Radiation-Associated Malignancies

ESSENTIAL INFORMATION

Key Differential Diagnosis Issues

- Classification of primary soft tissue neoplasms of chest wall determined by tissue of origin
- Differentiation between malignant and benign osseous neoplasms is critical
  - Malignancies frequently result in soft tissue mass formation
  - Benign neoplasms do not result in extraosseous soft tissue masses and typically exhibit nonaggressive imaging features
- Advantages of MR
  - Superior soft tissue contrast compared to CT
  - Optimal imaging modality for delineating extent of local disease
  - Enables differentiation of neoplasm from normal chest wall structures, infection, and inflammation
  - Enables better identification of residual or recurrent disease than CT in posttreatment assessment
- Limitations of MR
  - Limited utility for assessment of bone involvement and mineralization; operator dependent

Helpful Clues for Common Diagnoses

- **Soft Tissue**
  - Undifferentiated Pleomorphic Sarcoma
    - Soft tissue mass
      - T1WI: Isointense to muscle
      - T2WI: Intermediate to high signal intensity; iso- to hyperintense to fat
    - Myxoid components
      - T1WI: Low signal intensity
      - T2WI: High signal intensity
    - High collagen content: Low signal intensity on all sequences
    - Hemorrhage: Variable signal intensity on all sequences
  - Neurofibroma
    - T1WI: Hypointense
    - T2WI: Hyperintense
    - T1 C+: Heterogeneous enhancement
  - Schwannoma
    - T1WI: Iso- or hypointense
    - T2WI: Heterogeneously hyperintense
    - T1 C+: Intense enhancement
  - Hemangioma
    - T1WI: Low or intermediate signal intensity; high signal intensity when fat is present
    - T2WI: High signal intensity
  - Lipoma
    - T1WI: High signal intensity
    - T2WI: Low signal intensity
    - Uniform loss of signal intensity on fat-suppression sequences; internal septations may be present
- **Osseous**
  - Chondrosarcoma
    - Cartilage background
      - T1WI: Iso- to hypointense to muscle
      - T2WI: Hyperintense to muscle
    - Mineralization: T1WI and T2WI: Hypointense to muscle
  - Myeloma
    - Untreated
      - T1WI: Hypointense to muscle
      - T2WI: Hyperintense to muscle
      - T1 C+: Enhancement
    - Treated
      - T1WI: Heterogeneous signal intensity
      - T2WI: Heterogeneous signal intensity
      - T1 C+: Heterogeneous enhancement
    - Inactive disease
      - T1WI: Hyperintense
      - T2WI: Hypointense
      - T1 C+: No enhancement
    - Extramedullary plasmacytoma
      - T1WI: Low signal intensity
      - T2WI: High signal intensity
      - T1 C+: Enhancement
  - Fibrous Dysplasia
    - T1WI: Low signal intensity
    - T2WI: Variable, low to high signal intensity
  - Osteochondroma
    - T1WI: Isointense to medullary cavity of affected bone
    - Cartilaginous cap
      - T1WI: Isointense to muscle

- T2WI: Hyperintense to muscle
  - Malignant transformation
    - Cartilage cap > 2 cm in adults or 3 cm in children
- **Metastatic Disease**
  - Frequently demonstrate imaging characteristics of primary malignancy

Helpful Clues for Less Common Diagnoses

- **Soft Tissue**
  - Elastofibroma Dorsi
    - T1WI: Isointense to muscle; regions of fat hyperintense
    - T2WI: Isointense to muscle
  - Fibromatosis
    - T1WI: Homogeneous low to intermediate signal intensity
    - T2WI: Heterogeneous (low, intermediate, &/or high signal intensity)
- **Osseous**
  - Osteosarcoma
    - Soft tissue component
      - T1WI: Hyperintense to muscle
      - T2WI: Iso- to hyperintense to muscle
      - T1 C+: Heterogeneous enhancement
    - Matrix mineralization: T1WI, T2WI hypointensity
  - Ewing Sarcoma
    - T1WI: Iso- or hyperintense to muscle; high signal intensity hemorrhage
    - T2WI: Heterogeneous and hyperintense to muscle
    - T1 C+: Intense enhancement
  - Giant Cell Tumor
    - T1WI: Low signal intensity
    - T2WI: High signal intensity
    - Fluid-fluid levels due to hemorrhage may be present
  - Aneurysmal Bone Cyst
    - T1W and T2WI: Heterogeneous signal
    - Thin rim of low signal intensity
    - Fluid-fluid levels due to hemorrhage may be present
- **Secondary Invasion**
  - MR superior to CT for identifying chest wall invasion
  - T1WI: Infiltration or disruption of normal extrapleural fat planes
  - T2WI and STIR: High signal intensity of parietal pleura and other chest wall structures
  - T1 C+: Enhancement of invasive tumor
  - Cine MR: Lesion attachment to chest wall

Helpful Clues for Rare Diagnoses

- **Soft Tissue**
  - Lymphoma
    - T1WI: Isointense to mildly increased signal intensity
    - T2WI: Hyperintense
  - Liposarcoma
    - Imaging features depend on histologic subtype
    - Well-differentiated liposarcoma
      - T1WI: High signal intensity
      - T2WI: Low signal intensity
      - T1 C+: Heterogeneous enhancement of nonadipose tissue; thick septa may enhance
    - Myxoid liposarcoma
      - T1WI: Moderately high signal intensity
      - T2WI: High signal intensity
- **Angiosarcoma**
  - T1WI and T2WI: Heterogeneous signal intensity
  - T1 C+: Intense enhancement
  - Malignant Peripheral Nerve Sheath Tumor
    - T1WI: Iso- or hyperintense to muscle
    - T2WI: Hyperintense to muscle
    - T1 C+: Heterogeneous enhancement
    - Findings suggestive of malignant transformation of neurofibroma
      - Loss of target, fascicular, and split fat signs; sudden change in size of lesion
      - Heterogeneous signal intensity due to necrosis &/or hemorrhage
- **Radiation-Associated Malignancies**
  - Soft tissue mass usually present, can enable differentiation of radiation-associated malignancy from benign osseous changes after radiation therapy

Hemangioma

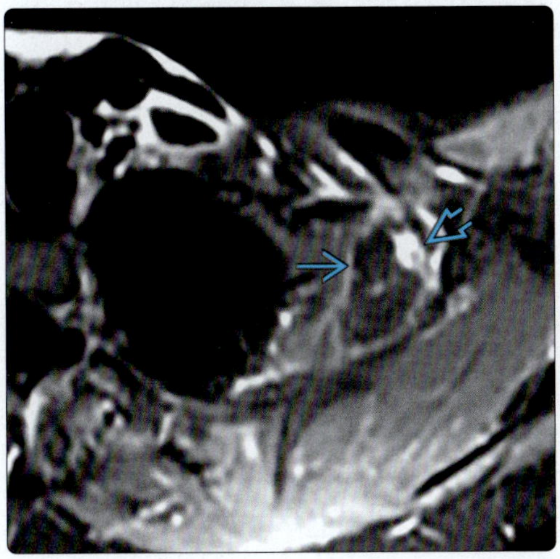

Hemangioma

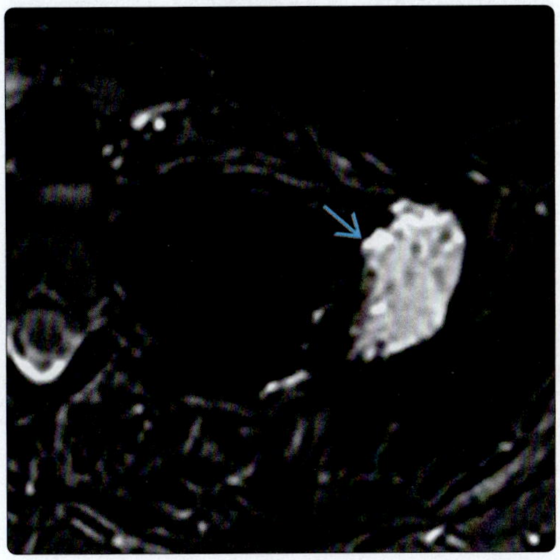

(Left) *Axial T1 C+ FS MR of a patient presenting with left chest wall pain demonstrates a soft tissue mass* → *in the left chest wall with regions of heterogeneous enhancement* ⇨. **(Right)** *Axial STIR MR of the same patient shows the lobular lesion with homogeneous high signal intensity* →. *Biopsy revealed hemangioma. Hemangiomas typically demonstrate high signal intensity on fluid-sensitive sequences but are more heterogeneous on T1WI due to the variable presence of fat.*

(Left) *Axial T1 MR of a patient with chondrosarcoma presenting with left chest wall pain shows a left anterior chest wall mass with signal intensity similar to the adjacent musculature →.* **(Right)** *Axial T1 C+ FS MR of the same patient shows linear and nodular peripheral enhancement but no internal foci of enhancement ⇒. Chondrosarcoma is the most common soft tissue primary malignancy involving the chest wall.*

Chondrosarcoma

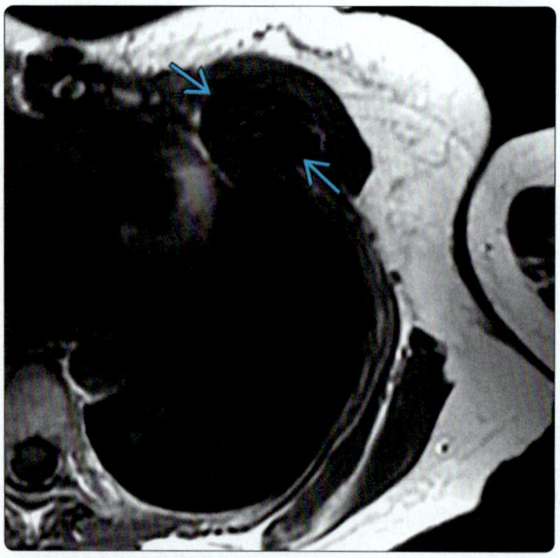

Chondrosarcoma

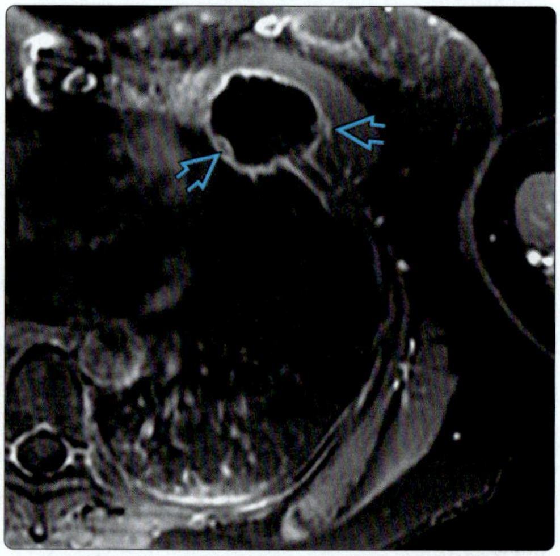

(Left) *Axial STIR MR of the same patient demonstrates high signal intensity within the mass → that is similar to the cerebrospinal fluid. Chondrosarcomas are characteristically hyperintense on fluid-sensitive sequences due to the high cartilage content.* **(Right)** *Axial T1 MR of a patient with multiple myeloma demonstrates an expansile rib lesion in the right chest wall that is similar in signal intensity to the adjacent musculature →.*

Chondrosarcoma

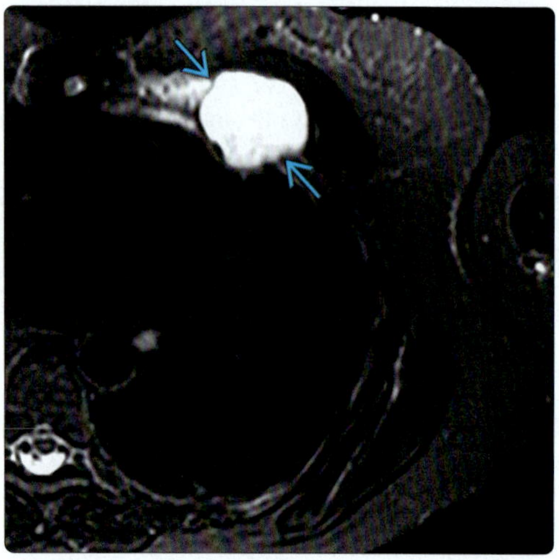

Myeloma

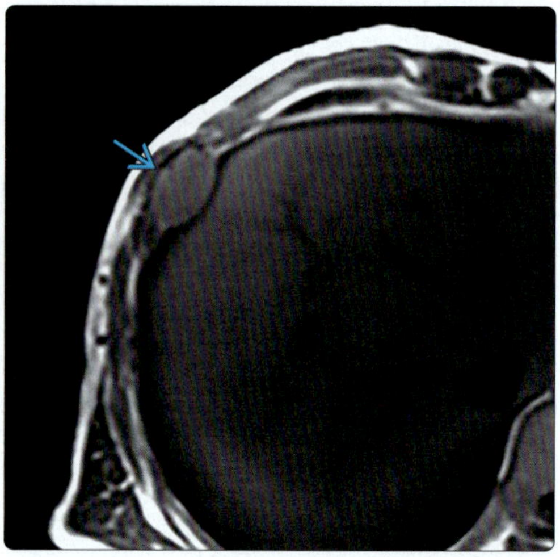

(Left) *Axial T1 C+ MR of the same patient demonstrates homogeneous high signal in the lesion representing enhancement →.* **(Right)** *Axial STIR MR of the same patient demonstrates homogeneous high signal intensity within the lesion →. Untreated myelomatous lesions typically demonstrate this appearance, with low signal intensity on T1WI, high signal intensity on T2WI, and enhancement following the administration of IV contrast.*

Myeloma

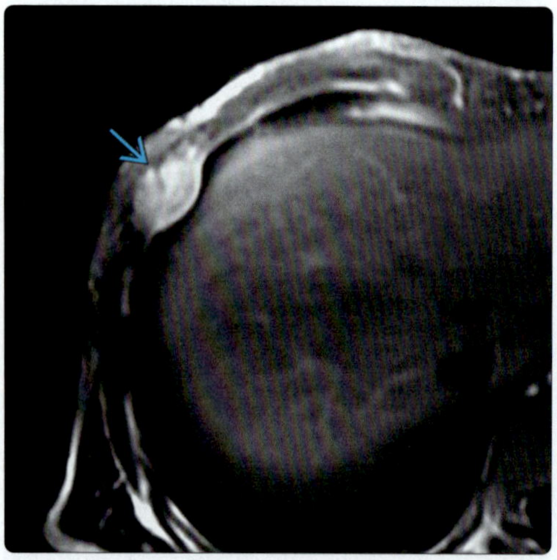

Myeloma

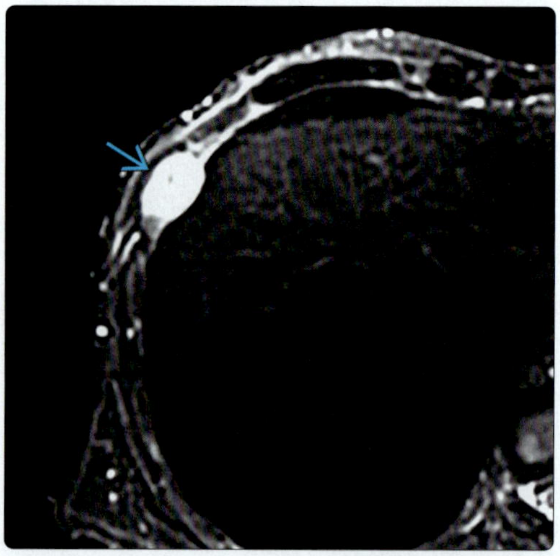

Aneurysmal Bone Cyst

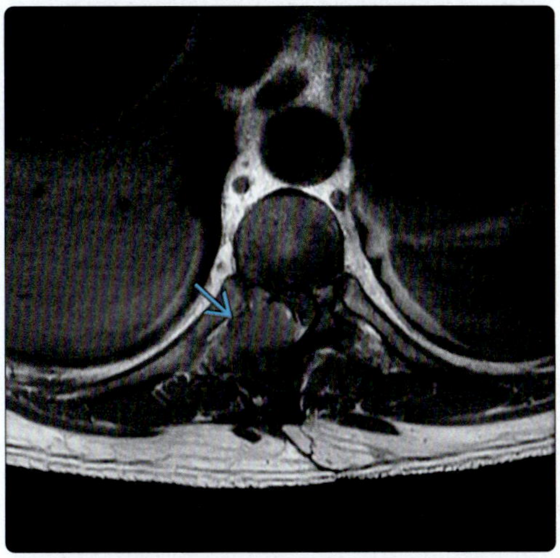

Aneurysmal Bone Cyst

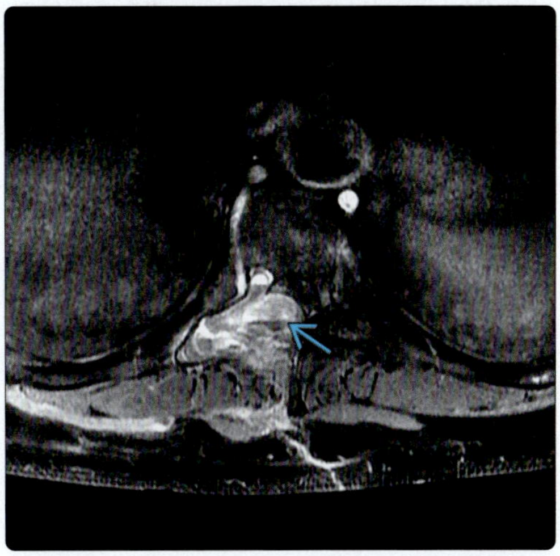

(Left) *Axial T1 MR of a patient with an aneurysmal bone cyst demonstrates an ill-defined mass in the lower thoracic spine that is higher in signal intensity than the adjacent musculature ➡.* **(Right)** *Axial T1 C+ FS MR of the same patient demonstrates regions of high signal intensity indicating enhancement. There is the suggestion of several fluid-fluid levels ➡.*

Aneurysmal Bone Cyst

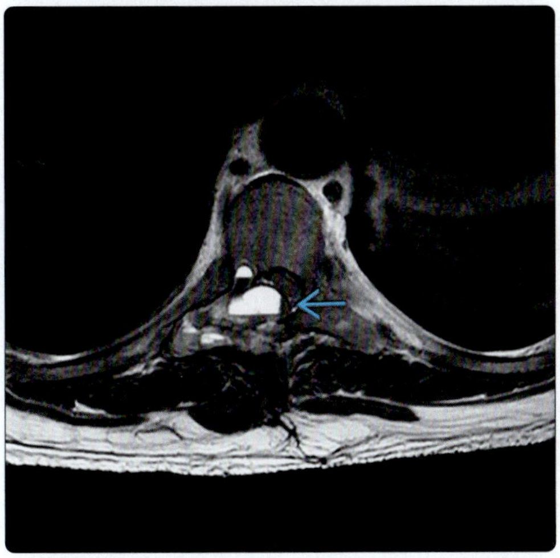

Secondary Invasion

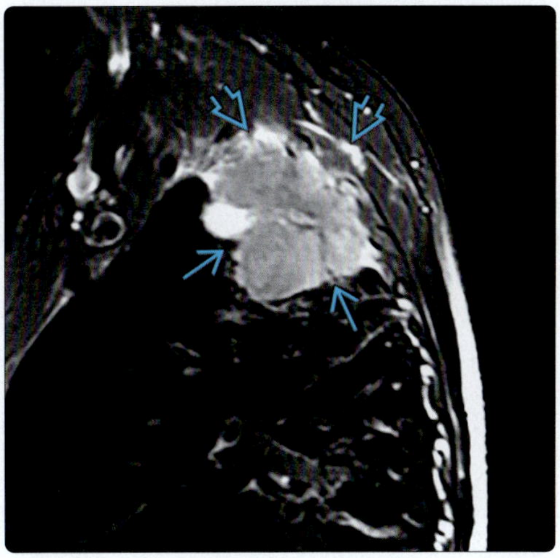

(Left) *Axial T2 MR of the same patient confirms the presence of multiple fluid-fluid levels ➡. Fluid-fluid levels are indicative of hemorrhage and may be present within giant cell tumors and aneurysmal bone cysts.* **(Right)** *Sagittal T1 C+ FS MR of a patient with a right upper lobe lung cancer demonstrates a homogeneously enhancing mass ➡ that results in multifocal invasion of the adjacent chest wall ➡.*

Liposarcoma

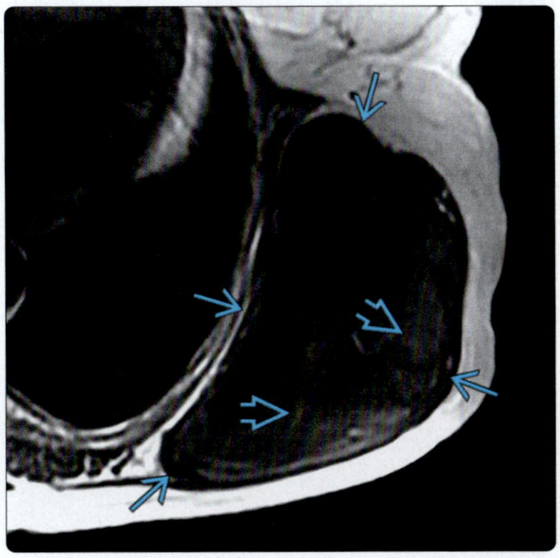

Liposarcoma

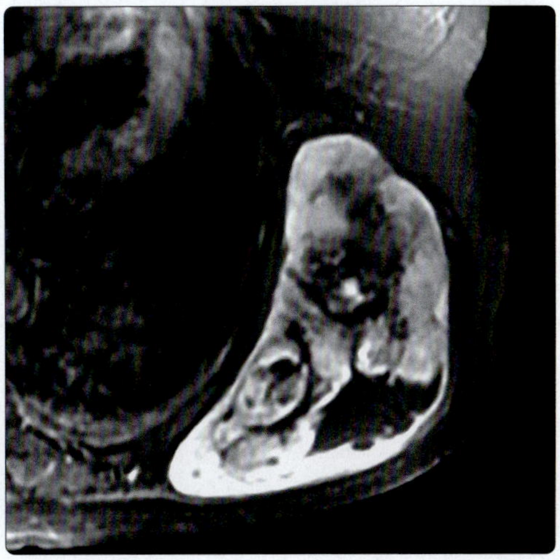

(Left) *Axial T1 MR of a patient with a liposarcoma demonstrates a large heterogeneous mass in the left chest wall ➡. Note the internal foci of high signal intensity representing fat ➡.* **(Right)** *Axial T1 C+ FS MR of the same patient shows extensive regions of high signal intensity within the mass indicating enhancement. The imaging features of liposarcoma vary with histology, as more aggressive lesions demonstrate less fat and more solid, enhancing components.*

SECTION 10

Heart

Approach to Heart

General Imaging Patterns

Modality-Specific Imaging Findings: Computed Tomography

Approach to Heart

Introduction

Cardiac imaging continues to expand in scope and has become central to the diagnosis and monitoring of many heart diseases. Simultaneously, advances in imaging technology have significantly increased not only the detailed cardiac anatomy visible, but also the detection and characterization of pathology previously hidden. The speed and spatial resolution of CT displays structural heart disease on even non-ECG-gated imaging of the chest. Novel MR sequences have expanded the role of this modality in cardiac imaging, enabling detection of subclinical myocardial disease.

Imaging Modalities

The imaging diagnosis of cardiac disease is an excellent example of the power of a multimodality approach. A mass may be incidentally discovered on echocardiography, precisely localized and anatomically delineated on CT, and tissue characterized on MR. These modalities are complementary, particularly in the evaluation of cardiac masses and heart failure of unknown etiology. For instance, cardiomyopathy may be determined to be nonischemic by a normal coronary CTA, characterized as infiltrative on MR, and deemed highly suspicious for sarcoidosis with FDG PET/CT.

Radiography

Chest radiography remains a frequent and important means of imaging the heart. Despite its poor specificity for cardiac pathology, this exam continues to play a role in the diagnosis of congestive heart failure, a common final pathway for many diseases. Left atrial enlargement may be suggested by the double density sign at the right heart border and splaying of the carina on the frontal radiograph and posterior protrusion of the posterior cardiac border on the lateral radiograph. The right atrium is very compliant and is often the most dilated chamber in very large hearts. Mitral annular calcification has a characteristic crescentic shape in the expected location of the mitral valve. Aortic valvular calcifications detected radiographically may suggest aortic stenosis before clinically apparent. Finally, hardware and postoperative complications may first be detected radiographically.

Echocardiography

Echocardiography is the most common dedicated cardiac imaging study, and many heart diseases are exclusively diagnosed and surveilled with this modality. With excellent temporal resolution, wide availability, and nonradiating imaging, this modality is certainly the first imaging recommendation when cardiac disease is suspected clinically or radiographically. Limited acoustic windows and operator dependence often necessitate CT or MR for definitive diagnosis or for problem solving suspected disease on echocardiography.

CT

From an imager's perspective, important cardiac findings are often incidentally discovered when imaging the chest or abdomen. For instance, coronary artery atherosclerotic calcifications are increasingly recognized on nongated CT of the chest, and this finding should be reported. The high sensitivity of CT for calcification also makes CT ideal for evaluation of valvular calcifications and calcification in masses. Fat attenuation may be detected within the myocardium on nongated CT, which may be a normal congenital finding, sequela of fibrofatty replacement in the setting of infarction, or fat within a cardiac mass.

ECG-gated CTA provides a comprehensive and noninvasive assessment of coronary artery anatomy and disease. From anomalies and plaque characterization to advanced applications, such as noninvasive fractional flow reserve CT, this modality has become an integral part of ischemic heart disease evaluation and risk stratification. ECG-gated cardiac CT is the gold standard for the preoperative evaluation of the aortic root or other valves in transcatheter valve replacement procedures while continuing its role as the modality of choice for postoperative valves, stents, and other metallic devices.

MR

MR has emerged as the gold standard for functional analysis of the heart and remains a key modality for detecting cardiomyopathies and for characterizing cardiac masses. The primary sequences employed in the most frequent clinical indications for cardiac MR are as follows:

- *Balanced steady-state free precession* allows a superior dynamic/cine assessment of cardiac function. Additionally, flow jets on this sequence can detect (but not truly quantify) valvular stenosis and regurgitation. An important consideration when analyzing these images is that contrast is dependent on a T2:T1 ratio. Therefore, tissue characterization on this sequence should be done with caution, and analysis of these sequences should focus on morphology and function.
- *Double inversion recovery* sequences may be T1 or T2 weighted, resulting in a black blood pool and allowing true tissue characterization. An important artifact to be aware of on this sequence is the hyperintense blood pool from slow-flowing blood, particularly in the trabeculations of the myocardium.
- *Phase-contrast* imaging uses bipolar gradients to measure phase shifts of moving spins proportional to their velocity. This allows quantification of flow volume and velocity of blood, a powerful tool when evaluating valvular heart disease and intracardiac shunts.
- *Late gadolinium enhancement (LGE)* inversion recovery sequences detect gadolinium that has accumulated in the interstitial/extracellular space of the myocardium, suggesting inflammation or fibrosis. Approximately 8-10 minutes after IV gadolinium administration, an optimum inversion time is selected to null the myocardium and detect enhancement. The patterns of LGE are associated with diseases with variable specificity. Subendocardial and transmural disease in a vascular territory is most consistent with ischemic cardiomyopathy. Midwall disease should raise the suspicion for infiltrative, nonischemic cardiomyopathies and myocarditis. Subepicardial disease is most frequently associated with myocarditis and sarcoidosis.

FDG PET/CT

FDG PET/CT identifies areas of pathologic glucose uptake and inflammation and has an emerging role in the detection and characterization of cardiac sarcoidosis when combined with perfusion imaging. 99mTc-pyrophosphate scanning has become an important tool for detecting amyloidogenic transthyretin protein specific cardiac amyloidosis.

Selected References

1. Expert Panel on Cardiac Imaging et al: ACR Appropriateness Criteria® suspected new-onset and known nonacute heart failure. J Am Coll Radiol. 15(11S):S418-31, 2018
2. Munden RF et al: Managing incidental findings on thoracic CT: mediastinal and cardiovascular findings. A white paper of the ACR incidental findings committee. J Am Coll Radiol. 15(8):1087-96, 2018

Coronary Artery Aneurysm

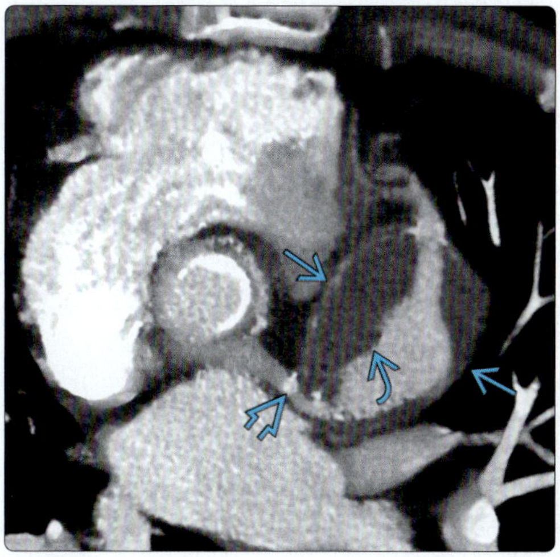

Papillary Fibroelastoma

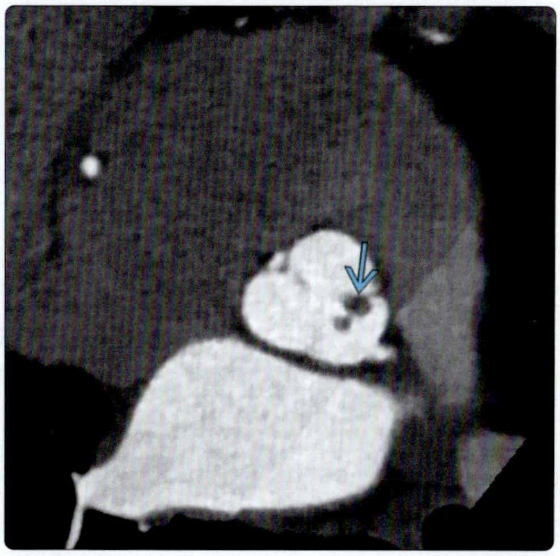

(Left) *ECG-gated MIP CTA reformatted short axis to the aortic valve of a patient status post aortic valve surgery shows a large aneurysm ➔ of the left anterior descending coronary artery. Note the eccentric thrombus ↷ in the aneurysm and atherosclerotic calcifications ⇒. Atherosclerosis is the most common cause of coronary artery aneurysm.* **(Right)** *ECG-gated CTA reformatted short axis to the aortic valve with papillary fibroelastoma shows a bilobed mass ➔ on the valve leaflet between the right and left coronary cusps.*

Cardiac Sarcoidosis

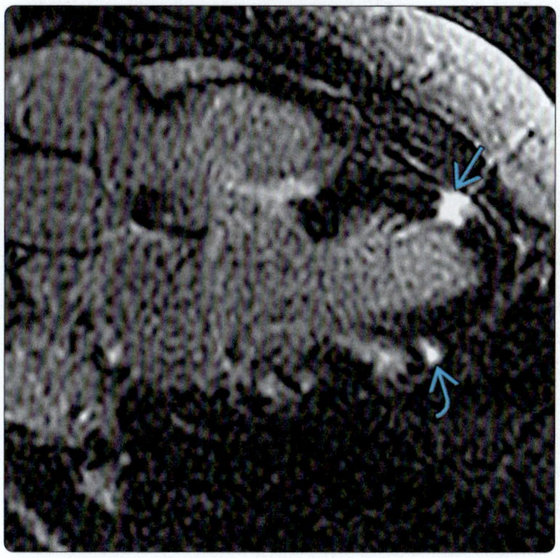

Cardiac Thrombus

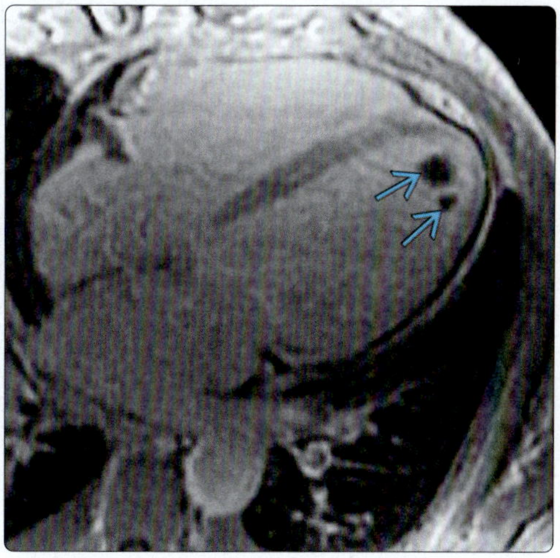

(Left) *Four-chamber late gadolinium enhancement (LGE) MR of a patient with sarcoidosis shows patchy midwall ➔ and subepicardial ↷ LGE, consistent with cardiac sarcoidosis. Cardiac MR is central to the diagnosis of many nonischemic cardiomyopathies.* **(Right)** *Inversion recovery (600 ms) 4-chamber MR of a patient with HIV cardiomyopathy shows 2 low-intensity masses ➔ in the cardiac apex, consistent with thrombus. Very long inversion times accentuate low-intensity thrombus.*

Cardiac Lymphoma

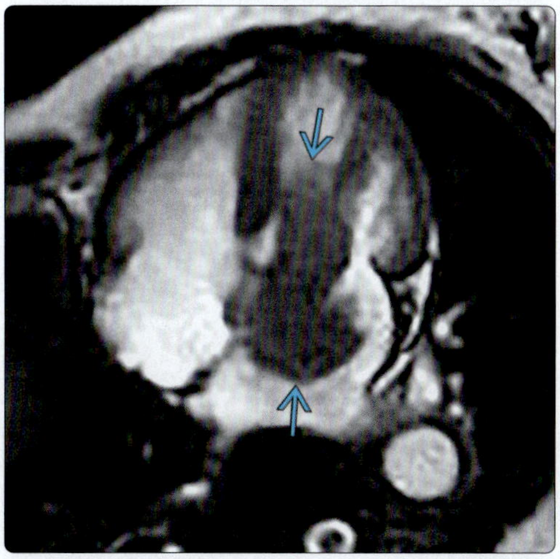

Cardiac Angiosarcoma

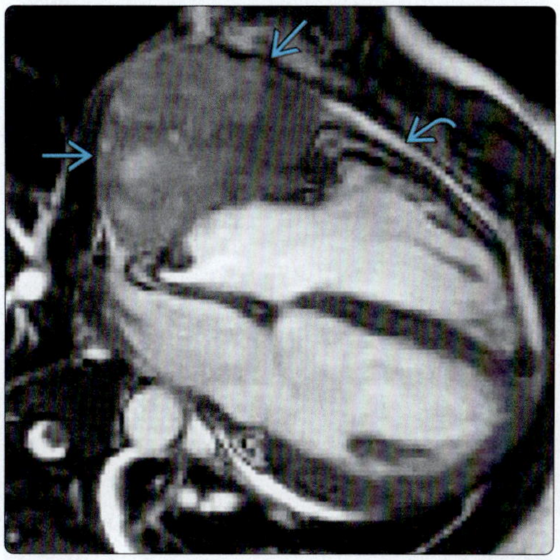

(Left) *Four-chamber balanced steady-state free precession (SSFP) MR of a patient with a history of dyspnea shows a large, lobulated mass ➔ in both the left atrium and left ventricle, spanning across the mitral valve, subsequently diagnosed with cardiac lymphoma.* **(Right)** *4-chamber SSFP MR of a patient with cardiac angiosarcoma shows a heterogeneous mass ➔ centered on the wall of the right ventricle and associated pericardial effusion ↷. Cardiac MR is an essential tool when evaluating cardiac masses.*

Left Atrial Enlargement

DIFFERENTIAL DIAGNOSIS

Common

- Left Heart Failure
- Mitral Valve Disease

Less Common

- Left-to-Right Shunt

Rare but Important

- Constrictive Pericarditis
- Restrictive Cardiomyopathy
  - Amyloidosis
  - Sarcoidosis
  - Hemochromatosis

ESSENTIAL INFORMATION

Key Differential Diagnosis Issues

- Radiography
  - Double density sign
  - Splaying of carina
  - Superior displacement of left mainstem bronchus
  - Posterior esophageal displacement
  - Enlarged left atrial appendage
- Anteroposterior diameter > 50 mm in men, > 45 mm in women
- Rightward displacement of interatrial septum suggests left atrial enlargement
- Normal volume = 22 ± 5 mL/m²

Helpful Clues for Common Diagnoses

- **Left Heart Failure**
  - Etiologies
    - Chronic ischemia
    - Diabetes
    - Chronic hypertension
  - Left ventricular enlargement with widening of mitral valve annulus
- **Mitral Valve Disease**
  - Stenosis
    - Coexistent edema suggests valve area is < 1 cm² (normal 4-6 cm²)
    - Calcified leaflets not to be confused with mitral annular calcification
    - Leaflet thickening
  - Regurgitation
    - May be secondary to widening of annulus in left ventricular enlargement or valvular disease
    - Often coexists with stenosis and calcified valve
    - Absence of calcifications suggests prolapse or ruptured papillary muscle

Helpful Clues for Less Common Diagnoses

- **Left-to-Right Shunt**
  - Qp:Qs ratio > 1
  - Ventricular septal defect does not cause left atrial enlargement unless large
  - Atrial septal defect only with Eisenmenger physiology in advanced age
  - Patent ductus arteriosus will also have left ventricular enlargement

Helpful Clues for Rare Diagnoses

- **Constrictive Pericarditis**
  - Etiologies
    - Pericarditis (including tuberculosis)
    - Prior cardiac surgery
    - Radiation to mediastinum
  - Tubular, bullet-shaped ventricles along with biatrial enlargement
  - Focal or diffuse pericardial thickening > 4 mm or calcification in presence of heart failure
  - Diastolic septal bounce accentuated during deep inspiration
- **Restrictive Cardiomyopathy**
  - Etiologies
    - Cardiac amyloidosis
    - Sarcoidosis
    - Hemochromatosis
  - Typically normal left ventricular volumes and preserved ejection fraction, along with atrial enlargement

Left Heart Failure

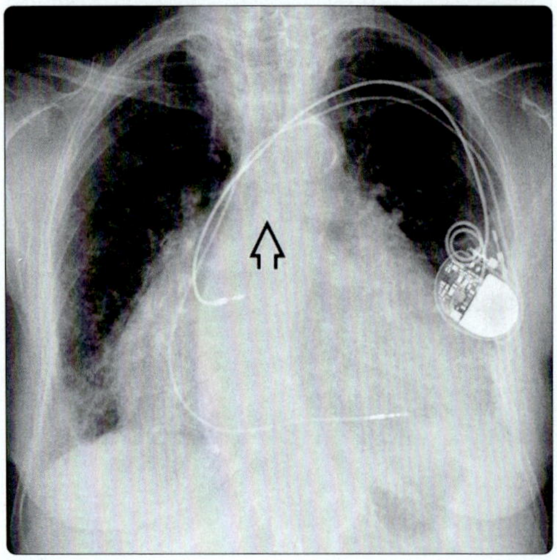

Left Heart Failure

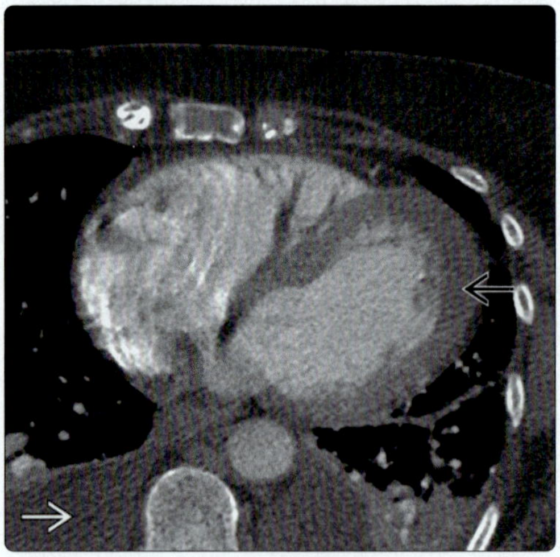

(Left) *Frontal radiograph shows marked cardiomegaly with left atrial and ventricular enlargement in a patient with heart failure. Note splaying of the carinal angle (normal < 90°) ⇨.* **(Right)** *Axial CECT of a patient with diastolic heart failure and left atrial enlargement from uncontrolled hypertension shows pleural effusion ➡ and concentric left ventricle thickening ⇨. Etiologies of left heart failure include chronic ischemia, diabetes, and chronic hypertension.*

Mitral Valve Disease

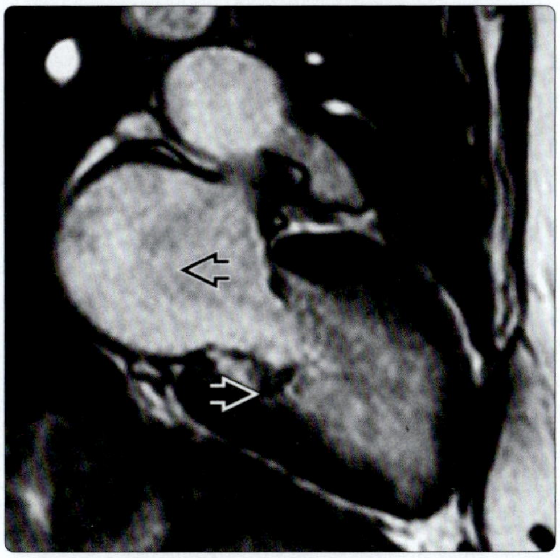

Mitral Valve Disease

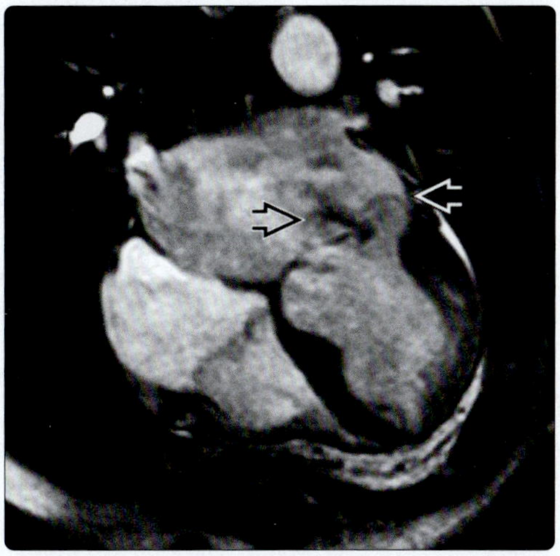

(Left) *Vertical long-axis bright-blood cine MR shows a calcified mitral valve with both mitral stenosis and regurgitation in a patient with rheumatic heart disease. Left atrial enlargement is present.* **(Right)** *Four-chamber bright-blood cine MR of the same patient shows prolapse of the mitral valve with a regurgitant jet. Mitral stenosis should be suspected when left atrial enlargement is present along with calcified leaflets and leaflet thickening.*

Mitral Valve Disease

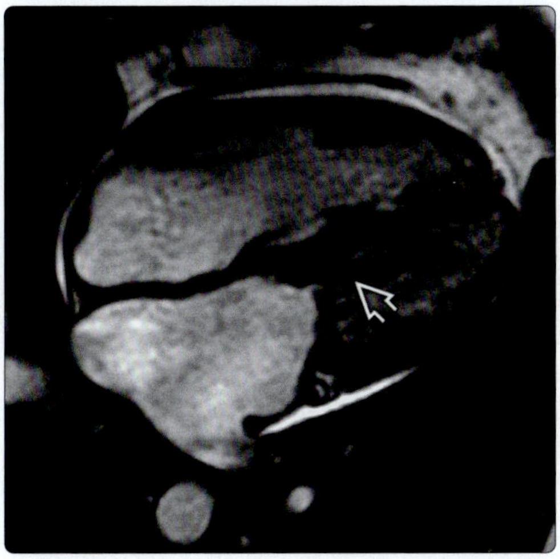

Left-to-Right Shunt

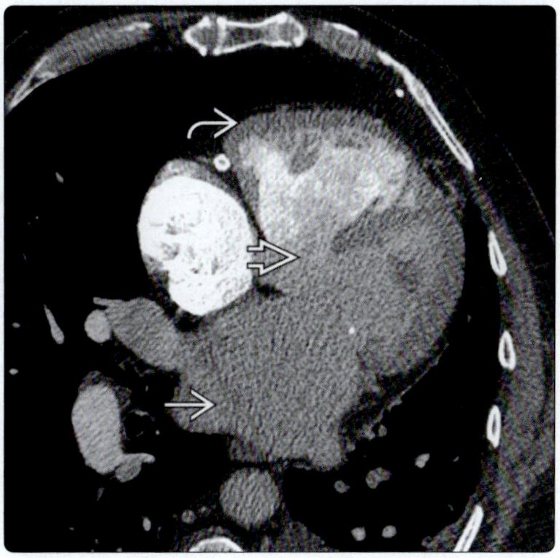

(Left) *Four-chamber bright-blood cine MR of a patient with mitral stenosis demonstrates a turbulent jet.* **(Right)** *Four-chamber CECT of a patient with a left-to-right shunt demonstrates a large membranous ventricular septal defect with left atrial enlargement. Right ventricular hypertrophy reflects long-standing elevated right-sided pressure. Ventricular septal defects typically do not cause left atrial enlargement unless they are large.*

Constrictive Pericarditis

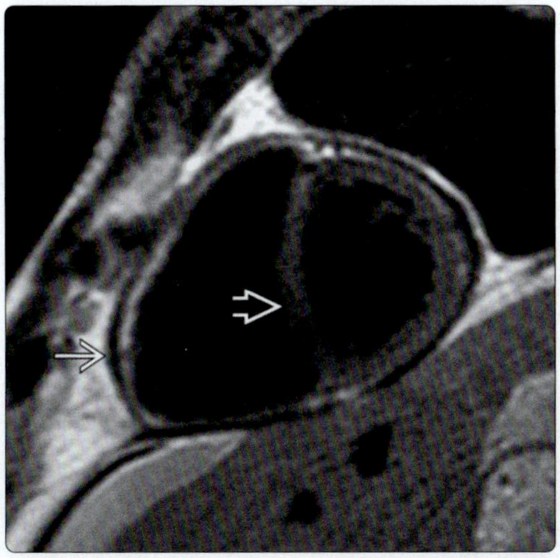

Restrictive Cardiomyopathy

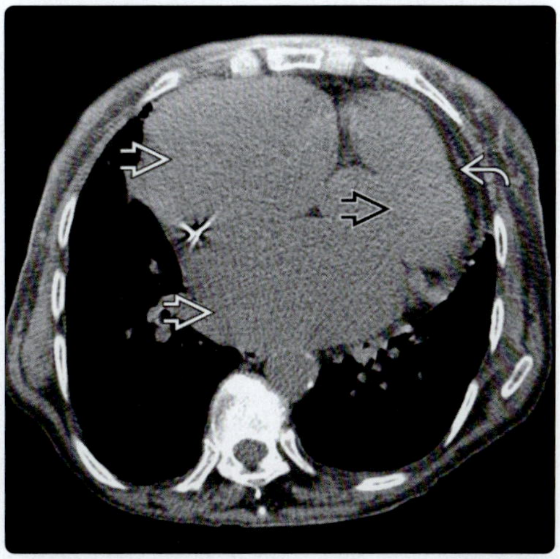

(Left) *Short-axis black blood mid-chamber MR shows pericardial thickening and flattening of the interventricular septum in a patient with constrictive pericarditis. Left and right atrial enlargement were also present.* **(Right)** *Axial NECT shows biatrial enlargement with small ventricles and a normal pericardium in a patient with restrictive cardiomyopathy from sarcoidosis. Normal left ventricular volumes and preserved ejection fraction along with atrial enlargement are typical.*

DIFFERENTIAL DIAGNOSIS

Common

- Pulmonary Hypertension
- Pulmonary Regurgitation
- Tricuspid Valve Disease

Less Common

- Left-to-Right Shunt

Rare but Important

- Right Atrial Mass
- Ebstein Anomaly

ESSENTIAL INFORMATION

Key Differential Diagnosis Issues

- Radiography
  - Rightward displacement of right lower heart contour
- CT/MR
  - End-diastolic volume (maximum volume) > 90 mL/m² highly specific for enlargement
  - Transverse diameter ≥ 67 mm for men and ≥ 64 mm for women

Helpful Clues for Common Diagnoses

- **Pulmonary Hypertension**
  - Secondary cause of right atrial enlargement
  - Pulmonary hypertension suggested by specific measurements
    - Aorta:PA ratio < 1:1
    - Main PA > 2.9 cm
- Pulmonary Regurgitation
  - Secondary cause of right atrial enlargement
  - Consider in patients with repaired tetralogy of Fallot
- **Tricuspid Valve Disease**
  - Commonly seen as result of widening of tricuspid valve annulus in setting of right ventricular enlargement
  - Other etiologies of regurgitation
    - Myxomatous degeneration, rheumatic heart disease in older population
  - Increased serotonin levels in carcinoid syndrome can generate fibrous tricuspid leaflet plaques that cause regurgitation

Helpful Clues for Less Common Diagnoses

- **Left-to-Right Shunt**
  - Qp:Qs > 1
  - Atrial septal defect
    - Bright-blood cine MR likely to show flow jet except in large atrial septal defect
  - Ventricular septal defect
    - Most common left-to-right shunt but often not hemodynamically significant or spontaneously closes by adulthood
  - Partial anomalous pulmonary venous return
    - Most commonly from right upper lobe to superior vena cava seen best on CT or MRA
    - Anomalous right upper lobe pulmonary venous return may coexist with sinus venosus atrial septal defect

Helpful Clues for Rare Diagnoses

- **Right Atrial Mass**
  - Myxoma
    - Soft, pliable mass
    - Connected to interatrial septum by thin stalk
    - MR
      - Intermediate to low signal on T1WI
      - High signal on T2WI
  - Angiosarcoma
    - Aggressive neoplasm typically arising from wall of right atrium
    - May invade chamber or pericardium
- **Ebstein Anomaly**
  - Apical displacement of septal and posterior tricuspid leaflets with atrialization of proximal right ventricle
  - Coexistent tricuspid regurgitation and stenosis common

Pulmonary Hypertension

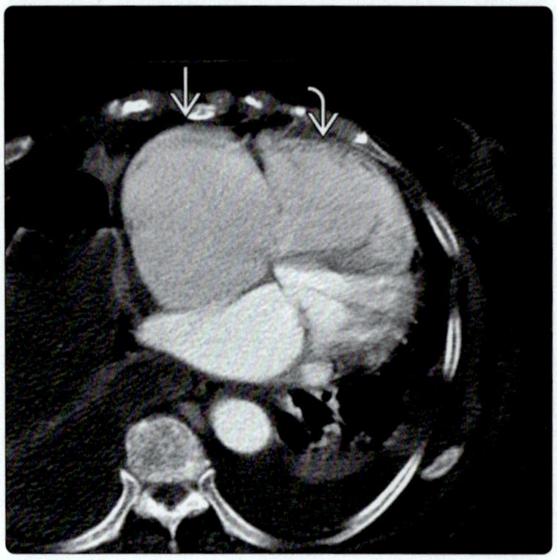

Tricuspid Valve Disease

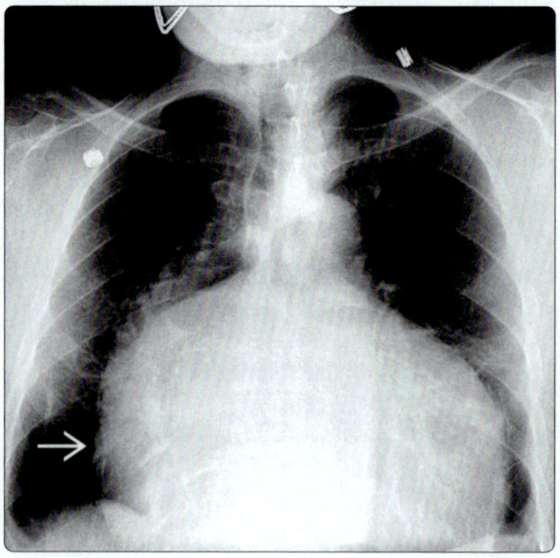

(Left) *Axial CECT demonstrates right atrial ➔ and right ventricular ➔ enlargement due to primary pulmonary hypertension and right heart failure. Left heart function is normal. On this admission, the patient presented with atrial fibrillation.* **(Right)** *Frontal radiograph shows enlarged cardiac silhouette in a patient with right atrial and right ventricular enlargement. Note marked lateral displacement of the right heart border ➔.*

Tricuspid Valve Disease

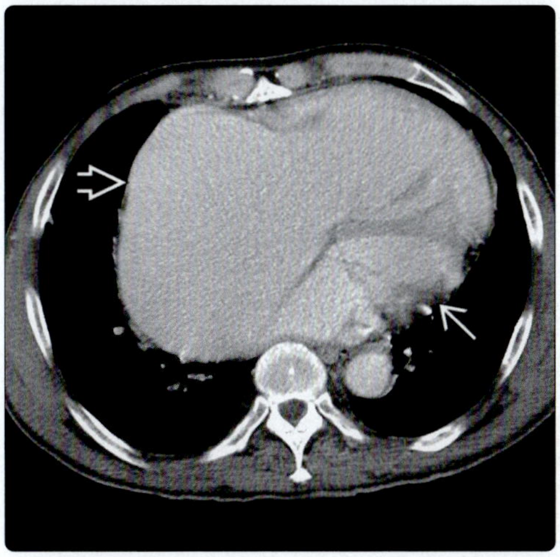

Tricuspid Valve Disease

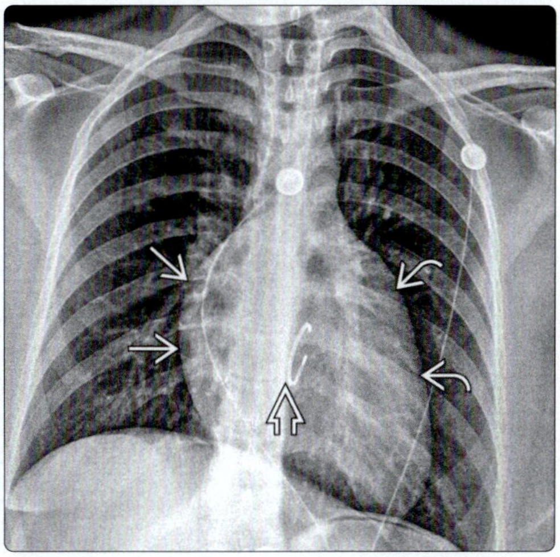

(Left) *Axial CECT of a patient with severe tricuspid regurgitation demonstrates marked right atrial enlargement. Note the massive right heart enlargement and normal left ventricle .* **(Right)** *Frontal radiograph of a patient with repaired pulmonary atresia and tricuspid regurgitation demonstrates displaced cardiac contours of both right atrial and right ventricular enlargement.*

Left-to-Right Shunt

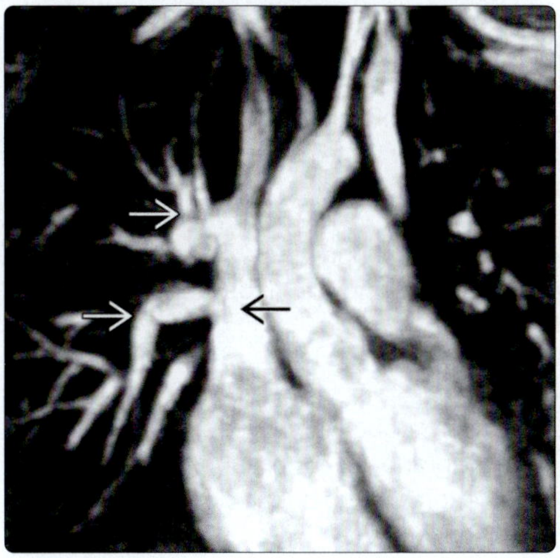

Left-to-Right Shunt

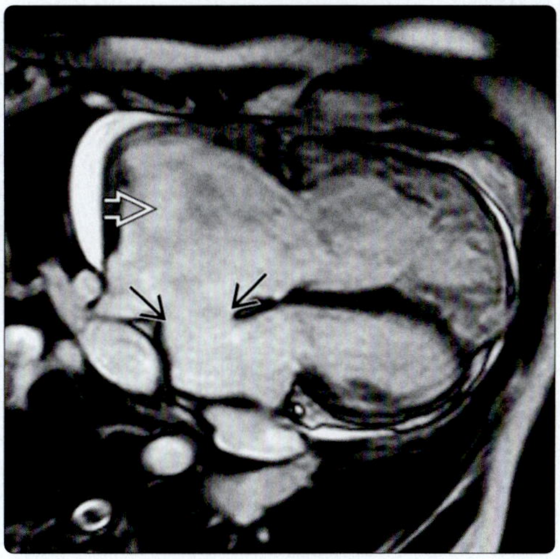

(Left) *3D MRA shows right upper lobe venous return entering the superior vena cava . Right atrial enlargement was present. This patient did not have a sinus venosus defect.* **(Right)** *Four-chamber cine MR shows a large atrial septal defect with right atrial enlargement . Note that no flow jet is present in this large atrial septal defect. Qp:Qs was 2.2. Left-to-right shunts, such as atrial septal defect and ventricular septal defect, may result in right atrial enlargement.*

Right Atrial Mass

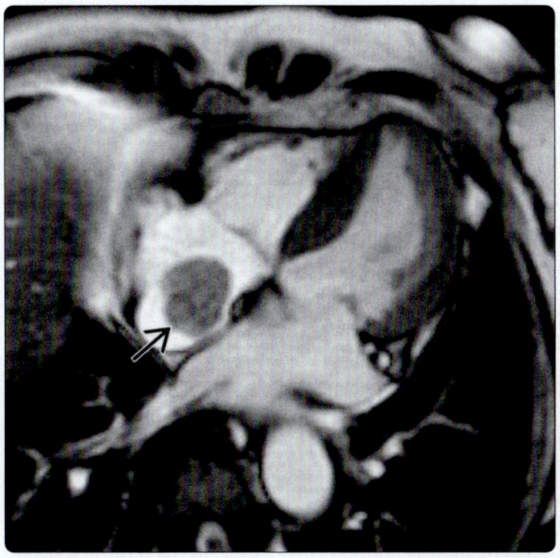

Ebstein Anomaly

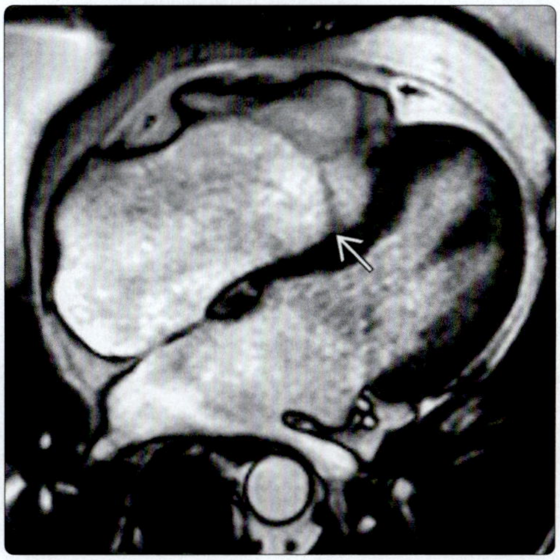

(Left) *Four-chamber cine MR shows a right atrial mass that attaches to the interatrial septum , representing a biopsy-proven right atrial myxoma. Although not in this case, these masses can obstruct the atrioventricular valve and cause chamber enlargement.* **(Right)** *Four-chamber cine MR shows downward displacement of the tricuspid leaflet , giving the appearance of an enlarged right atrium. This adult was an undiagnosed case of Ebstein anomaly with tricuspid regurgitation and an atrial septal defect.*

DIFFERENTIAL DIAGNOSIS

Common

- Heart Failure
- Aortic Regurgitation
- Mitral Regurgitation
- Acute Myocardial Infarction

Less Common

- Patent Ductus Arteriosus
- Coarctation of Aorta
- Idiopathic Dilated Cardiomyopathy
- Hypertrophic Cardiomyopathy
- Amyloidosis

Rare but Important

- Athlete's Heart
- Dilated Cardiomyopathy
  - Pregnancy-Induced
  - Alcohol-Induced

ESSENTIAL INFORMATION

Key Differential Diagnosis Issues

- Determination of left ventricular enlargement
  - Radiography
    - Normal cardiothoracic ratio
      - ≤ 0.5 on PA radiograph
      - ≤ 0.6 on AP radiograph at deep inspiration
    - Displacement of left heart border
      - Leftward
      - Downward
    - Left ventricle extending 2 cm posterior to border of inferior vena cava on lateral view
      - a.k.a. Hoffman-Rigler sign
  - CT/MR
    - Regarding left ventricular volume measurements
      - Best measured qualitatively, not quantitatively, when only axial planes are available
      - Reliable measurements require double oblique planes, usually short axis
    - Normal internal left ventricular diameter at base
      - 3.9-5.3 cm for females
      - 4.2-5.9 cm for males
    - Most reproducible
      - 2-dimensional Simpson rule of discs in short axis
      - 3D auto-segmented
    - Less reliable
      - Biplane method of Simpson rule and area length rule
    - Specific volumes are highly specific for pathology
      - > 130 mL in females
      - > 200 mL in males
- Determination of left ventricular wall thickness
  - Specific measurements are pathologic
    - End-diastolic wall thickness
      - > 1.2 cm
    - Left ventricular mass
      - > 104 gm/m² in females
      - > 119 gm/m² in males
- Pitfalls
  - Mimics of radiographic left ventricular enlargement
    - Pericardial effusion
    - Poor lateral positioning
    - Pericardial fat pad
  - Erroneous left ventricular size measurement
    - Misidentification of end-diastole
  - Cardiac volume may be affected by pre-imaging administration of medications
    - β blockers
    - Nitroglycerin

Helpful Clues for Common Diagnoses

- **Heart Failure**
  - Etiologies
    - Ischemic cardiomyopathy is most common
    - Diabetes
    - Hypertension
  - Imaging
    - EF < 40%
    - Multivessel coronary artery calcifications or stenosis
    - Evidence of prior infarct, subendocardial fat
    - Myocardium can be evaluated for evidence of hibernation
      - Retrospective gated CT or MR
    - Findings suggestive of ischemia
      - Subendocardial or transmural delayed enhancement present in coronary artery distribution
    - Findings suggestive of nonischemic etiologies
      - If delayed enhancement excludes subendocardial layer
- **Aortic Regurgitation**
  - Imaging
    - Bicuspid valve or calcified aortic valve
    - Incomplete coaptation of cusps during diastole
    - Regurgitant jet present on bright-blood MR
- **Mitral Regurgitation**
  - Imaging
    - Mitral valve calcifications
    - Dilated left atrium
    - Isolated right upper lobe edema
      - Rare manifestation
      - Results from regurgitant jet
- **Acute Myocardial Infarction**
  - Supporting clinical information
    - Troponin leak
    - ECG changes
    - Typical chest pain
  - Imaging
    - Enlarged cardiac silhouette compared to recent prior

Helpful Clues for Less Common Diagnoses

- **Patent Ductus Arteriosus**
  - Imaging
    - Initially, main pulmonary arteries are enlarged
    - Other vessels become enlarged later on
      - Left ventricle
      - Left atrium
      - Ascending aorta

- Left ventricular enlargement with dilated ascending aorta
  - Absence of valvular disease
- Best seen on gated CT or 3D MRA
- MR Qp:Qs ratio < 1:1

- **Coarctation of Aorta**
  - Associated with bicuspid valve
  - Imaging
    - Dilated intercostal collaterals
      - Represents hemodynamic narrowing
    - Potential pitfall
      - Pseudocoarctation of aorta: Tortuous arch without hemodynamic narrowing
    - Undiagnosed cases in adults often occur when narrowing distal to left subclavian take-off
- **Idiopathic Dilated Cardiomyopathy**
  - Age often < 60 years
  - Diagnosis of exclusion
    - Significant coronary artery occlusion
    - Myocarditis
  - Imaging
    - MR delayed enhancement
      - Present in ~ 40% of cases
      - Most commonly mid-myocardial
    - Specific measurements
      - EF < 40%
      - Fractional shortening < 25%
- **Hypertrophic Cardiomyopathy**
  - Variants
    - Asymmetric septal
    - Apical
    - Concentric
  - Differential diagnosis for concentric variant
    - Hypertensive heart disease/aortic stenosis
    - Amyloidosis
    - Sarcoidosis
  - Imaging
    - Left ventricular outflow tract view shows systolic anterior motion of mitral valve leaflet
    - Patchy mid-myocardial enhancement
      - Left ventricular thickening
      - Right ventricular insertion into left ventricle
- **Amyloidosis**
  - Patients typically > 65 years
  - Imaging
    - Increased left ventricular wall thickness
      - Poor or normal contractility
    - Diffuse subendocardial perfusion defect
    - Findings on delayed enhancement inversion recovery sequences
      - Equal relaxation times between blood pool and myocardium

Helpful Clues for Rare Diagnoses

- **Athlete's Heart**
  - Occurs in athletes who engage in prolonged aerobic activity
  - Imaging
    - End-diastolic volume > 0.15 in young patient with dilated heart suggests athlete's heart
    - Left ventricular volume will decrease following 3 months of de-conditioning
- **Pregnancy-Induced Dilated Cardiomyopathy**
  - Accompanying clinical history
  - Imaging
    - Left ventricular enlargement and hypokinesis
    - Follow-up imaging in 3 months may show resolution
- **Alcohol-Induced Dilated Cardiomyopathy**
  - Accompanying clinical history
  - Imaging
    - Left ventricular enlargement and hypokinesis
    - Follow-up imaging will show resolution if acute

Heart Failure

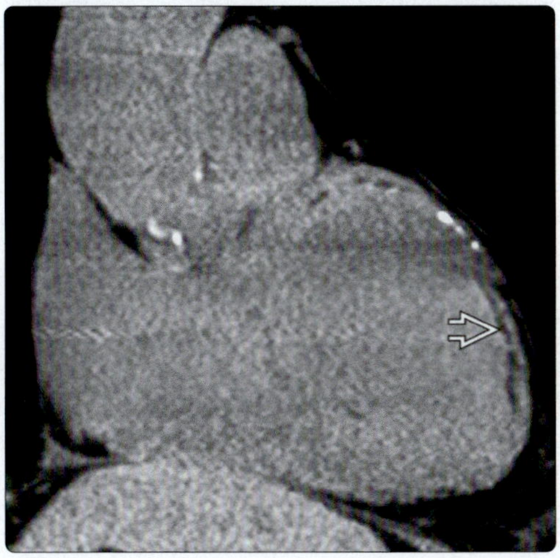

Heart Failure

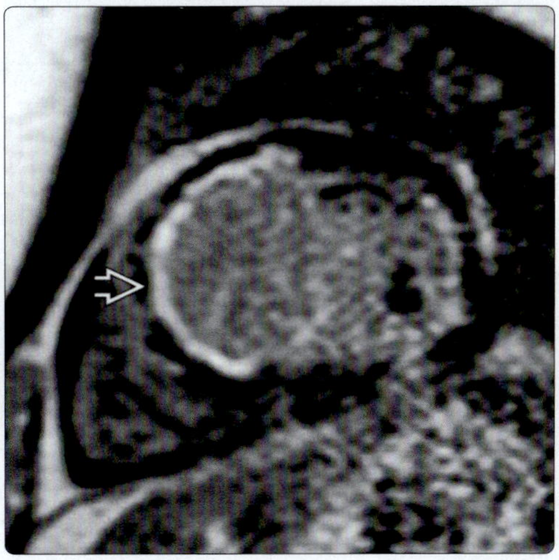

(Left) *Coronal oblique NECT of ischemic heart failure shows left ventricular enlargement with subepicardial fat ➡, predominantly in an LAD distribution, representing prior infarct.* **(Right)** *Short-axis inversion recovery MR through the mid-chamber of the left ventricle shows dilated left ventricle with late gadolinium enhancement in a LAD distribution ➡, compatible with ischemic cardiomyopathy.*

(Left) *Four-chamber bright-blood cine MR of a patient with history of longstanding, uncontrolled hypertension shows a mildly dilated left ventricle with diffuse wall thickening. This will eventually progress to an appearance indistinguishable from other dilated cardiomyopathies.* **(Right)** *Diastolic phase left ventricular outflow tract CECT shows a markedly dilated left ventricle without aortic valve disease. This patient had depressed ejection fraction and densely calcified coronary arteries, indicating ischemic cardiomyopathy.*

Heart Failure

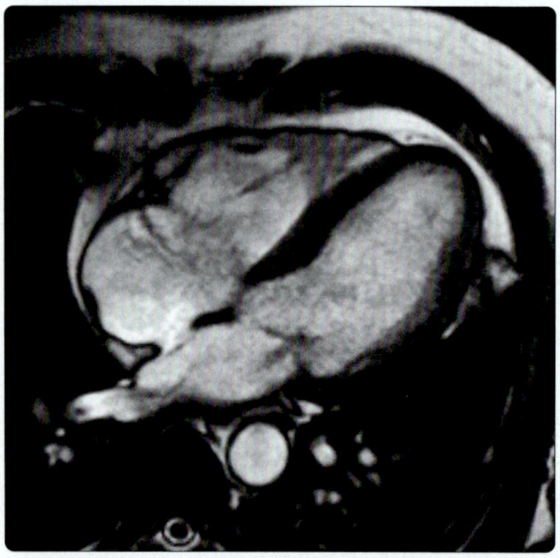

Heart Failure

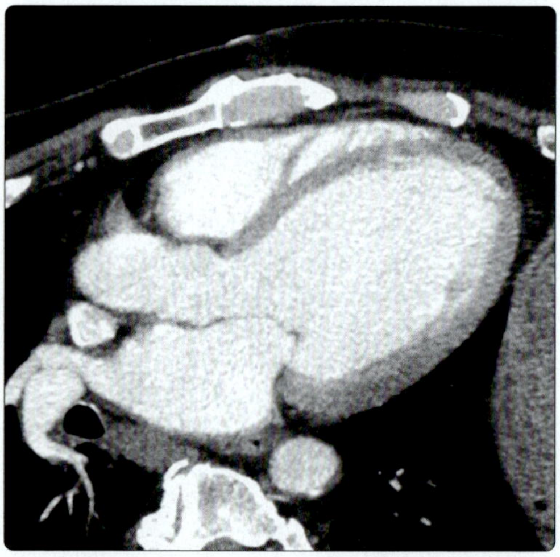

(Left) *Coronal cine MR of a patient with aortic regurgitation shows a turbulent jet originating at the aortic valve, directed toward the left ventricle ➔.* **(Right)** *Systolic phase left ventricular outflow tract cine MR of mitral regurgitation demonstrates low signal corresponding to regurgitation ➔ due to mitral valve prolapse. The prolapsing leaflet is seen ➔ with a regurgitant jet directed at the septum.*

Aortic Regurgitation

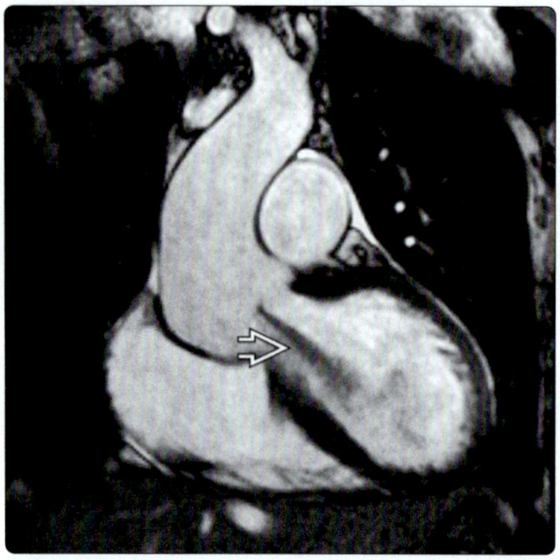

Mitral Regurgitation

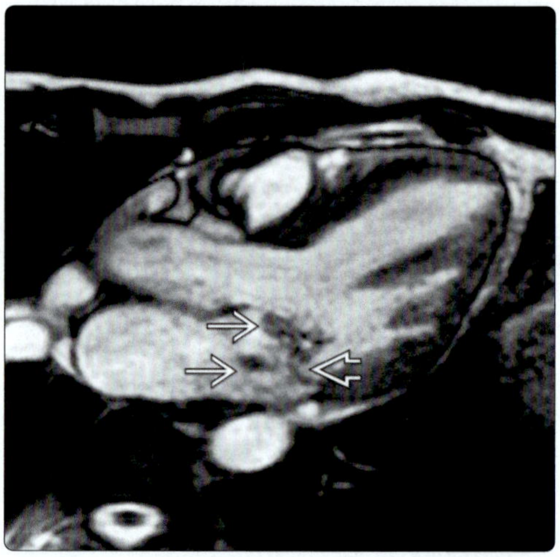

(Left) *Short-axis inversion recovery FSE MR through the left ventricle mid-chamber shows mid-myocardial LAD distribution late gadolinium enhancement ➔. Hypointense subendocardium indicates acute myocardial infarction-associated microvascular obstruction ➔.* **(Right)** *Axial oblique CTA shows a connection ➔ between the proximal descending aorta and the pulmonary artery, diagnostic of a patent ductus arteriosus. This left-to-right shunt resulted in left ventricular enlargement.*

Acute Myocardial Infarction

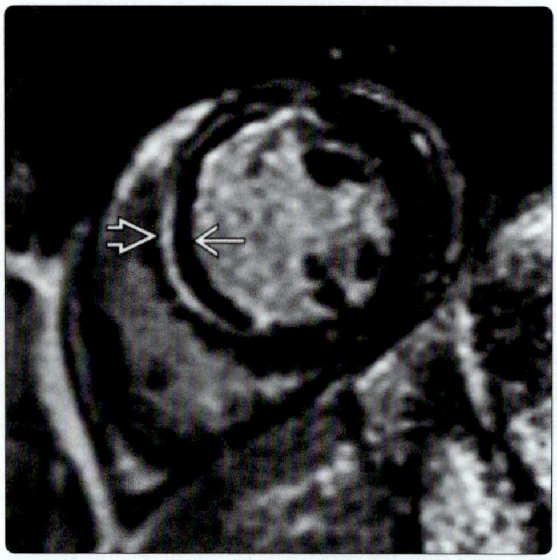

Patent Ductus Arteriosus

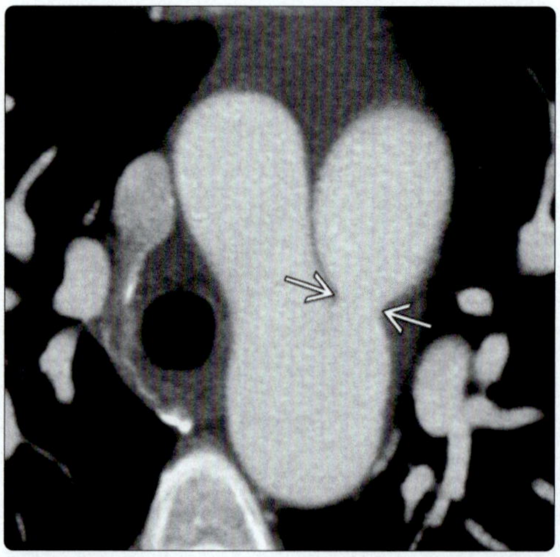

Patent Ductus Arteriosus

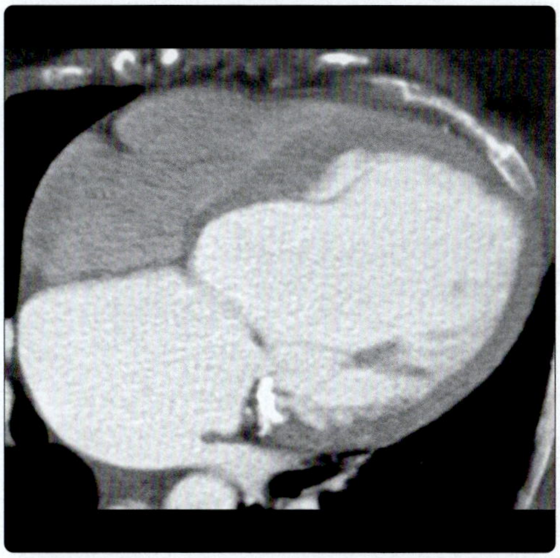

Coarctation of Aorta

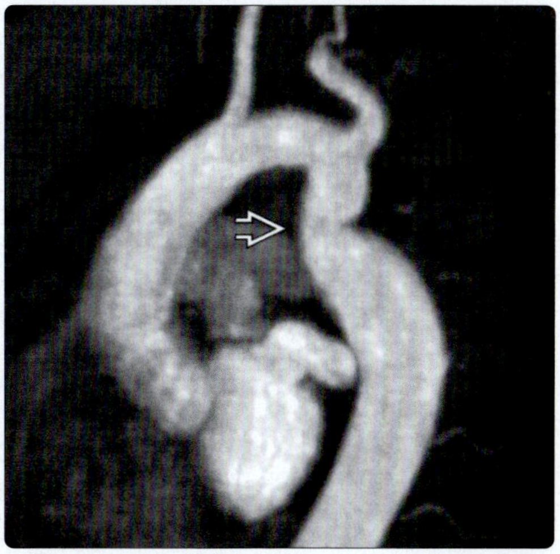

(Left) *Four-chamber CTA of a patient with patent ductus arteriosus shows dilation of the left atrium and left ventricle from chronic volume overload.* **(Right)** *Sagittal T1WI C+ FS MR shows focal narrowing distal to the left subclavian take-off ➔. The presence of intercostal collaterals and left ventricular enlargement indicated a hemodynamically significant stenosis, differentiating coarctation of the aorta from pseudocoarctation.*

Idiopathic Dilated Cardiomyopathy

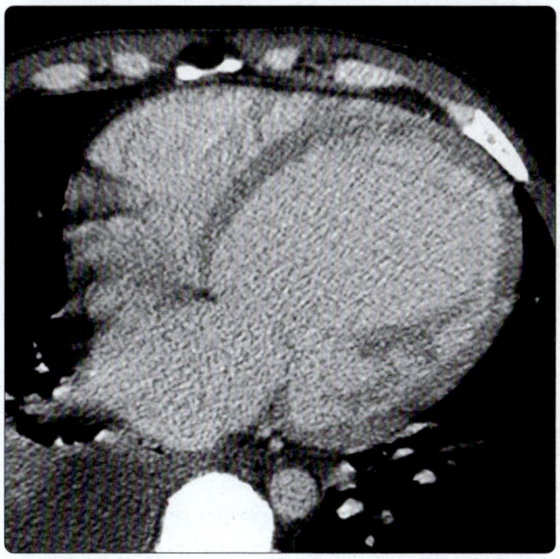

Idiopathic Dilated Cardiomyopathy

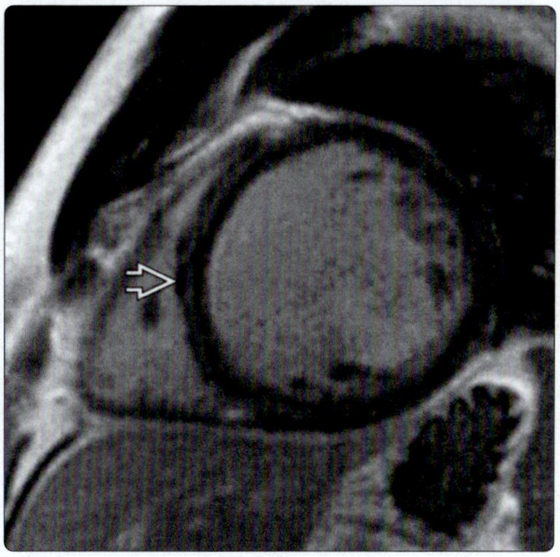

(Left) *Axial NECT of a 41-year-old man with symptoms of heart failure shows left ventricular dilation without coronary artery disease. The etiology of the cardiomyopathy was not found and a diagnosis of idiopathic dilated cardiomyopathy was made.* **(Right)** *Short-axis inversion recovery FSE MR shows septal mid-myocardial enhancement in a patient with idiopathic dilated cardiomyopathy ➔.*

Hypertrophic Cardiomyopathy

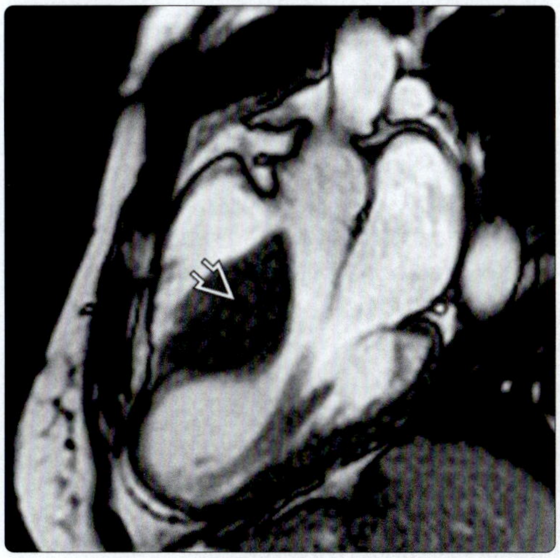

Amyloidosis

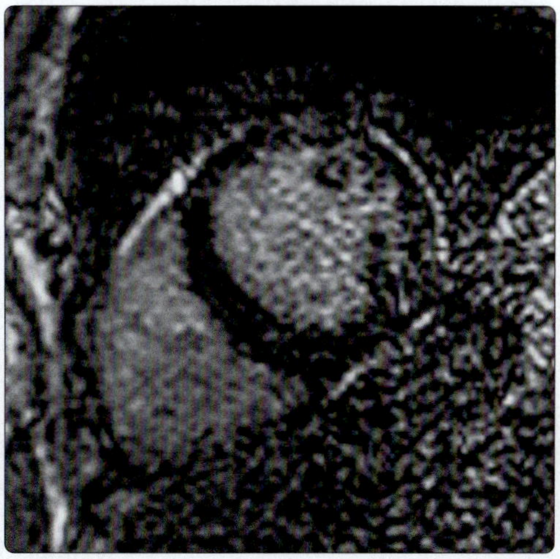

(Left) *Diastolic phase left ventricular outflow tract bright-blood cine MR of asymmetric variant hypertrophic cardiomyopathy shows asymmetric thickening of the interventricular septum at the base ➔.* **(Right)** *Short-axis inversion recovery FSE MR through the left ventricle mid-chamber 10 minutes after gadolinium injection shows near-equal relaxation of the blood pool and myocardium. This finding is caused by altered gadolinium concentration kinetics due to the presence of amyloid protein.*

DIFFERENTIAL DIAGNOSIS

Common

- Left Heart Failure
- Secondary Pulmonary Hypertension
- Right Heart Failure

Less Common

- Left-to-Right Shunt
- Right Heart Valvular Disease
- Primary Pulmonary Arterial Hypertension

Rare but Important

- Arrhythmogenic Right Ventricular Cardiomyopathy
- Congenital Heart Disease
  - D-Transposition of Great Vessels With Atrial Switch
  - Tetralogy of Fallot With Pulmonic Regurgitation or Stenosis

ESSENTIAL INFORMATION

Key Differential Diagnosis Issues

- Quantitative determination of right ventricular dilation
  - Normal end-diastolic volume
    - 75 ± 13 mL/m² for adolescent to adult
  - Best method of obtaining measurements
    - Bright-blood cine MR in axial or short axis plane
    - Retrospectively gated CT
- Radiographic signs of right ventricular enlargement
  - Frontal
    - Leftward displacement and flattening of left heart contour
  - Lateral
    - Filling of retrosternal clear space and posterior displacement of left ventricle
  - Flattening of interventricular septum only during diastole suggests volume overload
  - Flattening of interventricular septum during systole and diastole suggests pressure overload with or without volume overload
- Quantitative determination of right ventricular hypertrophy
  - Wall thickness > 5 mm suggests hypertrophy
  - Normal right ventricular free wall mass
    - 26 ± 5 g/m²
- Chest CT measurements for determination of right ventricular enlargement
  - Right ventricular transverse diameter
    - ≥ 60 mm for men
    - ≥ 57 mm for women

Helpful Clues for Common Diagnoses

- **Left Heart Failure**
  - Most common etiologies
    - Ischemic cardiomyopathy
    - Diabetes mellitus
  - Imaging
    - Multivessel coronary artery calcifications/disease
    - Left ventricular and atrial enlargement
    - Pulmonary edema
    - Prior myocardial infarction; left ventricular delayed enhancement, endomyocardial fat, or aneurysm
    - Diastolic heart failure more commonly associated with elevated left atrial pressure, left ventricle may be normal in size
- **Secondary Pulmonary Hypertension**
  - Pulmonary trunk > 2.8 cm if < 50 years, trunk:ascending aorta ratio > 1 if > 50 years
  - Right ventricular mass/(left ventricular + septum mass) > 0.6 suggests pulmonary hypertension
  - MR delayed contrast enhancement at right ventricular wall insertion into interventricular septum
  - Suspect if interstitial lung disease, COPD, or chronic pulmonary embolism
  - Suspect if mitral valve disease is present
    - Stenosis
      - Thickened, calcified leaflets
      - Diastolic jet on cine MR
    - Regurgitation
      - Widened mitral valve annulus
      - Mitral valve prolapse
      - Systolic jet directed towards left atrium on cine MR
- **Right Heart Failure**
  - Markedly enlarged right ventricle with relatively normal left ventricle
  - Right atrial enlargement
  - Enlarged inferior vena cava/superior vena cava and ascites
  - Ischemic cardiomyopathy suggested by proximal right coronary artery occlusive disease or left circumflex disease when left-dominant coronary anatomy present

Helpful Clues for Less Common Diagnoses

- **Left-to-Right Shunt**
  - Atrial septal defect (ASD)
    - 2nd most common left-to-right shunt but most likely to cause dilated right ventricle
    - Coexistent right atrial enlargement
    - MR bright-blood cine short axis or 4-chamber stack without skip throughout interatrial septum may show flow jet
    - Large ASD may not show flow jet on bright-blood cine
    - MR phase contrast determines main QpQs > 1
    - In cases of sinus venous ASD, look for partial anomalous pulmonary venous return
  - Ventricular septal defect
    - Most common left-to-right shunt but often not hemodynamically significant or spontaneously closes by adulthood
    - Best investigated with methods similar to ASD
  - Partial anomalous pulmonary venous return
    - Most commonly involves right upper lobe
- **Right Heart Valvular Disease**
  - Valvular calcifications indicate stenosis or regurgitation
  - Phase contrast MR to determine pressure gradients and regurgitant fractions most helpful
  - Isolated enlargement of left pulmonary artery suggests pulmonary stenosis
- **Primary Pulmonary Arterial Hypertension**
  - Pulmonary artery > 25 mmHg, pulmonary capillary wedge pressure < 15 mmHg, pulmonary vascular resistance > 2.4 mN x s/cm⁵
  - Absence of secondary cause of pulmonary hypertension

- Distinction between primary and secondary causes is critical, because therapeutic pulmonary vasodilators are deleterious in secondary causes
- Imaging findings suggesting primary pulmonary hypertension
  - Normal lung volumes and parenchyma
  - Normal left heart size and absence of valvular calcifications

Helpful Clues for Rare Diagnoses

- **Arrhythmogenic Right Ventricular Cardiomyopathy (ARVC)**
  - Diagnosis based on structural, histologic, electrocardiographic, arrhythmic, and genetic factors
  - Requires presence of sufficient major and minor criteria, many of which are not related to imaging; 2 major criteria, 1 major and 2 minor criteria, or 4 minor criteria required
  - Major criteria
    - Global or regional dysfunction and structural alterations
      - Severe dilatation of right ventricle and reduced right ventricular ejection fraction
      - Severe segmental dilatation of right ventricle
      - Localized right ventricular aneurysm
    - Tissue characterization
      - Fibrofatty replacement of right ventricular myocardium (established by endocardial biopsy)
    - Depolarization or conduction abnormalities
      - Epsilon waves
      - Prolonged QRS complex (> 110 msec)
    - Family history
      - Confirmed at autopsy or surgery
  - Minor criteria
    - Global or regional dysfunction and structural alterations
      - Mild dilatation of right ventricle and reduced right ventricular ejection fraction
      - Mild segmental dilatation of right ventricle
      - Regional right ventricular hypokinesia
    - Repolarization abnormalities
      - Inverted T waves
    - Depolarization or conduction abnormalities
      - Late potentials
    - Arrhythmias
      - Ventricular tachycardia with left bundle branch block and frequent excessive ventricular extrasystoles
    - Family history
      - Sudden death due to suspected ARVC
      - Family history on diagnostic criteria
  - MR features included in major and minor criteria
    - Major: Regional right ventricular akinesia or dyskinesia or dyssynchronous contraction and 1 of following: Ratio of end-diastolic volume:BSA 110 mL/m² (male) or 100 mL/m² (female) or ejection fraction < 40%
    - Minor: Regional right ventricular akinesia or dyskinesia or dyssynchronous contraction and 1 of following: Ratio of end-diastolic volume:BSA 100-110 mL/m² (male) or 90-100 mL/m² (female) or ejection fraction 40-45%
- **Congenital Heart Disease**
  - **D-Transposition of Great Vessels With Atrial Switch Repair**
    - Right ventricular hypertrophy and enlargement as result of acting as systemic ventricle
    - Prognosis and further therapy determined by changes in right ventricular function and size
  - **Tetralogy of Fallot (TOF) With Pulmonic Regurgitation or Stenosis**
    - Pulmonary regurgitation &/or stenosis in postrepair TOF patients
    - Right ventricular dilation severe in cases of pulmonary atresia
    - Regurgitant fraction best appreciated quantitatively with through-plane MR phase contrast of main pulmonary trunk

Left Heart Failure

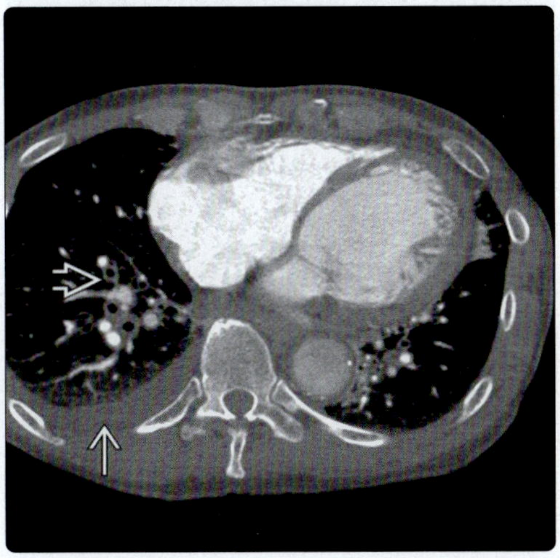

Secondary Pulmonary Hypertension

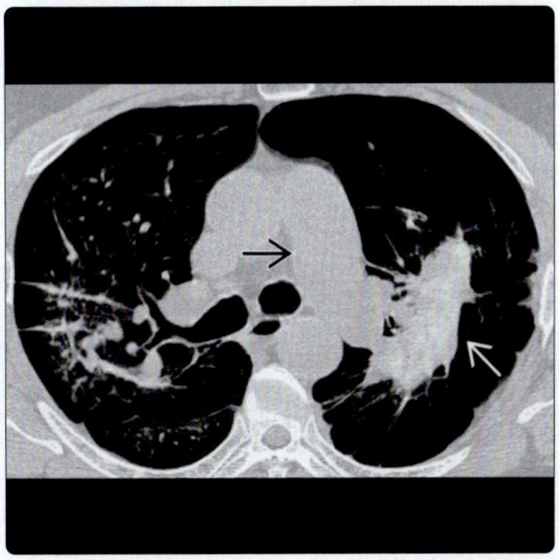

(Left) *Axial CECT of patient with heart failure exacerbation shows dilated left ventricle and right atrium. Additional views showed right atrial and right ventricular enlargement. Note pleural effusions* ➡ *and peribronchial edema* ➡. **(Right)** *Axial HRCT shows typical CT features of progressive massive fibrosis from talcosis. Note focal high-density opacities* ➡ *of progressive massive fibrosis as well as dilated left pulmonary artery* ➡ *from pulmonary hypertension, which can lead to right ventricular enlargement.*

(Left) *Axial HRCT shows honeycombing in idiopathic pulmonary fibrosis with an enlarged pulmonary trunk → reflecting secondary pulmonary hypertension, which can lead to right ventricular dilatation.* **(Right)** *Coronal CECT shows an enlarged pulmonary artery → and mosaic attenuation → in a patient with documented chronic pulmonary embolism (PE). Secondary pulmonary hypertension should be suspected when interstitial lung disease, COPD, or chronic PE are present.*

Secondary Pulmonary Hypertension

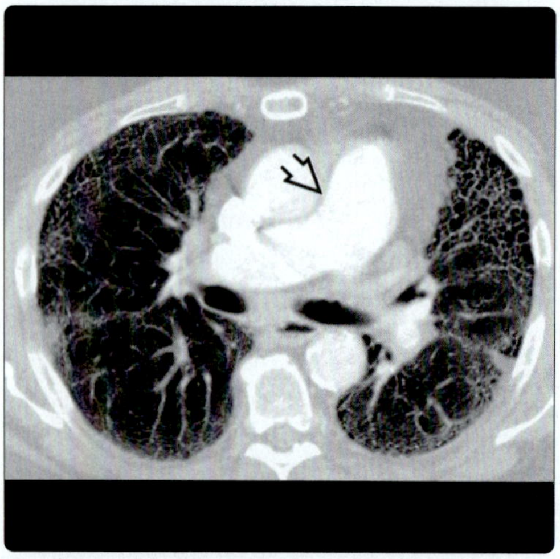

Secondary Pulmonary Hypertension

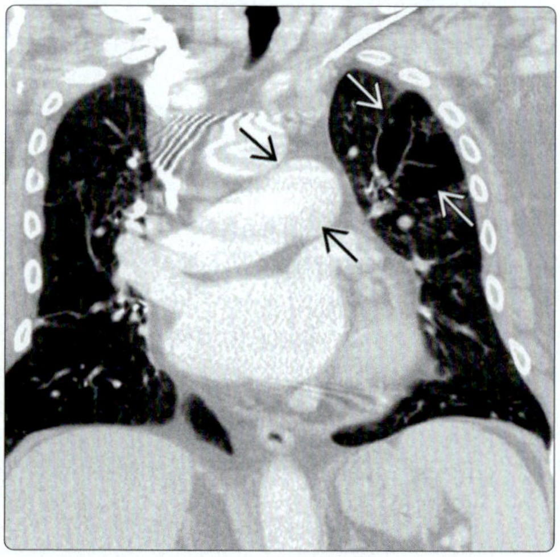

(Left) *Axial CECT shows a dilated pulmonary trunk → in a patient with Takayasu and pulmonary artery strictures →. This patient also had multiple branch vessel stenoses.* **(Right)** *Four-chamber cine MR shows turbulent mitral jet during diastole →. Left atrial enlargement is present. This patient had secondary pulmonary hypertension and right ventricular enlargement.*

Secondary Pulmonary Hypertension

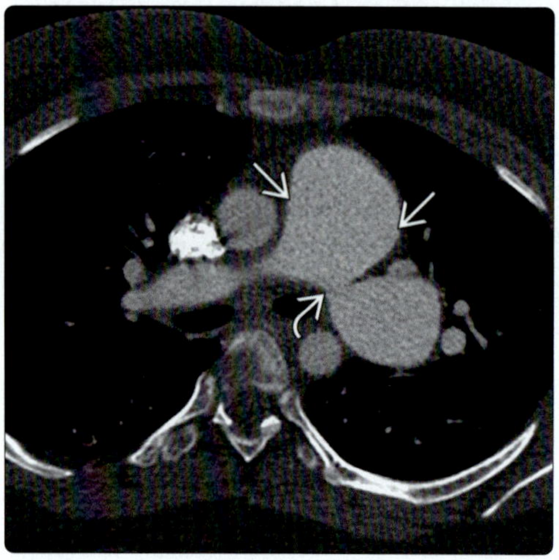

Secondary Pulmonary Hypertension

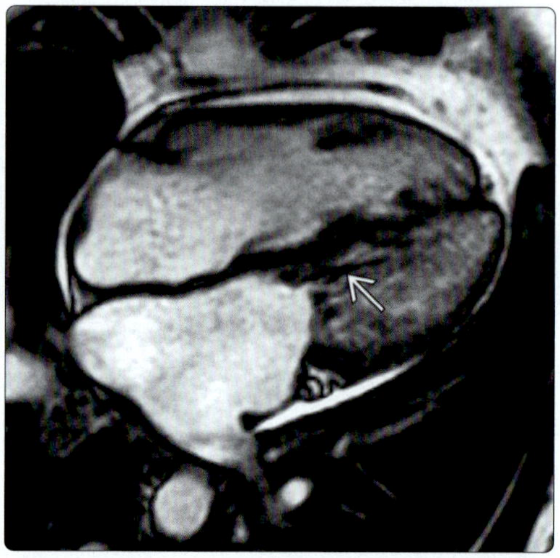

(Left) *Four-chamber cine MR demonstrates a large atrial septal defect with right atrial and ventricular enlargement →. Note that no turbulent jet was present because the atrial septal defect was so large.* **(Right)** *Axial CECT shows right atrial and right ventricular enlargement in a patient with tricuspid regurgitation. A regurgitant flow jet was also seen on MR. MR derived stroke volume and pulmonary artery forward flow was used to calculate the regurgitant fraction.*

Left-to-Right Shunt

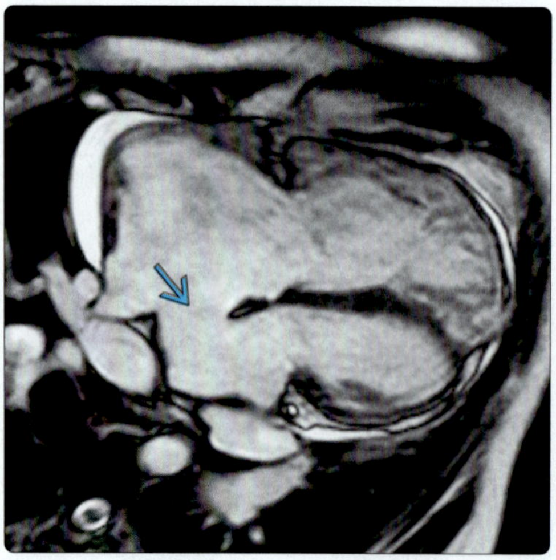

Right Heart Valvular Disease

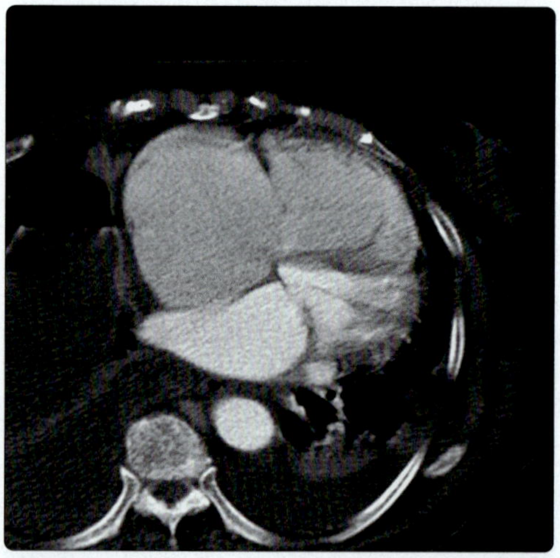

Right Heart Valvular Disease

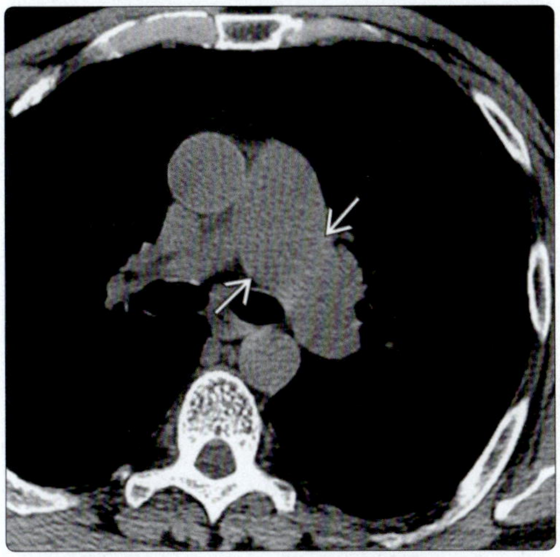

Primary Pulmonary Arterial Hypertension

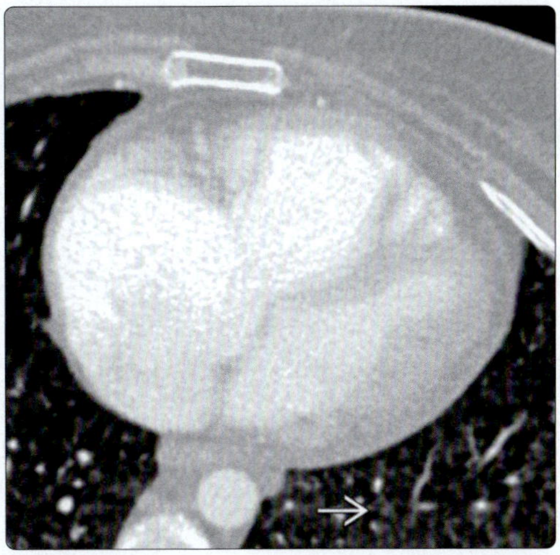

(Left) *Axial NECT shows isolated enlargement of the left main pulmonary artery* ➡. *This patient had pulmonary artery stenosis and right ventricular enlargement.* **(Right)** *Axial NECT shows right ventricular enlargement in a patient with pulmonary capillary hemangiomatosis. Note the poorly defined centrilobular ground-glass nodules* ➡.

Arrhythmogenic Right Ventricular Cardiomyopathy

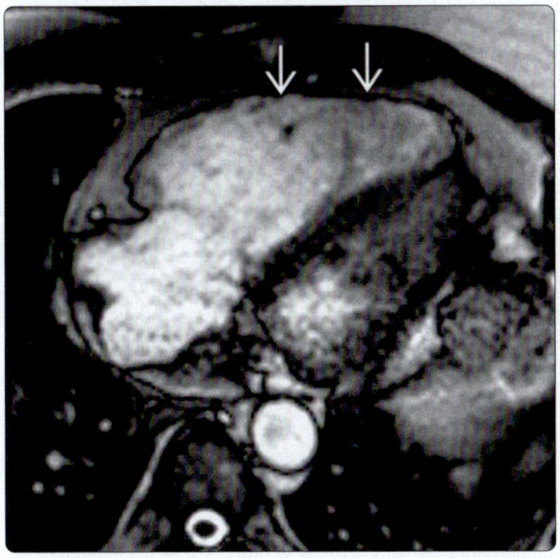

D-Transposition of Great Vessels With Atrial Switch

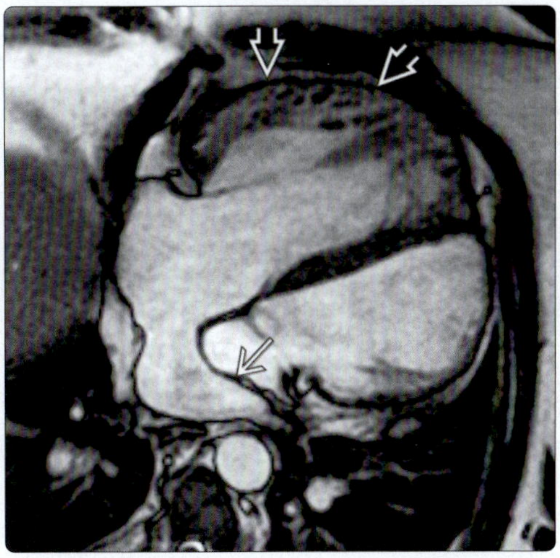

(Left) *Horizontal long axis cine MR shows severe right ventricular enlargement* ➡ *in a patient with arrhythmogenic right ventricular cardiomyopathy. This patient also had global hypokinesis. These findings represent major imaging criteria.* **(Right)** *Four-chamber cine MR of a patient with D-transpositions of the great vessels with atrial switch shows an atrial baffle* ➡. *The right ventricle supplies the systemic circulation, leading to dilatation and hypertrophy* ➡.

Tetralogy of Fallot With Pulmonic Regurgitation or Stenosis

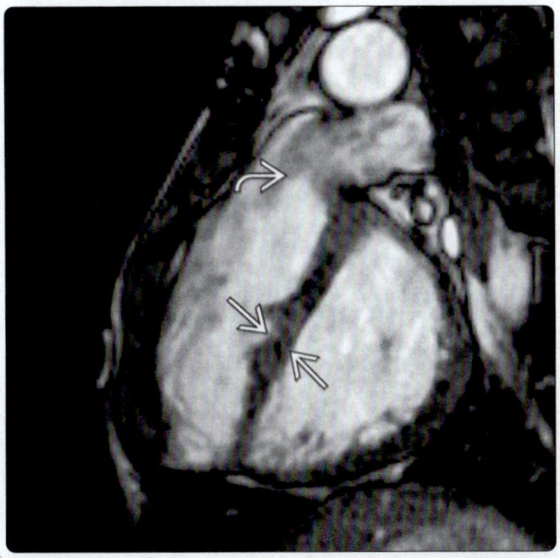

Tetralogy of Fallot With Pulmonic Regurgitation or Stenosis

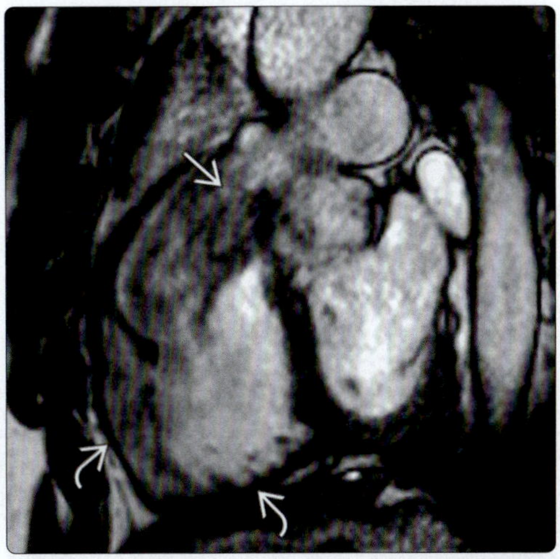

(Left) *Right ventricular outflow tract cine MR of a patient with corrected tetralogy of Fallot shows flattening of the interventricular septum* ➡ *and pulmonic regurgitation* ➡. *Flattening indicates increased right-sided pressure compared to the left ventricle.* **(Right)** *Right ventricular outflow tract bright-blood cine MR shows right ventricular dilation* ➡ *in a patient with tetralogy of Fallot and pulmonary regurgitation* ➡.

Wall Motion Abnormality

DIFFERENTIAL DIAGNOSIS

Common

- Acute Myocardial Infarction
- Postsurgical Septal Motion
- Nonischemic Cardiomyopathy

Less Common

- Ventricular Aneurysm

Rare but Important

- Constrictive Pericarditis

ESSENTIAL INFORMATION

Key Differential Diagnosis Issues

- 1st determination when wall motion abnormality (WMA) is suspected is whether it is regional or global
  - Regional WMA should raise suspicion for vascular etiology, specifically if in vascular territory
  - Global WMA is less specific, more frequently observed in nonischemic cardiomyopathies and myocarditis
- MR is gold standard for cardiac functional analysis and should be used when WMA is suspected
  - Cine steady-state free precession imaging best evaluates WMA, performed in short-axis and orthogonal planes
  - Segmental analysis of WMA based on 17-segment model
    - True apex best evaluated on long-axis planes
  - Global WMA requires experience, but can be suspected when ↓ systolic function and ↓ myocardial contractility

Helpful Clues for Common Diagnoses

- Acute Myocardial Infarction
  - Altered wall motion, particularly in response to stress, is 1 of the earliest signs of ischemic myocardium
  - Wall motion is typically segmental, in vascular territory, and most frequently hypokinetic or akinetic
  - Hibernating myocardium is viable, chronically ischemic myocardium with poor contractility
  - Stunned myocardium is reperfused myocardium that continues to demonstrate poor contractility
- Postsurgical Septal Motion
  - Also termed paradoxical septal motion
  - Systolic movement of interventricular septum toward right ventricle with normal thickness
  - May be due to altered movement within pericardium
- Nonischemic Cardiomyopathy
  - Infiltrated portions of myocardium may have WMA in regions of late gadolinium enhancement
  - Best documented in cases of hypertrophic cardiomyopathy and sarcoidosis
  - WMA is not in vascular territory
  - Takotsubo cardiomyopathy is catecholamine-mediated apical ballooning that resolves

Helpful Clues for Less Common Diagnoses

- Ventricular Aneurysm
  - Dyskinetic WMA defines aneurysm, can be subtle in postinfarct aneurysms of anterior wall and apex

Helpful Clues for Rare Diagnoses

- Constrictive Pericarditis
  - Exaggerated ventricular interdependence in pericardial constriction causes paradoxical septal motion
  - Occurs in early diastole, exaggerated in inspiration due to ↑ venous return to right heart

Other Essential Information

- Abnormal interventricular septal motion also observed in right ventricular pressure or volume overload and congenital heart disease
- Bundle branch blocks (left or right) may cause WMA of septum from abnormal sequence of ventricular activation
  - Normal myocardial thickness is key when differentiating this process from ischemia

SELECTED REFERENCES

1. Imazio M et al: Usefulness of cardiac magnetic resonance for recurrent pericarditis. Am J Cardiol. 125(1):146-51, 2020
2. Ali M et al: Advancements in the diagnostic workup, prognostic evaluation, and treatment of takotsubo syndrome. Heart Fail Rev. ePub, 2019

Acute Myocardial Infarction

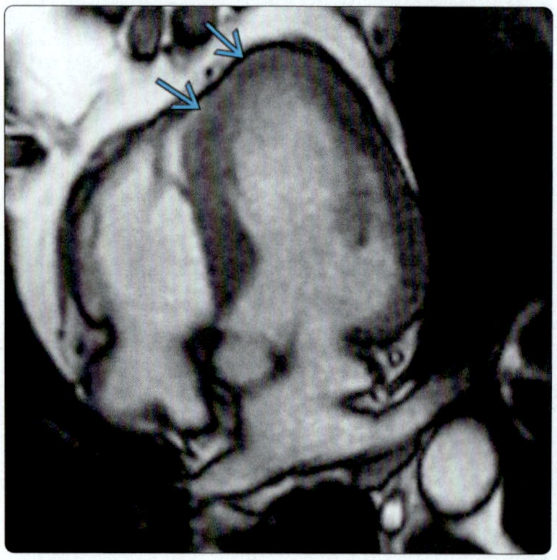

Acute Myocardial Infarction

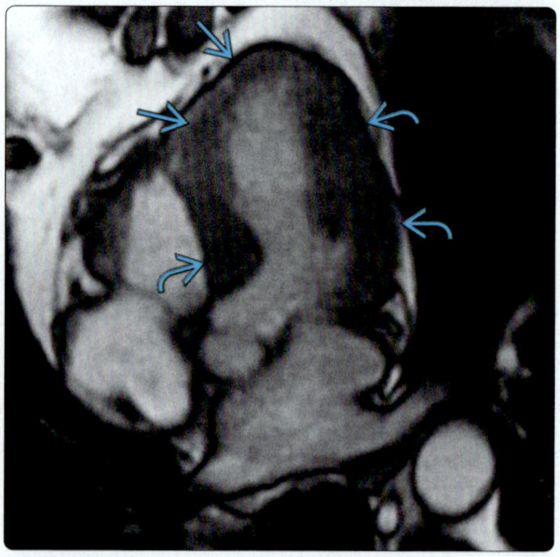

(Left) *Four-chamber steady-state free precession (SSFP) MR in end-diastole of a patient with acute chest pain shows subtle hyperintense signal* ➡ *of the apical and septal segments in a vascular territory most consistent with the left anterior descending coronary artery.* **(Right)** *Four-chamber SSFP MR in end-systole of the same patient shows akinesis* ➡ *of the high signal intensity segments while the remainder of the myocardium thickens and moves centrally* ➡*.*

Nonischemic Cardiomyopathy

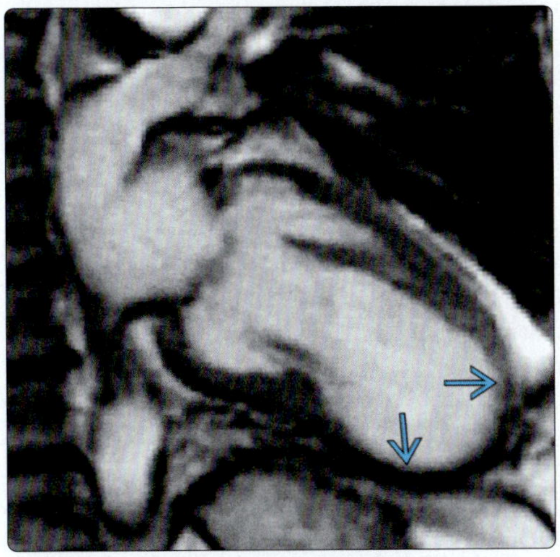

Nonischemic Cardiomyopathy

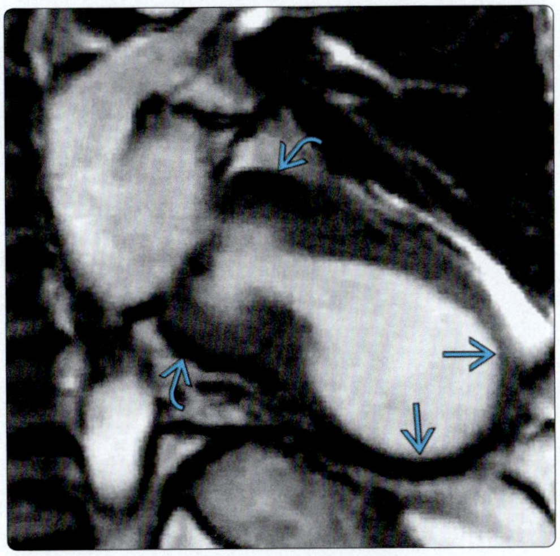

(Left) *Two-chamber SSFP MR in end-diastole of a patient with extreme emotional distress shows dilatation and thinning → of the left ventricular apex.* **(Right)** *Two-chamber SSFP MR in end-systole of the same patient shows apical ballooning/dyskinesis →, consistent with takotsubo cardiomyopathy. The base of the heart contracts and moves normally ↪. This catecholamine-induced cardiomyopathy must resolve before a diagnosis can confidently be made.*

Ventricular Aneurysm

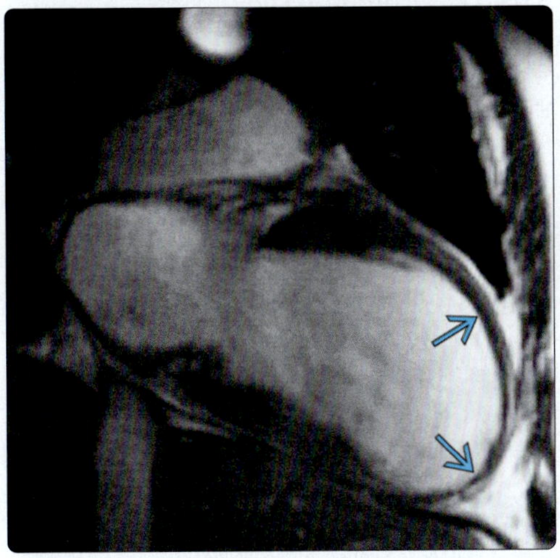

Ventricular Aneurysm

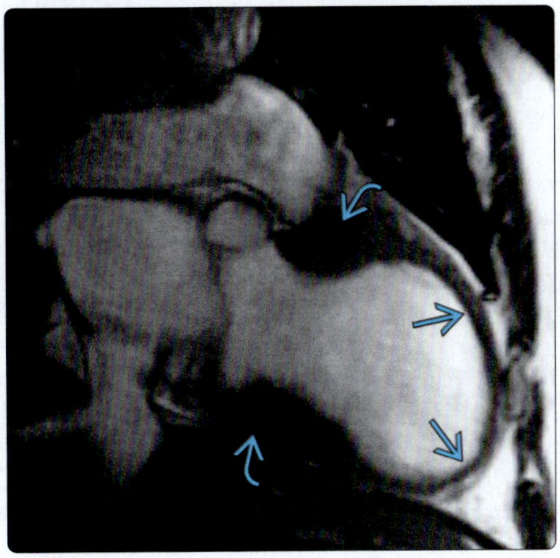

(Left) *Two-chamber SSFP MR of a patient with history of myocardial infarction shows thinning and chamber dilation → of the anterior wall and apex in a left anterior descending coronary artery distribution.* **(Right)** *Two-chamber SSFP MR of the same patient shows dyskinesis → of the thinned anterior and apical segments while the noninvolved segments ↪ contract and move centrally. Dyskinesis, thinning, and dilation define a postinfarction aneurysm.*

Constrictive Pericarditis

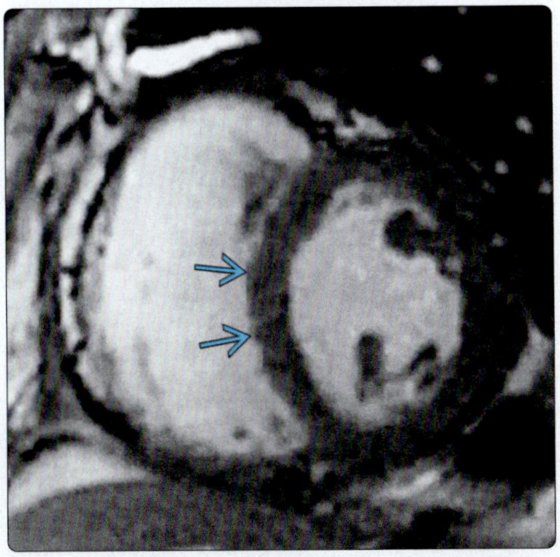

Constrictive Pericarditis

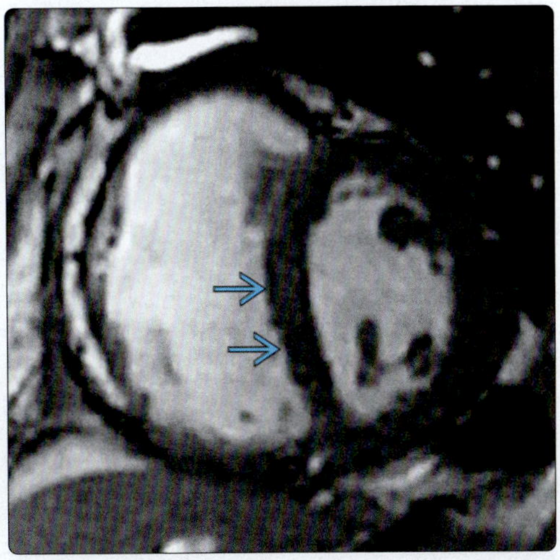

(Left) *Short-axis SSFP MR obtained during expiration of a patient with history of pericarditis shows qualitative dilation of the right heart and slight flattening of the interventricular septum → at end-diastole.* **(Right)** *Short-axis SSFP MR obtained at full inspiration of the same patient shows abnormal septal motion → toward the left ventricle in early diastolic filling. Exaggerated ventricular interdependence with inspiration is a sign of constriction.*

DIFFERENTIAL DIAGNOSIS

Common

- Hypertensive Heart Disease
- Aortic Stenosis
- Hypertrophic Cardiomyopathy
- Infiltrative Cardiomyopathy

Less Common

- Athlete's Heart

Rare but Important

- Cardiac Neoplasm

ESSENTIAL INFORMATION

Key Differential Diagnosis Issues

- Prevalence of left ventricular (LV) wall thickening 15-21%
- Myocardial thickness should be evaluated at end-diastole in short-axis plane
    - Generally 13-14 mm considered borderline thickened, and ≥15 mm considered abnormal
    - Apical segments may be overestimated in short-axis plane and suspected thickening should be confirmed in long-axis planes
- 1st decision should be whether thickened myocardium is focal or diffuse
    - Processes causing outflow tract obstruction or systemic arterial hypertension more likely to cause diffuse, concentric thickening of LV
    - Focal, asymmetric myocardial wall thickening is suspicious for infiltrative process or neoplasm
- LV hypertrophy independent risk factor of cardiac mortality

Helpful Clues for Common Diagnoses

- Hypertensive Heart Disease
    - Concentric LV wall thickening usually < 16 mm
    - Systolic function typically normal or mildly impaired
    - No late gadolinium enhancement (LGE)
- Aortic Stenosis
    - Aortic valve restriction causes elevated gradients across valve and increased LV pressures
    - LV wall thickening is usually concentric
- Hypertrophic Cardiomyopathy
    - Most common location of LV thickening is basal septum
        - Concentric, midcavity, apical variants less common
    - Typically, focal LV thickening > 15 mm
        - LV thickening > 30 mm high risk
    - LGE occurs most frequently in areas of most hypertrophy
        - Right ventricular insertion site LGE is characteristic
    - Increased FDG uptake may be present on FDG PET/CT
- Infiltrative Cardiomyopathy
    - Concentric LV thickening is characteristic of several entities causing deposition in myocardium
        - Hemochromatosis: LV thickening and low T2*
        - Amyloidosis: LV thickening and diffuse, subendocardial LGE, poor myocardial nulling
        - Sarcoidosis may cause acute myocardial thickening, often presenting with new arrhythmia (i.e., heart block)

Helpful Clues for Less Common Diagnoses

- Athlete's Heart
    - Endurance athletes can develop concentric LV thickening and dilatation of LV, left atrium, and right ventricle
    - No LGE, normal systolic and diastolic function
    - Regresses with modifications of physical activity

Helpful Clues for Rare Diagnoses

- Cardiac Neoplasm
    - Metastatic disease far more common than primary cardiac neoplasms, both may cause focal LV thickening
    - Pericardial effusion most common sign of malignancy
    - Right heart more suspicious for malignancy than left
        - Benign tumors and thrombus more common on left

SELECTED REFERENCES

1. Muntner P et al: Potential US population impact of the 2017 ACC/AHA High Blood Pressure Guideline. Circulation. 137(2):109-18, 2018
2. Stewart MH et al: Prognostic implications of left ventricular hypertrophy. Prog Cardiovasc Dis. 61(5-6):446-55, 2018

Hypertensive Heart Disease

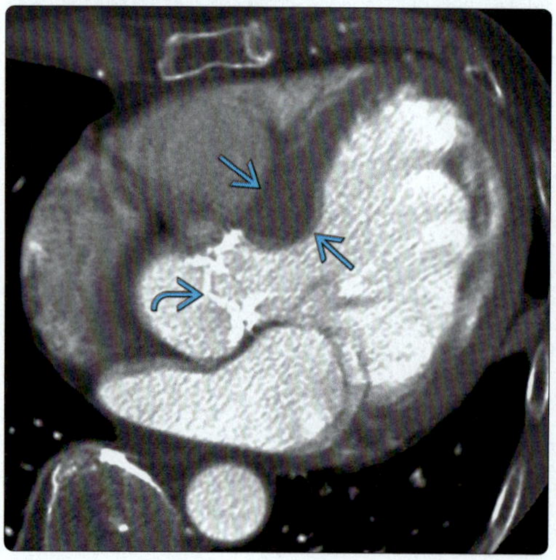

Hypertrophic Cardiomyopathy

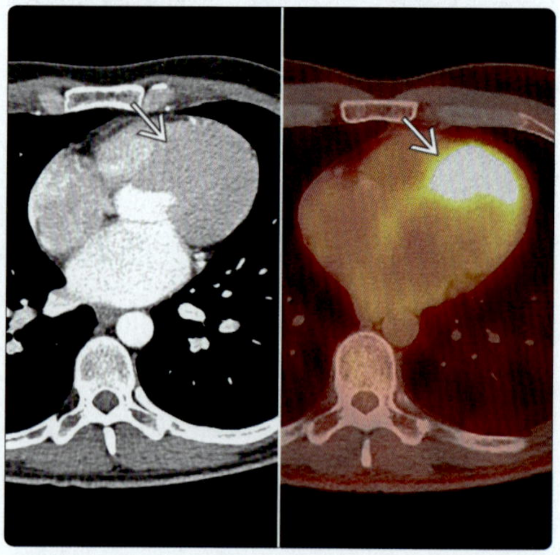

(Left) *Axial CECT of a patient with longstanding aortic stenosis shows left ventricular (LV) wall thickening at the basal septum ➔ and aortic valve calcification ➔. Aortic stenosis and hypertensive heart disease are common causes of LV wall thickening, typically concentric, although asymmetry is possible.* **(Right)** *Composite image of axial CECT (left) and fused axial FDG PET/CT (right) demonstrate mass-like thickening of the LV myocardium that is intensely FDG-avid ➔.*

Hypertrophic Cardiomyopathy

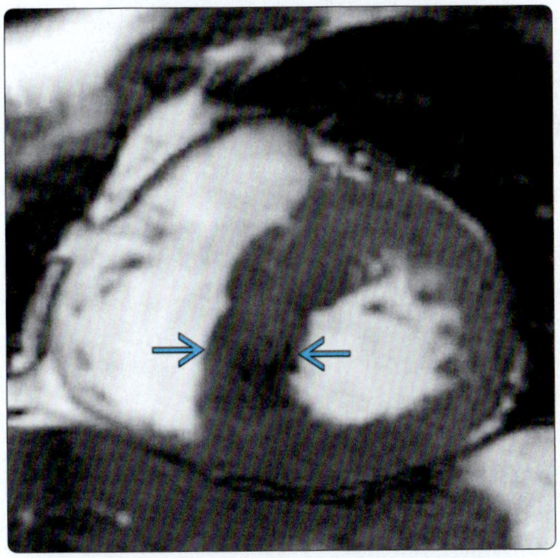

Hypertensive Heart Disease

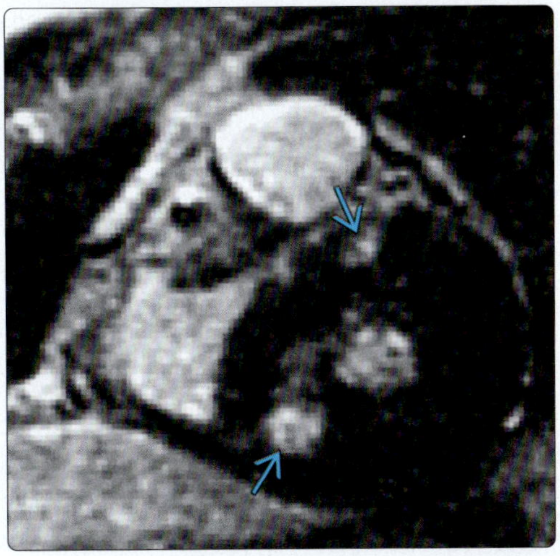

(Left) *Short-axis balanced steady-state free precession MR of a patient with hypertrophic cardiomyopathy (HCM) shows asymmetric thickening → of the basal septum. This is the most common site of thickening in HCM.* **(Right)** *Short-axis late gadolinium enhancement (LGE) MR of the same patient shows foci of midwall LGE → at the right ventricular insertion points to the LV. This pattern of LGE is characteristic of HCM. LV thickening > 15 mm is consistent with HCM and > 30 mm is a poor prognostic finding.*

Hypertrophic Cardiomyopathy

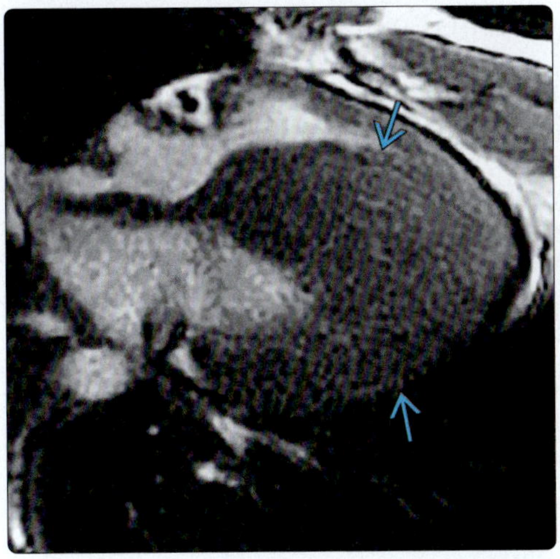

Hypertrophic Cardiomyopathy

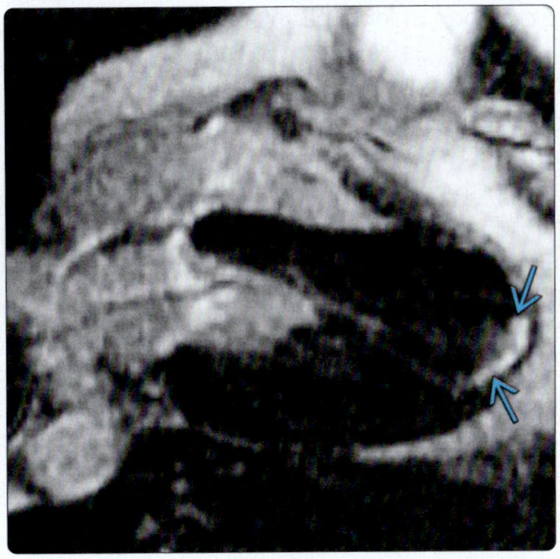

(Left) *Four-chamber steady-state free precession MR of a patient with apical variant HCM shows diffuse thickening → of the apical and mid segments, resulting in a spade-shaped morphology of the LV.* **(Right)** *Four-chamber LGE MR of the same patient shows focal midwall LGE → in the apex. This variant is more common in Asian patients and less commonly associated with LV outflow tract obstruction.*

Cardiac Neoplasm

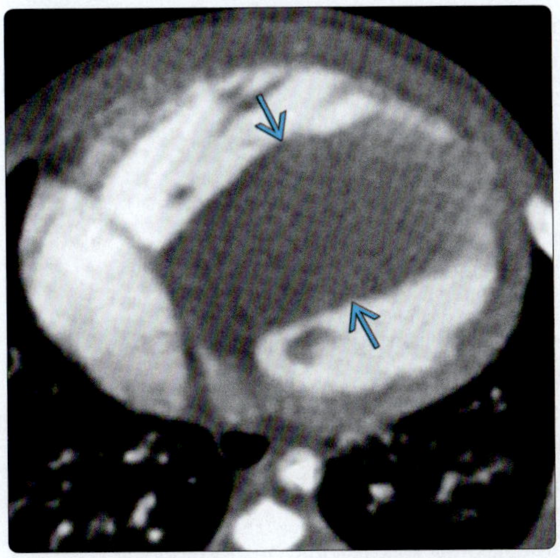

Cardiac Neoplasm

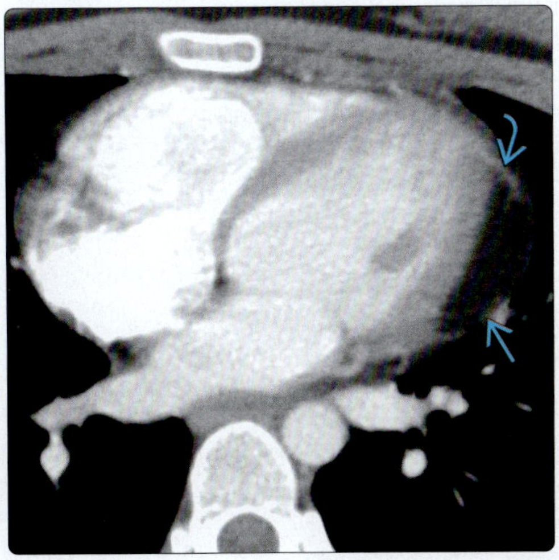

(Left) *Axial CECT of a 5-day-old infant with a heart murmur shows diffuse thickening → of the interventricular septum, subsequently diagnosed a cardiac rhabdomyoma.* **(Right)** *Axial CECT of a patient with tuberous sclerosis shows a fat-attenuation mass → in the LV, consistent with a cardiac lipoma. The myocardium of the LV envelopes the mass ↗, indicating cardiac origin. Neoplastic thickening of the myocardium is rare, and in the adult, metastatic disease should be the first consideration.*

DIFFERENTIAL DIAGNOSIS

Common

- Thrombus

Less Common

- Metastasis
- Myxoma
- Lipoma
- Angiosarcoma

Rare but Important

- Undifferentiated Pleomorphic Sarcoma
- Primary Cardiac Lymphoma
- Leiomyosarcoma
- Osteosarcoma
- Crista Terminalis

ESSENTIAL INFORMATION

Key Differential Diagnosis Issues

- Intracavitary thrombus is most common cardiac mass
- Cardiac metastases are more common than primary cardiac malignancies
- 75% of primary cardiac masses are benign
  - Myxoma is most common primary cardiac neoplasm
    - Typically originates in left atrium
- Angiosarcoma is most common primary cardiac malignancy
  - Typically originates in right atrium
- Enhancement on T1WI +C can help distinguish tumor thrombus from bland thrombus
- Primary cardiac malignancies, metastases, and tumor thrombus show increased FDG uptake on PET/CT

Helpful Clues for Common Diagnoses

- Thrombus
  - Most often involves left atrium (left atrial appendage)
    - Associated with atrial fibrillation, dilated left atrium, and mitral valve stenosis
  - Right atrial thrombus
    - Associated with indwelling catheter, atrial fibrillation, deep venous thrombus, and tricuspid valve stenosis
      - Complicates 10% of pulmonary embolism cases
    - Tumor thrombus
      - Most commonly associated with renal cell cancer, hepatocellular carcinoma, lung cancer, and melanoma
      - Associated with thrombus in inferior or superior vena cavae
  - CT
    - NECT: Hypodense mass with broad base; chronic thrombus may develop calcifications
    - CECT: No enhancement
  - MR
    - Signal intensity varies depending on age of thrombus
      - Acute: Intermediate signal on T1WI and T2WI
      - Subacute: T1 hypointense, T2 hyperintense
      - Chronic: T1 hypointense, T2 hypointense
      - T1WI +C (early and delayed): No enhancement
      - Tumor thrombus: Enhancement on T1WI +C

Helpful Clues for Less Common Diagnoses

- Metastasis
  - Cardiac metastases in 10-12% of patients with known malignancy
  - All age groups may be affected
  - Direct extension, hematogenous, lymphatic or transvenous spread
  - Most common primary neoplasms: Lung, breast, kidney, and liver cancers, melanoma
  - Right atrium most common location of solitary cardiac metastasis
  - CT
    - NECT: Hypodense mass
    - CECT: Heterogeneous enhancement
  - MR
    - T1WI: Low signal intensity; T2WI: High signal intensity
      - Melanoma: High signal intensity on T1WI
    - T1WI +C: Enhancement
- Myxoma
  - Most common primary cardiac neoplasm, 50% of all cases
  - Middle-aged adults (30-60 years), higher prevalence in women
  - Left atrium (60-75%), right atrium (15-20%)
  - Solitary, polypoid, ovoid, non-infiltrating tumor; smooth or lobular contours
    - Carney complex: Multiple recurrent cardiac/mucocutaneous myxomas, pigmented skin lesions, schwannomas, and endocrine neoplasms
  - Narrow or broad-based attachment to fossa ovalis
    - Prolapse through atrioventricular valves
  - CT
    - NECT: Hypodense lobular lesion, may exhibit calcification or necrosis
    - CECT: Heterogeneous enhancement
  - MR
    - T1WI and T2WI: Heterogeneous appearance secondary to hemorrhage, calcification, and necrosis
    - T1WI +C: Delayed, patchy enhancement
- Lipoma
  - Second most common benign cardiac neoplasm
  - All age groups may be affected
  - Solitary or multiple
    - Tuberous sclerosis: Multiple lipomas
  - CT
    - NECT: Well-defined encapsulated fat attenuation lesion
    - CECT: No enhancement
  - MR
    - T1WI and T2WI: High signal intensity
    - Fat saturation: Suppression of signal
    - T1WI +C: No enhancement
- Angiosarcoma
  - Most common primary cardiac sarcoma, 40% of all primary malignant neoplasms
  - Young adults (20-40 years), male predominance
  - 90% in right atrium
  - Single or multiple nodules or atrial mass infiltrating myocardium and pericardium

- Extension to superior or inferior vena cavae, pericardial effusion, &/or thickening
- Metastases in up to 80% patients at diagnosis
  - Most common sites: Lung, liver, bone, adrenal glands, and brain
- CT
  - NECT: Hypodense, irregular mass arising from right atrial free wall
  - CECT: Heterogeneous enhancement
- MR
  - T1WI and T2WI: Heterogeneous mass with intrinsic low, intermediate, or high signal intensity
  - T1WI +C: Peripheral enhancement, intralesional flow voids represent vascular channels

Helpful Clues for Rare Diagnoses

- Undifferentiated Pleomorphic Sarcoma
  - Most common in left atrium
  - Adults (30-40 years)
  - CT
    - NECT: Hypodense atrial mass
    - CECT: Heterogeneous enhancement on CECT
  - MR
    - T1WI: Heterogeneous, isointense; T2WI: Heterogeneous, high signal intensity
    - MR +C: Peripheral enhancement
- Primary Cardiac Lymphoma
  - Immunocompromised patient, B-cell lymphoma, less frequent than secondary lymphoma
  - Most common in right atrium
  - Large nodular mass with frequent pericardial thickening &/or effusion
    - May extend along pericardium, may encase coronary arteries and aortic root
    - Myocardial infiltration
  - CT: Hypodense or isodense relative to myocardium
    - NECT: Hypodense or isodense relative to myocardium
    - CECT: Mild enhancement
  - MR
    - T1WI: Hypo- or isointense; T2WI: Hyper- or isointense
- Leiomyosarcoma
  - Adults (40-50 years)
  - Posterior wall of left atrium (70%), right atrium (15-20%)
  - Invasion of pulmonary veins or mitral valve
  - CT
    - NECT: Irregular or lobular low-attenuation mass
    - CECT: Filling defects represent invasion of pulmonary veins
    - Pericardial effusion
  - MR
    - T1WI: Heterogeneous, isointense; T2WI: Heterogeneous, hyperintense
    - T1WI+C: Peripheral enhancement
- Osteosarcoma
  - Adults (50-60 years)
  - Location varies with type of neoplasm
    - Primary osteosarcoma: Left atrium
    - Metastasis: Right atrium
  - CT
    - NECT: Low-attenuation broad-based mass, dense calcifications
    - CECT: Invasion of atrial walls, valves, and pulmonary veins
  - MR
    - T1WI: Isointense; low-signal areas due to calcification
    - T1WI+C: Enhancement
- Crista Terminalis
  - Smooth fibromuscular crescentic structure in posterior right atrial wall
  - CT: Focal, low-density crescentic shape in right atrium
  - MR: Isointense to myocardium on T1WI and T2WI

SELECTED REFERENCES

1. Lichtenberger JP 3rd et al: MR imaging of cardiac masses. Top Magn Reson Imaging. 27(2):103-11, 2018
2. Kassop D et al: Cardiac masses on cardiac CT: a review. Curr Cardiovasc Imaging Rep. 7:9281, 2014

Thrombus

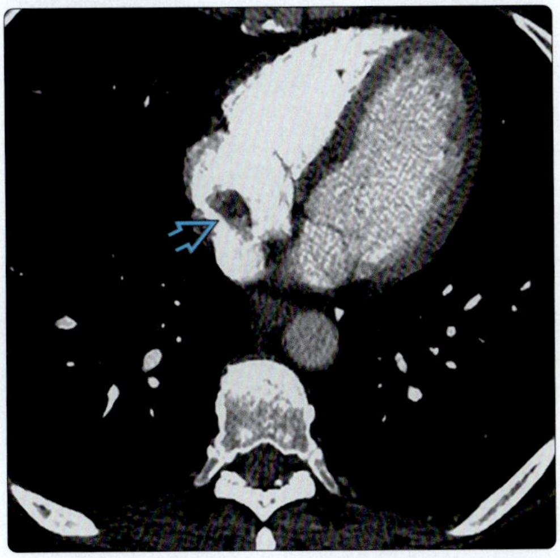

Thrombus

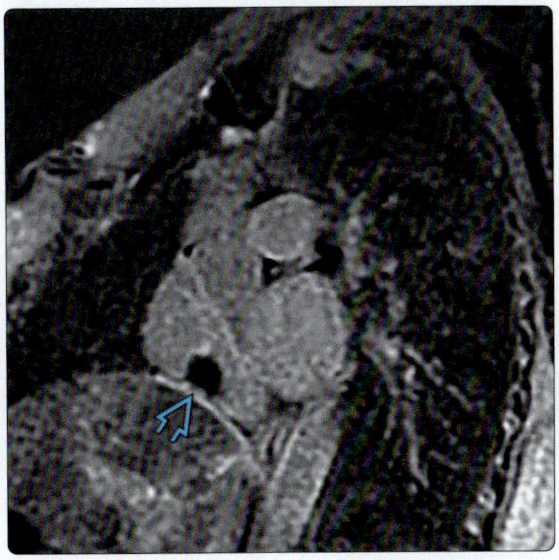

(Left) *Axial CECT of a 68-year-old woman with lung cancer and an indwelling catheter shows a crescent-shaped soft tissue lesion ➡ in the right atrium suspicious for intracardiac thrombus.* **(Right)** *Sagittal oblique delayed enhanced MR of the same patient shows a rounded low-signal lesion arising from the floor of the right atrium without contrast enhancement ➡ consistent with intracardiac thrombus. Absence of delayed contrast enhancement in an intracardiac lesion is highly suggestive of thrombus.*

(Left) *Axial CECT of a 32-year-old man with poorly-differentiated thyroid cancer shows a polylobular mass ⇨ in the right inferior pulmonary vein and adjacent left atrium. Note bilateral enlarged peribronchial lymph nodes ➡ consistent with lymph node metastases.* **(Right)** *Fused axial FDG PET/CT of the same patient shows increased FDG uptake in the right inferior pulmonary vein and atrial mass ⇨ consistent with tumor thrombus. Tumor thrombus is typically seen in renal and hepatocellular carcinomas, lung cancer, and melanoma.*

Thrombus

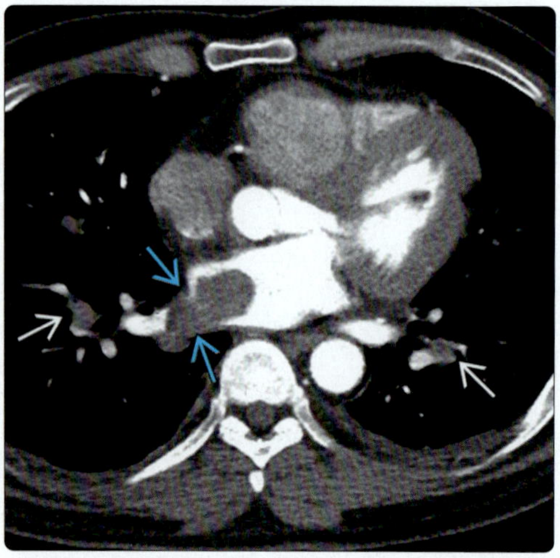

Thrombus

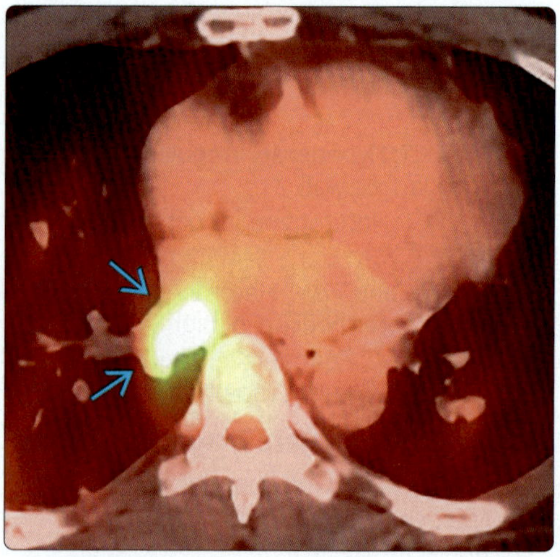

(Left) *Axial CECT of a 58-year-old woman with metastatic uterine sarcoma shows a large mass ⇨ in the right atrium consistent with a metastasis. A pulmonary metastasis ⇨ is also present in the left lower lobe. The right atrium is the most common location of solitary cardiac metastasis.* **(Right)** *Axial CECT of a 55-year-old man with metastatic bladder cancer shows a well-defined mass ⇨ in the posterior left atrium consistent with metastasis. Cardiac metastases are the most common malignant cardiac masses.*

Metastasis

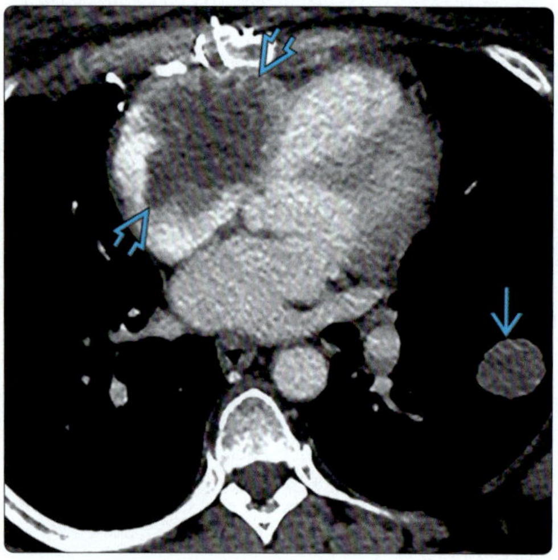

Metastasis

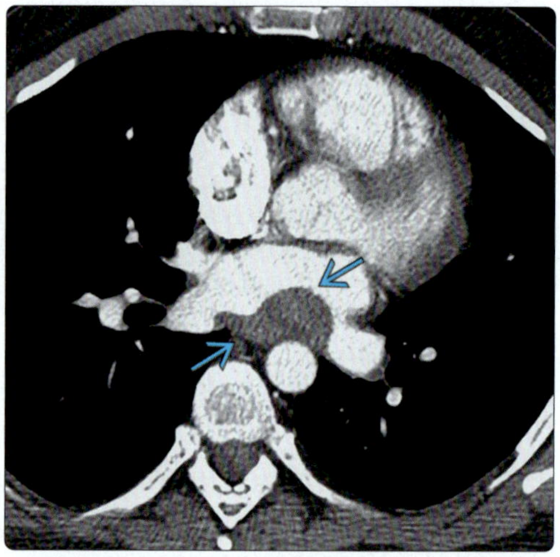

(Left) *Axial CECT of an asymptomatic 61-year-old man without a history of known malignancy shows a well-defined hypodense left atrial soft tissue nodule ⇨ attached to the interatrial septum.* **(Right)** *Coronal CECT of the same patient shows the well-defined hypodense left atrial soft tissue nodule ⇨. Biopsy confirmed the diagnosis of left atrial myxoma. Myxomas are the most common benign cardiac neoplasms, and the vast majority arise in the left atrium typically from a stalk attached to the fossa ovalis.*

Myxoma

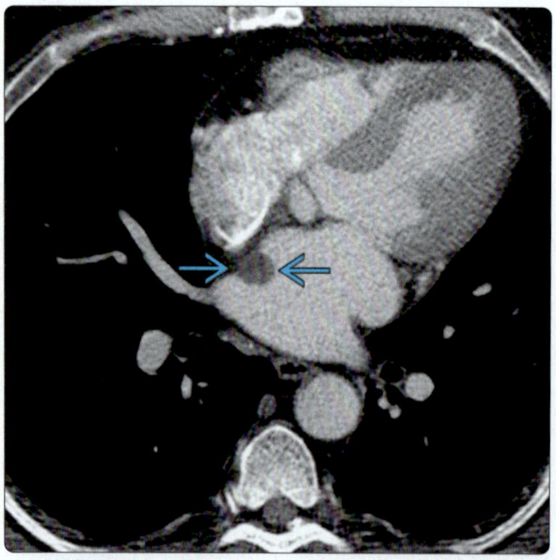

Myxoma

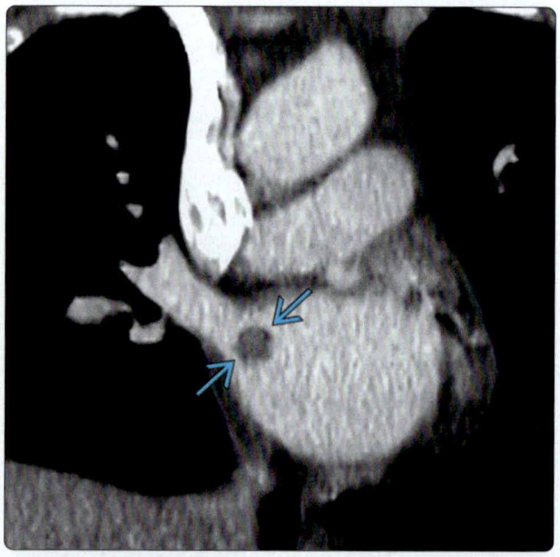

Metastasis

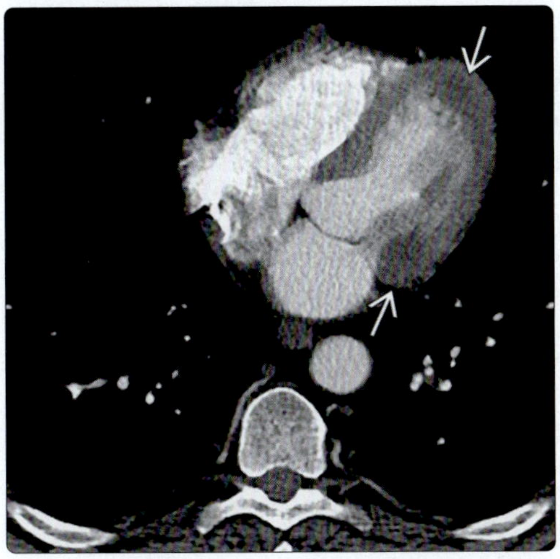

Metastasis

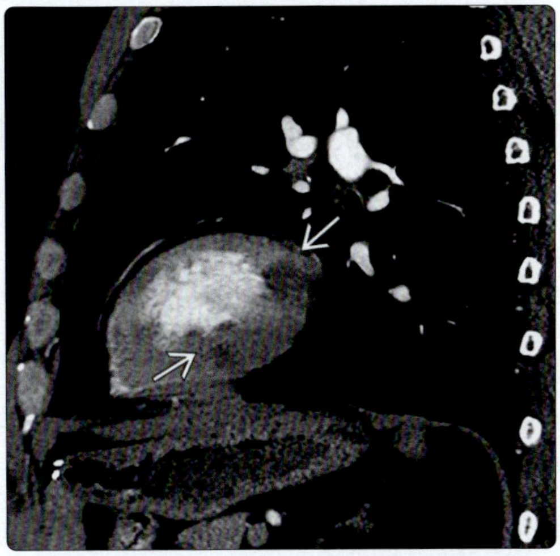

(Left) *Axial CECT of a 42-year-old man with sacral chordoma demonstrates low-attenuation lesions in the left ventricular myocardium, consistent with metastases. This patient also had osseous and pulmonary metastases (not shown).* **(Right)** *Coronal CECT of the same patient confirms the presence of intramural metastases. Left ventricular metastases are secondary to hematogeneous spread of malignant cells or tumor invasion via pulmonary veins.*

Fibroma

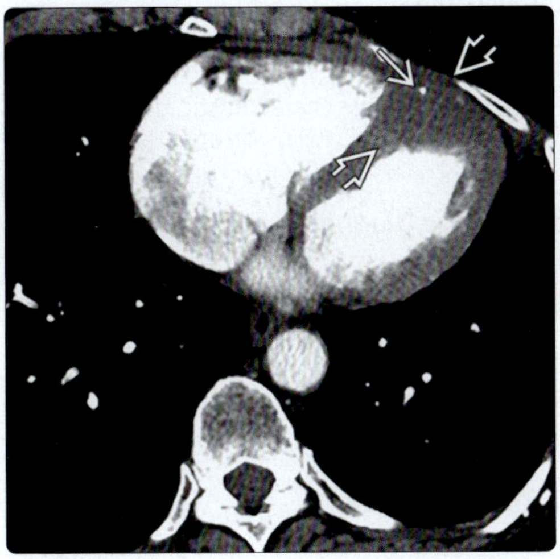

Fibroma

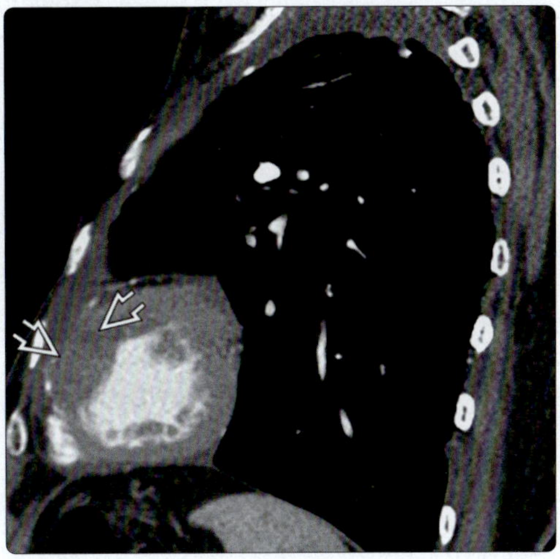

(Left) *Axial CECT of a 57-year-old woman with history of breast cancer shows a hypodense mass in the interventricular septum with a small eccentric calcification.* **(Right)** *Sagittal CECT of the same patient shows the presence of a mass, biopsy demonstrated as fibroma. Fibroma is more common in young adults or the pediatric population and usually presents as a mass in the interventricular septum or left ventricular free wall.*

Angiosarcoma

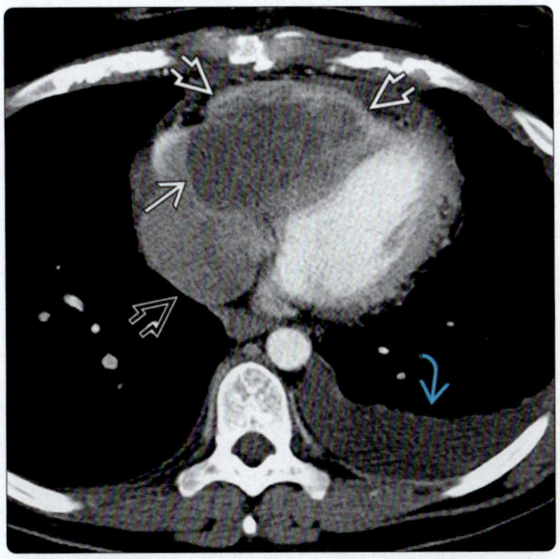

Angiosarcoma

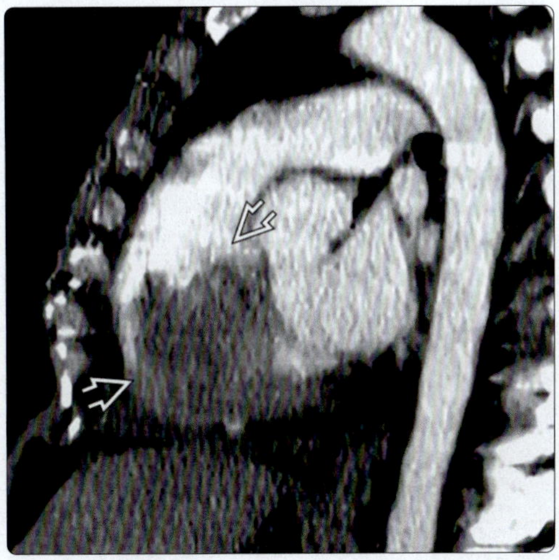

(Left) *Axial CECT of a 32-year-old woman with right ventricular angiosarcoma who presented with right heart failure shows a large right ventricular mass, which is extending into the right atrium and causes distension of the inferior vena cava. Note the left pleural effusion.* **(Right)** *Sagittal CECT of the same patient shows a large mass occupying the right ventricle. Biopsy demonstrated angiosarcoma. The right ventricle is the 2nd most common site of presentation of angiosarcoma after the right atrium.*

DIFFERENTIAL DIAGNOSIS

Common

- Thrombus
- Vegetation
- Mitral Annular Calcification

Less Common

- Papillary Fibroelastoma

Rare but Important

- Myxoma

ESSENTIAL INFORMATION

Key Differential Diagnosis Issues

- Masses discovered on cardiac valves are usually non-neoplastic in origin
  - Valve masses questioned on echocardiography frequently require cardiac-gated CT or MR for confirmation and further work-up
  - Degenerative disease may cause valve leaflet thickening and mitral annular disease, mimicking masses
  - Imaging differentiation of infectious vegetation and thrombus is usually not possible
    - Thrombus most frequently involves left atrium and mitral valve or complicates valve replacement in aortic or mitral position
    - Vegetations are usually in right heart, involving tricuspid or pulmonic valve
- Primary valve masses are rare, usually incidental
  - Papillary fibroelastoma typically involves aortic valve > mitral valve
  - Cardiac myxoma is most common primary cardiac tumor, but valve origin is uncommon

Helpful Clues for Common Diagnoses

- **Thrombus**
  - Intracardiac thrombus usually seen in patients with atrial fibrillation, usually involving left heart valves
  - Thrombus may secondarily involve cardiac valve, most frequently mitral valve
  - Prosthetic valves at increased risk for valve thrombus
    - Echocardiography is sensitive for small thrombus, but cardiac-gated CT better for prosthetic valve complications, including thrombus
- **Vegetation**
  - Cardiac valve vegetations are observed in infectious endocarditis, usually involving right heart valves
  - IV drug users and septic patients at increased risk for infectious endocarditis and vegetations
  - Acute regurgitation from valve destruction is important complication that drives clinical management
  - Typically arises from tip of valve leaflet
- **Mitral Annular Calcification**
  - May mimic mitral valve mass on echocardiography
  - Characteristically densely calcified at mitral annulus
    - May be rim-calcified with central lower density material, termed "caseous"
  - Associated with cardiovascular disease and end-stage renal disease from altered calcium metabolism

Helpful Clues for Less Common Diagnoses

- **Papillary Fibroelastoma**
  - 2nd most common benign primary cardiac neoplasm after cardiac myxoma
  - Pedunculated valvular mass characteristic, usually on aortic side of aortic valve or atrial side of mitral valve
  - Typically more central to valve leaflet than vegetations

Helpful Clues for Rare Diagnoses

- **Myxoma**
  - Most common primary cardiac neoplasm
  - Typically low-attenuation intracavitary mass near fossa ovalis
  - Rarely involves valves, may prolapse across mitral valve when pedunculated

SELECTED REFERENCES

1. Lichtenberger JP 3rd et al: MR imaging of cardiac masses. Top Magn Reson Imaging. 27(2):103-11, 2018
2. Maleszewski JJ et al: Pathology, imaging, and treatment of cardiac tumours. Nat Rev Cardiol. 14(9):536-49, 2017

Thrombus

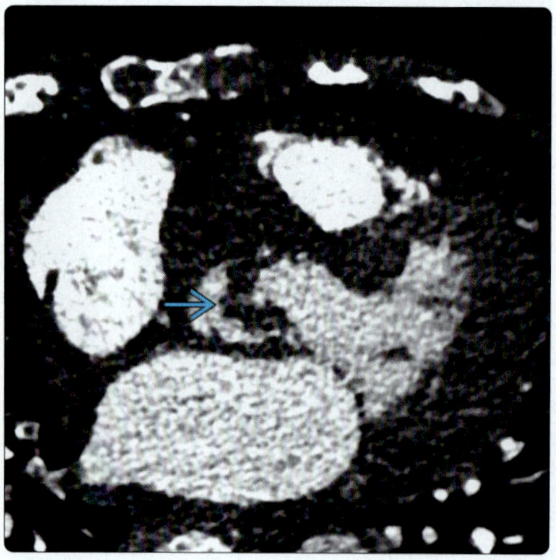

Thrombus

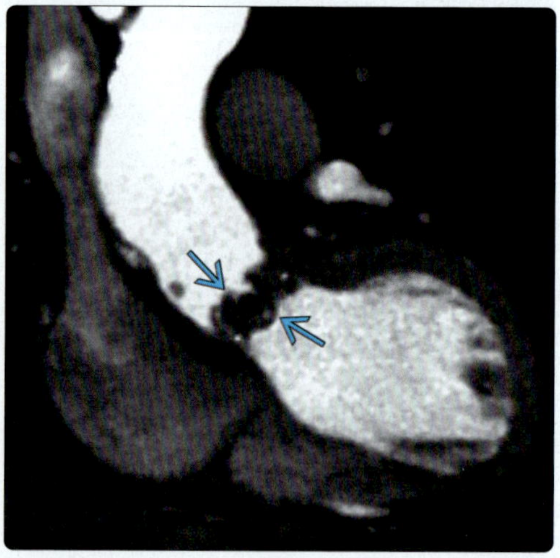

(Left) *Axial CECT of a patient status post bioprosthetic aortic valve replacement shows a low-attenuation mass* ⇒ *encompassing the prosthetic aortic valve leaflets, consistent with thrombus.* **(Right)** *Coronal reformatted CECT of the same patient shows low-attenuation mass-like thickening* ⇒ *of the bioprosthetic aortic valve, involving both the aortic and ventricular surface of the valve leaflet. Cardiac-gated CT is the preferred modality to evaluate prosthetic valve complications.*

Vegetation

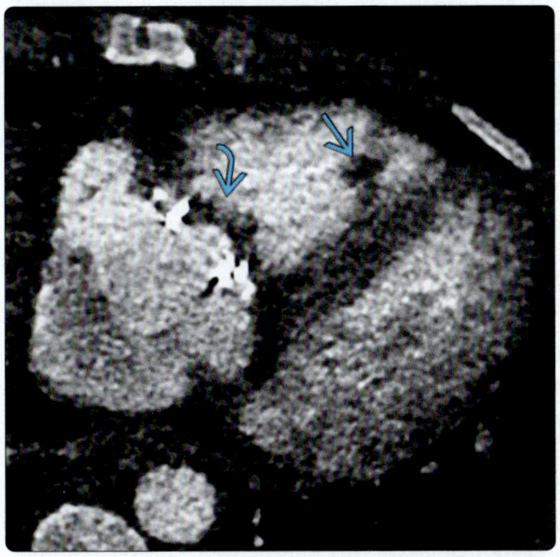

Mitral Annular Calcification

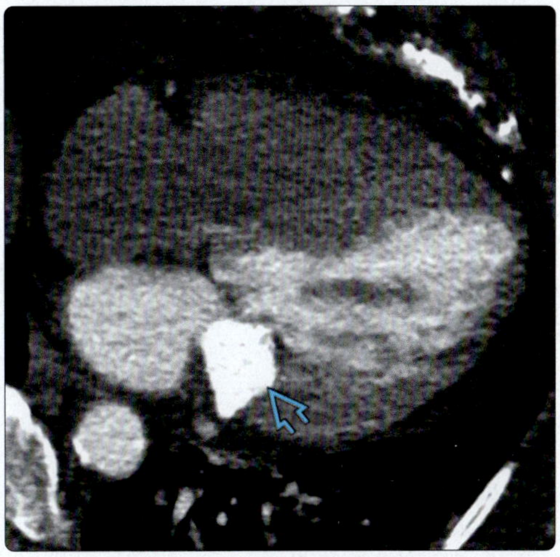

(Left) *Axial cardiac-gated CECT of a patient with endocarditis status post tricuspid valve replacement shows a low-attenuation mass of the tricuspid valve and an additional mass along the trabeculations of the right ventricle consistent with vegetations.* **(Right)** *Axial CECT of a patient with a suspected cardiac mass on echocardiography shows calcified mass-like thickening of the mitral valve annulus, consistent with mitral annular calcification.*

Mitral Annular Calcification

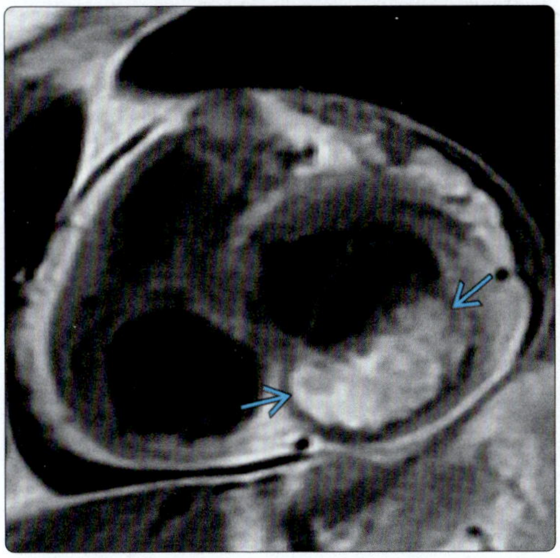

Papillary Fibroelastoma

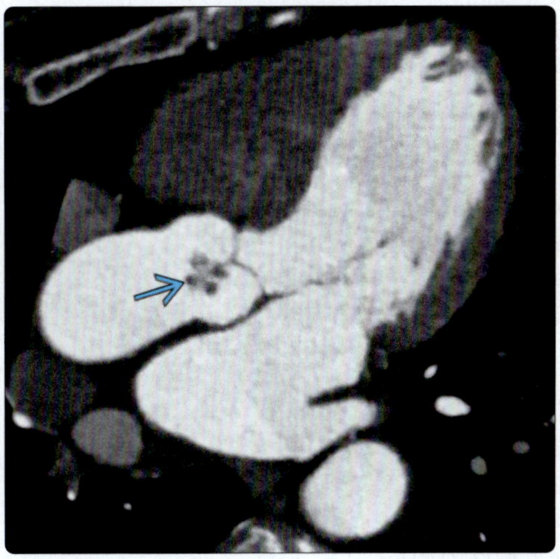

(Left) *Short-axis double inversion recovery T2-weighted MR of a patient with mitral annular calcification shows a hyperintense mass of the mitral annulus, consistent with caseous mitral annular calcification. This process is associated with cardiovascular disease and end-stage renal disease.* **(Right)** *Three-chamber reformatted CECT of a patient with papillary fibroelastoma shows a pedunculated mass attached to the aortic surface of the aortic valve. Neoplasms involving the left heart are typically resected.*

Myxoma

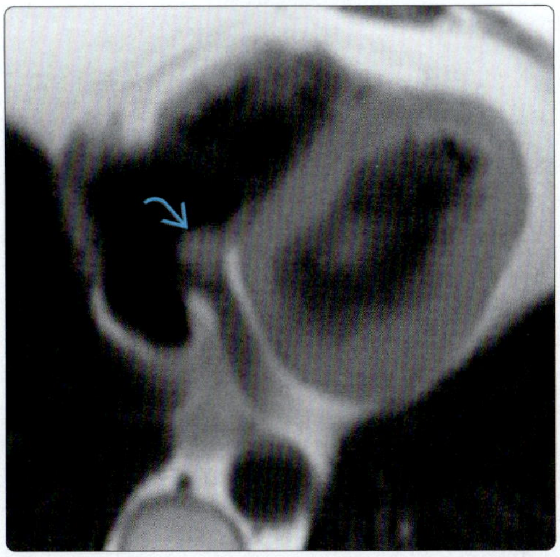

Myxoma

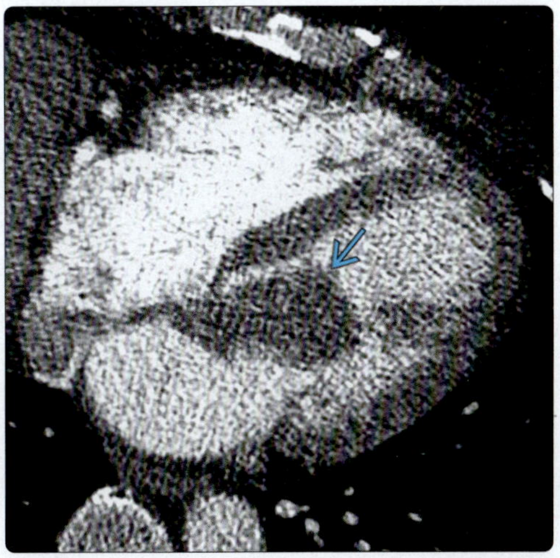

(Left) *Axial double inversion recover T2W MR of a patient with papillary fibroelastoma shows a focal mass at the base of the tricuspid valve. Papillary fibroelastoma more commonly arises from the central portion of the valve, whereas vegetations typically involve the valve leaflet tips.* **(Right)** *Four-chamber reformatted CECT shows a homogeneous myxoma centered on the anterior mitral valve leaflet. Pedunculated myxomas may prolapse across the mitral valve during diastole.*

DIFFERENTIAL DIAGNOSIS

Common

- Mitral Annular Calcification
- Calcified Thrombus

Less Common

- Mitral Stenosis

Rare but Important

- Cardiac Neoplasm

ESSENTIAL INFORMATION

Key Differential Diagnosis Issues

- Other than mitral annular calcifications, true atrial calcifications are rare and should be closely interrogated
- CT is most sensitive modality for calcification
  - NECT is probably best test to avoid contrast-mixing artifacts and artifact from dense contrast in atria

Helpful Clues for Common Diagnoses

- Mitral Annular Calcification
  - Common degenerative finding on radiography and CT
    - > 35% of elderly population
    - ~ 40% of end-stage renal disease patients
  - May mimic mass on echocardiography, requiring further evaluation with CT or MR
  - Characteristically C-shaped, near posterior leaflet
  - Although confined to mitral annulus, may be large and protrude into or involve atrium and myocardium
  - May be centrally low-attenuating from necrotized calcium and liquefaction necrosis
- Calcified Thrombus
  - Thrombus is most common intracardiac mass
  - Thrombus within cardiac chambers may calcify, particularly when chronic and large
    - Calcification typically in peripheral aspect of thrombus; may be stippled, laminated, or central
  - When in left atrium, most frequently complicating chronic atrial fibrillation and mitral stenosis

Helpful Clues for Less Common Diagnoses

- Mitral Stenosis
  - 1st consideration in mitral stenosis is rheumatic heart disease causing valve thickening and calcification
  - Left atrial enlargement and left atrial wall calcifications are characteristic of this entity
  - Restricted leaflet opening during cine image
    - Anterior leaflet may dome during diastolic opening, posterior leaflet may be relatively immobile

Helpful Clues for Rare Diagnoses

- Cardiac Neoplasm
  - Metastatic disease is far more common than primary cardiac tumors
    - Osteosarcoma in young patients may calcify when metastatic to heart
  - Most common primary cardiac tumor with associated calcification is cardiac myxoma
    - Calcification rare in left atrial myxoma but present in ~ 50% of right atrial myxomas
    - Must be differentiated from thrombus
      - Acute thrombus does not enhance
      - Stalk-like attachment to interatrial septum, prolapse across valve characteristic of myxoma
  - Primary cardiac osteosarcoma is rare, though well-described, entity representing 3-9% of cardiac sarcomas
    - Calcifications may be present

Other Essential Information

- Pericardial calcifications near atria may be mistaken for atrial calcification
- End-stage renal disease patients have high rate of incidental calcification in wall of atria of unknown clinical significance

SELECTED REFERENCES

1. Wunderlich NC et al: Rheumatic mitral valve stenosis: diagnosis and treatment options. Curr Cardiol Rep. 21(3):14, 2019
2. Shekar C et al: Calcification of the heart: mechanisms and therapeutic avenues. Expert Rev Cardiovasc Ther. 16(7):527-36, 2018

Mitral Annular Calcification

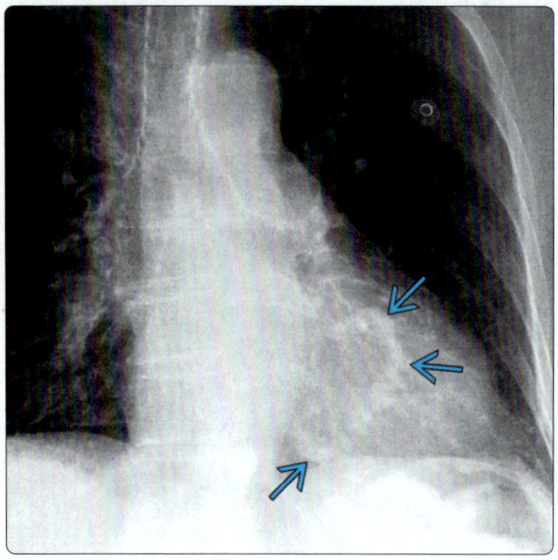

Mitral Annular Calcification

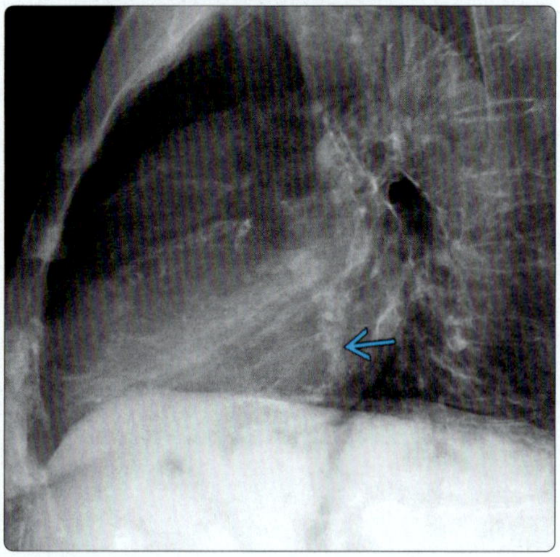

(Left) *PA chest radiograph of a patient with end-stage renal disease shows curvilinear calcification ➔ in a C-shape in the expected location of the mitral annulus.* **(Right)** *Lateral chest radiograph of the same patient shows curvilinear calcification ➔ confirmed to be located in the region of the mitral annulus. Although benign, mitral annular calcifications may mimic a mass on echocardiography and require CT for confirmation. These calcifications may involve the atrial myocardium.*

Mitral Annular Calcification

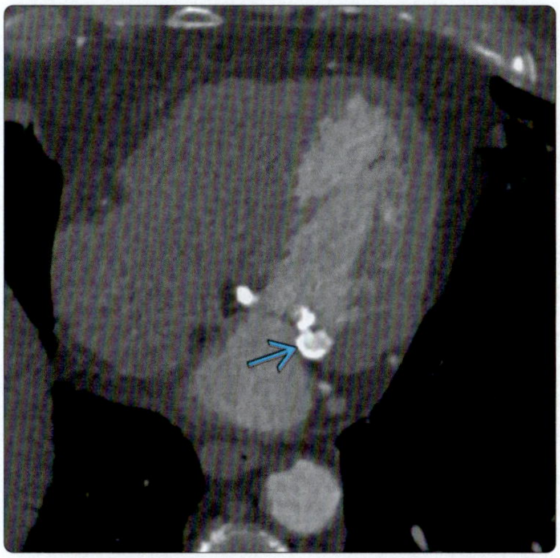

Mitral Annular Calcification

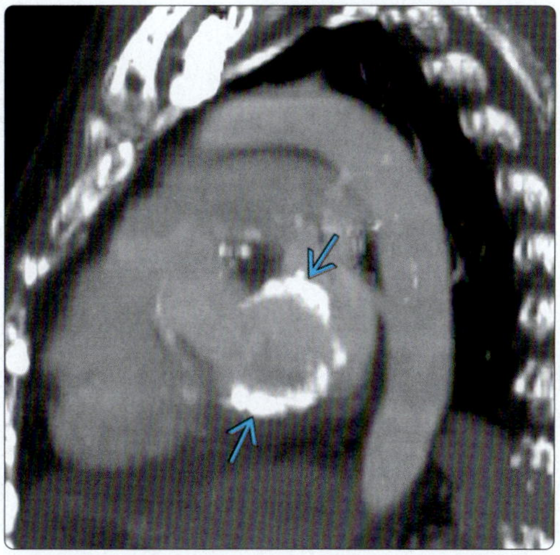

(Left) *Axial CECT of a patient with end-stage renal disease shows dense mitral annular calcification (MAC) → extending into the left atrial myocardium near the posterior mitral valve leaflet. MAC may contain central caseous material and be termed caseous MAC.* **(Right)** *Oblique sagittal MIP CECT of the same patient shows dense, C-shaped calcification → in mitral valve annulus. CT is very sensitive for calcification, and NECT may be sufficient to make a diagnosis of MAC as a problem-solving tool.*

Mitral Annular Calcification

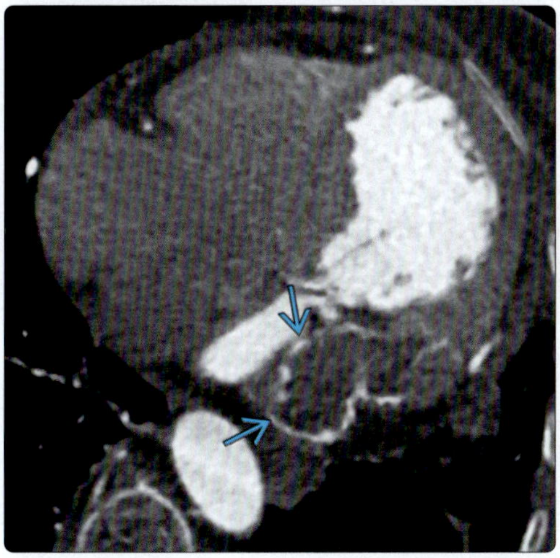

Calcified Thrombus

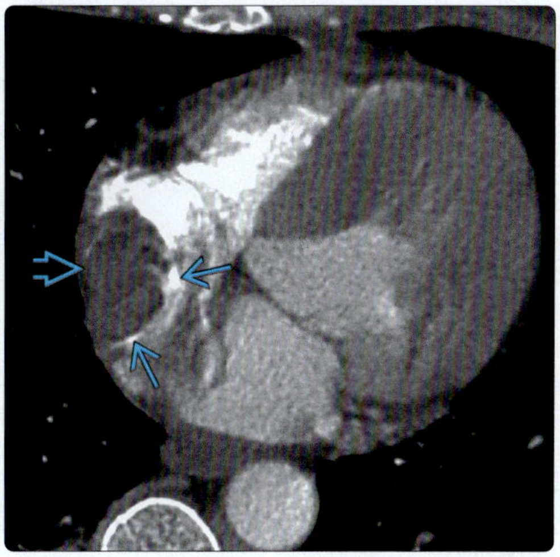

(Left) *Axial CECT of a patient with caseous MAC shows an incidentally noted, peripherally calcified mass → along the mitral valve annulus extending into the left atrial wall. The low-attenuation central component contains necrotized calcium and liquefaction necrosis.* **(Right)** *Axial CECT of a patient with right atrial thrombus shows a mass ⇨ in the right atrium containing foci of peripheral calcification →. Chronic thrombus may calcify, typically peripherally.*

Mitral Stenosis

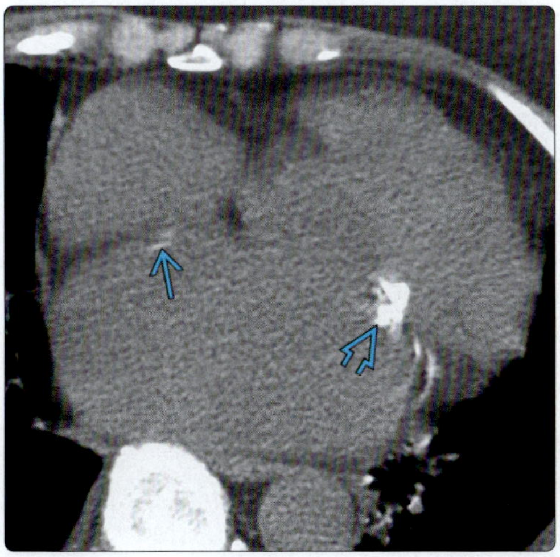

Cardiac Neoplasm

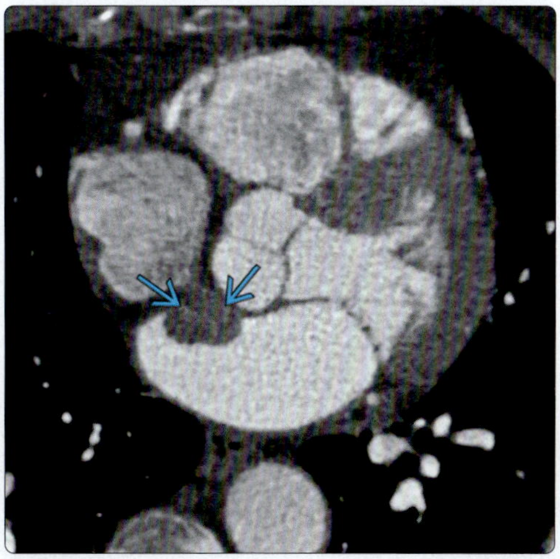

(Left) *Axial NECT of a patient with rheumatic heart disease shows dense calcification of the mitral valve leaflets ⇨ and linear calcification in the left atrial wall →. Mitral leaflet calcification, left atrial enlargement, and left atrial wall calcifications are suspicious for rheumatic heart disease and mitral stenosis.* **(Right)** *Axial CECT with cardiac gating of a patient with left atrial myxoma shows a lobulated mass along the interatrial septum with fine linear internal calcifications →, more common in right atrial myxomas.*

DIFFERENTIAL DIAGNOSIS

Common

- Chronic Myocardial Infarction
- Ventricular Aneurysm/Pseudoaneurysm
- Myocarditis

Less Common

- Rheumatic Heart Disease

Rare but Important

- Cardiac Neoplasm

ESSENTIAL INFORMATION

Key Differential Diagnosis Issues

- Dystrophic calcifications are most common cause of ventricular calcifications
  - Entities include prior myocardial infarction, aneurysm, myocarditis, and trauma
- Myocardial calcifications may be "metastatic" when associated with chronically elevated serum calcium levels
  - Most common in end-stage renal disease, hyperparathyroidism, osseous metastasis, myeloma

Helpful Clues for Common Diagnoses

- Chronic Myocardial Infarction
  - 8% of cases calcify 6 years after infarction
  - Most commonly occurs in anterior wall and apex
  - Linear myocardial/subendocardial calcification in vascular territory highly specific for chronic infarction
    - May also see subendocardial fibrofatty metaplasia
- Ventricular Aneurysm/Pseudoaneurysm
  - True aneurysms contain all myocardial layers, although thinned and dyskinetic
    - More common in anterior wall and apex
  - Calcification common in left ventricular apical aneurysms
  - Often associated with chronic thrombus in aneurysm
  - Ventricular pseudoaneurysms are rupture of ventricular wall contained by epicardium or pericardium
    - Characterized by dyskinesis, narrower neck than aneurysm sack, and usually post infarction
    - High risk of spontaneous rupture
    - More common in inferior wall
- Myocarditis
  - Calcification may complicate prior/healed myocarditis
  - Viral etiologies most frequent, such as Parvovirus B19
  - Suspected in younger patients with myocardial calcifications without other explanation
  - Extensive left ventricular calcification reported after sepsis, form of dystrophic calcification

Helpful Clues for Less Common Diagnoses

- Rheumatic Heart Disease
  - Often presents clinically years to decades after infection
  - Characterized by atrial calcification, left atrial enlargement, and mitral valve calcifications
  - Left ventricular myocardial calcifications less common

Helpful Clues for Rare Diagnoses

- Cardiac Neoplasms
  - Metastatic disease is far more common than primary tumors of heart
    - Among ventricular metastases, osteosarcoma and treated disease, such as lymphoma, likely to calcify
  - Cardiac myxoma rarely occurs in ventricles but may calcify in this location
  - Primary cardiac osteosarcoma may calcify
    - More common in atrium, ventricular invasion reported

Other Essential Information

- Degenerative aortic valve calcifications may extend into left ventricular outflow tract, important to note in transcatheter aortic valve replacement planning
- Linear left ventricular subendocardial calcification on chest CT may indicate missed infarction

SELECTED REFERENCES

1. Kimura Y et al: Massive biventricular myocardial calcification in a patient with fulminant myocarditis requiring ventricular assist device support. Intern Med. 58(9):1283-6, 2019

Ventricular Aneurysm/Pseudoaneurysm

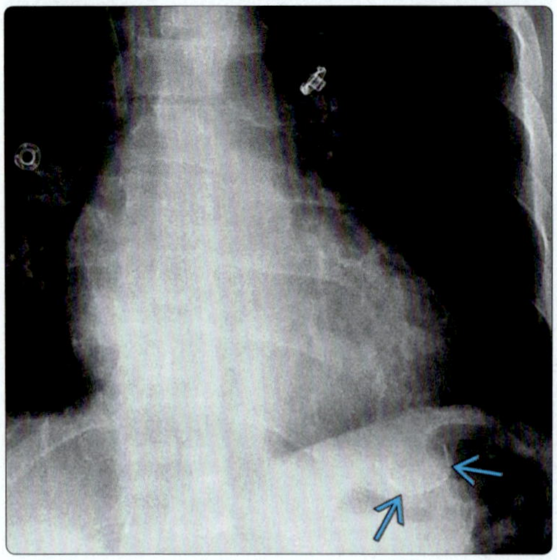

Ventricular Aneurysm/Pseudoaneurysm

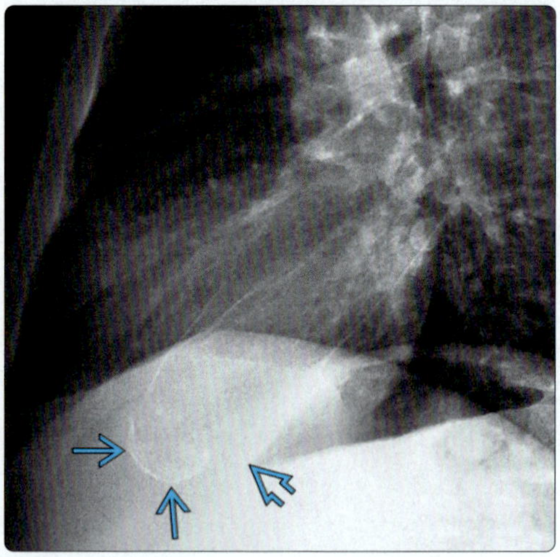

(Left) *PA chest radiograph of a patient with chronic chest pain shows curvilinear calcification* ➔ *projecting over the left upper quadrant, in the expected location of the true cardiac apex.* **(Right)** *Lateral chest radiograph of the same patient shows the curvilinear calcification* ➔ *to be superior to the anterior aspect of the left hemidiaphragm* ➔, *confirming cardiac location. Calcifications of this morphology and location are suspicious for a cardiac aneurysm.*

Ventricular Aneurysm/Pseudoaneurysm

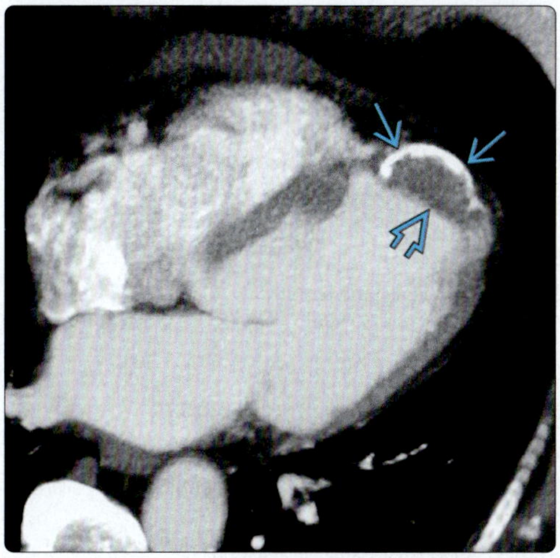

Ventricular Aneurysm/Pseudoaneurysm

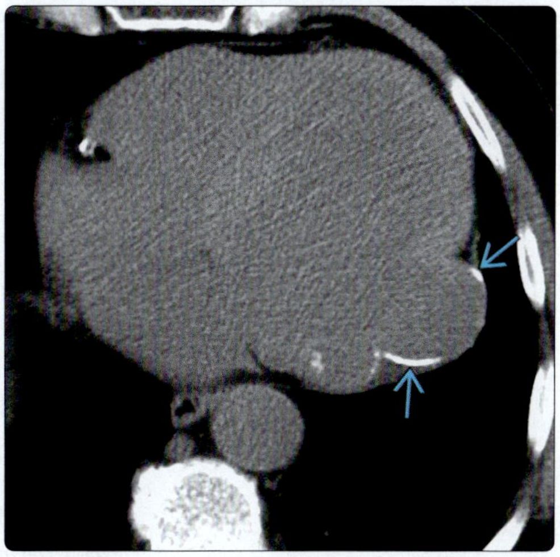

(Left) *Axial CECT of a patient with history of myocardial infarction shows a wide-mouth left ventricular aneurysm with curvilinear calcification* → *and internal thrombus* ⇒*. Postinfarct aneurysms most commonly involve the anterior wall and apex.* **(Right)** *Axial NECT of a patient with history of myocardial infarction shows curvilinear calcification* → *outlining a ventricular pseudoaneurysm with narrow neck. The inferior and lateral walls are more frequently involved by pseudoaneurysm than true aneurysm.*

Ventricular Aneurysm/Pseudoaneurysm

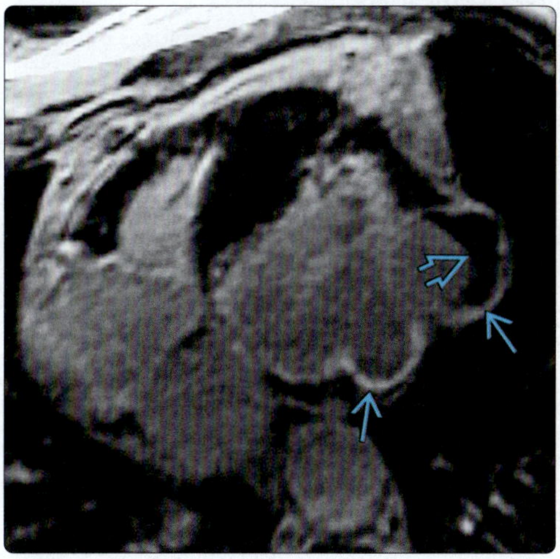

Myocarditis

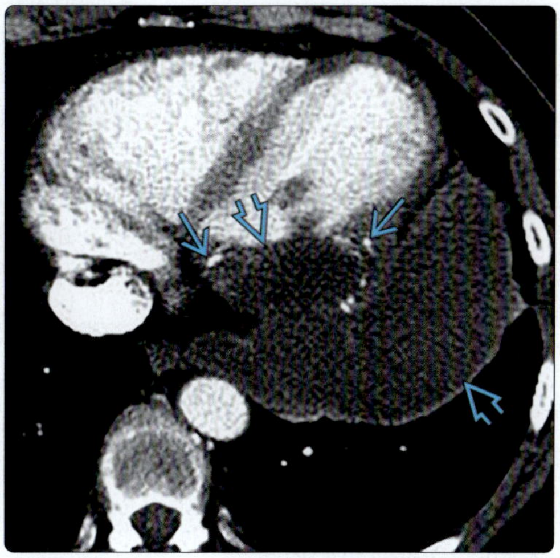

(Left) *Four-chamber late gadolinium enhancement (LGE) MR of the same patient shows enhancement of the pseudoaneurysm walls* → *with central low signal intensity, consistent with thrombus* ⇒*.* **(Right)** *Axial CECT of a patient with chronic chest pain and myocarditis shows punctate calcifications* → *in the left ventricular wall with large cysts* ⇒ *in the chamber that extend to the pericardial space, consistent with echinococcal abscess.*

Rheumatic Heart Disease

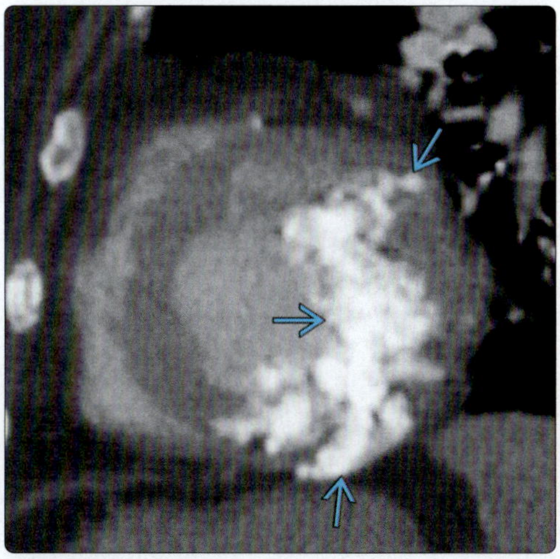

Rheumatic Heart Disease

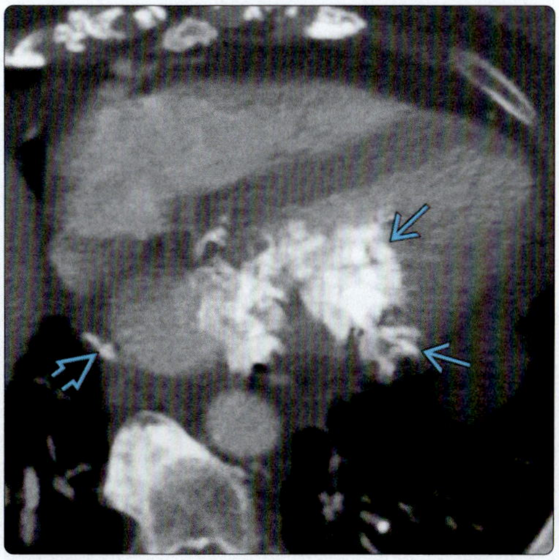

(Left) *Oblique sagittal MIP reformatted CECT of a patient with history of rheumatic heart disease shows extensive left ventricular calcification* →*.* **(Right)** *Axial CECT of the same patient shows extensive calcification* → *of the left ventricular myocardium. Left atrial calcification* ⇒*, left atrial enlargement, and mitral valvular calcifications are characteristic of rheumatic heart disease, which may present years to decades after infection. Extensive postinfectious calcification in the myocardium is also seen in patients with sepsis.*

DIFFERENTIAL DIAGNOSIS

Common

- Aortic
  - Aortic Stenosis
  - Bicuspid Aortic Valve

Less Common

- Mitral
  - Mitral Stenosis
  - Mitral Annular Calcification

Rare but Important

- Tricuspid
  - Tricuspid Stenosis

ESSENTIAL INFORMATION

Key Differential Diagnosis Issues

- Aortic valvular calcification detected on radiography may indicate aortic stenosis before clinically apparent
- CT is most sensitive modality for detecting valvular calcifications in any location
  - Clinical significance of small amounts of valvular calcification discovered incidentally on CT is unknown
  - ECG-gated CT may be superior to echocardiography for detecting bicuspid aortic valve when heavily calcified

Helpful Clues for Common Diagnoses

- **Aortic Stenosis**
  - Most commonly degenerative calcification secondary to inflammatory process similar to atherosclerosis
  - When degenerative, begins at base of valve leaflet, progresses toward tips
    - Rheumatic heart disease characterized by commissural fusion, which is less common in degenerative valvular disease
  - ECG-gated CT may show restricted valve leaflet opening
  - Degree of calcification important component of transcatheter aortic valve replacement planning
    - Valve leaflet, annulus, and left ventricular outflow tract
    - Valve calcification can be quantified on ECG-gated CT using calcium scores
- **Bicuspid Aortic Valve**
  - Most common congenital cardiovascular malformation
  - 2 physiologic cusps, determined on cine imaging
    - Congenital fusion of 2 cusps in morphologically trileaflet valve evidenced by raphe
    - Congenitally morphologic bileaflet valve less common
  - Acquired fusion may be secondary to rheumatic heart disease or degenerative disease
  - Valve predisposed to thickening and calcification

Helpful Clues for Less Common Diagnoses

- **Mitral Stenosis**
  - Rheumatic heart disease is most important differential consideration
  - Characterized by progressive dilation of left atrium
  - Left atrial wall calcification and mitral valve calcification are important diagnostic clues for this diagnosis
- **Mitral Annular Calcification**
  - Degenerative process of mitral valve annulus
  - Must differentiate from mitral valvular calcification

Helpful Clues for Rare Diagnoses

- **Tricuspid Stenosis**
  - Characterized by valve calcification and thickening with associated right atrial enlargement
  - Rheumatic heart disease is 1st diagnostic consideration

SELECTED REFERENCES

1. Wunderlich NC et al: Rheumatic mitral valve stenosis: diagnosis and treatment options. Curr Cardiol Rep. 21(3):14, 2019
2. Lichtenberger JP 3rd et al: MR imaging of thoracic aortic disease. Top Magn Reson Imaging. 27(2):95-102, 2018

Aortic Stenosis

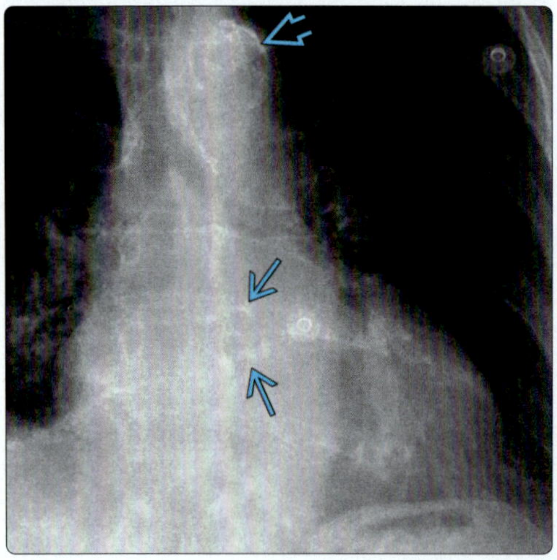

Aortic Stenosis

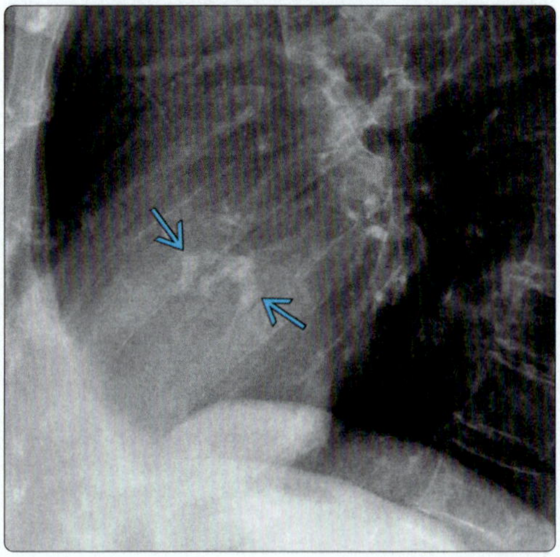

(Left) *PA chest radiograph of an asymptomatic patient with aortic stenosis shows valve leaflet calcification ➡ in the expected location of the aortic valve. Aortic arch calcification is also present, suggesting atherosclerotic disease ➡.* **(Right)** *Lateral chest radiograph of the same patient with asymptomatic aortic stenosis shows valve leaflet calcification ➡. Detecting valve calcification on radiographs often indicates significant valve disease and suggests possible subclinical aortic stenosis.*

Aortic Stenosis

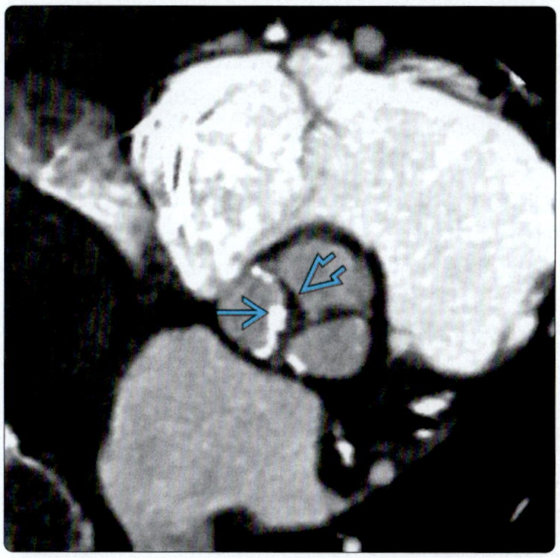

Aortic Stenosis

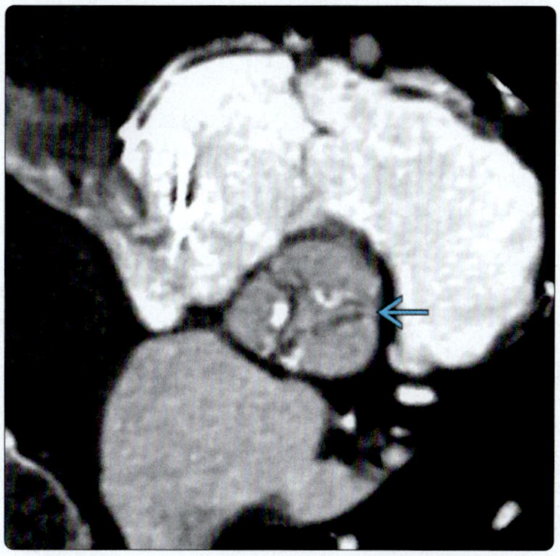

(Left) *Double oblique reformatted ECG-gated CECT short axis to the aortic valve in diastole of a patient with aortic stenosis shows trileaflet thickening ⇨ and calcification →. CT is very sensitive for calcification, and detecting small amounts of aortic valve calcification incidentally on CT does not carry the same significance as radiographically detected calcification.* **(Right)** *CECT of the same patient in systole shows restricted valve leaflet opening. Note that the commissures → are stenosed but not fused.*

Aortic Stenosis

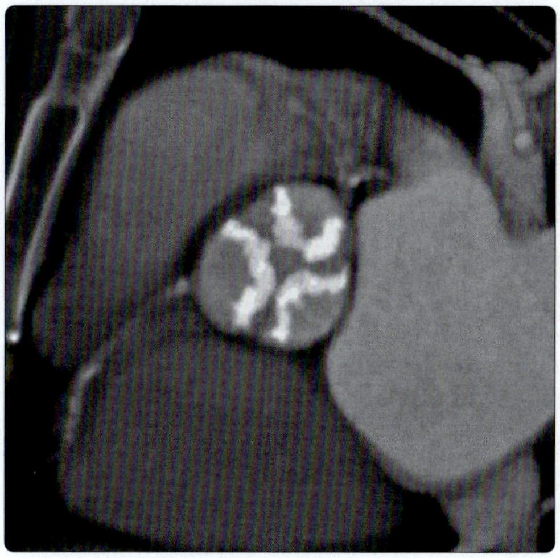

Bicuspid Aortic Valve

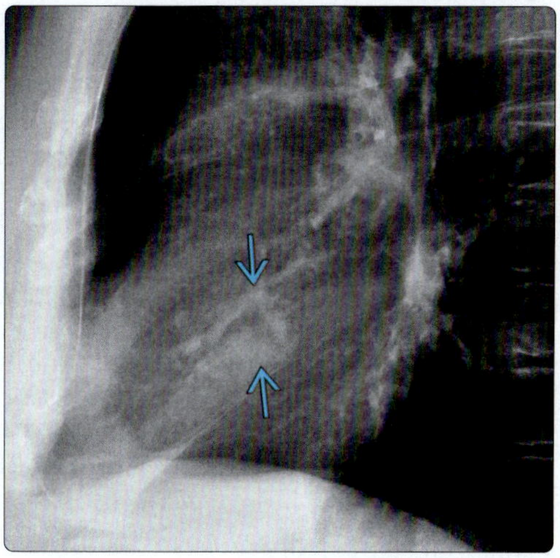

(Left) *Maximum intensity projection (MIP) reformatted CECT short axis to the aortic valve of a patient with aortic stenosis shows the extent of aortic valve calcification. Agatston scores of aortic valve calcification correlate well with degree of aortic stenosis.* **(Right)** *Lateral chest radiograph of a young patient with bicuspid aortic valve (BAV) and aortic stenosis shows extensive aortic valve calcification → in a fish mouth morphology.*

Bicuspid Aortic Valve

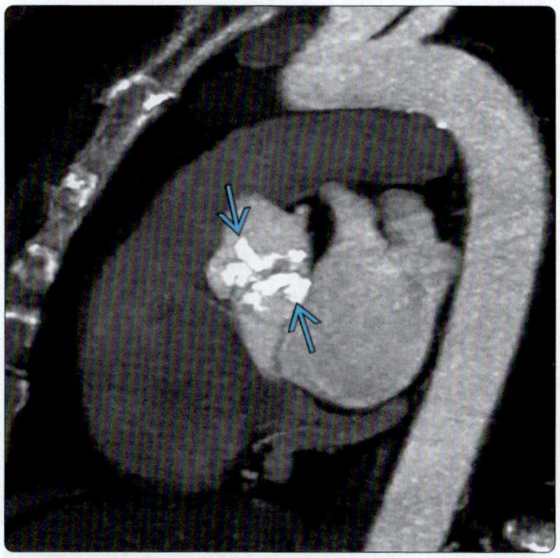

Mitral Stenosis

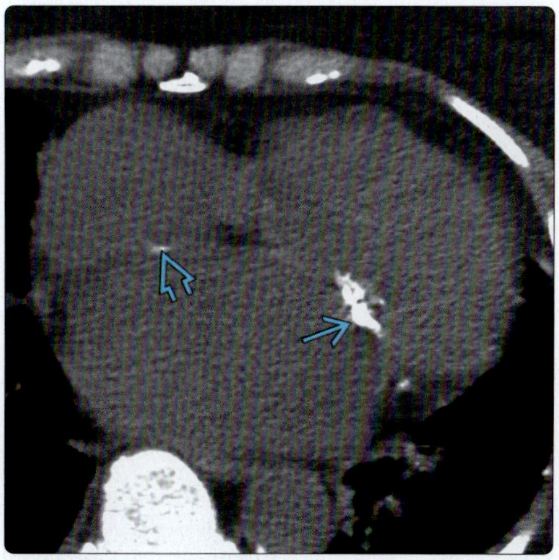

(Left) *Sagittal MIP CECT of a patient with BAV and aortic stenosis shows aortic valve calcification →. BAV should be considered in patients less than 70 years old with severe aortic valve disease and aortic stenosis.* **(Right)** *Axial NECT of a patient with mitral stenosis due to rheumatic heart disease shows extensive mitral valvular calcification →, left atrial enlargement, and left atrial wall calcification ⇨. Mitral valve calcification should be distinguished from mitral annular calcification.*

Coronary Artery Anomaly

DIFFERENTIAL DIAGNOSIS

Common

- Retroaortic Left Circumflex Artery (LCx)
- Interarterial Right Coronary Artery (RCA)

Less Common

- Interarterial Left Main/Left Anterior Descending (LAD) Artery
- Coronary Artery Fistula

Rare but Important

- Prepulmonic LAD
- Anomalous Left Coronary Artery From Pulmonary Artery (ALCAPA)

ESSENTIAL INFORMATION

Key Differential Diagnosis Issues

- Must determine if anomalous coronary courses between aorta and pulmonary artery, termed "interarterial"

Helpful Clues for Common Diagnoses

- **Retroaortic LCx**
  - Most common coronary artery anomaly
  - LCx originates from right cusp or RCA
  - Courses posterior to aortic root before entering left atrioventricular groove
  - Not hemodynamically significant
- **Interarterial RCA**
  - RCA originates from left cusp, left main, or shares common ostium with left main, then is interarterial
  - Necessary to assess for intramural course (within wall of aorta)
    - Intramural course usually < 1 cm in length
    - Slit-like ostium, small-caliber proximal segment
    - Parallels circumference of aortic wall
  - Weaker association with sudden cardiac death (compared with interarterial left coronary artery)
  - If symptoms are present (syncope, arrhythmias, chest pain, or sudden cardiac death), surgery is considered

Helpful Clues for Less Common Diagnoses

- **Interarterial Left Main or Left Anterior Descending (LAD) Artery**
  - Arises from right cusp, RCA, or shared ostium with RCA
  - Follows interarterial course (between ascending aorta and left main pulmonary artery)
  - Strong association with sudden cardiac death
  - When diagnosed, surgery is usually recommended
- **Coronary Artery Fistula**
  - Anomalous drainage of coronary artery with cardiac chamber or central venous structure
  - Most commonly involving RCA
  - Commonly drains into RV, RA, SVC, PA, or coronary sinus
  - Fistulous vessel is diffusely dilated and tortuous
  - Large fistulas may cause coronary steal, distal ischemia
  - Symptoms may include chest pain, syncope, arrhythmia
  - When symptomatic, treatment options include surgical ligation or embolization

Helpful Clues for Rare Diagnoses

- **Prepulmonic LAD**
  - LAD coursing anterior to main PA or right ventricular outflow tract
  - Common in patients with tetralogy of Fallot
  - Surgical risk during sternotomy
- **Anomalous Left Coronary Artery From Pulmonary Artery (ALCAPA)**
  - LM originates from main pulmonary artery
  - Effectively left-to-right shunt
  - Typically, all of coronary tree is tortuous and dilated
  - Most diagnosed early in life as shunt, leads to ischemia and early myocardial infarction
  - Surgical management is warranted

SELECTED REFERENCES

1. Agarwal PP et al: Anomalous coronary arteries that need intervention: review of pre- and postoperative imaging appearances. Radiographics. 37(3):740-57, 2017

Retroaortic Left Circumflex Artery (LCx)

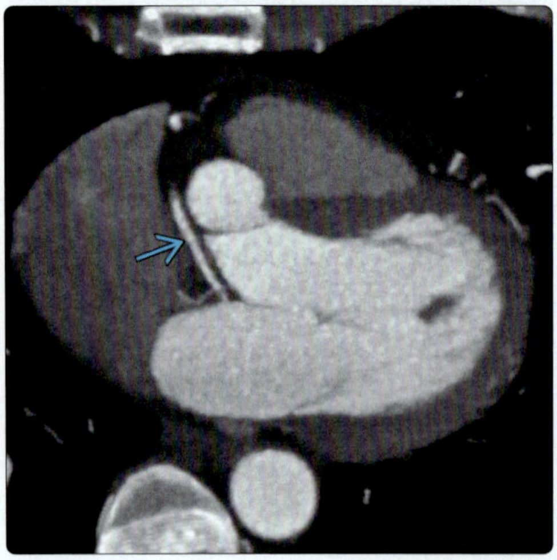

Retroaortic Left Circumflex Artery (LCx)

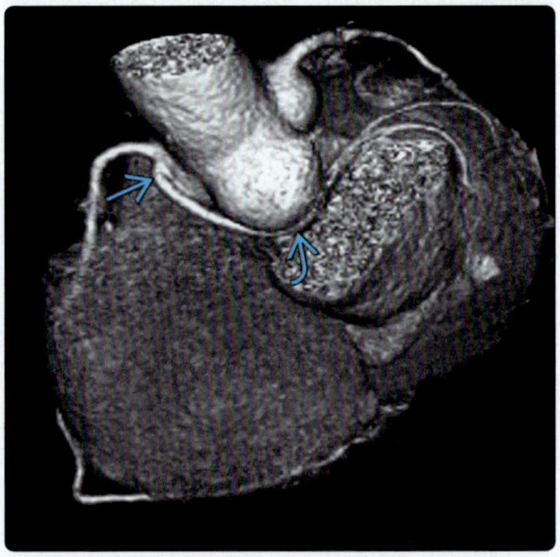

(Left) *Axial 6-mm MIP reformatted image from a coronary CTA of a patient with atypical chest pain shows a retroaortic left circumflex coronary artery (LCx) ➙.* **(Right)** *3D reconstructed coronary CTA of the same patient shows origin of the LCx ➙ from the right coronary cusp and subsequent retroaortic course ➙ to end in the left atrioventricular groove. This is the most common coronary artery anomaly, and it is not hemodynamically significant.*

Retroaortic Left Circumflex Artery (LCx)

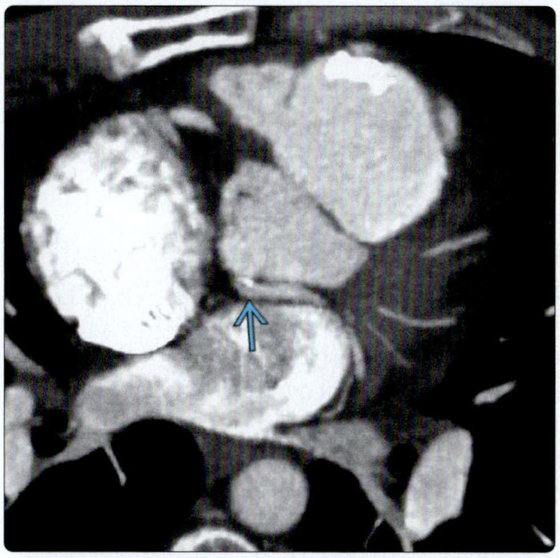

Interarterial Right Coronary Artery (RCA)

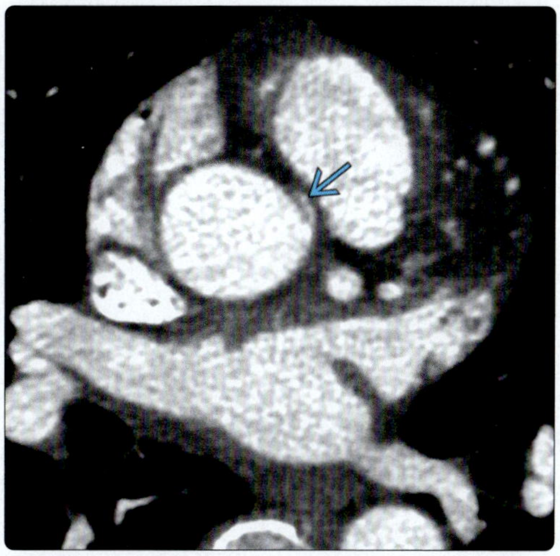

(Left) *Oblique 6-mm MIP reformatted image from a coronary CTA of a patient with atypical chest pain shows anomalous origin of the LCx from the noncoronary cusp. This artery assumes a retroaortic course to the left atrioventricular groove.* **(Right)** *Axial coronary CTA of a patient with exertional chest pain shows acute angle and slit-like orifice of the right coronary artery (RCA) originating from the superior aspect of the left coronary cusp, consistent with an intramural course.*

Interarterial Left Main/Left Anterior Descending (LAD) Artery

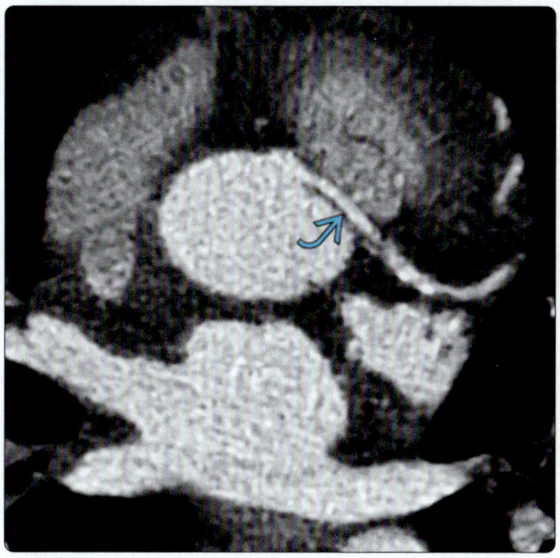

Interarterial Left Main/Left Anterior Descending (LAD) Artery

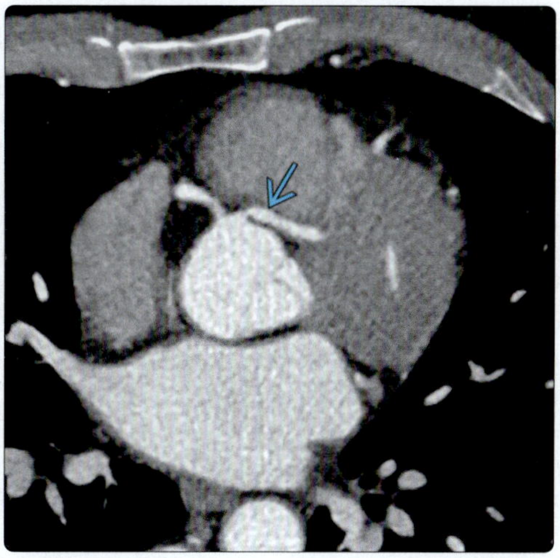

(Left) *Oblique reformatted image from a coronary CTA of a patient with chest pain shows interarterial course of the left main coronary artery originating from the right coronary cusp.* **(Right)** *Axial coronary CTA of a patient with chest pain shows a common origin of the right and left main coronary arteries and subsequent interarterial course of the left main coronary artery. This morphology has a strong association with sudden cardiac death, and surgical correction is often recommended.*

Coronary Artery Fistula

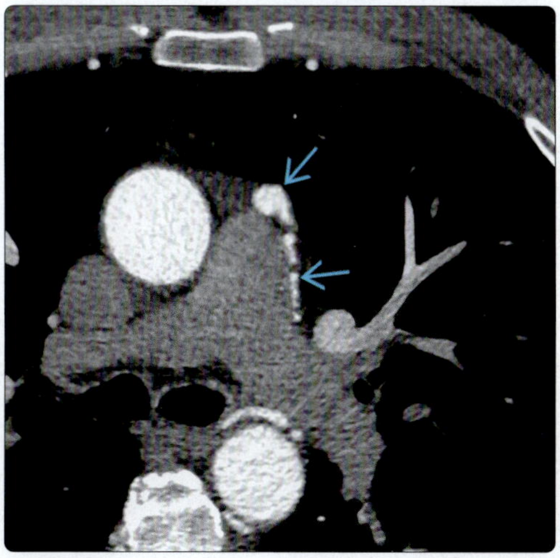

Anomalous Left Coronary Artery From Pulmonary Artery (ALCAPA)

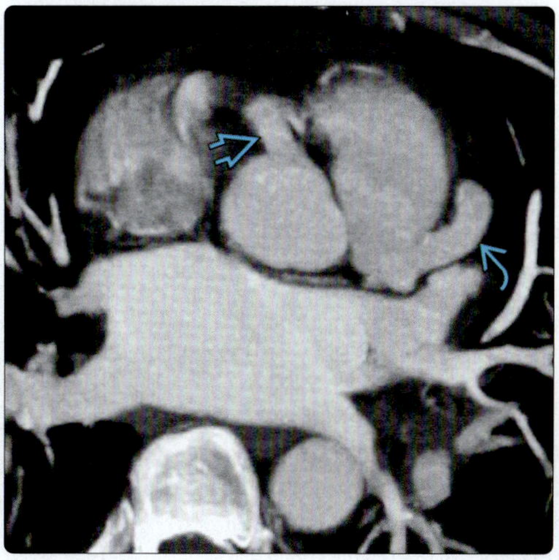

(Left) *Axial coronary CTA of a patient with atypical chest pain shows fistulous, tortuous arteries along the left aspect of the pulmonary artery. Large fistulas may cause coronary steal and be symptomatic.* **(Right)** *Axial 8-mm MIP reformatted image from a coronary CTA of a patient with chest pain shows anomalous origin of the left main coronary artery from the pulmonary artery. The right coronary is dilated and tortuous. Cases are often diagnosed in childhood with early myocardial infarction.*

DIFFERENTIAL DIAGNOSIS

Common

- Ischemic Cardiomyopathy
- Cardiac Sarcoidosis
- Myocarditis
- Hypertrophic Cardiomyopathy
- Nonischemic Dilated Cardiomyopathy

Less Common

- Cardiac Amyloidosis

Rare but Important

- Arrhythmogenic Right Ventricular Dysplasia

ESSENTIAL INFORMATION

Key Differential Diagnosis Issues

- Gadolinium collects in extracellular space in regions of fibrosis or myocardial edema
  - Typically imaged at 10 minutes post-injection to allow clearance from normal tissue
  - Inversion time for myocardium determined prior to late gadolinium enhancement (LGE) image acquisition
- 1st decision when LGE is detected on cardiac MR is to determine pattern
  - Subendocardial enhancement raises possibility of myocardial infarction
    - Confirm recognizable vascular territory in left ventricle (LV)
      - Left anterior descending (LAD): Anterior segments
      - Left circumflex (LCx): Lateral segments
      - Right coronary artery (RCA): Septal segments
    - Diffuse subendocardial LGE may indicate amyloidosis
  - Mid-myocardial (midwall) LGE typically indicates infiltrative process of myocardium
    - Cardiac sarcoidosis most frequently distributed in basal septum and LV free wall
    - Hypertrophic cardiomyopathy most frequently affects basal septum in areas of most hypertrophy
  - Subepicardial LGE frequently observed in myocarditis
  - Transmural disease can occur with ischemic cardiomyopathy and infiltrative disease
  - Diffuse disease most often observed in infiltrative disease and myocarditis
- Many common diseases exhibit varied patterns of LGE, but infarction almost always involves subendocardium

Helpful Clues for Common Diagnoses

- **Ischemic Cardiomyopathy**
  - LGE accumulates in areas of myocardial edema or fibrosis
    - Subendocardium is end-organ blood supply territory
    - Recognizable vascular territory in LV
    - Transmurality corresponds to segmental viability
  - Transmurality of LGE in cases of myocardial infarction has important prognostic and management implications
    - If LGE is < 50% of wall thickness → high likelihood of functional segmental recovery after revascularization
  - Central hypointense region in area of myocardial infarction may indicate microvascular obstruction
    - Poor prognostic sign, associated with adverse cardiovascular events
    - Differentiate from hemosiderin, which is low signal intensity on T2WI
  - Associated cardiac MR findings in ischemic cardiomyopathy
    - Regional or global wall motion abnormality and systolic thickening, decreased ejection fraction (EF)
    - Increased T2 signal intensity from muscular edema
    - Reduced subendocardial 1st pass perfusion in coronary territory
    - Evaluate for aneurysm and intracardiac thrombus
      - Aneurysm characterized by myocardial thinning and dyskinesis on cine imaging
      - Thrombus may show progressive loss of signal intensity on inversion recovery scout imaging
      - Chronic thrombus may be thin/eccentric, may appear to enhance peripherally
- **Cardiac Sarcoidosis**
  - LGE observed in patients with sarcoidosis is typically mid-myocardial in basal septum and LV free wall
    - Patchy disease is characteristic
    - Up to 10% may have subendocardial involvement mimicking coronary disease
    - When > 20% of LV involved, higher risk of death
    - Almost all patients with adverse events have LGE
  - Associated cardiac MR findings in cardiac sarcoidosis
    - High signal intensity on T2WI indicates myocardial edema in acute phase
    - Wall motion abnormality in non-coronary distribution
    - Mediastinal lymphadenopathy and lung disease are important extra-cardiac features
  - Most patients do not have cardiac symptoms
    - Conduction abnormality is common presentation
      - Complete heart block highly suggestive
      - Sustained or non-sustained ventricular tachycardia
    - Congestive heart failure less common
- **Myocarditis**
  - Clinical presentation ranges from subclinical to acute heart failure, usually viral
  - When symptomatic, can present with chest pain, ↑ cardiac enzymes
    - May be preceded by viral syndrome
  - LGE in myocarditis typically patchy, pattern is subepicardial or transmural
    - Subepicardial or transmural LGE component of Lake Louise consensus criteria
    - Lateral wall is most commonly affected
    - LGE may be diffuse in severe myocarditis
      - Diffuse, septal, and mid wall LGE associated with adverse cardiac events in myocarditis
  - Occurs in nonvascular territory
  - Pericardium may be involved in myopericarditis
- **Hypertrophic Cardiomyopathy (HCM)**
  - LGE detected in patients with known HCM is associated with sudden cardiac death
    - Often focal in hypertrophied segments, may be diffuse
    - Characteristically in anterior and posterior septum at RV insertion sites
    - "Extensive" when LGE in > 15% of myocardium

- Marker of high risk, often requiring implantable cardioverter-defibrillator
- Hypertrophied segments of myocardium > 15 mm, or ratio of hypertrophied segments:nonhypertrophied > 1.3
- Asymmetric LV hypertrophy is most common form, concentric or RV involvement (1/3 cases) less common
  - Basal septum most common (60% of HCM)
  - Midventricular HCM associated with apical aneurysm and thrombus formation
  - Apical variant has spade-like LV cavity
  - Mass-like HCM may mimic cardiac mass
  - Concentric HCM in 5% of cases
    - LGE in concentric HCM not commonly observed in mimics of HCM, such as hypertensive heart disease, athlete's heart, and aortic stenosis
- Left ventricular outflow tract obstruction observed on MR in 30%, most commonly when basal septum involved
  - Gradient > 50 mm Hg considered obstructive in LVOT
  - Systolic anterior motion of anterior mitral valve leaflet due to high-velocity jet across LVOT
- Typically ↑ EF, ↓ end-systolic volume
- Papillary muscle hypertrophy/anomaly observed in HCM
- Autosomal dominant with incomplete penetrance and variable expressivity in most cases
  - Genotype-positive family members screened and surveilled on imaging

- **Nonischemic Dilated Cardiomyopathy**
  - LV dilation with systolic dysfunction (EF < 55%)
    - Coronary disease, conditions such as myocarditis, iron overload, and sarcoidosis should be excluded
    - Right ventricle (RV) may also be involved
    - MR-derived quantitative LV volumes gold standard
  - Midwall septal pattern of LGE (midwall stripe) in ~ 30%
    - Typically basal and mid segments
    - LGE associated with major adverse cardiac events
      - Presence used as guide for implantable cardioverter-defibrillator placement
  - Increased prevalence and worse prognosis in African Americans and men
    - 25% of dilated cardiomyopathy may be genetic

Helpful Clues for Less Common Diagnoses

- **Cardiac Amyloidosis**
  - Extracellular accumulation of fibrillar protein deposits, can involve any portion of heart
  - Circumferential subendocardial LGE is characteristic
    - Finding optimal myocardial nulling time on T1 scout images typically difficult from altered T1 kinetics
    - May be diffuse ± RV or atrial involvement
    - On LGE, blood pool appears dark secondary to rapid clearance from circulation
      - When suspicion is high, acquire LGE at 5 minutes
  - Associated MR findings: Concentric LV thickening, biatrial enlargement, thickening of RV and atria if involved

Helpful Clues for Rare Diagnoses

- **Arrhythmogenic Right Ventricular Dysplasia (ARVD)**
  - Fibrofatty replacement predominantly involving RV thought to be secondary to mutation of desmosomal protein gene
    - 2010 International Task Force Criteria does not include LGE as major or minor criterion
  - LGE present in RV free wall in 2/3 of cases
    - LV may be involved, although septal LGE is unusual
  - Associated cardiac MR findings in ARVD
    - RV dilation and decreased function
    - RV wall motion abnormality and aneurysms
    - RV thickened trabeculations

SELECTED REFERENCES

1. Amano Y et al: Cardiac MR imaging of hypertrophic cardiomyopathy: techniques, findings, and clinical relevance. Magn Reson Med Sci. 17(2):120-31, 2018
2. Bulluck H et al: Cardiovascular magnetic resonance in acute ST-segment-elevation myocardial infarction: recent advances, controversies, and future directions. Circulation. 137(18):1949-64, 2018
3. Gandjbakhch E et al: Clinical diagnosis, imaging, and genetics of arrhythmogenic right ventricular cardiomyopathy/dysplasia: JACC state-of-the-art review. J Am Coll Cardiol. 72(7):784-804, 2018
4. Romano S et al: Cardiac MRI for detection of cardiac sarcoidosis. Radiology. 288(3):659, 2018

Ischemic Cardiomyopathy

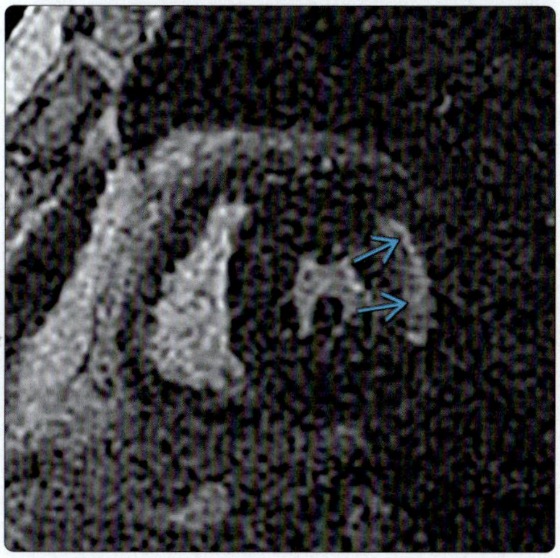

Ischemic Cardiomyopathy

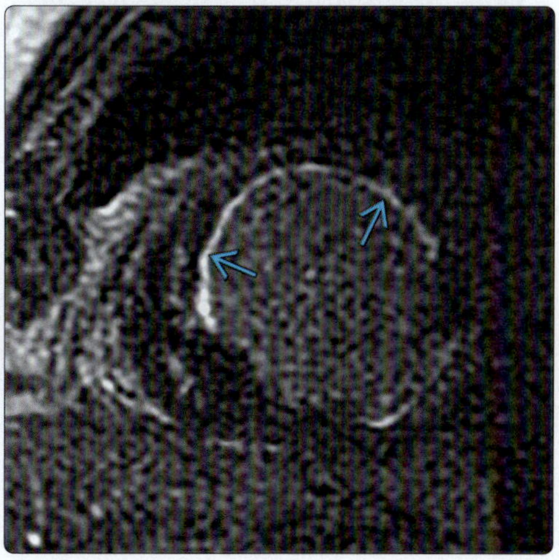

(Left) *Short-axis LGE image of a patient with acute myocardial infarction shows subendocardial enhancement* ➙ *in the left circumflex coronary artery distribution.* **(Right)** *Short-axis LGE image of a patient with chronic myocardial infarction shows subendocardial enhancement* ➙ *in the left anterior descending coronary artery distribution with associated myocardial thinning. When subendocardial LGE is encountered, the next determination should be whether the LGE follows a recognized vascular territory.*

(Left) *Short-axis LGE image of a patient with acute myocardial infarction shows transmural enhancement of the septal wall with central hypointense region, consistent with microvascular obstruction.* **(Right)** *Four-chamber LGE image of the same patient shows the extent of the transmural infarction extending from base to apex with linear hypointense central region, consistent with microvascular obstruction. This finding in cases of acute infarction is a poor prognostic sign.*

Ischemic Cardiomyopathy

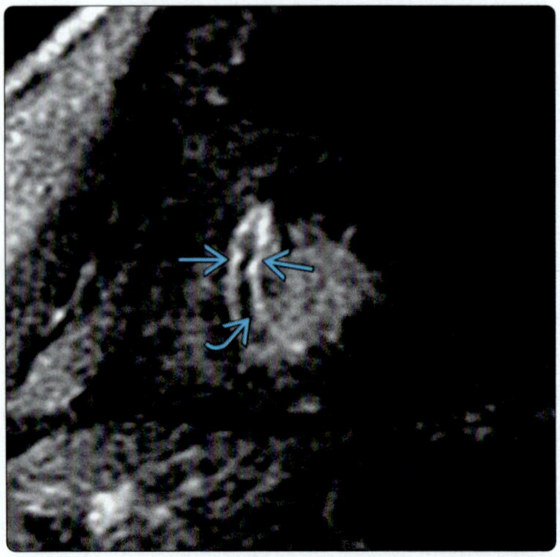

Ischemic Cardiomyopathy

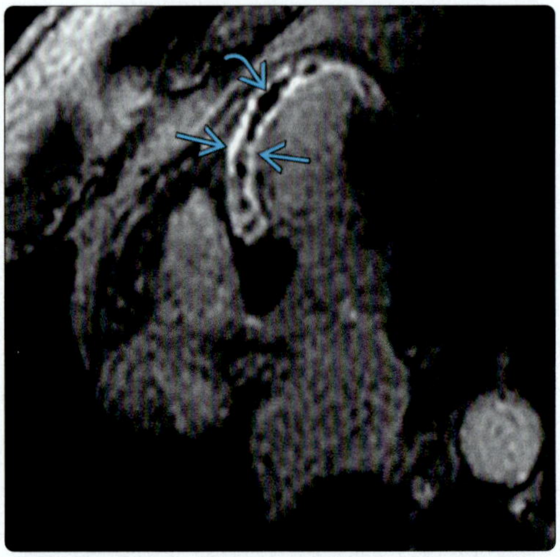

(Left) *Short-axis LGE image of a patient with sarcoidosis shows patchy mid-myocardial enhancement in the lateral and septal segments. Patchy right ventricular free wall enhancement is also present.* **(Right)** *Short-axis LGE image of a patient with myocarditis shows subepicardial enhancement in the inferior segments. Patchy mid-myocardial and subepicardial patterns of LGE are characteristic of cardiac sarcoidosis and myocarditis, respectively, although imaging appearance is variable and may overlap.*

Cardiac Sarcoidosis

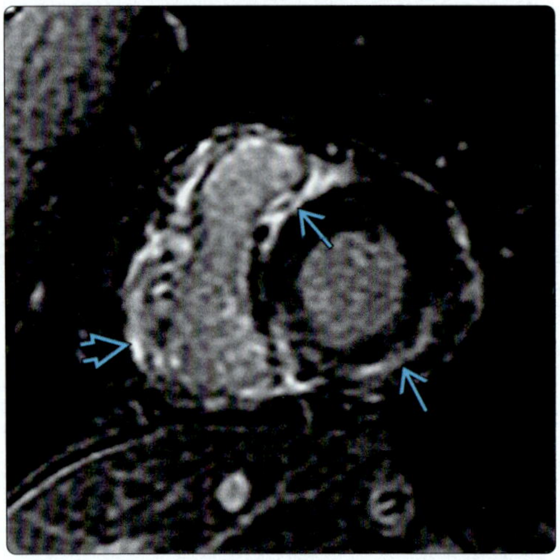

Myocarditis

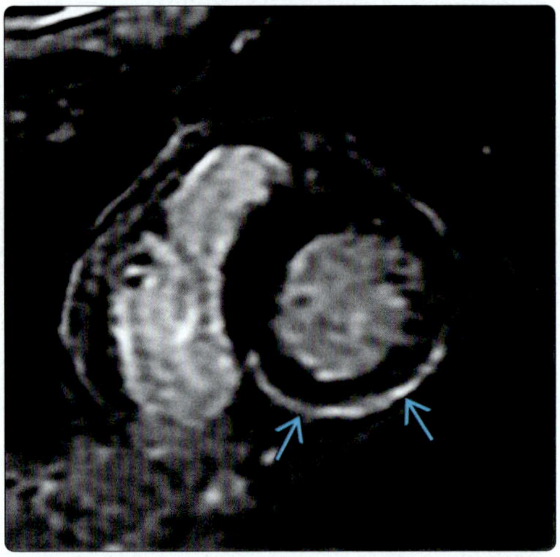

(Left) *Short-axis LGE image of a patient with hypertrophic cardiomyopathy (HCM) shows severe, asymmetric thickening of the septal segments with patchy mid-myocardial enhancement. Enhancement at the right ventricle insertion sites is characteristic of HCM.* **(Right)** *Four-chamber LGE image of a patient with apical HCM shows patchy mid-myocardial enhancement and asymmetric thickening of the apical segments of the left ventricle resulting in a spade-shaped morphology.*

Hypertrophic Cardiomyopathy

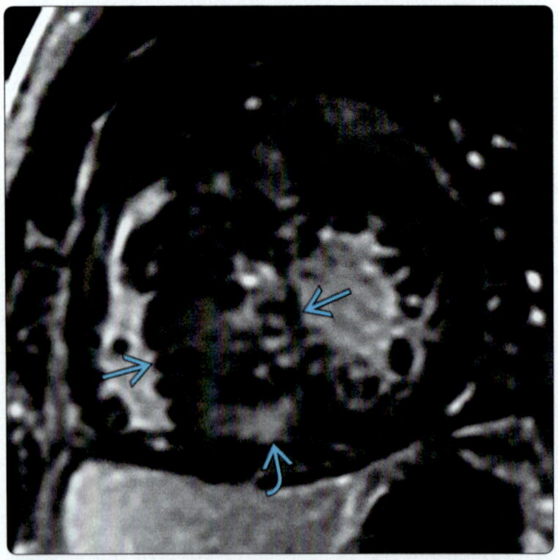

Hypertrophic Cardiomyopathy

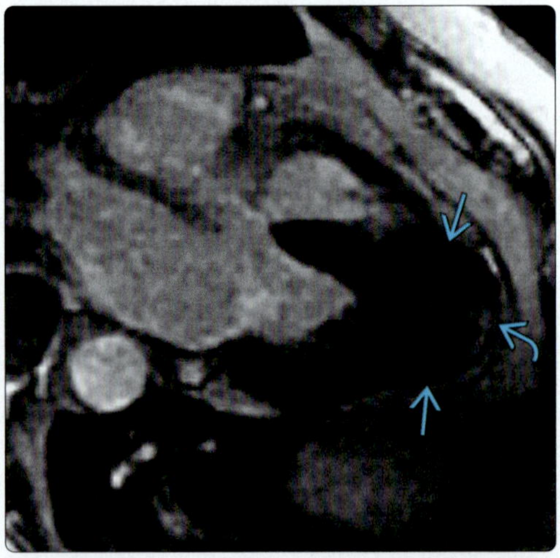

Nonischemic Dilated Cardiomyopathy

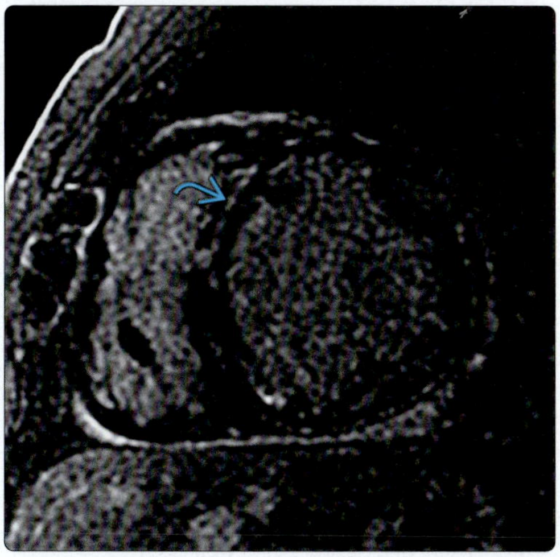

Nonischemic Dilated Cardiomyopathy

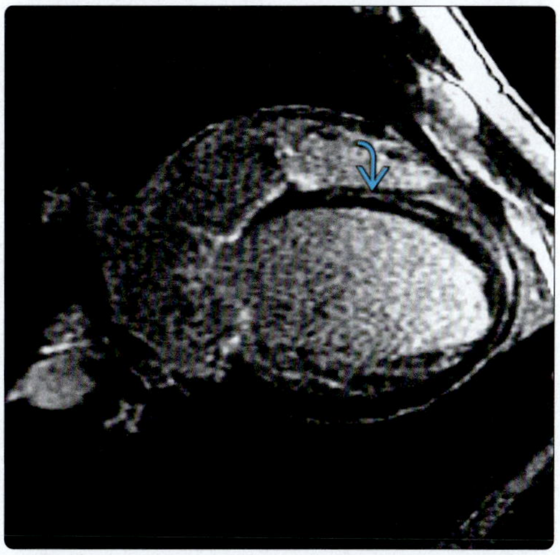

(Left) *Short-axis LGE image of a patient with dilated cardiomyopathy (DCM) shows linear mid-myocardial enhancement in the anteroseptal segment, a characteristic finding in DCM.* **(Right)** *Four-chamber LGE image of a patient with DCM shows the extent of the mid-myocardial stripe of enhancement and dilated left ventricle. Coronary disease and other causes of cardiomyopathy must be excluded to arrive at a diagnosis of nonischemic DCM.*

Cardiac Amyloidosis

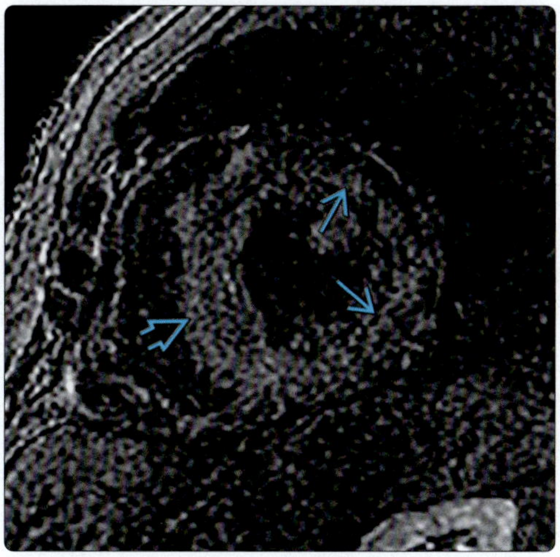

Cardiac Amyloidosis

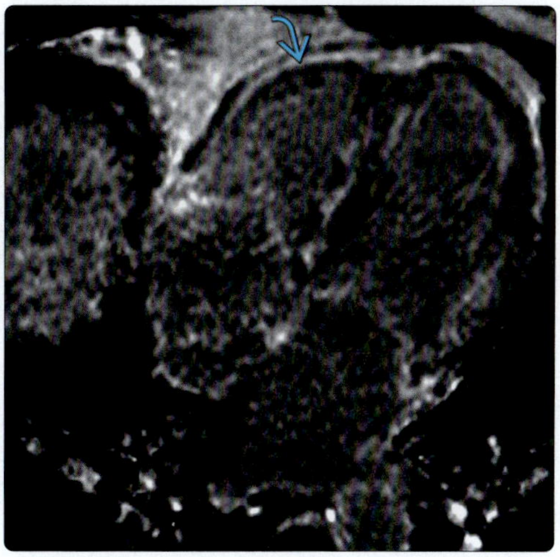

(Left) *Short-axis LGE image of a patient with cardiac amyloidosis shows transmural and diffuse subendocardial enhancement. The blood pool is black, and the inversion recovery time for myocardium is not optimal, clues to the diagnosis of cardiac amyloidosis.* **(Right)** *Four-chamber LGE image of a patient with cardiac amyloidosis shows diffuse left ventricular and right ventricular thickening and enhancement. Biatrial enlargement is an associated cardiac MR finding in this diagnosis.*

Arrhythmogenic Right Ventricular Dysplasia

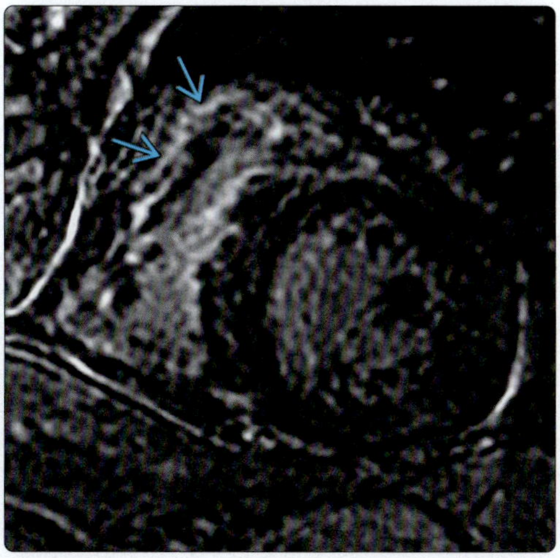

Arrhythmogenic Right Ventricular Dysplasia

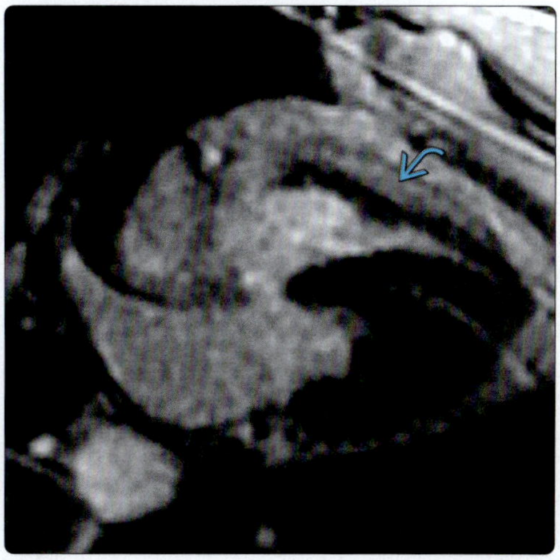

(Left) *Short-axis LGE image of a patient with arrhythmogenic right ventricular dysplasia (ARVD) shows right ventricular enhancement.* **(Right)** *Four-chamber LGE image of a patient with ARVD shows thickening and enhancement of the right ventricular free wall. While LGE is usually present in 2/3 cases of ARVD, it is not a major or minor task force criterion for this diagnosis. Wall motion abnormalities, aneurysms, and RV dilation are important imaging criteria. Fat in the right ventricle is not specific for ARVD.*

SECTION 11

Pericardium

Approach to Pericardium

General Imaging Patterns

Modality-Specific Imaging Findings: Computed Tomography

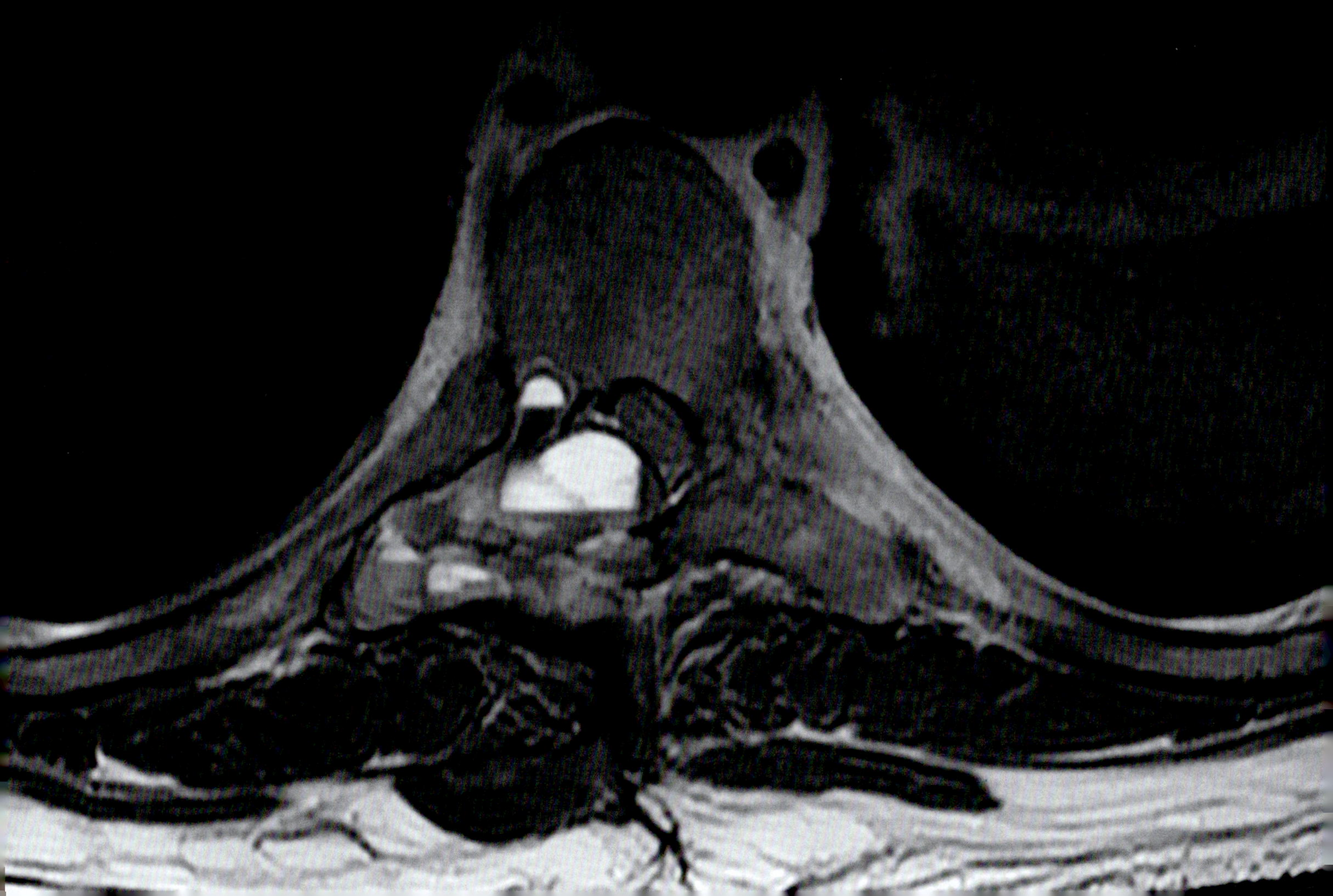

Introduction

Many infectious, inflammatory, and neoplastic diseases affect the pericardium, and this anatomic structure also serves as an important clue to cardiac diseases. Clinical symptoms attributable to the pericardium are frequently nonspecific, and accurate diagnosis often depends on noninvasive imaging techniques.

Anatomy

The pericardium is a double-layered, fluid-containing sac that surrounds the heart and proximal great vessels. The visceral pericardium is a serosal surface lining the heart and proximal great vessels. The parietal pericardium has both an outer fibrous and inner serosal surface. The serosal surfaces of the pericardium are composed of a contiguous layer of mesothelial cells, forming the pericardial sac.

Several recesses of the pericardium are recognized mimickers of lymphadenopathy or other mediastinal pathology, including the pulmonary vein recesses, which may mimic hilar lymph nodes, and the superior aortic recess, which may mimic aortic disease.

Imaging Modalities

Radiography

Pericardial effusion can be detected on radiography as a short interval change in the size and contour of the cardiac silhouette. Broadening at the base of cardiac silhouette on an upright frontal radiograph from the pericardial effusion sagging within the pericardiac sac has been likened to a pliable water bottle on a surface. On the lateral chest radiograph, a pericardial effusion may be detected as an opaque stripe between the relatively lucent epicardial fat posteriorly and mediastinal fat anteriorly (the Oreo cookie sign).

Pericardial calcifications may be visible on radiography but are occasionally difficult to differentiate from myocardial calcification. When visible on radiography, pericardial calcifications are highly suspicious for constrictive pericarditis. Pneumopericardium may be visible in cases of trauma or fistula formation with the gastrointestinal tract.

Echocardiography

Echocardiography remains the first imaging study typically employed in the evaluation of pericardial disease. Pericardial effusion and associated cardiac physiologic consequences of tamponade and constriction are rapidly assessed with this modality. Furthermore, echocardiography can guide diagnostic or therapeutic pericardiocentesis.

CT

The entire pericardium may be evaluated rapidly with CT, and CECT may show enhancement of the pericardium suspicious for inflammatory, infectious, or neoplastic disease. Considering that the pericardium is a thin structure in the normal state (≤ 3 mm), visibility of the pericardium itself is suspicious for thickening and enhancement. Moreover, the visceral pericardium is only a serosal layer of mesothelial cells such that seeing this layer is abnormal. Pericardial effusion, although nonspecific, is the most common sign of cardiac malignancy, and enhancing pericardial nodules are a more ominous finding for metastatic disease to the heart.

Calcification can be better localized to the pericardium on CT than radiography, although the significance of this finding is less well understood given the high sensitivity of CT for calcification. This finding is common after cardiac surgery, prior pericardial infection (specifically tuberculosis), prior radiation, and in patients with uremia.

MR

The primary advantages of MR over CT for pericardial disease are the detection of pericardial enhancement and the physiologic study of the heart in response to pericardial effusion or pericarditis. Advanced imaging techniques, such as myocardial tagging with grid-like saturation bands, can evaluate adhesions of the parietal pericardium to the visceral pericardium and epicardium.

MR has a defined role in the diagnosis and characterization of pericardial tumors, and the tissue contrast ability of this modality makes it ideal to evaluate the extent of tumor infiltration into the myocardium and mediastinal structures.

Cardiac Catheterization

Despite advances in the diagnostic ability of echocardiography, CT, and MR, invasive hemodynamics may still be required in equivocal cases of pericardial constriction.

Challenging Concepts

Pericardial Tamponade

The pericardial sac can accommodate large volumes of fluid if acquired gradually, most notably in cases of lupus pericarditis. However, rapid accumulation of pericardial fluid is not tolerated well, resulting in compression of cardiac chambers and impedance of venous return to the right heart. Echocardiography, CT, and MR showing collapse of the right atrium for > 1/3 of the cardiac cycle is sensitive and specific for tamponade. Left atrial collapse is specific but not sensitive for tamponade, which is not directly correlated to the size of effusion. Other associated findings include ventricular interdependence and enlargement of the inferior vena cava.

Pericardial Constriction

Constrictive pericarditis is difficult to differentiate from restrictive cardiomyopathy clinically. Important echocardiographic signs include diastolic septal motion, respiratory phasic shift of the interventricular septum, enlargement of the inferior vena cava, and myocardial tethering. Confirmatory CT and MR findings include thickened &/or calcified pericardium, tubular morphology of the ventricles, and sigmoid-shaped interventricular septum. The atria are often bilaterally enlarged. Exaggerated ventricular interdependence is evidenced by bowing of the interventricular septum toward the left ventricle in inspiration, when intrathoracic pressure are decreased and there is increased venous return to the right ventricle.

Pericardial Tumors

Metastatic disease is far more common than primary pericardial tumors, and the most sensitive sign for pericardial malignancy is a pericardial effusion. Lung, breast, lymphoma, and mediastinal tumors are the most frequent primary tumors to metastasize to the heart and pericardium, while primary malignant tumors of the pericardium are sarcomas and mesothelioma. Enhancing pericardial nodules with a pericardial effusion are suspicious for neoplastic pericardial disease.

Selected References

1. Kligerman S: Imaging of pericardial disease. Radiol Clin North Am. 57(1):179-99, 2019
2. Rajiah P et al: MRI of the pericardium. Radiographics. 39(7):1921-2, 2019

Pericardial Calcification

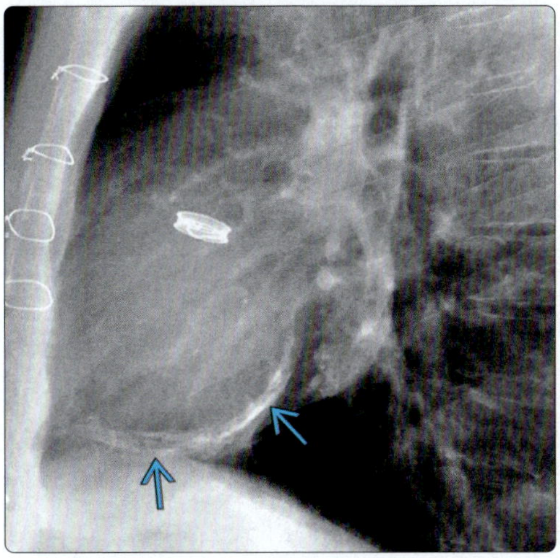

Pericardial Calcification

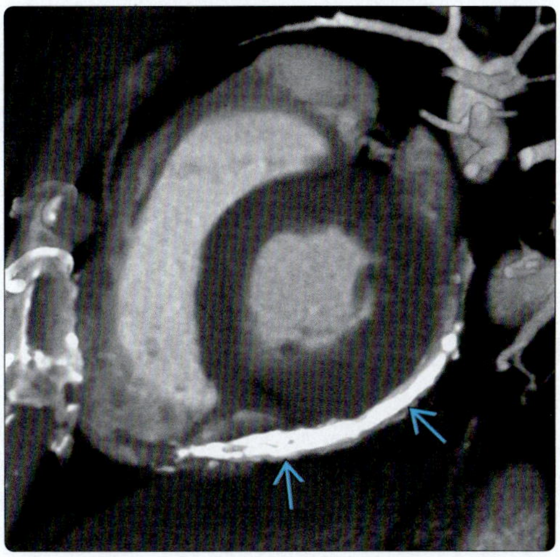

(Left) *Lateral chest radiograph of a patient status post remote aortic valve replacement shows curvilinear calcification along the posterior and inferior aspect of the heart. Pericardial calcification visible on radiographs should raise the suspicion for constrictive pericarditis.* **(Right)** *Oblique sagittal MIP reformatted CECT of the same patient shows the extent of pericardial calcification. The most common cause of pericardial calcification in developed countries is prior cardiac surgery.*

Pericarditis

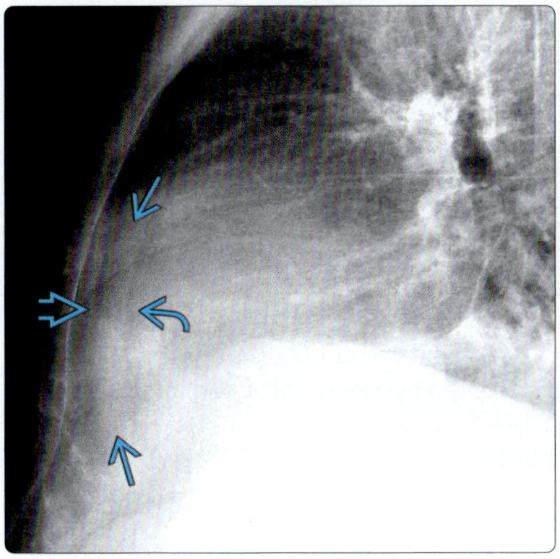

Pericarditis

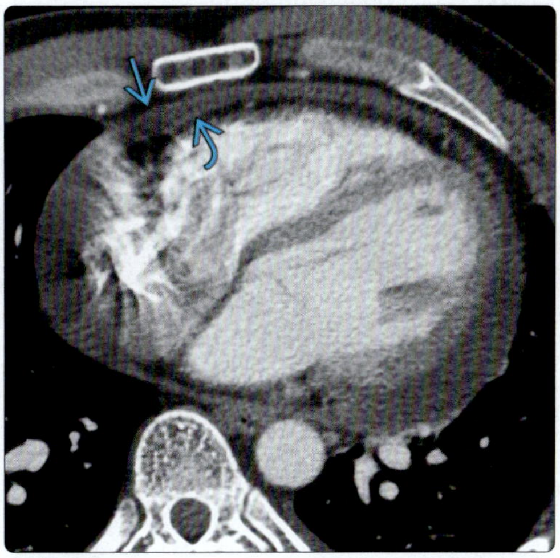

(Left) *Lateral chest radiograph of a patient with infectious pericarditis shows an opaque stripe representing pericardial effusion between the relatively lucent epicardial fat and mediastinal fat, the Oreo cookie sign.* **(Right)** *Axial CECT of a patient with chest pain and infectious pericarditis shows a moderate circumferential pericardial effusion with thickening and enhancement of the parietal and visceral pericardium. Visible pericardial layers are suspicious for thickening and enhancement.*

Cardiac Sarcoma

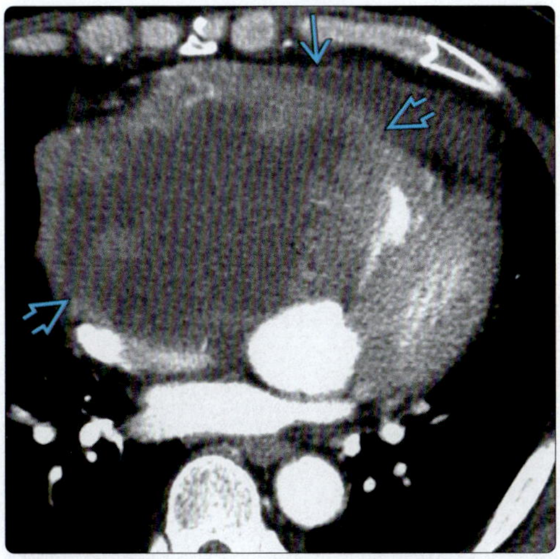

Constrictive Pericarditis

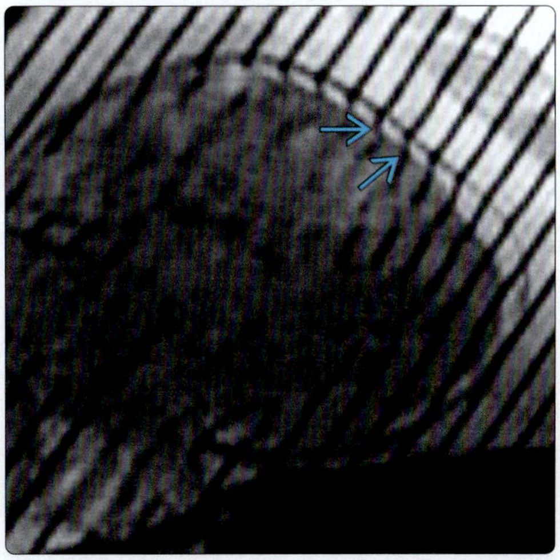

(Left) *Axial CECT of a patient with a cardiac sarcoma shows a moderate pericardial effusion with enhancing parietal pericardium tented outward by the mass, an important clue for cardiac origin of this tumor.* **(Right)** *Four-chamber myocardial tagging MR of a patient with constrictive pericarditis shows linear saturation bands that are continuous across the pericardium and the epicardium, indicative of adhesion. In the normal pericardium, these lines would be discontinuous during the cardiac cycle.*

DIFFERENTIAL DIAGNOSIS

Common

- Inflammatory Pericarditis
- Infectious Pericarditis
- Malignancy
- Pericardial Effusion (Mimic)

Less Common

- Iatrogenic
- Uremic Pericarditis

ESSENTIAL INFORMATION

Key Differential Diagnosis Issues

- Normal pericardial thickness < 2 mm
  - Pericardial thickness ≥ 6 mm is highly specific
  - Thickening may be focal, commonly adjacent to atrioventricular groove
- Pericarditis is often accompanied by effusion
- MR
  - Normal: Low signal on T1WI, T2WI; no enhancement on T1 C+
  - Abnormal: Low signal on T1WI, high signal on T2WI; enhancement on T1 C+
- Pericardial thickening + heart failure symptoms = constrictive pericarditis
  - Pericardial calcifications commonly present
  - Imaging of constrictive physiology
    - IVC:descending aorta ratio ≥ 2; SVC:descending aorta ratio ≥ 1; coronary sinus dilation; ascites
    - Biatrial enlargement with normal-sized, tubular-shaped ventricles
    - Septal bounce with respiratory variation in septal wall motion

Helpful Clues for Common Diagnoses

- **Inflammatory Pericarditis**
  - Pericardial friction rub, fever; response to NSAIDs
  - Rapid accumulation of serous or serosanguineous pericardial fluid; increasing risk of tamponade
  - **Post Myocardial Infarction (MI)**
    - Larger MI and lack of reperfusion therapy increases risk
    - Immediate form: Within 1 week
    - Late form: > 1 week post infarct
      - Associated with recurrent bouts of pericarditis, fever (Dressler syndrome)
  - **Connective Tissue Disease**
    - Rheumatoid arthritis and systemic lupus erythematosus (50% of patients)
  - **Idiopathic Pericarditis** (diagnosis of exclusion)
- **Infectious Pericarditis**
  - In developed world, viral and bacterial etiologies are most common
  - In developing countries, tuberculosis remains major etiology of pericarditis
- **Malignancy**
  - Lung cancer, breast cancer, and lymphoma
  - ~ 5% of presenting pericarditis: Undiagnosed malignancy
  - Nodular pericardial thickening and enhancement
  - Hemorrhagic effusions common; high signal on T1WI
- **Pericardial Effusion (Mimic)**
  - Small pericardial effusion on CT may mimic thickening
  - Fluid in pericardial recesses or pooling in dependent pericardium

Helpful Clues for Less Common Diagnoses

- **Iatrogenic**
  - Postpericardiotomy syndrome
    - Febrile illness secondary to inflammatory reaction involving pleura and pericardium
  - History of surgical incision of pericardium
  - May be complicated by aseptic loculated, simple, &/or hemorrhagic effusions
- **Uremic Pericarditis**
  - Patients with chronic renal dysfunction on dialysis or acute renal failure
  - Fibrinous pericarditis caused by accumulated toxins; resolves after dialysis
  - Hemorrhagic effusion is common

Inflammatory Pericarditis

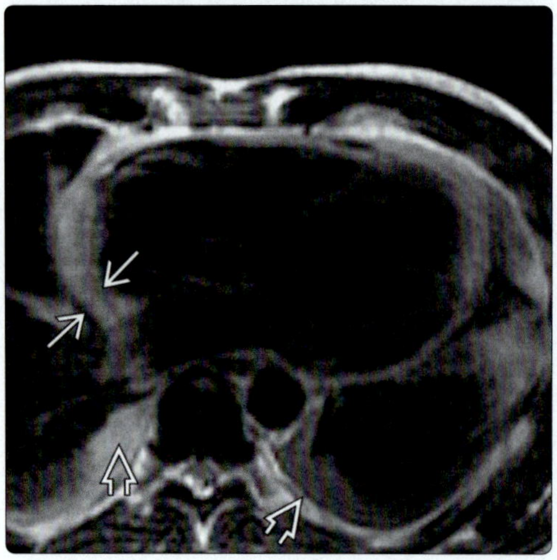

Inflammatory Pericarditis

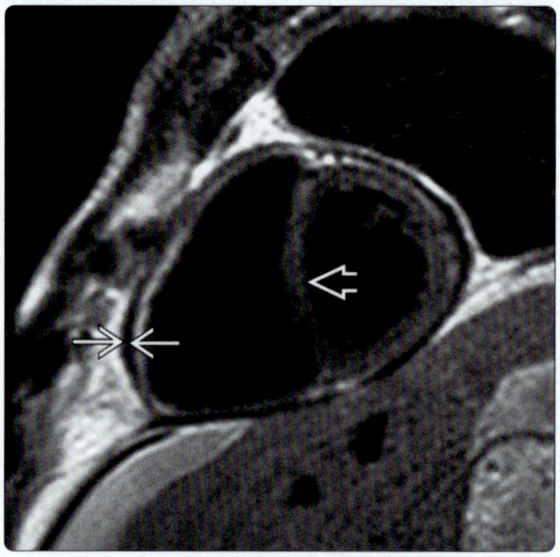

(Left) *Axial black blood MR of a patient with Still disease and symptoms of pericarditis demonstrates pericardial fluid and thickening ➔. Bilateral pleural effusions are also present ➔.* **(Right)** *Short axis black blood MR of a patient with remote pericarditis now presenting with pericardial constriction shows pericardial thickening ➔. Note flattening of the interventricular septum ➔. Inflammatory pericarditis often results in rapid accumulation of serous or serosanguineous pericardial fluid, which increases the risk of tamponade.*

Infectious Pericarditis

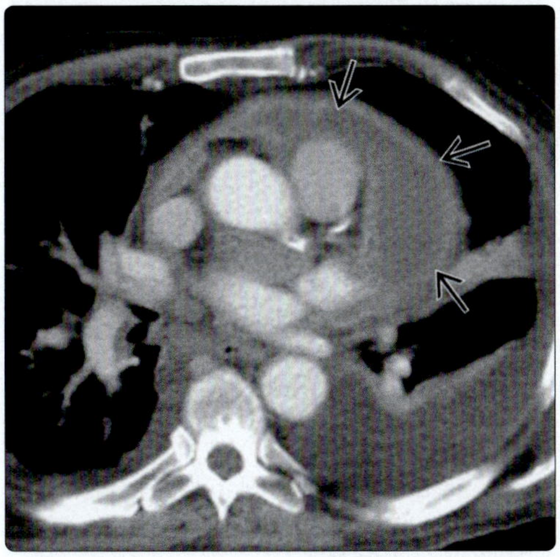

Malignancy

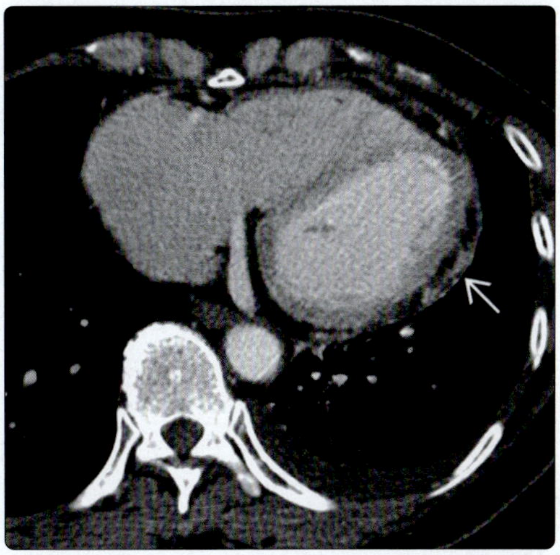

(Left) *Axial CECT demonstrates a large, multiloculated pericardial fluid collection with thickening and enhancement of the pericardium ➔. Fluid from a pericardiocentesis eventually revealed tuberculosis.* **(Right)** *Axial CECT of a patient with biopsy-proven metastasis to the pericardium shows nodular thickening of the pericardium ➔. Nodular pericardial thickening is concerning for malignancy as nonmalignant pericardial thickening is typically smooth.*

Pericardial Effusion (Mimic)

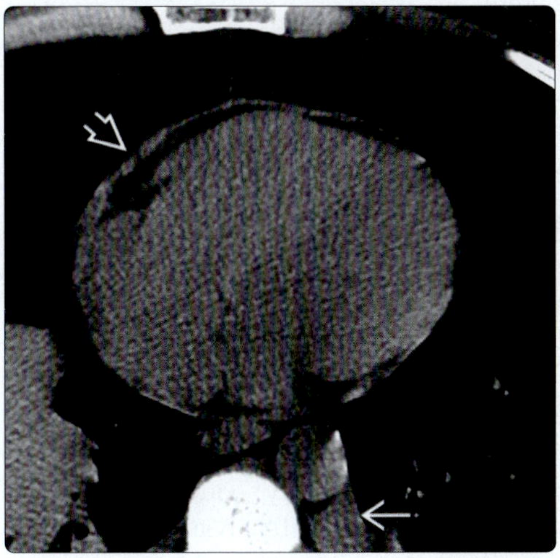

Pericardial Effusion (Mimic)

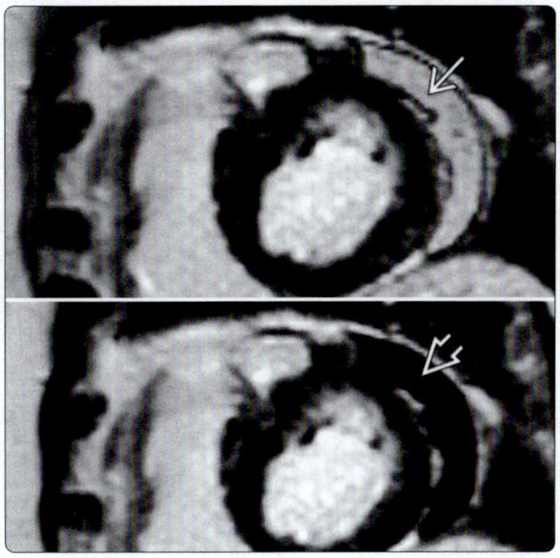

(Left) *Axial NECT demonstrates a small amount of fluid in the pericardial space mimicking smooth pericardial thickening ➔. This small amount of fluid later resolved. Note the small left pleural effusion ➔.* **(Right)** *Short axis magnitude (top) and phase preserved (bottom) inversion recovery MR demonstrate pericardial fluid that can be identified as high signal on magnitude images ➔ and low signal on phase preserved images ➔. Fluid in the pericardial recesses or pooling in the dependent pericardium may mimic effusion.*

Iatrogenic

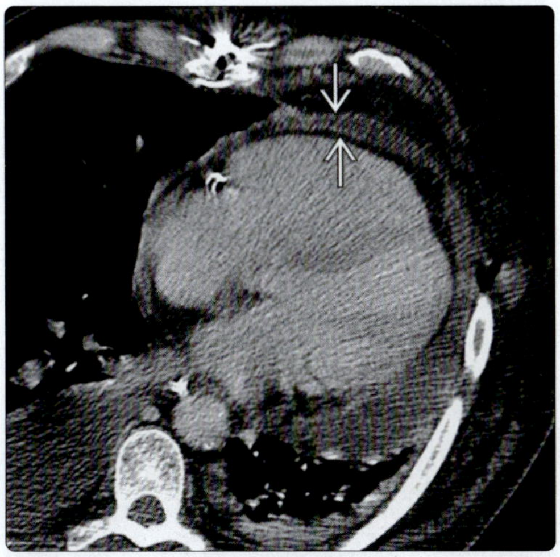

Uremic Pericarditis

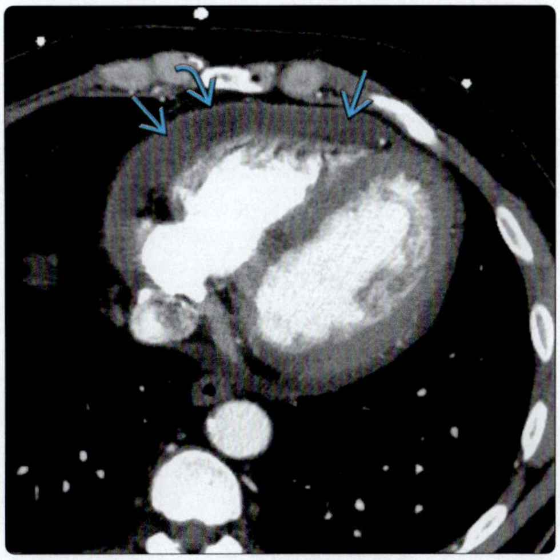

(Left) *Axial CECT of a patient status post cardiac surgery demonstrates mild pericardial thickening and enhancement as well as a small effusion ➔. Pericardial thickening following surgery may be complicated by aseptic loculated, simple, &/or hemorrhagic pericardial effusions.* **(Right)** *Axial CT angiogram of a patient with chronic renal failure and chest pain shows a small to moderate pericardial effusion ➔ as well as mild pericardial thickening and enhancement ➔ due to uremic pericarditis.*

DIFFERENTIAL DIAGNOSIS

Common

- Post Surgical
- Post Radiation
- Post Pericarditis
  - Infection
  - Uremia
  - Autoimmune
- Idiopathic

Less Common

- Post Hemopericardium

Rare but Important

- Malignancy: Metastasis

ESSENTIAL INFORMATION

Key Differential Diagnosis Issues

- Pericardial calcification: Can be incidental but should be regarded as concerning for constrictive pericarditis
  - 30% of pericardial calcifications associated with constrictive physiology
- Constrictive pericarditis often associated with pericardial calcification; 20% without calcification
  - Constrictive physiology: Dilated IVC, SVC, atria, tubular ventricles, and hepatic vein contrast reflux; cine MR shows septal flattening and septal bounce (paradoxical initial diastolic movement toward left ventricle)
- Calcification features or distribution are limited in identifying etiology; history most helpful

Helpful Clues for Common Diagnoses

- **Post Surgical**
  - Any cardiac surgery with pericardial violation may lead to inflammation and pericardial calcification
- **Post Radiation**
  - Acute and chronic forms of radiation pericarditis can lead to calcification
  - Radiotherapy must exceed 40 Gy, dose most commonly delivered for Hodgkin lymphoma or lung cancer
  - Chronic pericarditis does not occur before 6 months; may be asymptomatic, can lead to constrictive physiology
- **Post Pericarditis**
  - **Infection**
    - Pericardial tuberculosis is uncommon in developed countries but remains most common cause of pericardial calcification worldwide
      - Characteristically thick, irregular, amorphous calcifications predominantly over anterior and inferior RV
    - Viral pericarditis is common but calcification rarely develops
  - **Uremia**
    - Pathophysiology unclear; accumulation of toxic metabolites, nitrogen waste products, fluid overload, and electrolyte imbalance
    - Pericardial effusion, pericardial thickening and enhancement; may result in pericardial calcifications
  - **Autoimmunity**
    - Serositis is common in autoimmunity; longstanding serositis may lead to pericardial calcification and constrictive physiology
- **Idiopathic**: Diagnosis of exclusion; often result of undiagnosed viral infection

Helpful Clues for Less Common Diagnoses

- **Post Hemopericardium**
  - History of trauma, pseudoaneurysm (e.g., chamber perforation with pacemaker leads), malignancy, or surgery

Helpful Clues for Rare Diagnoses

- **Metastasis**
  - Much more common than primary neoplasms
  - Nodular pericardium with coexistent hemopericardium
  - Lung cancer, breast cancer, and lymphoma account for 75% of cases

Post Surgical

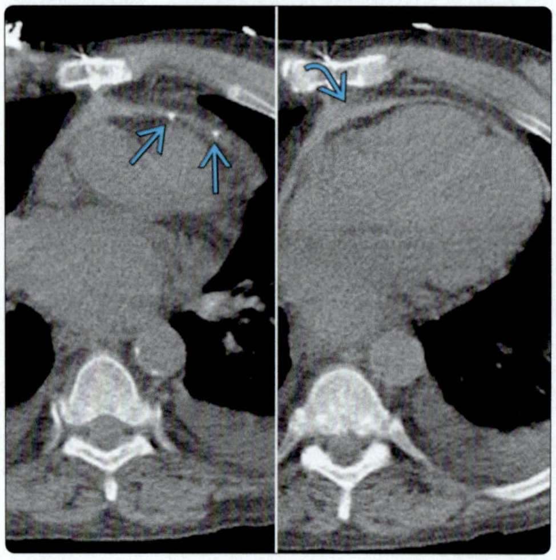

Post Surgical

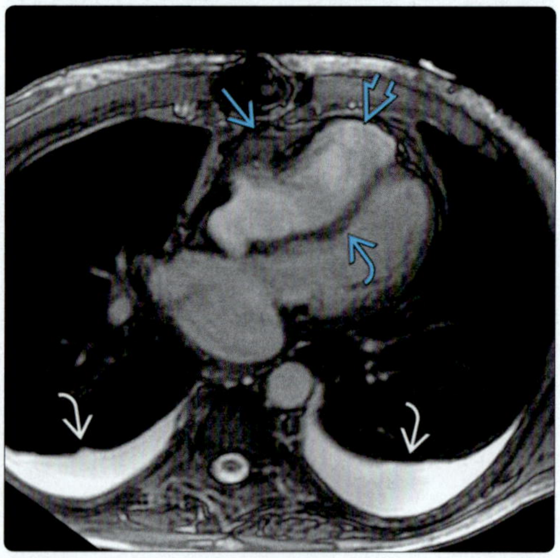

(Left) *Composite image with axial NECT at different levels of a patient with a history of heart transplant with constrictive pericarditis is shown. Note calcifications ➙ with marked pericardial thickening ➙.* **(Right)** *Axial SSFP cardiac MR of the same patient shows anterior pericardial calcification. Note pericardial thickening ➙, mildly dilated right ventricle ➙ with inversion of the interventricular septum ➙. Also note bilateral pleural effusions ➙, a common ancillary finding often seen in pericardial constriction.*

- Patients may be asymptomatic or present with symptoms secondary to catecholamine secretion (palpitations, chest pain, angina, headache)
- Most commonly arise adjacent to left atrium or anterior to aortic root
- CT
  - Intense enhancement, central area of necrosis
- MR
  - T2WI: High signal intensity
  - T1 MR +C: Intense enhancement

- **Hemangioma**
  - Arises from visceral pericardium
  - CT
    - NECT: Heterogeneous lesion with foci of calcification
    - CECT: Intense enhancement
  - MR
    - T1WI: Intermediate signal intensity
    - T2WI: High signal intensity
    - T1 MR +C: Nodular areas of enhancement, progressive filling on delayed images

Helpful Clues for Rare Diagnoses

- **Primary Pericardial Mesothelioma**
  - Most common primary malignancy of pericardium
  - Occurs more frequently in men than in women, 5th-7th decades of life
  - No clear association with asbestos exposure
  - CT
    - Heterogeneous enhancing mass involving visceral and parietal pericardium
      - May debut as large pericardial effusion with posterior development of pericardial nodules and thickening
      - Lymph node and lung metastases identified in 50% of cases
  - MR
    - Useful for identifying invasion of heart
    - MR+C: Heterogeneous enhancing mass, encasement of heart
    - Cine MR provides information regarding diastolic impairment
- **Primary Pericardial Sarcoma**
  - Uncommon neoplasms with very poor prognosis
  - Histologic subtypes: Angiosarcoma, synovial sarcoma, fibrosarcoma, liposarcoma, and undifferentiated sarcoma
    - Angiosarcoma and synovial sarcomas are most common sarcomas
      - Angiosarcoma frequently arises in region of atrioventricular groove
  - CT
    - Large, enhancing mass associated with hemopericardium
  - MR
    - T1WI: Heterogeneous signal intensity depending on extent of hemorrhage and necrosis
    - T2WI: High signal intensity
- **Lymphoma**
  - Extranodal lymphoma, usually high-grade B-cell type; can be associated with HIV infection
  - More common in men; 2:1 (M:W)
  - CT
    - Nodules or masses with heterogeneous enhancement, pericardial effusion frequently hemorrhagic (high attenuation)
  - MR
    - T1WI: Low signal intensity
    - T2WI: Iso- to hyperintense signal
- T1 MR +C: Heterogeneous postcontrast delayed enhancement

SELECTED REFERENCES

1. Maleszewski JJ et al: Neoplastic pericardial disease. Cardiol Clin. 35(4):589-600, 2017
2. Tower-Rader A et al: Pericardial masses, cysts and diverticula: a comprehensive review using multimodality imaging. Prog Cardiovasc Dis. 59(4):389-97, 2017

Pericardial Cyst

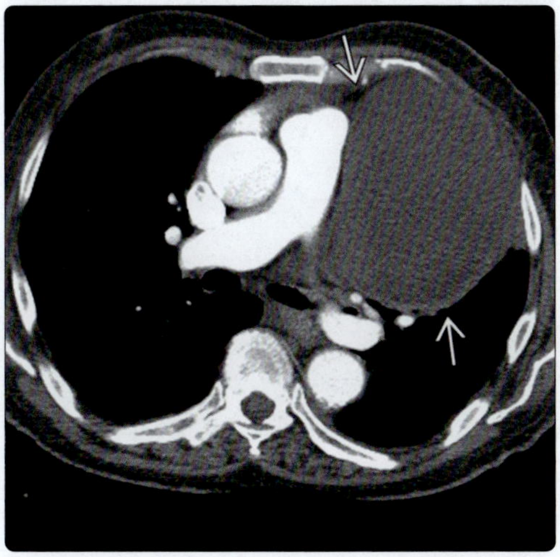

Pericardial Cyst

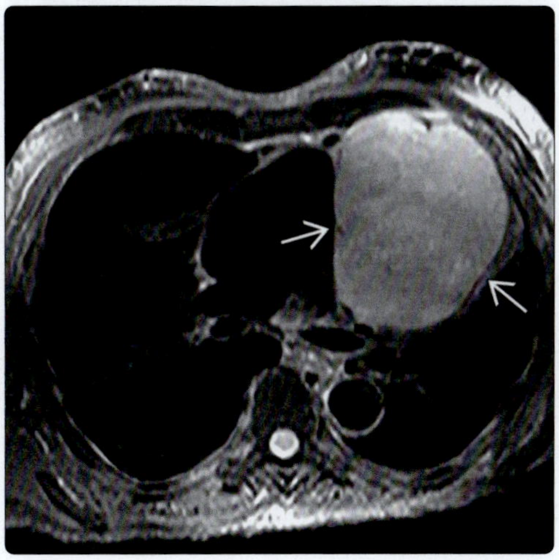

(Left) *Axial CECT of a 72-year-old man with pericardial cyst shows a well-defined fluid attenuation mass* ➔ *located along the anterosuperior aspect of the pericardium.* **(Right)** *Axial T2WI FS MR of the same patient shows a homogeneous high-signal lesion* ➔ *consistent with a pericardial cyst. Most commonly, pericardial cysts are located in the right anterior cardiophrenic angle, followed by the left costophrenic angle.*

Pericardial Metastases

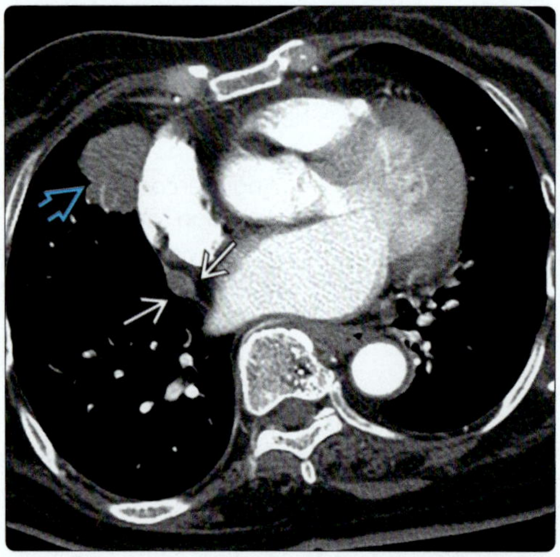

Pericardial Metastases

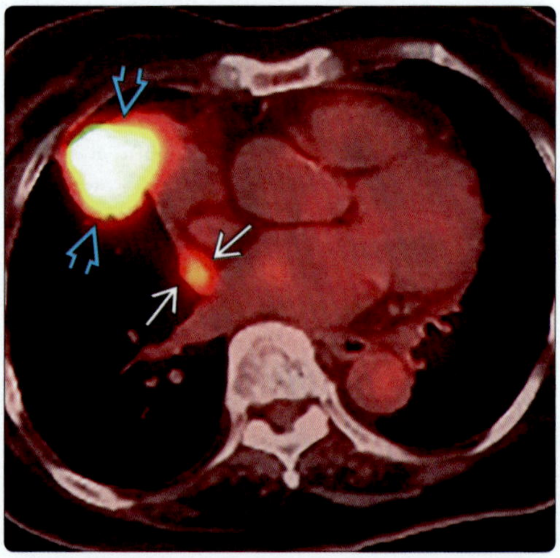

(Left) *Axial CECT of a 67-year-old woman with squamous cell carcinoma of the lung ➔ shows a small nodule along the pericardium ➔ consistent with a metastasis.* **(Right)** *Fused axial PET/CT of the same patient demonstrates increased FDG uptake within the primary lung malignancy ➔ and the metastatic pericardial nodule ➔. Lung and breast cancer are the most common primary malignancies associated with pericardial metastases.*

Pericardial Metastases

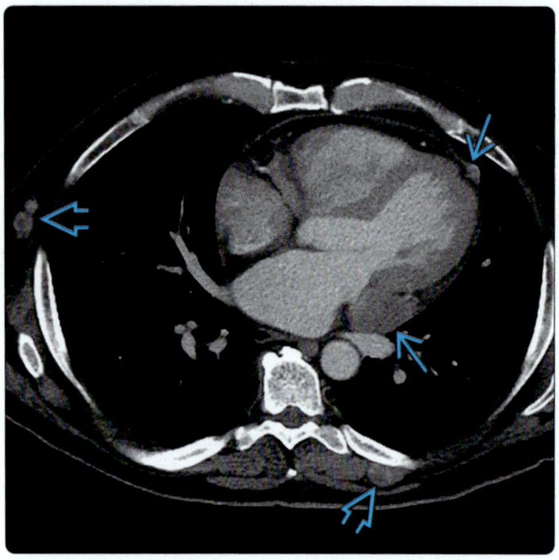

Lipoma

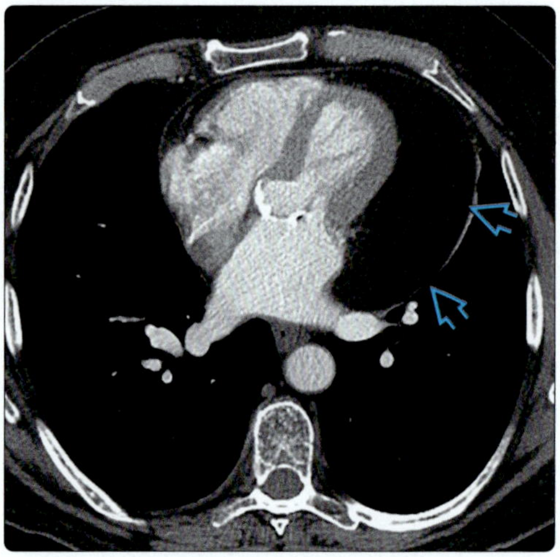

(Left) *Axial CECT of a 57-year-old man with renal cell carcinoma shows pericardial metastases ➔. Note metastases in the chest wall ➔. Pericardial metastases usually occur late in the course of a neoplasm and typically there is metastatic disease at other sites.* **(Right)** *CECT of a 73-year-old woman shows a homogeneous fat-attenuation mass in the pericardial space ➔ consistent with a lipoma. Lipomas are the most common benign tumors of the pericardium.*

Paraganglioma

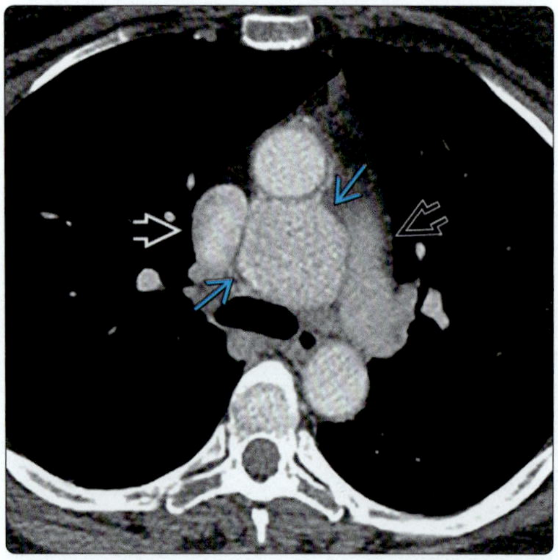

Paraganglioma

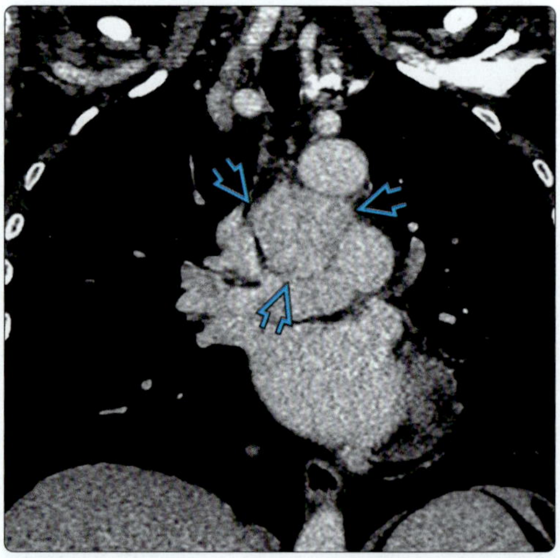

(Left) *Axial CECT of a 61-year-old woman with mediastinal paraganglioma shows a large hyperenhancing mass in the pericardial space ➔ between the superior vena cava ➔ and the left pulmonary artery ➔.* **(Right)** *Coronal CECT of the same patient shows intense contrast enhancement in the lesion ➔. Patients with paragangliomas may present with symptoms secondary to catecholamine excretion resulting in palpitations, diaphoresis, headache, and hypertension.*

Primary Pericardial Mesothelioma

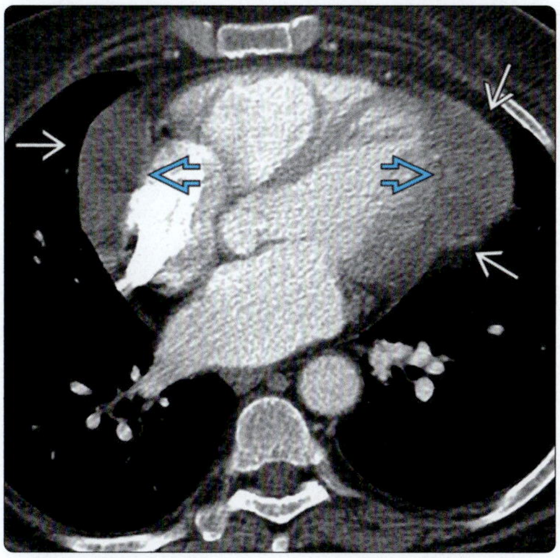

Primary Pericardial Mesothelioma

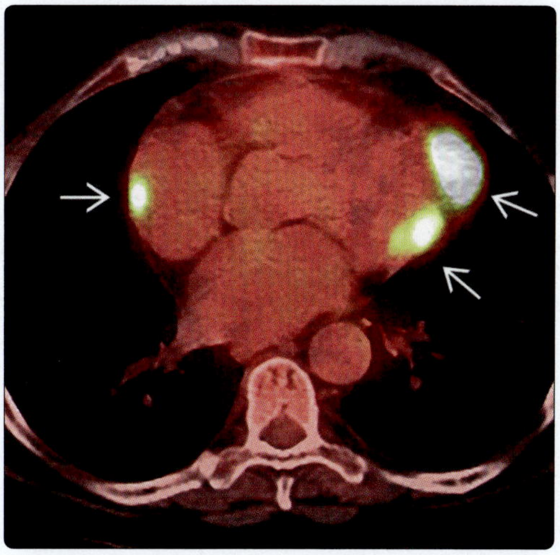

(Left) *Axial CECT of a 69-year-old man with pericardial mesothelioma shows pericardial masses within the pericardial space. There is loss of the pericardial fat plane along the right atrium and left ventricle.* **(Right)** *Fused axial FDG PET/CT of the same patient demonstrates increased FDG uptake within the pericardial masses. Biopsy confirmed mesothelioma. Pericardial mesothelioma is the most common primary malignancy affecting the pericardium.*

Primary Pericardial Sarcoma

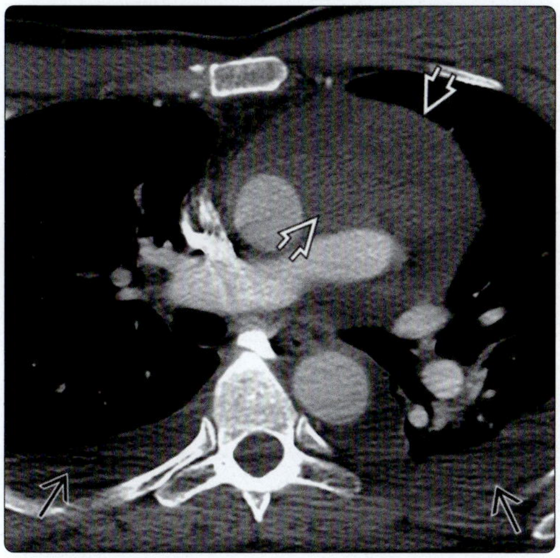

Primary Pericardial Sarcoma

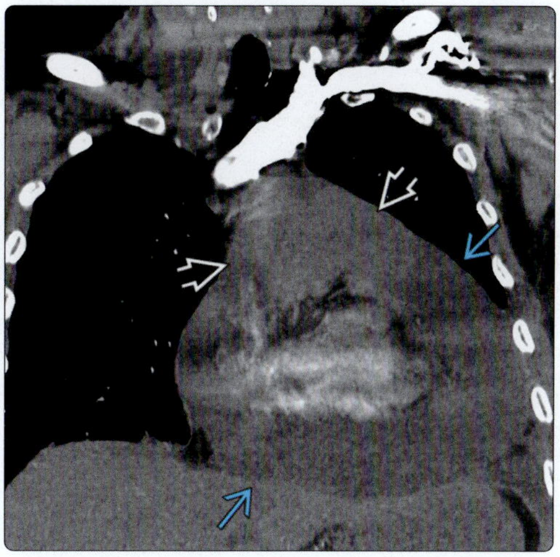

(Left) *Axial CECT of a 64-year-old woman with pericardial sarcoma who presented with shortness of breath shows a large pericardial effusion and an ill-defined soft tissue pericardial mass. Note bilateral pleural effusions.* **(Right)** *Coronal CECT of the same patient shows the mass in the anterior aspect of the pericardial space and a large pericardial effusion. Biopsy confirmed the diagnosis of synovial sarcoma. Synovial sarcoma and angiosarcoma are the most common sarcomas of the pericardium.*

Primary Pericardial Sarcoma

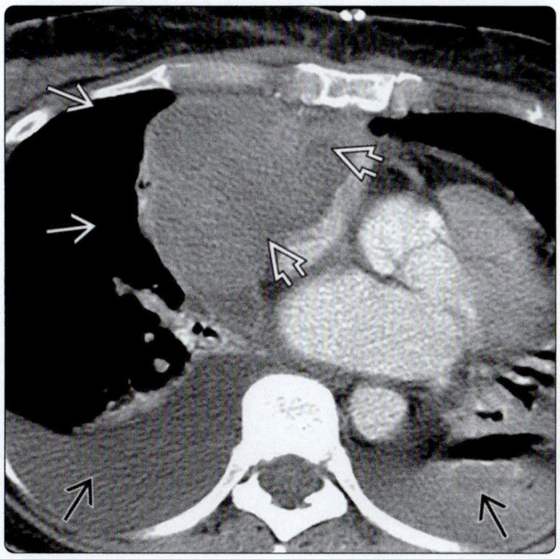

Lymphoma

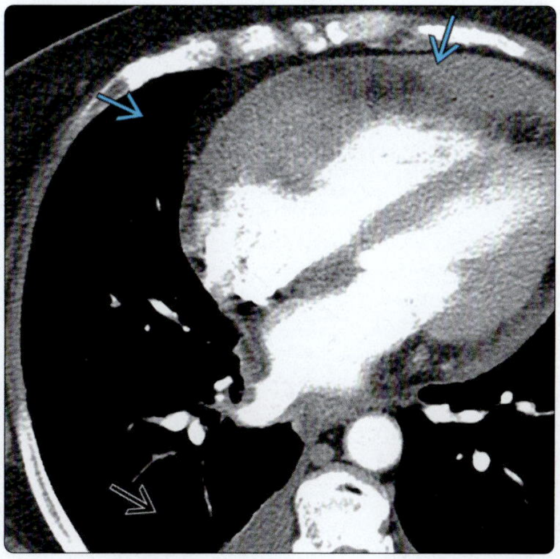

(Left) *Axial CECT of a 51-year-old man with pericardial angiosarcoma shows a heterogeneous pericardial mass compressing the right heart. Note the presence of bilateral pleural effusions. The prognosis of patients with pericardial sarcomas is very poor.* **(Right)** *Axial CECT of a 59 year old with pericardial B-cell lymphoma shows soft tissue masses within the pericardium. Note the presence of a small right pleural effusion. B-cell lymphoma is the most common primary pericardial lymphoma.*

INDEX

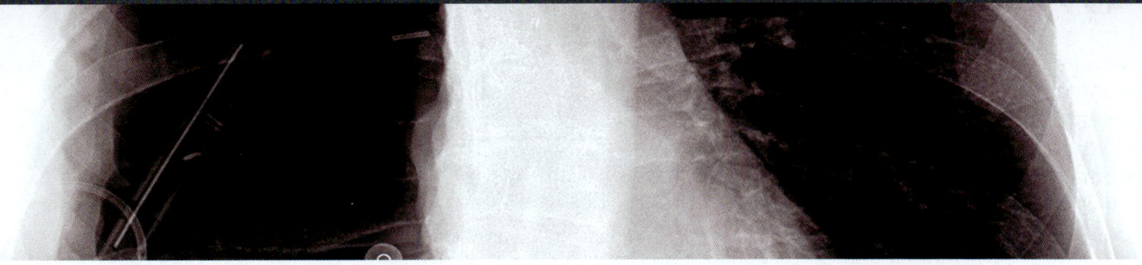

A

INDEX

INDEX

B

INDEX

C

INDEX

INDEX

INDEX

D

E

INDEX

F

G

I

INDEX

K

INDEX

L

P

INDEX

INDEX

R

INDEX

T